Congestive Heart Failure

Jeffrey D. Hosenpud   Barry H. Greenberg

Editors

Congestive Heart Failure

Pathophysiology, Diagnosis, and Comprehensive Approach to Management

With 327 Figures

Provided as an Educational Service By...

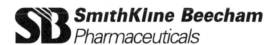 SmithKline Beecham
Pharmaceuticals

BOEHRINGER
MANNHEIM
THERAPEUTICS

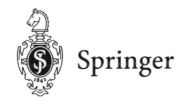 Springer

Jeffrey D. Hosenpud, M.D.
Division of Cardiology
Oregon Cardiac Transplant Program
Oregon Health Sciences University
Portland, OR 97201-3098
USA

Barry H. Greenberg, M.D.
Division of Cardiology
Oregon Health Sciences University
Portland, OR 97201-3098
USA

Library of Congress Cataloging-in-Publication Data
Congestive heart failure: pathophysiology, diagnosis, and
　　comprehensive approach to management/Jeffrey D. Hosenpud, Barry H.
　　Greenberg, editors.
　　　　p.　cm.
　　Includes bibliographical references and index.
　　ISBN 0-387-94017-0 (alk. paper).—ISBN 3-540-94017-0 (alk.
paper)
　　1. Congestive heart failure.　I. Hosenpud, Jeffrey D.
II. Greenberg, Barry H.
　　[DNLM:　1. Heart Failure, Congestive—physiopathology.　2. Heart
Failure, Congestive—diagnosis.　3. Heart Failure, Congestive—
therapy.　WG 370 C7513　1993]
RC685.C53C665　1993
616.1′29—dc20　　　　　　　　　　　　　　　93-12887

Printed on acid-free paper.

Production coordinated by TechEdit Production Services and managed by Francine McNeill; manufac-
turing supervised by Vincent Scelta.
Typeset by Asco Trade Typesetting Ltd., Hong Kong.
Printed and bound by Edwards Brothers, Inc., Ann Arbor, MI.
Printed in the United States of America.

9 8 7 6 5 4 3 2

ISBN 0-387-94017-0 Springer-Verlag New York Berlin Heidelberg
ISBN 3-540-94017-0 Springer-Verlag Berlin Heidelberg New York

Contents

Contributors

WILLIAM T. ABRAHAM, M.D., Fellow, Division of Cardiology, University of Colorado, Denver, CO 80262, USA

THOMAS AMIDON, M.D., Associate Professor of Medicine; Associate Director, Coronary Care Unit, Division of Cardiology, University of California, San Francisco, CA 94143, USA

JOHN AU, M.A.C.P., F.R.C.S., Research Associate, LVAD Technology Clinic, Detroit, MI 48235, USA

MARGARET E. BILLINGHAM, M.D., M.B., B.S., F.R.C.Path., Professor of Pathology, Department of Pathology, Stanford University Medical Center, Stanford, CA 94305, USA

REDMOND P. BURKE, M.D., Fellow, Cardiac Surgery, Harvard Medical School, Department of Surgery, Brigham and Women's Hospital, Boston, MA 02115, USA

BLASE A. CARABELLO, M.D., Professor of Medicine, Department of Medicine, Division of Cardiology, Medical University of South Carolina, Charleston, SC 29425, USA

RAUL R. CARDONA, M.D., Research Associate, Sinai Hospital; Research Associate, LVAD Technology Clinic, Detroit, MI 48235, USA

JAY N. COHN, M.D., Professor of Medicine, Cardiovascular Division, University of Minnesota Medical School, Minneapolis, MN 55455, USA

LAWRENCE H. COHN, M.D., Professor of Surgery, Harvard Medical School; Chief, Division of Cardiac Surgery, Brigham and Women's Hospital, Boston, MA 02115, USA

WILSON S. COLUCCI, M.D., Associate Professor of Medicine, Brigham and Women's Hospital, Boston, MA 02115, USA

MARK A. CREAGER, M.D., Associate Professor of Medicine, Harvard Medical School; Director of Vascular Diagnostic Lab, Brigham and Women's Hospital, Boston, MA 02115, USA

MICHAEL J. DOMANSKI, M.D., Clinical Trials Branch, National Heart, Lung and Blood Institute, Bethesda, MD 20892, USA

DAVIS C. DRINKWATER, M.D., Associate Professor of Surgery, UCLA School of Medicine, Department of Surgery, Division of Cardio-Thoracic Surgery, Center for the Health Sciences, UCLA Medical Center, Los Angeles, CA 90024, USA

JOHN A. FARMER, M.D., Associate Professor of Medicine, Baylor College of Medicine, Houston, TX 77030, USA

RICHARD I. FOGEL, M.D., Cardiology Fellow, Boston University School of Medicine, Arrhythmia Services, University Hospital, Boston City Hospital, Boston, MA 02118, USA

PAUL S. FREED, M.D., Senior Biomedical Engineer, LVAD Technology Clinic, Detroit, MI 48235, USA

REKHA GARG, M.D., M.S., Scientific Project Officer, Clinical Trials Branch, National Heart, Blood and Lung Institute, Bethesda, MD 20892, USA

THOMAS A. GOLPER, M.D., Professor of Medicine, Kidney Diseases Program, University of Louisville, Louisville, KY 40292, USA

SCOTT H. GOODNIGHT, M.D., Professor of Medicine and Clinical Pharmacology, Clinical Pathology, Oregon Health Sciences University, Portland, OR 97201-3098, USA

RICHARD GORLIN, M.D., Senior Vice President, Ambulatory Program, George Baehr, Professor of Medicine, Mount Sinai Medical Center, New York, NY 10029, USA

STEPHEN S. GOTTLIEB, M.D., Associate Professor of Medicine, University of Maryland, Baltimore, MD 21201, USA

BARRY H. GREENBERG, M.D., Professor of Medicine, Division of Cardiology, Oregon Health Sciences University, Portland, OR 97201-3098, USA

GARRIE J. HAAS, M.D., Assistant Professor of Medicine, Ohio State University, Columbus, OH 43210-1228, USA

CONSTANTINE A. HASSAPOYANNES, M.D., Associate Professor of Medicine, Division of Cardiology, Dorn Veteran's Hospital, Columbia, SC 29201, USA

RAY E. HERSHBERGER, M.D., Assistant Professor of Medicine, Oregon Cardiac Transplant Program, Oregon Health Sciences University, Portland, OR 97201-3098, USA

ALAN T. HIRSCH, M.D., Vascular Medicine Program, Cardiovascular Division, University of Minnesota Medical School, Minneapolis, MN 55455, USA

CHRISTIE B. HOPKINS, M.D., Associate Professor of Medicine, University of South Carolina, Columbia, SC 29203, USA

JEFFREY D. HOSENPUD, M.D., Professor of Medicine, Head, Cardiac Transplant Medicine, Oregon Cardiac Transplant Program, Oregon Health Sciences University, Portland, OR 97201-3098, USA

ADRIAN KANTROWITZ, M.D., Professor of Surgery, Center for Surgical Research, Sinai Hospital of Detroit, Detroit, MI 48235, USA

RALPH A. KELLY, M.D., Assistant Professor of Medicine, Cardiovascular Division, Brigham and Women's Hospital, Boston, MA 02115, USA

MARVIN A. KONSTAM, M.D., Professor of Medicine and Radiology, Division of Cardiology, Tufts University New England Medical Center Hospitals, Boston, MA 02111, USA

JOEL KUPFER, M.D., Staff Cardiologist, Cedars–Sinai Medical Center, Los Angeles, CA 90024, USA

HILLEL LAKS, M.D., Professor, and Çhief Cardiothoracic Surgery; Director, Heart and Heart/Lung Transplant Program, UCLA Medical Center, Los Angeles, CA 90024, USA

CARL V. LEIER, M.D., Professor of Medicine and Pharmacology, Ohio State University Hospitals, Columbus, OH 43210-1228, USA

JAY W. MASON, M.D., Professor of Medicine, Chief, Division of Cardiology, University of Utah Medical Center, Salt Lake City, UT 84132, USA

BARRY MASSIE, M.D., Professor of Medicine, Veteran's Affairs Hospital, San Francisco, CA 94121, USA

ELI MILGALTER, M.D., Department of Cardiothoracic Surgery, Jerusalem, Israel

ROGER M. MILLS, M.D., College of Medicine, University of Florida, Gainesville, FL 32610-0277, USA

MARK J. MORTON, M.D., Professor of Medicine, Division of Cardiology, Oregon Health Sciences University, Portland, OR 97201-3098, USA

WILLIAM P. NELSON, M.D., Professor of Medicine, University of South Carolina, Columbia, SC 29203, USA

ALAN S. NIES, M.D., Executive Director of Clinical Pharmacology, Merck Research Labs, Rahway, NJ 07065-0914, USA

JOHN B. O'CONNELL, M.D., Professor and Chairman, Department of Medicine, University of Mississippi Medical Center, Jackson, MS 39216, USA

MILTON PACKER, M.D., Professor of Medicine and Head of Division of Circulatory Physiology, Columbia Presbyterian, New York, NY 10032, USA

WALTER E. PAE., M.D., Professor of Surgery; Director of Cardiac Transplantation, Division of Cardiothoracic Surgery, Milton S. Hershey Medical Center, Pennsylvania State University, Hershey, PA 17033, USA

CARL PEPINE, M.D., Professor of Medicine/Co-Director, Division of Cardiology; Chief of Cardiology, Veterans Administration Medical Center, Division of Cardiovascular Medicine, University of Florida, Gainesville, FL 32610-0277, USA

WILLIAM S. PEIRCE, M.D., Professor of Surgery, Division of Cardiology, Pennsylvania State University, Milton S. Hershey Medical Center, Hershey, PA 17033, USA

PHILIP J. PODRID, M.D., Associate Professor of Medicine, Boston University School of Medicine, Arrhythmia Service, University Hospital, Boston, MA 02118, USA

HUBERT POULEUR, M.D., Ph.D. Professor of Medicine, University of Louvain School of Medicine, B-1200 Brussels, Belgium

REED D. QUINN, M.D., Research Fellow, Division of Artificial Organs, Department of Surgery, Milton S. Hershey Medical Center, Hershey, PA 17033, USA

STANLEY A. RUBIN, M.D., Attending Cardiologist, Chief of Cardiology, Cardiology Department, Long Beach Veterans Administration Medical Center, Long Beach, CA 90822, USA

ROBERT W. SCHRIER, M.D., Professor and Chairman, Department of Medicine, University of Colorado, Denver, CO 80262, USA

RALPH SHABETAI, M.D., Chief, Division of Cardiology, San Diego School of Medicine, University of California, Veteran's Administration Hospital, San Diego, CA 92161, USA

NORMAN SHARPE, M.D., F.R.A.C.P., F.A.C.C., Associate Professor of Medicine, Department of Medicine, Auckland Hospital, Auckland 1, New Zealand

THOMAS W. SMITH, M.D., Professor of Medicine, Cardiovascular Division, Brigham and Women's Hospital, Boston, MA 02115, USA

THERESE TORDJMAN-FUCHS, M.D., Director, Electrophysiology Laboratory, Boston University School of Medicine, Arrhythmia Service, University Hospital, Boston City Hospital, Boston, MA, 02118, USA

JAMES E. UDELSON, M.D., Director, Nuclear Cardiology Laboratory, Co-Director, Heart Failure/Cardiac Transplant Service, Associate Professor of Medicine and Radiology, Tufts University New England. Medical Center Hospital, Boston, MA 02111, USA

BARRY F. URETSKY, M.D., Associate Professor of Medicine, University of Pittsburgh, Presbyterian University Hospital, Pittsburgh, PA 15213, USA

JEAN-LOUIS VINCENT, M.D., Ph.D., Professor of Medicine, Department of Intensive Care, Erasme University Hospital, 1070 Brussels, Belgium

JAMES B. YOUNG, M.D., Professor of Medicine, Multi-Organ Transplant Center, Baylor College of Medicine, Houston, TX 77030, USA

SALIM YUSUF, M.D., M.B.B.S., F.R.C.P., D.Phil., Director of Cardiology, HGH–McMaster Clinic, Hamilton General Hospital, McMaster University, Hamilton, Ontario, Canada L8L 2X2

Part I
Historical Perspectives

1
Evolution of Concepts of Myocardial Function in the Treatment of Congestive Heart Failure in Man

Richard Gorlin, Jeffrey D. Hosenpud, and Barry H. Greenberg

Over the past 50 years, our understanding of cardiac function in normal and pathophysiologic states has evolved considerably. Not surprisingly, this has resulted in a great many changes in the way that we approach the management of patients with congestive heart failure (CHF). It seems fitting, then, in this introductory chapter of a new textbook on CHF, to provide a brief overview of some of these changes and to draw the important connection between advances in basic science and those in clinical medicine.

Appreciation of myocardial function in man has been an evolutionary process. It has depended on two elements: conceptual and technological advances and the adaptation of animal experiments to man. This chapter considers how conceptual advances could be adapted to man only through major technological advances. The latter permitted either access to critical information, as with the use of cardiac catheterization to determine pressure and flow or the *capability* to *measure* and record data such as cardiac volumes as a function of time, through dynamic imaging.

The clinical rewards of understanding basic pathophysiologic mechanisms begin with practical measures that have helped to evaluate myocardial function. Guiding these have been three concepts that govern much of what we do even today: the characterization of the heart as a pump, analysis of cardiac regulation in terms of force, velocity, and length, and the distinction between systolic and diastolic function.

We are so familiar with measures of myocardial function today, that it is hard to imagine that in the 1950s it was considered a remarkable advance when Hellems and his co-workers[1] first measured pulmonary capillary wedge pressure in order to estimate the filling pressure of the left ventricle. How the human ventricle contracted and the significance of its size were unknown. We would not have known what to do with that information if we had had it. In addition, as a direct result of our better understanding of myocardial function

and the relatively easy access to measurements such as ejection fraction, we can now diagnose more accurately the presence and cause of CHF, predict the clinical course with some degree of certainty, and most important, guide therapies directed at treating this syndrome.

Our early understanding of how heart function was regulated stemmed from the work of late 19th century investigators, culminating in the critical research of Starling.[2] These early experimental observations emphasized the role of stretching of the muscle fiber with consequent release of energy and augmented force of contraction. It remained for the animal investigations of Wiggers,[3] Katz,[4] Sarnoff,[5] and others to put into true perspective other aspects of control of ventricular function, including heart rate, blood pressure, and inotropic stimulation. It was not until the 1950s that Braunwald et al.[6] confirmed Starling's law of the heart in man.

Both technical and conceptual advances have contributed to our understanding of myocardial function. Conceptually, it was from the 1930s to 1950 that the circulatory consequences of heart failure were gradually being defined in man. For example, the contrasting concepts of backward and forward failure emerged.[7,8] The first was based on clinical observation, and the second was based on the fact that for the first time it was possible to study renal physiology in man.

Harrison stated in 1935[7]:

The clinical manifestations of congestive heart failure are due to "back pressure." . . . Dyspnea is a result of back pressure from the left side of the heart and edema . . . dependent on pressure from the right.

Heart failure was thought to be a mechanical disorder: The heart did not pump and empty adequately, and as a result the manifestations were due solely to back pressure and congestion. Dyspnea was a result of back pressure from the left side of the heart, and edema was dependent on elevated pressure from the right.

But with the advent of renal physiologic measure-

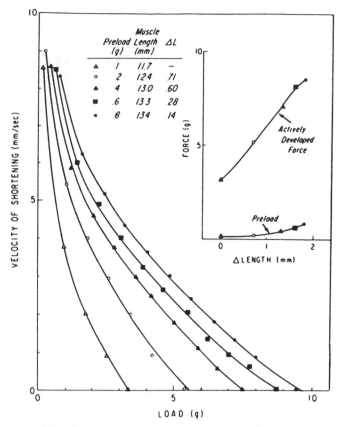

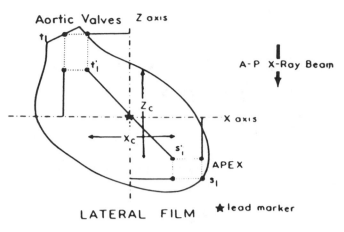

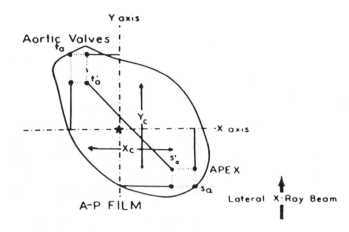

FIGURE 1.1. Effects of increasing initial muscle length on the force-velocity relation of the cat papillary muscle. Initial velocity of shortening has been plotted as a function of load for five different muscle lengths. Reproduced, with permission, from Sonnenblick EH. Series elastic and contractile elements in heart muscle: changes in muscle length. *Am J Physiol.* 1964;207:1330–1338.

FIGURE 1.2. The original geometrical methods and standardization used by Dodge and co-workers to quantify left ventricular volume. Reproduced, with permission, from Dodge HT et al. The use of biplane angiocardiography for the measurement of left ventricular volume in man. *Am Heart J.* 1960;60:762–776.

ments and the understanding of sodium exchange metabolism, renal plasma flow, and tubular function, Warren and Stead[8] in 1944 proposed another concept: forward failure. They pointed out that edema may develop in congestive failure because the kidneys do not excrete salt and water normally. This led to increased extracellular and intravascular volume, and finally to increased venous pressure. The shift in emphasis, of course, stimulated intense investigation of intrarenal mechanisms responsible for fluid retention and resulted in an appreciation of the important role of neurohormonal factors in salt and water retention in heart failure. This information supplied a rational basis for selecting powerful diuretics that act on specific sites in the nephron and the combining of diuretics that act on different sites to achieve specific purposes such as enhanced diuresis or preservation of potassium. It also helped stimulate interest in drugs that could inhibit some of the neurohormonal pathways that are activated in CHF.

Another important conceptual advance was made in understanding the cardiac aspects of heart failure when the heart was analyzed as a muscle. This emanated from the work of Abbott and Mommaerts,[9] followed by Sonnenblick,[10] who described the biophysical characteristics of contractile elements of isolated cardiac muscle (Fig. 1.1). These and other workers ultimately applied these principles to the overall contraction of the intact heart. This was accomplished through advances in imaging[11] (Fig. 1.2) and in integration with hemodynamics. This permitted the differentiation between abnormalities of the myocardium and abnormalities of the loading conditions of the heart. In analogy to force, velocity, and length, one could characterize regulation of the heart as dependent on afterload, preload, contractility, and heart rate and thus begin to rationalize ways in which the heart could be controlled[10,12] (Fig. 1.3). Much of this rested on fundamental studies of force, velocity, and length of muscle. These concepts

COMPENSATORY MECHANISMS FOR
REDUCED EFFECTIVE CARDIAC OUTPUT

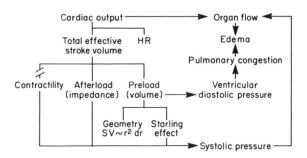

FIGURE 1.3. Flow diagram demonstrating that cardiac output is a function of heart rate and effective stroke volume while the latter is dependent on contractility, afterload, and preload. Preload in turn is a function of both a simple volumetric effect and increased force delivered by fiber stretching, the Starling effect. The portion of the diagram to the right shows how flow and pressure influence congestion and edema.

have largely faded from clinical view, but they have left their progeny, for example, in understanding distinctions between loading of the muscle and the regulation of cardiac contraction.

That leads naturally to characterizing the heart as a pump as well as a muscle. There are two major issues here: The first is the independence, as well as the interdependence, of the two ventricles.[13] The concept was long in coming that the two ventricles could function either separately or together under different conditions, depending on the common septum and the overall pericardial constraints. Second was the simple act of defining the cardiac chamber, which depended on quantitative time-related radiography: volume, shape, and wall dimension, which had not been studied, now were available as a continuum. Rushmer[13] used cineangiograms of the cardiac chambers throughout the cardiac cycle in animals and observed things that had not been thought about before. But it is the integration of all this that is essential. Dynamic cardiac imaging was put together with hemodynamics in order to define the heart as a pump as well as a muscle.

The cardiac cycle is probably the most important feature for us to delineate. While intertwined, systole and diastole make separate contributions both in health and disease. The first aspect is, obviously, impaired contractility. For clinical purposes the best marker for this is the ejection fraction. Initially, residual volume fraction had been used in experimental physiology to identify the poorly contractile ventricle. Its reciprocal, ejection fraction, emerged in clinical studies in the 1960s.[15] A second refinement appeared with the description of diastolic dysfunction, when the heart fails to fill appropriately.[16] The presumed causes are decreased diastolic relaxation (end-systolic) and diminished dia-

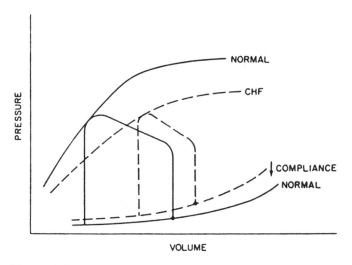

FIGURE 1.4. Pressure-volume curves for both the normal and the failing heart. Differences in compliance also are illustrated. The pressure-volume loop for the patient with heart failure shifts to the right and upward owing to a reduced pressure-volume relationship during systole and an increased pressure-volume relationship during diastole. Reproduced, with permission, from Grossman W. Diastolic dysfunction and congestive heart failure. *Circulation.* 1990;81(suppl III):III-1. Copyright by the American Heart Association.

stolic compliance, resulting in alterations in the pressure/volume/time relationships in diastole (Fig. 1.4).

Either systolic or diastolic dysfunction can result in low output, high filling pressure, and the potential for clinical congestive failure. Figure 1.5 represents the two disparate effects of the Starling mechanism and of altered distensibility on cardiac performance. The two broad forms of abnormality, that is, hypertrophy (center panel) versus dilation (right panel), are compared with normal (left panel). The upper set of curves represents the Starling relationship of stroke work to end-diastolic volume, whereas the lower set depicts compliance or the relationship of end-diastolic filling pressure to end-diastolic volume.

Under normal circumstances, as filling volume increases so does cardiac work. The compliance curve is so flat that filling pressure does not approach "pulmonary edema" levels. When hypertrophy or any other pathological state that increases wall stiffness is present, the Starling relationship is unaffected but increases in volume sufficient to maintain or increase cardiac force or work now may lead to unacceptably high filling pressures. Conversely, when filling pressures are normal, end-diastolic volume is usually too low to provoke an adequate myocardial response.

When dilatation occurs, as with any chronic volume load or damage to myocardium, the Starling curve is flat and cardiac work does not increase in response to volume. Filling pressure will be a function of the abnormal but often flat compliance curve. Combinations of

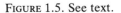
FIGURE 1.5. See text.

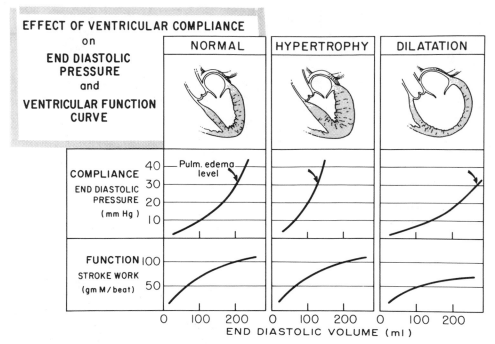

the two extremes of systolic and diastolic dysfunction often occur simultaneously as a result of various disorders of the myocardium and their interactions with loading conditions. In the past, most therapeutic approaches have been aimed toward correction of abnormalities resulting from systolic dysfunction. It is clear that in the future greater attention will have to be

directed toward understanding and treating diastolic abnormalities.

The last concept to enter the complex of myocardial function is that of asynergy[17] (Fig. 1.6). Ventricular contraction, from end-diastole to end-systole, is neither uniform nor necessarily symmetrical, especially with disease or with ectopic impulse formation. Zones of

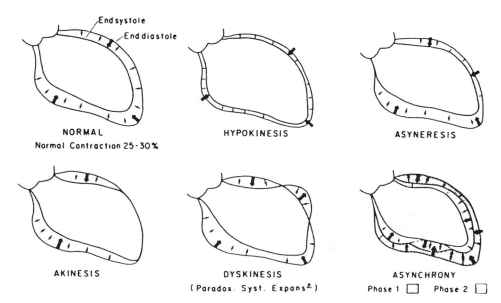

FIGURE 1.6. Silhouettes of ventricular contraction in the right anterior oblique projection from the original publication describing myocardial asynergy. Hypokinesis is self-explanatory, whereas asyneresis describes asymmetrically diminished contractile effort. Akinesis describes a zone of myocardium that exhibits no contraction, whereas dyskinesis is frank expansion (paradox. syst. expansion) during systole. Asynchrony describes a temporal disorder of contraction that vitiates a coordinated contraction and thus reduces stroke volume. Reproduced, with permission, from Herman MV et al. Localized disorders in myocardial contraction. *N Engl J Med.* 1967;277:225.

myocardium may not contract (akinesis), or there may be temporal disorder of systole so that the contraction is asynchronous. *Patterns* of contraction are as important as the *extent* of contraction. An asynchronous contraction is as serious a "pump" problem as frank hypokinesis.

How have these lessons been applied to clinical cardiology? The prognostic value of ejection fraction was first demonstrated in the early 1970s.[18] In a 1-year follow-up of 144 patients with coronary artery disease, reduction in ejection fraction was found to be a powerful predictor of subsequent mortality. Many studies use the ejection fraction as a measure of systolic contractile loss. The Vasodilators in Heart Failure Trial (VHeFT) showed mortality to correlate with the degree of depression of the ejection fraction.[19] This was true whether or not the patients had clinical congestive failure.

Does this tell the physician everything that needs to be known about the patient? No. In the registry of the SOLVD trial,[20] those with ejection fractions less than .29 were much more at risk of death than those with higher ejection fractions. Rate of hospitalization in heart failure patients, on the other hand, remained a consistent 12% to 16%, irrespective of ejection fraction.

In addition to ejection fraction, two other measures are exceedingly useful. These are cardiac size and cardiac shape. The larger the volume of the ventricle[21,22] and the rounder the heart,[23] the higher the mortality.

Improvement in therapy can be predicted from the physiologic principles. It is no coincidence that the use of vasodilators came into prominence almost simultaneously with the development of a flow-directed right heart catheter that allowed easy access to measurements of intracardiac pressures and flow. In this case, technical development helped familiarize researchers and clinicians with the prominent role of peripheral vasoconstriction in the pathophysiology of CHF. It soon became clear that vasodilator drugs could dramatically improve cardiac function in this setting. A series of a recent clinical trials,[19,24,25] which have shown that this kind of therapy can improve both survival and the rate of progression of CHF, serve as the latest examples of the powerful and rapid impact of basic science on clinical medicine.

Summary

Understanding myocardial function in man has been an evolutionary process. What is important is to know that the conceptual advances often proceed parallel with technological advances. The melding of basic muscle force-velocity-length concepts with the clinical physiological equivalents has been crucial. The integration of pressure and flow with dynamic quantitative imaging has been absolutely essential. As a result, we have gained a remarkable ability to prognosticate about our patients as well as to diagnose and to evaluate therapy.

References

1. Hellems HK, Haynes FW, Dexter L, Kinney TD. Pulmonary capillary pressure in animals estimated by venous and arterial catheterization. *Am J Physiol.* 1948;155:98–105.
2. Starling EH. Linacre Lecture on the Law of the Heart given at Cambridge, 1915. 27 pp. London, Longmans, 1918.
3. Wiggers CJ. *Modern Aspects of the Circulation in Health and Disease.* Philadelphia: Lea and Febiger; 1923.
4. Katz LN. The performance of the heart. (The Lewis A. Conner Memorial Lecture). *Circulation.* 1960;21:483–498.
5. Sarnoff SJ. Myocardial contractility as described by ventricular function curves; observations on Starling's law of the heart. *Physiol. Rev.* 1955;35:107–122.
6. Braunwald E, Frye RL, Aygen MM, Gilbert JW. Studies on Starling's law of the heart III. Observations in patients with mitral stenosis and atrial fibrillation on relationships between left ventricular end-diastolic segment length, filling pressure, and characteristics of ventricular contraction. *J Clin Invest.* 1960;39:1874–1884.
7. Harrison TR. *Failure of the Circulation.* Baltimore: Williams & Wilkins; 1935.
8. Warren JV, Stead EA Jr. Fluid dynamics in chronic congestive heart failure. An interpretation of the mechanisms producing the edema, increased plasma volume and elevated venous pressure in certain patients with prolonged congestive failure. *Arch Intern Med.* 1944;73:138–147.
9. Abbott BC, Mommaerts WFHM. Study of inotropic mechanisms in the papillary muscle preparation. *J Gen Physiol.* 1959;42:533–551.
10. Sonnenblick EH. Force-velocity relations in mammalian heart muscle. *Am J Physiol.* 1962;202:931–939.
11. Dodge HT, Hay RE, Sandler H. Pressure-volume characteristics of the diastolic left ventricle of man with heart disease. *Am Heart J.* 1962;64:503–511.
12. Gorlin R, Sonnenblick EH. Regulation of performance of the heart. *Am J Cardiol.* 1968;22:16–23.
13. Bemis CE, Serur JR, Borkenhagen D, Sonnenblick EH, Urschel CW. Influence of right ventricular filling pressure and dimension. *Circ Res.* 1974;34:498–504.
14. Rushmer RF. *Cardiovascular Dynamics.* Philadelphia: Saunders; 1961.
15. Gorlin R, Rolett EL, Yurchak PM, Elliott WC. Left ventricular volume in man measured by thermodilution. *J Clin Invest.* 1964;43:1203–1221.
16. Grossman W. Diastolic dysfunction and congestive heart failure. *Circulation.* 1990;81(suppl III):III-1–III-7.
17. Herman MV, Heinle RA, Klein MD, Gorlin R. Localized disorders in myocardial contraction. Asynergy and its role in congestive heart failure. *N Engl J Med.* 1967;277:222–232.
18. Cohn PF, Gorlin R, Collins JJ, Cohn L. The left ventricular ejection fraction as a prognostic guide in the surgical

treatment of coronary and valvular heart disease. *Am J Cardiol.* 1974;34:135–141.

19. V-HeFT Study. Effect of vasodilator therapy on mortality in chronic congestive heart failure. *N Engl J Med.* 1986;314:1547–1552.

20. The SOLVD Investigators. Effect of enalapril on survival in patients with reduced left ventricular ejection fractions and congestive heart failure. *N Engl J Med.* 1991; 325:293–302.

21. White HD, Norris RM, Brown MA, Brandt PWT, Whitlock RML, Wild CJ. Left ventricular end-systolic volume as the major determinant of survival after recovery from myocardial infarction. *Circulation.* 1987;76:44–51.

22. Hammermeister KE, Chikos PM, Fisher LL, Dodge HT. Relationship of cardiothoracic ratio and plain film heart volume to late survival. *Circulation.* 1979;59:89–95.

23. Douglas PA, Morrow R, Ioli A, Reichek N. Left ventricular shape, afterload and survival in idiopathic dilated cardiomyopathy. *J Am Coll Cardiol.* 1989;13:311–315.

24. The SOLVD Investigators. Effect of enalapril on mortality and the development of heart failure in asymptomatic patients with reduced left ventricular ejection fractions. *N Engl J Med.* 1992;327:685–691.

25. The SAVE Investigators. Effect of captopril on mortality and morbidity in patients with left ventricular dysfunction after myocardial infarction. *N Engl J Med.* 1992;327:669–677.

Part II
Pathophysiology of Congestive Heart Failure

2
Overview of Pathophysiology of Clinical Heart Failure

Jay N. Cohn

The syndrome of clinical heart failure (CHF) is growing in incidence and importance as our population ages. It has become one of the most common illnesses accounting for hospital admissions and physician visits in people over the age of 65 years. But despite its frequency and its well known manifestations, it remains a poorly understood, inadequately treated, and surprisingly lethal disease process. Since it represents the common pathway of progression of nearly all forms of heart disease, it is intuitive that recognition, pathophysiology, and management might differ depending on etiologic factors. This heterogeneity of the clinical syndrome adds to the complexity of its pathophysiology. This chapter addresses pathophysiologic mechanisms that impact on the diagnosis and treatment of heart failure. A number of recent studies and reviews have dealt extensively with this subject.[1-10]

The diagnosis of clinical heart failure is based on a constellation of signs and symptoms that may be recognized at the bedside or may require more precise quantitation by laboratory tests. When confronted with the full-blown clinical syndrome in a patient with known preexisting heart disease, the diagnosis is simple. Thus, the patient presenting with pedal edema, pulmonary congestion, an enlarged heart with a loud S3, jugular venous distention, and a tachycardia with a small pulse volume can clearly be identified as a patient with congestive heart failure. On the other hand, a patient presenting with complaints of exertional fatigue but without edema or congestion and with only minor cardiac findings represents a considerably more subtle presentation of the syndrome. The latter patient would need visualization of the heart and possibly a formal exercise test before the diagnosis could be established. If this latter patient were demonstrated to have a dilated and poorly contractiled left ventricle and if his/her exercise capacity were clearly diminished on a standard stress test, then the diagnosis of heart failure would be justified. Since congestion was not part of the clinical pic-ture in this patient, however, the term "congestive heart failure" would be inappropriate and should be replaced by the more general phrase, clinical heart failure.

There are four major clinical manifestations of heart failure that need to be understood. These include left ventricular dysfunction, exercise intolerance, sodium retention with edema and congestion, and ventricular arrhythmias.

Left Ventricular Dysfunction

Most cardiac disorders in our society exert their primary effect on the left ventricle. Thus, impairment of left ventricular function should be considered a prerequisite for diagnosing heart failure. Quantitation of the severity of left ventricular dysfunction is complicated by the variety of measurements that can be made. Left ventricular ejection fraction, which represents the stroke volume divided by the end-diastolic volume, is a commonly employed noninvasive measurement that can be performed either by echocardiography, by radionuclide techniques, or by ventriculography utilizing dye injected into the left ventricle. Any of these methods can provide a quantitation of the ejection fraction. This measurement quantitates systolic pump function but provides little insight into baseline cardiac output or the presence of symptoms. Indeed, symptoms of heart failure can exist in patients with a normal ejection fraction, and a very low ejection fraction can exist in the absence of symptoms. Therefore, the demonstration of the magnitude of left ventricular dysfunction should be viewed primarily as a diagnostic test to establish the presence of heart disease and a potentially useful prognostic marker for the disease.

Diastolic dysfunction of the ventricle also may lead to symptoms of heart failure. Although the most common form of diastolic dysfunction is the one that coexists with systolic dysfunction and merely contributes to the elevated ventricular filling pressure, there may be a considerable reservoir of patients who have primary diastolic dysfunction without evidence of poor systolic emptying of the ventricle. This diastolic dysfunction is manifested by an inappropriately high end-diastolic pressure for the given end-diastolic volume. Since noninvasive techniques to assess ventricular diastolic function are considerably less precise than those to define systolic function, the presence and magnitude of this disorder as a contributor to the syndrome of heart failure is as yet poorly understood.

It appears that all diseases that affect the myocardium may eventuate in impaired systolic and/or diastolic function. Coronary artery disease may develop initially as a regional wall motion abnormality that can contribute to poor systolic emptying, but in later stages of the disease there may be global systolic dysfunction as well as impaired diastolic filling. Similarly, cardiomyopathies may exhibit global systolic dysfunction at an early stage of the disease but often there may be regional heterogeneity in the degree of systolic dysfunction. Diastolic dysfunction may coexist with the systolic dysfunction. In diseases associated with ventricular hypertrophy, such as hypertension and aortic stenosis, wall thickening may impair diastolic function but fibrosis and structural alterations in the myocardium may eventuate in systolic dysfunction as well. Valvular regurgitation such as aortic or mitral insufficiency precipitates a volume overload of the left ventricle that initially may be compensated by increased systolic emptying. But eventually structural and functional changes in the myocardium and interstitium contribute to impairment of both systolic and diastolic function.

Although the degree of systolic dysfunction as defined by left ventricular ejection fraction bears a poor relationship to symptoms of heart failure, the magnitude of depression of ejection fraction appears to serve as a powerful guide to prognosis. In most large scale trials the lower the initial left ventricular ejection fraction the shorter the life expectancy.

Exercise Intolerance

The primary clinical manifestation of heart failure is reduction of exercise capacity. Exertional dyspnea or fatigue are hallmarks of the disease that usually lead the patient to seek medical attention. Although traditional thinking has assumed that the degree of exercise intolerance should be correlated with the degree of left ventricular dysfunction, that is not the case in most clinical trials. The problem with the symptom of exercise intolerance is that it depends on a variety of factors including motivation of the patient, blood flow to exercising skeletal muscle, gas exchange in the pulmonary vasculature, the filling pressure of the right and left

ventricle, and metabolic factors both in skeletal muscle and in the myocardium. Thus, it is hardly surprising that the degree of cardiac dilatation as reflected by the depression of left ventricular ejection fraction does not serve as a sensitive marker for exercise intolerance.

Quantitation of exercise capacity can be carried out on a bicycle or treadmill in an exercise laboratory. When gas exchange is monitored as well, it is possible to characterize the patient on the basis of oxygen consumption achieved at the time anaerobic metabolism occurs as well as the oxygen consumption reached at the time exercise is terminated because of dyspnea or fatigue. The test also allows for the identification of individuals who cease exercising before the onset of anaerobic metabolism apparently for reasons unrelated to cardiac dysfunction. Thus, an exercise test, particularly with gas exchange measurement, can confirm the diagnosis of heart failure and quantitate the severity of the disability.

A conceptual and practical problem with laboratory stress tests is that they usually are designed as progressive tests to a maximally tolerated load. Although it might intuitively be assumed that maximum exercise capacity would correlate with the comfort in performing submaximal exercise, that relationship has not been established in patients with heart failure. Since fatigue and dyspnea that limit daily activity usually result from repeated submaximal exercise, it would be helpful to have quantitative submaximal tests available for evaluating patients with heart failure. A number of approaches to this problem currently are being evaluated.

Sodium Retention

Renal retention of sodium may be an early manifestation of left ventricular dysfunction. The mechanism of this sodium retention is not entirely understood, but may relate both to abnormalities of renal perfusion and of tubular function. Contributors to the renal perfusion abnormalities may include activation of neural and endocrine factors that contribute directly to renal vasoconstriction and may influence glomerular filtration rate and peritubular pressure.

To a certain extent the sodium retention of heart failure may be viewed as a compensatory mechanism initiated by a fall in cardiac output. Enhanced intravascular volume would thus augment ventricular filling and theoretically increase cardiac output by virtue of the Frank Starling mechanism. But the sodium retention soon becomes an important contributor to symptoms. The enhanced systemic venous pressure leads to edema formation in the dependent portions of the body and the elevated pulmonary venous pressure leads to pulmonary congestion and exertional dyspnea. The congestive symptoms may be enhanced further by impairment of lymph flow resulting from the elevated right atrial pressure. Consequently, increased atrial pressure sets into motion a number of events that will precipitate and perpetuate tissue fluid accumulation: (a) increased venous pressure leading to transudation out of the capillary bed, (b) decreased lymph flow aggravating tissue fluid accumulation, (c) valvular regurgitation that may further increase atrial pressure, and (d) decreased renal sodium excretion by virtue of catecholamine, angiotensin, and vasopressin-induced renal vasoconstriction and inhibited tubular reabsorption not adequately counteracted by activation of atrial natriuretic peptide secretion.

The marked variation in the degree of sodium retention among different individuals with left ventricular dysfunction leads to a varied clinical presentation. In some patients edema may be the first manifestation of heart failure even in the absence of much fatigue. In others quite severe left ventricular dysfunction and exertional fatigue may exist in the absence of sodium retention or congestion. This unexplained variability raises the possibility that other factors play a role in the complex internal mechanisms determining the ability to excrete a salt load.

Ventricular Arrhythmias

Premature ventricular depolarizations and runs of nonsustained ventricular tachycardia commonly are observed in patients with left ventricular dysfunction. These ventricular arrhythmias usually are asymptomatic and are detected by ambulatory Holter monitoring. Since sudden death is a common terminal event in patients with heart failure, the role of these ventricular arrhythmias in the genesis of this presumed arrhythmic death needs to be carefully evaluated.

A variety of mechanisms may contribute to the high density of ventricular arrhythmias in the setting of heart failure. Myocardial hypertrophy and ventricular dilatation appear to be important risk factors in the development of arrhythmias, possibly because of reentry mechanisms related to structural changes in the ventricle or to alterations of channel function that may influence local transmembrane potential. The role of metabolic abnormalities and of neurohormonal activation also must be considered in the genesis of these arrhythmias.

Although the presence of ventricular arrhythmias may influence prognosis independently, it is apparent that the major determinants of life expectancy in patients with heart failure relate to left ventricular dysfunction rather than to the presence or absence of the ventricular arrhythmias. Consequently, the most prudent approach at the moment is to view these arrhythmias as manifestations of the heart failure and to focus on management of the heart failure rather than the arrhythmias.

Compensatory Responses in Clinical Heart Failure

In response to the primary disease process affecting the left ventricle, a number of systems appear to be activated leading to systemic and cardiac effects. The activation of these diverse systems may account for many of the symptoms of heart failure and may contribute importantly to the progression of the syndrome. Although these responses may be viewed as compensatory in nature, many of them are or become counterregulatory and lead to adverse effects.

Neuroendocrine Stimulation

Activation of neurohormonal vasoconstrictor systems is a hallmark of the heart failure syndrome. Activation of the sympathetic nervous systems appears to be an almost invariable accompaniment of heart failure and is even observed in patients with left ventricular dysfunction who have no symptoms of heart failure. This activation can be documented by the presence of high circulating levels of norepinephrine and by the measurement of increased sympathetic nerve traffic. The afferent stimulus for activating the sympathetic nervous system has not been well defined, but it probably involves baroreceptor function as well as chemoreceptor activation, possibly through metabolic changes in skeletal muscle.

The renin-angiotensin system is variably altered in patients with heart failure but occasionally may be strikingly stimulated. The weak correlation observed between plasma norepinephrine and plasma renin activity raises the likelihood that the sympathetic nervous system is not the major determinant of renin secretion in heart failure. Since renal baroreceptors appear to remain active in patients with heart failure, hypotension may be one stimulus for renin activation. Sodium retention and diuretic therapy also may contribute during the course of therapy for heart failure. Vasopressin, the third potent endogenous vasoconstrictor system, also is frequently elevated in patients with heart failure, usually to levels about twice normal. Osmolality does not appear to be the major stimulus for this vasopressin release and thus hemodynamic factors may play a key role. The interaction between the sympathetic nervous system, the renin-angiotensin system, and the vasopressin system may further influence the degree of activation of these hormonal systems.

A more recently studied hormonal system that is activated in heart failure and is dependent on the degree of ventricular dilatation is atrial natriuretic factor (ANF).

This peptide hormone secreted from the atria—and perhaps also from dysfunctional ventricles—exhibits a modest vasodilator effect that may be designed as a compensation for the vasoconstrictor hormone stimulation already described. Unfortunately, however, ANF is a relatively weak vasodilator and appears not to overcome adequately the vasoconstriction associated with heart failure. The diuretic effect of ANF also appears to be quite modest, particularly in patients with heart failure who have had sustained stimulation from the hormone. ANF also inhibits neurohormonal stimulation. Consequently, it may be viewed as a counterregulatory system not potent enough to counteract the vasoconstriction and antinatriuresis of heart failure.

Ventricular Hypertrophy and Remodeling

Whether ventricular hypertrophy precedes dilatation or dilatation precedes hypertrophy probably depends on the nature of the cardiac disease. Inevitably, however, these two pathological processes coexist. Progressive ventricular dilatation can be recognized clinically by echocardiographic measurements or by a reduction in left ventricular ejection fraction. This chamber enlargement must result either from elongation of the myofibrils by addition of sarcomeres longitudinally or by slippage of fibers in a remodeling process. In either case, however, the enlarged chamber will increase the radius of curvature and increase wall stress, a physical stimulus to myocardial hypertrophy. Thus, chamber enlargement and wall thickening are interactive processes that can be set into motion by myocardial damage or by an increase in workload.

The hypertrophy and remodeling of the ventricular chamber may depend on both load and hormonal influences. The relative importance of these two physiologic determinants of hypertrophy is difficult to define since interventions usually influence both factors. Pharmacologic approaches to inhibition of these processes is clearly a high priority in current mechanistic studies.

A critical issue is whether the compensatory dilatation and hypertrophy should be viewed as a favorable or an unfavorable response to left ventricular dysfunction. Traditional thinking suggests that the expanded end-diastolic volume is a useful response to maintain stroke volume in the face of a reduced wall motion. Similarly, hypertrophy can be viewed as compensatory to restore ventricular mass toward normal in view of loss of functioning myocardium. On the other hand, the dilatation, if left unchecked, leads to a strikingly enlarged chamber size, which of necessity results in a reduction of global wall motion. Similarly, the hypertrophy is associated with collagen growth, perfusion inadequacy, and myosin changes that may adversely affect left ventricular systolic and/or diastolic function. Indeed, it is possible that the remodeling process is a

major determinant of progression of the heart failure syndrome and its premature mortality.

Vasoconstriction

Increase in tone of the systemic vasculature is an expected finding in patients with heart failure. This tone increase is reflected in an increase in calculated systemic vascular resistance, a reduction in vascular compliance, and alterations in regional distribution of blood flow. Venoconstriction is reflected in an increase in venous tone, a decrease in venous capacitance, and an increase in the fraction of blood volume contained in the central circulation. These peripheral vascular changes result in an increase in impedance to left ventricular ejection and an increase in preload to the ventricle that contributes to dilatation and may contribute to ventricular remodeling.

The mechanism of vasoconstriction in heart failure probably is multifactorial. Activation of the sympathetic nervous system, the renin-angiotensin system, and vasopressin may contribute to an increase in vascular tone but attempts to correlate vasoconstriction with the degree of activation of these systems has been disappointing. Endothelial dysfunction may play an independent role in contributing to the changes in vascular tone. Preliminary studies suggest that endothelial-derived vascular relaxation is impaired in patients with heart failure, and this endothelial dysfunction may contribute to a reduction in arterial compliance and an increase in arterial resistance. Other local hormonal abnormalities also may contribute to tissue-mediated vasoconstriction independent of the systemic neuroendocrine measurements.

The role of the increase in systemic vascular tone in the natural history of heart failure has received considerable attention in recent years. Drugs that exert a relaxing effect on the arterial and venous circulation produce profound improvements in left ventricular function and appear also to exert a favorable effect on the course of the disease. However, the long-term benefits of these vasodilator drugs on exercise tolerance and survival may well relate to actions above and beyond their vasodilator actions. Consequently, some vasodilator drugs do not appear to share the favorable long-term benefits in this syndrome, whereas other vasodilators with even less vascular actions appear to have favorable long-term effects.

A feature of the peripheral circulation that has been less well explored in heart failure is the possibility that structural changes contribute to the increased impedance that imposes a load on the left ventricle. Vasoconstrictor substances often exert mitogenic effects that lead to vascular growth and remodeling. It is possible that some of the vascular changes observed in heart failure, much like those observed in hypertension, result

FIGURE 2.1. The interaction of various pathophysiologic mechanisms that lead to clinical heart failure.

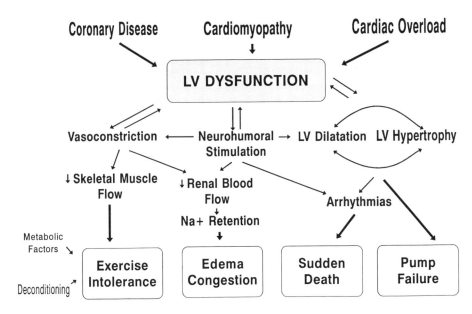

from structural alterations that may reverse more slowly than functional changes in response to drug therapy. Thus, growth inhibition as well as vasodilation may be critical for the long-term benefit of vasodilator drugs in this syndrome.

Integrated Pathophysiologic Mechanisms

The complex processes that initiate left ventricular dysfunction and contribute to symptoms and progression of the syndrome involve hemodynamic, metabolic, neuroendocrine, and structural changes. It is hardly surprising, therefore, that multiple therapeutic agents are being explored for their efficacy in this syndrome and that polypharmacy is gradually becoming the standard approach to treatment. The diversity of the syndrome also accounts for the multiple therapeutic endpoints that may be used in evaluating severity and therapeutic efficacy in the syndrome. Thus, symptom relief, improvement in ventricular function, relief of sodium retention, and prolongation of life all may be viewed as potentially independent endpoints for therapeutic response.

The interaction of these various pathophysiologic mechanisms is depicted in Figure 2.1. Despite the apparent complexity of this diagrammatic representation, it still may be oversimplified. Furthermore, it stresses only the macrophysiology and disregards the molecular and cellular aspects that are critical to the understanding of the disease process. Adrenergic receptor function, cyclic AMP generation, G protein abnormalities, calcium flux in cardiac and vascular smooth muscle, myocardial mechanics, electrical abnormalities in con-

duction tissue, and a host of other events at the cellular and subcellular level remain to be explored.

The rapid advances made in the past decade in our understanding of this syndrome, however, lead to optimism that new insights will have a significant impact on prognosis. It is becoming clear that the progressive nature of heart failure with its impairment of life style and premature death results in large part from processes in the myocardium and peripheral vasculature that can be prevented. The heart is a remarkable organ that appears to compensate rather effectively for acute loss of muscle function. It is this very compensation, however, that may lead to adverse long-term effects. The agenda for the next decade is to gain new understanding of the regulatory and counterregulatory mechanisms that contribute to the compensation and subsequent decompensation in this disease. Only then will we be able to develop therapeutic strategies that can arrest the process at the stage of modest cardiac impairment. Optimism is in order that this fundamental insight into the process will be accomplished and the approach to heart failure in the 21st century will be prevention rather than treatment.

References

1. Cohn JN. Current therapy of the failing heart. *Circulation*. 1988;78:1099–1107.
2. Cohn JN. Treatment by modification of circulatory dynamics. *Hosp Pract*.1984,9:37–51.
3. Cohn JN, Archibald DG, Francis GS. Veterans Administration Cooperative Study on vasodilator therapy of heart failure: Influence of prerandomization variables on the reduction of mortality by treatment with hydralazine and isosorbide dinitrate. *Circulation*. 1987;75:IV49–IV54.
4. Cohn JN, Johnson G. Heart failure with normal ejection

fraction: the V-HeFT Study. *Circulation*. 1990;81 (suppl III):III-48–III-53.

5. Cohn JN, Rector TS. Prognosis of congestive heart failure and predictors of mortality. *Am J Cardiol*. 1988;62:25A–30A.

6. Finkelstein SM, Cohn JN, Collins RV, Carlyle PF, Shelley W. Vascular hemodynamic impedance in congestive heart failure. *Am J Cardiol*. 1985;55:423–427.

7. Francis GS, Cohn JN. Heart failure: mechanisms of cardiac and vascular dysfunction and the rationale for pharmacologic intervention. Reviews. *FASEB J*. 1990;4:3068–3075.

8. Pfeffer MA, Braunwald E. Ventricular remodeling after myocardial infarction. *Circulation*. 1990;81:1161–1172.

9. Rector TS, Olivari MT, Levine TB, Francis GS, Cohn JN. Predicting survival for an individual with congestive heart failure using the plasma norepinephrine concentration. *Am Heart J*. 1987;114:148–152.

10. Sullivan MJ, Knight JD, Higginbotham MB, Cobb FR. Relation between central and peripheral hemodynamics during exercise in patients with chronic heart failure. *Circulation*. 1989;80:769–781.

3
The Molecular and Cellular Biology of Heart Failure

Joel Kupfer and Stanley A. Rubin

The annals of science are a dazzlingly lighted hall which can only be reached by passing through a long and ghastly kitchen.
Claude Bernard

The clinician's knowledge and perspective of heart failure has evolved concomitantly with the scientific investigation of the cardiovascular system. This is no accident of coincidence, but rather the purposeful adoption and adaptation by physicians of new information and insight developed through research from the basic and clinical sciences. If a previous clinical era of knowledge about heart failure was characterized by the contemporary information gleaned from research into pathology, and the present by physiology and biochemistry, then most assuredly the next will be strongly influenced by molecular and cellular biology. Molecular biology is a collection of methods and resources that are used to study the structure, function, and regulation of genes, whereas cellular biology is those that are used to study cell processes and functions. These methods and resources are not a discipline, but rather are a set of tools that are readily available as a mechanism of inquiry into the structure and function of the cardiovascular system by anatomists, biochemists, physiologists, and clinicians.

Our goal in this chapter is to provide the reader with the basic concepts and knowledge of some molecular and cellular science. We then apply this knowledge to some of the contemporary information concerning the molecular basis of cardiac function and hypertrophy. Finally, we suggest how this burgeoning knowledge may be applied to the diagnosis and treatment of heart failure.

A Primer of Molecular and Cellular Biology

"What is the secret of life?" I asked.
"Protein," the bartender declared.
"They found out something about protein."
—*Cat's Cradle*, Kurt Vonnegut

Proteins Are a Focus of Research in Molecular and Cellular Biology

Molecular and cellular biology is the study of cellular structure and function. These disciplines narrow attention to individual proteins (and their genes) and their relationship to specific cellular processes. For example, within the cell membrane of the heart are specific proteins that perform essential structural, receptor, and channel functions necessary for generation of action potentials and electromechanical coupling. Additional sets of proteins coordinate the contractile machinery of the cell through the myofilaments and provide energy through the metabolic machinery of the mitochondrion. Still others orchestrate the life cycle of the cell.

Proteins consist of single or multiple polypeptide chains. In their simplest form, each polypeptide chain represents a linear biopolymer assembled from covalently linked amino acids. Despite this deceiving simplicity, functional polypeptides are obtained only after complex folding into specific secondary, tertiary, and quaternary structures takes place. Specific patterns of higher structure (e.g., alpha-helix or beta-pleated sheet) are determined by the chemical and electrical interactions between neighboring amino acids and the sequence in which they are ordered in the polypeptide chain. More specifically, secondary structure refers to the folding of segments of polypeptides into regular repeating structures such as an alpha-helix or beta-pleated sheet. Tertiary structure represents the folding and interweaving of these secondary structures, and all other noncovalent interactions into a three-dimensional structure. Quaternary structure refers to noncovalent interactions that bind several polypeptide chains together.

The sequence in which amino acids are incorporated into a growing polypeptide chain is determined by specific nucleotide sequences within the DNA of the gene, which is the basic unit of information within the chromosomes of the cell. Because there are 20 amino acids, each with distinct chemical properties and nearly an infinite way of ordering them, there is tremendous potential for functional diversity.

It turns out that protein function is more closely related to these advanced structural forms rather than the simple primary structure of linear biopolymers of amino acids. This does not mean that the ordering of amino acids is unimportant. But that protein function is more closely determined by the biophysical properties of the complete structure: this in turn being a function of the amino acid sequence and the information encoded at the gene level. This is because the interactions between proteins and ions are largely biophysical, and determined by such surface features as pockets of specific size, shape, and charge. For example, amino acid substitutions that retain the basic elements of charge and pH may not interfere with important structural domains and protein function is left intact. On the other hand, substitution of a single amino acid that results in a change in the tertiary structure may interfere with protein function; for example, the substitution of valine for glutamate at position 6 of the hemoglobin B chain substantially impairs its oxygen carrying capacity and causes sickle cell anemia.

A Paradigm Shift in the Study of Proteins

Proteins are difficult to isolate and to study. For the first twothirds of the 20th century, the "protein problem" was attacked by direct isolation and identification. Thus, the standard paradigm for scientific research of proteins was established. But this traditional approach has been revolutionized by the development of the biology and the biotechniques of molecular biology.

The modern era of molecular biology began with the elucidation of the double-stranded structure of the gene's DNA. In simplest form, DNA is a linear polymer of four nucleotides: G (guanine), A (adenine), T (thymidine) and C (cytosine). The self-complementary organization of the two nucleic acid strands into 2 double helical structure as proposed by Watson and Crick immediately suggested a mechanistic relationship between DNA structure, reduplication, and ultimately protein synthesis. The process of synthesizing mRNA from the gene sequence is called transcription and the process of synthesizing the polypeptide from the message is called translation. Sometimes the term "expression" is also used as a surrogate for the gene transcriptional process or the protein translational process. Below, we will outline the process of gene and protein expression and explore some of its subtleties later in the chapter.

The subsequent development of the tools of molecular biology permitted molecular science to approach proteins other than by direct means: study the sequence of the DNA of the gene and/or the sequence of the mRNA and the primary structure of the protein can be deduced without isolation of the protein itself. When this molecular approach first identifies gene structure and is then applied to deduce a protein sequence, it is called "cloning". When this approach is applied to discovering the genetic basis of a heritable trait or disease, it is called "reverse genetics". In either case, the concept and application have been so powerful and productive that it has substantially altered the way in which science is conducted. Thus, a paradigm shift has occurred in the study of cell biology.

Gene and Protein Expression

The essence of a cell is to grow and develop into a functional entity capable of performing specific tasks. To accomplish this, cells must synthesize proteins. The protein content of a cell or the amount of a specific protein is determined by the balance between the rate of synthesis and degradation. Because proteins are so vital to cellular function, a variety of mechanisms have evolved to regulate tightly and couple protein synthesis to the metabolic needs of the cell. This is a highly complex process involving a coordinated effort between nuclear transcriptional events and cytoplasmic translational processing. Each point in this process is subject to regulation.

Transcription and Gene Structure

The process of protein synthesis begins in the nucleus with the faithful reproduction of the nucleic sequence of the DNA of the gene into mRNA. At first glance the linear nucleotide sequence of a gene appears amorphous. However, studies in the past 20 years show that each gene is divided into important groupings of nucleotides organized into exons and introns. Exons are stretches of nucleotides of various lengths that ultimately link together to form the mature strand of mRNA. They are interrupted by stretches of nucleotides called introns. Before these exons and introns are reached, there is an upstream region of the gene called the promoter. This is the binding site of RNA polymerase, the enzyme responsible for gene transcription, as well as other proteins that regulate the expression of the gene. RNA polymerase moves along the gene faithfully copying the DNA sequence into an early inmature RNA transcript in which U (uracil) is substituted for T. The nascent RNA strand is then further processed by removal of intronic region and splicing of exons back together. While the basic process of transcription is known, the specific mechanisms and biochemistry remain elusive. The mature mRNA is then transported from the nucleus to the cytoplasmic polyribosomes, where it directs protein synthesis.

Translation and the Apparatus of Protein Synthesis

Translation, which is the process of protein synthesis, involves the binding of mRNA to specific sites on the protein synthetic machinery called the ribosomes, which are composed of ribosomal RNA (rRNA) in association with about 140 different proteins. Together, these structures participate in the regulation of protein synthesis. Under special denaturing conditions ribosomes can be separated by high speed ultracentrifugation into two subfragments: a small 40S fragment and a larger 60S fragment.

In the cytoplasm of living cells, free ribosomes come together to form large aggregations known as polyribosomes, which are the site of protein synthesis. The first step in this process is called initiation, and involves binding of the mRNA to the 40S subunit of the ribosome. It is regulated by proteins located near the 40S site (initiation factors). After successful binding the mRNA moves across the surface of the ribosome and is read three nucleotides (a codon) at a time. Each codon carries the information of the genetic code that specifies the ordering of amino acids into the growing peptide. The sequential addition of amino acids is called peptide chain elongation and is also regulated by a set of ribosomal-based proteins (elongation factors).

Translational regulation of protein synthesis represents a vital mechanism that adjusts how efficiently peptides are elaborated. Ribosomal initiation and elongation proteins play a key role by enhancing or inhibiting each step in the process. In turn, the activity of these proteins, because they are distal targets of signal transduction pathways, integrate the process of translational regulation into the general metabolic responses of the cell.

Regulation of Gene Expression

The cytoplasmic ribosomal factories of protein synthesis require the information transmitted from DNA to mRNA. A protein is made only in response to the presence of the specific message that encodes it. This phenomenon, of the regulation of the transmission of information from DNA to mRNA, is vitally important because it determines which proteins are made and which are not. In turn, this determines the cell phenotype, a term that encompasses all the behavior of a cell, including its differentiation, development, growth, and specific functions. For example, muscles, including the heart, are able to form contractile units because genes responsible for specific myosin, actin, and other myofilament proteins have been turned on. In contrast, the level or quantity of the protein actually produced in a cell, and sometimes its function, depends on many

factors, some of which are described in greater detail below in our discussion of cardiac hypertrophy.

One of the great quests of molecular biology is to understand how genes are regulated: how they turn on and turn off. It is no surprise that, here too, proteins have a crucial role. The proteins to which we refer are a new class, not previously considered, that do not conveniently fit into roles traditionally visualized as we consider the structure and function of the cell. These proteins are called *trans*-acting factors, or transcriptional regulators. They bind to those special upstream regions of DNA within the gene (discussed above). Perhaps as a tongue-in-cheek corollary to classical chemistry, the regions of DNA sequences to which *trans*-acting factors bind are known as *cis*-acting gene elements. The precise mechanism by which transcriptional regulatory factors work is largely unknown, but it is thought to involve a configuration change within this DNA regulatory region. Ultimately, transcription of mRNA requires synthesis by the action of the enzyme RNA polymerase. A particular *trans*-acting factor in concert with its target *cis*-acting gene element may increase or decrease the binding and activity of this polymerase and thereby regulate gene transcription.[1]

There are many types of transcriptional regulatory proteins, some of which share a common structural motif. The zinc binding finger is one class of structural motif and defines the shape of a protein containing a repeating amino acid sequence that is folded into a fingered structure coordinated by a zinc ion. Zinc finger–like proteins have the ability to bind to a specific DNA sequence by fitting between the grooves of the helix and thereby regulating gene function. We will return to this motif of transcriptional regulators when we discuss the thyroid hormone receptor and its regulation of myosin heavy chain as well as the effect of certain oncogenes on cell growth. The substantial unraveling of this complex process of gene regulation will, perhaps, be molecular biology's finest moment at the end of the 20th century.

The Cell Cycle

Cell division occurs in all tissues, but its timing and repetition within a particular tissue and even within the various cell types of a multicellular organ is a complex story, which the cell is only grudgingly revealing. During fetal growth and development dividing myocytes pass through the cell cycle, but during maturity are mitosis-arrested. Proteins, including transcriptional regulators, have an important role in cell division. Understanding these phenomena has important implications for cardiac growth and the hypertrophic response to cardiac disease.

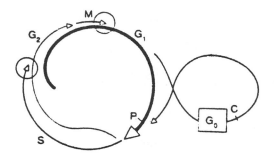

FIGURE 3.1. The cell cycle and its phases. Quiescent cells (G_0, *right side*) are transformed into competent cells by the action of hormones and polypeptide growth factors and progress into G_1. Competent cells progress in the cycle after they are stimulated by additional growth factors. Provided that all nutritional and metabolic criteria are satisfied, cells will progress to the P point of G_1 and are committed to DNA synthesis (S). Cells then progress through G_2 into mitosis (M) with resultant cell division. On repeat cycles, cells need not go through competency again and G_1 activities may begin during the previous cycle (i.e., G_2). Additionally, G_2 may overlap with S. Reproduced, with permission, from ref. 4 Copyright 1989 by the AAAS.

The process of cell division can be conceptualized as a cycle composed of discrete phases (Fig. 3.1). The most fundamental cycle consists of five sequential phases: G_0-G_1-S-G_2-M.[2,3] During each phase specific biochemical events take place. Based on well established experimental data, the "competency-progression" model of cellular division has evolved.[4] In this model, quiescent resting cells (phase G_0) initially are rendered competent to enter the cell cycle by the binding of factors, including hormones and polypeptide growth factors. Their effect is early and rapid, and brings about necessary phenotypic changes that allow the cell to progress through G_1. Part of the induction of competency includes the rapid transcription of a set of early response genes. Because many of these early genes are oncogenes, a link between regulated growth processes and neoplastic transformation was immediately suggested. Cells then progress through a number of G_1 subphases before entering the S phase, where DNA synthesis (duplication of the genome) occurs. Successful passage through G_1 and ultimate commitment to S phase depends on the synthesis of specific enzymes and other proteins that insure that nutritional and metabolic criteria are met. Should these criteria not be fulfilled, cells will become fixed (restricted) in G_1 and eventually cycle back to G_0.[3] After a certain point cells become fully committed to DNA reduplication and enter S phase even in the presence of protein synthesis inhibition. Cells then rapidly enter a second phase (G_2) before undergoing mitosis (phase M), in which

karyokinesis (division of the nucleus) and cytokinesis (division of the cytoplasm) results in two daughter cells. A cell may then become quiescent (G_0) or continue in the cycle by reentering stage G_2. Of the entire time spent in the cycle, about half is covered during G_1, highlighting the important regulatory function of this phase. We will return to some aspects of the cell cycle during our discussion of myocyte growth and hypertrophy.

A Framework for Examining Heart Failure Through Basic Science

Heart failure is defined as inadequate cardiac function to meet the metabolic demands of the body. Although heart failure is not synonymous with pump dysfunction, in most patients it is the predominant cause. The various etiologies of diseases leading to pump dysfunction are well described and increasingly mature in their developed knowledge. However, the mechanisms coupling the disease etiology to the cardiac pathophysiology are only partially understood. This is especially true during the chronic forms of heart disease. For example, the basis for an immediate decrease in cardiac function after myocardial infarction caused by atherosclerotic coronary heart disease appears self-obvious: loss of cardiac muscle impairs cardiac function. However, it is less clear as to why subsequent deterioration of cardiac function sometimes occurs in the absence of additional ischemia or infarction. What accounts for cardiac dilatation and a further decrease of pump performance? In a similar manner, a sudden pressure overload of arterial hypertension may impose an afterload mismatch on left ventricular performance, which immediately results in heart failure. But, what is the role of cardiac hypertrophy in the chronically hypertensive heart and why does pump performance sometimes not return to normal, or even deteriorate, after blood pressure has normalized?

One contemporary framework for describing the molecular and cellular mechanisms of cardiac adaptation to disease and devolution into heart failure is that of Meerson: when challenged by a load that occurs because of disease, the heart passes through stages of hyperfunction followed by load normalization and ultimately decompensation.[5] In the first stage, the framework proposes that the burden imposed by the disease process, unless it overwhelms the heart and causes immediate failure, is met by a state of increased function of the contractile apparatus and the supporting metabolic machinery (IFS, or intense function of structures). If this burden persists, a second stage occurs in which the synthetic apparatus of the myocytes increases its functions and results in cell hypertrophy. This normalizes the workload across an enlarged myocyte and collectively across the heart. But, according to the hypothesis, a long-term penalty incurred by this adaptation is the maintenance of the bloated protein and metabolic machinery of the cell by the genetic apparatus. In the third stage, unable to perform this task indefinitely, the cell fails to maintain its infrastructure and contractile performance declines. Without discussing the limitations of this framework, it does focus our attention on two enduring areas of research into the basic mechanisms of heart failure: the contractile machinery and the hypertrophied myocardium.

During these stages, the heart has at its disposal four basic and well known mechanisms to enhance its mechanical pumping ability in the face of an imposed additional hemodynamic burden. First, short-term changes in cardiac performance can occur through the Frank-Starling mechanism in which changes of preload are coupled to changes of stroke volume. Second, myocardial contractility can be directly affected by the particular structural form and energetics of proteins found in the contractile apparatus. Third, myocardial hypertrophy increases the number of contractile units and thereby augments force development. Fourth, myocardial contractility also can be augmented by a number of circulating and locally released molecules that act through the adrenergic receptors, ion channels, and sarcolemmal and sarcoplasmic reticulum, whose ultimate influence is modulation of the contractility through the availability of calcium at the level of the contractile proteins.

Each of the processes described above represents cornerstones in the pathophysiology of heart failure, and each are based on specific molecular mechanisms. In the material that follows we have chosen to focus on two aspects: first, the molecular genetics of contractile proteins, because the greatest advances in cardiac molecular biology have been in this area and second, cardiac hypertrophy, because this represents a universal response to increased hemodynamic load and diverse disease processes.

The Ultrastructural Basis of Contraction

The Sarcomeric Filaments

The heart is composed of a syncytium of longitudinally arranged myocytes with interspersed elements of connective tissue and blood vessels. Within each myocyte are parallel sets of serially connected contractile units known as sarcomeres, each separated by Z lines (Fig. 3.2). The sarcomere is composed of contractile, regulatory, and structural proteins arranged into thick and

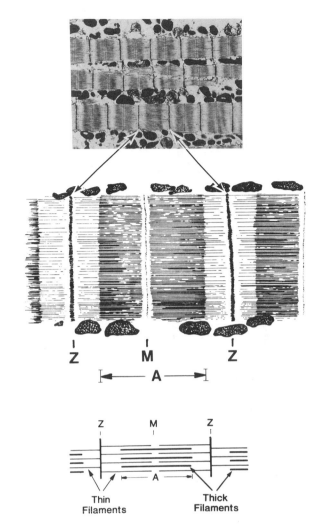

FIGURE 3.2. Ultrastructure of the Sarcomere. Details are progressively enlarged from top to bottom in the figure. **Top**: Electron photomicrograph (*EM*) of cardiac myocyte showing the registration of the sarcomeres. Dark circular structures between the parallel arrangements of sarcomeres are mitochondria. **Middle**: Schematic of a single sarcomere showing the arrangement of filaments and locations of the Z and M lines and the A band. **Bottom**: Exploded view of the sarcomeric filaments. This schematic explains the structural organization of the sarcomere and the basis for its appearance on EM. The thin filaments are attached at the Z lines, which bound the sarcomere on either end. The thick filaments constitute the central A band. The M line is the middle of the sarcomere, which is free of the thin filaments and comprised from overlap of the thick filaments (refer to Fig. 3.3 for further details of thick and thin filament architecture). EM courtesy of Michael Fishbein, M.D.

thin filaments.[6] The thick filaments anchored at the M line are globular filamentous strands of two types of myosin. discussed below (Fig. 3.3A). The thin filaments anchored at the Z lines contain three important groups of proteins and project inward, toward the M line (Fig. 3.3B). These filaments are composed of actin molecules

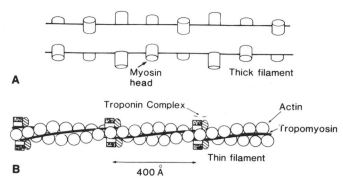

A

B 400 Å

FIGURE 3.3. Molecular structure of the thick and thin filaments. **A:** The globular heads of the thick filament myosin face toward the thin filaments and contain the enzymatic and actin-combining centers. **B:** The thin filament actin is normally prevented from binding to the myosin head by the troponin-tropomyosin complex. The tropomyosin protein is wound around the fibrous actin strand. The three proteins of the troponin complex interact with the tropomyosin at the active site of the actin. Modified with permission from ref. 6. Copyright by Cambridge University Press.

polymerized into a double helix. Running in the major groove of this double helix are tropomyosin (Tm) molecules arranged as dimers in a continuous head-to-tail coiled coil conformation stabilized by disulfide bridges. Each Tm dimer is associated with a troponin regulatory complex (Tn) composed of three proteins—troponin I (TnI), troponin C (TnC), and troponin T (TnT)—

distributed along the Tm molecule at approximately 400-A intervals. The Tm-Tn complex regulates the interactions between thick and thin filaments by modulating the calcium sensitivity of the contractile apparatus.

The power for contraction is provided by the thick filaments, also known as myosin filaments. These structures consist of myosin heavy chains associated with smaller proteins called myosin light chains. These structures are anchored to the M line and project symmetrically outward (e.g., in both directions) to form an interdigitating network of overlapping thin and thick filaments. On electron microscopy this overlapping region appears as a dense band known as the A band (Fig. 3.2). In addition to being a filamentous structure, this molecule has small globular heads located at regular intervals that reach out and form cross-bridges with neighboring actin filaments during the contraction cycle (Fig. 3.3). Sarcomere shortening is achieved when the myosin heads anchored by their rod portions to the M line pull oppositely directed thin filaments along with their attached Z lines toward the centrally located M line. The cycling of cross-bridges between attached and unattached states produces a sliding of thin filaments along myosin molecules and is the basis for contraction for all known striated muscles (Fig. 3.4). The entire process is energized by the hydrolysis of adenosine phosphate (ATP) by an ATPase localized to the head region of myosin heavy chain.[7] Electromechanical coupling between action potential and tension genera-

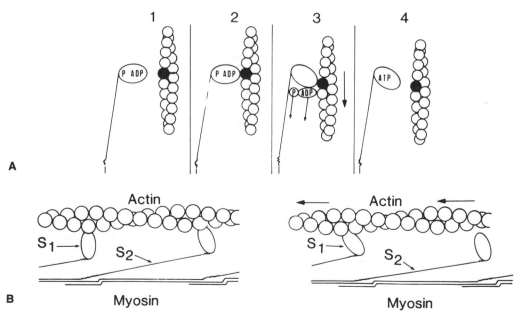

FIGURE 3.4. Biochemical basis of the sliding filament hypothesis of contraction. **A:** Hydrolysis of ATP into ADP and phosphate (P) permits the binding of the myosin head to the active site of actin on the thin filament and the cycle is completed by uptake of another ATP (sequences 1–4). **B:** This binding is associated with bending of the myosin head

(left), which generates force and shortens the sarcomere. During a single cardiac contraction, the myosin heads are recycled as they attach, bend, move the thin filaments, release, and bind again to another active site on the actin (right). Reproduced, with permission from ref. 7.

tion in the myocyte is initiated when depolarization triggers Ca^{2+} release from intracellular compartments, such as the sarcoplasmic reticulum, and increases the calcium concentration in the cytoplasm and especially around the contractile proteins.[6]

The Proteins of the Contractile Apparatus

Before 1977, the myosin of the cardiac thick filaments was thought to have a single molecular form. Therefore, the biochemistry of myosin was not linked with cardiac function or its changes in intact animal models subject to hormonal or hemodynamic manipulation.[8] For example, the typical muscle mechanics data of ventricular hypertrophy or failure would show depressed hemodynamic function (Fig. 3.5). However, the basis for this change did not appear to involve the contractile proteins themselves, even though other explanations were not supported. This enigma was resolved when investigator, employing a slightly different separation technique, showed that the myosin molecule was really composed of three different but closely related isoforms.[9]

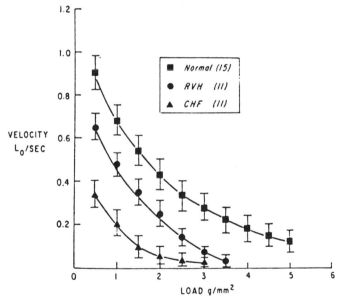

FIGURE 3.5. Muscle performance with cardiac hypertrophy and failure. Force-velocity diagram of papillary muscle function shows a decrease in response to increasing hemodynamic workloads imposed on a chronic animal model. Here, pulmonary artery banding of the cat resulted in groups of animals with right ventricular hypertrophy and heart failure. The basis for these results was believed to be mediated by biochemical events not involving the contractile proteins. However, discovery of the cardiac myosi isoforms largely resolved the basis for this altered contractility. Reproduced, with permission, from ref. 8. Copyright by the American Heart Association.

Named in accordance with their rate of migration on a protein gel, the V1, V2, and V3 myosin isoforms suggested that structural differences might have biochemical and physiological importance. Indeed, this and subsequent investigations showed that the ATPase activity of the V1 isoform was nearly three times the ATPase activity of the V3 isoform. Physiological studies also showed that the maximum speed of contraction of isolated unloaded muscle strips and denuded fibers correlated with the distribution of myosin isoforms (Fig. 3.6): increased contractility occurred with a higher fraction of V1 myosin and decreased contractility occurred with a higher fraction of V3 myosin.[10,11] Although both myosins can generate equivalent units of tension, it takes the V3 form (slower ATPase) longer to achieve the desired result. However, the price paid for high velocity contraction with V1 myosin is poor efficiency of ATP utilization and higher oxygen consumption.

Subsequent studies of cardiac myosin in the rat revealed that the myosin isoform (V1, V2, or V3) was developmentally regulated and responsive to hormonal (especially thyroid hormone) and hemodynamic manipulation.[12] These findings heralded the beginning of cardiovascular molecular biology and opened the door to a decade's worth of molecular investigations, initially of myosin and subsequently of the other proteins of the contractile apparatus.

Myosin Heavy Chain

Myosin is best described as a molecular motor that transduces chemical energy into a mechanical force. Myosin is a ubiquitous protein found in muscle and nonmuscle cells (nonsarcomeric myosin), such as yeast and ameba, where it is used to power secretory and lysosomal vesicle transport, cytoplasmic streaming, motility, and chemotaxis. The vectorial nature of muscle contraction requires that sarcomeric myosin incorporate the catalytic properties of an ATPase protein with a structural motif that transfers chemical energy into a useful mechanical force. Because of this unique feature and its ubiquitous nature, there has been great interest in myosin; detailed molecular analysis of myosin has proved extremely valuable in contributing to our understanding of how this molecule functions. A further discussion of the molecular analysis of myosin function is provided at the end of this section.

Myosin Substructure

Myocardial thick filaments are a hexameric structure consisting of two large myosin heavy chains (MHC), each with a mass of about 200,000 daltons (Da) and two pairs of smaller myosin light chains (MLC) with molecular masses ranging between 16,000 and 30,000 Da.[13] In vitro, the MLCs can be dissociated from the

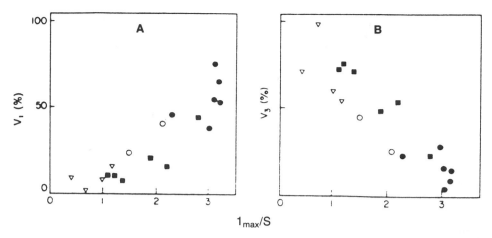

FIGURE 3.6. Myosin isoform effect on contractile function. The speed of unloaded contraction ($1_{max}/s$) of a papillary muscle in the rat correlates with the fraction of myosin isoform. The papillary muscles were obtained from juvenile controls (*closed circles*), mature controls (*open circles*), cardiac hypertrophy induced by abdominal aortic constriction (*closed rectangles*), and hypophysectomized rats (*open triangles*). These models produced a substantial variation in the fraction of myosin and the speed of contraction. The higher the fraction of the V1 myosin, the greater the speed of contraction. The higher the fraction of V3 myosin, the lesser the speed of contraction. These data confirmed the relationship between myosin isoform and contractile properties of the heart. Reproduced, with permission, from ref. 10. Copyright by Academic Press Inc. (London).

larger MHCs so that the latter can be studied independently. The two MHCs form a characteristic dimeric structure consisting of a thick filamentous rod region, followed by a flexible hinge region, beyond which the two polypeptide chains become partially dissociated to form free-floating globular heads (Fig. 3.7).

Each of myosin's structural domains perform vital functions and possess unique characteristics. The thick filamentous rod portion of myosin gives the molecule a stabilizing backbone during tension generation. The interweaving packing of rods must satisfy several structural criteria to maintain functional integrity.[14] First, on adjacent sides of the M line, where there are no globular heads, rods pointing in opposite directions are assembled back to back (e.g., antiparallel). It is this portion of the molecule, because it is anchored to the M line, that stabilizes the sarcomere during the contraction cycle. Second, in the A band rods now must be packed parallel to form a cylindrical array of heavy chain fibers with proper orientation and spacing of globular heads without interrupting the alpha-helical nature of the tail, which gives the molecule its resiliency. Last, fiber construction must orient the flexible hinge region so that the head can rotate freely during contraction.

Molecular Diversity: Myosin Is a Multigene Family

At least 10 to 15 different and distinct myosin genes have been identified.[15–18] All have the same basic structure described above: a globular head, hinge, and cylindrical rod. In the heart only two MHC genes are

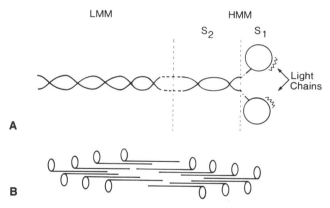

FIGURE 3.7. Structure of the myosin (thick) filament. **A:** Myosin is a dimer of two myosin heavy chains, each with a globular head and a fibrous, intertwined tail. Attached to each head are a pair of light chains. When digested by proteolytic enzymes, it yields a globular head fragment, called the S1 fragment or its almost identical fragment, called heavy meromyosin (*HMM*) a midportion called S2, and a tail portion called light meromyosin (*LMM*). **B:** The thick filament of the sarcomere is composed of myosin molecules packed in a parallel and antiparallel arrangement around the M line (Fig. 3.2).

expressed and encode for two physiologically distinct polypeptides (alpha and beta) with different ATPase activity.[15] In man these two genes are found in tandem on chromosome 14.[19] Skeletal and other types of muscle express other myosin genes that in humans are located on chromosome 17.[20,21] Complete character-

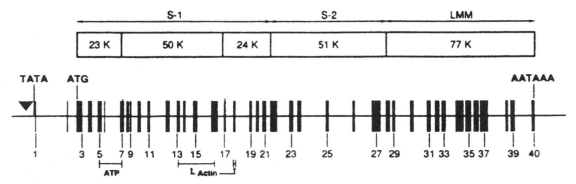

FIGURE 3.8. Structure of the human beta-MHC gene. The bottom portion of the diagram spans the 22.8 kilobases of the gene and consists of 40 exons and 39 introns and the adjacent 5' promoter region. The first two and last exons code for the 5' and 3' untranslated sequences, respectively, of the mRNA, whereas the remainder are protein coding sequences. The start of translation is marked in the third exon by "ATG," the universal initiator codon for the amino acid methionine. In the 5' flanking region of the gene, the "TATA" sequence orients RNA polymerase, the enzyme responsible for transcription. The gene domains that code for the protein sequences responsible for ATP and actin binding are shown below. Above are the corresponding peptide fragments and molecular weight of the MHC protein obtained by proteolytic digestion to Fig. 3.7). Reproduced, with permission, from ref. 23. Copyright by Academic Press.

ization of the genomic structure of the alpha and beta MHC genes has provided us with a better understanding of the molecular evolution of MHC, its function, and its regulation. For human beta MHC the complete gene is 22.8 kbp, which is rather large when one considers that the transcribed portion that constitutes the mRNA is only 6 kbp.[22,23] Forty exons encode the 1935 amino acids of the beta MHC polypeptide. Within the gene are regions that perform vital functions, such as binding to actin and binding and hydrolysis of ATP (Fig. 3.8). Comparison of subregions of the gene to other species, both vertebrate and invertebrate, reveals significant homology (discussed below).

In the preceding sections we have alluded to the three-form diversity of cardiac myosin proteins: the V1, V2, and V3 isoforms isolated by protein electrophoresis. Having elucidated the molecular genetics of myosin, an explanation of the origin of these protein isoforms could be offered. As shown in Figure 3.9, it turns out that the V1 isomyosin represents the dimeric product of two alpha-MHCs (alpha homodimer), the V3 isomyosin the dimeric product of two beta-MHCs (beta homodimer), and V2 isomyosin a chimeric product containing one alpha and one beta MHC polypeptide (heterodimer). In addition, each of the myosin isoforms contains a pair of myosin light chains (discussed below), but these additional polypeptides determine neither the separation of the isoforms nor their activity. Because the ATPase activity of the alpha polypeptide is greater than beta, it follows that the ATPase activity of V1 is greater than V2, which is greater than V3. The contractility of a particular muscle preparation therefore will be determined by the predominant isomyosin present in its thick filaments.

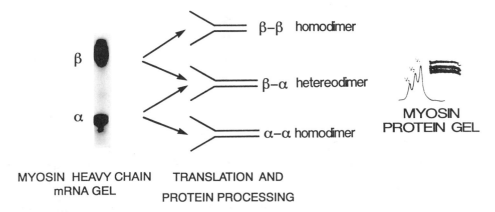

FIGURE 3.9. Molecular basis of myosin. Two myosin heavy chain genes, alpha and beta, encode closely related but different transcripts—the alpha- and beta-mRNAs (*left*). The translation products of these two transcripts form the three proteins isoforms (*center*), which are dimers of two peptides, called V1, V2, and V3 myosin according to their separation on protein gel electrophoresis (*right*).

Myosin Expression in the Rat

During fetal life, the V3 myosin protein is the predominant isoform present in the ventricles due to high levels of beta-myosin gene expression.[24,25] Shortly after birth there is a rapid increase in alpha gene expression and a corresponding rise in alpha-MHC synthesis. Concomitantly beta gene expression is downregulated so that the predominant fiber type throughout the juvenile period and adult life is the V1 fiber.[25,26] However, reemergence of an increasing fraction of beta MHC and V3 myosin is seen during senescence.[27]

Part of the explanation for these developmental changes is caused by the postnatal surge in thyroid hormone levels. In rodent and small animal studies, thyroid hormone has been found to have a dominant enhancing effect on alpha-gene expression.[28–31] Prenatally, fetal thyroid hormone levels are subphysiologic and alpha-gene expression is correspondingly low. Shortly after birth there is a surge in thyroid hormone levels to adult levels and concomitant activation of alphagene expression, and progressive switching off of beta-gene expression. While this observation had been noted for many years, the molecular mechanisms only recently have been elucidated.

MHC Gene Regulation by Thyroid Hormone

Thyroid hormone action is mediated by a thyroid hormone receptor located in the nucleus. When bound by its ligand this receptor has the unique property of functioning as a transcription regulatory factor by binding to specific nucleotide elements in the MHC genes. The thyroid hormone receptor is the protein product of a normal cellular protooncogene called c-erbA and shares homology with the v-erbA oncogene found in the erythroblastosis virus, which is responsible for leukemic transformation of red blood cells in chickens.[32] The c-erbA protooncogene is part of a superfamily of steroid hormone receptors, all of which are capable of regulating gene expression.[33] These receptors share homologous regions of protein function: the N-terminal portion binds to a *cis*-acting DNA element and transcriptionally regulates genes and the carboxy terminal portion binds to a particular steroid or thyroid hormone.

The MHC genes share structural features characteristic of all genes. Genes can be viewed as containing several DNA regions. The portion responsible for making mRNA, and subsequently the protein, is called the coding region and is composed of exons. In most cases it takes several exons to make a protein and usually these exons are separated by noncoding regions of DNA called introns (Fig. 3.10). During transcription introns are removed and the exons are sequentially spliced together.

Upstream from the first exon (toward the 5′ end) is another region of DNA that is also part of the gene, but is responsible for regulating gene activity. This area is called the 5′-flanking region and contains a promoter element that gives the gene polarity by orienting RNA polymerase; it also contains stretches of nucleotides (*cis*-acting elements, see primer) that can enhance or silence gene expression when bound by appropriate protein factors.

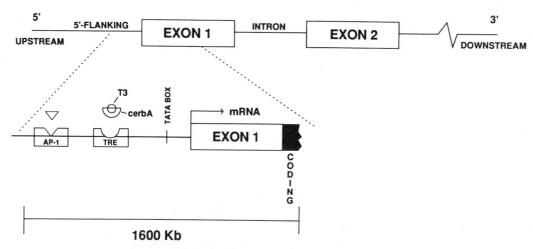

FIGURE 3.10. The general structure of a gene. Genes are composed of exons and introns as well as flanking regions. Initially, all exons and introns are transcribed. Subsequent processing in the nucleus splices out the introns and leaves the mature mRNA, which is then transported to the ribosomes located in the cytoplasm. Flanking regions contain nucleotide sequences which regulate gene transcription. Typically, the 5′ flanking region (*left*) contains the promoter, which binds RNA polymerase near the nucleotide sequence known as the "TATA" box and instructs the enzyme to begin transcription immediately 3′ (*right*). Further upstream (5′) of the TATA box are additional nucleotide sequences called enhancer and silencer elements. These *cis*-acting elements bind *trans*-acting proteins that modify binding of the RNA polymerase and thereby modify transcriptional activity. Examples of *cis*-elements include the TRE (thyroid response element, described in the text), which binds the thyroid receptor, and the AP-1 site, which binds the protein products of certain nuclear oncogenes.

The Thyroid Response Element

It turns out that the 5′-flanking region of the MHC genes contain *cis*-acting elements capable of binding the thyroid hormone receptor.[29,34,35] These thyroid hormone response elements (TRE) represent a family of consensus sequences found in the 5′-flanking region of many genes. One example of a TRE is the palindromic nucleotide sequence (same DNA bases when read from the other strand of the DNA duplex in the opposite direction)—TCAGGTCATGACCTGA. It is the presence of these *cis*-acting elements within the alpha-MHC gene that is the basis for the developmental regulation of myosin and the associated increase in alpha-MHC gene expression as thyroid hormone levels rise.

The action of the receptor is, in general, as follows: The unoccupied receptor has a dominant negative effect on gene transcription. Binding of the ligand to the carboxy terminal domain of the receptor leads to a conformational change that allows the protein to interact with TRE consensus elements and activate transcription. Interestingly, binding of the thyroid hormone receptor to the TRE of the two MHC genes causes opposing effects on gene expression: a decrease of beta and an increase in alpha transcription.[30] The basis for these opposite effects is not well understood, but may indicate that TRE action on gene transcription may be modified by other *trans*-acting factors.

Hemodynamic Models of MHC Gene Regulation

MHC gene expression also can be regulated by hemodynamic stimuli resulting in functional adaptation of the heart. A variety of different models have been used to demonstrate the effect of cardiac loading on myocardial performance and myosin gene expression. In all these models a similar pattern of gene expression emerges[25]: hemodynamic load leads to an increase in beta expression and a decrease in alpha expression. The result is a switch from the fiber type containing V1 myosin isoform to the V3 form and a commensurate decrease in intact muscle contractility (again review Fig. 3.5). In contrast, one model of hemodynamic load—exercise—is associated with an actual small increase of alpha and decrease of beta MHC.[36] Regardless of these hemodynamic changes, thyroid hormone retains its predominant effect on MHC gene expression. This has been demonstrated in experimental models in which beta-gene expression induced by increased hemodynamics stress has been shut off by supraphysiological doses of thyroid hormone, despite continued load and further hypertrophic development.[37]

Still unresolved is the transcriptional regulation of MHC on the basis of these hemodynamic models. In each of these models there is no change in circulating thyroid hormone level and, as yet, no other transcriptional regulatory factors or *cis*-acting elements have clearly been identified to account for this behavior.

Myosin Gene Expression in Humans: Important Distinctions

The discovery of MHC isoforms and their biochemical and physiological implications lead almost immediately to an analysis of human cardiac tissue. The results were somewhat of a surprise and a disappointment. The developmental regulation of MHC in human hearts is similar to that of small animals where alpha MHC is predominant. However, this effect is short-lived in the ventricles, where beta MHC and V3 myosin are vastly predominant throughout the remainder of life and in the presence of a wide variety of physiological and pathological states.[38] The mechanism of this species difference in the developmental regulation of ventricular myosin is somewhat of a puzzle because the gene regulatory regions of the human alpha and beta MHC gene appear to have, like the rodent, a TRE that should make them responsive to thyroid hormone. Indeed, transfection (artificial insemination of DNA into cells) of human alpha MHC gene regulatory regions that have been linked to reporter genes into rat myocytes shows that the human gene can respond to triiodothyronine (T$_3$) stimulation.[39] Work in this area has continued and it is likely that other transcriptional regulatory factors in the human myocardium will be discovered to account for these differences in gene expression.

In contrast, the human atria show a pattern of MHC gene and protein expression somewhat different than and more reminiscent of small animal studies. There is a balance of V1 and V3 protein that is shifted to V3 by a variety of disorders that cause elevated left heart filling pressures and/or work overload, such as mitral stenosis or arterial hypertension.[40] Because the origin of these proteins is both the alpha and beta MHC genes, this raises the intriguing question of tissue-specific control of gene expression even within the heart. Of immediate interest, mutations in the MHC genes have been discovered in patients with familial hypertrophic cardiomyopathy. This has opened a new vista for the molecular basis of cardiovascular disease, which is discussed below in the section on the Application of Molecular and Cellular Science to the Management of Heart Failure.

Molecular Analysis of Myosin: Assembly and Function

Evolutionary Analysis of Myosin

Molecular and genetic analysis have provided useful insight into myosin structure-function relationships. The complete cloning and characterization of myosin genes from many different organisms and different tissues has provided a means to map important structure-function domains by directly comparing nucleotide and amino acid sequences. Interestingly, sequence analysis between yeast and mammalian myosin indicates that myosin gene duplication probably occurred before species differentiation.[41] These studies show that specific domains of the molecule, even from distantly related organisms, are highly homologous, implying evolutionary conservation of functionally important domains. Evolutionary conservation of important structural or functional domains of a protein can occur in several ways. In its simplest form, stretches of genes contain identical or nearly identical nucleotide sequences that code for similar amino acid sequences. Examples of conserved nucleotide sequences, even from unrelated genes, are plentiful and in some cases are so prevalent that they are referred to as consensus sequences because they have analogous functions in all genes. Usually such sequences are involved in regulating gene expression or encoding structural motifs that subserve a common function. More complicated forms of conservation occurs when divergent nucleotide sequences encode for protein domains that share biophysical properties that modify secondary and tertiary structures within protein folding. Both of these patterns of homology are recognized to be present in all myosin genes and are believed to be important for filament assembly, orientation, and spacing of globular heads.

Application of Molecular Techniques to Elucidate Myosin Function

Before the widespread availability of molecular biological and cloning technologies, functionally important regions of myosin had been identified by analyzing the biochemical and biophysical properties of myosin subfragments generated by proteolytic digestion. All myosins are very sensitive to protease digestion by trypsin and papain, which cut the molecule into characteristic fragments. Initial digestion separates the molecule into a head-containing fragment known as heavy meromyosin (HMM) and a rod-containng fragment known as light meromyosin (LMM).[14,42] These represent the amino terminal and carboxy terminal portions of the molecule, respectively.

Light Meromyosin

Knowledge of the complete sequence of LMM provided a way to understand how the amino acid sequence (i.e., its primary structure) determines the self-association of tail regions into filamentous structures. Comparison of the primary structures of nonmuscle and muscle LMM reveals significant repeating patterns of homology that encode information shared by alpha-helical proteins and for proper parallel alignment of filaments. The primary structure of all LMM fragments

contain a repeating unit consisting of seven amino acid residues with hydrophobic residues at positions 1 and 4.[14,43] This structure is believed to be responsible for the formation of the alpha-helical coiled coil that characterizes the rod. Superimposed on this structure are repeating units of 28 amino acid residues creating an alternating pattern of positive and negative charges, believed to play a role in interfilament interaction.[14,43,44] The largest repeating subunit is composed of 196 amino acid residues and is thought to determine the packing of filaments into a cylindrical array with regularly spaced heads.[14,43,44]

A more recent approach for elucidating structure-function relationships of myosin is to express portions of the molecule in bacterial cells and then study the properties of the resulting protein fragments. To accomplish this, pieces of cDNA encoding specific and usually short regions of the molecule are ligated to plasmid vectors that can entire *Escherichia coli* and use the bacterial host to duplicate many copies of the foreign protein, which are then isolated and studied. There are several advantages of this approach over studying tryptic digestion products. First, cDNA sequences are easier to isolate and smaller regions of the molecule can be studied since endonuclease restriction sites are more frequent then proteolytic cleavage sites in the corresponding protein. Second, specific regions of sequences can be mutated and their functional role mapped out by studying the effects of these mutations on function. Last, because large amounts of protein are synthesized by the bacteria, isolation and subsequent analysis are facilitated.

Using this technology, the cloning of LMM cDNA fragments into bacterial expression factors has provided new insights into filament formation. Such studies reveal that only specific regions of LMM can form filamentous and paracrystalline structures when expressed in *E. coli*.[45,46] For adult human skeletal MHC it appears that information specified within the 430 amino acids of the carboxy terminus are necessary for filament formation.[47] These data show that amino acids near the carboxy terminus play a role in determining how LMM fragments interact and in initiating the coiling process that proceeds toward the amino end of LMM.

Heavy Meromyosin

HMM can be digested into two subfragments: the hinge-containing region (subfragment S-2) and the globular head regions (subfragment S-1). Further digestion of S-1 produces three subfragments (25 kDa, 50 kDa, and 20 kDa) that have been identified to contain ATPase activity as well as ATP and actin binding domains. Comparison of head regions from different myosins reveals long stretches of conserved amino acids, indicating that these regions are important functional domains. Subfragment analysis reveals that the 25-kDa subfragment contains the ATP binding site located between amino acid residues 170 and 214 (the amino terminal position is residue 1). This region is similar to other ATP binding proteins and contains a stretch of amino acids, GESGAGKT, found in all myosins.[41,43,44] The 20-kDa fragment has several highly conserved regions including a strong actin binding site mapped to residues 700 to 720 and two sequential reactive thiol groups (SH1 and SH2) that modify ATPase activity.[48] The intervening 50-kDa segment of HMM contains several conserved regions that have not been assigned a definite functional role. One region of this segment near the 20-kDa junction may participate in actin binding. In addition, there are two highly conserved loop regions that are thought to be responsible for folding the head region and juxtapositioning the reactive thiols near the ATP binding and ATPase sites. Recombinant myosin head fragments capable of binding regulatory light chains (see below) and actin-activated ATPase activity also have been expressed successfully in *E. coli*.[49,50]

Myosin Light Chain

The other protein of the thick filament is the myosin light chain (MLC). Each myosin head is associated with a pair of nonidentical light chains. The cardiac MLCs are classified by different naming schemes into two groups: alkali (also called essential or nonphosphorylatable, and the band of the protein electrophoresis numbered according to position in the gel as MLC 1) and regulatory (or phosphorylatable, MLC-2). The function of the light chains in the cardiac myosin is not clear because, although associated with the head of the MHC, the alkali light chains do not modify the ATPase activity of isolated myosin and the regulatory light chains only have been shown to activate ATPase activity and contraction in smooth muscle and nonmuscle cells.

MLCs also are encoded by a multigene family that are differentially expressed in atrium and ventricle, and developmentally regulated.[51] The ventricular alkali MLC-1 also is expressed in adult skeletal muscles, whereas the atrial form is expressed only in the heart. Furthermore, in the rat heart the ventricular MLC-1 is confined to expression in the ventricle, but the atrial MLC-1 is expressed not only in the atrium but also in the fetal and early neonatal ventricle.[52] This implies that birth initiates a process in the rat heart whereby expression of the atrial isoform becomes confined to the atrium. Although changes in the pattern of expression of the MLC 1 in adult rat hearts have not been seen in the few hemodynamic models in which it has been studied, limited human studies of pathological hemodynamic overload have shown the expression of ventricular MLC 1 in the atria.[53] The parallel observations of

expression have been made in the human heart concerning atrial and ventricular MLC 2.[54] In addition, studies of rat myocyte cultures stimulated by alpha-adrenergic agents and in vivo models of hypertension have shown increased levels of MLC 2 transcription and content. These studies suggest that the MLCs may provide an excellent model system to study transcriptional mechanisms of contractile protein gene expression. However, the functional significance of these changes awaits elucidation of the biochemical and physiological role of the MLCs. In some ways, this evolving story demonstrates that the information gleaned from molecular studies of the gene may run well ahead of other disciplines that confer cardiac structure and function and represents the dynamic nature of the science. This is also true for our next discussion, the proteins of the thin filament.

The Proteins of the Thin Filament

As described above, the thin filament is composed of actin, tropomyosin, and troponin. Molecular studies of these proteins have demonstrated the two different mechanisms by which contractile protein diversity is achieved: expression of a particular gene from a multigene family and/or alternative splicing of the immature message from a single gene to achieve more than one mature mRNA.[16]

Structure and Function of the Thin Filament

Contractile apparatus actin is about 1 μm long and is a filamentous structure (filament or F actin) that is a self-assembled double helical array of actin monomers (globular or G actin). Tropomyosin (Tm) is a coiled-coil helical dimer about 40 nm long and may be associated with actin along the helical grooves of the actin double strand. Troponin is a complex of three proteins: TnC, TnI, and TnT. These three thin filament proteins regulate striated muscle contraction. The current model of cardiac contraction requires movement of tropomyosin in order to uncover the active site on actin in order to effect actomyosin interaction, which leads to hydrolysis of ATP and the development of tension and shortening. The troponin complex modulates this activity through the binding of Ca^{2+} released during excitation. TnT binds to tropomyosin and to the other troponins; the TnI protein inhibits actin activation of myosin in the absence of Ca^{2+}, whereas the TnC protein conveys the calcium signal to the filament.

Contractile Actin

There are two genes on different chromosomes that encode contractile filament actin, and they are the alpha-skeletal and alpha-cardiac forms. The proteins encoded by these genes differ only by four amino acids, two of which are at the amino terminal end, the region that interacts with myosin during contraction. As suggested by their name, each isoform is predominant in its nominal tissue in small animals, such as rats. However, small amounts of alpha-skeletal actin appear in the fetal cardiac ventricle and are reexpressed in many of the hemodynamic models that result in myosin isoform switching.[55] In contrast, a recent report on the human heart demonstrates that whereas cardiac actin is predominant in utero and in the first few months of life, skeletal actin comprises the majority isoform thereafter.[56] Because of the small differences between the isoforms, there is the lingering question of contractile protein effects. In addition, the regulation of the isogene expression is of interest because of the complex aspects of transcription regulatory proteins and *cis*-acting DNA elements on genes.[57]

Tropomyosin and the Troponins

The alpha and beta tropomyosins, which undergo developmental expression in the myocardium, are the product of two genes and their variants also are alternatively spliced. The embryonic cardiac ventricle contains predominantly beta tropomyosin, whereas the adult is entirely alpha. However, a hemodynamic overload causes reexpression of some fraction of beta. Similar to the adult ventricle, the atria are entirely alpha tropomyosin.[16]

The troponins—TnC, TnI, and TnT—are the products of three different genes. Alternative splicing of TnT results in many mature mRNAs and related, but not identical, protein products that are expressed in response to developmental, tissue-specific, and physiological stimuli.[58] Both TnI and TnC do not undergo alternative splicing and appear as the single transcript and protein products of their respective genes.

Cardiac Development, Growth, and Hypertrophy

Cardiac Development

Perhaps the most obvious and predictable behavior observed in a living organism is its life cycle: development, growth, adaptation, and aging. These processes also are true for the heart. Cellular and molecular biology have added a substantial increment of information to our knowledge of these processes, and now are increasingly being applied to the heart. Our goal in this next section is to review these phenomena with a view toward the inclusion of newer information.

Determinants of Striated Muscle Cell Differentiation

The heart, just like skeletal muscle, is derived from the embryonic mesoderm and develops substantially in con-cert with, and perhaps on signals from, the splanchnic mesoderm. The molecular basis for skeletal muscle differentiation recently has been elucidated. Unfortunately, similar insights into cardiac myocyte differentiation have not progressed in parallel, highlighting the fact that whereas skeletal and cardiac muscle share many properties, the molecular senetic programs governing their differentiation are distinct. Nevertheless, the landmark identification of the signals that lead to the differentiation of other striatec myocytes should be reviewed.

A valuable model of muscle cell development was provided by examination of how primitive cells, not committed to skeletal cell lineage, differentiate to become skeletal muscle.[59] Previous experimentation had shown that exposure of pluripotential cell lines to certain drugs permitted their differentiation into precursor striated muscle cells.[60] These drugs were known to alter DNA through the common mechanism of methylation: a nonspecific process that affects transcription. Based on these observations, it was postulated that there existed a specific subset of regulatory genes particularly sensitive to methylation, that when activated, resulted in muscle differentiation. These genes subsequently were cloned by a process called differential gene expression, in which the opportunity to focus on the activities of differences in gene expression between similar cells or tissues—representing few in number—is exploited.[61]

The differences that they found are exemplified by a gene called myoD. The activity of this gene is necessary and sufficient to switch a cell, not yet committed to differentiation, to evolve into a skeletal muscle cell. For this reason, the myoD gene is thought of as a master switch that, when activated, sets in motion a cascade of events leading specifically to myoblastic differentiation. The protein product of this gene functions analogously to other transcriptional regulatory proteins. In contrast to the "zinc finger" motif of DNA binding by the thyroid hormone receptor (discussed above), the myoD protein shares structural homology to other "leucine finger" transcription factors. In striated muscle precursors, myoD protein appears to act as a transcriptional regulatory factor on an intermediary set of genes that regulate the expression of the set of genes that code for proteins that provide the characteristic muscle phenotype, such as contractile actin, myosin, and muscle creatine kinase.

The cloning and purification of myoD set off a flurry of activity directed at identifying similar regulatory genes in cardiac muscle. However, cardiac specific homologs of myoD or myoD-like genes have not been identified, suggesting that cardiac myocyte differentiation is a more complex process than skeletal myoblast differentiation. Indeed, identification and isolation of primitive cardiac myoblast cells (undifferentiated myocytes) has proved elusive. Recent work in this area has focused on the regulation of induction of cardiac-specific contractile proteins in azathioprine-treated cardiac fibroblasts,[62] the induction of cardiac-specific proteins in dimethylsulfoxide-treated embryonal carcinoma cell lines (Pl9), and on growth factor control of cardiac-specific gene transcription[63] Successful identification of the molecular regulation of cardiac differentiation will have far reaching influence on the biology of cardiac development and on therapeutic options in heart disease.

Prenatal Cardiac Development

During intrauterine life cardiac growth occurs through replication and division (i.e., hyperplasia) of both myocytes and nonmyocyte cells, such as endothelial cells, smooth muscle cells, and fibroblasts. Morphologically, fetal and neonatal right and left ventricles have nearly identical cavity dimensions, weights, and myocyte size,[64] indicating that developmental growth processes are uniform for both ventricles, and emphasizing that non-workload stimuli are predominant determinants of this early growth. However, when a hemodynamic burden is added, the fetal heart is capable of hypertrophy. Thus, pathways for transduction of volume and pressure information into biochemical signals is a property of the developing heart. It should be noted that even at the fetal stage the heart is a well differentiated structure. Indeed, many of the proteins and properties that characterize the juvenile, and even the adult, heart are already present in fetal myocytes.

The Cell Cycle in Prenatal Cardiac Growth

Although ubiquitous during fetal development, the molecular regulation of myocyte division is not well defined. The hallmark of cellular hyperplasia is increasing mass on the basis of cellular multiplication, requiring the reduplication of cellular DNA followed sequentially by nuclear and cytoplasmic division. The morphological, biochemical, and genetic events associated with cell division can be described by a series of related, but temporally discrete, phases known as the cell cycles (refer again to Fig. 3.1), which we outlined in the "Primer" at the beginning of this chapter and can be found in excellent reviews.[2]

In general, successful transition through each phase is a prerequisite for continuation through the cycle and a complex array of regulatory mechanisms ensure that initiation of later events occurs sequentially. However, mammalian cells differ considerably in the degree to which these controlling checkpoints are active. For example, rodent cell lines can reenter the cell cycle even in the absence of mitosis (resulting in serial DNA doublings without cell division), whereas human cells generally are inhibited from subsequent cycling if mitosis does not occur.[65] Recent data correlate these differences with the modulation cf specific cell cycle genes and their proteins, such as cyclin B and p34cdc2, which appear to collect the clumped DNA of the resting cell

(G_0) into the organized metaphase chromosomes of the dividing cell (M).[66,67] In addition, it should be noted that the above model most accurately describes post embryonic cell division of adult cells such as hepatocytes. However, more complex cycles can occur and recent data show that embryonic cycles lack G_1 and G_2 phases (and of course their attendant regulatory mechanisms) and essentially cycle between M and S.[2]

There is some preliminary evidence to suggest that at least two factors may contribute to fetal myocyte growth through hyperplasia. First, as in the case of other proliferating cells, circulating endocrine factors as well as locally derived and acting paracrine factors probably play important regulatory roles. Recent data suggest that paracrine action of insulin-like growth factors, particularly type 2 (IGF-II), may be especially important during fetal stages of development[68] In addition, a role for proto-oncogene regulation of the cell cycle in neonatal cells also may be postulated based on a number of lines of evidence. These include the participation of oncogenes in the cell cycle in a variety of dividing cells and tissues, the finding that some proto-oncogenes are expressed in the heart during fetal life, and the recent demonstration that the overexpression of c-myc in a transgenic model leads to hyperplasia of cardiac tissue.[69] We will return to each of these themes below.

Postnatal and Juvenile Growth and Development

Three important phenomena characterize postnatal development: permanent withdrawal from the cell cycle, phenotype maturation, and hypertrophy. Because both juvenile and adult cardiac cells are permanently postmitotic, hypertrophy becomes the dominant, and perhaps only, mechanism for the cardiac growth in response to physiological and pathological stimuli. Although fetal myocytes are fully differentiated, phenotype maturation does occur after birth.[70] This process consists of formation of discrete cellular organelles, which appeared amorphous only during prenatal life, as well as the switching to adult patterns of contractile gene expression. Both hemodynamic and humoral factors appear to have important roles in postnatal cardiac development of the myocyte.

The Role of Mechanical Load in Juvenile Development

The transition from hyperplastic to hypertrophic growth patterns appears to be correlated with the increasing circulatory pressures and volumes that occur at birth. A feature of the normal developing heart is the impressive increases in left ventricular wall thickness compared to the relative atrophy of the right ventricle. Experimental studies of neonatal rabbit hearts have shown higher rates of fractional protein and myosin synthesis in the left ventricle compared to the right side.[71] This relative

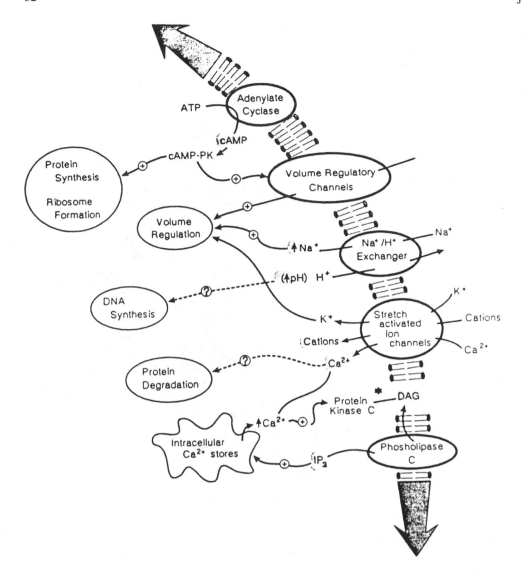

FIGURE 3.11. The cell membrane as a mechanotransducer. Five membrane-located proteins are proposed as responsive to mechanical forces. These include ion channels, porters, and second messengers. As a result of cell signaling, changes in transcription, translation, and protein degradation may result in cell growth because of a net increase in protein content. Reproduced, with permission, from ref. 72. Copyright by FASEB.

developmental hypertrophy of the left ventricle is apparent early after birth and is undoubtedly a consequence of higher left-sided pressures; it thereby highlights the intriguing but unresolved question of how mechanical loads are, in general, transduced and more specifically coupled to protein synthesis and growth.[72]

There are at least five candidate membrane mechanotransducers: adenylate cyclase, ion channels, volume regulatory channels, Na+/H+ exchanger, and enzymes involved in phosphatidylinositol turnover (Fig. 3.11). For example, increased aortic pressure through unidentified pathways activates membrane adenylate cyclase, leading to increased intracellular cyclic adenosine monophosphate (cAMP) levels, which in turn acts as a second messenger for enhancing myocardial protein synthesis.[73] Distal targets for cAMP may include gene regulatory sequences, ribosomal initiation, and elongation factors. Additionally, stretch-activated ion channels may operate by similar signaling pathways.[74] In particular, membrane cytoskeletal elements such as the dystrophin protein may be important mechanotransducing elements. We will return to the dystrophin protein

when we discuss muscular dystrophy in our section on Applications of Molecular Biology below.

The Role of Humoral Factors in Juvenile Development

Growth hormone (GH) is a polypeptide secreted by the anterior pituitary. The experiments of nature involving growth hormone deficiency or unresponsiveness (dwarfism in animals and humans) as well as the opposite effects of GH excess (acromegaly) demonstrate the important trophic actions of this hormone on body and cardiac growth. Limited experimental data exist on the molecular and cellular effects of GH on the heart and the myocyte. For example, there have been only a few studies on the protein synthetic effects of GH on the isolated animal heart or in myocyte tissue culture.[75] Intact animal studies suggest the importance of GH on the promotion of cardiac growth, but are confounded by concomitant effects on hemodynamics.[76,77] Regardless of its specific mechanism, GH has important trophic effects on the heart, which also play a supplementary role in the response of the heart to hemodynamic stimuli.

The thyroid hormones (T_3 and T_4) exert powerful metabolic effects on many tissues, including the heart. These hormones also are under the control of the anterior pituitary through the actions of thyroid-stimulating hormone (TSH) on the thyroid gland. Thyroid hormone effects are mediated through binding to the thyroid hormone receptor. Its mechanism of action has been studied extensively and was discussed above in the section on thyroid action on MHC gene expression. Here we make note of its structural differences from its retroviral offspring, the v-erbA oncogene. The oncogene is missing sequences that code for the portion of the protein that binds thyroid hormone, and is therefore unresponsive to the hormone. However, the protein's DNA binding domain remains intact.[78] As such, it blocks erythroid differentiation in chickens, and therefore prevents red cell differentiation, which then leads to erythroleukemia. From this we infer that the c-erbA protooncogene, with its thyroid binding domain intact, may stimulate differentiation of cells in the presence of T_3, an inference that has been supported by experimental studies of its effects and that of an analogous system: the retinoic acid and retinoic acid receptor system.

The specific role of T_3 in cardiac growth has been studied extensively and is easy to discern in experimental systems. In contrast to GH, which promotes cardiac growth in the context of proportional body growth, T_3 has specific trophic effects on the heart that result in myocyte hypertrophy in the absence of any gain in body mass. However, it has not been possible to resolve or separate the direct humoral effects from the secondary hemodynamic effects (i.e., heart rate and blood pressure) of T_3 on cardiac hypertrophy.

There are at least three pathways by which the humoral effects of T_3 could modulate cardiac growth. In addition to its role in the transcriptional regulation of the MHC genes, T_3 also regulates other genes, including expression of G-binding proteins.[79] Regulation of G-binding proteins may have important implications for determining adrenergic responsiveness (G-binding proteins) and they have been shown to effect cardiac growth in a wide variety of models ranging from tissue culture to the intact animal.[80,81] As discussed below, T_3 also regulates ribosomal synthesis rates, an important step in protein synthesis. Recently, a third mechanism for the cardiac trophic actions of T_3 has been identified showing that T_3, but not GH, increases paracrine/autocrine cardiac IGF-I gene expression.[82]

Neuroendocrine Effects on Juvenile Cardiac Development

Before the maturation of molecular and cellular biology and its application to the cardiovascular system, a wide variety of biochemical, pharmacological, and physiological studies established the importance of catecholamines as trophic hormones in the process of cardiac growth and hypertrophy. Previous findings of these studies include the role of adrenergic innervation of the myocardium at the time of birth for the switch from nyperplastic to hypertrophic growth patterns.[83] A number of investigators also showed that blocking or destruction of the adrenergic nervous system postnatally suppressed much of cardiac growth.[81]

Cardiac Hypertrophy

Cardiac hypertrophy represents one of the most important physiologically adaptive responses to increased functional demands on the heart. Mechanically, myocardial hypertrophy unloads the overburdened heart by adding new contractile units, thus distributing tension across a greater cellular mass. In this sense, hypertrophy is viewed as a benevolent and corrective response because it normalizes excessive forces and reduces the mechanical work performed per sarcomere. While this is certainly true from a hemodynamic perspective, it is now clear that sustained hypertrophy represents a myopathic process characterized by biochemical and metabolic defects that eventually have a deleterious effect on both systolic and diastolic mechanical performance and that translate to decreased patient survival. Indeed, the poor prognostic significance of cardiac hypertrophy and its association with accelerated cardiac mortality and morbidity (sudden death and myocardial infarction) have been clearly established.[84] However, the nature and timing of when the myopathic process begins to prevail over that conferred by the beneficial hemodynamic manifestations is not understood, but appears to be correlated with the duration of the hemodynamic insult and the intrinsic synthetic capacity of the heart.

Etiology

The most common etiology of left ventricular hypertrophy (LVH) is in response to excessive mechanical work, usually resulting from volume overload (as in mitral and aortic insufficiency) or pressure overload (as in aortic stenosis and hypertension). However, numerous and diverse other conditions result in cardiac and myocyte hypertrophy, including most cardiac diseases that damage the heart, even if they do not impose an obvious increase in the workload of the heart. For example, an important but uncommon cause of cardiac hypertrophy is familial hypertrophic cardiomyopathy (FHC), which is further discussed in the Applications section of the chapter. We have discussed the changes in expression of the beta MHC gene and its primary effects on myocardial performance above, but here we note the secondary, but important, effects on cardiac and myocyte hypertrophy. Two other systemic conditions, acromegaly (excessive production of GH) and hyperthyroidism, also are uncommon, but important, causes of LVH because they provide insight into the regulation of cardiac development and growth by circulating endocrine factors. All of these processes are marked by excessive cardiac mass and myocyte hypertrophy, which, in the long-term, frequently leads to progressive deterioration in cardiac function.

Morphology and Physiological Adaptations

There is no single definition of hypertrophy that satisfies inquiry into all basic and clinical studies. For the clinician, hypertrophy is defined as an increase in cardiac mass, whereas basic scientists define it as an increase in cell volume and mass on the basis of enhanced protein synthesis in the absence of proliferation. Clinical subtypes of hypertrophy include the gross morphological appearance of the hypertrophied heart, which is very much influenced by the manner in which hypertrophy developed. Under conditions of pure pressure overload, such as occurs in aortic stenosis, the increase in systolic wall stress leads to concentric hypertrophy characterized by a disproportionate increase in wall thickness compared to ventricular internal cavity dimensions. The immediate consequence of this is a reduction of peak systolic stress as pressure is distributed across a greater thickness. This relationship is expressed in the well known Laplace equation. Because stress is a major determinant of cardiac metabolism, hypertrophy decreases the energy requirement per unit mass of myocardium. However, it should not be overlooked that the process of adding additional myofibrillar units is itself an energy-consuming process.

Eccentric hypertrophy is seen characteristically in volume-overloaded states and is marked by progressive dilatation of the left ventricular (LV) cavity. The contractile and metabolic consequences of this type of response are more complex, but include optimization of Frank-Starling stretch-tension mechanisms and the normalization of wall stress and energy requirements through sarcomere hypertrophy. It is important to understand that these distinctions, frequently are blurred in clinical disorders, and may represent secondary changes in response to other myocardial adaptations.

In addition to changes in systolic function with hypertrophy, there also may be changes in diastolic function. Diastolic ventricular stiffness increases linearly with left ventricular wall thickness.[85] There are at least three explanations for this: The first is simply the change in stiffness of the ventricular wall as the myocytes hypertrophy and the wall thickens: a thick material is stiffer than a thin material of the same composition. The second is the change of material properties of the wall when fibrosis occurs along with or as a consequence of the

hypertrophy. The third is the physiological abnormalities of hypertrophied myocyte function. We will subsequently review some of the changes in sarcoplasmic reticulum and Ca^{2+} handling that have been observed in hypertrophied myocytes.

Cellular and Ultrastructural Response to a Hypertrophic Stimulus

Detailed ultrastructural analysis of the normal and hypertrophied myocyte has proved useful in providing a conceptual framework from which to understand the subcellular consequences of hypertrophy. Detailed electron microscopic analysis has shown that in many forms of experimental hypertrophy there is an increase in myocardial cell volume, expansion of myofibrils, and increased mitochondrial numbers.[86-88] However, when compared to control conditions it appears that the myofibrillar fraction increases disproportionately to the mitochondrial fraction. This has led to the suggestion that the hypertrophied myocyte is unable to supply sufficient oxidative production of ATP, thereby leading to eventual metabolic exhaustion. Experimental evidence supporting and refuting this point exist. Measurements of ATP levels in the chronically hypertrophied myocardium have not revealed substantial deterioration. However, these experiments are sensitive to the type of hemodynamic model used, how quickly the hypertrophy develops, and the methodology employed to measure intracellular purines. One explanation for the nondepletion of ATP stores views the switch to beta-MHC gene expression as an energy-optimizing adaptation because of its inverse relationship to ATPase activity and more efficient speed of contraction. However, it should not be overlooked that the process of adding new myofibrillar proteins requires ATP and that cells, in general, require more energy to develop and sustain increased protein mass.

Membranous components of the myocyte are responsible for the transport of nutrients and ions. The myocyte has two abundant membranous structures, sarcolemma (plasma membrane) and sarcoplasmic reticulum (SR), each subserving vital specialized functions. The latter organelles are responsible for storage, release, and uptake of intracellular calcium. The flux of calcium across these membranes is central for the appropriate trigger of contraction and relaxation. Abnormal intracellular calcium concentrations are one of the hallmarks of the failing human myocardium.[89] Recent data suggest that depressed activity of the sarcoplasmic reticulum (SR) Ca-ATPase (an enzyme that transports calcium from the cytoplasm up an electrochemical gradient into the SR) may be responsible for altered intracellular handling and calcium overload.[90] Additionally, as myocyte volume increases the surface area volume ratio declines. This potentially could limit sarcolemma transport of nutrients and ions vital to excitation-contraction coupling. However, recent patch clamping studies suggest that sarcolemmal transport of Ca^{2+} and other ions is normal in pressure overloaded myoytes, suggesting that there is upregulation of the enzymes and protein carriers responsible for ion transport.[91]

Substantial changes in other cell types and in the extracellular matrix of the myocardium also contribute to mechanical dysfunction. Fibroblast proliferation and increased deposition of extracellular matrix collagen are observed in some experimental models and clinical conditions.[92,93] Quantitation of specific collagen mRNA levels suggests that increased collagen synthesis may constitute an early response to pressure overload.[94] Exuberant extracellular matrix production may further impair transport of metabolites and oxygen between the capillary and myocyte. However, the degree of fibrosis is highly variable and is most correlated with late stages of cardiac failure. Early during the hypertrophic process when there is clear evidence of depressed contractile behavior, fibrosis and fibroblast proliferation are minimal.[95] Therefore, fibroblastic proliferation and extracellular matrix fibrosis appear to contribute minimally to the early pathophysiolgic evolution of heart failure at this stage.

With continual hemodynamic overload the synthetic capacity of the myocyte may be exhausted and this could lead to accelerated myocardial necrosis. Progressive proliferation of fibroblasts and accelerated deposition of extracellular matrix, perhaps arising from the autocrine action of locally released cytokines and polypeptide growth factors, appears to be temporally associated with myocyte necrosis.[96] Mechanically this results in stiffening and thinning of the ventricle wall, which in turn increases wall stress. Thus, a vicious cycle is established in which increasing hemodynamic burden, primarily by ventricular dilatation, perpetuates myocardial necrosis and fibrosis, ultimately leading to clinical deterioration.

In summary, it appears that pressure hypertrophy causes a specific and exaggerated expansion of contractile elements (myofibrils) and of calcium release and storage elements (SR) out of proportion to any increased volume. These changes highlight the early increase of protein synthetic capacity of the overloaded myocyte. Although these studies are interesting and perhaps even provide some insight into specific regional differences between normal and hypertrophied myocytes, they are not specific for particular underlying etiologies of cardiac disease, nor do they reveal the mechanism of the pathophysiologic evolution of the heart failure. This is one of the reasons that endomyocardial biopsy has not flourished as a principal cardiac diagnostic tool. The utility of morphologic examination is enhanced when a specific disease and his-

tological pattern can be correlated, such as in serial biopsies of the transplanted heart when monitoring for rejection.

The Molecular and Cellular Basis of Cardiac Hypertrophy

There has been much research focusing on identifying the cellular and biochemical basis for hypertrophy and the progressive deterioration in cardiac function that follows. Initially, research focused primarily on the role of mechanical and humoral factors on cardiac development and hypertrophy, and more specifically on rates of protein synthesis and degradation. Subsequently this work was expanded to include mechanisms by which hemodynamic and hormonal stimuli are coupled to biochemical effectors such as second messengers, and the regulation of ion channels and intracellular calcium metabolism and handling. More recently, research has focused on the potential role of transient proto-oncogene expression in signal transduction and transcriptional regulation. Last, there is growing interest in the role of polypeptide growth factors and their receptors as potential autocrine mediators of hypertrophy. As yet no satisfactory pathologic, mechanical, electrophysiologic, or biochemical study has isolated a specific abnormality that can be mechanistically coupled to hypertrophy and progressive functional deterioration of the heart. Perhaps the only exception to this observation is the linking of depressed maximal contractile velocity to specific alterations in the predominant isoform of myosin expressed. However, in humans this mechanism has little relevance since MHC isoform switching does not occur to any significant degree in the ventricle.

The Importance of Protein Synthesis

The most basic definition of cardiac hypertrophy is increased myocardial muscle mass, principally due to enlargement of myocytes (hypertrophy) but also increased numbers of nonmyocyte cellular elements (i.e., hyperplasia). Numerous studies employing DNA labeling techniques during pressure or volume overload have established that cellular proliferation is confined to nonmyocyte elements, principally fibroblasts.[93] Based on this evidence, it must be concluded that at the cellular level the hallmark of cardiac hypertrophy is expansion of existing myocyte mass through increased protein content and synthetic capacity. Because acceleration of synthetic rates consumes energy, all eukaryotic cells tightly regulate rates of protein synthesis. Protein synthesis depends on three important processes, each of which has unique regulatory mechanisms at its disposal: (a) transcriptional activation and posttranscriptional

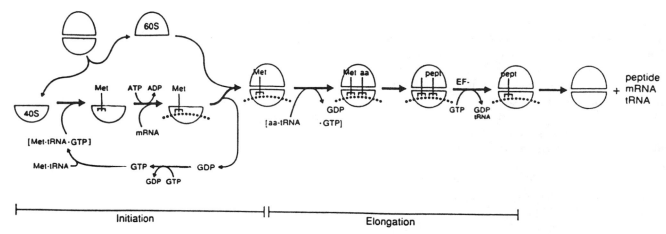

FIGURE 3.12. Peptide chain initiation and elongation. Translation is initiated by the binding of methionine-tRNA-GTP complex (*Met-tRNA-GTP*) and charging of the 40S ribosome, which consumes energy from the hydrolysis of GTP and ATP. Peptide chain elongation occurs by the sequential addition of amino acids (*aa*) complexed to their respective tRNA-GTP complex (*aa-tRNA-GTP*). This process is controlled by addi- tional ribosomal proteins called elongation factors (*EF*). For each amino acid added to the growing chain, a GTP is hydrolyzed to GDP, which is subsequently recycled for further use. Reproduced, with permission, from ref. 100. Copyright by the American Society for Biochemistry and Molecular Biology.

stabilization of protein encoding mRNA, (b) total ribosomal content and the fraction actually contained in protein synthesizing polyribosomes, and (c) regulation of peptide chain initiation and elongation. Although we described the principles of each of these mechanisms in the primer, their specific coordination in myocyte hypertrophy is discussed below.

Regulation of Protein Synthesis

Protein synthesis rates (Ks) can be determined both in vivo and in vitro. In general, this involves measuring the rate of incorporation of a specific radiolabeled amino acid into protein relative to total tissue weight, total protein, or specific protein (fractional synthesis rate). For muscle, phenylalanine, tyrosine, or leucine are the preferred amino acids because their slow rates of metabolism limit problems with recycling of degradation products. Unequal compartmentalization of radiolabeled precursor can result in differences between the specific activities of extra- and intracellular pools, leading to erroneous calculations of protein synthesis rates. This problem is circumvented if the perfusate concentration of the radioactive tracer is raised to a concentration where it has been shown that the specific activities of the extracellular, intracellular, and tRNA-bound pools are equivalent. Under these conditions, the perfusate-specific activity can be used to calculate directly rates of protein synthesis,[97] Alternatively, fractional rates of protein synthesis can be determined using a dual-isotope labeling technique. This protocol is particularly useful for measuring Ks in tissue cultures.[98] The most important technical pitfall of all these methods is accurate determination of the specific

activity of the precursor tRNA pool. Simple assumption of equilibration between intracellular and extracellular pools is not satisfactory and could lead to gross underestimates of protein synthesis rates since charging of the tRNA pool with the labeled isotope is delayed.

The synthetic capacity is grossly estimated by determining the relative content of the RNA and protein pools (i.e., mg RNA/g of protein, Cs). The efficiency with which proteins are synthesized (Ke) reflects how well a fixed quantity of ribosomes is able to translate mRNA and can be estimated by dividing Ks by Cs (mg of protein per unit time/mg of RNA). Ke primarily reflects regulation at the ribosomal level and in particular is strongly dependent on peptide chain initiation and elongation. These measurements are crude at best, but they can be performed in vivo and in vitro, and are helpful in narrowing experimental focus to important rate-limiting steps.[99]

Ribosomal Regulation of Protein Synthesis

Ribosomal control of protein synthesis primarily takes place during translation, the complex process of initiation and elongation of the peptide chain[100] (Fig. 3.12) Initiation always begins with the ribosomal recognition of the universal start-of-translation nucleotide sequence of the mRNA: the ATG codon. This triplet nucleotide sequence codes for methionine (met). Amino acids are ferried to the ribosome by transfer RNAs (tRNAs). Peptide chain initiation begins when the Met-tRNA-GTP complex binds to the 40S subunit of the ribosome. Initiation factor 2 (eIF-2) is the principle regulatory protein involved in this event and comprises three subunits: alpha, beta, and gamma. The eIF-2 protein binds with GTP and Met-tRNA to form a ternary complex. After the successful incorporation of Met-tRNA into the 40S subunit, the remaining eIF-2-GDP complex is displaced from the ribosome. Another factor, eIF-2B, aids in the recycling of eIF-2 by displacing GDP and replacins it with GTP.

It is now known that phosphorylation on serine-51 of the alpha subunit of eIF-2 represses protein synthesis by preventing this recycling step. Phosphorylation of eIF-2 phosphorylation is, in turn, controlled by protein serine kinases (enzymes that phosphorylate serine amino acids incorporated into a protein) and protein phosphatases (enzymes that dephosphorylate amino acids incorporated into a protein).[101] Activation of these enzymes is part of the general signal transduction process and biochemical cascade initiated by binding of growth factors and mitogens to their receptors, thereby integrating the regulation of protein synthesis into the general metabolic responses of the cell. Double-stranded RNA activated-kinase (DAI) and hemin-regulated inhibitor (HRI) are two important serine kinases specific for eIF-2. Interestingly, HRI activity may be repressed by certain isoforms of heat shock proteins (HSP), specifically the 68-kDa isoform.[100] This may be one mechanism whereby the transient expression of HSP fits into regulating myocardial protein synthesis in several models of hypertrophy.

After successful charging of 40S with Met-tRNA, selection and binding of mRNA takes place. This process appears to be regulated by at least three different ribosomal proteins (initiation factors) that are responsible for uncoiling (melting) and promoting binding of mRNA to the 40S subunit. This process depends on ATP hydrolysis. Within the 40S subunit is a large protein structure (S6 ribosomal protein) that contains specific mRNA binding regions. Binding of mRNA to this protein is controlled by phosphorylation on at least five serine residues. Protein S6 phosphorylation appears to be responsive to growth factors, mitogens, and insulin, suggesting that this protein is a distal target for signal transduction pathways activated during proliferation and hypertrophy. S6 protein kinase is directly responsible for phosphorylating the S6 protein. Activation of this kinase is in turn regulated by another serine kinase: microtubule-associated protein kinase 2 (MAP-2). Recent data reveal that MAP-2 kinase (a serine kinase) can be activated by insulin-dependent and other tyrosine kinase receptor–dependent factors.[102,103]

Peptide chain elongation takes place as the mRNA moves across the ribosome and amino acids, brought to the ribosome by tRNA, are incorporated into the protein. This process is controlled by additional sets of ribosomal proteins or elongation factors. Of these, elongation factor 2 (EF-2) is induced rapidly by insulin and its state of phosphorylation is dependent on a calcium-dependent protein kinase: Ca^{2+}-calmodulin–

dependent protein kinase III.[104,105] These characteristics make this eEF-2 an attractive candidate for regulating muscle protein synthesis.

Myocardial Hypertrophy and Protein Synthesis

A variety of experimental models have been employed to measure rates of protein synthesis and degradation. This has included in vivo measurements of whole heart protein synthesis, the use of Langendorff-perfused hearts, and recently, dissociated neonatal myocyte cultures. Each of these models has important strengths and limitations. In vivo models are well suited for looking at the influence of hormonal manipulations and their interactions with pressure-or volume-overloaded models. However, secondary hemodynamic effects arising from hormonal depletion or excess make it difficult to establish mechanistic relationships. The Langendorff model attempts to overcome this problem by allowing the investigator to manipulate left ventricular pressure and workload and to study the acute effects of drugs under controlled hemodynamic conditions. This particular methodology has been useful to study the acute effects of ventricular pressure, stretch, and beating on protein synthesis. Compared to in vivo experiments, this is a more accurate method because it avoids complicated in vivo measurements of protein synthesis rates where exact determination of the specific activity of precursor pools is complicated by whole body distribution of the radioisotope. Tissue culture models offer the best opportunity of establishing a mechanistic understanding of how myocardial protein synthesis is regulated, but it is difficult to extrapolate these results into meaningful physiological conclusions.

Animal and Whole Heart Models

In vivo studies in adult animals have shown the importance of normal levels of thyroid hormone and growth hormone on the maintenance of cardiac weight. Hypophysectomy in the adult animal quickly leads to cardiac atrophy.[76] In juvenile hypophysectomized rats, growth hormone repletion only partially restores cardiac weight, whereas T_3 replacement seems to promote full recovery.[106] Thyroid hormone excess results in significant increases in cardiac mass and a 22% to 24% increase in total protein synthesis rates, compared to placebo treatment.[107,108] This has been shown both in vivo and by short-term treatment before mounting of the heart in a perfusion apparatus. Catecholamines have been shown to have a permissive role in the development of cardiac hypertrophy.[109–111] In vitro models have extended these observations to show direct effects cf catecholamines on cardiac protein synthesis in whole heart preparations.[112,113] By comparison, acute increases in intraventricular or aortic pressure result in about a 40% to 60% increase in protein synthesis rates.[114,115] Insulin also has profound effects on protein synthesis and content.[115,116] Regardless of the specific model and methodology employed, it is generally agreed that increases in protein synthetic capacity predominate over decreases in protein degradation as the basis for an increase of protein content.[117]

Tissue Culture Models

Most of this work now has been extended to neonatal myocyte culture models. These offer an excellent opportunity to study myocyte cell biology, trophic actions of hormones, and growth factors in the absence of confounding hemodynamic influences. Exposure of serum-deprived myocytes to isoproterenol or norepinephrine significantly stimulate myocyte hypertrophy as measured by cell volume, cell surface area, and accelerated protein synthesis.[112,113] These agents also specifically promote synthesis of myofibrillar proteins with little or no effect on DNA synthesis or protein degradation. This response appears to be specifically mediated through the alpha$_1$-adrenergic receptor since prazosin and phentolamine block norepinephrine NE-stimulated protein synthesis, whereas propranolol and yohimbine have no effect.[118] Mechanical activity in the form of synchronous contraction, independent of serum or other growth factors, also is a potent stimulus for protein synthesis.[113,119] Pathways for adrenergic stimulation of protein synthesis can be dissociated from mechanical activity since exposure to propranolol inhibits synchronous contraction but has no effect on norepinephrine-induced protein synthesis. Additionally, thyroid hormone, insulin, and IGF-1 also have been shown to increase protein synthesis in myocyte cultures.[99,120] The important aspect of all these studies is that they show that myocyte protein synthesis can be regulated independent of hemodynamic load through activation of specific receptors.

Mechanisms Regulating Protein Synthesis

Accelerated protein synthesis can arise from enhanced capacity, greater translational efficiency, or a combination of the two. Under most physiologic conditions, rates of protein synthesis are proportional to the concentration of total cellular RNA (85% of which is ribosomal RNA), concentration and half-life of mRNA, and the availability of polyribosomal complexes. Availability of myofibrillar mRNA and polyribosomes have not been shown to constitute important rate-limiting steps in cardiac protein synthesis. Transient expression of transcriptional regulatory oncogenes in response to hypertrophic stimuli recently has been demonstrated and undoubtedly plays an important step in signal transduction.

Transcriptional Control

During hypertrophy increased ribosomal content and ribosomal protein synthesis is a common finding that usually precedes increases in protein synthesis. Availability of polyribosomes does not appear to be a rate-limiting step since the proportion of polyribosomes is unaffected by T$_3$ treatment or imposition of a hemodynamic burden.[108,121,122] Furthermore, general increases in mRNA levels and, specifically, expression of myofibrillar mRNA result after hypertrophic stimulation. Resumption of contraction in depolarized myocytes accelerates rRNA synthesis and stimulates cell growth.[119,123] Taken together, these data suggest that faster protein synthesis depends on rapid increases in ribosomal content (i.e., increased rRNA transcription) and elevated levels of specific mRNAs, leading to enhanced synthetic capacity.

Translational Control

The cascade of biochemical events initiated by hypertrophic stimuli can directly affect translational efficiency through phosphorylation-dependent pathways that are part of the signal transduction process. Such a mechanism need not necessarily require enhanced transcriptional activation. Insulin, for example, promotes cardiac protein synthesis primarily by increasing translation efficiency. In other cell types, insulin and IGF-I have been shown to be capable of enhancing translation by phosphorylating ribosomal S6 protein through MAP-2 kinase– and S6 kinase–dependent pathways. In addition, catecholamine-induced protein synthesis does not appear to be blocked by actinomycin (an inhibitor of transcription), suggesting posttranscriptional (mRNA stability) and translational regulation of protein synthesis.[112] Taken together, it is likely that myocardial protein synthesis in response to hypertrophic stimuli is regulated both by increased capacity (transcriptional) and enhanced efficiency (translational). The predominating mechanism likely will depend on the nature of the trophic signal and the distal targets of its signal transduction pathway.

The Relation Between Myocyte Phenotype and Hypertrophy

The relationship, if any, between permanent exit from the cell cycle, hypertrophy, and emergence of the mature cardiac phenotype also is not known. It is thought that the protein synthetic capacity needed to result in pressure hypertrophy requires reversion to a fetal phenotype. This perspective is based on the coupling of two phenomenologic sets of data: (a) reemergence of fetal isoforms of MHC, MLC and actin, (b) transient expression of several protooncogenes, specifically c-fos and c-myc.[124–127] However, no mechanistic data exist to couple these events to protein synthesis, whereas a substantial body of data demonstrates that reemergence of the fetal phenotype is not a prerequisite of growth. For example, postnatal and juvenile cardiac growth are the most prominent forms of hypertrophy that all developing hearts undergo, and yet neither fetal isoforms of contractile proteins nor fetal oncogenes are expressed. Indeed, reemergence of the beta-MHC gene (the fetal isoform) is a property of the aging rat and rabbit heart, in which most of the data pertaining to contractile isoforms in hypertrophy have been derived; yet it would be paradoxical to label this transition as "fetal".[26–28] Moreover, the protein synthetic capacity of myocytes isolated from senescent rats is not depressed compared to younger cohorts.[128] Last, data derived from heterotopic transplanted hearts show that hypertrophy and changes in contractile gene expression can be functionally uncoupled.[129,130] Moreover, in large animal species and humans, beta-MHC is the predominant isoform in the ventricle throughout normal postnatal life (except during the first few weeks after birth) and has not been shown to undergo any regulation during hypertrophy.[26,27] Therefore, we suggest that the weight of available experimental evidence does not support a causal link between reemergence of a fetal phenotype (as measured in terms of contractile proteins) and the ability to undergo hypertrophy.

Second Messengers and Signal Transduction

There is a very complex pathway between signals received at the surface of the cell, such as mechanical stretch or hormones, and the intracellular response of the cell. Study of both the intact cardiac muscle of humans and animals and myocyte tissue culture models of cardiac hypertrophy has provided a means to study this pathway, which links signals received at the cell surface, receptor activation, second messengers, and the control of gene expression and protein synthesis.

Adrenergic Signaling

Activation of alpha-adrenergic receptors results in a cascade of cytosolic and nuclear events that can potentially regulate protein synthesis. Characteristic receptor-associated events include intracellular alkalinization, changes in ion fluxes, release of intracellular stores of Ca^{2+}, modulation of cAMP, and protein kinase C (PKC), phoshotidyl inositol degradation, and activation of nuclear transcription factors (i.e., protooncogenes). Within the cardiac sarcolemma are numerous membrane-associated proteins that are coupled to adrenergic receptors and effect many of the changes referred to above. This includes G-binding proteins, GTPase proteins, phospholipase C-gamma, phosphoinositol 3'-kinase, and several membrane and cytoplasmic oncogenes such as c-ras and c-raf.

Other Signals

Intracellular Ca^{2+}, cAMP, and PKC have been shown to regulate myocardial protein synthesis.[105,131,132] Contractile activity (i.e., beating) is not a requirement to maintain synthetic capacity if hearts are treated with agents that increase cAMP levels. Moreover, inhibition of cAMP induction abolishes stretch-induced increases in protein and ribosomal synthesis rates, but does not affect insulin-dependent increases, again highlighting dual regulatory pathways for myocardial protein synthesis.[122] Recent data have shown that ribosomal S6 protein can be phosphorylated by cAMP-dependent pathways leading to enhanced mRNA binding and faster rates of protein synthesis. In addition, many genes have cis- acting regulatory regions that contain cAMP responsive elements (CRE)—elements that promote enhanced transcription when activated.

Activation of PKC also has been shown to induce directly myocyte protein synthesis. Treatment of myocytes with tetradecanoyl phorbol acetate (TPA) results in increased protein synthesis and rapid induction of the oncogenes c-fos, c-jun and egr-1.[131] TPA, also known as tumor promoting agent, is a potent mitogen for other cell lines and an activator of PKC. In contrast to adrenergic receptors, PKC is an intracellular serine-threonine protein kinase and represents an alternative hypertrophic pathway. As in the case of cAMP, ribosomal S6 also is a distal target of PKC-dependent pathways. In addition, PKC also rapidly induces expression of nuclear transcription factors. Thus, both nuclear events and cytoplasmic protein phosphorylations are distal targets of cAMP and PKC. This again suggests two levels of protein synthesis regulation: a nuclear level dependent on transcriptional activation and a translational level dependent on enhanced efficiency of protein synthesis.

Oncogenes and Transcriptional Regulation

We frequently have referred to oncogenes and protooncogenes in previous sections of this chapter. Oncogenes are genes that first were identified in certain tumor viruses as the basis for their oncogenicity. For example, we mentioned above the v-erbA oncogene as the tumorigenic gene of the avian erythroblastosis virus. Subsequently, the origins of these viral genes were found to be the remnants of mutated eukaryotic (such as mammalian and human) qenes whose normal function in the cell is, in many cases, the control and participation in the cell cycle and response to growth factors. In order to distinguish these two genes, the latter is sometimes called a cellular (c) or protooncogene. For example, the likely origin of v-erbA is the protooncogene c-erbA, a variety of thyroid hormone receptor. The generic term "oncogene" frequently is used to refer to either the viral or cellular gene, leaving it to the reader to distinguish between them according to the context of usage. There is a profusion of names as a result of a burgeoning number of oncogenes and protooncogenes that have been discovered: the names are the delight of molecular biologists and the bane of the occasional user. In addition, it is necessary to distinguish the gene (lower case letters) from the protein product of the gene (capital letters); usually this is best understood in the context of the sentence in which it is used.

Oncogenes Expressed in the Heart

Numerous protooncogenes are expressed in fetal, neonatal, and adult myocardium. Many of these are developmentally, hormonally, and functionally regulated. Shown in Table 3.1 is a partial list of typical oncogenes that have been identified in the heart. Notable among these are c-Ha-ras and c-raf, both of which appear to be constitutively expressed in high copy number in fetal and adult myocardium.[126] c-RAF is a cytoplasmic threonine/serine protein kinase that participates in transduction of mitogenic signals.

Ras oncogenes are membrane-associated G-binding/GTPase proteins and are structurally similar to the G-binding proteins that are coupled to adrenergic receptors.[133,134] Ras proteins belong to a family of polypeptides that have been linked to growth regulation and abnormal proliferation. Localized point mutations in these genes have been correlated with certain known cancers and abnormal growth regulation in experimental systems. Recent data suggest that certain ras mutations alter expression of cytokines that participate in and contribute to hyperplasia.[135]

Other growth-related oncogenes also expressed in the heart include c-sis and c-src, which express the PDGF-B chain and a membrane-associated tyrosine kinase receptor, respectively. Sis does not appear to be developmentally regulated, whereas src expression is high during the fetal and neonatal periods and then is downregulated in adult myocardium.[126] Both of these genes participate in growth control in other cell lines. The specific function of these oncogenes in heart is unknown but may be related to myocyte differentiation.

The nuclear oncogenes c-fos, c-myc, c-jun and the nuclear protein egr-1 are expressed in a wide variety of tissues and cell lines after trophic or mitogenic stimulation.[136-138] For those cells that are capable of reentering the cell cycle, induction of these genes appears to be necessary, but not always sufficient for entry and progression through G1.[139,140] In the heart these same oncogenes are induced transiently and differentially by growth factors and other trophic stimuli.[141-143] Because induction is rapid (within minutes to the first several hours) and does not require intervening protein synthesis, these oncogenes are called early or primary response genes. Their kinetic profile and independence from protein synthesis suggests that expression/induction requires specific factors already present within the cell and awaiting activation. These oncogenes undoubtedly couple transmembrane signaling to transcriptional regulation. A recent transgenic model of c-myc overexpression has shown the permissive role of this oncogene in cardiac hyperplasia.[69]

How expression of nuclear oncogenes is mechanistically coupled to transcriptional regulation is just becoming understood. Perhaps the prototype for this is transcriptional regulation by AP-1, a TPA-inducible protein, and cooperation between the protein products of c-fos and c-jun in conferring activity to AP-1.[144,145] AP-1 protein is a nuclear transcription acting factor that recognizes a specific *cis*-acting element with a particular nucleotide sequence (TGACTCA) found in promoters and enhancers of many genes. It turns out that the active component of AP-1 is composed of FOS and JUN heterodimers and that TPA regulation of AP-1–inducible genes is through expression of fos and jun oncogene families.

Nuclear oncogene proteins have specific structural motifs that allow them to bind and interact with DNA. Structural motifs on JUN include a leucine zipper for promoting dimerization and DNA binding, a basic region adjacent to the leucine zipper for stabilizing DNA binding, and a proline-rich region that is required for transcriptional activation. Other members of the jun family, including jun B and jun D, also are TPA-

TABLE 3.1. Oncogenes.

Nuclear transcription factors	
Structural motif	*Name*
Leucine zipper	fos, jun
Helix-loop-helix	myc
Zinc finger	erbA
Other	myb
Membrane-associated	
Biochemical class	*Name*
Tyrosine kinase	src, abl
G-protein associated	Ha-ras
Cytoplasmic	
Biochemical class	*Name*
Protein serine kinase	raf
Humoral growth factor	
	Name
PDGF B chain	sis

responsive, and their protein products can form homodimers or heterodimers among themselves or with FOS. Although all can bind to AP-1 sites, only specific forms can actually activate transcription, whereas others may in fact be antagonistic.

FOS also is a nucleoprotein that is part of the activated AP-1 protein. It was shown subsequently that FOS and JUN interact to form heterodimers that confer transcriptional activity to AP-1. Like JUN, FOS has a leucine zipper and an adjacent basic motif that give it the structural ability to interact with JUN. However, FOS cannot form homodimers so that by itself it possesses no transcriptional activity. Within the 5'-flanking region of the c-fos gene is another *cis*-acting element called a serum response control element (SRE) that binds an inducible serum response factor (SRF) and activates transcription of c-fos.[146] It turns out that phosphorylation of SRF by c-raf activates this factor causing it to be translocated to the nucleus where it, in turn, activates c-fos. Raf activation is linked to receptor-mediated events such as tyrosine phosphorylation and PKC activation. Thus, cooperation between oncogenes is an integral part of the signal transduction process. Together FOS and JUN interact to activate AP-1. It is believed that FOS stabilizes or increases the transcriptional activity of JUN.

Application of Molecular and Cellular Science to the Management of Heart Failure

The burgeoning information supplied by cellular and molecular biology holds substantial promise for the management of heart failure. This is a promissory note, as yet unfulfilled. In the final section of this chapter, we would like to suggest how this information may be applied to etiology, pathophysiology, and treatment of congestive heart failure.

Application to Etiology

Heart failure is a pathophysiological syndrome in search of an etiology. Perhaps the simplest mistake that can be made in the management of heart failure is an inability to obtain an etiological diagnosis. However, even the best of clinical acumen can have a limited impact if the sophistication of the etiological diagnosis is limited. For some disorders the understanding of the basis of the disease is limited. Some of these disorders appear to have a molecular basis and we will summarize briefly what is known about these below.

In molecular terms, "etiology" is synonymous with "gene defect." Gene disorders come in two sizes: single gene and multigene defects. Many diseases of the cardiovascular system appear to be multigenetic in etiology, implying that more than one gene defect is responsible for the disorder. Examples of these include very common problems, such as hypertension and garden variety atherosclerosis. which compose much of the epidemic of cardiovascular disease of the developed countries. For these disorders, we currently assume that DNA mutations—changes in the nucleotide sequence—occur in a group of genes that leads to minor qualitative or quantitative protein changes that collectively account for the disease, perhaps with an important interaction of environmental factors (e.g., smoking, diet, and exercise in the development of atherosclerotic coronary heart disease). It is difficult to isolate and identify multiple genes that interact to form the etiology of a disease and so genetic progress has been slow. To define these diseases, we either will need to understand how to determine multiple gene linkage from the pattern of inheritance, or how to assemble many single gene defects into the montage of a complicated disease.

In contrast, a single gene disease (usually) has a clear pattern of inheritance that allows it to be recognized as a heritable disorder: autosomal dominant, autosomal recessive, or sex-linked. There is an additional and unusual set of genetic disorders involving the mitochondrial genome, which has its own rules of inheritance. Molecular identification of these disorders is comparatively straightforward by the tools of cloning or reverse genetics.

Numerically, these single-gene disorders appear to be the exception rather than the rule in our cardiovascular disease epidemic probably because of two seemingly contradictory reasons: lethality or benignity. One explanation for the paradox of either of these two ends of the spectrum is as follows. The altered protein of a single-gene defect may be so functionally important that it extinguishes embryonic life and therefore leaves no evidence of a clinical disease. At the opposite pole, the altered protein of a single gene disease may be so functionally unimportant that it causes no clinically apparent disease. It is only when the consequences of the mutation are mild at onset and subsequently progressive, or delayed during the lifetime, that clinically important disease becomes apparent.

In the causes of genetic disorders, as in life-in-general, Murphy's law prevails: anything that can go wrong, will go wrong. Single-gene diseases have thus far been shown to be a result of mutations in the protein-coding portion of the gene. In a simplified classification scheme, these mutations generally appear as one of two varieties: point and deletional. A point mutation causes a change of a single nucleotide base pair in the gene sequence. This results in a change of the mRNA and may cause a change in an amino acid of the translated protein sequence. As discussed at the beginning of this chapter, protein structure and function

TABLE 3.2. Cardiac diseases secondary to single gene defects.

Disorder	Mode of inheritance	Gene
Familial hypertrophic cardiomyopathy	Autosomal dominant	Myosin heavy chain (?)
Duchenne's muscular dystrophy	Sex-linked recessive	Dystrophic
Long Q-T syndrome	Autosomal dominant Autosomal recessive	C-Ha-ras (?)
Mitochondrial myopathies	Maternal (mitochondrial)	Cytochrome oxidase and others
Carnitine deficiency	Autosomal recessive and unknown	1° Carnitine transporter (?) 2° Acyl transferases

may be affected substantially by even a change in a single amino acid in a protein. A deletional mutation causes the loss of a stretch of the gene sequence and thereby a substantial deletion in the mRNA and translated protein. This is likely to have important functional consequences. Examples of both of these mutations can be found in a few cardiovascular disorders whose basis only recently has been elucidated.

Perhaps the first single-gene disorder of the cardiovascular system to be identified was familial hypercholesterolemia, which is an autosomal recessive disorder caused by one or more mutations in the (low density lipoprotein) (LDL) receptor, the membrane protein found on liver cells responsible for the uptake and cellular internalization of the (LDL) particle.[147] This well established story will not be repeated here, but serves as a paradigm of the intersection of molecular science with clinical medicine. Instead, we will review briefly a few diseases in which very recent studies have shed some light on the basis of the disorder (Table 3.2). Subsequently in this section, we will turn our attention to the enigmatic disorder of viral cardiomyopathy in order to illustrate the contributions of molecular biology to unraveling other etiologies of heart disease.

Familial Hypertrophic Cardiomyodathy

The evolving story of the search for the familial hypertrophic cardiomyopathy (FHC) gene is extremely important because it marks the first cardiac disease in which clinicians, geneticists, and molecular biologists can clearly communicate. A hereditable disorder, FHC is passed as an autosomal dominant trait but with variable degrees of penetrance. The hallmark of this disorder is cardiac hypertrophy in affected family members, especially of the left ventricle, in the absence of other known humoral or hemodynamic conditions that lead to hypertrophy. There are a number of additional

clinical, physiologic, and pathologic features including a risk of sudden death, ventricular arrhythmias, increased contractility of the ventricle, and paradoxically, heart failure. Previous names used for this entity, such as idiopathic hypertrophic subaortic stenosis or asymmetrical septal hypertrophy, emphasized physiologic or pathologic features, but actually shed little light on the etiology of the disease. However, the application of reverse genetics has focused attention on chromosomal location 14ql (chromosome 14, the first cytogenetic band below the centromere) in large kindreds of families with FHC.[148,149] This chromosome locus is close to the gene location of the MHC genes, whose gene and protein structure are described earlier in this chapter.

Recent studies have suggested that mutations in the beta-MHC gene may be responsible for some families with FHC. The first mutation described in a single large family kindred showed a missense mutation in exon 13 of the beta-MHC gene in affected family members.[150] This resulted in a change of an amino acid in a highly evolutionarily conserved region of the globular head of the myosin. Speculation, but no firm evidence, has suggested that this abnormal gene leads to an altered MHC protein, which leads to cardiac hypertrophy and the other clinical manifestations. Although the genetic studies are clear about the mutational event in the MHC gene, it is less clear how this change leads to the disease state. Especially perplexing is the earlier protein studies of FHC, which suggested no change in the structure or function of myosin proteins.[151] Additional studies of FHC patients have shown other single missense mutations located throughout the beta-MHC gene, further complicating interpretation of this extraordinary finding (C. Seidman, *personal communication*).

The importance of this discovery may allow identification of family members, prenatal screening, and determination of the etiology of sporadic cases of cardiac hypertrophy whose basis is unknown. It also should permit the development of newer strategies for a disease whose treatment is most difficult.

Duchenne's Muscular Dystrophy

The muscular dystrophies are a set of heritable skeletal muscle disorders and include some diseases with cardiac involvement manifested by myopathy, arrhythmias, and conduction system disturbance. Duchenne's is a sex-linked recessive disease, which means that the gene defect occurs on the X chromosome and is maternally transmitted. One half of the male offspring of a carrier mother will be affected, because the only copy of the gene transmitted from parents to male offspring is the defective allele (gene copy) of the maternal X chromosome. Female offspring also have a 50% chance of obtaining one copy of the muscular dystrophy gene from one of the X chromosomes of their mother;

however, they will be only carriers because of inheritance of a normal gene obtained from the other X chromosome of the (normal) father.

This disorder was originally considered to be two disorders which included not only the severe form of dystrophy, but also a milder disease called Becker's. However, the gene and protein basis for this disorder recently have been identified.[152,153] and one of the surprises has been that the two disorders represent phenotype differences based on the severity of mutation of the dystrophin gene.

The largest gene identified to date in the human genome the dystrophin gene, spans over 2 million nucleotide bases. Within the exons of the DNA are buried the coding sequence of the dystrophin protein, which will translate into a very large protein with a molecular mass of about 400 kDa. Once synthesized in the cytoplasm of the muscle cell, the protein is localized to the cell membrane and is believed to be a cytoskeletal filament that is involved in and somehow maintains the integrity of the sarcolemma. During the very long search for the cause of Duchenne's, it was not possible to isolate the dystrophin protein, probably because it is present in very small amounts. Reverse genetic techniques were used to identify the dystrophin gene locus and to "walk" along the chromosome until a new gene was recognized and demonstrated to be the source of the disorder.

The mutation in both Becker's and Duchenne's is a deletion in the gene. In the extreme, the message and/or its ability to be translated is so defective that no protein is produced at all and the result is Duchenne's, the severe form of the disease. Alternatively, the deletion in the gene is smaller, which results in reduced synthesis of the partially defective protein of Becker's, the milder form of the disease. Techniques have been developed that permit diagnosis of the affected patient, prenatal screening, and carrier testing. The possibility for treatment is clear but elusive: replace the defective gene with a correct copy or with a surrogate that will serve the vital membrane function of dystrophin. The time course for the development of such treatment is unknown.

Long Q-T Syndrome

Communication between the extracellular milieu and the response of a target cell is referred to as cell signaling. The components of such a system include receptors on the target cell, which are coupled to G proteins whose effect is to activate membrane enzymes, such as adenylate cyclase or protein kinases C and A. These membrane enzymes, which act as second messengers, are activated through the hydrolysis of GTP, which is the function of the "G proteins," and also the basis for their name: guanine nucleotide binding proteins. Re-

cently it has been shown that G protein activation of membrane enzymes causes phosphorylation, and thereby regulation, of some ion channels.[154] As a result of their activity, G proteins may modulate Na^+, Ca^{2+}, and K^+ ion channels and thereby alter the action potential. Receptors coupled to G proteins include the adrenergic and cholinergic receptors. The G protein family is large and includes members that are known oncogenes and protooncogenes, such as the ras group (again refer to Table 3.1). However, unlike other members of the G proteins, the pathway of signal transduction of the ras protooncogenes has not been identified clearly and their role in modulation of ion channel activity is more speculative. However, a recent study in the molecular genetics of the long Q-T syndrome (LQTS) has focused attention on the relationship between ras and ion channels.

The LQTS includes some patients with a recognized familial inheritance pattern. Affected individuals have a prolonged QT interval on their electrocardiogram, usually in excess of a heart rate corrected value of about 0.45 s. There are two forms of this syndrome: the Romano Ward syndrome, which is an autosomal dominant disorder, and the Jervell and Lange-Nielson syndrome, which is autosomal recessive. The latter disorder includes hearing impairment. There is a very large variation in the clinical phenotype of this syndrome, which includes some patients who develop recurrent fainting and sudden death due to ventricular tachycardia and ventricular fibrillation. Episodes of ventricular arrhythmias can occur as a result of increased sympathetic tone, with symptoms appearing during exercise or anxiety; this also can be simulated with an infusion of catecholamines. Recently it has been reported that the gene locus in one of these LQTS families is the c-Ha-ras protooncogene, which is located on chromosome 11p.[155] Because of the increasing physiologic evidence of modulation of ion channels by G proteins, a mutation in a ras protooncogene is an interesting candidate for the cause of the LQTS. However, the exact mutation responsible for this syndrome remains to be elucidated and the results of family screening await further confirmation. In addition to this defining the basis of this rare syndrome, these results point the way to additional studies on the mechanisms of cardiac arrhythmogenesis, which is a major cause of morbidity and mortality in cardiac disease.

Mitochondrial Myopathy and the Other Genome

Evidence for a deficiency of energy production has long been speculated as a basis for cardiomyopathy. Impairment could affect myocardial performance in at least the two ways, both of which have been the broad theme of earlier sections of this chapter: diminished energy for the contractile apparatus and for maintenance of protein synthesis. It is also possible that energy depletion occurs as a secondary phenomenon in the myocyte of the failing heart. However, measurement of ATP levels in the failing hearts of humans and of experimental models has not conclusively demonstrated a decrease. ATP is synthesized from the oxidation of foodstuffs, the final steps of which are under the control of the proteins of oxidative phosphorylation located on the inner mitochondrial membrane. From a historical perspective of the role of mitochondria in the cell, the possibility of a primary impairment of energy production based on abnormalities of the proteins of oxidative phosphorylation appeared to be implausible, because it was thought that such an impairment would result in widespread and severe organ dysfunction that would be incompatible with maintenance of life. However, the discovery of specific disorders of the mitochondrial genome have changed that viewpoint.

Recent evidence has emerged that there is a rare group of disorders in which ATP synthesis is impaired—the mitochondrial myopathies. The basis for these disorders is a gene mutation in one or more of the 80 or so proteins of the inner mitochondrial membrane that form the five complexes of oxidative phosphorylation. Most of these proteins are coded by genes located on the chromosomes of the nucleus; however, a DNA mutation in one of these has not yet been definitively demonstrated. In contrast, the separate and small mitochondrial genome contains genes for only 15 of these proteins, as well as genes for its own translation apparatus including rRNAs and tRNAs. The heritable basis for a disorder of the mitochondrial genome is distinctly different from the rules of heredity that we outlined at the beginning of this section. Because mitochondria have their own genome and are present at fertilization only in the ovum (the cytoplasm of the sperm is too sparse to accommodate their presence), mitochondrial genes are inherited only from the mother.

Disorders of the mitochondrial DNA have been identified that usually involve deletions in a "hot spot" of this small genome. All of these deletional syndromes involve ophthalmoplegia, and in advanced stages may include cardiac involvement such as dilated cardiomyopathy or conduction system defects, as can occur in the mitochondrial myopathies (MM), Kearns-Sayre syndrome (KSS), myoclonic epilepsy and ragged red fibers (MERRF), and lactic acidosis and stroke-like episodes (MELAS).[156–158] It is now simple to screen for these disorders because large deletions of a gene segment change the pattern of "restricted" or cut-up pieces of the DNA. When DNA (including mitochondrial DNA) is harvested from cells and cleaved into fragments with specialized proteins known as restriction enzymes, the fragments can be separated on a sieving matrix and sorted according to size and pattern. This cut-and-paste method of identifying mutations in molecular biology is called restriction mapping, and the changes in the appearance of different pieces of cleaved DNA reveals a distinct pattern called RFLPs, restriction fragment length polymorphisms, which provide a visual clue to DNA mutations.

Developmental mutations also may occur in the mitochondrial genome, because DNA repair mechanisms, normally present in the nucleus, are not available in the mitochondrion. For example, recent data suggest that subpopulations of human cardiac mitochondria, which contain deletional mutations of DNA, appear with aging and infarction.[159,160] It is speculated that these changes could be responsible for deterioration of cardiac function in response to aging. The relevance of these observations requires physiological inquiry because it would appear as if substantial quantitative abnormalities of ATP production would be required to change the metabolism of the myocyte. Indeed, the entire field of the molecular biology of oxidative phosphorylation, including examination of nuclear and mitochondrial genes, is under active investigation.

Carnitine Deficiency

Although disorders of carnitine metabolism are classified in some textbooks as a mitochondrial disorder, based on the metabolic locus of the problem, this group of diseases appears to involve gene mutations in the nuclear genome. Carnitine is a small molecule that is both synthesized by the liver and kidney and absorbed from the gastrointestinal tract from a variety of food sources; the molecule is transported in the blood and actively taken up by cells of the body (especially muscle) and located in the mitochondria. Carnitine is a shuttle that transports fatty acids from the cytoplasm of the cell into the inner mitochondrial membrane for oxidation. Since the primary fuel of the heart is fatty acids, the cardiac effect of carnitine deficiency leads to an early childhood or juvenile cardiomyopathy, which may have either a dilated and/or hypertrophied appearance and on tissue section shows characteristic perinuclear fat droplets.

The primary disorder takes two forms: a systemic disorder, which shows widespread liver, neurological, and metabolic manifestations, and a narrower phenotype muscular disorder.[161,162] Both forms show low carnitine levels in tissues; however, the former is probably due to abnormalities of kidney reuptake of carnitine from urine filtrate, whereas the latter probably is due to abnormalities of a muscle cell transport molecule. Both kidney and and muscle transporters have not yet been identified, and it is likely that elucidation of their gene and protein structure and function will provide considerable information about this disease. A more common form of carnitine deficiency is the secondary disorder that occurs as a result of deficiencies of the group of enzymes called acyl transferases. This disorder leaves carnitine complexed to fatty acids as acyl-carnitine, which results in excess excretion in the urine and which also results in tissue deficiency. Both of these disorders appear to be hereditary, although their genetics are poorly understood. However, biochemical tests are available, including prenatal screening, which can demonstrate reduced tissue and blood levels in the primary form of the disease and aminoaciduria in the secondary forms. Currently the only treatment available is dietary supplementation of carnitine, which appears to have beneficial, but selective, effects on patients.

Viral Cardiomyopathy

Although not a heritable disorder, viral cardiac infections that lead to heart failure have been opened to the possibility of detection by molecular techniques. It is our opinion that clinically significant viral infections of the heart are a rare and largely unproven etiologic entity because of the absence of conclusive criteria for diagnosis as well as in depth knowledge of disease pathogenesis. This diagnosis is made in the presence of symptomatic heart disease accompanied by objective changes in the electrocardiogram (ECG) and diminution of cardiac function. These criteria include exclusion of other etiologies and inclusion of nonspecific criteria such as a rise in viral titer during observation of the disease. Morphological and ultrastructural examination of heart biopsy tissue may show myocyte damage, fibrosis, and/or inflammation, but usually does not confirm a viral infectious agent—except perhaps in cytomegalic virus with its characteristic inclusion bodies. A few viruses, among them the enteroviruses, are major candidates as etiological agents. One criterion for infection is the presence of the infectious agent in tissue, but viral agents rarely are cultured from heart tissue and even their presence in tissue culture may be suspect and considered a contaminant. Molecular techniques, such as polymerase chain reaction, recently have been used to identify the presence of portions of enterovirus genomes from myocardial biopsies of patients with congestive cardiomyopathy, which suggests a viral presence, and perhaps etiology, in their illness.[163,164] These first studies require confirmation and need further refinement with studies of expression of viral proteins in myocardial cells and cellular and molecular studies on pathogenesis.

Application to Pathophysiology

In addition to defining the proximate cause of disease, molecular and cell biology should make a substantial contribution to defining the pathophysiology of many of the causes of heart failure.

The Final Common Pathway of Heart Failure

Meerson postulated that heart failure could start from a diverse group of illnesses that had a common denominator of myocardial injury and subsequently devolved to heart failure by a common series of molecular mechanisms that lead to inadequate myocardial function.[5] The search for these factors has become a holy grail in heart failure research and there are many mechanisms that have been proposed to account for these changes, including functional and structural changes in the myocardium. Current thinking includes changes in gene expression as a result of humoral or mechanical signals that act on the myocyte, or accumulated damage or even mutatior, to sensitive gene structures. Whether or not these will pass muster, the molecular and cellular tools to raise hypotheses and answer questions are now available. For example, it is now possible to take small samples of myocardium, such as endomyocardial biopsies of the human heart, and quantitate the level of a particular mRNA through a recently developed technique called polymerase chain reaction. In the failing human heart, decreases in the mRNA level of phospholamban (a protein that regulates the Ca^{2+} pump of the sarcoplasmic reticulum and helps to induce relaxation) and increases in atrial natiuretic peptide (a protein with vasodilator and diuretic properties) were found.[165] In general, substantial changes in the level of message are associated with changes of protein level and, therefore, functional changes in the myocardium may be expected (but are not proven) by these findings. These techniques will be applied in depth to both catalog and hopefully classify changes in myocardial gene expression. Ultimately, the mechanisms and importance of these changes will be elucidated.

Another important contribution that can be made to pathophysiology is the basis for cardiac hypertrophy and the further adaptation of the heart in response to hypertrophy. Characterizing the pattern and timing of gene expression in hypertrophy is a beginning to this process.[16] Clearly, however, an understanding of the control of gene expression and the cellular consequences of that expression is at the very root of this problem.

Atherosclerotic Coronary Heart Disease

Coronary heart disease (CHD) due to atherosclerosis is the predominant cause of cardiovascular morbidity in the Western world. A small fraction of patients with CHD have familial hypercholesterolemia, which causes premature atherosclerosis. However, even in this disorder the pathogenesis between abnormalities of lipid metabolism and the development of atherosclerosis is unresolved. For most CHD patients without obvious severe lipid metabolism disorders, the disorder is an enigma.

Built on a foundation of a century of basic and clinical studies, recent molecular and cellular techniques have been applied to study the pathogenesis of atherosclerosis.[166] After experimental injury to the endothelial surface of the arterial blood vessel wall there is lipid accumulation, macrophage and platelet adhesion to the surface wall, and smooth muscle cell migration to and proliferation at the subintima during the early stages of atherogenesis.

The role of proliferation and migration of the normally medially positioned vascular smooth muscle cells recently has been emphasized. Vascular smooth muscle cells. normally in the contractile phenotype, are predominantly at resting phase G_0 in the cell cycle. In response to growth factors elaborated by the macrophage and those made available from the blood and its formed elements after intimal damage, the smooth muscle cell assumes a synthetic phenotype, migrates into the subintimal position of the vessel, and reenters the cell cycle. The principal signal for changes in the smooth muscle cell population of the blood vessel wall appears to be platelet-derived growth factor (PDGF),[167] but also includes the transforming growth factors (TGF), fibroblast growth factor (FGF) and epidermal growth factor (EGF). These factors are the cellular homologs of viral oncogenes, and their eulects on cells represent still another aspect of the discussion that we initiated earlier on the thyroid hormone receptor. The resultant cellular proliferation and increase of extracellular matrix begins a complex event that results in vascular obstruction. The details of this process, from initiating events in the vascular wall through thrombotic occlusion of the obstructed vessel, should be elucidated more clearly by molecular and cellular techniques, and this will permit the development of effective therapeutic strategies.

Inflammation and Rejection

The process that leads to destruction of myocytes and the accumulation of collagen and other extracellular matrix proteins, and ultimately to heart failure, is unknown for inflammatory heart disease. A number of seemingly divergent disorders, including exposure to heavy metals, drugs, and toxins and autoimmune diseases may lead to a similar pathological and physiological picture. Perhaps the most immediately promising forum for the study of cardiac injury is transplantation rejection and accelerated transplant atherosclerosis. At present, the basis of acute rejection is believed to be a cellular phenomenon, with perhaps a lesser role attributed to humoral response except in hyperacute rejection. It now appears possible to characterize not only the T-cell lymphocytes of the rejection response, but also the pattern of gene expression of these cells and that of the myocardium. Although the incidence of graft rejection has markedly declined due to immunosuppressive treatment, the incidence of graft atherosclerosis has not changed and is now the most common cause of cardiac graft failure. The concept of immune-mediated atherogenesis as the basis for graft atherosclerosis in heart transplantation is controversial. In contrast, at least one type of injury is characterized by smooth muscle cell proliferation with varying degrees of lipid accumulation and mononuclear cell infiltrates.[168] which suggests a similar pathogenesis to restenosis after angioplasty.

Application to Treatment

The era of molecular biology–driven treatment options for cardiac disease was launched with the application of recombinant DNA to produce drugs for the thrombolytic therapy of acute myocardial infarction. Although the entire number of drugs currently available from recombinant DNA techniques is small, the opportunity to manufacture protein drugs in great quantity and purity and to modify and redesign drugs to greater therapeutic advantage has occupied great attention. Recently, the therapeutic horizons have been expanded by novel attempts at gene therapy: the introduction of a replacement gene for a defective one in somatic (working) cells of an organ; or, even the placement of a novel therapeutic gene in the body to combat disease. In at least one cardiovascular disease, familial hypercholesterolemia. a proposal to replace the defective LDL receptor gene in the liver with a correct copy currently is under study. These first attempts at recombinant drug and gene therapy presage important and widespread therapeutic advances in cardiovascular medicine. As a final—and somewhat speculative—note to this chapter, we would like to focus on the therapeutic possibilities for the the failing myocardium (Table 3.3).

Rethinking the Basis for Cardiac Contractility

The basis for the control mechanisms of cardiac contractility has undergone considerable revision with dis-

TABLE 3.3. Cellular and molecular therapeutic possibilities for the failing heart.

Problem	Possible solution
Cardiac contraction	Expression of MHC isoforms
	Altered cell signaling of calcium and/or adrenergic receptors
	Intracardiac expression of a drug that increases contractility
Inadequate myocardial mass	Stimulate existing myocytes to hypertrophy/divide
	Alter phenotype of fibroblasts or other nonmyocyte cells
	Implant primitive precursors of myocytes into the myocardium

coveries of the molecular basis of the contractile proteins and their physiological significance, especially myosin. Before this, physiological and pharmacological paradigms of control of contractile function focused on the modulation of Ca^{2+} in the contractile apparatus as the final common pathway. Experimentally and clinically, myocyte calcium can be influenced by many factors such as the activity of the adrenergic receptors through cAMP, the membrane Na^+-K^+ ATPase in conjunction with the Na^+, Ca^{2+} exchanger, and the extracellular level of ionic calcium.[169,170] Control of Ca^{2+} may yet prove to be a productive approach in the treatment of heart failure. However, other options now may be considered based on modulation of the proteins that control the flux and level of calcium or on control of the quantity or isoforms of proteins of the contractile apparatus.

At the top of this list is the attractive hypothesis that cardiac contractility could be increased by changing MHC gene expression with an increase of alpha-MHC with the higher ATPase activity and faster velocity of contraction of V1 myosin protein (see our earlier discussion of myosin biochemistry). Because the human ventricle predominantly expresses beta-MHC and V3 myosin in both healthy hearts and heart failure, this would appear to be an attractive mechanism for improving cardiac function. The feasibility of this molecular intervention is strengthened by the increasing knowledge of the control of gene expression, such as the effects of thyroid hormone (see Developmental and Thyroid Hormone Effects on MHC). However, enthusiasm for this approach is tempered by the energetic costs imposed by V1 myosin: isometric contraction requires more energy because cross-bridge cycling splits ATP at a faster rate during maintenance of tension.[171] The failing myocardium may be vulnerable with respect to the supply of energy, and therefore this additional factor would have to be considered in a therapeutic switch of myosin. Further, the most obvious candidate to increase alpha-MHC expression also is the poorest: thyroid hormone. This is because the systemic effects of the hormone and its requirements for increased tissue metabolic demands cannot be met by the failing heart. In fact, it may be remembered that only a generation ago induction of hypothyroidism was considered as a possible therapy for end-stage heart failure. This approach still may be viable when the mechanisms of MHC gene transcription are fully elucidated. For example, control of gene-enhancer elements that increase alpha-MHC transcription by non–thyroid hormone factors may be possible, along with additional therapy that allows the myocardium to cope with the altered metabolic requirements.

Other approaches should be considered. It also may be possible to control a different aspect of MHC as a therapy for heart failure: increase the total level of MHC gene expression and the myosin proteins. Analysis of the parameters of muscle mechanics suggests that increasing the total level of myosin, without a change in the ratio of V1/V3, would increase maximum developed force without a concomitant increase of maximal velocity of shortening.[172] These effects would be similar to that which occurs with enhanced preload of the Starling effect, but without the negative attributes of increased diastolic volume and wall tension. Additionally, neither the contractility of the ventricle nor the energetic requirements for a similar level of tension development would increase. However, maximal tension development, which is a major determinant of cardiac output, should increase. A recent study of the failing human myocardium showed that beta-MHC gene expression was unchanged,[165] which suggests that investigators may consider the possibility of breaking the status quo and increasing the level of myosin gene and protein expression.

Repair, Replacement, and Augmentation of the Myocardium

Although heart failure in its fully developed and pernicious phase is truly a systemic disorder, there is no doubt that therapeutic efforts solely directed at correcting cardiac function will restore health: witness the resolution of heart failure with successful cardiac transplantation. Therefore, in addition to specific treatments that are highly recommended for specific etiologies, the molecular promise of repair of the damaged myocardium is tantalizing. The questionable classification of observations of "restoring the fetal phenotype of gene expression" in experimental models of cardiac hypertrophy should be refocused on an important therapeutic goal: restoration of cellular hyperplasia. Loss of functioning myocytes is a common denominator of heart failure, and the ability to increase the pool of the functioning myocytes should be a major priority in molecular and cellular research. What cannot be accomplished in large scale by cardiac transplantation because of many serious limitations should be accomplishable by regrowing myocardial cells. The current generation of molecular studies on hypertrophy of the myocyte are a prelude to two different approaches: studies on the ontogeny of the cell cycle of the myocyte and studies on the phylogeny of the myocyte.

It is currently unknown why the myocyte is arrested in G_0 of the cell cycle (see Cell Cycle). When the oncogenes and growth factors that control the myocyte growth and development are uncovered, it may be possible to move myocytes from the resting stage and back into cell division as a way of restoring myocardial mass. With a better understanding of progenitor cells of the myocardium, it also may be possible to coax immature cells into differentiated myocytes. This could occur in at least two ways. First, nonmyocyte cells currently within the heart may be metamorphosed into myocytes. Preliminary data suggest that cardiac fibroblasts have some limited potential to express myofibrillar proteins[173] and one may extend this observation to imagine that those cells that comprise the remnant of myocardial damage from a number of sources may prove to be its rebirth. Still another possibility is seeding of the myocardium with cells nurtured in vitro and that have the potential to divide and proliferate when seeded in the myocardium. The source of these cells may be the patient's myocardium itself, other cell types from the affected individual, or possibly fetal source with the pluripotential capability of differentiating into mature, working myocytes.

Summary

One goal of this chapter was to convey our enthusiasm about the information content of cellular and molecular biology and its prospects for application to cardiovascular disease. We have briefly outlined important basic concepts about molecular and cellular science. Building on the vocabulary and ideas of this basic science, we discussed the physiology and pathophysiology of cardiac contractile proteins and the process of cardiac growth and hypertrophy. In the final section, we reviewed the current attempts and indicated some future prospects for the integration of this information into the treatment of heart failure.

The reader may sense a dichotomy between the basic science knowledge currently being generated by molecular and cellular science and its application to the treatment of cardiovascular diseases and their important manifestations, such as heart failure. The pathway between the integration of the two is uncertain, but the possibilities are predictable. We see three different paradigms by which this information will become integrated.

The first is a classical model of trickle-down basic science. In this tried and true method, the information from basic science becomes accessible, focused, and relevant to clinical medicine and, perhaps with adaptation, is applied to the practice of medicine. The second also has classical roots, but is acknowledged less frequently as a mechanism of change in the practice of medicine: the seizing of an undeveloped idea by clinicians and its application to a medical problem even when the basic science is rudimentary or fragmented. This paradigm frequently is accompanied by narrow and defined investigations of basic science that supplement the preparedness of the clinical application. Cardiovascular medicine in the last quarter of this 20th century has been particularly adept at this course, such as with the introduction of thrombolytic therapy to acute myocardial infarction and coronary angioplasty to

myocardial ischemia. The third is, perhaps, a subset of the second. When clinicians push the envelope of medical practice frequently they discover phenomena that are complex and poorly understood. For example, the above-cited angioplasty has spawned the important and perplexing finding of restenosis. Such phenomena are fertile soil for basic investigation. This inversion of the pyramid of knowledge from its normal position of basic to clinical is increasingly frequent and important. In this chapter, we hope to have provided sufficient information for clinicians to appreciate and become enthused by the developments that will occur as basic science and clinical medicine interact and perhaps to initiate one or more of these paradigms as they improve on the management of heart failure.

Dedication

This chapter is dedicated in honor of, and with love and affection to, our student Afroditi Davos.

References

1. Mitchell PJ, Tijan R. Transcriptional regulation in mammalian cells by sequence-specific DNA binding proteins. *Science*. 1989;245:371–378.
2. Cross F, Roberts J, Weintraub S. Simple and complex cell cycles. *Annu Rev Cell Biol* 1989;5:341–395.
3. Pledger WJ, Stiles CD, Antoniades HN, et al. An ordered sequence of events is required before BALB/c-3T3 cells become committed to DNA synthesis. *Proc Natl Acad Sci USA*. 1978;75:2839–2843.
4. Pardee AB. G_1 events and regulation of cell proliferation. *Science*. 1989;246:603–608.
5. Meerson FZ. The myocardium in hyperfunction, hypertrophy and heart failure. *Circ Res*. 1969;25(suppl 2): 1–163.
6. Perry SV. The control of muscular contraction. *Symp Soc Exp Biol*. 1973;27:531–550.
7. Holmes KC. The myosin cross-bridge, as revealed by structure studies. In: Riecker G, et al., eds. *Myocardial Failure*. Berlin: Springer-Verlag; 1977:16–27.
8. Spann JF, Braunwald E, Buccino RA, et al. Contractile state of cardiac muscle obtained from cats with experimentally produced ventricular hypertrophy and heart failure. *Circ Res*. 1967;19(2):341–354.
9. Hoh JFY, McGrath PA, Hale PT. Electrophoretic analysis of multiple forms of rat cardiac myosin: effects of hypophysectomy and thyroxine replacement. *J Mol Cell Cardiol*. 1977;10:1053–1076.
10. Schwartz K, Lecarpentier Y, Martin JL, et al. Myosin isoenzymic distribution correlates with speed of myocardial contraction. *J Mol Cell Cardiol*. 1981;13:1071–1075.
11. Ebrecht G, Rupp H, Jacob R. Alterations of mechanical parameters in chemically skinned preparations of rat myocardium as a function of isoenzyme pattern of myosin. *Basic Res Cardiol*. 1982;77:220-234.
12. Mercadier J-J, Lompre A-M, Wisnewsky C, et al.

Myosin isoenzymic changes in several models of rat cardiac hypertrophy. *Circ Res*. 1981,49:525–532.

13. Lowey S, Slayter HS, Weeds, et al. Substructure of the myosin molecule. I Subfragments of myosin by enzymatic degradation. *J Mol Biol*. 1969;42:1–29.

14. McLachlan AD. Structural implications of the myosin amino acid sequence. *Annu Rev Biophys Bioeng*. 1984; 13:167–189.

15. Mahdavi V, Periasamy M, Nadal-Ginard B. Molecular characterization of two myosin heavy chain genes expressed in the adult heart. *Nature*. 1982;297:659–664.

16. Nadal-Ginard B, Mahdavi V. Molecular basis of cardiac performance. *J Clin Invest*. 1989;84:1693–1700.

17. Leinwand LA, Fournier REK, Nadal-Ginard B, et al. Multigene family for sarcomeric myosin heavy chain in mouse and human DNA: localization on a single chromosome. *Science*. 1983;221:766–768.

18. Wydro RM, Nguyen HT, Gubits RM, et al. Characterization of sarcomeric myosin heavy chain genes. *J Biol Chem*. 1983;258:670-678.

19. Mahdavi V, Chambers AP, Nadal-Ginard B. Cardiac a- and b-myosin heavy chain genes are organized in tandem. *Proc Natl Acad Sci USA*. 1984;81:2626–2630.

20. Matsuoka R, Yoshida MC, Kanda N, et al. Human cardiac myosin heavy chain gene mapped withion chromosome region. *Am J Med. Genet*. 1989;32:279–284.

21. Saez LJ, Gianola KM, McNally EM, et al. Human cardiac myosin heavy chain genes and their linkage in the genome. *Nucleic Acids Res*. 1987;15:5443–5457.

22. Liew CC, Sole MJ, Yamauchi-Takihara K, et al. Complete sequence and organization of the human cardiac beta-myosin heavy chain gene. *Nucleic Acids Res*. 1990;18(12)3647–3651.

23. Jaenicke T, Diederich KW, Haas W, et al. The complete sequence of the human beta myosin heavy chain gene and a comparative analysis of its product. *Genomics*. 1990;8:194–206.

24. Bouvagnet P, Neveu S, Montoya M, et al. Developmental changes in the human cardiac isomyosin distribution: an immunohistochemical study using monoclonal antibodies. *Circ Res*. 1987;61:329–336.

25. Izumo S, Lompre A-N, Matsuoka R, et al. Myosin heavy chain messenger RNA and protein isoform transitions during cardiac hypertrophy. *J Clin Invest*. 1987; 79:970–977.

26. Lompre AM, Mercadier JJ, Wisnewsky C, et al. Species- and age-dependent changes in the relative amounts of cardiac myosin isoenzymes in mammals. *Dev Biol*. 1981;84:286–290.

27. Banerjee SK, Wiener J. Effects of aging on atrial and ventricular human myosin. *Basic Res Cardiol*. 1983; 78:685–694.

28. Lompré AM, Nadal-Ginard B, Mahdavi V. Expression of the cardiac venticular a- and b-myosin heavy chain genes is developmentally and hormonally regulated. *J Biol Chem*. 1984;259:6437–6446.

29. Gustafson TA, Bahl JJ, Markham BE, et al. Hormonal regulation of myosin heavy chain and alpha-actin gene expression in cultured fetal rat heart myocytes. *J Biol Chem*. 1987;262:13316–13322.

30. Izumo S, Nadal-Ginard B, Mahdavi. All members of the MHC multigene family respond to thyroid hormone in a highly tissue-specific manner. *Science*. 1986;231:597–600.

31. Mahdavi V, Lompre AM, Chambers AP, et al. Cardiac myosin heavy chain isozymic transitions during development and under pathological conditions are regulated at the level of mRNA availability. *Eur Heart J* 1984;5:181–191.

32. Lazar MA, Chin WW. Nuclear thyroid hormone receptors. *J Clin Invest*. 1990;86:1777–1782.

33. Evans RM. The steroid and thyroid hormone receptor superfamily. *Science*. 1988;240:889–895.

34. Gustafson TA, Markham BE, Bahl JJ, et al. Thyroid hormone regulates expression of a transfected alpha-myosin heavy-chain fusion gene in fetal heart cells. *Proc Natl Acad Sci USA*. 1987;84:3122–3126.

35. Dillman WH. Biochemical basis of thyroid hormone action in the heart. *Am J Med*. 1990;88:626–630.

36. Scheuer J, Malhotra A, Hirsch C, et al. Physiologic cardiac hypertrophy corrects contractile protein abnormalities associated with pathologic hypertrophy in rats. *J Clin Invest*. 1982;70:1300–1305.

37. Morgan HE, Gordon EE, Kira Y, et al. Biochemical mechanisms of cardiac hypertrophy. *Annu Rev Physiol*. 1987;49:533–543.

38. Mercadier JJ, Bouveret P, Gorza L, et al. Myosin isoenzymes in normal and hypertrophied human ventricular myocardium. *Circ Res*. 1983;53:52–62.

39. Tsika RW, Bahl JJ, Leinwand LA, et al. Thyroid hormone regulates expression of a transfected human alpha-myosin heavy-chain fusion gene in fetal rat heart cells. *Proc Natl Acad Sci USA*. 1990;87:379–383.

40. Gorza L, Mercadier JJ, Schwartz K, et al. Myosin types in the human heart. *Circ Res*. 1984;54:694–702.

41. Warrick HM, DeLozanne A, Leinwand LA, et al. Conserved protein domains in a mysoin heavy chain gene from dictyostelium discoideum. *Proc Natl Acad Sci USA*. 1986,83:9433–9437.

42. Nyitray L, Mocz G, Szilagyi L, et al. The proteolytic substructure of light meromyosin. *J Biol Chem*. 1983; 258:13213–13220.

43. Warrick HM, Spudich JA. Myosin structure and function in cell motility. *Annu Rev Cell Biol*. 1987;3:379–421.

44. Swynghedauw B. Developmental and functional adaptation of contractile proteins in cardiac and skeletal muscles. *Physiol Rev*. 1986;66:710–749.

45. Leinwand LA, Sohn R, Frankel SA, et al. Bacterial expression of eukaryotic contractile proteins. *Cell Motil Cytoskel*. 1989;14:3–11.

46. DeLozanne A, Berlot CH, Leinwand LA, et al. Expression in Escherichia coli of a functional dictyostelium myosin tail fragment. *J Cell Biol*. 1987;105:2999–3005.

47. O'Halloran TJ, Ravid S, Spudich JA. Expression of dictyostelium myosin tail segments in *escherichia coli*: domains required for assembly and phosphorylation. *J Cell Biol*. 1990;110:63–70.

48. McNally EM, Kraft R, Bravo-Zehnder M, et al. Full-length rat alpha and beta cardiac myosin heavy chain sequences. *J Mol Biol*. 1989,210:665–671.

49. Manstein DJ, Ruppel KM, Spudich JA. Expression and

characterization of a functional myosin head fragment in dictyostelium discoideum. *Science*. 1989;246:656–658.

50. McNally EM, Goodwin EB, Spudich JA, et al. Co-expression and assembly of myosin heavy chain and myosin light chain in *escherichia coli*. *Proc Natl Acad Sci USA*. 1988;85:7270–7273.

51. Barton PJR, Buckingham ME. The myosin alkali light chains and their genes. *Biochem J*. 1985;231:249–261.

52. Rovner AS, McNally EM, Leinwand LA. Complete cDNA sequence of rat atrial myosin light chain 1: patterns of expression during development and with hypertension. *Nucleic Acids Res*. 1990;18:1581–1586.

53. Hirzel HO, Caspar R, Tuchschmid, et al. Relationship between myosin isoenzyme composition, hemodyamics, and myocardial structure in various forms of human cardiac hypertrophy. *Circ Res*. 1985;57:729–740.

54. Cummins P. Transitions in human atrial and ventricular myosin light- chain isoenzymes in response to cardiac-pressure-overload-induced hypertrophy. *Biochem J*. 1982;205:195–204.

55. Schiaffino S, Samuel JL, Sassoon D, et al. Nonsynchronous accumulation of alpha skeletal actin and beta myosin heavy chain mRNAs during early stages of pressure-overloaded-induced cardiac hypertrophy. *Circ Res*. 1989;64:937–948.

56. Boheler KR, Carrier L, de la Bastie D, et al. Skeletal actin mRNA increases in the human heart during ontogenic development and is the major isofrom of control and failing adult hearts. *J Clin Invest*. 1991;88: 323–330.

57. Gustafson TA, Kedes L. Identification of multiple proteins that interact with functional regions of the human cardiac alpha-actin promoter. *Mol Cell Biol*. 1989; 9:3269–3283.

58. Breitbart RE, Nadal-Ginard B. Developmentally induced, muscle-specific trans factors control the differential splicing of alternative and constitutive troponin T exons. *Cell*. 1987;40:793–803.

59. Weintraub H, Davis R, Tapscott S, et al. The myoD gene family: nodal point during specification of the muscle cell lineage. *Science*. 1991,251:761–766.

60. Constantinides PG, Taylor SM, Jones P. Phenotype conversion of cultured mouse embryo cells by aza pyrimidine nucleosides. *Dev Biol*. 1978;66:57–71.

61. Davis RL, Weintraub H, Lasser AB. Expression of a single transfected cDNA converts fibroblasts to myoblasts. *Cell*. 1987;51:987–1000.

62. Eghbali M, Tomek R, Woods C, et al. Cardiac fibroblasts are predisposed to convert into myocyte phenotype: specific effect of transforming growth factor beta. *Proc Natl Acad Sci USA*. 1991;88:795–799.

63. Parker TG, Packer SE, Schneider MD. Peptide growth factors can provoke "fetal" contractile protein gene expression in rat cardiac myocytes. *J Clin Invest*. 1990;85:507–514.

64. Anversa P, Olivetti G, Loud AV. Morphometric study of early postnatal development in the left and right ventricular myocardium of the rat. *Circ Res*. 1980;46: 495–502.

65. Kung AL, Sherwood SW, Schimke RT. Cell line-specific differences in the control of cell cycle progression in the

66. Wittenberg C, Sugimoto K, Reed S. G_1-specific cyclins of S. cerevisiae: cell cycle periodicity, regulation by mating pheromone, and association with the p34cdc28 protein kinase. *Cell*. 1990;62:225–231.

67. O'Farrell PH, Edgar BA, Lakich D, et al. Directing cell division during development. *Science*. 1989;246:635–640.

68. Engelmann GL, Boehm KD, Haskell JF. Insulin-like growth factors and nenonatal cardiomyocyte development: ventricular gene expression and membrane receptor variatlons in normotensive and hypertensive rats. *Mol Cell Endocrinol*. 1989;63:1–14.

69. Erikson T, Allard MF, Sreenan CM, et al. The c-myc proto-oncogene regulates cardiac development in transgenic mice. *Mol Cell Biol*. 1990;10:3709–3716.

70. Ueno H, Perryman MB, Roberts R, et al. Differentiation of cardiac myocytes after mitogen withdrawal exhibits three sequential states of the ventricular growth response. *J Cell Biol*. 1988;107:1911–1918.

71. Robinson ME, Samarel AM. Regional differences in in-vivo myocardial protein synthesis in the neonatal rabbit heart. *J Mol Cell Cardiol*. 1990;22:607–618.

72. Watson PA. Function follows form: generation of intracellular signals by cell deformation. *FASEB J*. 1991;5:2013–2019.

73. Zimmer HG, Pfeffer H. Metabolic aspects of the development of experimental cardiac hypertrophy. *Basic Res Cardiol*. 1986;81:127–137.

74. Morris CE. Mechanosensitive ion channels. *J Membr Biol*. 1990;112:93–107.

75. Mowbray J, Davies JA, Bates DJ, Jones CJ. Growth hormone and cyclic nucleotides and rapid control of translation in heart muscle. *Biochem J*. 1975,152(3):583–592.

76. Beznak M. Effect of growth hormone preparations on cardiac hypertrophy and blood pressure of hypophysectomized rats. *Am J Physiol*. 1956;184:563–568.

77. Rubin SA, Buttrick P, Malhotra A, Melmed S, Fishbein M. Cardiac physiology, biochemistry and morphology in response to excess growth hormone in the rat. *J Mol Cell Cardiol*. 1990;22:429–438.

78. Damm K, Thompson CC, Evans RM. Protein encoded by v-erbA functions as a thyroid-hormone receptor antagonist. *Nature*. 1989;339:593–597.

79. Rapiejko PJ, Watkins DC, Ross M. Thyroid hormones regulate G-protein beta-subunit mRNA expression in vivo. *J Biol Chem*. 1989;26:16183–16189.

80. Simpson P, McGrath A, Savion S. Myocyte hypertrophy in neonatal rat heart cultures and its regulation by serum and by catecholamines. *Circ Res*. 1982;51:787–801.

81. Ostman-Smith I. Cardiac sympathetic nerves as the final common pathway in the induction of adaptive cardiac hypertrophy. *Clin Sci*. 1981,19:265–272.

82. Kupfer JM, Rubin SA. Regulation of IGF-I expression during juvenile cardiac growth by thyroid and growth hormone in the hypophysectomized rat. *J Cell Biochem*. 1991;15C(suppl):170.

83. Claycomb WC. Biochemical aspects of cardiac muscle differentiation. *J Biol Chem*. 1976;19:6082–6089.

84. Kannel WB, Gordon T, Castelli WP, et al. Electrocar-

diographic left ventricular hypertrophy and risk of coronary heart disease. *Ann Intern Med.* 1970;72:813–822.

85. Grossman W, McLaurin LP, Stefadouros MA. Left ventricular stiffness associated with chronic pressure and volume overload. *Circ Res.* 1974;47:567–574.

86. 34 Page E, McCallister LP. Quantitative elctron microscopic description of heart muscle cells. *Am J Cardiol.* 1973;31:172–181.

87. Anversa P, Beghi C, Kikkawa Y, et al. Myocardial infarction in rats. *Circ Res.* 1986;58:26–37.

88. Anversa P, Ricci R, Olivetti G. Quantitative structural analysis of the myocardium during physiologic growth and induced cardiac hypertrophy: a review. *J Am Coll Cardiol.* 1986;7:1140–1149.

89. Gwathmey JK, Copelas L, MacKinnon R, et al. Abnormal intracellular calcium handling in myocardium from patients with end-stage heart failure. *Circ Res.* 1987, 61:70–76.

90. Nagai R, Zarain-Herzberg A, Brandl CJ, et al. Regulation of myocardial Ca^{2+}-ATPase and phospholamban mRNA expression in response to pressure overload and thyroid hormone. *Proc Natl Acad Sci USA.* 1989; 86:2966–2970.

91. Keung EC. Calcium current is increased in isolated adult myocytes from hypertrophied rat myocardium. *Circ Res.* 1989,64:753–763.

92. Weber KT, Janicki JS, Shroff SG, et al. Collagen remodeling of the pressure-overloaded, hypertrophied nonhuman primate myocardium. *Circ Res.* 1988;62:757–765.

93. Skosey JL, Zak R, Martin AF, et al. Biochemical correlates of cardiac hypertrophy. *Circ Res.* 1972;31:145–157.

94. Chapman D, Weber KT, Eghbali M. Regulation of fibrillar collagen types I and III and basement membrane type IV collagen gene expression in pressure overload rat myocardium. *Clin Res.* 1990;67:787–794.

95. Low RB, Stirewalt WS, Hultgren P, et al. Changes in collagen and elastin in rabbit right-ventricular pressure overload. *J Biochem.* 1989;263:709–713.

96. Benjamin IJ, Jalil JR, Tan LB, et al. Isoproterenol-induced myocardial fibrosis in relation to myocyte necrosis. *Circ Res.* 1989;65:657–670.

97. McKee EE, Cheung JY, Rannels DE, et al. Measurement of the rate of protein synthesis and compartmentation of heart phenylalanine. *J Biol Chem.* 1978,253:1030–1040.

98. Clark WA Jr, Zak R. Assessment of fractional rates of protein synthesis in cardiac muscle cultures after equilibrium labeling. *J Biol Chem.* 1981;256:4863–4870.

99. Sugden PH, Fuller SJ. Regulatlon of protein turnover in skeletal and cardiac muscle. *Biochem J.* 1990;273:21–37.

100. Hershey JWB. Protein phosphorylation controls translation rates. *J Biol Chem.* 1989;264:20823–20826.

101. Sarre TF. The phosphorylation of eukaryotic initiation factor 2: a principle of translational control in mammalian cells. *Bio Systems.* 1989;22:311–325.

102. Sturgill TW, Ray LB, Erikson E, et al. Insulin-stimulated MAP-2 kinase phosphorylates and activates ribosomal protein S6 kinase II. *Nature.* 1988; 334(6184):715–718.

103. Boulton TG, Gregory JS, Jong S-M, et al. Evidence for insulin-dependent activation of S6 and microtubule-associated protein-2 kinases via a human insulin receptor/v-ras hybrid. *J Biol Chem.* 1990;265:2713–2719.

104. Levenson RM, Nairn AC, Blackshear PJ. Insulin rapidly induces the biosynthesis of elongation factor 2. *J Biol Chem.* 1989;264:11904–11911.

105. Brostrom CO, Brostrom MA. Calcium-dependent regulation of protein synthesis in intact mammalian cells. *Annu Rev Physiol.* 1990;52:577–590.

106. Rubin SA. Juvenile heart growth is optimized by the coordinate action of both thyroid and growth hormones. *Clin Res.* 1990;38:91A.

107. Sanford CF, Griffin EE, Wildenthal K. Synthesis and degradation of myocardial protein during the development and regression of thyroxine-induced cardiac hypertrophy in rats. *Circ Res.* 1978;43:688–694.

108. Siehl D, Chua BHL, Lautensack-Belser N, et al. Faster protein and ribosome synthesis in thyroxine-induced hypertrophy of rat heart. *Am J Physiol.* 1985;248:C309–C319.

109. Ostman-Smith I. Cardiac sympathetic nerves as the final common pathway in the induction of adaptive cardiac hypertrophy. *Clin Sci.* 1981;19:265–272.

110. Raum WJ, Laks WW, Garner D, Swerdoff RS. alpha-adrenergic receptor and cyclic AMP alterations in the canine ventricular septum during long-term norepinephrine infusion: implications for hypertrophic cardiomyopathy. *Circulation.* 1983;68:693–699.

111. Rubin SA, Fishbein MC. Effect of chemical sympathectomy on cardiac hypertrophy and hemodynamics following myocardial infarction in the rat. *Am J Cardiovasc Pathol.* 1990;3:45–53.

112. Fuller SJ, Caitanaki CJ, Sugden PH. Effects of catecholamines on protein synthesis in cardiac myocytes and perfused hearts isolated from adult rats. *Biochem J.* 1990;266:727–736.

113. Simpson P. Stimulation of hypertrophy of cultured neonatal rat heart cells through an alphal-adrenergic receptor and induction of beating through an alpha1- and beta1-adrenergic receptor interaction. *Circ Res.* 1985;56:884–894.

114. Xenophontos XP, Gordon EE, Morgan HE. Effect of intraventricular pressure on protein synthesis in arrested rat hearts. *Am J Physiol.* 1986;251:C95–C98.

115. Smith DM, Sugden PH. Effects of pressure overload and insulin on protein turnover in the perfused rat heart. *Biochem J.* 1987;243:473–479.

116. Rannels DE, Kao R, Morgan HE. Effect of insulin on protein turnover in heart muscle. *J Biol Chem.* 1975;250:1694–1701.

117. Gordon EE, Kira Y, Demers LM, et al. Aortic pressure as a determinant of cardiac protein degradation. *Am J Physiol.* 1986;250:C932–C938.

118. Meidell RS, Sen A, Henderson SA, et al. Alpha$_1$-adrenergic stimulation of rat myocardial cells increases protein synthesis. *Am J Physiol.* 1986;251:H1076–H1084.

119. McDermott PJ, Morgan HE. Contraction modulates the capacity for protein synthesis during growth of neonatal heart cells in culture. *Circ Res.* 1989;64:542–553.

120. Carter WJ, van de Weijden Benjamin h'S, Faas FH. Effect of thyroid hormone on protein turnover in cultured cardiac myocytes. *Am J Physiol*. 1987;252:C323–C327.

121. Chua BH, Russo LA, Gordon EE. Faster ribosome synthesis induced by elevated aortic pressure in rate heart. *Am J Physiol*. 1987, 252:C323–C327.

122. Watson PA, Haneda T, Morgan HE. Effect of higher aortic pressure on ribosome formation and cAMP content in rat heart. *Am J Physiol*. 1989; 256:C1257–C1261.

123. McDermott PJ, Rothblum Li, Smith SD. Accelerated rates of ribosomal RNA synthesis during growth of contracting heart cells in culture. *J Biol Chem*. 1989; 264:18220-18227.

124. Komuro 1, Kurabayashi M, Takaku F, et al. Expression of cellulzr oncogenes in the myocardium during the development stage and pressure-overloaded hypertrophy of the rat heart. *Circ Res*. 1988;62:1075–1079.

125. Starksen NF, Simpson PC, Bishopric N, et al. Cardiac myocyte hypertrophy is associated with c-myc proto-oncogene expression. *Proc Natl Acad Sci USA*. 1986; 83:8348–8350.

126. Claycomb WC, Lanson NA Jr. Proto-oncogene expression in proliferating and differentiating cardiac and skeletal muscle. *Biochem J*. 1987;247:701–706.

127. Izumo S, Nadal-Ginard B, Mahdavi V. Protooncogene induction and reprogramming of cardiac gene expression produced by pressure overload. *Proc Natl Acad Sci USA*. 1988;85:339–343.

128. Biggs RB, Booth FW. Protein synthesis rate is not suppressed in rat heart during senescence. *Am J Physiol*. 1990;258:H207–H211.

129. Klein I, Hong Chull. Effects of thyroid hormone on cardiac size and myosin content of the heterotopically transplanted rat heart. *J Clin Invest*. 1986;77:1694–1698.

130. Korecky B, Zak R, Schwartz K, Aschenbrenner V. Role of thyroid hormone in regulation of isomyosin composition, contractility, and size of heterotopically isotransplanted rat heart. *Circ Res*. 1987;60:824–830.

131. Dunnmon PM, Iwaki K, Henderson SA, et al. Phorbol esters induce immediate-early genes and activate cardiac gene transcription in neonatal rat myocardial cells. *J Mol Cell Cardiol*. 1990;22:901–910.

132. Xenophontos XP, Warson PA, Chua BHL, et al. Increased cyclic AMP content accelerates protein synthesis in rat heart. *Circ Res*. 1989;65:647–656.

133. Robishaw JD, Foster KA. Role of G proteins in the regulation of the cardiovascular system. *Annu Rev Physiol*. 1989;51:229–244.

134. Santos E, Nebreda AR. Structural and functional properties of ras proteins. *FASEB J*. 1989;3:2151–2163.

135. Demetri GD, Ernst TJ, Pratt ES, et al. Expression of ras oncogenes in cultured human cells alters the transcriptional and posttranscriptional regulztion of cytokine genes. *J Clin Invest*. 1990;86:1261–1269.

136. Reed JC, Alpers JD, Nowell PC, et al. Sequential expression of protooncogenes during lectin-stimulated mltogenesis of normal human lymphocytes. *Proc Natl Acad Sci USA*. 1986;83:3982–3986.

137. Herschman HR. Primary response genes induced by growth factors and tumor promoters. *Annu Rev Biochem*. 1989;60:281–319.

138. Frick KK, Womer RB, Scher CD. Platelet-derived growth factor-induced c-myc RNA expression. *J Biol Chem*. 1988;263:2948–2952.

139. Kelly K, Cochran BH, Stiles CD, et al. Cell-specific regulation of the c-myc gene by lymphocyte mitogens and platelet-derived growth factor. *Cell*. 1983;35:603–610.

140. Heikkila R, Schwab G, Wickstrom E, et al. A c-myc antisense oligodeoxynucleotide inhibits entry into s phase but not progress from g0 to g1. *Nature*. 1987,328:445–449.

141. Komuro I, Kurab2yashi M, Takaku F, et al. Expression of cellular ocogenes in the myocardium during the developmental stage and pressure-overloaded hypertrophy of the rat heart. *Circ Res*. 1988;62:1075–1079.

142. Moalic JM, Bauters C, Himbert D, et al. Phenylephrine, vasopressin and angiotensin iI as determinants of proto-oncogene and heat-shock protein expression in adult rat heart and aorta. *J Hypertension*. 1989;7:195–201.

143. Iwaki K, Sukhatme VP, Shubeita HE, et al. alpha- and beta-andrenergic stimulation induces distinct patterns of immediate early gene expression in neonatal rat myocardian cells. *J Biol Chem*. 1990;265:13809–13817.

144. Curran T, Rauscher FJ, Cohen DR, et al. Beyond the second messenger: ocogenes and transcription factors. *Cold Spring Harbor Symposia on Quantitative Biology*. 1988;53:769–777.

145. Lewin B. Oncogenic conversion by regulatory changes in transcription factors. *Cell*. 1991;64:303–312.

146. Norman C, Runswick M, Pollock R, et al. Isolation and properties of cDNA clones encoding SRF, a transcription factor that binds to c-fos serum response element. *Cell*. 1988;55:989–1003.

147. Brown MS, Goldstein JL. A receptor-mediated pathway for cholesterol homeostasis. *Science*. 1986;232:34–47.

148. Jarcho JA, McKenna hl, Pare JAP, et al. Mapping a gene for familial hypertrophic cardiomyopathy to chromosome 14ql. *N Engl J Med*. 1989;321:1372–1378.

149. Hejtmancik JF, Brink PA lowbin J, el al. Loczlization of gene fon familial hypertrophic cardiomyopathy to chromosome 14ql in a diverse US population. *Circulation*. 1991;83:1552–1557.

150. Geisterfer-Lowrance AAT, Kass S, Tanigawa G, et al. A molecular basis for familial hypertrophic cardiomyopathy: a beta cardiac myosin heavy chain gene missense mutation. *Cell*. 1990;62:999–1006.

151. Schier JJ, Adelstein RS. Structural and enzymatic comparison of human cardiac muscle myosins isolated from infants, adults, and patients with hypertrophic cardiomyopathy. *J Clin Invest*. 1982;282:816–825.

152. Hoffman EP, Brown RH, Kunkel LM, et al. Dystrophin: the protein product of the Duchenne muscular dystrophy locus. *Cell*. 1987,51:919–928.

153. Koenig M, Hoffman EP, Bertelson CJ, et al. The cDNA of the muscular dystrophy gene. *Cell*. 1987;50:509–517.

154. Brown AM, Birnbaumer L. Ionic channels and their regulation by G protein subunits. *Annu Rev Physiol*. 1990;52:197–213.

155. Keating M, Atkinson D, Dunn C, et al. Linkage of a

cardiac arrhythmia the long QT syndrome, and the Harvey ras-1 gene. *Science*. 1991;253:704–706.

156. Holt IJ, Harding AE, Morgan-Hughes JA. Deletions of muscle mitochondrial DNh ir, patients with mitochondrial myopathies. *Nature*. 1988;331:717–719.

157. Wallace DC, Zheng X, Lott MT, et al. Familial mitochondrial encephalomyopathy (MERRF): genetic, pathophysiological, and biochemical characterization of a mitochondrial DNA disease. *Cell*. 1988;55:601–610.

158. Shoffner JM, Lott MT, Voljavec AS, et al. Spontaneous Kearns-Sayre/chronic external opthalmoplegia plus syndrome associated with a mitochondrial DNA deletion: a slip-replication model and metabolic therapy. *Proc Natl Acad Sci USA*. 1989;86:7952–7956.

159. Cortopassi GA, Arnheim N. Detection of a specific mitochondrial DNA deletion in tissues of older humans. *Nucleic Acids Res*. 1990;18:6927–6933.

160. Corral-Debrinski M, Stepien G, Shoffner JM, et al. Hypoxemia is associated with mitochondrial DNA damage and gene induction. *JAMA*. 1991;266:1812–1816.

161. Breningstall GN. Carnitine deficiency syndrome. *Pediatr Neurol*. 1990;6:75–81.

162. Editorial. Carnitine deficiency. *Lancet*. 1991;335:631–633.

163. Jin O, Sole MJ, Butany JW, et al. Detection of enterovirus RNA in myocardial biopsies from patients with myocarditis and cardiomyopathy using gene amplification by polymerase chain reaction. *Circulation*. 1990:82:8–16.

164. Weiss LM, Movahed LA, Billingham ME, et al. Detection of coxsackievirus B3 RNA in myocardial tissues by the polymerase chain reaction. *Am J Pathol*. 1991;138:497–503.

165. Feldman AS, Ray PE, Silan CMt et al. Selective gene expression in failing human heart. *Circulation*. 1991;83:1866–1872.

166. Ip JH, Fuster V, Badimon l. et al. Syndromes of accelerated atherosclerosis: role of vascular inJury and smooth muscle cell proliferation. *J Am Coll Cardiol*. 1990;15:1667–87.

167. Ross R, Raines EW, Bowen-Pope DF. The platelet derived growth factor. *Cell*. 1986;46:155–69.

168. Demetris AJ, Zerbe T, Banner B. Morphology of solid organ allograft arteriopathy;identification of proliferating intimal cell populations. *Transplant Proc*. 1989;21:3667–3669.

169. Lakatta EG. Excitation contraction coupling in heart failure. *Hosp Prac*. 1991;26(July 15):85–98.

170. Homcy CJ. The beta adrenergic signaling pathway in the heart. *Hosp Prac*. 1991;26(May 15):43–50.

171. Alpert N, Mulieri L. Hect, mechanics, and myosin ATPase in normal and hypertrophied heart muscle. *Fed Proc*. 1982;41:192–158.

172. Winegrad S. Membrane control of force generation. In Fozzard HA, et al, eds. *The Heart and Cardiovascular System*. New York: Raven Press; 1986:703–730.

173. Eghbali M, Tomek R, Woods C, et al. Cardiac fibroblasts are predisposed to convert into myocyte phenotype: specific effect of transforming growth factor beta. *Proc Natl Acad Sci USA*. 1991;88:795–799.

4
Abnormalities in Cardiac Contraction: Systolic Dysfunction

Blase A. Carabello

To sustain life, the heart must pump a cardiac output adequate to supply the tissues' needs for nutrients. In providing this perfusion, the ventricles must generate enough pressure to overcome the resistance offered by the systemic and pulmonary circulations. This vital function of the heart as a pump is best described by Ohm's law as it applies to the circulation where $BP = CO \times TR$, where BP = blood pressure, CO = cardiac output, and TR = total resistance. Cardiac output in turn is maintained by the cyclical contraction and relaxation of the ventricles that generate pressure and propel blood forward. If the heart fails to perform its function, failure can only occur in three ways: (a) failure of proper cycle generation, i.e., arrythmia, (b) failure to relax properly (diastolic dysfunction), or (c) failure to contract properly (systolic function). This chapter addresses systolic dysfunction. It defines the components of systolic mechanics and ways of measuring abnormalities of these components in the overall assessment of systolic dysfunction.

Determinants of Cardiac Output

Cardiac output is the product of the volume ejected from either ventricle during one beat (stroke volume) and the heart rate. Stroke volume is obtained by measuring cardiac output using a variety of means (e.g., Fick, dye dilution, and thermodilution) and dividing by heart rate or by analyzing cardiac images to obtain end-diastolic and end-systolic volumes. Certainly maintenance of an adequate stroke volume is important to the patient, but obtaining the value for stroke volume gives little information about overall cardiac function or about whether systolic dysfunction exists. For instance, in hemorrhagic shock the underfilled ventricles have a greatly reduced stroke volume even though the ventricles themselves may be perfectly normal. Conversely, in dilated cardiomyopathy a left ventricle ejecting only

20% of an end-diastolic volume of 400 cc maintains a normal stroke volume (80 cc) despite what is obviously severe systolic dysfunction.

To evaluate systolic function one must take into account the four basic properties that determine stroke volume: preload, afterload, contractility, and myocardial mass. Stroke volume varies directly with preload and contractility and inversely with afterload. Additionally, the innate size (mass) of the muscle composing the ventricle is a key determinant of stroke volume; that is, an elephant's heart produces a greater stroke volume than a rat's heart regardless of preload, afterload, or contractility. Further, when the myocardium is overloaded by requirements to generate excess pressure or volume, the major form of long-term compensation is the development of hypertrophy. When the stress is a volume overload, new sarcomeres are laid down in series, producing an increase in myocardial mass as well as chamber volume (eccentric hypertrophy). When the stress is a pressure overload, new sarcomeres are laid down in parallel, producing increased wall thickness (concentric hypertrophy), which increases myocardial mass but not chamber volume. In evaluating overall cardiac function, myocardial mass and hypertrophy must be considered together with preload, afterload, and contractility. For instance, in aortic stenosis the left ventricle may be able to develop a systolic pressure of 270 mm Hg by a doubling of left ventricular mass. However, even though the pressure-generating ability of the entire chamber is increased, individual units of myocardium actually may have depressed contractility.[1,2]

Preload and Measures of Preload

The Frank-Starling law of the heart indicates that as end-diastolic volume and diastolic sarcomere stretch increase, force generation increases.[3] According to the sliding filaments theory, increased force generation

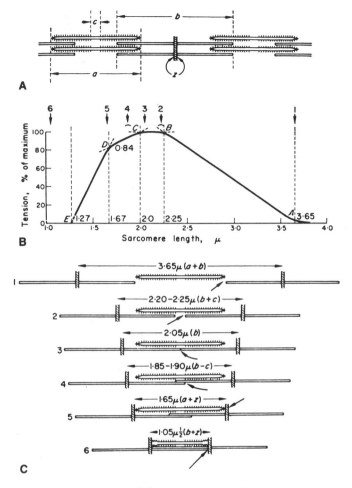

FIGURE 4.1. Top panel (A) is a schematic of a sarcomere. The thin filaments (actin) are attached at the Z band. The length of two actin filaments as they extend from the Z band is denoted by a small letter "b." The length of a thick filament (myosin) is denoted by a small letter "a." Tension is correlated with sarcomere stretch in panels B and C. Position number 1 shows extreme sarcomere stretch where neither actin filament can interact with the myosin filament and thus tension development is zero. Situations 2 and 3 demonstrate situations of maximum actin myosin overlap and thus tension production is maximal. In situations 4 and 5, the sarcomere has been shortened such that the actin filaments overlap one another, preventing cross-bridge attachment in the overlapping areas reducing tension development. In position 6 there is complete actin overlap preventing any cross-bridging with the myosin and the tension development again is zero. Reproduced with permission from Braunwald E, Ross J Jr, Sonnenblick EH, eds. *Mechanisms of Contraction of the Normal and Failing Heart.* 2nd ed. Boston: Little, Brown; 1972:77.

occurs with increased sarcomere stretch up to 2.2 μm. At this sarcomere length, the thin actin filaments are stretched to a configuration allowing maximal cross-bridge interaction with the thick myosin filaments (Fig. 4.1).[4,5] The term "preload" is intimately linked to the Frank-Starling concept, although no exact definition of preload is universally accepted. Most authorities define

preload as the actual sarcomere stretch that exists at the end of diastole. However, others define preload as the force that causes this sarcomere stretch. This difference in definition can lead to real discrepancies in the concept of preload. For instance, in hypertrophic states where ventricular compliance can be reduced, increased diastolic distending force actually may cause less than normal sarcomere stretch.[6] In this case, is preload increased or decreased? Since it is the actual presystolic sarcomere stretch that affects systolic contraction, I favor end-diastolic sarcomere length as the most precise definition of preload. Thus, in the case above, preload is reduced despite increased filling pressure. Unfortunately, defined in this way, preload is difficult to evaluate except in research settings where actual sarcomere length can be obtained. In clinical practice preload is inferred from end-diastolic pressure, end-diastolic stress, or end-diastolic dimension or volume. Each has its inherent limitation in the assessment of preload. For instance, an end-diastolic pressure of 15 mm Hg might cause near-maximum sarcomere stretch in one patient with a compliant ventricle and much less sarcomere stretch in another patient with a less compliant ventricle. In these two patients the same end-diastolic pressure produces different preload (sarcomere stretch). End-diastolic stress, which takes into account geometry and chamber thickness, examines the force producing sarcomere stretch. Although more sophisticated, it shares the same limitations as end-diastolic pressure. A given end-diastolic stress will stretch the sarcomeres to a greater degree in more compliant ventricles than in less compliant ventricles. Fortunately, both end-diastolic pressure and end-diastolic stress may be used as relative indicators of preload if compliance in a given patient has not changed. Thus, although one cannot be certain what the sarcomere stretch is in a given patient, if end-diastolic pressure is increased from 15 to 20 mm Hg it is likely that preload has increased unless compliance has become reduced.

End-diastolic dimension or volume is obviously in part dependent on sarcomere stretch. As stretch goes up, end-diastolic dimension (or volume) also must go up. However, if eccentric cardiac hypertrophy has intervened, more sarcomeres stretched to a lesser degree produce the same end-diastolic dimension as fewer sarcomeres stretched to a greater degree in the normal heart. Thus, neither dimension nor volume is a precise measurement of preload. Like end-diastolic pressure or stress, end-diastolic dimension or volume can be used as relative indicators of preload. If end-diastolic dimension in a given patient is increased acutely, it is certain that preload has increased. On the other hand, if in the same patient a volume overload has been interposed and end-diastolic dimension is examined 3 months after volume overloading, an increased diastolic dimension could be due to either increased preload, eccentric hypertrophy (increased number of series sarcomeres), or both.

In summary, sarcomere stretch probably is the best definition for preload since it is this property that is one of the key determinants of systolic function. However, no precise, easily obtained method is available for determining this property. End-diastolic pressure, stress, dimension, and volume if increased acutely in a given patient usually indicate that preload is increased. Unfortunately, because compliance differs from ventricle to ventricle and because the presence of eccentric cardiac hypertrophy may alter end-diastolic length or volume independent of sarcomere stretch, none of these measures can be used as an absolute measure of preload when comparing one patient or one ventricle to another.

Afterload and Measures of Afterload

Afterload is the force that the ventricular myocardium must overcome in order to shorten. It is the force that resists contraction. As this force increases, a ventricle of given strength will be less capable of overcoming the force and will shorten less completely to a greater end-systolic dimension or volume. Thus, evaluation of afterload is important in assessing overall ventricular performance. For instance, under high afterload, a ventricle of normal strength may be unable to shorten normally and thus appear to have depressed function. This situation has been termed "afterload mismatch".[7] It can cause the erroneous judgment that ventricular muscle strength is reduced when in fact excess afterload is the cause for the poor ventricular performance.

Peripheral resistance, systolic pressure, systolic stress, and systolic impedance all have been used to assess afterload. Total peripheral resistance has several limitations as an indicator of afterload. Mathematically,

$$\text{peripheral resistance} = \frac{\text{mean arterial pressure}}{\text{cardiac output}}.$$

In turn,

$$\text{mean arterial pressure} = \frac{2 \times \text{diastolic pressure} + \text{systolic pressure}}{3}.$$

Thus, mean arterial pressure is predominantly determined by a diastolic property. Consequently, total peripheral resistance makes a significant departure from the definition of afterload—the systolic force against which the heart contracts. While flow occurs only during systole in the proximal aorta, in the periphery flow is less pulsatile and is present during both systole and diastole. Since most of the peripheral resistance occurs distally at the arteriolar level, some of the flow opposed by this resistance occurs during diastole. Thus, total

peripheral resistance is inherently limited as an indicator of afterload by dependence on a diastolic factor. This is probably a key reason why Lang and his colleagues have demonstrated that there may be significant discrepancies between total peripheral resistance and other more succinct indicators of afterload.[8]

Systolic pressure also is used as an indicator of afterload. Since pressure is equal to force divided by area, systolic force is incorporated in the expression of pressure and thus systolic pressure does relate to afterload. Pressure is an expression of the total force that the ventricle must overcome and thus systolic pressure represents chamber afterload. However, pressure is not normalized for the myocardial mass present. If ventricular hypertrophy is present, there is more muscle to bear the load. In this case normalization for the amount of myocardium present is needed to examine afterload on individual muscle fibers in assessing myocardial strength. Here, examination of wall stress is a better indicator of myocardial load than pressure. Wall stress in its simplest definition is stated by the Laplace relationship: $\text{stress} = (p \times r)/2h$, where $p = \text{pressure}$, $r = \text{radius}$, and $h = \text{thickness}$. Stress normalizes the pressure in the ventricle for its radius and thickness and thus examines the force that a unit of myocardium must generate during systole in order to shorten.

While wall stress examines forces occurring in the ventricle itself, stress neglects coupling with vasculature, which is the actual source of the resistance (afterload) against which the ventricle must contract. In this respect, aortic impedance is a useful indicator of afterload. Descriptively, aortic impedance is the vascular resistance against which the ventricle contracts in systole and differs from total peripheral resistance, which as noted above is both a systolic and diastolic phenomenon. Impedance can be measured by examining the Fourier analysis of the instantaneous relationship between systolic aortic pressure and flow. Unfortunately, impedance loses its usefulness as a descriptor of afterload in aortic stenosis or in situations such as mitral regurgitation where ejection from the left ventricle into more than one chamber occurs. During mitral regurgitation, ejection from the ventricle occurs both into the left atrium as well as into the aorta and thus aortic impedance only examines partial afterload. In many severe cardiac diseases, ventricular dilatation leads to some mitral regurgitation and diminishes impedance as a useful tool for measuring afterload.

Contractility

Contractility is the ability of the myocardium to develop force independent of loading conditions. In essence, it is the strength of the ventricle. It is this property that is best related to prognosis. Diseases that lead to a reduction in contractility lead to progressive cardiovascular deterioration and eventually to death. Thus, it is not surprising that there have been multiple attempts to measure this prognostic property in both experimental and clinical settings. However no "contractilometer" exists; that is, there is no simple, precise way to measure ventricular contractility. The ideal index of contractility should be independent of preload, afterload, and myocardial mass but also should be sensitive to small changes in inotropic state. No currently available index entirely fulfills these criteria. The following is a review of some of the indices of contractility that have been employed and an examination of their assets and limitations.

Isovolumic Indices of Ventricular Contractility

As the name implies, isovolumic indices examine ventricular contraction during the period of isovolumic systole; that is, after the atrioventricular valves have closed but before the semilunar valves have opened. The cornerstone of the isovolumic indices of contractile function is the rate of change of ventricular pressure (P) development (dp/dt). In theory, this rate of change reflects the velocity of contractile element shortening before the elastic elements are stretched to the point where they cause overall ventricular shortening (the point at which the semilunar valves open and volume is ejected from the ventricle). Examination of left ventricular dp/dt/P (velocity of shortening) at various pressures before the opening of the aortic valve can be used to extrapolate to the velocity that might have occurred if no pressure was present in the ventricle.[9] This property, termed V_{max}, is equivalent to the maximum velocity of contractile element shortening if no load was present (Fig. 4.2); originally it was thought to be a good indicator of contractile function. V_{max} is sensitive to changes in contractile state.[10] However, some dependence on preload and the need to extrapolate to a theoretical, unconfirmable state reduced enthusiasm for its use.[11] Further, the index was unable to separate patients with clear contractile dysfunction from normal persons in two important clinical studies, obviously raising questions about the clinical usefulness of V_{max} as an accurate index of contractile function.[12,13]

Ejection Phase Indices of Contractile Function

The ejection phase indices of contractile function examine ventricular performance from end-diastole to end-systole. The two most popular such indices are ejection fraction and the mean velocity of circumferential fiber shortening. Ejection fraction is equal to the stroke volume divided by the end-diastolic volume. Descriptively, it is the percentage of the end-diastolic volume that is ejected during systole. As such, it does not ex-

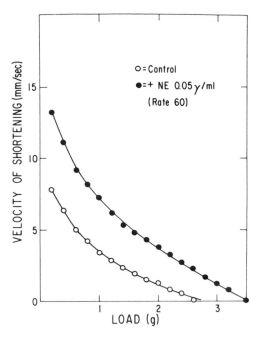

FIGURE 4.2. Velocity of shortening of a papillary muscle is plotted against load in the control state and in the presence of norepinephrine at several different loads. Extrapolation of these curves to zero load would give the velocity of shortening at zero load (V_{max}). Norepinephrine (*NE*) obviously increased V_{max}, indicating increased contractility. Reproduced with permission from Braunwald E, Ross J Jr, Sonnenblick EH, eds. *Mechanisms of Contraction of the Normal and Failing Heart.* 2nd ed. Boston: Little, Brown; 1972:49.

amine force generation (which is part of the definition of contractility) but rather examines the global shortening performance of the ventricle. Ejection fraction has two major advantages as an index of contractile function. First, in a large variety of clinical and experimental circumstances it has been an excellent prognostic indicator of outcome and thus has clinical relevance.[14] Second, it is easy to obtain and dimensionless and thus can be applied to virtually any patient or experimental subject. Its major drawback (besides the theoretic consideration that it does not examine force generation) is that it is not dependent only on contractility (the property one wishes to measure) but is also dependent on preload and afterload.[15,16] This fact may cause ejection fraction to lead to erroneous conclusions regarding contractility. For example, in mitral regurgitation where preload is greatly increased and afterload is normal or reduced,[17,18] ejection fraction is enhanced by these favorable loading conditions and will overestimate contractility.[19] Conversely, in aortic stenosis where afterload may be increased, ejection fraction may be reduced by afterload mismatch rather than by depressed contractility and thus ejection fraction may underestimate contractile function in this disease.[20]

The mean velocity of circumferential fiber shortening

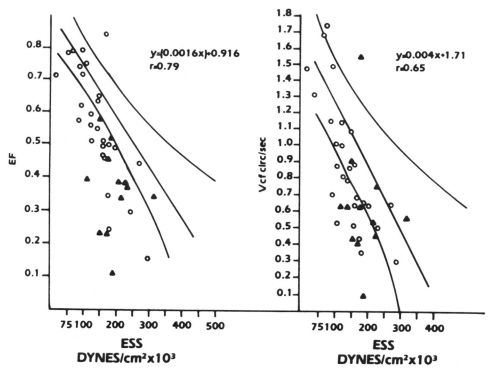

FIGURE 4.3. Ejection fraction (*EF, left hand panel*) and the mean velocity of circumferential fiber shortening (*Vcf, right hand panel*) is plotted against end-systolic stress (*ESS*). The slope of the normal relationship and the 95confidence limits are demonstrated. Patients with valvular disease who had a satisfactory outcome at surgery (○) and those patients with a poor outcome (▲) are plotted against the normal relationships. As can be seen, most patients with a poor outcome fell down and to the left of the normal relationship indicating that they had reduced contractile function prior to surgery. Reproduced with permission from Carabello et al., ref. 27.

is defined as the shortening fraction divided by ejection time [(EDD − ESD)/(EDD × ET), where EDD = end-diastolic dimension, ESD = end-systolic dimension, and ET = ejection time]. This index is less preload dependent than ejection fraction.[21] However, like ejection fraction, the mean velocity of circumferential fiber shortening (V_{cf}) also is afterload dependent.

Afterload-Corrected Ejection Phase Indices

Since ejection fraction and V_{cf} are afterload dependent, plotting them against existing afterload (Fig. 4.3) helps correct for the afterload present. As shown, ejection fraction and V_{cf} are inversely but linearly related to afterload (wall stress). A given individual can be plotted against the normal ejection fraction–end-systolic stress or V_{cf}–end-systolic stress relationship to examine contractile function.[1,22] A patient whose plot is downward and to the left of this relationship demonstrates decreased ejection performance for a given amount of afterload. In this circumstance, excess afterload cannot explain reduced ejection performance (since excess afterload is not present) and the reduced ejection performance is thus likely due to reduced contractile func-

tion. This relationship has been used in many studies effectively to imply contractile function. However, to date no universal slope, intercept, and confidence intervals for these relationships have been agreed on. Therefore, each laboratory must develop its own relationship from normal persons against which patients will be plotted.

End-Systolic Indices of Contractility

End-Systolic Volume

End-systolic volume or dimension is dependent on contractile state, afterload, and left ventricular myocardial mass but is not dependent on preload.[23] Therefore by examining end-systolic dimension or end-systolic volume instead of the entire ejection phase, preload is removed as a confounding influence in the determination of contractile function. Not surprisingly, in disease states where preload is exaggerated such as in aortic and mitral regurgitation, end-systolic volume or end-systolic dimension have been valuable indicators regarding the timing of surgery.[24–27] As end-systolic

TABLE 4.1. Published studies comparing various indexes of cardiac function.

Reference	No. of subjects	Index examined	Disease	Conclusions
30	8 dogs	PSP/ESVI ESS/ESVI	Pacing CMP	Correlated will with resting EF, afterload independence an advantage over EF
29	7 dogs	MSVR	—	Ratio increased appropriately with inotropic state, but ratio was afterload dependent—varying directly with afterload
31	11 patients	PSP/ESV	S/P CABG	Ratio was preload independent but increased if afterload increased
32	11 patients	ESS/ESVI	Sickle cell anemia	Ratio correlated well with slope of the ESPVR
33	11 patients	ESS/ESVI	Hypertension	Ratio correlated well with slope of the ESPVR
19	21 patients	ESS/ESVI	MR	Ratio was prognostic of outome and superior to EF
27	37 patients	ESS/ESVI	Valvular HD	Ratio predictive of outcome in MR but not for AS or AR
34	76 patients	PSP/ESVI	MR	Low PSP/ESVI associated with increased mortality but EF was superior in predicting overall clinical outcome
35	33 patients	PSP/ESVI	CAD	Failure of ratio to increase with exercise correlated with the extent of CAD
36	30 patients	PSP/ESV	CAD	Ratio was depressed at rest in 71% of patients with CAD and depressed with exercise in 95%
37	243 patients	PSP/ESV	CAD	Ratio 84% sensitive to CAD during exercise but not superior to EF
38	20 patients	PSP/ESV	CAD	Ratio responded appropriately to increased inotropic state but was inferior to ESPVR in assessing contractility

AR = aortic regurgitation; AS = aortic stenosis; CABG = coronary artery bypass grafting; CAD = coronary artery disease; CMP = cardiomyopathy; EF = ejection fraction; ESPVR = end-systolic pressure-volume relationship; ESS = end-systolic stress; ESV = end-systolic volume; ESVI = end-systolic volume index; HD = heart disease; MR = mitral regurgitation; MSVR = maximum stress/volume ratio; PSP = peak systolic pressure; S/P = status post.

dimension or volume increases there is a proportionately less favorable prognosis, presumably because contractile function is increasingly depressed. The implication of increased end-systolic volume is that the weaker ventricle is unable to contract as completely as a stronger ventricle and thus it remains larger at the end of systole.

The End-Systolic Stress-Volume Ratio

As noted above, end-systolic volume is preload independent but remains dependent on contractile function, afterload, and overall heart size. I and others have attempted to correct end-systolic volume for the afterload present at the end of systole by making a ratio of end-systolic stress to end-systolic volume index.[19,28] The concept behind the ratio is that a stronger ventricle will contract to a smaller volume against the same afterload than a weaker ventricle. Thus, the denominator of the ratio will be smaller and the ratio itself consequently larger. By incorporating afterload into the index it seemed that this ratio might better assess contractility than end-systolic volume alone. Unfortunately, the index is still somewhat afterload dependent.[29] Table 4.1 lists some of the studies in which the ratio of end-systolic stress to volume or end-systolic pressure to volume has been used and the relative success of the index.[19,27–38] We have found it particularly useful in predicting the outcome of patients undergoing surgery for mitral regurgitation, where it has superior predictive accuracy to end-systolic volume alone.[19,27]

Time-Varying Elastance and the Slope of End-Systolic Pressure-Volume Relationship

As afterload increases, a ventricle of given contractile function will be less able to overcome the afterload and thus will remain larger at a given time in systole.[23] Progressive increases in afterload produce a nearly linear increase in volume. By matching the afterload, volume coordinates from multiple variably loaded beats, one can develop the slope of the afterload/volume relationship. As demonstrated in Figure 4.4, beginning at the QRS and proceeding through systole, the slope (elastance) of the relationship of pressure (chamber afterload) and volume increases progressively until it reaches a maximum value (E_{max}) at the end of systole. Thus, elastance varies with time from the beginning of systole. Elastance also varies with contractile state. Maximum elastance increases as contractile function increases, indicating that for any given incremental change in pressure (Δy) the resultant increase in volume (Δx) is less, resulting in a steeper slope.[39] The time-varying method for assessing contractile function is cumbersome to develop as it requires the assessment of pressure and volume at multiple times during systole and synchronization of these times from multiple variably loaded beats. However, maximum elastance occurs at end-systole where the pressure and volume coordinates usually are coincident with the upper left-hand corner of the ventricular pressure volume curve (Fig. 4.5).[40] These coordinates usually are closely related to dicrotic notch pressure and end-ejection volume, which

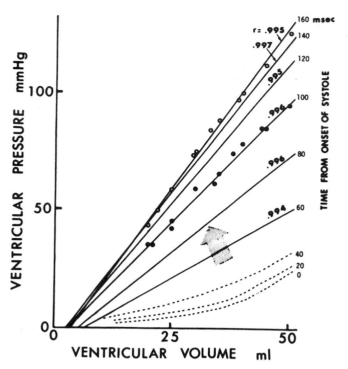

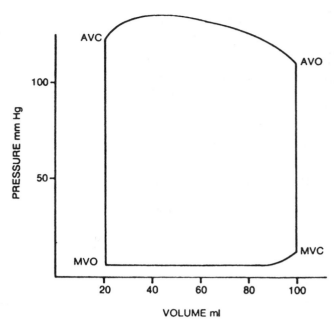

FIGURE 4.4. Ventricular pressure is plotted against ventricular volume in an isolated ventricle at several different afterloads (ventricular pressures) beginning at 60 ms from the onset of systole to the point at which the slope of the relationship is maximal (E_{max}) at 160 ms after the onset of systole. Reproduced with permission from Sagawa K, Suga H, Shoukas AA, Bakalar KM. End-systolic pressure/volume ratio: a new index of ventricular contractility. *Am J Cardiol.* 1977;40:748.

FIGURE 4.5. A left ventricular pressure volume loop is demonstrated. MVO = mitral valve opening; MVC = mitral valve closure; AVO = aortic valve opening; AVC = aortic valve closure. End systole defined as E_{max} usually corresponds with the upper left hand corner (*AVC*), obviating the need for development of the entire time varying elastance relationship to determine E_{max}. Reproduced with permission from Carabello BA. Cardiac catheterization. In: Parmley WW, Chatterjee K, eds. *Cardiology, vol. 1, Physiology, Pharmacology, Diagnosis.* Philadelphia: JB Lippincott; 1990: 11.

therefore often can be used to represent the values for pressure and volume at E_{max}, obviating the time variation analysis. By plotting the coordinates of the upper left-hand corners of the pressure volume loops from multiple variably loaded beats, as shown in Figure 4.6, the slope of the end-systolic pressure volume relationship (ESPVR) can be obtained. As with maximum elastance, steeper slopes indicate increased contractile performance (Fig. 4.6). It is clear that the slope of the end-systolic/pressure volume relationship is accurate in assessing acute changes in contractility.[23,39] However, this relationship has several limitations. First, although in general usage the relationship is considered linear, some curvilinearity of the relationship has been demonstrated.[41,42] Further, the curvilinearity may produce a relatively convex shape at high contractility states and a relatively concave shape at low contractility states.[42] The effects of these changes of the slope on the predictability of the relationship have yet to be defined. Second, the pressure-volume relationship examines the performance of the chamber as a whole because the afterload (pressure) is the afterload on the chamber and is not normalized to the amount of myocardium present. To overcome this problem, the stress-volume rela-

tionship can be used. In this relationship the term "fiber elastance" is indicative of the afterload-volume relationship normalized to the mass of myocardium available to generate force.[29,43,44] Both the pressure-volume and stress-volume relationships unfortunately are dependent on ventricular size.[45] The slope of any relationship is defined as a change in the y axis term divided by the change in the x axis term. In a rat, a change in end-systolic pressure of 10 mm Hg might yield a change in end-systolic volume of 0.1 cc. The slope of this relationship would then be 100 mm Hg/cc. In a human, a similar change in pressure might yield a 3-cc change in end-systolic volume, yielding a slope of 3.33 mm Hg/cc. It is unlikely that the contractile function of the rat is 30 times higher than that of the human but rather it is the small size of the rat compared to the human that causes a relatively smaller change in volume for any change in pressure. Less dramatic but important differences exist within the same species.[46] Thus, some method for normalizing this relationship for size is needed but none has yet been agreed on. Some investigators have multiplied the slope by the end-diastolic volume present at the time the slope was obtained.[43,47] However, end-diastolic volume is affected not only by the number of

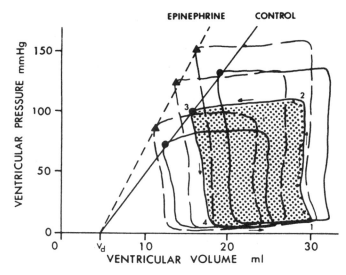

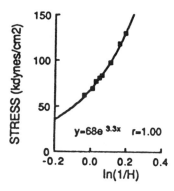

FIGURE 4.6. Pressure-volume loops from differently after-loaded beats are demonstrated in the isolated ventricle. As afterload increases, end-systolic volume increases as the ventricle shortens less completely against increasing load. The end-systolic pressure/volume relationship (*ESPVR*) is plotted using the coordinates of the upper left hand corner of these loops in the control state (●) and during the present of epinephrine (▲). Epinephrine increased inotropic state allowing the ventricle to shorten more completely at any given increase in afterload producing a steeper slope of the ESPVR. Reproduced with permission from Suga et al., ref. 23.

FIGURE 4.7. End-systolic stress is plotted against end-systolic strain (represented as ln(1/H), where H = wall thickness) from multiple variably-loaded beats. The exponential constant relating stress (y) to strain (x) is 3.3, which is the stiffness constant, the indicator of contractility. Reproduced with permission from Nakano et al., ref. 49.

sarcomeres present but also by the stretch of those sarcomeres (preload). Thus, volume correction may lead to overcorrection. Other investigators have suggested normalizing for myocardial mass since the intended correction is to normalize for the number of sarcomeres present.[48]

Last, end-ejection may become uncoupled from end-systole in pathologic states such as mitral regurgitation. In such instances, the upper left-hand corner of the pressure-volume loop may no longer represent end-systole, necessitating the more cumbersome isochronal assessment of E_{max}.

End-Systolic Stiffness

Recently, end-systolic stiffness has been proposed as a load- and size-independent index of contractility.[16,49] Stiffness is defined as the change in strain (ϵ) produced by a change in stress ($d\sigma/d\epsilon$). Strain is the change in length, area, or volume in reference to some baseline length, area, or volume (e.g., $\Delta L/L_0$, where L = length) and thus is a dimensionless property. As such, it is not affected by heart size. By examining the relationship of change in stress to the change in strain, the constant k (stiffness constant) relating these two variables can be obtained (Fig. 4.7). Increased end-systolic stiffness indicates end-systolic contractility. Recently, this index has

been demonstrated to vary appropriately with the maneuvers that are known to change inotropic state and also has been demonstrated to be independent of preload and ventricular size.[49] The exact place of this index in the armamentarium of contractility indexes has yet to be determined.

The above end-systolic relations require the definition of load and volume at multiple different afterloads. This need makes them difficult to apply to sick patients and makes it unlikely that these measures will gain widespread clinical usage. However, they will continue to be useful in experimental investigations of contractility.

Recruitable Stroke Work

Stroke work is the area under the ventricular pressure volume curve during a cardiac cycle. Either increased ventricular pressure or volume will increase stroke work. Thus, stroke work partially takes into account changes in preload and afterload. By increasing preload (here defined as end-diastolic volume) the amount of stroke work that the ventricle can perform is increased.[50] The relationship of end-diastolic volume to stroke work has been proposed as an index of contractile function. As shown in Figure 4.8, a calcium-mediated increase in contractile state produced more recruitable stroke work for a relatively smaller increase in end-diastolic volume than at baseline. Thus, the relationship was able to detect an increase in inotropic state. This index has been demonstrated to be relatively load insensitive and sensitive to changes in inotropic state. However, the effects of intervening left ventricular hypertrophy on recruitable stroke work has not yet been defined. Since hypertrophied ventricles should be able to do more stroke work than normal ventricles, it is not clear how myocardial contractility

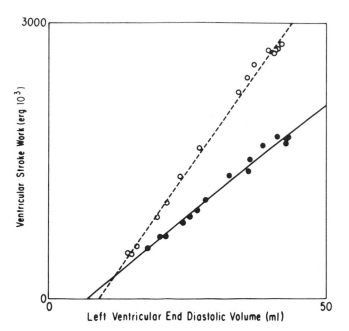

FIGURE 4.8. Ventricular stroke work is plotted against left ventricular end-diastolic volume in the control state (●) and after calcium infusion (○). The increased slope after calcium infusion indicates that more stroke work was performed at a lower preload (end-diastolic volume) consistent with increased contractility. Reproduced with permission from Glower et al., ref. 50.

cated finite element models analyzing segmental contractile function have been employed; however, their complexity precludes routine use. Clinically, segmental wall motion alone is generally used to imply regional contractile function. The assumption made in doing so is that afterload and preload are homogeneous throughout the ventricle and regional wall motion deficits therefore can be judged to reflect regional impairment of contractile function. While this assumption is not always true, it is fair to say that impaired regional shortening fraction usually indicates impaired regional contractile function.

Integration of Ventricular Mechanics in Assessing Cardiac Function

Interpreting cardiac performance at any given time requires a cautious analysis of preload, afterload, contractile function, and intervening hypertrophy. No simple way exists to accomplish this. Left ventricular function curves that can be derived from data obtained from a Swan-Ganz catheter can be used to analyze overall cardiac function but give no information about which components of function are involved. Two cardiac function curves plotting stroke volume against wedge pressure (as could be obtained from measurements made by a Swan-Ganz catheter) are demonstrated in Figure 4.9. An acute change from curve A to curve B often is misinterpreted as an increase in contractile function. While an increase in contractile function could cause this change, the same changes could be affected by several other mechanisms. An acute improvement in left ventricular compliance as might occur with the relief of ischemia would allow a greater end-diastolic volume at any wedge pressure producing increased stroke volume at any given wedge pressure, and thereby causing the improvement from curve A to curve B. Likewise, a reduction in afterload would permit enhanced stroke volume (by reducing end-systolic volume) at any given

can be assessed using this relationship in hypertrophic states. It is likely that some correction for the presence of hypertrophy will need to be made, but this awaits further investigation.

A relative comparison of the indices of contractile function is shown in Table 4.2.

The foregoing discussion of contractility and indexes of contractility deal with the ventricle as if the disease processes affect it globally. However, some diseases, most notably coronary disease, affects the ventricle segmentally—severely disrupting contractile function in some areas while not affecting other areas. Sophisti-

TABLE 4.2. Dependencies of various indexes of contractility.

Index	Affected by changes in:			
	Contractility	Preload	Afterload	Myocardial mass
dp/dt	+++	+	++	0
V_{max}	+++	+	+	0
Ejection fraction	++	++	+++	0
V_{cf}	++	+	+++	0
ESV	++	0	++	++
Ess/ESVI	++	0	+	++
ESPVR	++	+	0	++
$d\sigma/d\epsilon$	+++	0	0	0
Recruitable stroke work	++	0	0	?

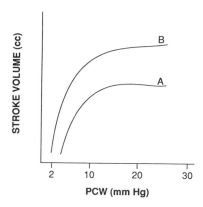

FIGURE 4.9. Two cardiac function curves from one patient are demonstrated. The change from **A** to **B** indicates enhanced cardiac performance, which could be caused by an increase in contractility, an increase in compliance, a reduction in afterload, the development of hypertrophy, or a combination of these elements.

TABLE 4.3. Hemodynamics and mechanics in aortic regurgitation.

	Base	AAR	CCAR	CDAR
EDV (cc)	150	180	270	300
ESV (cc)	50	50	70	150
Ejection fraction	.67	.72	.74	.50
Regurgitant fraction	0	.50	.50	.50
TSV (cc)	100	130	200	150
FSV (cc)	100	65	100	75
LVP mm HG	120/10	120/50	180/20	170/40
AoP mm Hg	120/80	120/60	180/70	170/70
Preload	nl	↑↑↑	↑↑↑	↑↑↑
Afterload	nl	nl	↑	↑↑
Contractility	nl	nl	nl	↓
LVH	Absent	Absent	↑↑↑	↑↑↑

AAR = acute aortic regurgitation; AoP = aortic pressure; Base = baseline state; CCAR = chronic compensated aortic regurgitation; CDAR = chronic decompensated aortic regurgitation; EDV = end-diastolic volume; ESV = end-systolic volume; FSV = forward stroke volume; LVH = left ventricular hypertrophy; LVP = left ventricular pressure; TSV = total stroke volume; nl = normal.

wedge pressure, again producing the change from curve A to curve B without any change in contractile function. If these two curves were observed at points in time far removed from one another, the development of left ventricular hypertrophy also could accomplish the change in curves from A to B without any change in contractile function. Thus, while left ventricular function curves are useful in assessing overall changes in cardiac function referring to such curves as "Frank-Starling curves" or contractility curves clearly is not accurate.

Examples of the Integration of Systolic Mechanics in Assessment of Left Ventricular Systolic Function

Example 1: Aortic Regurgitation

Acute Aortic Regurgitation

In acute aortic regurgitation as might occur in staphylococcal destruction of an aortic leaflet, there is an abrupt volume overload on the left ventricle as it becomes filled both from the left atrium and from aortic regurgitation during diastole. The results of the acute aortic regurgitation are to increase left ventricular filling pressure and to decrease effective forward stroke volume. This results in congestive heart failure as the increased filling pressure causes pulmonary congestion and the reduced effective forward stroke volume leads to reduced tissue perfusion. Acutely, pulse pressure is not greatly widened since high left ventricular diastolic filling pressure helps to maintain diastolic aortic pressure and eccentric cardiac hypertrophy has not yet had

time to augment the increase in total stroke volume. As shown in Table 4.3, an examination of systolic mechanics at this point shows that contractile function and afterload remain normal. Preload is increased greatly as the increased left ventricular filling pressure increases sarcomere stretch. Increased preload is a compensatory mechanism that helps increase total left ventricular stroke volume, a portion of which helps compensate the fall in forward stroke volume. However, this compensatory mechanism is not adequate to fully restore normal forward cardiac output.

Chronic Compensated Aortic Regurgitation

Whereas most patients subjected to the above events will require immediate aortic valve replacement, an occasional patient either will not require it because congestive heart failure does not occur or is deemed not a surgical candidate. Such a patient may then adapt to his chronic aortic regurgitation and become chronically compensated. As shown in Table 4.3, eccentric cardiac hypertrophy now has occurred, which increases left ventricular end-diastolic volume. Preload is still increased but because total myocardial volume also has increased, left ventricular filling pressure can be relatively less. Contractility is still normal. Increased left ventricular volume and increased total stroke volume increase forward stroke volume. The increased total stroke volume also increases left ventricular systolic pressure. Increased pressure combined with increased radius increases systolic wall stress (afterload), which opposes ventricular contraction leading to increased end-systolic volume. However, the increased preload offsets this afterload mismatch and ejection perform-

TABLE 4.4. Systolic indexes as predictors of outcome in chronic aortic regurgitation.

Index	Cutoff for good outcome	Reference
End-systolic dimension	< 55–60 mm	24, 52
End-systolic volume	< 110 cc/m²	27, 56
Ejection fraction	> .45	52
Shortening fraction	.23–.27	24, 52

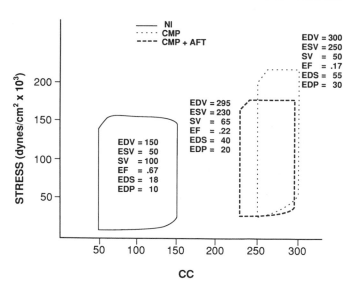

FIGURE 4.10. Stress volume loops from a normal (*nl*) person and a patient with dilated cardiomyopathy (*CMP*) before and after afterload reduction therapy (CMP + AFT) are demonstrated. EDP = end-diastolic pressure, EDV = end-diastolic volume; EDS = end-diastolic stress; EF = ejection fraction; ESV = end-systolic volume; SV = stroke volume.

ance remains normal. During the chronic compensated phase, increased preload together with eccentric cardiac hypertrophy allows for normalization of forward stroke volume and a return toward normal filling pressure. Under these circumstances the patient should be relatively asymptomatic.

Chronic Decompensated Aortic Regurgitation

Although volume overload may be tolerated for a long period of time, eventually contractile function fails. At this point the patient enters a chronic decompensated phase. The reduction in contractility produces an increase in end-systolic volume, reducing total and forward stroke volumes and ejection fraction (Table 4.3). There is further cardiac dilatation, which increases left ventricular radius, which further increases afterload, impairing left ventricular function. Left ventricular filling pressure is reelevated.

If the left ventricular dysfunction is mild or of short duration, aortic valve replacement can lead to improvement in ventricular performance.[51,52] Improved ventricular performance after correction of aortic regurgitation probably results from afterload reduction (as ventricular radius and pressure return toward normal) as well as restoration of contractility.[51,53–55] If left ventricular dysfunction is severe or prolonged, left ventricular performance remains depressed after surgery. Table 4.4 is a partial list of systolic indexes that have proved useful in predicting outcome for this disease.

Example 2: Idiopathic Dilated Cardiomyopathy

The changes in left ventricular mechanics produced by idiopathic dilated cardiomyopathy are demonstrated in the stress volume loops depicted in Figure 4.10. Compared to normal, the patient with idiopathic dilated cardiomyopathy has a much lower ejection fraction, a much larger left ventricle, and higher afterload (wall stress) than normal. While single stress-volume loops do not enable the assessment of contractile function, one can infer that contractile function must be reduced severely since afterload is not elevated enough to cause this severe reduction in ejection fraction and preload is almost surely increased, which would act to increase

ejection fraction. This figure also demonstrates the mechanisms by which vasodilator therapy improves function in this condition. Afterload (wall stress − P·r/2h) is reduced when vasodilatation reduces resistance to ejection, thereby permitting the left ventricular radius to become smaller and wall thickening to increase. Systolic blood pressure also is reduced. The fall in pressure and radius components of the stress equation, together with increased thickening due to enhanced shortening, all act in concert to reduce afterload. Reduced afterload allows for greater ejection of blood from the left ventricle increasing cardiac output. Because the diastolic portion of the stress/volume relationship is on the steep part of its curve, diastolic stress (and diastolic pressure) can be reduced without significantly reducing end-diastolic volume. This allows for maintenance of the gain in stroke volume produced by afterload reduction while at the same time reducing pulmonary congestion.

Summary

In the complete assessment of systolic function in any given patient, preload, afterload, contractility, and myocardial mass should be evaluated. Unfortunately this is not practical in everyday clinical practice. Contractility is a key determinant of prognosis in most cardiac diseases. However, measurements of contractile function in patients with cardiac disease are laborious and have not gained wide clinical acceptance. Since current indexes of contractile function require load manipulation for their development, these measures probably will continue to be limited to use as research tools. In the absence of an easily obtained clinical measure of contractile function, evaluation of ejection fraction often is substituted for evaluation of contractile function. In situations such as coronary disease where loading is relatively normal, ejection fraction closely follows contractile function and is useful in the assessment of contractility and prognosis. However, in conditions such as valvular heart disease where loading can be extremely abnormal, load must be taken into account. In such situations, use of preload-independent indices such as end-systolic volume or dimension may be superior to ejection phase indices in predicting outcome.

References

1. Carabello BA, Green LH, Grossman W, Cohn LH, Koster JK, Collins JJ Jr. Hemodynamic determinants of prognosis of aortic valve replacement in critical aortic stenosis and advanced congestive heart failure. *Circulation*. 1980;62:42–48.
2. Huber D, Grimm J, Koch R, Krayenbuehl HP. Determinants of ejection performance in aortic stenosis. *Circulation*. 1981;64:126–134.
3. Starling EH. *Linacre Lecture on the Law of the Heart*. London: Longmans, Green and Co. Ltd; 1915.
4. Gordon AM, Huxley AF, Julian FJ. Tension development in highly stretched vertebrate muscle fibres. *J Physiol*. 1966;184:143–169.
5. Spotnitz HM, Sonnenblick EH, Spiro D. Relation of ultrastructure to function in the intact heart: sarcomere structure relative to pressure volume curves of intact left ventricles of dog and cat. *Circ Res*. 1966;18:49–66.
6. Gaasch WH, Battle WE, Oboler AA, Banas JS Jr, Levine HJ. Left ventricular stress and compliance in man. With special reference to normalized ventricular function curves. *Circulation*. 1972;45:746–762.
7. Ross J Jr. Afterload mismatch and preload reserve: a conceptual framework for analysis of ventricular function. *Prog Cardiovasc Dis*. 1976;18:255–264.
8. Lang RM, Borow KM, Neumann A, Janzen D. Systemic vascular resistance: an unreliable index of left ventricular afterload. *Circulation*. 1986;74:1114–1123.
9. Wolk MJ, Keefe JF, Bing OHL, Finkelstein LJ, Levine HJ. Estimation of Vmax in auxotonic systoles from the rate of relative increase of isovolumic pressure: (dP/dt)/kP. *J Clin Invest*. 1971;50:1276–1285.
10. Mahler F, Ross J Jr, O'Rourke RA, Covell JW. Effects of changes in preload, afterload and inotropic state on ejection and isovolumic phase measures of contractility in the conscious dog. *Am J Cardiol*. 1975;35:626–634.
11. Grossman W, Haynes F, Paraskos JA, Saltz S, Dalen JE, Dexter L. Alterations in preload and myocardial mechanics in the dog and in man. *Circ Res*. 1972;31:83–94.
12. Peterson KL, Skloven D, Ludbrook P, Uther JB, Ross J Jr. Comparison of isovolumic and ejection phase indices of myocardial performance in man. *Circulation*. 1974; 49:1088–1101.

13. Kreulen TH, Bove AA, McDonough MT, Sands MJ, Spann JF. The evaluation of left ventricular function in man. A comparison of methods. *Circulation*. 1975; 51:677–688.
14. Cohn PF, Gorlin R, Cohn LH, Collins JJ Jr. Left ventricular ejection fraction as a prognostic guide in surgical treatment of coronary and valvular heart disease. *Am J Cardiol*. 1974;34:136–141.
15. Quinones MA, Gaasch WH, Alexander JK. Influence of acute changes in preload, afterload, contractile state and heart rate on ejection and isovolumic indices of myocardial contractility in man. *Circulation*. 1976;53:293–302.
16. Mirsky I, Tajimi T, Peterson KL. The development of the entire end-systolic pressure-volume and ejection fraction-afterload relations: a new concept of systolic myocardial stiffness. *Circulation*. 1987;76:343–356.
17. Wong CY, Spotnitz HM. Systolic and diastolic properties of the human left ventricle during valve replacement for chronic mitral regurgitation. *Am J Cardiol*. 1981;47: 40–50.
18. Wisenbaugh T, Spann JF, Carabello BA. Differences in myocardial performance and load between patients with similar amounts of chronic aortic versus chronic mitral regurgitation. *J Am Coll Cardiol*. 1984;3:916–923.
19. Carabello BA, Nolan SP, McGuire LB. Assessment of preoperative left ventricular function in patients with mitral regurgitation: value of the end-systolic wall stress–end-systolic volume ratio. *Circulation*. 1981;64: 1212–1217.
20. Gunther S, Grossman W. Determinants of ventricular function in pressure-overload hypertrophy in man. *Circulation*. 1979;59:679–688.
21. Nixon JV, Murray RG, Leonard PD, Mitchell JH, Blomqvist CG. Effect of large variations in preload on left ventricular performance characteristics in normal subjects. *Circulation*. 1982;65:698–703.
22. Colan SD, Borow KM, Neumann A. Left ventricular end-systolic wall stress-velocity of fiber shortening relation: a load-independent index of myocardial contractility. *J Am Coll Cardiol*. 1984;4:715–724.
23. Suga H, Sagawa K, Shoukas AA. Load independence of the instantaneous pressure-volume ratio of the canine left ventricle and effects of epinephrine and heart rate on the ratio. *Circ Res*. 1973;32:314–322.
24. Henry WL, Bonow RO, Borer JS, Ware JH, Kent KM, Redwood DR, McIntosh CL, Morrow AG, Epstein SE. Observations on the optimum time for operative intervention for aortic regurgitation. I. Evaluation of the results of aortic valve replacement in symptomatic patients. *Circulation*. 1980;61:471–483.
25. Borow KM, Green LH, Mann T, Sloss LJ, Braunwald E, Collins JJ, Cohn L, Grossman W. End-systolic volume as a predictor of postoperative left ventricular performance in volume overload from valvular regurgitation. *Am J Med*. 1980;68:655–663.
26. Zile MR, Gaasch WH, Carroll JD, Levine HF. Chronic mitral regurgitation: predictive value of preoperative echocardiographic indexes of left ventricular function and wall stress. *J Am Coll Cardiol*. 1984;3:235–242.
27. Carabello BA, Williams H, Gash AK, Kent R, Belber D, Maurer, A, Siegel J, Blasius K, Spann JF. Hemodynamic

predictors of outcome in patients undergoing valve replacement. *Circulation*. 1986;74:1309–1316.

28. Carabello BA. Ratio of end-systolic to end-systolic volume: is it a useful clinical tool? [Editorial]. *J Am Coll Cardiol*. 1989;14:496–498.

29. Wisenbaugh T, Yu G, Evans J. The superiority of maximum fiber elastance over maximum stress-volume ratio as an index of contractile state. *Circulation*. 1985;72:648–653.

30. Morgan DE, Tomlinson CW, Qayumi AK, Toleikis PM, McConville B, Jamieson WR. Evaluation of ventricular contractility indexes in the dog with left ventricular dysfunction induced by rapid atrial pacing. *J Am Coll Cardiol*. 1989;14:489–495.

31. Daughters GT, Derby GC, Alderman EL, Schwarzkopf A, Mead CW, Ingels NB Jr, Miller DC. Independence of left ventricular pressure-volume ratio from preload in man early after coronary artery bypass graft surgery. *Circulation*. 1985;71:945–950.

32. Denenberg BS, Criner G, Jones R, Spann JF. Cardiac function in sickle cell anemia. *Am J Cardiol*. 1983; 51:1674–1678.

33. Troy AD, Chakko CS, Gash AK, Bove AA, Spann JF. Left ventricular function in systemic hypertension. *J Cardiovasc Ultrasonogr*. 1983;2:251–257.

34. Ramanathan KB, Knowles J, Connor MJ, Tribble R, Kroetz FW, Sullivan JM, Mirvis DM. Natural history of chronic mitral insufficiency: relation of peak systolic pressure/end-systolic volume ratio to morbidity and mortality. *J Am Coll Cardiol*. 1984;3:1412–1416.

35. Dehmer GJ, Lewis SE, Hillis LD, Corbett J, Parkey RW, Willerson JT. Exercise-induced alterations in left ventricular volumes and the pressure-volume relationship: a sensitive indicator of left ventricular dysfunction in patients with coronary artery disease. *Circulation*. 1981; 63:1008–1018.

36. Wilson MF, Sung BH, Herbst CP, Lee RH, Brackett DJ. Evaluation of left ventricular contractility indexes for the detection of symptomatic and silent myocardial ischemia. *Am J Cardiol*. 1988;62:1176–1179.

37. Gibbons RJ, Clements IP, Zinsmeister AR, Brown ML. Exercise response of the systolic pressure to end-systolic volume ratio in patients with coronary artery disease. *J Am Coll Cardiol*. 1987;10:33–39.

38. El-Tobgi S, Fouad FM, Kramer JR, Rincon G, Sheldon WC, Tarazi RC. Left ventricular function in coronary artery disease. Evaluation of slope of end-systolic pressure-volume line (E_{max}) and ratio of peak systolic pressure to end-systolic volume (P/V_{es}). *J Am Coll Cardiol*. 1984;3:781–788.

39. Little WC, Cheng CP, Peterson T, Vinten-Johansen J. Response of the left ventricular end-systolic pressure-volume relation in conscious dogs to a wide range of contractile states. *Circulation*. 1988;78:736–745.

40. Kono A, Maughan WL, Sunagawa K, Hamilton K, Sagawa K, Weisfeldt ML. The use of left ventricular end-ejection pressure and peak pressure in the estimation of the end-systolic pressure-volume relationship. *Circulation*. 1984;70:1057–1065.

41. Burkhoff D, Sugiura S, Yue DT, Sagawa K. Contractility-dependent curvilinearity of end-systolic pressure-volume relations. *Am J Physiol*. 1987;252(*Heart Circ Physiol* 21):H1218–H1227.

42. Kass DA, Beyar R, Lankford E, Heard M, Maughan WL, Sagawa K. Influence of contractile state on curvilinearity of in situ end-systolic pressure-volume relations. *Circulation*. 1989;79:167–178.

43. Carabello BA, Nakano K, Corin W, Biederman R, Spann JF Jr. Left ventricular function in experimental volume overload hypertrophy. *Am J Physiol*. 1989;256(*Heart Circ Physiol* 25):H974–H981.

44. Corin WJ, Swindle MM, Spann JF Jr, Nakano K, Frankis M, Biederman RW, Smith A, Taylor A, Carabello BA. Mechanism of decreased forward stroke volume in children and swine with ventricular septal defect and failure to thrive. *J Clin Invest*. 1988;82:544–551.

45. Suga H, Hisano R, Goto Y, Yamada O. Normalization of end-systolic pressure volume relation and E_{max} of different sized hearts. *Jpn Circ J*. 1984;48:136–143.

46. Belcher P, Boerboom LE, Olinger GN. Standardization of end-systolic pressure-volume relation in the dog. *Am J Physiol*. 1985;249(*Heart Circ Physiol* 18):H547–553.

47. Berko B, Gaasch WH, Tanigawa N, Smith D, Craige E. Disparity between ejection and end-systolic indexes of left ventricular contractility in mitral regurgitation. *Circulation*. 1987;75:1310–1319.

48. Starling MR, Walsh RA, Dell' Italia LJ, Mancini GB, Lasher JC, Lancaster JL. The relationship of various measures of end-systole to left ventricular maximum time-varying elastance in man. *Circulation*. 1987;76:32–43.

49. Nakano K, Sugawara M, Ishihara K, Kanazawa S, Corin WJ, Denslow S, Biederman RWW, Carabello BA. Myocardial stiffness derived from end-systolic wall stress and the logarithm of the reciprocal of wall thickness: a contractility index independent of ventricular size. *Circulation*. 1990;82:1352–1361.

50. Glower DD, Spratt JA, Snow ND, Kabas JS, Davis JW, Olsen CO, Tyson GS, Sabiston DC Jr, Rankin JS. Linearity of the Frank-Starling relationship on the intact heart: the concept of preload recruitable stroke work. *Circulation*. 1985;71:994–1009.

51. Bonow RO, Rosing DR, Maron BJ, McIntosh CL, Jones M, Bacharach SL, Green MV, Clark RE, Epstein SE. Reversal of left ventricular dysfunction after aortic valve replacement for chronic aortic regurgitation: influence of duration of preoperative left ventricular dysfunction. *Circulation*. 1984;70:570–579.

52. Carabello BA, Usher BW, Hendrix GH, Assey ME, Crawford FA, Leman RB. Predictors of outcome in patients with aortic regurgitation and left ventricular dysfunction: a change in the measuring stick. *J Am Coll Cardiol*. 1987;10:991–997.

53. Bonow RO, Dodd JT, Maron BJ, O'Gara PT, White GG, McIntosh CL, Clark RE, Epstein SE. Long-term serial changes in left ventricular function and reversal of ventricular dilatation after valve replacement for chronic aortic regurgitation. *Circulation*. 1988;78:1108–1120.

54. Taniguchi K, Nakano S, Kawashima Y, Sakai K, Kawamoto T, Sakaki S, Kobayashi J, Morimoto S, Matsuda H. Left ventricular ejection performance, wall stress, and contractile state in aortic regurgitation before and after aortic valve replacement. *Circulation*. 1990;82:798–807.

55. Carabello BA. Aortic regurgitation. A lesions with similarities to both aortic stenosis and mitral regurgitation [Editorial]. *Circulation*. 1990;82:1051–1053.

56. Taniguchi K, Nakano S, Hirose H, Matsuda H, Shirakura R, Sakai K, Kawamoto T, Sakaki S, Kawashima Y. Preoperative left ventricular function: minimal requirement for successful late results of valve replacement for aortic regurgitation. *J Am Coll Cardiol*. 1987;10:510–518.

5
Abnormalities in Cardiac Relaxation and Other Forms of Diastolic Dysfunction

Hubert Pouleur

In 1651, William Harvey wrote: "I saw the heart and its auricles begin to move, to contract and to relax . . . The motion and action of the heart is a kind of swallowing and transfusion of the blood from the veins into the arteries . . . "[1] In this vivid description, Harvey made it clear that the heart had two separate functions: the systolic function and the diastolic function.

The systolic function is the active process by which the cardiac chambers empty and eventually ensure the perfusion of all organs. The diastolic function also is a complex and active process, by which the myocardium returns to its precontractile state and by which the cardiac chambers will be able to "swallow" blood flowing from the venous bed.

Heart failure traditionally is associated with ventricular systolic dysfunction. However, impaired left ventricular diastolic function is common in ischemic heart disease, left ventricular hypertrophy, and congestive cardiomyopathy.[2-14] These impairments may result from one of several causes[15,16]:

alterations in the passive viscoelastic properties of the ventricular walls (i.e., hypertrophy, scarred tissue, and alterations in the type and amount of collagen in the interstitial matrix)

the persistence throughout diastole of actin-myosin interactions due to abnormalities in the active relaxation process (i.e., calcium reuptake by the sarcoplasmic reticulum and calcium efflux)

mechanical interference between the cardiac chambers and the pericardium.

Ultimately, all these alterations have a common pathophysiological consequence: they reduce left ventricular distensibility and increase cardiac filling pressure. Such an increase in cardiac filling pressure may induce pulmonary congestion and subendocardial ischemia. A reduction in left ventricular distensibility limits the effectiveness of the Starling mechanism and influences systolic performance at rest and during exercise. These abnormalities, therefore, play an important role in the pathophysiology of heart failure.[16]

In recent years various clinical interventions have been shown to improve this phase of the cardiac cycle. Objective assessment of diastolic function in patients with heart failure is now possible and treatment may be adapted accordingly. The purpose of this chapter is to help physicians and cardiologists in making such a diagnosis and in taking the appropriate therapeutic steps.

The Determinants of Diastolic Distensibility in Health and Disease

When the diastolic function of the left ventricle is normal, the distensibility of the chamber is such that, at end-diastole, the sarcomeres within the myocytes may be stretched near the top of their length-tension curve by an end-diastolic pressure of less than 12 mm Hg (or a wall stress no greater than 70 ± 20 kdyne/cm^2). Thus, a normal diastolic function provides optimal use of the priming effect of the Starling mechanism in the absence of pulmonary or systemic venous congestion.[17]

The walls of the cardiac chambers, like all living biological material, exhibit complex physical characteristics such as plasticity, hysteresis, and viscosity: the characterization of their physical properties is complicated by the heterogeneous materials (membranes, sarcomeres, nuclei, coronary vessels, valves, etc.) that form the walls. Fortunately, for practical purposes, the main factors that determine the distensibility of the ventricle are sufficient (Table 5.1).

There are several approaches to the study of these factors. In experimental conditions, the entire pressure/volume relationship of the left and right ventricles can be determined in the isolated arrested heart with or without pericardium. Much theoretical work has been applied to the mathematical characterization of these relationships, the simplest being the index of com-

TABLE 5.1. Factors influencing the left ventricular diastolic pressure/volume relationship.

Primary
Passive physical properties of ventricular walls
  Thickness of ventricular wall
  Composition of ventricular wall (e.g., fibrotio scar tissue,
    ultrastructure of the collagen matrix, amyloid)
  Viscous properties
  Elastic recoil
Active relaxation process
  Sympathetic stimulation Ca^{2+} repumplog
  Heart rate   Capacity of Ca^{2+}
  Loading conditions   Total Ca^{2+} load
  Metabolism   Sensitivity of troponin to Ca^{2+}
Pericardial properties and mechanical interference between cardiac
  chambers

Secondary
  Pleural pressures
  Coronary perfusion pressure
  Aortic root pressure
  Mitral value elasticity
  Inertia, temperature, oedema
  Activation sequence

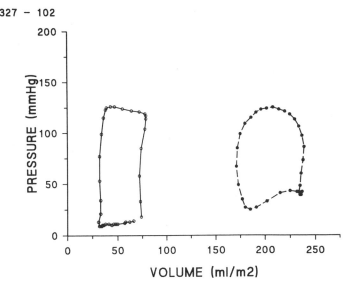

327 − 102

FIGURE 5.1. Typical pressure/volume loops in patients with a normal left ventricular function and in a patient with congestive heart failure.

pliance derived from the change in volume per change in pressure (dV/dP). However, these relationships cannot be obtained clinically. They are of limlted use because they describe only one aspect of diastolic function (the fully relaxed myocardium studied under static conditions), whereas diastolic filling is a dynamic process in which rate of myocardial relaxation, recoil forces, arterial pressure, coronary perfusion, and atrial contraction all interact continuously. In patients, the best approach to the assessment of diastolic function is to determine the pressure/dimension relationship (Fig. 5.1).

During cardiac catheterization, high fidelity left ventricular pressure is recorded, and left ventricular volume or diameter is obtained simultaneously by cineangiography, calibrated radionuclide angiography, or echocardiography.[18–21] These techniques enable the determination of indices of the rate of myocardial relaxation such as the time constant of the rate of pressure fall during isovolumetric relaxation, as well as various indices of ventricular distensibility and regional synchrony. Diastolic pressure/volume relationships, similar to those depicted in Figure 5.1, are used in the following sections to illustrate how the various determinants of diastolic function affect the dynamic left ventricular cor. ,ance. The use of noninvasive methods to assess diasiolic function is discussed later in this chapter.

Passive Physical Properties of Left Ventricular Walls

Under this heading, we consider the passive viscoelastic propertles of the ventricular wall when the myocytes are

fully relaxed; that is, when actin-myosin links are no longer present. The passive stiffness of the wall is determined mainly by the highly complex collagen matrix of the heart. In several pathologic conditions, particularly in pressure-overload hypertrophy, an extensive remodeling of the collagen network occurs, which increases myocardial stiffness. This reorganization, which involves both the type and total amount of collagen present in the heart, has been studied extensively by Weber and Janicki,[22,23] who described: " . . . (a) a reactive interstitial fibrosis where a greater number of intermuscular spaces were occupied by fibrillar often times thicker collagen; (b) a meshwork of collagen fibres that surrounded myocytes; and (c) in a late phase of established hypertrophy a reparative fibrosis that consisted of collagen fibres bridging the void created by myocyte loss."

Such alterations in collagen matrix are not present in physiologic forms of hypertrophy such as during growth, and there is increasing evidence that the angiotensin system is at least partially responsible for this detrimental reorganization of "the heart skeleton". Indeed, continuous infusion in rats of angiotensin II at doses too low to raise arterial pressure leads after 2 days to myocyte necrosis and fibroblast proliferation and, after 14 days, to a myocardial fibrosis characteristic of renovascular hypertension.[22] The role of angiotensin II and aldosterone in promoting interstitial fibrosis has been confirmed in other experimental models; the effects of angiotensin-converting enzyme (ACE) inhibitors in preventing these ultrastructural changes also have been established.[22,24] Thus, there now is a wide body of experimental evidence indicating

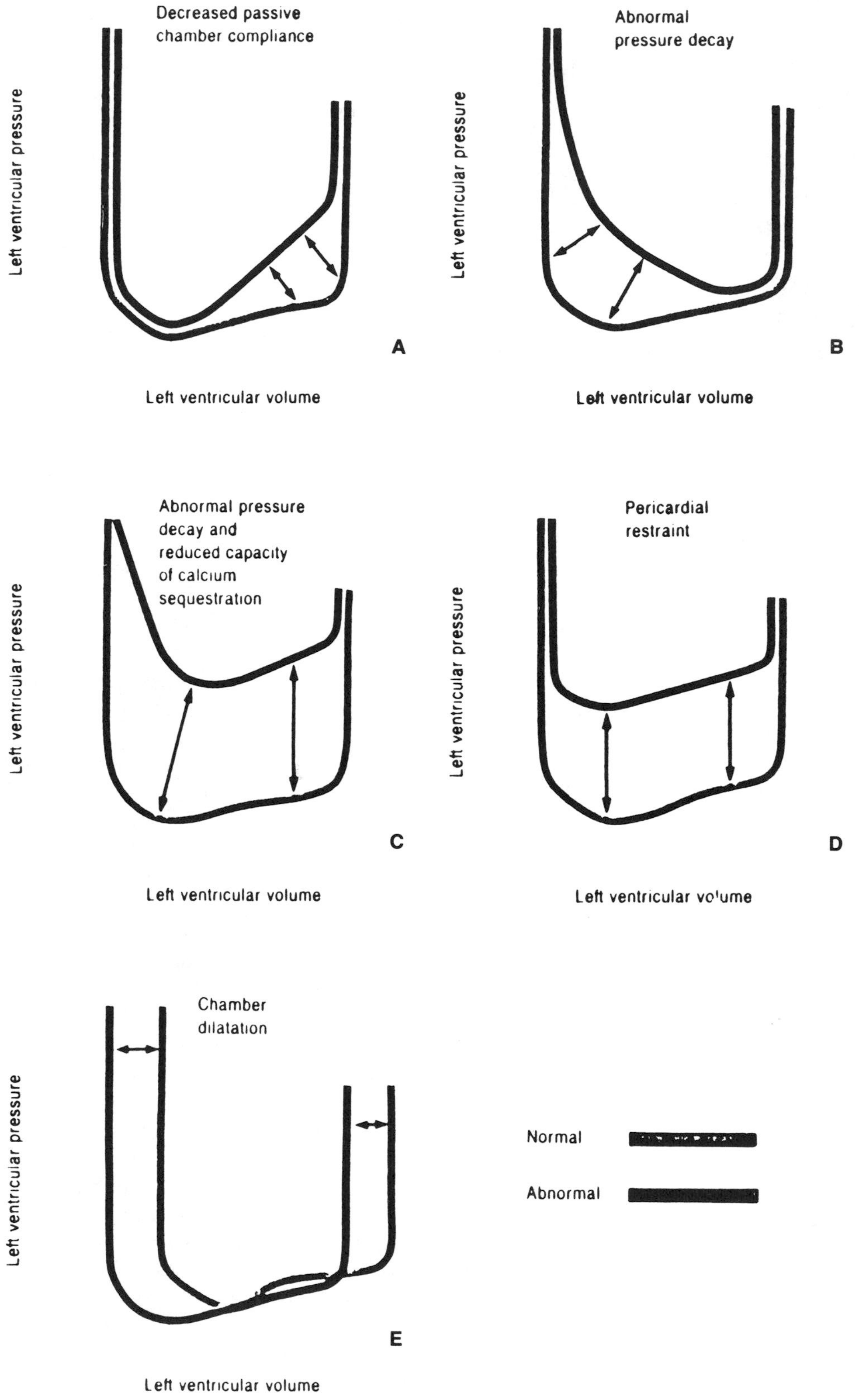

FIGURE 5.2. Schematic representation of the changes in diastolic pressure/volume relation in various types of diastolic dysfunction. **A**: Decreased passive chamber compliance. **B**: Impaired rate of relaxation. **C**: Impaired rate of relaxation and reduced capacity of calcium sequestration. **D**: Increased pericardial restraints. **E**: Chamber dilatation.

that the renin-angiotensin-aldosterone system may directly affect the connective tissue of the heart and hence affect both its systolic and diastolic performance. Moreover, in hypertrophy with heart failure, the increased fibrosis is accompanied by a reduction in the coronary reserve of the subendocardial layers.[25,26] The type of collagen remodeling observed in pressure-overload hypertrophy, together with the concentric hypertrophy, leads to an increase in passive stiffness of the left ventricle (Fig. 5.2A).

In ischemic heart disease, increased fibrosis and of course extensive scarring after myocardial infarction also have been described, but little is known of the passive diastolic stiffness of the left ventricle in ischemic heart failure or in idiopathic dilated cardiomyopathy. In these cases, progressive left ventricular (LV) dilatation is the rule (Fig. 5.1, 5.2E) and the rupture of some components of the collagen matrix might occur.[23] It is quite possible, therefore, that from a therapeutic viewpoint, the challenges could be quite different in pressure overload and in volume overload types of hypertrophy.

The Pericardium and the Mechanical Interference Between the Cardiac Chambers

It has been known for a long time that the pericardium may acutely limit the distensibility of the ventricles. In heart failure with an elevated right atrial pressure and an enlarged right ventricle, the left ventricular distensibility may be reduced further by a septum displacement and by an increase in pericardial constraints[27,28] (Fig. 5.2D). The sodium and water retention induced by the activation of the renin-angiotensin-aldosterone system eventually will increase the blood volume and the right-sided filling pressures and dimensions. This is thus another mechanism by which, indirectly, the renin-angiotensin system will reduce the distensibility of the left heart. Importantly, the rise in filling pressure caused by fluid retention triggers another vicious circle. The diastolic stretch of the fibers is, indeed, augmented and this constitutes one of the stimuli for hypertrophy and fiber slippage.

The administration of vasodilators, such as nitroprusside or nitroglycerin, increases venous capacitance and lowers the right atrial pressure. This is accompanied by a downward shift of the diastolic pressure/volume relationship, which is no longer observed when the pericardium is removed.[27] The intravenous infusion of an ACE inhibitor like benazeprilat, which induces some venous pooling, also causes a downward shift of the pressure/volume relationship.[29] As shown in Figure 5.3, this improvement in distensibility is particularly marked in some patients with more severe heart failure. Konstam et al.,[30] using radionuclide angiography, have been able to demonstrate that the largest improvement in diastolic

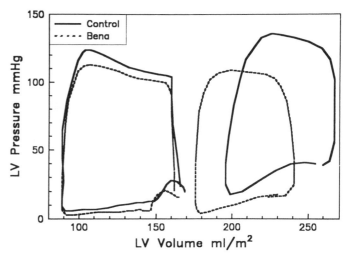

FIGURE 5.3. Typical pressure/volume loops before and after acute ACE inhibition with benazeprilat in a patient with mild (*left*) or severe (*right*) ventricular dysfunction. In both cases, there was a downward shift of the diastolic pressure/volume relationship, indicating improved distensibility; this effect, however, was more marked in the patient with severe ventricular enlargement.

function after intravenous ACE inhibition occurred in the patients with the largest right ventricles, thereby demonstrating the clinical relevance of the mechanisms described above. Finally, during prolonged administration of ACE inhibitors, alone or with diuretics, blood volume and right-sided pressure will be reduced further and the diastolic dysfunction may improve accordingly.

The Active Relaxation Process

Another factor that affects diastolic distensibility of the myocardium is the active relaxation process. Active tension is generated during systole when the myoplasmic free calcium concentration is increased, allowing the binding of calcium ions to troponin and thus formation of actin-myosin cross-linkages. During diastole, several active, energy-dependent processes are necessary to reduce myoplasmic calcium concentration and to remove calcium from its troponin binding sites.[31,32]

Thus, during diastole the calcium that entered the cell through the slow channels during the plateau of the action potential is extruded through a calcium pump and via the sodium-calcium exhange mechanism. Simultaneously, calcium released from intracellular stores (mainly from the sarcoplasmic reticulum but probably also from the mitochondria) is actively resequestered against a concentration gradient.

These delicate biochemical processes are controlled by multiple neurohormonal and intracellular feedback loops. When the active relaxation process is impaired, troponin-calcium interactions and cross-linkage cycling persist during part of, or throughout, the whole diastolic period. In this case, the left ventricular pressure decay is slowed and myocardial distensibility is reduced (Figs. 5.2B, C).

Among the multiple regulatory mechanisms controlling myocardial relaxation, three are particularly important from a practical viewpoint: the sympathetic nervous system, the energy supply, and the effects of heart rate.

Sympathetic Regulation of Myocardial Relaxation

In addition to increasing the force and speed of contraction, stimulation of myocyte β_1-adrenoceptors by noradrenaline (or any other full agonist) shortens the duration of the action potential and of the mechanical systole, and accelerates the speed of relaxation. These effects of catecholamines are mediated through the intracellular messenger cyclic adenosine monophosphate (cAMP), which triggers a cascade of enzyme phosphorylations in the sarcoplasmic reticulum (increasing the rate of calcium pumping), in the contractile apparatus (decreasing sensitivity of troponin to calcium), and in receptor-operated channels of the sarcolemma (shortening the action potential). These relaxatory effects are enhanced or prolonged by agents that inhibit the destruction of cAMP by phosphodiesterase.

By promoting both systolic and diastolic function, sympathetic stimulation plays a key role in the physiological adaptation of the heart to exercise, and acts as a compensatory mechanism in the presence of myocardial dysfunction such as myocardial infarction or cardiomyopathy. Conversely, β_1-adrenoceptor blockade or the myocardial denervation that may occur in areas adjacent to transmural myocardial necrosis will impair relaxation. It also is well known that prolonged or excessive β_1-adrenoceptor stimulation results in downregulation of these receptors.[33] In this setting, β_1-adrenoceptors either are sequestered below the sarcolemma or uncoupled from adenylate cyclase, the enzyme that generates cAMP. This phenomenon has been observed in cultured myocytes, in animal experiments, and in myocardium obtained from patients with end-stage heart failure. Although no quantitative evaluation of relaxation has been provided in these studies, it is likely that β_1-adrenoceptor downregulation results in depression of the myocardial relaxation rate. Finally, the slowing in relaxation seen in the aging heart also might be associated with an age-related uncoupling of the β_1-adrenoceptor.[34]

Energy Supply and Active Relaxation

Movement of ions against concentration gradients through the sarcolemma, the sarcoplasmic reticulum, or the mitochondrial membrane is an energy-consuming

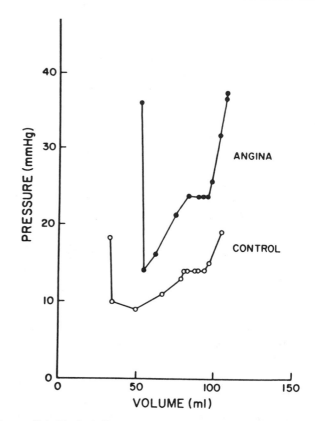

FIGURE 5.4. Typical diastolic pressure/volume relationships before and after angina pectoris. Reproduced from *Eur J Cardiol* 1978;7:239–249, with permission.

process. Factors that prevent adequate high energy phosphate synthesis will depress relaxation, although other parameters, such as intracellular pH, also may affect relaxation. Ischemic heart disease is the most common clinical situation in which alterations in energy supply are responsible for alterations in intracellular calcium homeostasis and impaired relaxation.

The most severe reductions in myocardial distensibility are observed immediately after the classical form of "high demand" angina pectoris[35] (Fig. 5.4), but some impairment of relaxation is found in most patients with coronary artery disease, even in the absence of clinical signs of ischemia.[36] Indeed, it is now well established that myocardial ischemia is not an all-or-nothing phenomenon, and that silent ischemia and anaerobic metabolism in the myocardium are common in patients with coronary stenoses.[37,38]

Thus, in ischemic heart disease, regional metabolism and energy production may be permanently abnormal because of chronically reduced perfusion ("hibernating myocardium"), or because of incomplete recovery from previous ischemic episodes ("stunned myocardium"). Relaxation is impaired in these zones because of cellular calcium overload, a decreased rate of calcium uptake by the sarcoplasmic reticulum or, perhaps, by a reduced capacity for calcium uptake by other intracellular structures. Accordingly, diastolic stiffness is increased and, if the area involved is sufficiently large, the stiffness of the ventricle itself is increased. This hypothesis is supported by the observed correlation between the amount of myocardium with reduced perfusion (estimated by thallium scintigraphy), the alterations in diastolic function at rest or after pacing-induced angina, and metabolic markers of ischemia such as lactate or alanine production.[39,40]

It is also noteworthy that impaired diastolic relaxation appears to be a more sensitive marker of chronic ischemia than systolic dysfunction. This observation indirectly supports recent data suggesting that the high energy phosphate used for relaxation comes from different metabolic pathways from those used for contraction.

Myocardial ischemia also might play a role in the relaxation abnormalities observed in hypertensive or idiopathic hypertrophic cardiomyopathy, dilated cardiomyopathy, aortic stenosis, or chronic volume overload hypertrophy. Even in the absence of coronary artery disease, it is possible that the alterations in subendocardial perfusion caused by hypertrophy and fibrosis could be severe enough to cause ischemic diastolic dysfunction during exercise.[25,26] Myocardial ischemia may be present particularly in the subendocardium, because of elevated diastolic wall stress and because of the mismatch between myocyte hypertrophy and microvasculature growth.[10,41] Myocardial ischemia related to vasospasm or thrombosis in the microvasculature also has been reported in some experimental models of heart failure.

In addition, there is now growing evidence that calcium handling is impaired in hypertrophy,[10,42] probably because of a relative reduction in the number of calcium pumps on the sarcoplasmic reticulum[43] and that the renin-angiotensin system also could modify these active processes. Lorell et al.,[44] indeed, observed that angiotensin I infusion in isolated rat hearts caused a dose-dependent increase in isovolumic left ventricular end-diastolic pressure in the hearts with pressure-overload hypertrophy but not in the control hearts. Hypertrophied hearts also showed a greater ACE activity. These authors concluded that the intrinsic cardiac renin-angiotensin system is stimulated in pressure-overload hypertrophy and that this may contribute to altered diastolic function as well as to the promotion of hypertrophy. These preliminary results therefore also suggest a direct role of the local ACEs and of the angiotensin receptors on the myocytes in regulating both the active relaxation process and the hypertrophy process.

Effects of Heart Rate on Myocardial Relaxation

An increase in frequency of stimulation, for example by atrial pacing, shortens the duration of the action potential and accelerates myocardial relaxation by mechanisms that still are poorly understood. Consequently, during exercise, relaxation rate is normally improved by two mechanisms: β_1-adrenoceptor stimulation and tachycardia. More rapid relaxation is essential when

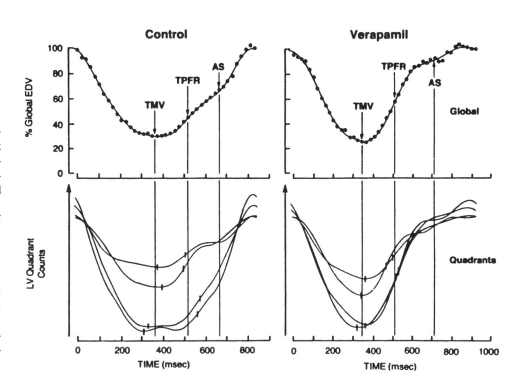

FIGURE 5.5. Regional left ventricular asynchrony in a patient with hypertrophic cardiomyopathy studied at rest by radionuclide angiography before and after oral verapamil therapy. In control, a large dispersion of regional time to minimum volume (*TMV*) and of time to peak filling rate (*T PFR*) is noted, together with a large contribution of atrial systole (*AS*) to the total end-diastolic volume (*EDV*). These abnormalities are improved by verapamil. Reproduced from ref. 27, with permission.

heart rate rises because during tachycardia, systole occupies a greater proportion of the cardiac cycle.

In the normal exercising heart, beating at less than 170 beats/min, the diastolic pressure/volume relation usually is unaffected by this reduction in diastolic interval. Above 170 beats/min, complete relaxation may no longer occur, causing an elevated ventricular pressure for any given volume.[45] If myocardial relaxation is impaired at rest, this phenomenon will occur at a lower heart rate and will be responsible for an inappropriate rise in left ventricular filling pressure during exercise or for a fall in end-diastolic volume.

Other Factors

Many other factors affect diastolic function. Relaxation is a load-dependent phenomenon[46] and any afterload increase may contribute to slow relaxation. The right atrial pressure also influences the left ventricular distensibility by a sort of "erectile venous effect."[47] Again, this is another factor by which fluid retention will impair diastolic distensibility. Finally, it must be realized that in many patients, particularly those with coronary artery disease and idiopathic hypertrophic cardiomyopathy, the severity of the alteration in diastolic properties may vary from one area of the ventricle to the other. This nonuniformity of diastolic function will be expressed clinically as a regional asynchrony of filling[48] (Fig. 5.5). When the areas involved are large enough, impaired diastolic distensibility also results.[21,49]

Diastolic Dysfunction and Heart Failure

Diastolic dysfunction may cause clinical symptoms of heart failure by three mechanisms[50]:

by increasing cardiac filling pressure at rest or during exercise
by preventing cardiac output from rising adequately during exertion
by reducing cardiac output at rest.

The following section examines these three mechanisms and the corresponding clinical situations in detail, before considering how diastolic dysfunction leads to events that trigger further deterioration of left ventricular pump function.

Increased Atrial Pressure as a Cause of Heart Failure

The various forms of diastolic dysfunction depicted in Figure 5.2 have a common pathophysiological conse-quence: the left ventricular distensibility is reduced. During part, or throughout the whole of diastole, filling pressure must increase in order to maintain a constant ventricular volume. Accordingly, to preserve cardiac output in the presence of reduced dynamic left ventricular compliance, pressure increases within the left ventricle, the left atrium, and the pulmonary capillaries and heart failure results.

In some instances, additional driving pressure is provided by an increased force of contraction from the left atrium. Clinical studies have shown the importance of this "booster" effect of atrial contraction for the optimal use of the Starling mechanism after acute myocardial infarction or in hypertrophic cardiomyopathy.[51,52] Moreover, atrial fibrillation is known to worsen symptoms of heart failure in these clinical conditions. The atrial contribution to the total end-diastolic volume also increases with age to compensate for the impaired distensibility of the aging heart.

In most cases, however, the atrial contribution is insufficient to compensate entirely for the impaired dynamic compliance and the left atrial pressure will increase not only at the a wave but also during the rapid filling and diastasis. Furthermore, during long-standing or severe left ventricular diastolic dysfunction, this atrial booster effect frequently appears to weaken or to be insufficient, particularly in ischemic heart disease.[53]

Impaired Exercise Tolerance

Reduced exercise tolerance is the most common symptom of heart failure but there is a poor correlation between objective measurements of physical capacity (such as maximal oxygen uptake) and the indices of systolic function.[54–56] Several mechanisms have been proposed to explain the lack of correlation between systolic function and exercise duration, including metabolic, peripheral, and respiratory factors.

Changes in ventricular relaxation and filling on exercise recently have attracted interest, and there is now increasing evidence that impaired diastolic filling might be one of the major determinants of the poor adaptation to exercise in many heart failure patients.[56–62] Except at low exercise levels, the increase in cardiac output during exercise in normal, untrained individuals is brought about largely by an increase in heart rate and myocardial contractility.[59] Although ejection time is reduced, the positive inotropic effect of increased sympathetic activity and the reduction in peripheral resistance allow the ejection rate to rise and end-systolic volume to decrease, so that stroke volume is maintained or slightly increased.

Simultaneously, left ventricular filling time becomes shorter, falling to 100 ms/beat when the heart rate reaches 150 beats/min.[59] Adequate ventricular filling

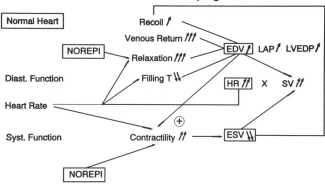

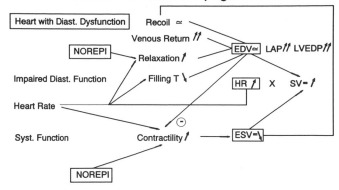

FIGURE 5.6. Schematic representation of the mechanisms involved in the increase in cardiac output during upright exercise in the presence of a normal heart. Despite the reduction in filling time during tachycardia, left ventricular filling is maintained up to high heart rate and end-diastolic volume increases slightly, whereas rises in filling pressure remain moderate. Systolic performance improves because of sympathetic activation, tachycardia, and use of the Frank-Starling mechanism. Thus, high values of cardiac output can be achieved by means of improved stroke volume and high heart rate. *Recoil* = recoil forces; Norepi = norepinephrine; EDV = end-diastolic volume; LAP = left atrial pressure; LVEDP = left ventricular end-diastolic pressure; Filling T = filling time; SV = stroke volume; ESV = end-systolic volume.

FIGURE 5.7. Schematic representation of the cardiac adaptation during upright exercise in the presence of diastolic dysfunction. The example selected is a severe case in which diastolic distensibility would already be depressed at rest. Despite large increases in filling pressure, end-diastolic volume is unchanged (or might eventually decrease if tachycardia increased) and systolic performance improves less than in normal. The result is an impaired rise in cardiac output high filling pressures. Abbreviations same as in Fig. 5.6.

under these conditions depends on increasing the mean filling rate during diastole far above that normally achieved during ejection. The mechanisms involved in this adaptation in the normal heart are shown in Figure 5.6. This compensation is impaired particularly in the aging heart and in the heart with a reduced contractile reserve, which is largely dependent on the Starling mechanism to maintain stroke volume during exercise.[58,62]

Under these adverse conditions, factors that determine the size of the ventricle during diastole will directly control the maximal cardiac output. If the dynamic compliance of the ventricle is already abnormal at rest or poorly adapts during exercise, filling rates will be too slow to achieve adequate filling and cardiac output will not rise normally despite large increases in left atrial and pulmonary capillary pressure (Fig. 5.7). This situation will be exacerbated even if the right ventricular pump function improves more than the left during exercise. In these cases, even if the patient may seem to stop because of poor skeletal muscle perfusion and resulting lactic acidemia, instead of dyspnea, the primary determinant of exercise capacity will be diastolic filling, in a situation not unlike mitral stenosis.

In summary, although many uncertainties remain regarding the underlying mechanisms, striking abnormalities of left ventricular filling may be demonstrated at

rest and during exercise in patients with impaired exercise tolerance and left ventricular hypertrophy, ischemic cardiomyopathy or other dilated cardiomyopathies. In many of these patients, these abnormalities in diastolic function enable a better prediction of exercise tolerance than that provided by indices of systolic function. This suggests that diastolic dynamic compliance and, in particular, the ability to achieve rapid ventricular filling are important determinants of functional capacity.

Diastolic Dysfunction in Severe Heart Failure

Except for certain situations such as cardiac tamponade or constrictive pericarditis, in severe heart failure with reduced cardiac output at rest, the cardiac chambers usually are markedly enlarged and systolic and diastolic function are compromised (e.g., because of subendocardial ischemia, angiotensin effects on load and relaxation, pericardial effect, etc.). Thus, even in this setting, diastolic dysfunction impairs pump function by preventing adequate sarcomere stretch (if calcium is not completely sequestrated) or by causing the mechanical interference between the dilated cardiac cavities and the pericardium. During exercise, the mechanisms discussed in the previous section also will come into play.

Heart Failure Progression

In many cases of pressure or volume overload, the deterioration of the left ventricular function that ultimately leads to refractory congestive heart failure is a slow, gradual process. Analysis of the remodeling process of the left ventricle that occurs after acute myocardial infarction has indicated that diastolic dysfunction could be the trigger for this relentless progression from mild to severe heart failure.[63,64] The increase in filling pressure and diastolic wall stress will progressively remodel and dilate the ventricular cavity: there is fiber slippage and viscous creep in the wall (Fig. 5.2), whereas the elevated diastolic wall stress stimulates an eccentric hypertrophy similar to that caused by volume overload. As already discussed, breaks in the collagen matrix also may occur in this setting, facilitating the vicious circle of dilatation. Although hemodynamic improvement sometimes accompanies this early remodeling, in other cases ventricular dilatation may continue and lead to severe heart failure.[63]

In such cases, deleterious feedback mechanisms may be present that are independent of the progression of the coronary artery disease. The first of these is reduced coronary perfusion. Coronary perfusion occurs mainly in diastole and all factors that increase intramural pressure will increase the extravascular components of coronary vascular resistance. In the presence of slow myocardial relaxation and elevated wall stress during diastole, coronary perfusion is reduced, particularly in the subendocardial layers. Hypertrophy of the ventricular wall or coronary artery disease will further reduce perfusion. Myocardial ischemia impairs relaxation (as previously discussed) and depresses contractile function, which also creates the conditions to further remodeling.

Another detrimental mechanism is related to cavity enlargement and eccentric hypertrophy, which leads to an increase in radius of curvature. Consequently, the wall stress (which is directly proportional to pressure and radius) increases out of proportion with the ability of the myocytes to shorten against it, a situation defined by Ross as the "afterload mismatch."[65] The result of these two mechanisms is a gradual deterioration of the left ventricular pump function, eventually leading to decreased systemic perfusion. At this stage, stimulation of the renin-angiotensin system and a marked increase in sympathetic activity are the rule, with possible β_1-adrenoceptor downregulation leading to severe congestive heart failure.

If left ventricular remodeling, triggered by increased diastolic wall stress, is associated with long-term deleterious hemodynamic changes, then attempts to decrease wall stress may attenuate this process, limit progressive ventricular dilatation, and offset any resulting adverse hemodynamic consequences.[66-68] Consequently, sustained reductions in systolic and diastolic wall stress may soon become an important therapeutic goal if the undergoing controlled clinical trials confirm the above hypotheses.

Clinical Assessment of Diastolic Function and the Relative Importance of Systolic and Diastolic Dysfunction in Heart Failure

Unlike systolic pressure and systolic wall stress, which may be evaluated noninvasively, left ventricular filling pressure and diastolic wall stress cannot be measured or even estimated without cardiac catheterization. Invasive techniques are necessary to analyze the various factors responsible for diastolic dysfunction and to examine the pressure/volume relationship. Nevertheless, in routine clinical practice, cardiologists still require simpler and less expensive means to diagnose diastolic dysfunction.

Noninvasive Assessment of Left Ventricular Diastolic Function

Because left ventricular diastolic pressure cannot be measured noninvasively, most of the noninvasive indices are derived from the analysis of left ventricular filling dynamics.[2,3,5,69-74] Slow relaxation or reduced myocardial distensibility is associated with the delayed opening of the mitral valve, and the maximal rate of filling of the left ventricle during the rapid filling period is reduced. If the atrial contribution is increased, an increase in filling rate will occur during this phase of the cardiac cycle. Perhaps the oldest method for evaluating diastolic function is cardiac auscultation. The gallop sound S3 corresponds to the sounds generated by the sudden impact of the mitral flow against poorly distensible left ventricular walls. Similarly, the gallop sound S4 is generated by the pressure wave of atrial contraction against stiff walls, and indicates an increased atrial contribution to left ventricular filling.

The use of apexcardiography to study diastolic filling has been superseded by radionuclide angiography and, more recently, by pulsed Doppler echocardiographic analysis of mitral flow. From the time-activity curve obtained from multiple-gated acquisition scanning, it is possible to derive not only the ejection fraction but also the peak filling rate during rapid filling and the time to peak filling rate. With appropriate acquisition techniques, it is even possible to calculate the atrial contribution to total diastolic filling. These techniques have yielded important results in the assessment of diastolic dysfunction, particularly in hypertrophic cardiomyopathy in patients with coronary artery disease, and in hypertensive heart disease.

The combination of echocardiography with pulsed Doppler analysis of the mitral flow provides another elegant means of determining the duration of the isovolumic relaxation period, the peak velocity during rapid filling, and the blood velocity during atrial filling. If the cross-sectional area of the mitral anulus is established, absolute flow rates may be calculated. Recent studies have shown a good correlation between the filling rates determined using angiographic techniques, radionuclide ventriculography, and pulsed Doppler echocardiography.[72,73]

Unfortunately, the indices of diastolic function derived from the study of filling dynamics are influenced not only by the ventricular distensibility but also by the heart rate and by the pressure gradient between the atrium and the ventricle.[74] Thus, in severe heart failure with markedly elevated left atrial pressure, the peak filling rate may remain within normal limits despite the presence of significant alterations in diastolic function (i.e., false negative results). Because of these problems, the ACC/AHA Task Force on clinical application of echocardiography recommended caution in the use of echo Doppler indices for clinical purposes.[75] Still, in the presence of heart failure symptoms, an echo Doppler study may yield valuable information to confirm a diagnosis of "diastolic heart failure." A preserved global systolic shortening, the presence of well established diagnostic criteria for hypertrophic cardiomyopathy or for restrictive cardiomyopathy, or the presence of a definite reduction in early peak filling rate will strongly direct the diagnosis toward diastolic heart failure. Thus, in many cases, an echocardiographic examination will be very useful for detecting resting alterations in diastolic function. Hence, cardiologists already have sensitive methods for detecting diastolic dysfunction noninvasively. Provided that the technical and physiological limitations of the tools and of indices used are recognized, there are few problems in correctly diagnosing left ventricular diastolic dysfunction in most patients. And, of course, the gray area that may remain always can be sorted out by more invasive diagnostic studies.

Importance of Distinguishing Diastolic from Systolic Heart Failure

Recent advances have enabled the differentiation of systolic and diastolic dysfunction. This has led to the identification of a subgroup of patients with clinical congestive heart failure despite relatively well preserved systolic function.[76–80] In one study, over a 3-month sampling period, 42% of the patients with a clinical diagnosis of congestive heart failure referred to a nuclear cardiology laboratory were found to have intact systolic function.[76] In another study of 188 patients with congestive heart failure,[77] 36% of patients had a radionuclide ejection fraction greater than 45%; these patients had a greater incidence of systemic hypertension than the remaining patients and diastolic dysfunction was the main cause of their symptoms. Another interesting finding of this study was the presence of diastolic dysfunction in all patients with congestive heart failure who also had a depressed ejection fraction. A review of a large data base of patients with definite clinical criteria of congestive heart failure also found a 38% to 40% incidence of patients with a left ventricular ejection fraction above 40%.[78]

Recently, the pressure/volume relationship and the various indices of systolic and diastolic function were reviewed at our institution in a group of patients with myocardial infarction. Forty three percent of the patients with an angiographic ejection fraction above 45% had a reduction in exercise tolerance together with a significant upward shift of diastolic pressure/volume relationship.[62] Again, this proportion is close to the percentage reported in two previous studies.

The Veterans' Administration Heart Failure Trial (V-HeFT) also identified a subgroup of patients with heart failure and normal or preserved ejection fraction.[79] Long-term prognosis appeared to be relatively favorable for this subgroup, but this may not always be the case. Indeed, patients with normal ejection fraction but with acute pulmonary edema after myocardial infarction formed a high-risk group, presumably because their diastolic dysfunction was related directly to severe coronary disease.[80] Recently, an increased mortality in women after myocardial infarction has been explained by a greater degree of diastolic dysfunction, probably related to hypertension and diabetes mellitus.[81]

Therapeutic Implications

The heart failure primarily caused by diastolic dysfunction does exist and may range in severity from mild to severe congestive heart failure. In contrast, heart failure caused solely by systolic dysfunction probably is extremely rare; there is always some degree of diastolic dysfunction that may contribute to the patient's symptoms or to the progression of the disease. This concept of diastolic heart failure and mixed heart failure has important therapeutic implications. In a randomized trial of digoxin versus placebo, only 14 of 25 patients improved clinically with digoxin. Nonresponders were characterized by the presence of less severe symptoms, smaller left ventricular dimensions, and a higher mean ejection fraction indicating that, as expected, patients with relatively minor systolic impairment did not benefit from pure inotropic support.[82] Similarly, the use of diuretics to reduce preload or afterload without simultaneously improving diastolic function may be of limited benefit. Even when contractility is severely depressed, the cardiologist also must consider interventions aimed at improving diastolic function and reducing filling pressures.[56] At the present time, no dogmatic guidelines can be laid out as few controlled trials have specifically examined the effects of therapeutic interventions susceptible to normalize left ventricular diastolic distensibility. Nevertheless, some rational approach is possible, and probably desirable, in treating these patients.

From a practical viewpoint, it is important to distinguish first the patients in whom heart failure is primarily caused by diastolic dysfunction from those with mixed systolic and diastolic abnormalities.

Heart Failure Caused Primarily by Diastolic Dysfunction

The typical example is the patient admitted in acute pulmonary edema and in whom, after stabilization of the clinical status, an echocardiographic or a radionuclide study reveals normal or near normal end-diastolic and end-systolic left ventricular dimensions and a high ejection fraction (classically above 50%). When pathologies such as acute myocardial infarction, mitral stenosis, or constrictive pericarditis have been ruled out, two important diagnostic options remain: severe ischemic heart disease and cardiomyopathy (hypertrophic or restrictive).

It is therefore important to remember that a subset of patients with severe coronary artery disease may have this form of heart failure as their main clinical manifestation. In such cases, coronary angiography and optimal revascularization are the obvious diagnostic and therapeutic steps to take.

If coronary artery disease is excluded, one is probably confronted with a hypertrophic cardiomyopathy or a restrictive cardiomyopathy. A history of hypertension is not uncommon in these patients and among the therapeutic options that have been shown to improve diastolic function and functional status in these settings, calcium antagonists rank first[83-85] (Fig. 5.5). Beta-blockers also may be useful in that they increase diastolic filling time, particularly during exercise. There is little data regarding the use of ACE inhibitors in this setting although in hypertensive cardiomyopathy, they might be useful. During long-term therapy, these agents may, like the calcium antagonists, perhaps be able to promote the regresslon of hypertrophy and induce some normalization of the collagen matrix.[86] The fact that both supraventricular and ventricular arrhythmias constitute a major risk factor in this population also must be remembered when optimizing therapy. Indeed, in this type of cardiomyopathy, the appearance of heart failure symptoms frequently coincides with the development of atrial fibrillation. The deterioration in diastolic filling is worse during atrial fibrillation than during regular tachycardia for several reasons. First, there is a loss of atrial "booster" effect. Second, the diastolic filling

time of the beats with a very short RR interval is extremely reduced. Third, in contrast to regular tachycardia in which a steady state between increased calcium influx and increased rate of calcium efflux is reached, there is in atrial fibrillation constant oscillations in the intracellular calcium load. These oscillations in intracellular calcium are caused by the incessant variation of the interval between beats and may result in an impaired rate of relaxation, in contrast to the regular tachycardia, which accelerates relaxation rate. The combination of these three mechanisms therefore causes a drastic reduction in left ventricular filling, thereby resulting in a reduced stroke volume despite elevated filling pressure.

Interestingly, most of these atrial fibrillations also could be a consequence of the primary abnormality in diastolic distensibility. Atrial hypertrophy, developed to compensate for the lack of adequate rapid filling, eventually provides the substrate for this arrhythmia.

Heart Failure with Mixed Systolic and Diastolic Dysfunction

In this category, I would consider first patients with clinical symptoms of mild to moderate heart failure. In our country, most of this population has had a myocardial infarction, whereas the patients with dilated cardiomyopathy represent the second most frequent etiology. Cardiac output generally is normal at rest in these patients, but cardiac filling pressures are significantly increased and cardiac chambers are enlarged.

Diuretics are perhaps the drugs used most commonly in the treatment of congestive heart failure. By reducing total blood volume, they decrease cardiac filling pressure. Their widespread use reflects the importance of the left ventricular filling pressure in causing symptoms of heart failure. Generally, however, the use of diuretic therapy does not improve cardiac output at rest nor its rise during exercise. Furthermore, in mild to moderate heart failure, diuretics activate the renin-angiotensin system, which may be detrimental. ACE-inhibitors are now used widely in this setting, and they have beneficial effects on mortality and morbidity[87] that even appear superior to those provided by ordinary vasodilators, like the combination of nitrates and hydralazine.[88]

The effect of ACE-inhibitors on left ventricular diastolic function has not been widely investigated in heart failure patients. Acutely, their action mimics that of nitrate vasodilators but their effects during long-term administration might be more complex.[64,66,67] The changes in left ventricular diastolic function induced by prolonged enalapril therapy were analyzed in 42 patients with an ejection fraction $\leq 35\%$ enrolled in the "Studies of Left Ventricular Dysfunction." Sixteen patients were randomized to placebo and 26 received enalapril. After an average follow-up of 12.4 months, there was evidence of a left ventricular dilatation and an increase in chamber compliance in the placebo group, whereas prolonged enalapril therapy was characterized by a decrease in left ventricular volume accompanied by a reduction in left ventricular chamber compliance. As the reduction in chamber compliance was also accompanied by a tendency for left ventricular mass and sphericity to improve, those changes were suggestive of a partial reversal of left ventricular remodeling by enalapril administration.

These data suggest that with conventional therapy for heart failure, there is a progressive deterioration of the left ventricular dysfunction, characterized by ventricular dilatation[89] and an increase in diastolic distensibility. ACE-inhibitors appear able to slow down or even partially reverse this progression.

The short-term administration of other vasodilators, particularly those with a balanced action on the venous and arterial beds, produces important downward shifts of the diastolic pressure/volume relationship in heart failure patients that appear to be related primarily to pericardial effects.[27] The decrease in afterload during vasodilator therapy also may improve the relaxation rate. Finally, as impaired diastolic function is frequently related to active or chronic ischemia, the improvement in the balance between oxygen supply and demand that may accompany vasodilator therapy also may play a role in the improvement of ventricular function. Thus, to treat these patients a role still has to be given to long-acting nitrates that reduce filling pressures and improve left ventricular distensibility by reducing pericardial restraints or myocardial ischemia. At least one study suggests that they influence prognosis favorably in these early forms of heart failure.[90]

When systolic dysfunction is severely impaired (ejection fraction <20%), the heart is generally markedly enlarged. The alterations in diastolic function are poorly characterized in this setting. Rupture in collagen tethers might occur[23] but myocyte hypertrophy, asynchrony, and impaired calcium handling are universally present. More research is needed in this area to clarify the long-term effects on diastolic function of the therapies classically used in these severe forms of heart failure.

In summary, studies of diastolic function in heart failure have revealed important information, not only regarding the contribution of this phase of the cardiac cycle to the hemodynamic abnormalities and symptoms of the syndrome but also regarding the role of diastolic dysfunction as a possible trigger for the progression of left ventricular dysfunction. The need for specific therapies to improve diastolic dysfunction has been stressed but more studies are still needed to clarify the effects of both traditional and newer therapies on this phase of the cardiac cycle.

Acknowledgment. The author thanks Ms. Isabelle Mottard for her careful secretarial assistance.

References

1. Harvey W. *An Anatomical Disputation Concerning the Movement of the Heart and Blood in Living Creatures.* Oxford: Blackwell; 1976:44–51.
2. Bonow RO, Bacharach SL, Green MV, et al. Impaired left ventricular diastolic filling in patients with coronary artery disease: assessment with radionuclide cineangiography. *Circulation.* 1981;64:315–323.
3. Bonow RO, Frederick TM, Bacharach SL, et al. Atrial systole and left ventricular filling in hypertrophic cardiomyopathy: effect of verapamil. *Am J Cardiol.* 1983; 51:1386–1391.
4. Grossman W, McLaurin LP, Rollett EL. Alterations in left ventricular relaxation and diastolic compliance in congestive cardiomyopathy. *Cardiovasc Res.* 1979;13:514–522.
5. Reduto LA, Wickmeyer WJ, Young JB, et al. Left ventricular diastolic performance at rest and during exercise in patients with coronary artery disease. Assessment with first-pass radionuclide angiography. *Circulation.* 1981;63: 1228–1237.
6. Papapietro SE, Coghlan HC, Zissermann D, Russell RO, Rackley CE, Rogers WJ. Impaired maximal rate of left ventricular relaxation in patients with coronary artery disease and left ventricular dysfunction. *Circulation.* 1979;59:984–991.
7. Rousseau MF, Veriter C, Detry JMR, Brasseur LA, Pouleur H. Impaired early left ventricular relaxation in coronary artery disease. Effects of intracoronary Nifedipine. *Circulation.* 1980;62:764–772.
8. Rousseau MF, Pouleur H, Detry JM, Brasseur L. Impaired left ventricular relaxation in patients with aortic or mitral regurgitation. *Am J Cardiol.* 1982;49:990.
9. Pouleur H, Rousseau MF, van Eyll C, Charlier AA. Assessment of regional left ventricular relaxation in patients with coronary artery disease: importance of geometric factors and changes in wall thickness. *Circulation.* 1984;69:696–702.
10. Lorell BH, Grossman W. Cardiac hypertrophy: consequences for diastole. *J Am Coll Cardiol.* 1987;9:1189–1193.
11. Peterson KL, Tsuji J, Johnson A, DiDonna J, LeWinter M. Diastolic Left ventricular pressure-volume and stress-strain relations in patients with valvular aortic stenosis and left ventricular hypertrophy. *Circulation.* 1978;58:77.
12. Eichhorn P, Grimm J, Koch R, Hess O, Carroll J, Krayenbuehl P. Left ventricular relaxation in patients with left ventricular hypertrophy secondary to aortic valve disease. *Circulation.* 1982;65:1395–1404.
13. Hess OM, Schneider J, Koch R, Bamert C, Grimm J, Krayenbuehl HP. Diastolic function and myocardial structure in patients with myocardial hypertrophy. Special reference to normalized viscoelastic data. *Circulation.* 1981;63:360–371.
14. Hess OM, Ritter M, Schneider J, Grimm J, Turina M, Krayenbuel HP. Diastolic stiffness and myocardial struc-

ture in aortic valve disease before and after valve replacement. *Circulation*. 1984;69:855–865.

15. Grossman W, Barry WH. Diastolic pressure-volume relations in the diseased heart. *Fed Proc*. 1980;39:148–155.

16. Grossman W. Diastolic dysfunction and congestive heart failure. *Circulation*. 1990;81-2:III1–III7.

17. Spotnitz HM, Sonnenblick EH. Structural conditions in the hypertrophied and failing heart. In: Mason DT, ed. *Congestive Heart Failure*. New York: York Medical Books; 1976:13–24.

18. Magorien DJ, Shaffer P, Bush CA, et al. Assessment of left ventricular pressure-volume relations using gated radionuclide angiography, echocardiography, and micromanometer pressure recordings. *Circulation*. 1983;67:844–853.

19. McKay RG, Aroesty JM, Heer GV, et al. Left ventricular pressure-volume diagrams and end-systolic pressure-volume relations in human beings. *J Am Coll Cardiol*. 1984;3:301–312.

20. Ludbrook PA, Byrne JD, Kurnik PB, McKnight RC. Influence of reduction of preload and afterload by nitroglycerin on left ventricular diastolic pressure-volume relations and relaxation in man. *Circulation*. 1977;56:937–943.

21. Pouleur H, Rousseau MF, van Eyll C, Gurné O, Hanet C, Charlier AA. Impaired regional diastolic distensibility in coronary artery disease: relations with dynamic left ventricular compliance. *Am Heart J*. 1986;112:721–728.

22. Weber KT, Janicki JS. Angiotensin and the remodelling of the myocardium. *Br J Clin Pharmacol*. 1989;28:141S–150S.

23. Weber KT. Cardiac interstitium in health and disease: the fibrillar collagen network. *J Am Coll Cardiol*. 1989;13-7:1637–1652.

24. Brilla CG, Pick R, Tan LB, Janicki JS, Weber KT. Remodeling of the rate right and left ventricles in experimental hypertension. *Circ Res*. 1990;67:1355–1364.

25. Hittinger L, Shannon RP, Bishop SP, Gelpi RJ, Vatner SF. Subendomyocardial exhaustion of blood flow reserve and increased fibrosis in conscious dogs with heart failure. *Circ Res*. 1989;65:971–980.

26. Vatner SF, Shannon R, Hittinger L. Reduced subendocardial coronary reserve. A potential mechanism for impaired diastolic function in the hypertrophied and failing heart. *Circulation*. 1990;81:(III)8–14.

27. Ross J Jr. Acute displacement of the diastolic pressure-volume curve of the left ventricle: role of the pericardium and the right ventricle. *Circulation*. 1979;59:32–37.

28. Ludbrook PA, Byrne JD, McKnight RC. The influence of right ventricular hemodynamics on left ventricular pressure-volume relations in man. *Circulation*. 1979;59:21–28.

29. Rousseau MF, Gurné O, van Eyll C, Benedict CR, Pouleur H. Effects of benazeprilat on left ventricular systolic and diastolic function and neurohumoral status in patients with ischemic heart disease. *Circulation*. 1990;81:III-123–129.

30. Konstam MA, Kronenberg MW, Udelson JE, et al. Effect of acute angiotensin converting enzyme inhibition on left ventricular filling in patients with congestive heart failure. Relation to right ventricular volumes. *Circulation*. 1990;81:III-115–122.

31. Katz AM. Cellular mechanisms in congestive heart failure. *Am J Cardiol*. 1988;62:3A–8A.

32. Opie LH, Nayler W, Gevers W. Calcium fluxes. In: Opie L, ed. *The Heart*. Orlando: Grune & Stratton; 1984:88–97.

33. Bristow MR, Ginsburg R, Umans V, et al. β_1- and β_2-adrenergic-receptor subpopulations in nonfailing and failing human ventricular myocardium: coupling of both receptor subtypes to muscle contraction and selective β_1-receptor down-regulation in heart failure. *Circ Res*. 1986;59:297–309.

34. Lakatta EG. Excitation-contraction. In: Weisfeldt ML, ed. *The Aging Heart*. New York: Raven Press; 1980:77–100.

35. Mann T, Goldberg S, Mudge GH, Grossman W. Factors contributing to altered left ventricular diastolic properties during angina pectoris. *Circulation*. 1979;59:14–20.

36. Pouleur H, Rousseau MF. Regional diastolic dysfunction in coronary artery disease: clinical and therapeutic implications. In: Grossman W, Lorell BH, eds. *Diastolic Relaxation of the Heart*. Boston: Martinus Nijhoff Publishing; 1988:245–254.

37. Wisneski JA, Gertz EW, Neese RA, Gruenke LD, Craig JC. Dual carbon-labeled isotope experiments using D-(6-^{14}C)glucose and L-(1,2,3-^{13}C$_3$)lactate: a new approach for investigating human myocardial metabolism during ischemia. *J Am Coll Cardiol*. 1985;5:1138–1146.

38. Gertz EW, Wisneksi JA, Neese R, Bristow JD, Searle GL, Hanlon JT. Myocardial lactate metabolism: evidence of lactate release during net chemical extraction in man. *Circulation*. 1981;63:1273–1279.

39. McKay RG, Aroesty JM, Heller GV, et al. The pacing stress test reexamined: correlation of pacing-induced hemodynamic changes with the amount of myocardium at risk. *J Am Coll Cardiol*. 1984;3:1469–1481.

40. De Kock M, Melin JA, Pouleur H, Rousseau MF. Alterations in myocardial metabolism and function at rest in stable angina pectoris: relations with the amount of exercise-induced Thallium-201 perfusion defect. *Cathet Cardiovasc Diagn*. 1986;12:391–398.

41. Marcus ML, Harrison DG, Chilian WM, et al. Alterations in the coronary circulation in hypertrophied ventricles. *Circulation*. 1987;75(suppl I):I19–I25.

42. Morgan JP, Erny RE, Allen PD, Grossman W, Gwathmey JK. Abnormal intracellular calcium handling, a major cause of systolic and diastolic dysfunction in ventricular myocardium from patients with heart failure. *Circulation*. 1990;81-2:III21–III32.

43. de la Bastie D, Levitsky D, Rappaport L, et al. Function of the sarcoplasmic reticulum and expression of its Ca^{2+}-ATPase gene in pressure overload-induced cardiac hypertrophy in the rat. *Circ Res*. 1990;66:554–564.

44. Lorell BH, Schunkert H, Grice WN, Tang SS, Apstein CS, Dzau VJ. Alteration in cardiac angiotensin converting enzyme activity in pressure overload hypertrophy. *Circulation*. 1989;80:II-297. Abstract.

45. Weber KT, Janicki JS, Shroff SG. The heart as a mechanical pump. In: Weber KT, Janicki JS, eds. *Cardio-*

Pulmonary Exercise Testing. Philadelphia: Saunders; 1986:34–76.

46. Brutsaert DL, Housmans PR, Goethals MA. Dual control of relaxation. Its role in the ventricular function in the mammalian heart. *Circ Res*. 1980;47:637–652.

47. Watanabe J, Levine MJ, Bellotto F, Johnson RG, Grossman W. Effect of coronary venous pressure on left ventricular diastolic distensibility. *Circ Res*. 1990;67:923–932.

48. Bonow RO. Regional left ventricular nonuniformity. Effects on left ventricular diastolic function in ischemic heart disease, hypertrophic cardiomyopathy, and the normal heart. *Circulation*. 1990;81(III):54–65.

49. Hanet C, Rousseau MF, van Eyll C, Pouleur H. Effects of nicardipine on regional diastolic left ventricular function in patients with angina pectoris. *Circulation*. 1990; 81:III-148–154.

50. Braunwald E, Ross J, Sonnenblick EH. Heart failure. In: *Mechanisms of Contraction of the Normal and Failing Heart*. Boston: Little, Brown and Company; 1976:309–356.

51. Matsuda Y, Toma Y, Ogawa H, et al. Importance of left atrial function in patients with myocardial infarction. *Circulation*. 1983;67:566–571.

52. Linderer T, Chatterjee K, Parmley WW, Sievers RE, Glantz SA, Tyberg J. Influence of atrial systole on the Frank-Starling relation and the end-diastolic pressure-diameter relation of the left ventricle. *Circulation*. 1983; 67:1045–1053.

53. Pouleur H, van Eyll C, Cheron P, Hanet C, Charlier AA, Rousseau MF. Changes in left ventricular filling dynamics after long-term xamoterol therapy in ischemic left ventricular dysfunction. *Heart Failure*. 1986;2:176–184.

54. Franciosa JA, Park M, Levine TB. Lack of correlation between exercise capacity and indexes of resting left ventricular performance in heart failure. *Am J Cardiol*. 1981;47:33–39.

55. McKirnan MD, Sullivan M, Jensen D, Froelicher VF. Treadmill performance and cardiac function in selected patients with coronary heart disease. *J Am Coll Cardiol*. 1984;3:253–261.

56. Packer M. Abnormalities of diastolic function as a potential cause of exercise intolerance in chronic heart failure. *Circulation*. 1990;81(III):78–86.

57. Balfour IC, Arensman FW, Eubig C, Garrido M, Jones C. Abnormal ventricular filling in sickle cell anemia. *J Am Coll Cardiol*. 1987;9:58A.

58. Kitzman DW, Higginbotham MB, Cobb FR, Sheikh KH, Sullivan MJ. Exercise intolerance in patients with heart failure and preserved left ventricular systolic function: failure of the Frank-Starling mechanism. *J Am Coll Cardiol*. 1991;17:1065–1072.

59. Oldershaw PJ, Dawkins KD, Ward DE, Gibson DG. Diastolic mechanisms of impaired exercise tolerance in aortic valve disease. *Br Heart J*. 1983;49:568–573.

60. Pouleur H, Hanet C, Rousseau MF, van Eyll C. Relation of diastolic function and exercise capacity in ischemic left ventricular dysfunction. Role of β-agonists and β-antagonists. *Circulation*. 1990;82(I):89–96.

61. Cuocolo A, Sax FL, Brush JE, Maron BJ, Bacharach SL, Bonow RO. Left ventricular hypertrophy and impaired diastolic filling in essential hypertension. *Circulation*. 1990;81-3:978–986.

62. Rodeheffer RJ, Gerstenblith G, Becker LC, Fleg JL, Weisfeldt ML, Lakatta EG. Exercise cardiac output is maintained with advancing age in healthy human subjects: cardiac dilatation and increased stroke volume compensate for a diminished heart rate. *Circulation*. 1984;69:203–213.

63. McKay RG, Pfeffer MA, Pasternak RC, et al. Left ventricular remodeling after myocardial infarction: a corollary to infarct expansion. *Circulation*. 1986;74:693–702.

64. Pfeffer JM, Pfeffer MA, Braunwald E. Influence of chronic captopril therapy on the infarcted left ventricle of the rat. *Circ Res*. 1985;57:84–95.

65. Ross J Jr. Afterload mismatch and preload reserve: a conceptual framework for the analysis of ventricular function. *Progr Cardiovasc Dis*. 1976;18:255–264.

66. Sharpe N, Smith H, Murphy J, Hannan S. Treatment of patients with symptomless left ventricular dysfunction after myocardial infarction. *Lancet*. 1988:256–259.

67. Pfeffer MA, Lamas GA, Vaughan DE, Parisi AF, Braunwald E. Effect of captopril on progressive ventricular dilatation after anterior myocardial infarction. *N Engl J Med*. 1988;319:80–86.

68. Pouleur H, van Eyll C, Hanet C, Cheron P, Charlier AA, Rousseau MF. Long-term effects of xamoterol on left ventricular diastolic function and late remodeling: a study in patients with anterior myocardial infarction and single-vessel disease. *Circulation*. 1988;77:1081–1089.

69. Inouye I, Massie B, Loge D, Topic N, Silverstein D, Simpson P, Tubau J. Abnormal left ventricular filling: an early finding in mild to moderate systemic hypertension. *Am J Cardiol*. 1984;53:120–126.

70. Takenaka K, Dabestani A, Gardin JM, Russell D, Clark S, Allfie A, Henry WL. Pulsed Doppler echocardiographic study of left ventricular filling in dilated cardiomyopathy. *Am J Cardiol*. 1986;58:143–147.

71. Takenaka K, Dabestani A, Gardin JM, et al. Left ventricular filling in hypertrophic cardiomyopathy: a pulsed Doppler echocardiographic study. *J Am Coll Cardiol*. 1986;7:1263–1271.

72. Rokey R, Kuo LC, Zoghbi WA, Limacher MC, Quinones MA. Determination of parameters of left ventricular diastolic filling with pulsed Doppler echocardiography: comparison with cineangiography. *Circulation*. 1985;71:543–550.

73. Spirito P, Maron BJ, Bonow RO. Noninvasive assessment of left ventricular diastolic function: comparative analysis of Doppler echocardiographic and radionuclide angiographic techniques. *J Am Coll Cardiol*. 1986;7:518–526.

74. Ishida Y, Meisner JS, Tsujioka K, et al. Left ventricular filling dynamics: influence of left ventricular relaxation and left atrial pressure. *Circulation*. 1986;74:187–196.

75. Fisch C, Beller GA, DeSanctis RW, et al. ACC/AHA guidelines for the clinical application of echocardiography. *Circulation*. 1990;82(6):2323–2345.

76. Soufer R, Wohlgelernter D, Vita NA, et al. Intact systolic left ventricular function in clinical congestive heart failure. *Am J Cardiol*. 1985;55:1032–1036.

77. Dougherty AH, Naccarelli GV, Gray EL, Hicks CH, Goldstein RA. Congestive heart failure with normal systolic function. *Am J Cardiol.* 1984;54:778–782.

78. Marantz PR, Tobin JN, Wassertheil-Smoller S, et al. The relationship between left ventricular systolic function and congestive heart failure diagnosed by clinical criteria. *Circulation.* 1988;77:607–612.

79. Cohn JN, Johnson G, Veterans Administration Cooperative Study Group. Heart failure with normal ejection fraction. The V-HeFT study. *Circulation.* 1990;81(III):48–53.

80. Warnowicz MA, Parker H, Cheiltin MD. Prognosis of patients with acute pulmonary edema and normal ejection fraction after acute myocardial infarction. *Circulation.* 1983;67(2):330–334.

81. Tofler GH, Stone PH, Muller JE, et al. Effects of gender and race on prognosis after myocardial infarction: adverse prognosis for women, particularly black women. *J Am Coll Cardiol.* 1987;9:473–482.

82. Lee DC, Johnson RA, Bingham JB, et al. Heart failure in outpatients: a randomized trial of digoxin versus placebo. *N Engl J Med.* 1982;306:699–705.

83. Bonow RO, Rosing DR, Bacharach SL, et al. Effects of verapamil on left ventricular systolic function and diastolic filling in patients with hypertrophic cardiomyopathy. *Circulation.* 1981;64:787–796.

84. Setaro JF, Schulman DS, Black HR, LaCroix M, Zaret BL, Soufer R. Congestive heart failure, intact systolic function, and abnormal diastolic filling: improvement with verapamil in a placebo-controlled trial. *Circulation.* 1988;78:II-204.

85. Lorell BH, Paulus WJ, Grossman W, Wynne J, Cohn PF. Modification of abnormal left ventricular diastolic properties by nifedipine in patients with hypertrophic cardiomyopathy. *Circulation.* 1982;65:499–507.

86. Frishman WH, Skolnick AE, Strom JA. Effects of calcium entry blockade on hypertension-induced left ventricular hypertrophy. *Circulation.* 1989;80:151–161.

87. The SOLVD Investigators. Effect of enalapril on survival in patients with reduced left ventricular ejection fractions and congestive heart failure. *N Engl J Med.* 1991; 325:293–302.

88. Cohn JN, Johnson G, Ziesche S, et al. A comparison of enalapril with hydralazine-isosorbide dinitrate in the treatment of chronic congestive heart failure. *N Engl J Med.* 1991;325:303–310.

89. Konstam MA, Rousseau MF, Kronenberg MW, et al. Effects of the angiotensin converting enzyme inhibitor enalapril, on the long-term progression of left ventricular dysfunction in patients with heart failure. *Circulation.* 1992;86:431–438.

90. Cohn JN, Archibald DG, Ziesche S, et al. Effect of vasodilator therapy on mortality in chronic congestive heart failure. Results of a Veteran Administration Cooperative Study. *N Engl J Med.* 1986;314:1547–52.

6
Cardiac Remodeling in Congestive Heart Failure

Norman Sharpe

The structural and functional changes that occur in heart failure have long been studied. However, it is only relatively recently that the term "cardiac remodeling" has been introduced, as the complexity and importance of the regional and global changes in ventricular size, shape, and composition that occur in heart failure have become better understood. Cardiac or ventricular remodeling denotes structural changes that occur in ventricular chamber size, wall thickness, and composition after myocardial damage. The regional and global topographic changes that occur after myocardial infarction have been the subject of most studies, but it is also relevant to consider the myocardial changes that occur in other forms of heart failure with pressure or volume overload.

Linzbach[1] in 1960 refuted the earlier concept that myocardial fibers were "overstretched" in heart failure (myogenic dilatation), by demonstrating that sarcomere length was the same in normal, hypertrophied, and pathologically dilated hearts. He concluded that the dilatation of these hearts must involve plastic structural changes within the myocardium and rearrangements of muscle fibers (Fig. 6.1). He compared the mobilizable residual volume of the physiologically dilated athlete's heart with the fixed residual volume of plastic dilatation and concluded that such structural dilatation was the morphologic substrate of the decompensated heart (Fig. 6.2). He explained cardiac insufficiency in strictly mechanical terms with the available cross-sectional area of contracting muscle too small for the increased volume of the ventricle. Thus, Linzbach's early quantitative morphologic approach to heart failure resulted in the recognition of afterload mismatch as a central factor in the progression of cardiac remodeling and failure. Whatever the underlying cause of heart failure, there is commonly a prolonged period before the occurrence of clinically manifest congestive heart failure during which ventricular remodeling occurs, initially as an adaptive compensatory process with varying degrees of ventricular dilatation and hypertrophy, but leading to progressive ventricular dysfunction. The poor prognosis of advanced clinical congestive heart failure has recently led to consideration of earlier intervention during the phase of symptomless ventricular dysfunction and treatment directed at modifying the process of ventricular remodeling.

Myocardial Tissue Changes After Experimental Infarction

Morphologic studies by Anversa et al.[2] have provided detailed information on the changes in myocardial tissue occurring in response to experimental infarction. Three days after acute myocardial infarction produced in rats by left coronary artery ligation, compensatory hypertrophy was demonstrated in the surviving left ventricular myocardium. Hypertrophy of left ventricular myocytes resulted from increases in cell length and diameter, changes considered characteristic of combined pressure and volume-overload hypertrophy. Morphometric analysis of the microvasculature demonstrated inadequate adaptation of the capillary vasculature to the myocardial hypertrophy. Thus, greater ventricular workload was not supported by proportionate expansion of the capillary bed, a possible limiting factor for recovery in the infarcted heart.

Similar experimental studies[3] have shown a correlation between the size of infarction and the degree of hypertrophy present at 5 weeks after myocardial infarction, although the hypertrophy plateaued in the group with the largest infarcts. In this group it appeared that hypertrophy was unable to compensate for the myocardial loss from more extensive infarction.

Anversa et al.[4] more recently also have studied myocyte characteristics at 40 days after coronary occlusion and compared the findings with their earlier study at 3 days. Whereas in the first studies at 3 days it was

84

Norman Sharpe

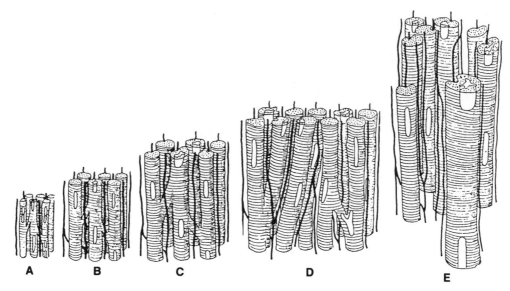

FIGURE 6.1. Growth of six heart muscle fibers and their capillaries in the myocardium of the left ventricle. Weights in parentheses. **A**: Infant (heart, 15 g; left ventricle, 7 g). **B**: Adult (heart, 300 g; left ventricle, 100 g). **C**: Athlete (heart, 500 g; left ventricle, 200 g). **D**: Concentric pressure hypertrophy: the same group of muscle fibers after longitudinal cleavage (heart, 650 g; left ventricle, 400 g). **E**: Decompensation. Eccentric hypertrophy. Structural dilatation. Some muscle fibers have disappeared. The surviving muscle fibers show compensatory hypertrophy with rearrangement. Between the muscle fibers is scar tissue (heart, 900 g; left ventricle, 500 g). Reprinted, with permission, from Linzbach AJ. *Am J Cardiol.* 1960;5:370–382.

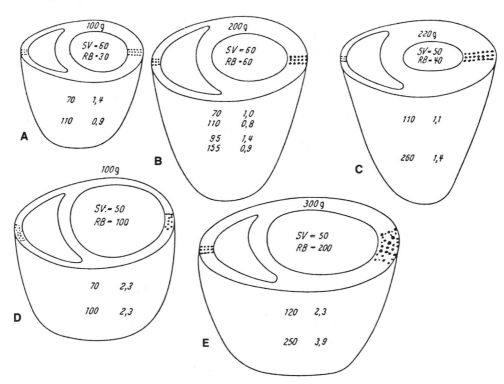

FIGURE 6.2. Relationship between heart muscle mass (figures in parentheses), chamber volume, and tension. **A**: Normal person (300 g). **B**: Athlete (500 g). **C**: Concentric hypertrophy due to hypertension (550 g). **D**: Plastic structural dilatation (300 g). **E**: Eccentric hypertrophy (650 g). Black dots on figure illustrate relative distribution and numbers of fibers on cross section. SV = stroke volume, RB = residual volume. Numbers on surface of cross section = weight of ventricle. Numbers on ventricular surface = *left*, diastolic and systolic pressures; *right*, force of tension in 10^5 dynes cm^{-2}. Reprinted, with permission, from Linzbach AJ. *Am J Cardiol.* 1960;5:370–382.

found that acute infarcts affecting approximately 50% of the ventricle were associated with a 28% enlargement of surviving myocytes of the left ventricle, at 40 days there was a 78% increase. Thus, myocyte growth is an early event that continues through the reparative phase tending to compensate for the loss of muscle mass and function. However, at the subcellular level there was a reduction in mitochondria: myofibril volume ratio in large infarcts indicating disproportionate growth and lack of a balanced reactive response, which might be important in limiting the functional capacity of the hypertrophied muscle cells. The deficit in capillary adaptation noted earlier also was present at 40 days, with the capillary luminal surface area and oxygen diffusion distance being more greatly compromised in the presence of large infarcts, abnormalities considered likely to increase vulnerability to subsequent ischemia.

Myocardial Growth Factors and Remodeling

While the myocardial tissue changes observed after experimental infarction have been explained in mechanical terms and attributed to altered wall stress, recent progress in cell biology has indicated that alteration of gene expression and synthesis of myocardial proteins is relevant to remodeling and may occur in response to various tissue growth factors. This new perspective is consistent with the paradigmatic shift that has occurred in cardiovascular research, as in many other areas, from basic organ physiology to cell biochemistry and biophysics and gene expression.[5] Catecholamines, and more importantly angiotensin II (Table 6.1), have been studied in this context and there is increasing evidence for the role that angiotensin II may play a role as a stimulus for hypertrophy in both the heart and vasculature.[6,7] Several cellular oncogenes have been invoked in this process. One particular cellular oncogene, the mas oncogene, has been reported to encode a functional angiotensin receptor able to mediate the action of angiotensin II to increase cytosolic calcium,[8] although this has not been demonstrated in the heart. The growth-promoting effects of angiotensin II involve interaction between cytosolic calcium and activated protein kinase C, which result in induction of the nuclear protooncogene c-fos. The c-fos product appears to accelerate transcription and plays a central role in protein synthesis in smooth[9] and cardiac muscle.[10] Thus, angiotensin II may act not only as a pressor agent but also as an important growth factor and may mediate the effects of various stimuli to produce hypertrophy in the overloaded heart. The potential importance of cardiac angiotensin in modulation of myocyte growth and hypertrophy has been emphasized by the demonstration

TABLE 6.1. Paradigms in cardiovascular regulation: the role of angiotensin II.

Organ physiology	Vasopressor
	Blood pressure regulation
Cell biochemistry and biophysics	Promotion of smooth muscle contraction
	Ca^{2+} fluxes
Gene expression	Increased vascular and myocardial growth and hypertrophy

Adapted from Katz, *Am J Mol Cell Cardiol.* 1990; 22:729–747, with permission.

of a transient increase in angiotensinogen mRNA in noninfarcted left ventricle after experimental infarction.[11] From this perspective, the timing and progression of this process, from initial compensatory hypertrophy, which may be advantageous, to pathologic hypertrophy from sustained overload, which is detrimental,[12] is relevant when consideration is given to intervention, particularly with angiotensin converting enzyme (ACE) inhibition.

Attention has been focused predominantly on cardiac myocyte changes in myocardial failure; however, other abnormalities of myocardial structure may produce impaired contractile function while myocyte contractility is preserved. In the left ventricular hypertrophy related to hypertension, abnormal accumulation of fibrillar collagen occurs in the extracellular space, producing progressive interstitial and perivascular fibrosis, which causes abnormal myocardial stiffness and ventricular dysfunction.[13] It has been suggested that such cardiac fibroblast growth and enhanced collagen synthesis may result from elevated angiotensin II and aldosterone levels and also that other growth factors such as catecholamines, platelet-derived growth factor, and transforming growth factor beta also may play a role in hypertrophy of myocyte and nonmyocyte cells.[13] Improved understanding of these processes should also have implications for the prevention and regression of pathological hypertrophy and fibrosis.

Functional Changes After Experimental Infarction

Compensatory hypertrophy in surviving myocardium allows preservation of ventricular systolic function to some degree, depending on the extent of myocardial damage. Experimentally, ventricular systolic function has been related to infarct size in the rat. Small healed infarcts produced no detectable impairment of left ventricular function, moderate infarcts produced impaired performance with preload and afterload stress, and large infarcts impaired basal performance.[14] Changes in left ventricular diastolic pressure/volume relations also occur after myocardial infarction and although difficult to quantitate reliably in the clinical setting, have been demonstrated in patients in the acute and convalescent phases.[15,16] Experimental studies in the canine model have shown increased compliance immediately after experimental myocardial infarction and later reduced compliance during healing associated with improved systolic function.[17] More detailed studies in the rat model with a wider range of healed infarcts have demonstrated an increase in left ventricular diastolic volume at low transmural filling pressure that is related to infarct size with parallel shift of the diastolic pressure volume curve on the volume axis and close correlation of the degree of left ventricular dilatation with impaired systolic performance.[18] The morphologic changes in the infarcted and noninfarcted myocardium thus have very important functional significance, particularly with larger infarcts.

Infarct Expansion and Healing

After acute coronary occlusion in the clinical setting, there are various factors to consider at different times that may contribute to subsequent ventricular dilatation. Thrombolytic therapy may produce coronary reperfusion and limit infarct size. Early infarct expansion and later healing may be accompanied by compensatory hypertrophy in the noninfarcted region and progressive global dilatation, which may progress over the long term, the major stimulus being increased wall stress.

A sequential two-dimensional echocardiographic study of patients after acute transmural myocardial infarction demonstrated disproportionate dilatation and transmural thinning of the infarcted zone in 8 of the 28 patients studied.[19] This regional expansion was first observed as early as 3 days after infarction and was progressive during the 2 weeks of study. Infarct segment length increased 50%, producing a total left ventricular circumferential dilatation of 25%. Patients showing infarct expansion all had anterior infarcts and significantly greater 8-week mortality compared with the patients without expansion. The relationship of two-dimensional echocardiographic wall motion abnormality to morphologic evidence of myocardial infarction has been established from an autopsy study.[20] Two-dimensional echocardiographic evidence of regional wall motion abnormality was sensitive in detecting and localizing segmental pathologic myocardial lesions but overestimated their extent, possibly because of the proximity of morphologically normal segments to scar or the presence of reversible ischemia.

A distinction is required between infarct expansion and extension; that is, between disproportionate dilatation and thinning of the area of infarction not explained by additional myocardial necrosis and new myocardial necrosis.[21] Infarct extension appears to be a much less frequent event than expansion and generally will not further compromise cardiac function. Infarct expansion can mimic or possibly cause extension and commonly worsens cardiac function through ventricular dilatation.

Experimental studies in the rat infarct model have confirmed the early occurrence and progressive nature of infarct expansion.[22] A critical infarct size of 17% was necessary for significant expansion and the degree of expansion correlated with infarct size, occurring in 66% of the large series of transmural infarcts but in none of the few nontransmural infarcts. Infarct healing and preservation of a normal left ventricular contour was observed in only 20% of the infarcted hearts in the series.

Various cellular mechanisms for infarct expansion have been suggested, including myocyte necrosis and rupture, reduction in intercellular space, and stretching or slippage of myocytes.[23] Detailed histologic study of rat hearts with infarct expansion complemented by study of human hearts indicates that rearrangement of groups or bundles of myocytes with a decreased number of cells across the wall accounts for most of the wall thinning in the infarct zone and all the thinning of noninfarcted regions.[23] In the infarct zone, both cell stretch and loss of intercellular space occur, whereas in noninfarcted regions, cell slippage alone accounts for all thinning (Fig. 6.3).

The association of infarct expansion with larger, more transmural infarcts noted experimentally has been confirmed in a large patient autopsy analysis.[24] Infarcts with greater expansion had significantly more endocardial thrombus and endocardial fibroelastosis. Left ventricular hypertrophy and increased heart weight had a significant negative correlation with infarct expansion, which occurred more frequently in left anterior descending coronary artery distribution compared with the right coronary artery. From these findings it can be postulated that differences in the degree of normal segmental wall thickness related to radius of curvature and intramural tension explain the increased tendency for infarct expansion in the distribution of the left anterior descending coronary artery.[24] With left ventricular hypertrophy and increased wall thickness, infarcts tend to be less transmural and the apparent protection from expansion in the presence of hypertrophy may be due to a relatively smaller infarct size.

Global Ventricular Dilatation

Early infarct expansion and regional ventricular dilatation after myocardial infarction may be accompanied or followed by a phase of global ventricular dilatation occurring over subsequent months and involving both infarcted and noninfarcted segments (Table 6.2). This has been demonstrated from serial two-dimensional

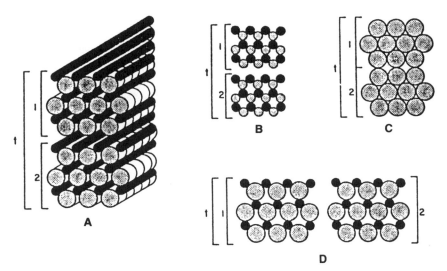

FIGURE 6.3. Schematic drawings of possible mechanisms of infarct expansion. **A**: Myocytes (*stippled cylinders*) and capillaries (*solid cylinders*) are shown as being arranged in discrete bundles (1 and 2). A is a three-dimensional perspective diagram of a hypothetical preinfarct ventricular wall. In subsequent panels, only the two-dimensional cross-sectional view is shown. For illustrative purposes, cross sections of only two bundles are shown composing the total wall thickness (*t*). **B**: With cell stretch, the total number of cells across the wall and capillary dimension remain unchanged, but a number of cells per unit length (cell density) increases as the wall thins. **C**: Collapse of the microvascular space results in tighter packing of the myocytes also producing an increase in cell density and hence wall thinning. **D**: With rearrangement of myocyte bundles, fewer cells make up the thickness of the wall, but the number of cells per unit length is unchanged. Reprinted, with permission, from Weisman et al. *Circulation*. 1988;78:116–201. Copyright by the American Heart Association.

TABLE 6.2. Ventricular dilatation after myocardial infarction

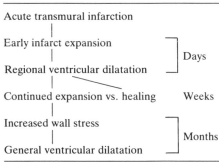

echocardiographic studies in a group of patients after transmural anterior myocardial infarction.[25] Patients showing early infarct expansion showed significant continuing dilatation during long-term observation up to 30 months in the infarcted anterior and noninfarcted posterior segments. In contrast, the patients without initial infarct expansion showed no significant later change in anterior or posterior segment length.

As indicated from earlier experimental animal studies,[2–4] remodeling of the entire left ventricle with volume-overload hypertrophy of noninfarcted segments also may occur during the early convalescent period and accompany infarct expansion. An angiographic study on admission and at 2 weeks in a group of patients with their first acute transmural anterior myocardial infarct treated successfully with thrombolytic therapy showed a significant increase in left ventricular volume over the 2-week period but a significant decrease in left ventricular filling pressure.[26] The volume increase correlated with infarct size as assessed by the extent of wall motion abnormality present acutely. Increased endocardial perimeter lengths were present in both infarcted and noninfarcted segments at 2 weeks. Lengthening of the endocardial perimeter in the ventricular wall without regional wall motion abnormality and wall thinning suggests a volume-overload hypertrophy with a net increase in myocardial mass of these segments and is analogous to the compensatory hypertrophy demonstrated early after acute myocardial infarction in experimental animal studies.[2–4] Such volume-overload hypertrophy results from series addition of sarcomeres in contrast to pressure-overload hypertrophy, where new myofibrils are added in parallel. It has been postulated that increased diastolic pressure and wall stress from volume overload leads to sarcomere replication in series with resultant chamber enlargement.[27] Such chamber enlargement accommodates the volume overload returning diastolic pressure to normal. The chamber enlargement also causes an increase in systolic wall stress, which results in slight wall thickening.

The volume-overload hypertrophy that occurs after myocardial infarction can be compared with the ventricular remodeling that occurs with cardiac conditions that cause chronic left ventricular pressure or volume overload, such as aortic stenosis or valvular regurgitation.[27] In these situations, overload is matched initially by appropriate hypertrophy but eventually in some cases, persisting hemodynamic overload and wall stress imbalance leads to pump failure. Thus, "adaptive" or "compensatory" hypertrophy may progress to pathologic concentric or eccentric hypertrophy as a result of systolic or diastolic wall stress imbalance. This hemodynamic interpretation of cardiac hypertrophy and failure is consistent with Linzbach's earlier morphologic interpretations.[1]

The demonstration of early significant left ventricular diastolic dysfunction assessed by radionuclide angiography within 24 hours of acute myocardial infarction, which occurred even in patients with preserved systolic function, further supports the suggestion that left ventricular dilatation and increased diastolic wall stress act as the primary stimuli for continued ventricular remodeling.[28] An increase in wall stress in infarcted and ischemic segments also has been demonstrated in patients with coronary artery disease studied by cardiac catheterization.[29] End-systolic wall stress was increased in infarcted and ischemic segments compared with normal matched segments. Residual wall stress at the end of isovolumic relaxation was increased both in infarcted areas and in noninfarcted areas perfused by stenosed arteries. However, whereas the rate of decrease in local stress in infarcted areas paralleled the rate of decrease in pressure, in ischemic areas the rate of decrease in stress was slower. While initial volume overload and increased wall stress may be matched by adequate hypertrophy, with the tendency to progressive dilatation, eventually mismatch occurs and heart failure becomes clinically manifest.[12,27]

The pattern of left ventricular dilatation after myocardial infarction can be quite variable. In a group of 57 patients with myocardial infarction, none of whom had thrombolysis, radionuclide evaluation showed approximately half of the patients to have a greater than 20% increase in left ventricular end-diastolic volume index from 2 weeks to 1 year after infarction.[30] A similar study with serial evaluation of left ventricular volume changes in 50 patients who did not receive thrombolysis showed a greater than 20% increase in left ventricular end-diastolic volume from day 2 to day 10 in 11 patients, and similar left ventricular dilatation from day 10 to 6 months in 10 other patients.[31] Among these 21 patients, progressive dilatation with serial volume increases on two or more occasions occurred in eight patients, all of whom had large anterior infarcts. Thus, approximately 40% of infarct survivors demonstrated significant ventricular dilatation within 6 months of infarction. Progressive dilatation was associated with deterioration in left ventricular function and increased 2-year mortality, in contrast to patients with dilatation who stabilized, who had a better clinical outcome.

TABLE 6.3. Ventricular remodeling after myocardial infarction.

Process	Intervention
Coronary occlusion	Restore infarct artery patency
Myocardial infarction	Restore infarct artery patency
Size	Optimise O$_2$ supply: demand
Transmural extent	Reduce regional wall stress
Reperfusion injury	Attenuate reperfusion injury
Myocardial infarct expansion Early/late	Reduce regional wall stress
Global ventricular dilatation and compensatory hypertrophy	Reduce wall stress and hypertrophy
Progressive ventricular dysfunction	Ventricular unloading
Recurrent ischemia/infarction Arrhythmias	Optimise O$_2$ supply: demand
Clinical congestive heart failure	Relieve congestion Block neurohormonal activation Improve myocardial contractility

Modification of Left Ventricular Remodeling

Various processes may contribute to ventricular remodeling at different stages from the time of coronary occlusion until the possible development of progressive ventricular dysfunction and clinical heart failure (Table 6.3). These processes are amenable to intervention at different times, the overall aim being to prevent significant ventricular dysfunction and heart failure and improve the long-term prognosis. The loading conditions of the ventricle and infarct artery patency are of central importance in influencing ventricular remodeling and eventual outcome.

Increased Afterload

Afterload changes during acute myocardial infarction may have important effects not only on myocardial ischemia and infarct size but also on ventricular remodeling. Early transient increases in afterload have been shown to produce relative infarct expansion and thinning and slow the early phase of infarct healing in dogs.[32] The duration of hypertension induced by methoxamine infusion required for this was relatively brief (4 hr) and topographic differences were determined at 7 days postinfarction. Further studies of the effects of sustained increase in afterload from aortic banding in the rat also have shown increased infarct expansion independent of infarct size.[33] Patients with hypertensive left ventricular hypertrophy are known to have increased morbidity and mortality after infarction.[34] Autopsy studies have shown a correlation between a history of systemic hypertension and infarct expansion and rupture.[35,36] Thus, afterload reduction

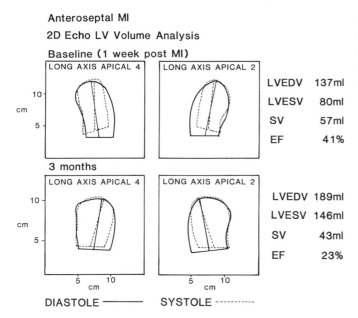

Anteroseptal MI

2D Echo LV Volume Analysis

Baseline (1 week post MI)

LONG AXIS APICAL 4   LONG AXIS APICAL 2

LVEDV   137ml
LVESV   80ml
SV   57ml
EF   41%

3 months

LONG AXIS APICAL 4   LONG AXIS APICAL 2

LVEDV   189ml
LVESV   146ml
SV   43ml
EF   23%

DIASTOLE ———   SYSTOLE ----------

FIGURE 6.4. Two-dimensional echocardiograms from a patient 1 week and 3 months after transmural anteroseptal infarction and showing global ventricular dilatation and severe ventricular dysfunction. Left ventricular end-diastolic, end-systolic, and stroke volumes and ejection fraction derived from a Simpson's rule method combining the four-chamber and two-chamber area outlines are shown for each study. The extensive segmental akinesis and dyskinesis evident initially is followed by considerable global dilatation.

early in the course of myocardial infarction may have important effects on left ventricular remodeling through reduced infarct expansion as well as through limitation of infarct size.

Exercise

Experimental studies have varied in their conclusion as to the effects of exercise on myocardial infarct size and healing, although the different forms and intensity of exercise applied probably account for the disparities reported. Rats subjected to 40 min of swimming exercise daily from 7 to 21 days after coronary artery occlusion showed thinning of the transmural scar compared with control.[37] Similar exercise in the same animal model but started 24 hr after coronary occlusion and continued for 7 days followed by 2 weeks of rest produced even more marked relative thinning of myocardial scar.[38] However, infarcted rats subjected to more moderate daily treadmill exercise for 1.5 hr for 1 week from the day of coronary ligation did not show a detrimental effect on infarct expansion.[39] Such experimental findings from this infarct model of single vessel disease may have limited relevance to patients with multivessel disease.

The view that exercise training might be injurious to patients with extensive transmural infarction has been

supported by a clinical study of patients with anterior Q wave myocardial infarction.[40] In a two-dimensional echocardiographic study, a group of patients were identified with greater initial akinesia/dyskinesia (greater than 18% left ventricular asynergy). This group developed increased asynergy, infarct expansion and thinning, and reduced ejection fraction compared with controls during 12 weeks of low-level exercise started 15 weeks after infarction (Fig. 6.5). The relatively late expansion observed was attributed to further increase in wall stress due to the increased afterload of exercise and possible increased contractile pull of the adjacent nonasynergic segments. The extent of initial asynergy determining later expansion with exercise in this study is consistent with the data from animal studies that suggest a similar critical infarct size for acute expansion.

Infarct Artery Patency

Infarct artery patency may confer a beneficial effect on ventricular remodeling and long-term survival through mechanisms other than early limitation of infarct size. The relation between perfusion of the infarct-related artery and changes in left ventricular volume and function during the month after a first myocardial infarct has been examined in a clinical study of 40 patients who did not receive thrombolysis.[41] Infarct artery perfusion was documented at predischarge angiography and left ventricular volumes assessed from radionuclide angiography within 48 hr of infarction and at 1 month. Left ventricular dilatation (greater than 20% increase in volume) occurred in all 14 patients without perfusion of the infarct-related artery compared with only 2 of 26 with perfusion due to subtotal occlusion or collateral vessels. Five patients with a decrease in left ventricular volume all had a perfused infarct artery. The degree of perfusion was a more important predictor of volume change than was infarct size assessed by peak creatine kinase or electrocardiographic QRS score. Thus, perfusion of the infarct related artery may be important in preventing continuing infarct expansion and left ventricular dilatation. Reperfusion may preserve endocardial tissue and it is also possible that reperfused infarcts with contraction band necrosis may have higher tensile strength and reduced propensity to expansion than unperfused infarcts.[42]

A further study of the time course of left ventricular dilatation after myocardial infarction, which confirmed variable patterns of early, later, and progressive dilatation and showed greater dilatation in those with left anterior descending coronary artery occlusion, did not show any relationship of volume changes to reperfusion.[43] This was attributed to relatively late thrombolysis with delay between onset of symptoms and reestablishment of flow. Various other studies of thrombolysis and left ventricular function have clearly dem-

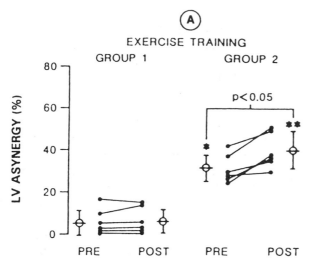

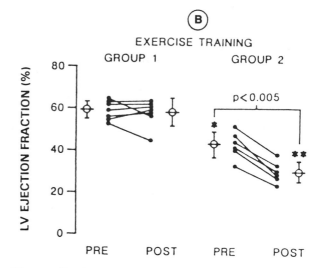

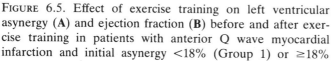

FIGURE 6.5. Effect of exercise training on left ventricular asynergy (**A**) and ejection fraction (**B**) before and after exercise training in patients with anterior Q wave myocardial infarction and initial asynergy <18% (Group 1) or ≥18%

(Group 2). *$p < .001$ group 2 vs. group 1 pretraining; **$p < .001$ group 2 vs. group 1 posttraining. Adapted with permission from Jugdutt BI et al. *J Am Coll Cardiol.* 1988;12:362-372.

onstrated benefit from myocardial reperfusion with reduced infarct size and associated improvement in regional and global ventricular function.[44-47] Reperfusion and patency of the infarct-related artery may thus determine not only a reduction in infarct size and propensity to early infarct expansion but also possible later benefits for ventricular remodeling and long-term survival.

Pharmacologic Intervention

Improved understanding of the process of ventricular remodeling and the prognostic importance of ventricular dilatation after myocardial infarction[48] have led to experimental and clinical studies of pharmacologic intervention for treatment of left ventricular dysfunction in the postinfarct period. As previously mentioned, thrombolysis and other measures are of proven value in the acute phase where the primary objective is limitation of infarct size and salvage of ischemic myocardium. Once infarct evolution has occurred, however, there is potential for intervention to minimize the sequelae of infarct expansion and ventricular dilatation and thus improve the long-term prognosis.

Intravenous nitroglycerin has been shown to limit infarct size, infarct expansion, other infarct-related complications, and mortality up to 1 year.[49] The beneficial effect of nitroglycerin on limiting infarct expansion was apparent from serial echocardiographic study during the first 2 to 3 days, suggesting early remodeling. Decreased preload and afterload were considered important contributing factors to this, although reduced infarct size and improved collateral flow also may have played a role.

There has been considerable interest in the effects of ACE inhibition on left ventricular remodeling. In rats studied 3 to 4 months after myocardial infarction, ventricular dilatation and depression of cardiac performance were demonstrated as a function of infarct size.[50] A continuum of heart failure was observed with progressive rise in left ventricular filling pressure and decrease in maximal forward output and ejection fraction as infarct size increased. Compensatory dilatation of the left ventricle allowed preservation of forward output at any filling pressure. Infarction of moderate and larger size reduced overall chamber stiffness. Captopril treatment improved forward output, reduced ventricular dilatation, and the change in ventricular chamber stiffness. Longer term studies in the same model showed survival inversely related to infarct size but improved with captopril treatment, particularly in animals with infarcts of moderate size.[51]

Clinical studies also have been carried out to study the effects of ACE inhibition after myocardial infarction. In a randomized double-blind trial,[52,53] the effects of captopril, frusemide, and placebo were studied in patients with asymptomatic left ventricular dysfunction (ejection fraction less than 45%) 1 week after Q wave myocardial infarction. Left ventricular volumes and function were assessed at intervals during the subsequent year using two-dimensional echocardiography. The frusemide and placebo groups showed significant increases in ventricular volumes with stroke volume index unchanged and ejection fraction slightly reduced, whereas the captopril group showed a significant reduction in left ventricular end-systolic volume index with stroke volume index and ejection fraction increased. At

12 months the difference in the change in ejection fraction from baseline between the captopril and other groups was about 10%.

Another study[54] randomized patients to captopril or placebo at a mean of 18 days after a first myocardial infarction. As in the former study, no patient had overt heart failure and all had ejection fraction less than 45%. End-diastolic volume increased in the placebo group during the year of treatment but not in the captopril group, although there was no significant difference between the groups. Dilatation was more evident in the placebo patients with an extensive wall motion abnormality or with an occluded infarct-related artery. In a subgroup of patients from this study,[55] the importance of left ventricular shape in determining exercise capacity was assessed and the interaction between left ventricular shape and captopril therapy evaluated. A greater shape distortion indicated by increasing left ventricular sphericity was associated with increased left ventricular volumes, decreased ejection fraction, and a larger abnormally contracting segment. Left ventricular sphericity index was the only independent predictor of exercise duration in the placebo group. Placebo-treated patients in the tercile with the most spherical ventricles had the lowest exercise capacity and highest heart failure and specific activity scores. Captopril-treated patients with the same baseline distortion of left ventricular shape did not show these shape-dependent changes in functional capacity.

It has been speculated that despite the expected fall in equatorial wall stress with changes in radius of curvature as the dilating ventricle assumes a more spherical shape, altered myocardial fiber orientation may be associated with increased stress per myocardial fiber.[56] The motion of endocardial landmarks in a normally contracting ventricle follows a pattern maximizing systolic mechanical advantage.[57] This pattern may be changed with apical distortion leading to loss of the mechanical advantage of orderly contraction of myocardial segments, which compromises global ventricular function more than expected from the extent of the infarct alone. These observations may explain the importance of left ventricular shape as a descriptor of left ventricular structure and function as well as outcome.

Whereas left ventricular dysfunction can be improved with ACE inhibition commenced 1 week after myocardial infarction or later, earlier intervention appears to provide greater benefit. In a double-blind study in patients with Q wave myocardial infarction but without clinical heart failure, treatment with captopril or placebo was commenced 24 to 48 hr after the onset of symptoms.[58] During 3 months of treatment, the placebo group showed significant increases in left ventricular volumes with ejection fraction unchanged. In contrast, the captopril group showed no change in left ventricular

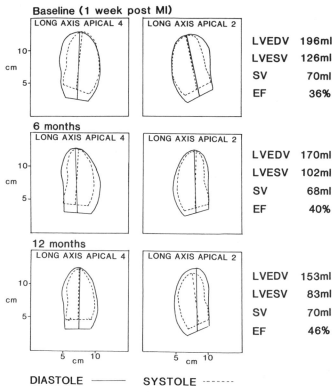

FIGURE 6.6. Serial two-dimensional echocardiograms from a patient after an extensive inferolateral infarction showing improved ventricular size and function during a year of treatment with the ACE inhibitor, captopril. (Methods and format as for Fig. 6.4)

end-diastolic volume index and a significant reduction in left ventricular end-systolic volume index with ejection fraction increased significantly. Most of the treatment benefit was evident during the first month. Comparison of the results of this study with those from the study where treatment was commenced 1 week after myocardial infarction[52,53] indicate a greater benefit from earlier treatment.

These clinical results are somewhat disparate from those of an experimental study in rats with myocardial infarction[59] where there was no difference in the benefit with immediate treatment commenced orally 2 hr after coronary ligation compared with delayed treatment started at 21 days when the animals' left ventricular performance, weight, and volumes were assessed after 4 months of treatment. These experimental data suggest that the primary effect of treatment may not be due to an effect on infarct expansion, which has been shown experimentally to have occurred in most large infarcts by 7 days.[60,61] Also, blockade of compensatory mechanisms activated at the time of infarction may not be desirable in the immediate postinfarct period, even though these mechanisms may be deleterious later. This possibility is supported by further experimental data that indicate that captopril therapy in chronically infarcted conscious rats improved cardiac function when treatment was started after completion of the healing process, but that early treatment had an adverse effect on function.[62] When captopril was given from 1 to 21 days during the healing period, cardiac output with volume loading was the same as in the untreated infarct control animals, but with heart rate increased and stroke volume reduced. While the rat model is useful for studies of left ventricular remodeling after myocardial infarction, patients with coronary artery disease may respond differently to ACE inhibition. Nevertheless, the timing of this treatment is obviously important clinically. Intervention after 24 hr appears practical and beneficial and more immediate treatment may increase the risk of hypotension with thrombolytic treatment and possibly compromise coronary perfusion.

The mechanism of improvement with ACE inhibition probably is related principally to the peripheral vasodilating effect and ventricular unloading; in this respect both preload and afterload reduction appear important.[63] There also may be additional beneficial effects on the coronary circulation[64,65] that are advantageous for remodeling. However, whereas coronary hemodynamic data have suggested a balanced effect of ACE inhibition on the coronary circulation, a recent clinical study in patients with heart failure and ischemia has indicated that such treatment may worsen ischemia as a result of hypotension and presumably compromised coronary perfusion.[66] Finally, ACE inhibition may have an important direct effect on myocardial tissue,[13,67,68] preventing inappropriate growth and hypertrophy stimulated by angiotensin II and other growth factors.

Remaining Questions

The process of left ventricular remodeling has now been studied extensively but a number of important questions remain to be answered. While the progression from initial compensatory hypertrophy to pathologic hypertrophy has been studied experimentally, this aspect of remodeling is not easily amenable to clinical study and remains poorly understood. Study of laboratory models of heart failure must be complemented by clinical investigation of the role of cardiac growth and hypertrophy in heart failure for a better understanding to be obtained.

With the gradual change of the myocardial infarction paradigm during the past decade from considerations of infarct size to infarct artery patency and further to early and late ventricular remodeling, there are now a number of therapeutic interventions that may be applied.

The benefits of early and late ventricular unloading and reduced wall stress have been demonstrated in terms of improved ventricular size and function. Recent data indicate that this can be translated into clinical benefit in terms of heart failure prevention and improved survival.[69] Large-scale studies currently in progress should provide further information on this most important aspect during the next several years, including refinement of dosage regimens and the timing of intervention.

Further clinical studies also are required to confirm the optimal timing of this type of intervention and particularly the value of treatment in combination with or immediately after thrombolysis. Assessment of the comparative and possibly additive effects of ACE inhibition, nitrates, and beta-blockade in the postinfarction period also is required.

References

1. Linzbach AJ. Heart failure from the point of view of quantitative anatomy. *Am J Cardiol.* 1960;5:370–382.
2. Anversa P, Loud AV, Levicky V, Guideri G. Left ventricular failure induced by myocardial infarction. I. Myocyte hypertrophy. *Am J Physiol.* 1985;17:H876–882.
3. Rubin SA, Fishbein MC, Swan HJC, Rabines A. Compensatory hypertrophy in the heart after myocardial infarction in the rat. *J Am Coll Cardiol.* 1983;1:1435–1441.
4. Anversa P, Loud AV, Levicky V, Guideri G. Left ventricular failure induced by myocardial infarction. II. Tissue morphometry. *Am J Physiol.* 1985;17:H883–H889.
5. Editorial. Angiotensin II: hemodynamic regulator or growth factor? *J Mol Cell Cardiol.* 1990;22:729–747.
6. Dzau VJ. Cardiac renin-angiotensin system. Molecular and functional aspects. *Am J Med.* 1988;84(suppl 3A)22–27.
7. Re RN. The cellular biology of angiotensin: paracrine, autocrine and intracrine actions in cardiovascular tissues. *J Mol Cell Cardiol.* 1989;21:(suppl V)63–69.
8. Jackson TR, Blair AC, Marchall J, Goedert M, Hanley MR. The mas oncogene encodes an angiotensin receptor. *Nature.* 1988;335:437–440.
9. Naftilan AJ, Pratt RE, Eldridge CS, Lin HL, Dzau VJ. Angiotensin II induces c-fos expression in smooth muscle via transcriptional control. *Hypertension.* 1989;13:706–711.
10. Izumo S, Nadal-Ginard B, Mahdavi V. Protooncogene induction and reprogramming of cardiac gene expression produced by pressure overload. *Proc Nat Acad Sci.* 1988;85:339–343.
11. Drexler H, Lindpaintner K, Lu W, Schieffer B, Ganten D. Transient increase in the expression of cardiac angiotensinogen in a rat model of myocardial infarction and failure. *Circulation.* 1989;80(suppl II):459.
12. Katz AM. Cardiomyopathy of overload. A major determinant of prognosis in congestive heart failure. *N Engl J Med.* 1990;322:100–110.
13. Weber KT, Brilla CG. Pathological hypertrophy and cardiac interstitium. *Circulation.* 1991;83:1849–1865.

14. Pfeffer MA, Pfeffer JM, Fishbein MC, et al. Myocardial infarct size and ventricular function in rats. *Circ Res.* 1979;44:503–512.

15. Diamond G, Forrester JS. Effect of coronary artery disease and acute myocardial infarction on left ventricular compliance in man. *Circulation.* 1972;45:11–19.

16. Bleifeld W, Mathey D, Hanrath P. Acute myocardial infarction. VI. Left ventricular wall stiffness in the acute phase and in the convalescent phase. *Eur J Cardiol.* 1974;2:191–198.

17. Kumar R, Hood WB Jr, Joison J, Norman JC, Abelman WH. Experimental myocardial infarction. II. Acute depression and subsequent recovery of left ventricular function: serial measurements in intact conscious dogs. *J Clin Invest.* 1970;49:55–62.

18. Fletcher PJ, Pfeffer JM, Pfeffer MA, Braunwald E. Left ventricular diastolic pressure–volume relations in rats with healed myocardial infarction. *Circ Res.* 1981;49:618–626.

19. Eaton LW, Weiss JL, Bulkley BH, Garrison JB, Weisfeldt ML. Regional cardiac dilatation after acute myocardial infarction. *N Engl J Med.* 1979;300:57–62.

20. Weiss JL, Bulkley BH, Hutchins GM, Mason SJ. Two-dimensional echocardiographic recognition of myocardial injury in man: comparison with postmortem studies. *Circulation.* 1981;63:401–408.

21. Hutchins GM, Bulkley BH. Infarct expansion versus extension: two different complications of acute myocardial infarction. *Am J Cardiol.* 1978;41:1127–1132.

22. Hochman JS, Bulkley BH. Expansion of acute myocardial infarction: an experimental study. *Circulation.* 1982; 65:1146–1450.

23. Weisman HF, Bush DE, Mannisi JA, Weisfeldt ML, Healy B. Cellular mechanisms of myocardial infarct expansion. *Circulation.* 1988;78:186–201.

24. Pirolo JS, Hutchins GM, Moore GW. Infarct expansion: pathologic analysis of 204 patients with a single myocardial infarct. *J Am Coll Cardiol.* 1986;7:349–354.

25. Erlebacher JA, Weiss JL, Eaton LW, Kallman C, Weisfeldt ML, Bulkley BH. Late effects of acute infarct dilatation on heart size. A two dimensional echocardiographic study. *Am J Cardiol.* 1982;49:1120–1126.

26. McKay RG, Pfeffer MA, Pasternak RC, et al. Left ventricular remodeling after myocardial infarction: a corollary to infarct expansion. *Circulation.* 1986;74:693–702.

27. Grossman W. Cardiac hypertrophy: useful adaptation or pathologic process? *Am J Med.* 1980;69:576–584.

28. Seals AA, Pratt CM, Mahmarian JJ, et al. Relation of left ventricular dilatation during acute myocardial infarction to systolic performance, diastolic dysfunction, infarct size and location. *Am J Cardiol.* 1988;61:224–229.

29. Pouleur H, Rousseau MF, Van Eyll C, Charlier AA. Assessment of regional left ventricular relaxation in patients with coronary artery disease: importance of geometric factors and changes in wall thickness. *Circulation.* 1984;69:696–702.

30. Gadsboll N, Hoilund-Carlsen PF, Badsberg JH, et al. Late ventricular dilatation in survivors of acute myocardial infarction. *Am J Cardiol.* 1989;64:961–966.

31. Jeremy RW, Allman KC, Bautovitch G, Harris PJ. Patterns of left ventricular dilatation during the six months after myocardial infarction. *J Am Coll Cardiol.* 1989; 13:304–310.

32. Hammerman H, Kloner RA, Alker KJ, Schoen FJ, Braunwald E. Effects of transient increased afterload during experimentally induced acute myocardial infarction in dogs. *Am J Cardiol.* 1985;55:566–570.

33. Nolan SE, Mannisi JA, Bush DE, Healy B, Weisman HF. Increased afterload aggravates infarct expansion after acute myocardial infarction. *J Am Coll Cardiol.* 1988; 12:1318–1325.

34. Rabkin SW, Mathewson FAL, Tate RB. Prognosis after acute myocardial infarction: relation to blood pressure values before infarction in a prospective cardiovascular study. *Am J Cardiol.* 1977;40:604–610.

35. Christensen DJ, Ford M, Reading J, Castle CH. Effect of hypertension on myocardial rupture after acute myocardial infarction. *Chest.* 1977;72:618–622.

36. Schuster EH, Bulkley BH. Expansion of transmural myocardial infarction: a pathophysiologic factor in cardiac rupture. *Circulation.* 1979;60:1532–1538.

37. Kloner RA, Kloner JA. The effect of early exercise on myocardial infarct scar formation. *Am Heart J.* 1983;106:1009–1013.

38. Hammerman H, Schoen FJ, Kloner RA. Short-term exercise has a prolonged effect on scar formation after experimental acute myocardial infarction. *Am J Coll Cardiol.* 1983;2:979–982.

39. Hochman JS, Healy B. Effect of exercise on acute myocardial infarction in rats. *J Am Coll Cardiol.* 1986; 7:126–132.

40. Jugdutt BI, Michorowski BL, Kappagoda CT. Exercise training after anterior Q wave myocardial infarction: importance of regional left ventricular function and topography. *J Am Coll Cardiol.* 1988;12:362–372.

41. Jeremy RW, Hackworthy RA, Bautovich G, Hutton BF, Harris PJ. Infarct artery perfusion and changes in left ventricular volume in the month after acute myocardial infarction. *J Am Coll Cardiol.* 1987;9:989–995.

42. Connelly CM, Vogel WM, Weigner AW. Effects of reperfusion after coronary artery occlusion on post-infarction scar tissue. *Circ Res.* 1985;57:562–577.

43. Warren SE, Royal HD, Markis JE, Grossman W, McKay RG. Time course of left ventricular dilatation after myocardial infarction: influence of infarct-related artery and success of coronary thrombolysis. *J Am Coll Cardiol.* 1988;11:12–19.

44. Serruys PW, Simoons ML, Suryapranata H, et al. Preservation of global and regional left ventricular function after early thrombolysis in acute myocardial infarction. *J Am Coll Cardiol.* 1986;7:729–742.

45. Sheehan FH, Doerr R, Schmidt WG, et al. Early recovery of left ventricular function after thrombolytic therapy for acute myocardial infarction: an important determinant of survival. *J Am Coll Cardiol.* 1988;12:289–300.

46. Touchstone DA, Beller GA, Nygaard TW, Tedesco C, Kaul S. Effects of successful intravenous reperfusion therapy on regional myocardial function and geometry in humans: a topographic assessment using two-dimensional echocardiography. *J Am Coll Cardiol.* 1989;13:1506–1513.

47. Marino P, Zanolla L, Zardini P (GISSI). Effect of

streptokinase on left ventricular modeling and function after myocardial infarction: the GISSI Trial. *J Am Coll Cardiol.* 1989;14:1149–1158.

48. White HD, Norris RM, Brown MA, Brandt PW, Whitlock RML, Wild CJ. Left ventricular end-systolic volume as the major determinant of survival after recovery from myocardial infarction. *Circulation.* 1987;76:44–51.

49. Jugdutt BI, Warnica W. Intravenous nitroglycerin therapy to limit myocardial infarct size expansion and complications. *Circulation.* 1988;78:906–919.

50. Pfeffer JM, Pfeffer MA, Braunwald E. Influence of chronic captopril therapy on the infarcted left ventricle of the rat. *Circ Res.* 1985;57:84–95.

51. Pfeffer MA, Pfeffer JM, Steinberg C, Finn P. Survival after an experimental myocardial infarction: beneficial effects of long-term therapy with captopril. *Circulation.* 1985;72:406–412.

52. Sharpe N, Murphy J, Smith H, Hannan S. Treatment of patients with symptomless left ventricular dysfunction after myocardial infarction. *Lancet.* 1988;i:255–259.

53. Sharpe N, Murphy J, Smith H, Hannan S. Preventive treatment of asymptomatic left ventricular dysfunction following myocardial infarction. *Eur Heart J.* 1990; 11:S147–156.

54. Pfeffer MA, Lamas GA, Vaughan DE, Parisi AF, Braunwald E. Effect of captopril on progressive ventricular dilatation after anterior myocardial infarction. *N Engl J Med.* 1988;319:80–86.

55. Lamas GA, Vaughan DE, Parisi AF, Pfeffer MA. Effects of left ventricular shape and captopril therapy on exercise capacity after anterior wall acute myocardial infarction. *Am J Cardiol.* 1989;63:1167–1173.

56. Gould KL, Lipscomb K, Hamilton GW, Kennedy JW. Relation of left ventricular shape, function and wall stress in man. *Am J Cardiol.* 1974;34:627–634.

57. Slager CJ, Hooghoudt TEH, Serruys P, et al. Quantitative assessment of regional left ventricular motion using endocardial landmarks. *J Am Coll Cardiol.* 1986;7:317–326.

58. Sharpe N, Smith H, Murphy J, Greaves S, Hart H, Gamble G. Early prevention of left ventricular dysfunction after myocardial infarction with angiotensin-converting-enzyme inhibition. *Lancet.* 1991;337:872–876.

59. Gay RG. Early and late effects of captopril treatment after large myocardial infarction in rats. *J Am Coll Cardiol.* 1990;16:967–977.

60. Hochman JS, Bulkley BH. Expansion of acute myocardial infarction: an experimental study. *Circulation.* 1982; 65:1446–1450.

61. Weisman HF, Bush DE, Mannisi JA, Bulkley BH. Global cardiac remodeling after acute infarction: a study in the rate model. *J Am Coll Cardiol.* 1985;5:1355–1362.

62. Schoemaker RG, Debets JJM, Struyker-Boudier HAJ, Smits JFM. Delayed but not immediate captopril therapy improves cardiac function in conscious rats, following myocardial infarction. *J Mol Cell Cardiol.* 1991;23:187–197.

63. Raya TE, Gay RG, Goldman S. The importance of venodilatation in the prevention of left ventricular dilatation after chronic large myocardial infarction in rats: a comparison of captopril and hydralazine. *Circ Res.* 1989; 64:330–337.

64. Daly P, Mettauer B, Rouleau JL, Cousineau D, Burgess JH. Lack of reflex increase in myocardial sympathetic tone after captopril: potential antianginal effect. *Circulation.* 1985;71:317–325.

65. Magrini F, Shimizu M, Roberts N, Fouad FM , Tarazi RC, Zanchetti A. Converting-enzyme inhibition and coronary blood flow. *Circulation.* 1987;75:S1168–1174.

66. Cleland JGF, Henderson E, McLenachen J, Findlay IN, Dargie HJ. Effect of captopril, an angiotensin-converting enzyme inhibitor, in patients with angina pectoris and heart failure. *J Am Coll Cardiol.* 1991;17:733–739.

67. Dzau VJ, Re RN. Evidence for the existence of renin in the heart. *Circulation.* 1987;75:S1134–1136.

68. Lindpaintner K, Kin M, Wilhelm MJ, et al. Intracardiac generation of angiotensin and its physiologic role. *Circulation.* 1988;77:S1-18.

69. Pfeffer MA, Braunwald E, Moye LA, et al. Effect of captopril on mortality in patients with left ventricular dysfunction after myocardial infarction—Results of the Survival and Ventricular Enlargement Trial. *N Engl J Med.* 1992;327:669–677.

7
The Role of the Pericardium in the Pathophysiology of Heart Failure

Ralph Shabetai

Physiology of the Pericardium

The major function of most organs is readily apparent and requires no deep knowledge of biology or physiology. However, whether or not the pericardium subserves an important function or, like the vermiform appendix, serves no useful purpose has been debated over the years and the debate continues. To state that all organs are enveloped in an invaginated serosal membrane containing a small amount of fluid, and that the heart is no exception, does not imply that the pericardium has no discernible effects on cardiac function. Indeed, since the turn of this century, researchers have reported experiments designed to determine whether or not the pericardium restrains cardiac volume, and if so to quantify this effect.

The pericardium is closely applied to the heart, embracing all the cardiac chambers except the posterior aspect of the left atrium, where the pulmonary veins enter. Furthermore, the volume of the unstressed pericardium is only slightly larger than the volume of its contents. This reserve volume, as it is sometimes called, allows for changes in the volume of the heart and intrapericardial great vessels that occur physiologically with alterations in posture, the fluctuations of the respiratory cycle, and variations in the state of hydration.

A key to understanding the physiology of the pericardium and its effects on the normal or enlarged heart is the pressure/volume and stress/strain relationships of the pericardium. These relationships may be constructed for pericardial tissue itself, or for the pericardium treated as a chamber. When considering pericardial stress/strain relationships, it is critical to take into account the time course of pericardial strain, because whereas the pericardium is highly resistant to acute stretch, it appears compliant when stretched over a period of weeks or months.

When pericardial tissue is subjected to acute biomechanical testing, the resulting curve has a characteristic J shape (Fig. 7.1).[1] Thus, minor strain produces little if any increase in pericardial stress. Additional stretching of the tissue produces the bend of the J, during which there is a measurable increase in pericardial stress that gradually increases. At the end of the bend, the curve becomes almost perpendicular, indicating that from that point onward, the pericardium is virtually inextensible. Most studies of the mechanical properties have been performed on canine pericardium,[2] but we also have studied the human tissue, which we found to be considerably thicker than canine pericardium and correspondingly less compliant.[3]

Pericardial chamber pressure-volume and stress-strain curves are performed in vivo, usually using a fresh post-mortem canine preparation with the heart enclosed in the pericardium (Fig. 7.1B). When, under these conditions, fluid is added to the pericardial space, a pressure-volume curve closely resembling the in vitro stress-strain curve is generated. Because it is difficult to measure accurately the thickness of the pericardium, it is difficult to generate accurate pericardial stress-strain curves in vivo. However, when this is attempted, this curve also closely resembles the in vitro pericardial stress/strain relationship.

Considering these curves, it is apparent that, from the clinical point of view, pericardial volume must be considered as the sum of the volume of pericardial fluid, the volume of the myocardium and great vessels together with the volume of the blood contained within them. Thus, the contact force between heart and pericardium can be increased by pathological changes in the pericardium, increased volume of pericardial fluid, or enlargement of the heart or great vessels.

Numerous functions have been ascribed, with varying degrees of experimental proof, to the pericardium.[4] It is thought that pericardial fluid serves as a lubricant permitting constant cardiac activity without damage to epicardium or pericardium. The presence of a thin film of

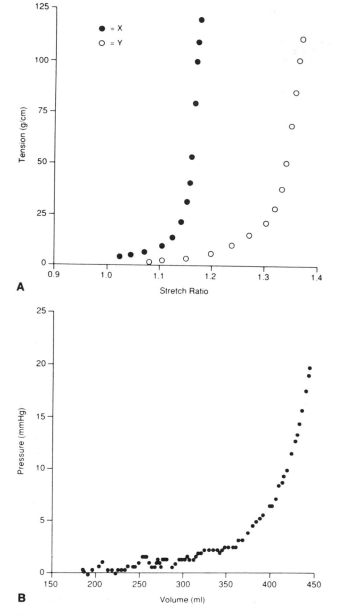

A

B

FIGURE 7.1. **A:** The stress/strain relation of pericardial tissue tested in vitro. The solid circles represent the data obtained when the tissue is stretched in the x direction and the open circles stretching in the y direction. The difference in the two curves indicates that pericardial tissue is anisotropic. Reprinted with permission from Lee et al. Biaxial mechanical properties of the pericardium in normal and volume overload dogs. *Am J Physiol.* 1985;249:H222. Copyright by the American Physiological Society. **B:** The pressure volume curve of canine pericardium tested in situ.

pericardial fluid could serve to equalize gravitational forces generated when the body experiences acceleration or deceleration.[5] It also has been suggested that the pericardium may help to integrate the stroke volumes of the left and right ventricles by limiting inspiratory in-

crease in right heart volume and expiratory decrease in left heart volume. Like other serous membranes, the pericardium may limit the spread of infection to the heart and may serve immunological functions.

The pericardial function most germane to heart failure is its role, or potential role, in restricting cardiac volume. This role should be considered separately for the normal heart, the acutely enlarged heart, and the chronically enlarged heart. So far as the normal heart is concerned, after numerous animal experiments and clinical investigations, many with conflicting results, a general consensus has been reached that when the heart, pericardium, and state of hydration are normal, a small degree of pericardial restraint can be demonstrated, but its magnitude is such that for all practical considerations, it can be ignored. However, when cardiac volume is rapidly increased, for instance by rapid intravenous fluid infusion sufficient to raise the left and right ventricular diastolic pressures several mm Hg, appreciable, physiologically significant restraint on the heart can be convincingly demonstrated, an observation having obvious significance for the pathophysiology of heart failure.

Several years ago, Ludbrook et al.[6] studied a number of patients with heart failure in the cardiac catheterization laboratory. By simultaneously recording left ventricular pressure and volume throughout diastole, they confirmed that in heart failure, the entire diastolic pressure/volume relation of the left ventricle is displaced upward on the pressure axis (Fig. 7.2). When these investigators administered nitroglycerin, they found that for any given pressure at any point in diastole, the corresponding pressure was lower, such that the entire diastolic pressure/volume relation was displaced downward. This observation suggested to us that the displacement of the curve could have been the manifestation of withdrawal of pericardial restraint. We hypothesized that when the nitroglycerin was administered to these patients, cardiac volume shrank as a consequence of venodilatation, thus disengaging the heart from the pericardium. Our hypothesis presumed that in these patients with severe heart failure being studied at cardiac catheterization, a significant proportion of the increase in ventricular diastolic pressure was borne by the pericardium; that is, were it possible to measure intrapericardial pressure under those circumstances, it would have been elevated, such that intrapericardial pressure would be only slightly less than ventricular diastolic pressure. A precedent for this hypothesis was to be found in the work of Holt et al.,[7] who showed in dogs that rapid infusion of dextran sufficient to cause a major increase in right atrial pressure and diastolic pressure in the two ventricles caused a large increase in intrapericardial pressure such that the change in transmural left and right ventricular diastolic pressures was substantially less than the change in these pressures re-

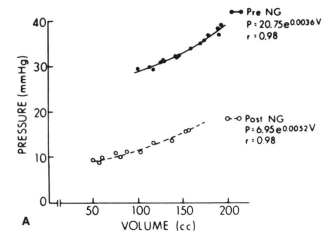

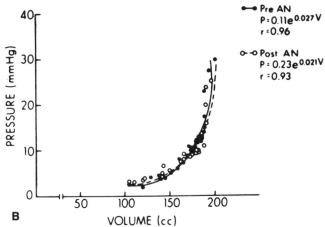

FIGURE 7.2. Left ventricular pressure-volume curves (**A**) before and after nitroglycerin (*NG*) and (**B**) before and after amyl nitrite (*AN*). Significant downward and leftward displacement of the pressure-volume curve occurs after nitroglycerin. In contrast, the diastolic pressure-volume curves before and after amyl nitrite are virtually superimposable. Reprinted with permission from Ludbrook et al. Influence of right ventricular hemodynamics on left ventricular diastolic pressure-volume relations in man. *Circulation.* 1979;59:21–31. Copyright by the American Heart Association.

ferred to atmospheric pressure (Fig. 7.3). Accordingly, we carried out an experiment to test this hypothesis.[8]

In chronically instrumented dogs, we measured left and right ventricular segment length as a surrogate for left ventricular diastolic volume, together with left ventricular pressure from the end of early rapid filling to the beginning of atrial systole; that is, during diastasis. We then rapidly infused a liter of dextran, which caused a dramatic shift up the pressure axis of the entire left ventricular diastolic pressure-volume curve, much as is seen in the cardiac catheterization laboratory when patients with acute heart failure, or an acute exacerbation of chronic heart failure, are studied. We then infused nitroprusside, which produced a dramatic fall of the entire curve down the pressure axis. In a number of these animals, we also measured intrapericardial pressure, confirming the observation of Holt et al.[7] that after volume infusion, intrapericardial pressure rose in parallel with ventricular diastolic pressure. Intrapericardial pressure fell in parallel with ventricular diastolic pressure when nitroprusside was infused. The dogs were then subjected to pericardiectomy and were restudied after a suitable period was allowed for recovery from the operation. Dextran infusion now produced a large increase in diastolic pressure, but no longer displaced the curve as a whole. Likewise, nitroprusside infusion in the pericardiectomized dogs produced a totally different effect from that seen when the agent was administered to dogs with the pericardium intact. Now, instead of shifting the curve downward, we found that left ventricular diastolic pressure fell because the pressure-volume data points followed the original diastolic pressure/segment length relationship (Fig. 7.4). In the dogs in which we had measured pericardial pressure, we

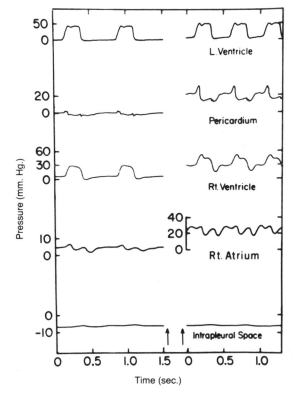

FIGURE 7.3. Data from Holt demonstrating the effect of transfusion on the pressure in the pericardial space, right ventricle, right atrium, left ventricle, and intrapleural space in a closed chest dog. Pressure was measured with a flat balloon. 1000 ml of 5% dextran was injected intravenously over a period of a few minutes. All pressures except the pleural pressure increased. The increased intrapericardial pressure reduced the effect of acute hypervolemia on transmural ventricular diastolic pressures. Reprinted with permission from Holt et al. Pericardial and ventricular pressure. *Circ Res.* 1960;8:1171–1181. Copyright by the American Heart Association.

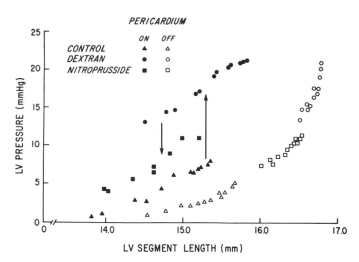

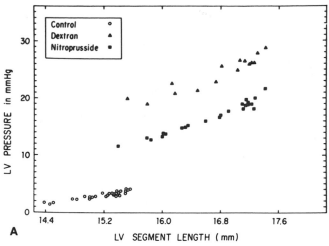

FIGURE 7.4. Left ventricular diastolic pressure-segment length relation before and after removal of the pericardium. With the pericardium intact, the curve obtained during acute volume loading is shifted upward. Sodium nitroprusside infusion lowered the curve downward toward the control position. After pericardiectomy, the pressure-segment length relation, during the same intervention, moved along a single curve. Reprinted with permission from Shirato et al. Alteration of the left ventricular diastolic pressure-segment length relation produced by the pericardium. *Circulation.* 1978;57:1191–1198. Copyright by the American Heart Association.

subtracted the pericardial effect mathematically by plotting left ventricular diastolic transmural pressure instead of absolute pressure against the segment length. Comparing the status control, versus dextran infusion, the effect of nitroprusside now yielded data indistinguishable from those obtained from dogs that had undergone pericardiectomy (Fig. 7.5). These and other studies make it quite clear that acute volume overload, such as may occur after rapid intravenous infusion, acute mitral[9] or aortic regurgitation, or acute heart failure, causes the heart to engage the pericardium strongly and thereby greatly increase pericardial pressure. Thus, when the heart is acutely dilated, the pericardium exerts a powerful, clinically important restraining effect on the size of the heart. The pericardium thus limits massive acute dilatation with its potentially disastrous effect on myocardial performance and the competency of the atrioventricular valves.

The next question that we asked was to what extent pericardial restraint on cardiac volume persists when cardiac dilatation develops more slowly and is chronic. To address this problem, we turned to a model of cardiac dilatation and hypertrophy that had been extensively studied in our laboratory, namely the infrarenal aortocaval shunt. An anastomosis of about 1 cm in length reliably produces cardiac dilatation and hypertrophy and eventually the animals develop edema, ascites, and a high venous pressure, although cardiac

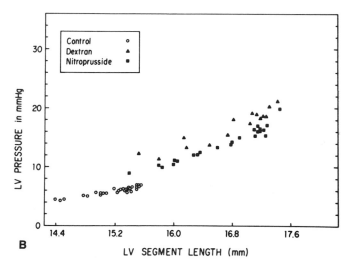

FIGURE 7.5. Pressure and segment length data from one of the dogs in the study illustrated by Fig. 7.4. Transmural left ventricular diastolic pressure (LVEDP minus pericardial pressure) is plotted on the ordinate for the same animal. When the influence of the pericardium on the pressure-segment length relation is thus subtracted, the points tend to fall along a single curve in a manner similar to that seen after pericardiectomy.

output is elevated. We studied dogs 30 days after creation of the aortocaval shunt using simultaneous measurements of left ventricular volume by cineangiogram and left ventricular diastolic pressure measured with a catheter-tipped transducer.[10] As expected, we found the left ventricular diastolic pressure/volume relation was significantly elevated on its pressure axis. When we infused nitroprusside, we obtained results similar to those in the acute experiment. That is, the entire diastolic pressure/volume relationship fell such that for any ventricular diastolic volume, the pressure was lower. We concluded that pericardial restraint persists at least into the subacute stage of cardiac dilatation.

LeWinter and Pavalec[11] examined this question, which is highly relevant to heart failure, in a different way, choosing to do an acute study and to examine end-diastolic left ventricular pressure/volume relationships rather than the relationship throughout the course of diastasis. They studied dogs about 10 days after the creation of an infrarenal aortocaval shunt and again about 45 days later. They obtained left ventricular end-diastolic pressure-volume data over a large series of rapidly changing ventricular diastolic volumes obtained at one extreme by applying occluders to the venae cavae, which were subsequently gradually released through normal volumes to volumes obtained after rapid dextran infusion. They then removed the pericardium and immediately again recorded left ventricular diastolic pressure-volume data over the same, or a similar, range of left ventricular volumes. This study showed that when dogs were studied soon after the creation of the shunt, pericardiectomy shifted the diastolic pressure-volume curve to the right, but when dogs were studied late, pericardiectomy had no discernible effect on the curve. These data were interpreted to mean that pericardial restraint persists into the subacute phase of cardiac dilatation, but gradually lessens and finally disappears.

The observation that, with time, pericardial restraint generated by cardiac enlargement dissipates, led to experiments designed to inquire into the mechanism of this adaptation.[12] For this experiment, control dogs and dogs with an aortocaval shunt were compared. In vivo pericardial pressure-volume curves demonstrated that the curve was greatly shifted to the right on its volume axis in dogs with a shunt (Fig. 7.6A). Post-mortem measurement of pericardial weight, surface area, and thickness indicated that the pericardium had hypertrophied in response to cardiac enlargement. However, when pericardial in vivo stress-strain curves were performed, no difference was detected on comparing the curves from normal dogs and those with cardiac enlargement. It was therefore concluded that pericardial adaptation to chronic cardiac enlargement took the form of pericardial hypertrophy with an increase in pericardial chamber compliance, but no change in its tissue compliance. However, the difficulty of obtaining satisfactory pericardial chamber stress-strain curves led us to retest the hypothesis using in vitro stretching of pericardial tissue obtained from dogs with chronic experimentally induced cardiac enlargement compared with normal dogs.[1] This more sensitive technique demonstrated that the pericardium of dogs with cardiac enlargement was distinctly more compliant than the pericardium of dogs with a normal heart (Fig. 7.6B). So it can now be stated that the pericardium adapts to chronic cardiac enlargement with lessening or even disappearance of increased pericardial restraint because the pericardium becomes larger and inherently more

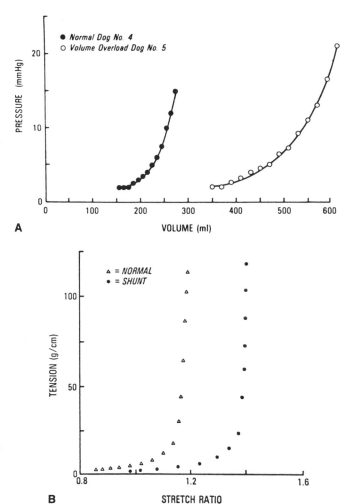

FIGURE 7.6. **A**: Pericardial pressure/volume relation from a normal dog and a dog with chronic volume overload, showing a rightward shift in the presence of cardiac enlargement. Reprinted with permission from Freeman and LeWinter. Pericardial adaptations during chronic cardiac dilation in dogs. *Circ Res.* 1984;54:298. Copyright by the American Heart Association. **B**: Stress/strain relation of pericardium from a normal dog and a dog after chronic volume overload. The tissue was stretched biaxially. Pericardial tissue from a dog with cardiac enlargement secondary to chronic volume overload shows a curve shifted to the right, because the tissue is more compliant after chronic stretching. Reprinted with permission from Lee et al. Biaxial mechanical properties of the pericardium in normal and volume overload dogs. *Am J Physiol.* 1985; 249:H222–H230. Copyright by the American Physiological Society.

compliant. These observations would suggest that in patients with chronic heart failure, in the absence of an acute exacerbation, pericardial restraint should not be greatly increased over normal.

The subject of pericardial restraint invariably introduces the troublesome topic of how restraint should be defined and measured. As every reader of this volume knows, cardiac and vascular pressures can be measured either via fluid-filled catheters attached to transducers or by catheter-tipped transducers. These devices measure liquid pressure, which has the important characteristic that it exerts a lateral force equal at all points. This characteristic means that, aside from small hydrostatic differences and, in the case of catheter-tipped transducers, gravitational effects, pressure measured anywhere within a chamber is identical. A problem arises, however, when the question is asked whether it is appropriate to consider the pericardial sac as a fluid-filled chamber, because in relation to the surface area of the heart and pericardium, the volume of pericardial fluid is small and somewhat unevenly distributed. Many investigators and clinicians consider that the pericardial space over much of the heart is not a real space, but rather a potential space. If that were the case, it could reasonably be argued that the pericardium would exert a direct contact force on the heart, not a pressure mediated by pericardial fluid.[13] It would then become inappropriate to use measurement of pericardial fluid pressure as a measure of pericardial contact force; that is, as the external pressure to calculate cardiac transmural pressure.

Ventricular Interaction

The left and right sides of the heart are arranged in parallel, but the circuit for flow is in series; pericardial reserve volume is modest, and the pericardium is not compliant. Acute dilatation of one side of the heart therefore encroaches to a greater or lesser extent on the other side, and this interaction is greatly strengthened by the pericardium.[14,15] Henderson and Prince demonstrated this interaction in an elegant series of experiments in 1914.[16] In patients with left heart failure, the severity of secondary right heart failure is highly variable, suggesting that in some cases, left ventricular enlargement causes the interventricular septum to bulge into the right ventricle, thereby distorting its shape and consequently impairing its function (Bernheim's syndrome). Ventricular interaction has been studied in the fresh post-mortem canine heart.[17] Pressure-volume curves of the left ventricle were performed with the right ventricle empty, or holding various fixed volumes of fluid. The study showed that increased right ventricular volume shifted the left ventricular pressure-volume curve to the left on its volume axis. This study was performed in hearts removed from the pericardium, demonstrating that ventricular interaction occurs even without the restraining influence of the pericardium. Subsequent studies showed that interaction is more pronounced when the pericardium is intact.[14,15] For instance, the strongest predictor of left ventricular diastolic pressure in a canine volume expansion model was right ventricular diastolic pressure, not left ventricular volume.[18] This relationship is tighter with the pericar-

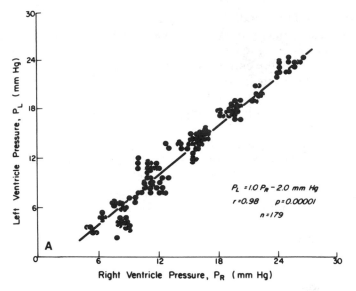

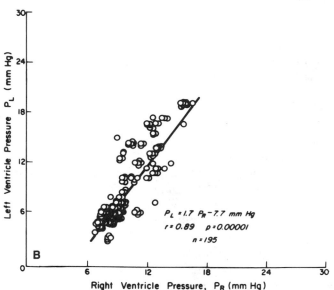

FIGURE 7.7. The effects of right ventricular diastolic pressure on left ventricular diastolic pressure. Left and right ventricular diastolic pressures correlate, although the correlation is significantly tighter with the pericardium closed (**A**) than with it open (**B**). Reprinted with permission from Glantz SA, Misbach GA, Moores WY, et al. The pericardium substantially affects the left ventricular diastolic pressure-volume relationship in the dog. *Circ Res.* 1978;42:433–441. Copyright by the American Heart Association.

dium closed, although it is still demonstrable with the pericardium open (Fig. 7.7).

In our laboratory we extended the observation of Taylor et al.[17] We also used the fresh canine post-mortem heart, but we did not open the pericardium.[15] We performed left heart pressure-volume curves with different fixed volume in the right heart. We also performed the converse experiment, filling the right heart while the left heart was maintained at various constant

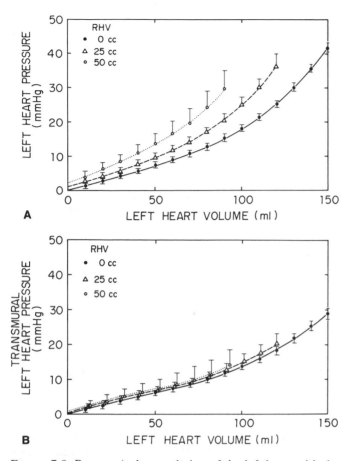

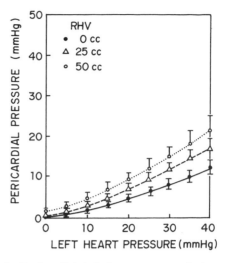

FIGURE 7.9. Pericardial left heart pressure/volume relation. Note that the pericardial left heart-pressure relation is shifted to the left and is steeper when the volume of the right heart is increased. Reprinted with permission from Hess et al. The role of the pericardium in interactions between the cardiac chambers. *Am Heart J.* 1983;106:1377–1383.

FIGURE 7.8. Pressure/volume relation of the left heart with the right heart empty (*closed circles, solid line*), with 25 ml in the right side (*open triangles, dashed line*) and with 50 ml in the right side (*open circles, dotted line*). **A:** The left heart pressure-volume relation. **B:** The transmural left heart pressure-volume relation. Note that the left heart pressure volume-relation becomes steeper with higher volumes in the right heart, whereas the transmural pressure-volume relation remains essentially unchanged. Reprinted with permission from Hess et al. The role of the pericardium in interactions between the cardiac chambers. *Am Heart J.* 1983;106:1377–1383.

volumes. During these experiments we also monitored intrapericardial pressure. We found that interaction between the cardiac chambers was evident regardless of which side of the heart was progressively filled and which maintained at constant volume (Fig. 7.8). Of particular relevance to the subject of this chapter, progressive filling of one side of the heart not only changed the diastolic pressure/volume relation of the other side, but also significantly raised intrapericardial pressure (Fig. 7.9). This effect also was illustrated by replotting the data substituting transmural pressure for absolute pressure. Replotting the data in this manner almost abolished the effect of the volume of the contralateral side of the heart on the pressure/volume relation of the side of the heart under study, once more illustrating that

chamber interaction is enhanced greatly by the pericardium (Fig. 7.8B). The study also confirms yet again that at normal cardiac volume, pericardial constraint is slight or absent, but comes increasingly into play in response to cardiac dilation. Santamore et al., who performed a number of important studies to prove and quantify ventricular interdependence, has more recently quantified the contribution of the pericardium to cardiac chamber interaction, and also has shown that, as expected, this interaction becomes extreme in cardiac tamponade[19] and constrictive pericarditis.[20]

The relevance of cardiac chamber interaction to heart failure is readily apparent. Although Bernheim's syndrome applies to chronic heart failure, it should be apparent from the foregoing that the phenomenon is more pronounced when chamber enlargement is relatively acute and in the presence of cardiac tamponade or constrictive pericarditis. Nevertheless, ventricular interaction has been cited as one mechanism of left ventricular dysfunction in cor pulmonale. Other causes include hypoxia, muscle bundles common to both ventricles, and undetected independent disease of the left heart.

Pericardial Pressure and Contact Force

In the experiments on ventricular interaction described in the preceding paragraphs, pericardial pressure was measured conventionally. However, further consideration of contact force is necessary before concluding this section. Contact force can be measured invasively by means of a flat balloon, which may be fluid-[21] or air-[22]

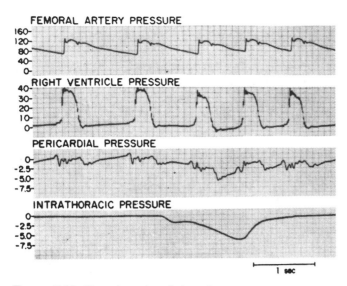

FIGURE 7.10. Pleural, pericardial, and vascular pressures measured in an intact sedated dog breathing spontaneously. Note the similarity in value and waveform comparing intrapericardial with intrapleural (thoracic) pressure. Reprinted with permission from Morgan et al. Relationship of pericardial to pleural pressure during quiet respiration and cardiac tamponade. *Circ Res.* 1965;16:493–498. Copyright by the American Heart Association.

filled, but is unstressed; that is, when the balloon has been filled, the pressure within it is atmospheric. The balloon is placed between the pericardium and myocardium over a ventricular surface to which it can conform. Pressure in the in situ balloon is then the pressure exerted by the heart and pericardium against each other. The magnitude and nature of this pressure and the manner in which it differs from conventionally measured pressure are of fundamental importance to the student of heart failure. When a conventional catheter is introduced into the pericardial cavity and pressure is measured during spontaneous respiration with the chest closed, pericardial pressure is slightly subatmospheric and close to intrapleural pressure[23] (Fig. 7.10). The respiratory variations in intrapericardial pressure track those of intrapleural pressure in the domain of time, but are slightly less in amplitude. Intrapericardial pressure measured in this manner also shows fluctuations related to the cardiac cycle. Minimal pericardial pressure corresponds with the ejection phase of systole and maximal pressure with end-diastole, but variation in this pattern may occur depending on the location of the catheter tip in the pericardial space. Conventionally measured liquid pressure within the pericardial space is lower than the diastolic pressure of either ventricle and thus lower than atrial pressure. Transmural atrial and transmural ventricular diastolic pressures are therefore substantial, amounting to several mm Hg. Typically, if the intrapericardial pressure were −3 mm Hg and the left and

right ventricular diastolic pressures 8 mm Hg and 4 mm Hg, their transmural diastolic pressures would be 11 mm Hg and 7 mm Hg, respectively.

Contact pressure measured from an intrapericardial balloon, however, is not subatmospheric, but is close to right atrial pressure.[13,21,24] This similarity of intrapericardial pressure and intracavity pressure means that when contact pressure is taken as the pressure external to the heart, transmural right ventricular diastolic pressure is close to zero over a broad range of right ventricular volumes, a calculation that influences estimation of right ventricular function and diastolic compliance. Furthermore, inherent in the concept of diastolic heart failure is that this syndrome may reflect reduced left ventricular diastolic compliance. Compliance is the change of volume resulting from a change of transmural pressure, but the transmural diastolic pressure of the left ventricle is appreciably less if pericardial pressure is taken to be the same as right atrial pressure, rather than subatmospheric. The difference becomes substantial in patients with right heart failure. Another basic difference from conventionally measured pressure is that contact pressure is not necessarily uniform around the heart.[25,26] Indeed, occlusion of one of the great arteries raises contact pressure over the ventricle that supplies it and lowers contact pressure over the opposite ventricle. Whether clinicians should consider pericardial constraint in terms of contact versus conventionally measured pressure is, to my mind, not settled. Before relegating conventional intrapericardial pressure to the category of an artifact, one should take into account that it is highly reproducible in magnitude and waveform in a large variety of animals, including humans, and that it increases appropriately in response to acute expansion of cardiac volume (Fig. 7.3) and to changes in external pressure such as the strain phase of a Valsalva maneuver, or when the hepatojugular reflux is elicited (Fig. 7.11). Finally, one should recall that transmural pressure represents distending force and thus determines preload. It is not easy to conceive that the right ventricle does not require a distending force of several mm Hg.[27,28]

A shift of the entire ventricular diastolic pressure-volume curve in response to volume loading or the administration of venodilating agents has been cited as evidence that pericardial constraint may be called into play when cardiac volume is rapidly increased by a substantial amount. In 1964 it was observed that the hemodynamics of subacute mitral regurgitation caused by rupture of the chordae tendinea bore a striking resemblance to those of constrictive pericarditis.[9] The authors posited that acute massive dilation of the left heart was prevented by the pericardium which, in consequence, exerted a greatly exaggerated restraint on all cardiac chambers. In these patients, right atrial, left atrial, and left ventricular diastolic pressures were equal.

FIGURE 7.11. **A**: Tracing made during cardiac catheterization of a patient who had a pericardial catheter in place for prior aspiration of pericardial effusion. During the strain phase of a Valsalva maneuver, pericardial and right atrial pressures are raised to 17 mm Hg. Upon release of the strain, both pressures dropped, the pericardial pressure falling below right atrial pressure. **B**: Superior vena caval pressure and blood flow velocity. Pressure is increased by the external force applied to elicit the hepatojugular reflux, but velocity is unchanged.

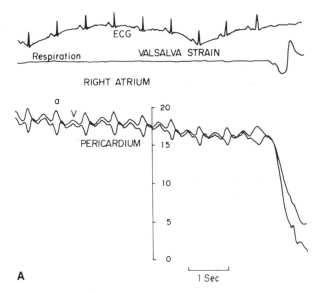

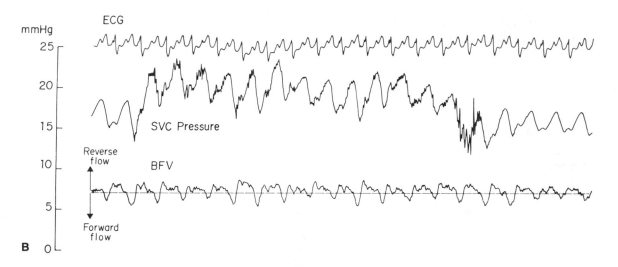

Furthermore, a dip and plateau configuration of ventricular diastolic pressures and a prominent y descent of atrial pressures were recorded in these patients, so that the hemodynamics mimicked constrictive pericarditis. This hemodynamic picture differs from that of chronic mitral regurgitation without right heart failure, in which the pericardium has had time to adapt to chronic stretch. Then, the left atrium and left ventricle dilate and their diastolic pressures fall, although not necessarily to normal. Therefore, in chronic mitral regurgitation, left ventricular diastolic pressure exceeds right, and neither ventricular diastolic pressure exhibits a dip and plateau configuration. Late in the course of mitral regurgitation, during episodes of acute right and left ventricular failure, the hemodynamics may again simulate constrictive pericarditis.

Equalization (tracking) of left and right ventricular diastolic pressures, especially during inspiration, at which time right heart volume is maximized, has been noted in the study of patients with heart failure of various etiologies and attributed to pericardial restraint.[29]

Exercise

The studies described so far were carried out with the patients or subjects lying at rest on a table. Data on how the volume of the individual cardiac chambers changes during the performance of upright exercise are difficult to come by, although it is generally agreed that left ventricular diastolic volumes increase and that increased stroke volume occurs more as a consequence of the Frank-Starling mechanism than of decreased end-systolic volume. It is likely that the failing left ventricle would dilate earlier, or to a greater extent, than the normal left ventricle. Janicki et al.[30] sought evidence for the development of pericardial restraint on cardiac volume in patients with heart failure performing upright exercise. Their hypothesis was that when the heart engaged the pericardium, the rate of rise of pulmonary wedge pressure would be the same as that of right atrial pressure and from that point on, stroke volume would fail to increase as exercise progressed. Thus, they sought the development of a hemodynamic response to exercise in patients with heart failure that would be highly comparable to that of patients with constrictive pericarditis. With left heart failure in the absence of pericardial constraint, one would anticipate a much steeper rise in pulmonary wedge pressure than in right atrial pressure and that the stroke volume would increase, although considerably less than in normal subjects. When Janicki et al.[30] analyzed their data, they found that their patients could be placed into three groups. In one, during the early stages of exercise, pulmonary wedge pressure rose steeply, right atrial pressure rose little if at all, and stroke volume increased; but when patients in this group continued to exercise, the higher workloads were characterized by the anticipated equal slopes of pulmonary arterial wedge and right atrial pressure increase. Coincident with the abrupt change in the relationship between the slopes of left and right atrial pressure rise, the previously increasing stroke volume became fixed. In another group, this evidence of pericardial restraint could be demonstrated throughout the whole exercise period; that is, right atrial and pulmonary wedge pressures rose equally from the beginning to the end of exercise, and stroke volume failed to increase at any stage of exercise. In the third group, evidence for pericardial restraint never appeared. In these patients, the slope of rise of pulmonary wedge pressure always exceeded that of right atrial pressure and stroke volume never became invariant. Which of these three patterns of response to exercise would be manifest failed to correlate with a number of the usual parameters used to assess the magnitude of left ventricular dysfunction and the severity of exercise impairment in patients with heart failure. In our laboratory we routinely measure right heart and systemic arterial pressures, arteriovenous oxygen difference, and expired air volume and gas content in patients considered for cardiac transplantation and in patients in whom it is difficult to assign dyspnea to a cardiac or pulmonary etiology. We have yet to encounter a patient in whom rate of rise of right atrial and pulmonary wedge pressures was the same.[31] Further information concerning the development of pericardial constraint during exercise in patients with heart failure may be forthcoming from the ongoing SOLVD study.

Evidence has been published for the development of pericardial constraint during the performance of treadmill exercise in normal experimental animals; that is, in the absence of heart failure. One of the most exciting such studies was that carried out by Stray-Gundersen et al.,[32] who reported that removing the pericardium from dogs allows them to achieve a 25% increase in

their maximum exercising cardiac output and oxygen consumption. We have confirmed this observation for the pig,[33] demonstrating a similar increase in both parameters. Our studies also showed that in the weeks after pericardiectomy, a progressive increase in left ventricular end-diastolic volume takes place and that furthermore, its pressure/volume relationship is shifted to the right along the volume axis. We could find no evidence for a decreased end-systolic volume, indicating that in normal animals, the enhanced cardiac performance does not result from increased contractility, as would be anticipated, but as would be anticipated from implementation of the Frank-Starling mechanism via increased left ventricular end-diastolic volume. Confirming the importance of the Frank-Starling mechanism after pericardiectomy, our study showed that for any given workload, the heart rate after pericardiectomy was lower than with the pericardium intact. Currently, we are using paced tachycardia-induced heart failure in pigs to determine the time course of pericardial restraint as cardiac size increases progressively and then returns to normal after cessation of pacing.

In summary, it is fair to state that pericardial restraint of cardiac volume is apt to become manifest in patients with heart failure. This constraint may be evident with the patient supine at rest, particularly in the presence of acute cardiac dilatation. One of its principal manifestations is downward displacement of the left ventricular diastolic-volume curve in response to reducing cardiac volume by means of venodilator treatment. In some patients, pericardial restraint may develop during exercise and may be a contributing factor to impaired cardiac performance during exercise. On the other hand, the pericardium may play a beneficial role in preventing excessive dilatation of the heart. Not surprisingly, these observations have given rise to the idea that in patients with severe end-stage heart failure who were not suitable for cardiac transplantation, pericardiectomy may be of benefit. However, most clinicians would oppose taking such a drastic step without stronger evidence that it would be beneficial, and indeed there are only a few anecdotal reports of patients with heart failure subjected to pericardiectomy in an attempt to alleviate symptoms of heart failure.

Compressive, Constrictive, and Restrictive Heart Disease

Excessive restraint of cardiac volume exerted by the pericardium may result from disease of the pericardium itself rather than from enlargement of the heart. Cardiac tamponade is a disorder in which venous return and ventricular diastolic filling are impeded by pericardial fluid under increased pressure compressing the cardiac chambers.[34] Circulation cannot be maintained for long if pericardial pressure exceeds pulmonary venous and systemic venous pressures. Therefore, these venous pressures reflexly rise to meet any pathological increase in pericardial pressure. Cardiac tamponade is fatal when pericardial pressure rises to a degree that cannot be met by an equal increase in the venous pressures.

Cardiac Tamponade

Although, as we have seen, controversy exists regarding the value of normal pericardial pressure and how it should be measured, from the clinical point of view, normal pericardial pressure can be regarded as between 2 and 3 mm Hg subatmospheric to 3 and 4 mm Hg above atmospheric, depending on whether it is measured with a conventional catheter transducer device, or with a flat unstressed balloon placed between the heart and pericardium. When fluid accumulates in the pericardial space, pericardial pressure increases. The extent of this increase in intrapericardial pressure depends on the volume of effusion and whether fluid accumulates slowly or rapidly in the pericardial space. In either case, systemic venous pressure increases and equilibrates with the intrapericardial pressure. Thus, even in its early stages, because of increased venous pressure, cardiac tamponade may simulate cardiac failure. When cardiac tamponade becomes severe, the increase in intrapericardial and venous pressures becomes quite substantial. Moderate cardiac tamponade is characterized by pressures in the range of 10 to 15 mm Hg and severe cardiac tamponade by pressures in the range of 20 to 30 mm Hg. At these higher pressures, cardiac volume is significantly compressed and, in consequence, stroke volume falls (Fig. 7.12). The heart rate increases in an attempt to sustain cardiac output. Finally, in the most advanced stages of cardiac tamponade, blood pressure falls. By this time, the patient is dyspneic, fatigued, and frequently anuric. The reader will appreciate that the clinical picture of cardiac tamponade has many features in common with cardiac failure. However, it must be emphasized that in cardiac tamponade, the ventricles are unloaded rather than overloaded and that in the vast majority of cases systolic function is entirely normal, indeed usually hyperkinetic.[35] Thus, although circulatory failure characterizes cardiac tamponade, the patient emphatically does not have heart failure. The distinction is important in understanding the pathophysiology of cardiac tamponade and thus its therapy.

Acute (Surgical) Cardiac Tamponade

Classical acute cardiac tamponade arises when blood accumulates rapidly in the pericardial space of a patient who does not have preexisting heart disease of any kind.[36] The normal pericardium, while it can stretch in

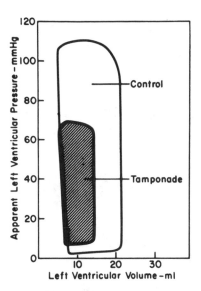

FIGURE 7.12. Pressure volume loops before and after experimental cardiac tamponade in a dog. (Apparent pressure means absolute, i.e., not transmural, pressure.) Note the elevated ventricular diastolic pressure and the reduction in end-diastolic volume and stroke volume. End-systolic volume is normal. Reprinted with permission from Craig et al. Pressure and volume changes of the left ventricle in acute pericardial tamponade. *Am J Cardiol.* 1968;22:65–74.

response to chronic strain such as that associated with normal growth, slowly developing cardiac enlargement or slowly accumulating pericardial effusion, is highly resistant to acute stretch by virtue of the nature of its pressure-volume curve. Thus, in acute cardiac tamponade such as may develop from a stab or bullet wound of the heart or from major blunt trauma, a relatively small volume of pericardial hemorrhage results in the rapid development of high pericardial pressure and severe cardiac tamponade. Severe acute cardiac tamponade also may develop in consequence of rupture into the pericardial space of an acute myocardial infarction or of an aortic aneurysm or dissecting hematoma, but here, the clinical picture may be modified by the preexisting cardiovascular disease.

The venous pressure in such patients is extremely elevated. Despite this elevation, and in contradistinction to many cases of heart failure, careful inspection of the jugular venous pressure reveals a small decline during inspiration. It also can be noted that the y descent of venous pressure is absent. This phenomenon occurs because, while cardiac tamponade is present throughout the cardiac cycle, it is least severe when cardiac volume is minimal; that is, during rapid ventricular ejection. Venous return to the heart therefore is limited to systole. Venous return in normal subjects is biphasic, with a peak coincident with the x descent of venous pressure and another peak coincident with its y descent[37] (Fig.

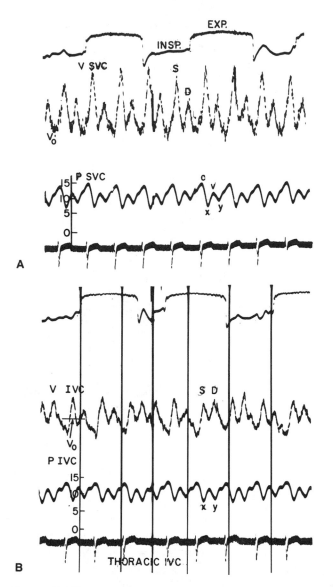

FIGURE 7.13. **A**: Blood flow velocity and pressure in the superior vena cava. Velocity was measured by an electromagnetic catheter tip transducer in the superior vena cava of a patient with mild congestive heart failure. V_0 indicates zero flow. VSVC and PSVC are velocity and pressure respectively in the superior vena cava. The dominant peak (S) is systolic and corresponds with the x descent of pressure. The second and smaller peak (D) corresponds with the y trough. **B**: Pressure and flow in the inferior vena cava of the same patient. Systolic and diastolic velocity peaks corresponding with x and y pressure troughs again are evident.

7.13). In cardiac tamponade, filling is confined to the period of ventricular ejection; therefore, no y descent is present.[38] At the bedside, it usually is a simple matter to distinguish the x descent of venous pressure from the y. The x descent is synchronous with the carotid pulse, whereas the y descent is out of phase with the carotid pulse. The distinction may not be easy in the most

severe cases when tachycardia and tachypnea are prominent.

Examination of the pulse reveals tachycardia and pulsus paradoxus. Pulsus paradoxus, despite its name, is not truly a paradoxical phenomenon, but rather an exaggeration of a normal phenomenon, a decline in arterial pressure during inspiration. In cardiac tamponade, this decline is much greater than normal and often is so pronounced that pulsus paradoxus is detected easily as a diminution in the amplitude of the pulse during inspiration. In the most severe cases, the pulse actually disappears altogether during inspiration. The term pulsus paradox was coined to describe the paradox of an apparently regular heart beat but an irregular pulse.[39,40]

The magnitude of pulsus paradoxus can be assessed by careful sphygmomanometry. The blood pressure cuff is inflated in the usual way several mm Hg higher than the level that renders the radial or brachial pulse impalpable throughout the respiratory cycle. While watching or palpating the chest to ascertain the phase of respiration, the cuff is slowly deflated. At first, the Karatkoff sounds are audible only during expiration but are inaudible during inspiration. As the cuff is slowly and steadily deflated, a point arises where the sounds are audible throughout the respiratory cycle. The difference in systolic pressure from the reading at which the sounds first become audible and are confined to expiration, to the reading at which the sounds are audible throughout the respiratory cycle, is the measure of pulsus paradoxus. When the physician is attempting to quantify pulsus paradoxus in this manner, the patient should not be instructed to breathe deeply; rather, the measurement should be made without asking the patient to modify breathing in any way. When assessing pulsus paradoxus simply by palpation, the phenomenon can be enhanced by having the patient breathe deeply and slowly, but the examiner must be familiar with the extent of change that can occur with this maneuver in normal subjects. If pulsus paradoxus is not evident in the radial artery, it often can still be appreciated in larger vessels such as the femoral or carotid. When cardiac tamponade is extreme, hypotension, which can be quite profound, develops. Under these circumstances, pulsus paradoxus may be difficult or impossible to detect. Cardiac activity may be difficult to feel, although it is important to appreciate that this sign is not always present. In some cases a pericardial friction rub is present. Here it must be emphasized that, contrary to popular belief, a loud pericardial friction rub is perfectly consistent with the presence of a large pericardial effusion.

Subacute and Chronic (Medical) Tamponade

Cardiac tamponade may develop in response to an accumulation of pericardial fluid that is considerably

FIGURE 7.14. Schema of hemodynamic changes during serial fluid withdrawals in a 22-year-old man with tamponade due to uremic pericarditis. Diagnostic levels of pulsus paradoxus persist as long as left ventricular end-diastolic pressure is equilibrated with pericardial pressure. Reprinted with permission from Reddy et al. Cardiac tamponade: hemodynamic observations in man. *Circulation*. 1978;58:265–272. Copyright by the American Heart Association.

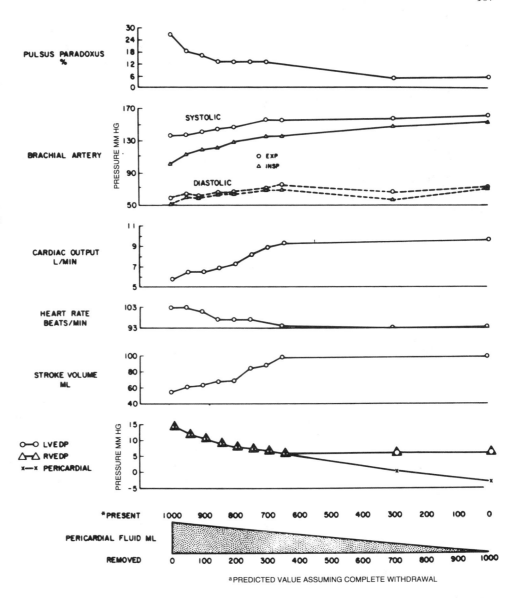

less rapid than the hemorrhagic pericardial effusions described in the preceding paragraphs. With the more gradual accumulation of pericardial fluid, the pericardium has more chance to accommodate. Pericardial pressure therefore rises more slowly, giving the pericardial effusion a chance to become larger.[41] Moderate pericardial effusion may occur in a matter of days or weeks. The severity of cardiac tamponade of this type varies from mild and barely detectable to severe and is a function of the size of the effusion and the speed of its development. Thus, in its early stages, the venous pressure may be elevated only to 5 to 8 mm Hg and the y descent may be attenuated rather than abolished. Blood pressure is well maintained, tachycardia may not be prominent, and even pulsus paradoxus may be absent in these milder forms of cardiac tamponade.

It should be apparent to the reader that cardiac tamponade cannot be defined by any particular level of pericardial pressure, but ranges from mild when the pericardial pressure is only 5 to 10 mm Hg, to moderate with a pericardial pressure in the range of 10 to 15 mm Hg, and severe when the pericardial pressure exceeds 15 mm Hg. For practical purposes, cardiac tamponade can be said to begin when pericardial pressure has risen to a value exceeding normal right atrial pressure. When this event occurs, right atrial and pericardial pressures are equal.[42] If cardiac tamponade worsens, right atrial and pericardial pressures rise equally and thus continue to be identical (Fig. 7.14). Eventually, these pressures rise to equal the left atrial and pulmonary wedge pressures. At this point in the development of cardiac tamponade, pressure in both atria, the diastolic pressure in both ventricles, the pulmonary wedge pressure, and the pulmonary arterial diastolic pressure equilibrate with the pericardial pressure. If cardiac tamponade continues to worsen, these equal pressures continue to rise and remain equal to each other. When medical cardiac tamponade becomes severe, its picture comes more and more to simulate that of surgical cardiac tamponade, although it must be recognized that in some of the patients, preexisting heart disease exists and therefore the cardiac chambers may be enlarged despite the presence of cardiac tamponade.

Etiology

Virtually any disorder of the pericardium can cause pericardial effusion and pericardial effusion of virtually any etiology can be the cause of cardiac tamponade. In medical patients in whom the differential diagnosis between cardiac tamponade and cardiac failure is most apt to apply, common etiologies include idiopathic or viral pericarditis including recurrent pericarditis, neoplasm, particularly bronchogenic and mammary carcinoma and lymphoma, renal dialysis, ionizing radiation, tuberculous pericarditis, and AIDS.[43]

Diagnosis

The key to diagnosis is a high index of suspicion that cardiac tamponade rather than cardiac failure may be the cause of dyspnea and elevated venous pressure, especially when there is, or has been, evidence of acute pericarditis or of a disorder likely to affect the pericardium. This suspicion is strengthened when clinical examination fails to reveal a murmur, third heart sound, or other evidence of cardiac disease, particularly when there is no apparent etiology for heart failure. Sometimes the diagnosis is first suggested by the appearance of cardiomegaly on a chest radiogram, particularly when a previous radiogram showing normal heart size is available. In contradistinction to congestive heart failure, the radiogram usually does not show the degree of pulmonary congestion anticipated in heart failure. However, in patients with heart failure with consequent dilatation of the right ventricle and tricuspid valve ring, pulmonary congestion may be minimal because the tricuspid incompetence provides a low impedance leak, preventing much of the right ventricular output from reaching the lung.

The electrocardiogram usually shows nothing more than nonspecific ST and T changes, although sometimes the characteristic widespread ST segment elevation characteristic of acute pericarditis may still be present. QRS voltage may be low, and in extreme cases, electrical alternans may be seen.[44] This phenomenon has been attributed to swinging of the heart within the pericardial fluid. Echocardiography in these cases shows excessive movement of the anterior wall and abnormal motion of the posterior wall, and most importantly, apparently congruous motion of the anterior and posterior walls of the heart during part of the cardiac cycle. In addition to translation, rotation occurs.[44,45] Feigenbaum et al. have suggested that cardiac displacement is so great that the heart cannot return to its original position before the beginning of the next cardiac cycle, so that the heart begins its next depolarization in a slightly altered physical position.[46] The following systolic contraction produces less displacement and the heart therefore returns to its original starting position. A large pericardial effusion apparently frees the heart from the constraints imposed by the lungs and the mediastinum, allowing it to rotate about its fixed attachments. Usually, cardiac motion within the pericardial sac has the same frequency as the heart rate, but when cardiac tamponade develops, cardiac motion becomes a fraction (usually $\frac{1}{2}$) of the heart rate.

The determinants of the frequency of cardiac motion in cardiac tamponade have not been fully determined, but they include the basic heart rate, the pressure in the pericardial fluid, the viscosity of the fluid, and its volume. The length of the arc along which the heart can move in systole is related to the volume of the pericardial effusion. If the arc length is less than the distance the heart can travel in one cardiac cycle, the frequency of cardiac motion is equal to the heart rate; if, on the other hand, arc length is longer, the frequency becomes a fraction of the heart rate.[44] Recently, a nonlinear dynamic model of electrical alternans in pericardial effusion and cardiac tamponade has been proposed.[47,48] A highly specific electrocardiographic sign of cardiac tamponade is alternation of the entire electrocardiogram, P, QRSST, and T. Like many other highly specific signs, this one is not sensitive.[49]

Echocardiography

It is seldom that recourse to the echocardiogram has to be had for the distinction between cardiac failure and cardiac tamponade. However, in atypical cases, the echocardiogram can be invaluable in this regard and in typical cases, the echocardiogram confirms the diagnosis by proving the presence of pericardial effusion, providing evidence of cardiac compression, and showing that heart disease is absent; for example, valvular abnormalities, global hypokinesis, chamber enlargement, and ventricular hypertrophy should not be evident in pure cardiac tamponade. In typical cases of cardiac tamponade, circumferential pericardial effusion is unequivocally demonstrated; in medical patients, the pericardial effusion usually is at least moderate in amount and often large. In acute surgical cardiac tamponade the effusion quite often is smaller, but nonetheless is unequivocal and usually global. The two most important echocardiographic signs of cardiac tamponade are right atrial compression[50] and right ventricular diastolic collapse.[51] The free wall of the right atrium is normally convex outward, but when it is compressed by pericardial fluid under increased pressure, the convexity straightens out and, in more severe cases, then becomes concave.[52] The geometry of the right ventricle is complex, so that it is often convenient to consider separately the inflow portion and the outflow portion. The M mode nicely demonstrates narrowing of the right ventricular outflow tract, an observation that was made before the advent of two-dimensional echocardiography.[53] The two-dimensional study shows that during early diastole, the cavity of the right ventricular outflow tract is narrowed. In the more severe cases, this narrowing is severe.[54,55] Furthermore, the more intense the cardiac tamponade, the longer the duration of right ventricular diastolic collapse. The subcostal and four chamber views, but sometimes the parasternal short axis view in the case of the right ventricle, usually are the optimal projections for evaluating right atrial compression and right ventricular diastolic collapse.[55]

It has been appreciated by physiologists and clinicians alike that the manifestations of cardiac tamponade are more profound when there is accompanying hypovolemia. In experimental cardiac tamponade produced in the intact canine model, it has been shown that right atrial compression, right ventricular diastolic collapse, hypotension, and low cardiac output all develop at lesser volumes of pericardial fluid and lower values of intrapericardial pressure when the dogs are rendered hypovolemic.[56] On the other hand, hypervolemia delays these manifestations of cardiac tamponade.[56]

In the final stages of cardiac tamponade, venous pressure cannot rise to meet the challenge of the increased intrapericardial pressure. Additionally, it has been suggested that extreme elevation of intrapericardial pressure compresses the epicardial coronary arteries, thereby adding myocardial ischemia to the burden of the failing circulation,[57] although these manifestations really exemplify the modus exitus in the final stages of cardiac tamponade. In other circumstances, however, the echocardiogram is invaluable as a means of confirming the presence of cardiac tamponade and the absence of heart failure. Thus, in typical cases, all cardiac valves appear normal in structure, although in elderly patients thickening of the aortic valve leaflets should not deter clinicians from making the diagnosis of cardiac tamponade. Significant stenosis of any valve is absent in all cases of typical cardiac tamponade. Likewise, one should not expect to encounter more than physiological regurgitation at any of the valve orifices. Reduced size of the left ventricle can give rise to pseudo-prolapse of the mitral valve. All the cardiac chambers are either normal or reduced in dimensions and ventricular wall thickness is either normal or slightly increased. Global systolic function of both ventricles usually is hyperkinetic but may be normal. Severely reduced systolic function usually indicates cardiac failure rather than cardiac tamponade as the cause of circulatory failure, although rarely it may indicate that a patient with severe cardiac tamponade is in extremis. Minor regional wall motion abnormality may be

observed, but is seldom sufficient to cause the clinician to give serious consideration to the diagnosis of cardiac failure secondary to ischemic heart disease. Exaggerated respiratory variation in the dimension of the ventricles as observed by M mode is a characteristic feature of cardiac tamponade.[58,59] During inspiration, enlargement of the right ventricular dimension and diminution of that of the left ventricle is seen to be a function of inspiratory curving of the interventricular septum causing it to bulge into the left ventricular cavity.[60] Doppler examination shows an abnormal increase in respiratory variation in aortic and pulmonary arterial blood flow velocity.[61] Doppler interrogation of venous flow confirms a large inspiratory increase in systemic venous return and decrease in pulmonary venous return. Abnormal respiratory variation in venous return and blood flow velocity in the great vessels appears early[62] and can be demonstrated before the advent of right atrial compression and right ventricular diastolic collapse, and certainly before pulsus paradoxus and the development of hypotension.

Cardiac Catheterization

Thoughtful clinical evaluation and satisfactory quality echocardiography almost always can establish the diagnosis of cardiac tamponade beyond reasonable doubt. Therefore, it is seldom necessary to perform cardiac catheterization simply to make the diagnosis of cardiac tamponade. However, right heart catheterization and monitoring of arterial blood pressure constitute an integral part of pericardiocentesis. It is standard clinical practice to confirm the presence of cardiac tamponade at the time of contemplated or actual pericardiocentesis by documenting the appropriate hemodynamic changes. In more complex cases, the procedure is done to evaluate complicating cardiac abnormalities. In this situation, both left and right heart cardiac catheterization, usually with coronary arteriography and ventriculography, is carried out. The crux of the diagnosis is equalization of relatively low pressures. It is therefore critically important that all pressure transducers be at the same height and that their calibration be identical. The right atrial pressure is elevated, the magnitude of the elevation depending on the severity of cardiac tamponade. In all but the mildest cases, the x descent is prominent, but the y descent is replaced by an upsloping wave that persists until the next a wave.[63] Systolic pulmonary hypertension in the absence of complicating pulmonary or cardiac disease is modest, usually around 40 mm Hg.[35] The right ventricular diastolic pressure is elevated to the same extent as the right atrial pressure and does not have a dip and plateau configuration[35] (Fig. 7.15). When the catheter is advanced to the pulmonary artery, it is observed that the pulmonary arterial diastolic pressure is equal to the right atrial pressure. The pul-

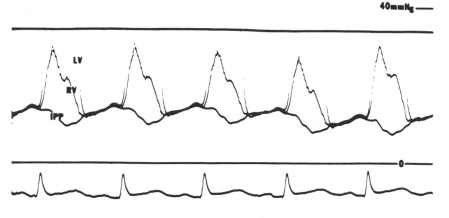

FIGURE 7.15. Ventricular pressure in a patient with cardiac tamponade. Simultaneous pressure recordings from the pericardium, right ventricle, and left ventricle in a patient with cardiac tamponade. The ventricular pressures were recorded by a catheter-mounted transducer. The two ventricular diastolic pressures and the pericardial pressure are elevated to approximately 15 mm Hg. No early ventricular diastolic dip of pressure or plateau of mid and late pressures is present. Reprinted with permission from Reddy et al. Cardiac tamponade: hemodynamic observations in man. *Circulation*. 1978;58:265–272. Copyright by the American Heart Association.

monary wedge tracing shows a pressure within 1 or 2 mm Hg of right atrial pressure. The pulmonary arterial wedge pressure tracing often is difficult to distinguish from the pulmonary arterial pressure tracing in patients with severe cardiac tamponade. Inspiration may cause a larger decline in pulmonary wedge pressure than in right atrial pressure so that equilibration between these two pressures may not be tight throughout the respiratory cycle (Fig. 7.16). The nature of the pressure tracing recorded from a systemic artery depends on the severity of cardiac tamponade. In mild cardiac tamponade, the tracing appears normal. In more severe tamponade, pulsus paradoxus characterized by an inspiratory decline in peak systolic pressure of at least 10 mm Hg and a significant reduction in pulse pressure is recorded. In the more severe cases, hypotension also is present. Stroke volume is greatly diminished, but the

reduction in cardiac output is partially offset by compensatory tachycardia.

When pericardiocentesis is to be carried out, the right heart catheter is withdrawn to the right atrium. As soon as the pericardial cavity has been entered, and before a significant amount of fluid has been aspirated, pericardial and right atrial pressures should be recorded simultaneously on equisensitive scales. The tracings are found to be virtually superimposable unless there is complicating right heart disease, pulmonary hypertension, or atypical localized cardiac tamponade. During inspiration a drop in both pericardial and right atrial pressure is observed. If a Cournand or similar catheter is employed instead of a balloon flotation catheter, it is impossible to engage the tip of the catheter against the apparent edge of the right atrium, as can easily be done when the pericardium is normal. The tip of the catheter

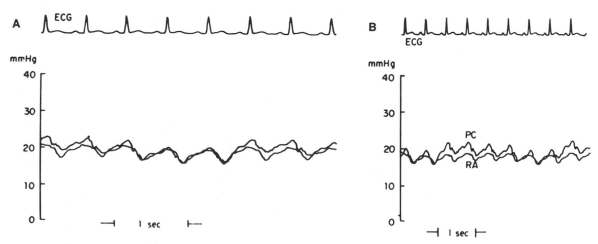

FIGURE 7.16. Tracings obtained during cardiac catheterization of a patient with severe cardiac tamponade. **A**: Right atrial and pericardial pressures are elevated to 20 mm Hg and are

virtually superimposable. **B**: The pulmonary capillary wedge pressure equilibrates with the right atrial, but does so more closely when the pressures are lower (inspiration).

in patients with pericardial effusion is separated from the edge of the cardiopericardial silhouette by the width of the pericardial effusion. If angiocardiography is carried out, straightening or concavity of the right atrium is demonstrated.[52] The optimal projection for evaluating this sign is the mild right anterior oblique. As contrast passes through the circulation, the hyperdynamic action of the ventricles during systole provides a striking contrast to the inactivity of the rest of the cardiopericardial silhouette.

Cardiac Tamponade in the Presence of Preexisting Heart Disease

Increasingly, the practice of internal medicine, especially in hospitalized patients, deals with the geriatric population. For this reason, a number of patients who have cardiac tamponade, particularly secondary to bronchogenic or mammary carcinoma, may have developed heart disease before the advent of pericardial effusion. The preexisting heart disease is commonly of ischemic or hypertensive origin, but cases with preexisting cardiomyopathy, congenital heart disease, or cor pulmonale also are encountered. Also, one may find cardiac tamponade in patients with coexisting pericardial and cardiac disease such as may occur in myopericarditis or AIDS and in patients recovering from cardiac transplantation or pulmonary endarterectomy for chronic pulmonary emboli.[64] Chronic renal disease, which in the present era often means patients undergoing chronic hemodialysis, is an important cause of cardiac tamponade in individuals who may have serious left ventricular dysfunction or cardiac failure due to a combination of adverse factors including hypertension, coronary artery disease, iatrogenic shunt, anemia, and if that debatable entity truly exists, uremic cardiomyopathy.[65] In cases of this kind, it is apparent that the clinical, electrocardiographic, radiographic, echocardiographic, and hemodynamic findings may be quite different from those found in patients with uncomplicated cardiac tamponade.

It was pointed out several years ago that preexisting left ventricular disease in which left ventricular end-diastolic pressure is severely elevated results in modification of the clinical picture of cardiac tamponade.[42] For example, if in a case of chronic renal disease with hypertension, the left ventricular end-diastolic pressure were elevated to 25 mm Hg and the right ventricular end-diastolic pressure were little if at all elevated, the advent of cardiac tamponade would be heralded by equilibration of the right atrial, right ventricular diastolic and pericardial pressures, but not the left ventricular diastolic pressure, which would remain considerably higher. In such a case, pulmonary arterial systolic hypertension may be greater than the customary 40 mm Hg and the pulmonary arterial diastolic pressure may

be higher than the right atrial and pericardial pressures, owing to pulmonary vascular constriction or obliteration. Furthermore, the high diastolic pressure within the left ventricle would remove the required condition of equal diastolic compliance of the two ventricles imposed by cardiac tamponade uncomplicated by preexisting heart disease, and therefore pulsus paradoxus and abnormal bowing of the intraventricular septum toward the left ventricle during inspiration would not occur. In these cases, the chest radiogram may show more evidence of pulmonary congestion than is anticipated in the usual case of cardiac tamponade and the electrocardiogram may well show left ventricular hypertrophy, left bundle branch block, or evidence of prior myocardial infarction. By the same token, although the echocardiogram would confirm a large pericardial effusion, left ventricular hypertrophy, dilatation, or regional wall motion abnormality may well be apparent as well.

In cases with severe preexisting right heart failure, right atrial compression and right ventricular diastolic collapse would be prevented by the high right-sided intracardiac pressures; also pulmonary hypertension would be out of all proportion to that anticipated in ordinary cardiac tamponade. In this situation, increased intrapericardial pressure would equilibrate with left ventricular diastolic pressure and pulmonary wedge pressure long before it equilibrated with right atrial and right ventricular diastolic pressure. Once more, pulsus paradoxus would be prevented. Under these circumstances, left atrial compression and left ventricular diastolic collapse, rather than right, might be observed.

In cases where cardiac tamponade complicating preexisting cardiac disease is suspected, cardiac catheterization and angiography are indicated. Interpretation of the data requires a clear understanding of the hemodynamics of cardiac tamponade and how they are modified by preexisting disease of the left or right side of the heart, or combined left and right heart failure.

Atypical Cardiac Tamponade

So far, we have considered classical cardiac tamponade and the modifications of the characteristic picture that emerge when cardiac tamponade is superimposed on preexisting heart disease, especially ventricular dysfunction or congestive heart failure. We have seen that the diagnosis of typical cardiac tamponade in the absence of confounding preexisting heart disease is a relatively straightforward matter, requiring only that the physician keep in mind the possibility of cardiac tamponade even though tamponade is less common than circulatory embarrassment secondary to cardiac dysfunction. When cardiac tamponade supervenes on established heart disease, even experienced and skilled clinicians find it difficult to apportion laboratory and clinical abnormalities appropriately between the pericardial and cardiac pathology.

Failure to diagnose cardiac tamponade correctly may lead to death or severe incapacitation, an outcome that has resulted in successful malpractice suits against physicians and hospitals. If rupture of a myocardial infarction or the aorta into the pericardial space is wrongly diagnosed as cardiogenic shock or acute myocardial infarction, failure to aspirate the pericardium may be compounded by the prescription of anticoagulant or thrombolytic therapy with fatal consequences.

The pathophysiology of patients receiving hemodialysis who have a pericardial effusion can be extremely complex. High jugular venous pressure may be a sign of tamponade, fluid overload, cardiac failure, or any combination and in any proportion. Hypotension in these patients may be a sign of advanced cardiac tamponade or of fluid depletion resulting from excessive treatment, or a combination of both. Hypertension may mask severe cardiac tamponade. The absence of pressure equilibration on the two sides of the heart and of pulsus paradoxus already has been commented on.

Cardiac Tamponade Complicating Cardiac Surgery

Cardiac tamponade is an important complication of cardiac surgery and unfortunately it is frequently atypical in presentation and therefore recognition often is late. Of all forms of cardiac tamponade, that complicating a prior operation on the heart is the most commonly missed. One does not have to seek far to discover why this is so. Tamponade may occur early when the patient is still in the intensive care unit.[66,67] Under these circumstances, the diagnosis is missed less often than when tamponade occurs later, after the patient has been transferred to a regular surgical ward. Cardiac tamponade is only one of many causes of dyspnea, hypotension, tachycardia, oliguria, and raised venous pressure after cardiac operation. Among the other more common causes are included severe preexisting myocardial insufficiency, inadequate intraoperative myocardial preservation, intraoperative myocardial infarction, malfunction of a valvular prosthesis, pulmonary embolism, or infection. In the early postoperative days, the patient may still be ventilated artificially and multiple drugs usually are being administered intravenously. When significant left ventricular dysfunction with an increased end-diastolic pressure was present preoperatively, pulsus paradoxus in cardiac tamponade is absent even after the patient has been removed from a mechanical ventilator.

When a patient is not recovering at the anticipated speed after a cardiac operation, particularly when dyspnea and raised venous pressure are evident, it is important to keep in mind the possible diagnosis of cardiac tamponade. First, more common causes for slow recovery or deterioration are considered. The possibility of myocardial infarction or ischemia is evaluated by standard electrocardiographic and enzymatic techniques. In addition to bedside evidence of left ventricular function, such as pulmonary crepitations, a new cardiac murmur or third heart sound, left ventricular function can be assessed by echocardiography or radionuclide ventriculography. Unless a readily apparent cause of the patient's difficulties is rapidly established, cardiac tamponade must be considered and, in most cases, this possibility must be checked by echocardiography.[68] It is most important not to be lulled into a false sense of security by the knowledge that the surgeon did not close the pericardium at the end of the intracardiac procedure, because cardiac tamponade occurs just as readily in patients in whom the pericardium was left open as it does in those in whom it was closed. This phenomenon occurs because the mediastinum acts as a false pericardium, so that when bleeding into the mediastinum occurs, cardiac tamponade develops exactly as it would if the bleeding were all intrapericardial.[67]

If the patient has postoperative cardiac tamponade, the echo-Doppler study should not demonstrate marked deterioration of cardiac function or striking dilatation of any cardiac chamber. Likewise, no new stenosis or regurgitation at any native or replaced valve orifice should be seen. Furthermore, one would not anticipate new abnormalities of regional wall motion, save for the paradoxical motion of the interventricular septum that characterizes the echocardiogram after cardiac surgery under cardiopulmonary bypass.[69] On the other hand, if the correct diagnosis is cardiac tamponade, pericardial effusion should be visualized. However, especially in the cases that occur later postoperatively, the effusion may not be circumferential, but may be localized in front of or behind the heart.[70] Also, the appearances may be somewhat atypical owing to clotting. While it is true that chronic hemorrhagic pericardial effusion fails to clot, evidence of clotting often is found when the fluid is examined early; that is, before the blood has become defibrinated. Most cardiac surgeons have a low threshold for the diagnosis of cardiac tamponade, and are willing to take the patient back to the operating room to explore the pericardium and mediastinum whenever they suspect bleeding or cardiac tamponade. In the first 1 to 3 postoperative days, taking a patient back to the operating room for cardiac tamponade that is not confirmed when the chest is explored is, and should be, a far more common event than missing the diagnosis of cardiac tamponade. Early postoperative hemorrhagic tamponade is caused by active bleeding into the pericardium or mediastinum, a truly surgical event to which surgeons are trained to react promptly and appropriately.

In most medical centers, when patients are discharged from the intensive care unit, they receive considerably less supervision from senior skilled members of the cardiac surgical team, because these individuals are busy in the operating room, in the intensive care unit, and with more acute cardiological problems. Any cardiologist who has spent much time at a medical center with a busy cardiac surgical program knows that it is not an uncommon experience to discover patients who are convalescing from cardiac surgery, but not recovering at the expected rate. Examination of these patients frequently shows that they are dyspneic, have crepitations or rales in the lung fields, edema, tachycardia, and raised venous pressure. Most often, these findings are manifestations of reversible postoperative myocardial dysfunction, insufficient treatment especially with diuretics, and fluid overload. Treatment usually is straightforward. Investigation may disclose other significant problems, such as valvular dysfunction, but may suggest the possibility of cardiac tamponade, a diagnosis that always must be borne in mind in these particular circumstances. Whenever cardiac tamponade is a reasonable diagnostic possibility, it is essential to evaluate the patient by echocardiography. If pericardial effusion is absent, the diagnosis may safely be dismissed. If a pericardial effusion is present, the differential diagnosis rests between a benign low pressure postoperative pericardial effusion,[71] cardiac tamponade due to delayed bleeding with reactive effusion, and the postpericardiotomy syndrome. For the reasons discussed earlier, pulsus pardoxus, when present, is a useful diagnostic sign, but its absence certainly does not rule out the diagnosis of tamponade. Likewise, the echocardiogram may be atypical. Adhesions between the sternum and the anterior surface of the heart may prevent right atrial compression and right ventricular diastolic collapse.[72] The effusion may be loculated and contain fibrin strands. There may be a single loculated effusion or there may be a more widespread effusion divided into several loculi. These are the circumstances under which the diagnosis of cardiac tamponade most frequently is overlooked, or not made until pericardial pressure has become extremely high and the patient is in danger of cardiac arrest. All too often, the first pericardiocentesis in cases of this kind has been carried out in the course of an unsuccessful cardiopulmonary resuscitation attempt.

I can think of no more important example than that given in the preceding paragraph of the importance of correctly distinguishing between heart failure and cardiac tamponade. The manifestations of heart failure and cardiac tamponade in a patient 2 or 3 weeks after cardiac operation are frighteningly similar, yet the treatment and pathophysiology are totally different. Prolonged attempts to treat cardiac tamponade with diuretics and vasodilators may end tragically. Likewise, surgical exploration of a patient who has severe myocardial failure carries the risk of increased morbidity and even mortality. Careful clinical and echocardiographic assessment combined with a sound knowledge of the atypical nature of cardiac tamponade in postoperative patients usually ensures the correct diagnosis. However, when serious doubt remains, surgical exploration is fully justified; indeed, is mandated.

Other Forms of Atypical Cardiac Tamponade

Effusive constrictive pericarditis is a syndrome[73] that will be discussed after the description of constrictive pericarditis. Low pressure cardiac tamponade[74] is tamponade occurring without major elevation of left and right ventricular diastolic pressures (Fig. 7.17) and must

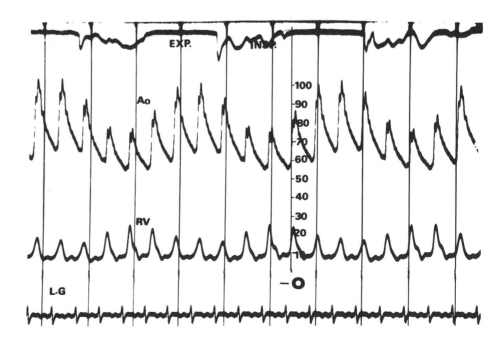

FIGURE 7.17. Low pressure cardiac tamponade: tracings from above down; the phase of respiration, the aortic pressure, right ventricular pressure, and the electrocardiogram. Note that although mild hypotension and severe pulsus paradoxus have developed, the right ventricular diastolic pressure is relatively low at 10 mm Hg. Note also absence of a dip and plateau configuration of right ventricular diastolic pressure. Reprinted with permission from Shabetai R., et al. Pulsus paradoxus. *Clin Invest.* 1965;44: 1882–1898. Copyright by the American Heart Association.

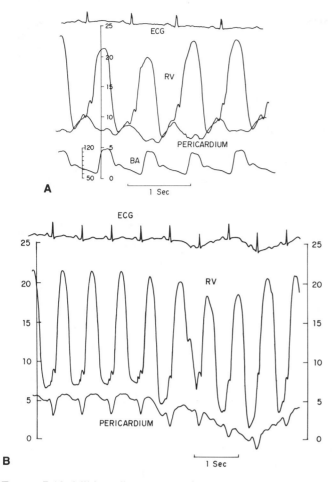

FIGURE 7.18. Mild cardiac tamponade. **A**: In comparison with low pressure cardiac tamponade illustrated in Fig. 7.17, the blood pressure is normal and pulsus paradoxus is absent. The left ventricular diastolic pressure is only slightly above normal, but cardiac tamponade is documented by the equalization of pericardial and right ventricular diastolic pressure. **B**: Tracings from the same patient after pericardiocentesis. The drop in right ventricular diastolic pressure is relatively modest, but there is now clear separation of pericardial from right ventricular diastolic pressure throughout the respiratory and cardiac cycles. Reprinted with permission from Shabetai R. *The Pericardium*. Philadelphia: Grune & Stratton; 1981.

be distinguished from mild or early cardiac tamponade, in which these pressures also are low (Fig. 7.18). Low pressure cardiac tamponade is severe cardiac tamponade in which only modest elevation of the left and right atrial or ventricular diastolic pressures is evident, when central blood volume is severely depleted from massive hemorrhage elsewhere or from overzealous diuretic treatment.

Treatment of Cardiac Tamponade

Whereas the major components of treatment of heart failure are to unload the heart with vasodilators and diuretics and perhaps to increase inotropy and baroreflex sensitivity with digitalis, the aims of treatment of cardiac tamponade are to restore or augment central blood volume and normal loading conditions. Removal of pericardial fluid is the correct treatment for most cases of cardiac tamponade. The fluid can be evacuated by pericardiocentesis or surgically, usually by the subxiphoid route. Which of these two routes is chosen depends to a large extent on the preferences and experience of the medical or surgical team in charge and, to some extent, the nature of the underlying illness. The surgical approach is preferable if there is need for a pericardial biopsy. Recently, pericardial drainage has been accomplished by what one may term percutaneous balloon pericardioplasty.[75] The rationale for this treatment is similar to that underlying creation of what is commonly but incorrectly called a pericardial window, and therefore has the same disadvantage, namely that the drainage site is not apt to remain open long term. The technique is therefore most applicable to patients with pericardial effusion that is not likely to recur. Another recent innovation is pericardioscopy,[76] a technique that is said to have utility in diagnosing the etiology of cardiac tamponade. However, the technique has not been widely employed; therefore its place, if any, remains to be established. Details of the technique of pericardiocentesis and subxiphoid pericardiotomy are beyond the scope of this chapter, which is to discuss the pericardium and its disorders in relation to heart failure.

Removal of pericardial effusion, while a standard treatment of cardiac tamponade, is not necessary in all cases. Mild cardiac tamponade that is not progressing may be observed carefully and fluid drainage postponed until evidence of increasing cardiac tamponade appears. In several such cases, fluid drainage is never required. Patients with acute idiopathic pericarditis frequently have an element of pericardial effusion that may be complicated by cardiac tamponade. If the tamponade is not severe, it is appropriate to place the patient on antiinflammatory therapy and observe closely for signs of regression or progression of cardiac tamponade. In the former case, removal of pericardial fluid is not warranted, either for diagnosis or treatment.[77]

Constrictive Pericarditis

Severe acute cardiac tamponade by virtue of tachycardia, dyspnea, hypotension, and raised venous pressure in some cases simulates acute left ventricular failure, and in others cardiogenic shock. Subacute cardiac tamponade, at least until the late stages, can simulate heart failure. In contrast, constrictive pericarditis frequently presents a clinical syndrome that can easily be mistaken for congestive heart failure.[78] The leading symptoms in the two conditions are the same: exertional dyspnea, fatigue, swelling, and palpitation. Also, many of the physical findings in patients with constrictive pericarditis are the same as those that characterize heart failure: raised jugular venous pressure, sinus tachycardia or atrial fibrillation, edema, hepatic enlargement, an early diastolic third heart sound, and hypotension. It is not surprising, therefore, that before constrictive pericarditis is recognized and treated, many cases are thought to have, and are treated for, congestive heart failure. Although hemodynamically, pulmonary venous and systemic venous pressures are elevated equally, clinically, systemic congestion often dominates and therefore the patient may be misdiagnosed as having severe right heart failure. Just as it is critically important to distinguish cardiac tamponade from heart failure, it is imperative to distinguish between heart failure and constrictive pericarditis, because the pathophysiology of the two conditions is diametrically opposed and the long-term treatment plan is radically different.

Dyspnea is a common complaint, but the usual presenting complaints are gain in weight, leg edema, and frequently increase in abdominal girth.[79] Examination rapidly confirms dyspnea, edema, and ascites. Furthermore, the liver is found to be considerably enlarged and sometimes tender. Hepatic pulsations, synchronous with the jugular pulse (Fig. 7.19), are readily seen and felt unless ascites is tense. This evidence of congestion may lead the physician to consider the diagnosis of cirrhosis of the liver and therefore to search for spider angiomata and jaundice. The search is quite commonly rewarded by finding both. The physician is now ready to confirm the diagnosis of hepatic cirrhosis and may order liver function studies; the results show an increase in the plasma concentration of bilirubin and hepatic enzymes. At this point, the diagnosis appears to be clinched, although on occasion, physicians order a hepatic biopsy and the biopsy has been read as confirming the clinical diagnosis of cirrhosis of the liver. The reader will readily appreciate the omission of any mention of the jugular venous pressure. Unfortunately, this omission may still occur in clinical practice. Had the venous pressure been evaluated when assessing severe systemic congestion and hepatic dysfunction, the diagnosis of primary liver disease would not have been made, but it would have been immediately apparent that the patient was suffering either from cardiac disease or pericardial disease. At that stage, the physician would begin to undertake the task of distinguishing between heart failure, tricuspid valve disease, and constrictive pericarditis. This differentiation would include right heart failure secondary to left heart failure, cor pulmonale, or less commonly a congenital malformation of the heart, the most likely congenital abnormality being atrial septal defect with pulmonary hypotension. Less common malformations causing right-heart failure in adults are Eisenmenger physiology associated with a large ven-

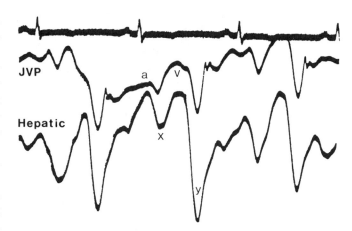

FIGURE 7.19. Simultaneous recordings of the jugular venous pulse (*JVP*) and hepatic pulsations in a patient with severe constrictive pericarditis. Reprinted with permission from Manga et al. Pulsatile hepatomegaly in constrictive pericarditis. *Br Heart J.* 1984;52:465–467.

tricular septal defect, a large atrial septal defect, or a large patent arterial duct.

In most patients with heart failure, which is best defined as symptomatic ventricular dysfunction, there is either intrinsic myocardial abnormality, or the ventricular chambers are subject to increased volume or pressure load, or both, and there is a myocardial abnormality causing systolic or diastolic ventricular dysfunction, or more usually a combination of the two. In the vast majority of cases of constrictive pericarditis, on the other hand, intrinsic myocardial function is normal,[78] but diastolic filling is impeded by the diseased pericardium. In constrictive pericarditis, pulmonary and systemic congestion, tachycardia, and low cardiac output are the results, not of heart failure, but of unloading the heart.

Combined systolic and diastolic ventricular dysfunction characterizes most cases of heart failure, but in some cases impaired systolic pumping predominates, whereas in others ventricular diastolic dysfunction, represented by strikingly increased ventricular diastolic pressure, dominates. Thus, ventricular diastolic dysfunction sufficient to produce severe pulmonary and systemic congestion is not the sole prerogative of constrictive pericarditis, but may occur in patients with what has been called diastolic heart failure.[80–83] The ability to assess left ventricular diastolic pressure and the rate and pattern of diastolic filling using noninvasive techniques has increased awareness of diastolic heart failure and has forced cardiologists to recognize that a significant proportion of patients with heart failure have relatively well preserved systolic function but severe diastolic dysfunction. Most often the diagnosis is first made when a patient presents with the classical symptoms of heart failure, but in whom, while the chest radiogram confirms severe pulmonary congestion, radiographic cardiac size is hardly if at all increased. This combination of findings leads to measurement of left ventricular ejection fraction, which is found to be normal or much less impaired than would have been anticipated considering the degree of pulmonary congestion. Echo-Doppler studies then confirm that the pattern of left ventricular filling during diastole is abnormal. In many of these cases, the deceleration time is greatly shortened, indicating a high left ventricular diastolic pressure.

Severe long-standing constrictive pericarditis must be distinguished from chronic heart failure, a distinction that can almost always be made easily by careful clinical and noninvasive laboratory evaluation. More difficult can be distinguishing between constrictive pericarditis and restrictive cardiomyopathy because a restrictive pattern of ventricular filling is common to both.

Restrictive cardiomyopathy is defined as a primary or secondary disease of the myocardium that generates clinical and hemodynamic findings that closely mimic constrictive pericarditis. The most common systemic myocardial disease causing restrictive cardiomyopathy is cardiac amyloidosis.[84] Cardiac hemochromatosis, when severe enough to produce clinical manifestations, usually results in dilated heart failure,[85] but restrictive cardiomyopathy also may occur.[86] Restrictive cardiomyopathy also is a feature of the recently transplanted heart,[87] but the configuration and level of systemic and pulmonary venous pressures gradually return to normal, although rarely the abnormality is permanent. A restrictive pattern also has been described in some cases of acute myocarditis.[88,89]

It has been stated already that the restrictive pattern may develop secondary to increased pericardial restraint when enlargement occurs acutely. The example furnished by subacute mitral regurgitation due to prior rupture of the chordae tendinea already has been cited.[9] To this may be added subacute tricuspid regurgitation in some patients with carcinoid syndrome. A restrictive pattern of ventricular filling also can be observed after acute right ventricular myocardial infarction.[90] Here, the restrictive pattern is ascribed to acute dilatation of the right ventricle. In idiopathic restrictive cardiomyopathy, an abnormal degree of fibrosis may be present,[91] but in some cases no pathological substrate can be identified.[92]

Here, it is pertinent to define the term "restrictive pattern" as abnormally rapid early ventricular diastolic filling, with abnormally slow or absent mid- and late-diastolic filling. Restricted filling may be a consequence of constrictive pericarditis, impaired ventricular diastolic compliance, or abnormal constraint imposed by the normal pericardium on an acutely dilated heart.

Clinical Features of Constrictive Pericarditis

For a full description, the reader is referred to appropriate texts,[93] because the purpose of the present chapter is to discuss constrictive pericarditis in the light of congestive heart failure and the differential diagnosis between the two.

Pericardial disease of almost any etiology can lead to constrictive pericarditis. Several decades ago tuberculous pericarditis was the most common cause of constrictive pericarditis in the Western hemisphere. At present, tuberculosis is the cause of constrictive pericarditis in undeveloped countries, but is now an uncommon cause in the West. In the current era, common causes of constrictive pericarditis include neoplasm, radiation, collagen vascular disease, and trauma. A significant proportion of cases remain idiopathic despite intensive workup, but it is possible that some of these result from old tuberculous pericarditis. Rheumatoid arthritis is an important collagen vascular cause of constrictive pericarditis[94] often necessitating surgical treatment.[95] An important, although now fortunately an uncommon, cause of constrictive pericarditis is prior cardiac operation. In general, the constrictive pericarditis seen today is less chronic than it was in the era of chronic tuberculous constrictive pericarditis.

Pathology

The pericardium is increased in thickness from the normal 1 to 3 mm. In subacute constrictive pericarditis as frequently encountered today, the pericardium may increase to only 5 or 6 mm in thickness, but in the more chronic versions, pericardial thickness may exceed a centimeter. Most of the increased thickness is owing to dense fibrosis, but additionally, there may be calcification. Calcification was common in tuberculous constrictive pericarditis, but is seen much less commonly in today's spectrum of etiology.

Pathophysiology

The thickened fibrotic and sometimes calcified pericardium becomes virtually noncompliant and therefore sets a limit to end-diastolic volume. At end-systole when the heart is at minimal volume, restriction of cardiac volume is absent and remains so until the end of the first third of diastole.[35] Thereafter, ventricular filling becomes increasingly impeded and therefore diastolic pressure increases rapidly until filling ceases abruptly and ventricular volume remains constant for the remaining two thirds of diastole. That no filling occurs during the latter two thirds of diastole is commonly inferred in the laboratory by documenting failure of ventricular diastolic pressure to increase from the end of the early rapid filling period until the onset of the next systole (Fig. 7.20). Examination of ventricular volume or dimensions throughout the cardiac cycle confirms that during the latter portion of diastole, ventricular volume is static throughout the latter two thirds of diastole. This absence of late ventricular diastolic filling means that ventricular filling in the first third of diastole must be abnormally rapid. Abnormally rapid filling is documented by a sharp dip of early diastolic pressure, as active ventricular expansion exceeds the rate of passive venous return. Exaggerated early rapid filling followed by a long diastasis accounts for the characteristic waveform of left and right ventricular diastolic pressure, the so-called dip and plateau or square root sign (Fig. 7.20). The nadir of the early rapid filling wave approaches 0 mm Hg and then climbs rapidly to an abnormally high level, the value of which depends on the severity of constriction. Thus, the plateau of late ventricular diastolic pressure is in the range of 20 mm Hg in severe cases and 10 mm Hg in milder cases. In almost all cases, all four cardiac chambers are equally constrained by the pericardial scar; thus, the plateaus of pressure in the two ventricles attain exactly the same value. Naturally, therefore, during diastasis left and right atrial pressures are equal to the ventricular diastolic pressures. Thus, as in cardiac tamponade, an important hemodynamic indicator of pericardial abnormality is that in late diastole, pressures are equal in both ventricles and the atria. Furthermore, as in cardiac tamponade, pulmonary wedge pressure and pulmonary arterial diastolic pressure also equilibrate quite closely with the ventricular diastolic pressure plateaus (Fig. 7.20). Rarely, constriction is less uniform, but takes the form of a band, so that mitral stenosis, tricuspid stenosis, or pulmonary stenosis may be mimicked, but the corresponding pressure gradients are caused by extrinsic compression, not primary valve disease.[96,97]

When the patient is dyspneic, pulmonary wedge pressure varies markedly during respiration, but the right atrial pressure is almost constant throughout the respiratory cycle. When this situation occurs, equilibration of wedge and right atrial pressures is limited to inspiration (Fig. 7.21).

Cardiac Catheterization

Cardiac catheterization is required in most cases of constrictive pericarditis. The purposes are to assess the severity, detect unrecognized concomitant disease of the heart or coronary arteries that may modify the pathophysiology or treatment, and in some cases, to help differentiate from restrictive cardiomyopathy.

Proof that filling pressures on the two sides of the heart are equal is crucial to the diagnosis; therefore, extra precautions must be taken to make this proof convincing. If the catheterization personnel are experi-

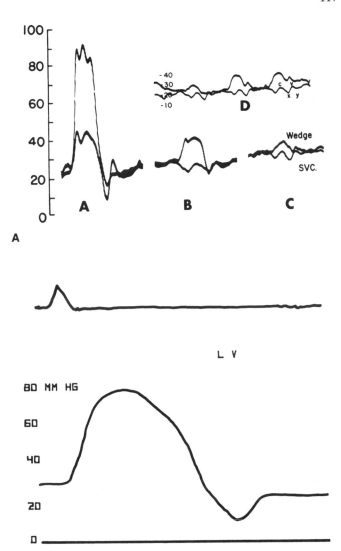

FIGURE 7.20. **A**: Tracings obtained during cardiac catheterization of a retired stock car driver who sustained a severe chest injury 2 years previously. *Panel A:* Simultaneously recorded left and right ventricular pressures. Note the dip and plateau and the artifact because fluid-filled catheters and transducers were used. *Panel B:* Simultaneously recorded pressures from the right ventricle and right atrium showing the correspondence of the early diastolic dip of ventricular diastolic pressure and prominent y descent of atrial pressure. *Panel C:* Simultaneously recorded pulmonary arterial wedge and superior vena caval pressures. *Panel D:* Simultaneously recorded pressures from the pulmonary artery and the right atrium. Note the agreement between the diastolic pressures during diastole. Reprinted with permission from Grossman W. *Cardiac Catheterization and Angiography.* Philadelphia: Lea & Febiger; 1980. **B**: Left ventricular pressure from a patient with severe constrictive pericarditis. A Millar transducer was used and the recording is a signal-averaged beat. Note the unmistakable early diastolic dip that remains well above zero and the smooth elevated plateau of mid and late diastolic pressure. Reprinted with permission from Shabetai R. *The Pericardium.* New York: Grune & Stratton; 1981.

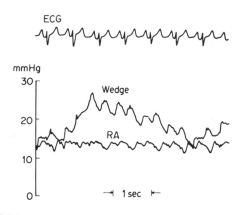

FIGURE 7.21. Simultaneous pressure recordings from a case of severe constrictive pericarditis. During inspiration, pulmonary wedge but not right atrial pressure, drops.

enced with catheter-tip transducers and use them frequently, this technique yields optimal results. Otherwise, the results will be more reliable when fluid-filled catheters and external transducers are used. In either case, the calibration of all transducers must be exactly the same. When conventional recording systems are employed, the transducers must be levelled at precisely the same height. Pressures should be recorded simultaneously, not sequentially when equilibration is the object of investigation. Ideally, pressures are measured via identical catheters rather than through the lumina of a double lumen catheter. The proximal lumen of the Swan-Ganz catheter is appreciably smaller than the distal, so damping characteristics are different. Extra care with filling and flushing catheters and transducers helps

to keep damping similar in all systems. Particularly useful combinations are right atrial plus pulmonary wedge pressure and right atrial plus left ventricular pressure. The two ventricular pressures also can be recorded together, but unless high fidelity catheter-tip transducers are used, artifact due to underclamping hinders evaluation of diastolic pressure equilibration, especially when the heart rate is fast. When left ventricular pressure is included in the combination, recordings should be made at both high and low gain settings to evaluate respiratory variations in systemic and pulmonary systolic pressure. Pulmonary wedge pressure serves as an excellent marker of the phase of respiration. Typically during inspiration, pulmonary wedge pressure drops, but right atrial pressure, except the y descent, is unaffected (Fig. 7.21).

The dip and plateau configuration is demonstrated in the recordings of left and right ventricular diastolic pressure in constrictive pericarditis (Figs. 7.15 and 7.20), but here it is important to emphasize that this finding often is simulated in cases without constrictive pericarditis or restrictive cardiomyopathy (Fig. 7.22). In these instances, artifact also is seen in the systolic portion of the ventricular tracing, especially near the peak. Fluctuations also are often present in mid- and late diastole. A substantially subatmospheric pressure dip, for example, more than 10 mm Hg, is almost always artifactual, whether or not the patient has constrictive percarditis (Fig. 7.20B). The right atrial pressure shows prominent x and y descents and no respiratory variation (Fig. 7.23), thus dlffering from that seen in cardiac tamponade (Figs. 7.17 and 7.18). The appearance of the coronary arteries also may be helpful in confirming constrictive pericarditis.[98]

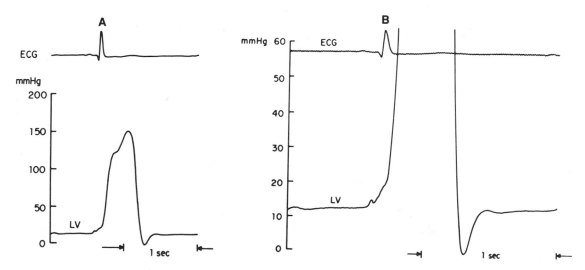

FIGURE 7.22. Left ventricular pressure tracings obtained during routine diagnostic cardiac catheterization of a patient with coronary artery disease, a normal pericardium, and no features suggestive of restrictive cardiomyopathy. The pressure tracings are underdamped and show a dip and plateau pattern that has nothing to do with constrictive or restrictive disease. A, low gain, B, high gain.

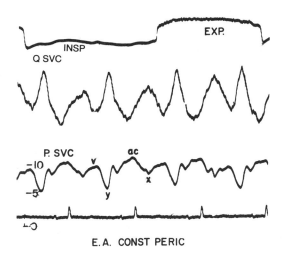

FIGURE 7.23. Tracings obtained during cardiac catheterization of a woman with mild constrictive pericarditis. Tracings from above down: phase of respiration, superior vena caval blood flow velocity (QSVC), superior vena caval pressure (PSVC), and the electrocardiogram. Although pressure elevation is mild, respiratory variation, except in the depth of the y descent, is absent. Note the prominent y descent. Blood flow velocity is not influenced by respiration and is bimodal corresponding with the x and y descents of pressure. Reprinted with permission from Shabetai R. *The Pericardium.* New York: Grune & Stratton; 1981.

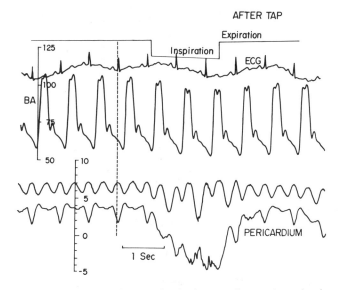

FIGURE 7.24. Recording made during cardiac catheterization of a patient with effusive constrictive pericarditis owing to bronchogenic carcinoma. A considerable volume of pericardial fluid had been aspirated, therefore the pericardial pressure had fallen below right atrial pressure. Observe that the right atrial pressure shows the typical wave form of constrictive pericarditis with absence of respiratory variation. Reprinted with permission from Shabetai R. *The Pericardium.* New York: Grune & Stratton; 1981.

Variants of Constrictive Pericarditis

Occult Constrictive Pericarditis

Constrictive pericarditis may be too mild to be easily recognized clinically or hemodynamically. The first publication on occult constriction[99] dealt with a series of patients with chest pain, many of whom had a history of remote pericarditis. Their hemodynamics at rest were normal, but upon a vigorous fluid challenge assumed the characteristics of constrictive pericarditis. When the patients were submitted to pericardiectomy, the surgeon observed that the heart appeared to be encased. The pathological specimen showed chronic inflammation.

Unfortunately, the fluid challenge test often is employed in patients in whom there is no sound reason to suspect pericardial disease. Furthermore, the results are usually equivocal and good control studies are lacking. Finally, if constrictive pericarditis is so mild that it takes a fluid challenge to diagnose it, it does not need to be treated by pericardiectomy. This author prefers to withhold diuretics until the patient has gained several pounds rather than perform acute volume loading as a means to facilitate the diagnosis in less severe cases.

Effusive Constrictive Pericarditis

As its name states, effusive constrictive pericarditis is a pericardial condition characterized by increased thickness and decreased compliance associated with a hemodynamically significant effusion.[73] The clinical and hemodynamic features are those of tamponade but imaging reveals the abnormal thickness and density of the pericardium. After removal of pericardial effusion the pericardial pressure returns to normal, but the right atrial pressure tracing does not, instead showing the M or W pattern and diminished respiratory variation typical of constrictive pericarditis (Fig. 7.24). When the central venous pressure fails to normalize after satisfactory pericardial drainage, the differential diagnosis includes underlying heart failure or tricuspid disease and effusive constrictive pericarditis. Elastic constrictive pericarditis refers to a form of constriction in which some degree of elasticity is retained by the pericardium despite significant pathological involvement. The hemodynamics are similar to those of classic constrictive pericarditis except that the ventricles enlarge and generate additional pressure and flow in response to appropriate atrial contraction. An example in which the stimulus was a correctly timed atrial contraction is shown in Figure 7.25.

Transient Constrictive Pericarditis

Constriction is usually permanent, but transient constriction may develop after acute pericarditis (Fig. 7.26).

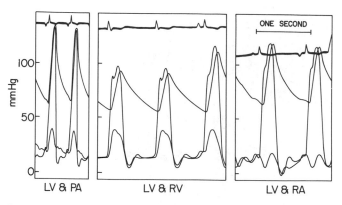

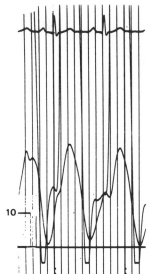

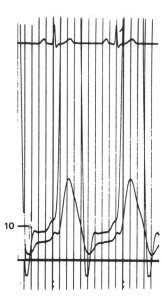

FIGURE 7.25. High fidelity pressure tracings in a patient with elastic constrictive pericarditis. The rhythm spontaneously varied between atrial ectopic (*Panel A*, first and second beats of *Panel B*, and second beat of *Panel C*) and sinus. After a properly coordinated atrial systole, left ventricular pressure and aortic pressure are considerably increased (third beat of panel B). Reprinted with permission from Gaasch et al. Left ventricular function in chronic constrictive pericarditis. *Am J Cardiol*. 1974;34:107–110.

FIGURE 7.26. Left and right ventricular pressure tracings in a patient who had transient constriction. On the left panel, the dip and plateau pattern is present and the two ventricular diastolic pressures are equal. On the righ panel all signs of constriction have disappeared. Reprinted with permission from Sagrista-Sauleda et al. Transient cardiac constriction: an unrecognized pattern of evolution in effusive acute idiopathic pericarditis. *Am J Cardiol*. 1987;59:961.

Treatment of Constrictive Pericarditis

The treatment is pericardiectomy, which should be as complete as possible while avoiding injury to the phrenic nerves. For reasons that are poorly understood, venous pressure may not return to normal for several weeks or even months[100] and ventricular systolic function may temporarily diminish.

Diuretics are useful in preoperative management, but should be used relatively sparingly. No attempt to clear all edema, still less to establish a normal venous pressure, should be made.

Improved techniques and the trend for constrictive pericarditis to be less chronic have combined to reduce the surgical risk appreciably.[101]

Differentiation Between Constrictive Pericarditis and Restrictive Cardiomyopathy

The therapeutic consequences of mistaking constrictive pericarditis and restrictive cardiomyopathy for each other are obvious. The distinction may be straightforward and obvious, difficult, or even impossible short of exploratory operation.

By definition, the patients have a myocardial abnormality that alters ventricular chamber compliance such that a restrictive filling pattern develops in the absence of hypertrophy, dilatation, pericardial disease, aortic stenosis, or hypertension. The clinical and hemodynamic features resemble, or may even be the same as, those of constrictive pericarditis. Some but by no means all patients with diastolic heart failure present the problem of the differential diagnosis between constrictive and restrictive heart disease. The history may furnish important clues, but by definition physical examination of the circulatory system does not. Noninvasive and catheterization studies may or may not be helpful. A history of tuberculosis, pericarditis, trauma, collagen vascular disease neoplasm, or prior cardiac surgery favors constrictive pericarditis. Absence of evidence for these disorders from the history or by current evaluation is not helpful either way. A history of amyloidosis or sarcoidosis favors myocardial disease, but absence of such a history is noncontributory. Prior radiation can induce mixed myocardial and pericardial disease. Examination of the heart and circulation, by definition, is not helpful, but important clues to systemic disease may be discovered by general clinical examination and routine laboratory tests. Heavy continuous calcification of the pericardium obviously points to constrictive pericarditis, but absence of pericardial calcification is equally consistent with either diagnosis. When the electrocardiogram shows major depolarization abnormalities such as bundle branch block or hypertrophy, or shows atrioventricular delay, myocardial disease is far more likely than pericardial disease, although the latter has been reported.[102] Nonspecific repolarization changes do not help to distinguish restrictive cardiomyopathy from constrictive pericarditis.

An abnormally dense and thick pericardium as imaged by ultrasound, magnetic resonance, or computerized tomography implicates the pericardium, but a

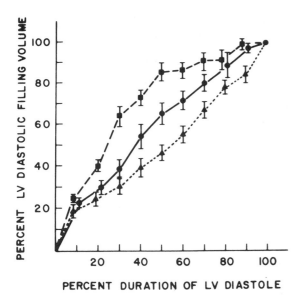

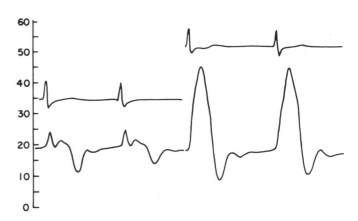

FIGURE 7.27. Composite left ventricular (*LV*) filling volume curves in seven normal control subjects (*solid lines*, *solid circles*), in four patients with restrictive amyloid cardiomyopathy (*broken line*, *solid triangles*), and in seven patients with constrictive pericarditis (*broken line*, *solid squares*). Data are expressed as mean ± standard deviation) percent left ventricular filling volume versus percent duration of left ventricular diastole. Reprinted with permission from Tyberg et al. Left ventricular filling in differentiating restrictive amyloid cardiomyopathy and constrictive pericarditis. *Am J Cardiol.* 1981;47:791.

FIGURE 7.28. Tracing recorded from a patient with amyloid restrictive cardiomyopathy. Note that the diastolic pressures in the right ventricle and atrium are identical to those characteristic of constrictive pericarditis. The data were recorded using a high fidelity (Millar) transducer. Reprinted with permission from Meaney et al. Cardiac amyloidosis, constrictive pericarditis and restrictive cardiomyopathy. *Am J Cardiol.* 1976;38:547.

normal appearance of the membrane does not rule out constrictive pericarditis, especially subacute and postoperative cases. The same interpretation applies to hemodynamic variables that in the past were thought to be important in the differential diagnosis.[103] Thus, while it remains true that severe pulmonary hypertension is not consistent with the diagnosis of constrictive pericarditis, and that a left ventricular diastolic plateau several mm Hg higher than right, strongly supports myocardial over pericardial disease, the finding of pulmonary arterial systolic pressure in the range of 40 to 50 mm Hg and equal diastolic pressure in both ventricles is equally consistent with either diagnosis. In some cases of restrictive cardiomyopathy, early diastolic ventricular filling is slow (Fig. 7.27), a finding that militates against constrictive pericarditis,[104] but once more, abnormally rapid early diastolic filling may be observed in both conditions. Likewise, a grossly abnormal endomyocardial biopsy is strong evidence against constrictive pericarditis, and whereas a normal biopsy strongly indicates the pericardium over the myocardium as the source of reduced compliance, it is not infallible.

Most students of restrictive and constrictive heart disease believe that the waveform of ventricular diastolic pressure is the same in both conditions, but one important investigator states that the typical dip and plateau

configuration is limited to constrictive pericarditis and is not seen in restrictive cardiomyopathy.[105] This finding corresponds with slower early ventricular filling in restrictive cardiomyopathy, but in the experience of this writer, ventricular diastolic filling and pressure patterns are both identical to those of constrictive pericarditis in many, and certainly the most difficult, cases of restrictive cardiomyopathy (Fig. 7.28).

The decision whether to explore the mediastinum in cases with mixed pericardial and myocardial disease, usually postradiation in etiology, can be difficult. When thoracic imaging discloses a thickened pericardium in patients who have been exposed to mediastinal radiation, hemodynamics confirm a restrictive filling pattern and the biopsy shows only mild radiation damage without extensive fibrosis, exploration is fully justified.

Echo-Doppler studies, carefully performed by individuals who are well trained and experienced, may be helpful. Respiratory variation in transvalvular blood flow velocity is more prominent in constrictive pericarditis than in restrictive cardiomyopathy and isovolumetric relaxation is slower.[106] In constrictive pericarditis the x descent and corresponding systolic surge of venous return are often more prominent than the y descent and early diastolic surge. It has been reported that this phenomenon is not present in restrictive cardiomyopathy, but in the opinion of this author, the pattern is identical to constrictive pericarditis in cases with amyloidosis presenting as restrictive cardiomyopathy. The ventricles are tightly coupled by severe constrictive pericarditis, but in restrictive cardiomyopathy ventricular coupling is, if anything, less than normal because of the stiff, noncompliant nature of the interventricular septum. Inspiratory increase in venous return can therefore generate excessive increases in right ventricular diastolic pressure without greatly affecting the left ventricle. This dissociation of the mechanics of the ventricles explains inspiratory decrease in the deceleration time of tricuspid blood flow velocity and ventriculoatrial regurgitation at the end of the early diastolic rapid filling period.

Summary

The pericardium exerts an important influence on cardiac, especially ventricular, diastolic function, and this influence becomes more pronounced when the heart enlarges, especially acutely. Compressive and constrictive pericardial heart disease have many clinical, hemodynamic, and metabolic features in common with heart failure, but should be considered differently, since usually the underlying myocardium is normal. Restrictive cardiomyopathy may be extremely difficult to distinguish from constrictive pericarditis, but usually can be achieved premortem and without exploratory operation.

References

1. Lee MC, Lewinter MM, Freeman G, Shabetai R, Fung YC. Biaxial mechanical properties of the pericardium in normal and volume overload dogs. *Am J Physiol.* 1985;249:H222–H230.
2. Rabkin SW, Hsu PH. Mathematical and mechanical modeling of stress-strain relationship of the pericardium. *Am J Physiol.* 1975;229:896–900.
3. Lee MC, Fung YC, Shabetai R, Lewinter MM. Biaxial mechanical properties of human pericardium and canine comparisons. *Am J Physiol.* 1987;253:H75–H82.
4. Freeman GL. The effects of the pericardium on function of normal and enlarged hearts. *Cardiol Clin.* 1990;8:579–586.
5. Banchero N, Rutishauser WJ, Tsakiris AG, Wood EH. Pericardial pressure during transverse acceleration in dogs without thoracotomy. *Circ Res.* 1967;20:65–77.
6. Ludbrook PA, Byrne JD, McKnight RC. Influence of right ventricular hemodynamics on left ventricular diastolic pressure-volume relations in man. *Circulation.* 1979;59:21–31.
7. Holt JP, Rhode EA, Kines H. Pericardial and ventricular pressure. *Circ Res.* 1960;8:1171–1181.
8. Shirato K, Shabetai R, Bhargava V, Franklin D, Ross J Jr. Alteration of the left ventricular diastolic pressure-segment length relation produced by the pericardium. *Circulation.* 1978;57:1191–1198.
9. Bartle SH, Hermann HJ. Acute mitral regurgitation in man. Hemodynamic evidence and observations indicating an early role for the pericardium. *Circulation.* 1967;36:839–851.
10. Shabetai R. *The Pericardium.* New York: Grune & Stratton; 1981;58–59.

11. LeWinter MM, Pavelec R. Influence of the pericardium on left ventricular end-diastolic pressure-segment relations during early and later stages of experimental chronic volume overload in dogs. *Circ Res.* 1982;50:501–509.
12. Freeman GL, LeWinter MM. Pericardial adaptations during chronic cardiac dilation in dogs. *Circ Res.* 1984;54:294–300.
13. Smiseth OA, Frais MA, Kingma I, et al. Assessment of pericardial constraint: the relation between right ventricular filling pressure and pericardial pressure measured after pericardiocentesis. *J Am Coll Cardiol.* 1986;7:307–314.
14. Janicki JS, Weber KT. The pericardium and ventricular interaction, distensibility and function. *Am J Physiol.* 1980;238:H494–H503.
15. Hess O, Bhargava V, Ross J Jr, Shabetai R. The role of the pericardium in interactions between the cardiac chambers. *Am Heart J.* 1983;106:1377–1383.
16. Henderson Y, Prince AL. Relative systolic discharges from the right and left ventricles and their bearing upon pulmonary congestion and depletion. *Heart.* 1914;5:217–226.
17. Taylor RR, Covell JW, Sonnenblick EH, Ross J Jr. Dependence of ventricular distensibility on filling of the opposite ventricle. *Am J Physiol.* 1967;213:711–718.
18. Glantz SA, Misbach GA, Moores WY, et al. The pericardium substantially affects the left ventricular diastolic pressure-volume relationship in the dog. *Circ Res.* 1978;42:433–441.
19. Santamore WP, Heckman JL, Bove AA. Right and left ventricular pressure-volume response to elevated pericardial pressure. *Am Rev Respir Dis.* 1986;134:101–107.
20. Santamore WP, Bartlett R, VanBuren SJ, Dowd MK, Kutcher MA. Ventricular coupling in constrictive pericarditis. *Circulation.* 1986;74:597–602.
21. Smiseth OA, Refsum, H, Tyberg JV. Pericardial pressure assessed by right atrial pressure: a basis for calculation of left ventricular transmural pressure. *Am Heart J.* 1984;108:603–605.
22. Mann D, Lew W, Ban-Hayashi E, Shabetai R, Waldman L, LeWinter MM. In vivo mechanical behavior of canine pericardium. *Am J Physiol.* 1986;251:H349–H356.
23. Morgan BC, Guntheroth WG, Dillard DH. Relationship of pericardial to pleural pressure during quiet respiration and cardiac tamponade. *Circ Res.* 1965;16:493–498.
24. Smiseth OA, Frais MA, Kingma I, Smith ER, Tyberg JV. Assessment of pericardial constraint in dogs. *Circulation.* 1985;71:158–164.
25. Smiseth OA, Scott-Douglas NW, Thompson CR, Smith ER, Tyberg JV. Non-uniformity of pericardial surface pressure in dogs. *Circulation.* 1987;75:1229–1236.
26. Hoit BD, Lew WY, LeWinter M. Regional variation in pericardial contact pressure in the canine ventricle. *Am J Physiol.* 1988;255:H1370–H1377.
27. Santamore WP, Constantinescu M, Little WC. Direct assessment of right ventricular transmural pressure. *Circulation.* 1987;75:744–747.
28. Slinker BK, Ditchey RV, Bell SP, LeWinter MM. Right heart pressure does not equal pericardial pressure in the potassium chloride-arrested canine heart in situ. *Circulation.* 1987;76:357–362.

29. Boltwood CM, Skulsky A, Drinkwater DC, et al. Intraoperative measurement of pericardial constraint; role in ventricular diastolic mechanics. *J Am Coll Cardiol*. 1986;8:1289–1297.

30. Janicki JS. Influence of the pericardium and ventricular interdependence on left ventricular diastolic and systolic function in patients with heart failure. *Circulation*. 1990;81(suppl 3):III15–III20.

31. Hammond HK, White FC, Bhargava V, Shabetai R. Heart size and maximal cardiac output are limited by the pericardium. *Am J Physiol*. 1992;263:(Heart Circ Physiol 32) H1675–H1681.

32. Stray-Gundersen J, Musch TI, Haidet GC, Swain DP, Ordway GA, Mitchell JH. The effect of pericardiectomy on maximal oxygen consumption and maximal cardiac output in untrained dogs. *Circ Res*. 1986;58:523–530.

33. Hammond HK, White FC, Bhargava V, Shabetai R. Pericardium limits utilization of the Starling mechanism during maximal exercise. *Circulation*. Supplement III 1990;82:III-697.

34. Shabetai R. Cardiac tamponade. In Shabetai R ed. *The Pericardium*. New York: Grune & Stratton; 1981.

35. Shabetai R, Fowler NO, Guntheroth WG. The hemodynamics of cardiac tamponade and constrictive pericarditis. *Am J Cardiol*. 1970;26:480–489.

36. Beck CS. Two cardiac compression triads. *JAMA*. 1935;104:714–716.

37. Brecher GA. *Venous Return*. New York: Grune & Stratton; 1956.

38. Shabetai R, Fowler NO, Fenton JC, Masangkay M. Pulsus paradoxus. *J Clin Invest*. 1965;44:1882–1898.

39. Reddy PS, Curtiss EI. Cardiac tamponade. *Cardiol Clin*. 1990;8:627–637.

40. Kussmaul A. Mediastino-pericarditis und den paradoxen. *Klin Wochenschr*. 1873;10:433–464.

41. Guberman BA, Fowler NO, Engel PJ, Gueron M, Allen JM. Cardiac tamponade in medical patients. *Circulation*. 1981;64:633–640.

42. Reddy PS, Curtiss El, O'Toole JD, Shaver JA. Cardiac tamponade: hemodynamic observations in man. *Circulation*. 1978;58:265–272.

43. Dacso CC. Pericarditis in AIDS. *Cardiol Clin*. 1990;8:697–699.

44. Usher BW, Popp RL. Electrical alternans: mechanism in pericardial effusion. *Am Heart J*. 1972;83:459–463.

45. Gabor GE, Winsberg F, Bloom HS. Electrical and mechanical alternation in perlcardial effusion. *Chest*. 1971;59:341–344.

46. Feigenbaum H, Zaky A, Grabhorn LL. Cardiac motion in patients with pericardial effusion: a study using reflected ultrasound. *Circulation*. 1966;34:611–619.

47. Goldberger AL, Shabetai R, Bhargava V, West BJ, Mandell AJ. Nonlinear dynamics, electrical alternans, and pericardial tamponade. *Am Heart J*. 1984;107:1297–1299.

48. Rigney DR, Goldberger AL. Nonlinear dynamics of the heart's swinging during pericardial effusion. *Am J Physiol*. 1989;257(Heart Circ Physiol 26):H1292–H1305.

49. Spodick DH. Acute cardiac tamponade: pathologic physiology, diagnosis and management. *Prog Cardiovasc Dis*. 1967;10:64–96.

50. Gillam LD, Guyer DE, Gibson TC, King ME, Marshal JE, Weyman AE. Hydrodynamic compression of the right atrium: a new echocardiographic sign of cardiac tamponade. *Circulation*. 1983;68:294–301.

51. Singh S, Wann LS, Schuchard GH, et al. Right ventricular and right atrial collapse in patients with cardiac tamponade—a combined hemodynamic and echocardiographic study. *Circulation*. 1984;70:966–971.

52. Spitz HB, Holmes JC. Right atrial contour in cardiac tamponade. *Radiology*. 1972;103:69–75.

53. Schiller NB, Botvinick EH. Right ventricular compression as a sign of cardiac tamponade: an analysis of echocardiographic ventricular dimensions and their clinical implications. *Circulation*. 1977;56:774–779.

54. Feigenbaum H. *Echocardiography*. Malvern, Penn: Lea and Febiger; 1986.

55. Hoit BD and Shabetai R. Pericardial disease. In: Pohost GM, O'Rourke RA, eds. *Principles and Practice of Cardiovascular Imaging*. Boston: Little, Brown; 1991:757–772.

56. Cogswell TL, Bernath GA, Wann LS, Hoffman RG, Brooks HL, Klopfenstein HS. Effects of intravascular volume state on the value of pulsus paradoxus and right ventricular diastolic collapse in predicting cardiac tamponade. *Circulation*. 1985;72:1076–1080.

57. Jarmakani JMM, McHale PA, Greenfield JC. The effect of cardiac tamponade on coronary hemodynamics in the awake dog. *Cardiovas Res*. 1975;9:112–117.

58. Settle HP, Adolph RJ, Fowler NO, Engel P, Agruss NS, Levenson NI. Echocardiographic study of cardiac tamponade. *Circulation*. 1977;56:951–959.

59. D'Cruz IA, Cohen HC, Prabhu R, Glick G. Diagnosis of cardiac tamponade by echocardiography: changes in mitral valve motion and ventricular dimensions, with special reference to paradoxical pulse. *Circulation*. 1975;52:(3)460–465.

60. Candell-Riera J. Tamponade and constriction: an appraisal of echocardiography and external pulse recordings. In: Soler-Soler J, Permanyer-Miralda G, Sagrista-Sauleda J, eds. *Pericardial Disease—New Insights and Old Dilemmas*. Dordrecht: Kluwer; 1988.

61. Appleton CP, Hatle LK, Popp RL. Cardiac tamponade and pericardial effusion: respiratory variation in transvalvular flow velocities studied by Doppler echocardiography. *J Am Coll Cardiol*. 1988;11:1020–1030.

62. Gonzales MS, Basnight MA, Appleton CP. Experimental pericardial effusion: relation of abnormal respiratory variation in mitral flow velocity to hemodynamics and diastolic right heart collapse. *J Am Coll Cardiol*. 1991;17:239–248.

63. DeCristofaro D, Liu CK. The haemodynamics of cardiac tamponade and blood volume overload in dogs. *Cardiovasc Res*. 1969;3:292–298.

64. Valantine HA, Hunt SA, Gibbons R, Billingham ME, Stinson EB, Popp RL. Increasing pericardial effusion in cardiac transplant recipients. *Circulation*. 1989;79:603–609.

65. Shabetai R, Rostand SG. Nephrogenic pericardial disease. In: O'Rourke RA, ed. *The Heart and Renal Disease. Contemporary Issues in Nephrology*. New York: Churchill-Livingstone; 1984:89–125.

66. Wickstrom PH, Monson BK, Helseth HK. Delayed postoperative bloody pericardial effusion. *Minnesota Med.* 1985;68:19–22.

67. Ellison LH, Kirsh MM. Delayed mediastinal tamponade after open heart surgery. *Chest.* 1974;65:64–66.

68. Hochberg MS, Merrill WH, Gruber M, McIntosh CL, Henry WL, Morrow AG. Delayed cardiac tamponade associated with prophylactic anticoagulation in patients undergoing coronary bypass grafting. Early diagnosis with two-dimensional echocardiography. *J Thorac Cardiovasc Surg.* 1978;75:777–781.

69. Akins CW, Boucher CA, Pohost GM. Preservation of interventricular septal function in patients having coronary artery bypass grafts without cardiopulmonary bypass. *Am Heart J.* 1984;107:304–309.

70. Fyke FE, Tancredi RG, Shub C, Julsrud PR, Sheedy PF. Detection of intrapericardial hematoma after open heart surgery: the roles of echocardiography and computed tomography. *J Am Coll Cardiol.* 1985;5:1496–1499.

71. Ikaheimo MJ, Huikuri HV, Airaksinen KE, et al. Pericardial effusion after cardiac surgery: incidence, relation to the type of surgery, antithrombotic therapy, and early coronary bypass graft patency. *Am Heart J.* 1988;116:97–102.

72. Kronzon I, Cohen ML, Winer HE. Cardiac tamponade by loculated pericardial hematoma: limitations of M-mode echocardiography. *J Am Coll Cardiol.* 1983;1:913–915.

73. Hancock EW. Subacute effusive-constrictive pericarditis. *Circulation.* 1971;43:183–192.

74. Antman EM, Cargill V, Grossman W. Low pressure cardiac tamponade. *Ann Intern Med.* 1979;91:403–406.

75. Palacios IF, Tuzcu EM, Ziskind AA, Younger J, Block PC. Percutaneous balloon pericardial window for patients with malignant pericardial effusion and tamponade. *Cathet Cardiovasc Diagn.* 1991;22:244–249.

76. Kondos GT, Rich S, Levitsky S. Flexible fiberoptic pericardioscopy for the diagnosis of pericardial disease. *J Am Coll Cardiol.* 1986;7:432–434.

77. Permanyer-Miralda G, Sagrista-Sauleda J, Soler-Soler J. Primary acute pericardial disease: a prospective series of 231 consecutive patients. *Am J Cardiol.* 1985;56:623–630.

78. Gaasch WH, Peterson KL, Shabetai R. Left ventricular function in chronic constrictive pericarditis. *Am J Cardiol.* 1974;34:107–110.

79. Wise DE, Conti CR. Constrictive pericarditis. *Cardiovasc Clin.* 1976;7:197–209.

80. Soufer R, Wohlgelernter D, Vita NA, et al. Intact systolic left ventricular function in clinical congestive heart failure. *Am J Cardiol.* 1985;55:1032–1036.

81. Gaasch WH. Congestive heart failure in patients with normal left ventricular systolic function: a manifestation of diastolic dysfunction. *Herz.* 1991;16:22–32.

82. Gaasch WH. Diastolic dysfunction of the left ventricle: importance to the clinician. *Adv Intern Med.* 1990;35:311–340.

83. Stauffer JC, Gaasch WH. Recognition and treatment of left ventricular diastolic dysfunction. *Prog Cardiovasc Dis.* 1990;32:319–332.

84. Meaney E, Shabetai R, Bhargava V, et al. Cardiac amyloidosis, constrictive pericarditis and restrictive cardiomyopathy. *Am J Cardiol.* 1976;38:547–556.

85. Dabestani A, Child JS, Eberhard H, et al. Primary hemochromatosis: anatomic and physiologic characteristics of the cardiac ventricles and their response to phlebotomy. *Am J Cardiol.* 1984;54:153–159.

86. Wasserman AJ, Richardson DW, Baird CL, Wyso EM. Cardiac hemochromatosis simulating constrictive pericarditis. *Am J Med.* 1962;32(Part 1)316–323.

87. Young JB, Leon CA, Short HD, et al. Evolution of hemodynamics after orthotopic heart and heart-lung transplantation: early restrictive patterns persisting in occult fashion. *J Heart Transplant.* 1987;6:34–43.

88. Katayama T, Iwamoto K, Ochi S, Honda Y, Shigematsu K. Restrictive cardiomyopathy following acute myocarditis—a case report. *Angiology.* 1990;41:76–81.

89. Schmaltz AA, Seitz KH, Schenck W, Both A, Kraus B. Restrictive cardiomyopathy as a late sequel of influenza A2 viral myocarditis. *Z Kardiol.* 1986;75:605–608.

90. Jensen DP, Goolsby JP, Oliva PB. Hemodynamic pattern resembling pericardial constriction after acute inferior myocardial infarction with right ventricular infarction. *Am J Cardiol.* 1978;42:858–861.

91. Siegel RJ, Shah PK, Fishbein MC. Idiopathic restrictive cardiomyopathy. *Circulation.* 1984;70:165–169.

92. Benotti JR, Grossman W, Cohn PF. Clinical profile of restrictive cardiomyopathy. *Circulation.* 1980;61:1206–1212.

93. Shabetai R. Constrictive pericarditis. In: Shabetai R. *The Pericardium.* New York: Grune & Stratton; 1981.

94. Thould AK. Constrictive pericarditis in rheumatoid arthritis. *Ann Rheum Dis.* 1986;45:89–94.

95. Burney DP, Martin CE, Thomas CS, Fisher RD, Bender HW. Rheumatoid pericarditis; Clinical significance and operative management. *J Thorac Cardiovasc Surg.* 1979;77:511–515.

96. Spodik DH. *Chronic and Constrictive Pericarditis.* New York: Grune & Stratton; 1964.

97. McGaff GJ, Haller JA, Leight L, Towery BT. Subvalvular pulmonary stenosis due to constriction of the right ventricular outflow tract by a pericardial band. *Am J Med.* 1963;34:142–146.

98. Alexander J, Kelley MJ, Cohen LS, Langou RA. The angiographic appearance of the coronary arteries in constrictive pericarditis. *Radiology.* 1979;131:609–617.

99. Bush CA, Stang JM, Wooley CF, Kilman JW. Occult constrictive pericardial disease. Diagnosis by rapid volume expansion and correction by pericardiectomy. *Circulation.* 1977;56:924–930.

100. Kloster FE, Crislip RL, Bristow JD, Herr RH, Ritzmann LW, Griswold HE. Hemodynamic studies following pericardiectomy for constrictive pericarditis. *Circulation.* 1965;32:415–424.

101. McCaughan BC, Schaff HV, Piehler JM, et al. Early and late results of pericardiectomy for constrictive pericarditis. *J Thorac Cardiovasc Surg.* 1985;89:340–350.

102. Levine HD. Myocardial fibrosis in constrictive pericarditis: electrocardiographic and pathologic observations. *Circulation.* 1973;48:1268–1281.

103. Schoenfeld MH, Supple EW, Dec GW Jr, Fallon JT,

Palacios IF. Restrictive cardiomyopathy versus constrictive pericarditis: role of endomyocardial biopsy in avoiding unnecessary thoracotomy. *Circulation.* 1987;75:1012–1017.

104. Tyberg TI. Goodyer AVN, Hurst VW III, Alexander J, Langou RA. Left ventricular filling in differentiating restrictive amyloid cardiomyopathy and constrictive pericarditis. *Am J Cardiol.* 1981;47:791–796.

105. Hirota Y, Kohriyama T, Hayashi T, et al. Idiopathic restrictive cardiomyopathy: differences of left ventricular relaxation and diastolic wave forms from constrictive pericarditis. *Am J Cardiol.* 1983;52:421–423.

106. Hatle LK, Appleton CP, Popp RL. Differentiation of constrictive pericarditis and restrictive cardiomyopathy by Doppler echocardiography. *Circulation.* 1989;357–370.

8
The Sympathetic Nervous System in Congestive Heart Failure

Wilson S. Colucci

The sympathetic nervous system (SNS) plays a pivotal role in the regulation of cardiovascular function, both in health and disease. Over the last 30 years the important role of the SNS in the syndrome of congestive heart failure has become apparent. The SNS can help to support cardiovascular function when cardiac performance is compromised, particularly in the acute phase after the onset of myocardial failure. Conversely, the SNS contributes to many of the pathophysiologic features of congestive heart failure, some of which may have a deleterious impact on the clinical course of patients. Furthermore, many current or investigational drug therapies for heart failure act, directly or indirectly, to affect SNS function at one level or another.

Sympathetic Nervous System Activity in Congestive Heart Failure

It is now accepted that SNS activity is increased in patients with congestive heart failure. This conclusion initially was based on the observation that urinary excretion and circulating plasma levels of norepinephrine (NE) were increased in patients with congestive heart failure.[1,2] In contrast to activation of the renin-angiotensin system, which frequently shows little or no relationship to the severity of hemodynamic dysfunction, plasma NE is directly related to the severity of hemodynamic dysfunction.[3]

An indirect measure of SNS activity is the plasma NE concentration, which reflects the net result of efflux of NE from the neuroeffector junction and its clearance from the plasma. Plasma NE can be increased because of increased nerve release, reduced local reuptake by neuronal and nonneuronal mechanisms in the neuroeffector junction, and/or a reduction in the metabolism of NE by systemic clearance mechanisms. Direct assessment of cardiac SNS activity in man is difficult. However, measurement of the electrical activity in the perineal nerve has demonstrated that heart failure is associated with an increase in sympathetic traffic to skeletal muscle.[4] Although direct measurements of cardiac sympathetic nerve traffic have not been made in patients with heart failure, the aorta/coronary sinus gradient of plasma NE is increased in patients with heart failure.[5] This net increase in the release of NE from the heart indicates an increase in the ratio of NE production to degradation, but does not clarify the relative importance of each process. Studies of NE turnover kinetics based on tracer quantities of [^{3}H]-NE have demonstrated that NE spillover from both the heart and kidneys is increased in patients with heart failure.[6]

The effects of increased SNS activity in heart failure may be both beneficial and detrimental. Acutely following the onset of myocardial failure, increased SNS activity plays an important role in supporting cardiovascular homeostasis. Symphatic activity increases cardiac output by increasing heart rate, contractility, and venous return. Blood pressure may be increased due to increased systemic vascular resistance, as well as the increase in cardiac output. Thus, the acute effect of sympathetic activation is to improve the perfusion of vital organs. If there is no subsequent improvement in myocardial function, the sustained support of the SNS may continue to be important on a long-term basis. However, in many cases it appears that the degree of sympathetic activation is excessive, or at least may have a deleterious effect. Thus, arterial and venous constriction and increased salt and water retention by the kidneys lead to increases in preload and afterload, and hence, increases in diastolic and systolic wall stresses, respectively. Increases in wall stress result in higher oxygen and energy requirements, and possibly may contribute to failure of the myocardial cell. Increased sympathetic activity may lead to arrhythmias and desensitization of the postsynaptic β-adrenergic receptor pathway. Increased sympathetic activity also may contribute to activation of other neurohumoral systems such as the reninangiotensin system, which in turn may contribute to increases in preload and afterload. Finally, it is now apparent that several neurohormones, including NE and angiotensin II, may act directly on myocardial cells to cause cell hypertrophy and phenotypic alterations, which may be deleterious.

The goal of the subsequent discussion is to review the current understanding of SNS function in heart failure, to consider the role of the SNS in the pathophysiology and clinical course of patients with heart failure, and to consider the implications of abnormal SNS activity with regard to therapeutic interventions.

General Organization of the Sympathetic Nervous System

Efferent SNS activity to the cardiovascular system is under the control of both higher regulatory centers within the central nervous system and reflex mechanisms involving cardiopulmonary baroreceptors located in the heart, great vessels, and lungs. Efferent sympathetic nerves innervate virtually all aspects of the cardiovascular system. At the peripheral nerve ending, electrical impulses cause release of the neurotransmitter, NE. NE release from nerve endings is also under local regulation by substances that act on the peripheral nerve ending.[7] The local concentration of NE in the neuroeffector junction is regulated further by the relationship between neurotransmitter release and reuptake/metabolism.[6] NE released from nerve endings, plasma NE due to spillover from other tissues/organs, and plasma epinephrine secreted by the adrenal medulla act on α- and β-adrenergic receptors located on essentially all end-organs (e.g., myocardium, vascular smooth muscle). Stimulation of these adrenergic receptors results in the production of a variety of second messengers such as calcium, cyclic adenosine monophosphate (cAMP), and cyclic guanosine monophosphate (cGMP), and as a consequence, results in changes in myocardial and vascular smooth muscle function. Both the number of adrenergic receptors and the efficiency of their coupling to second messenger pathways can be regulated under a variety of physiologic and pathophysiologic conditions.

For the sake of clarity, it is convenient to simplify the regulation of SNS function into three general components: (a) regulation of SNS efferent nerve activity, (b) regulation of NE release, reuptake, and local concentration, and (c) regulation of end-organ receptors and tissue responsiveness. There is evidence that heart failure is associated with alterations in each of these components.

Regulation of Sympathetic Nervous System Efferent Activity

SNS activity is regulated by cardiovascular centers located in the brain stem, from which neurons descend in the spinal cord to interact with preganglionic neurons that innervate sympathetic ganglia and the adrenal medulla. Release of acetylcholine from preganglionic neurons results in stimulation of postganglionic neurons emanating from the sympathetic ganglia and constitute peripheral sympathetic nerves. The activity of the cardiovascular centers within the brain stem, in turn, is under the influence of both higher cortical centers and reflex pathways associated with a variety of mechanoreceptors and baroreceptors within the heart, blood vessels, and lungs. Increases in mean arterial or pulse pressure, or increased atrial and/or ventricular filling pressures and distention normally cause activation of cardiopulmonary and arterial baroreceptors, thereby resulting in inhibition of SNS outflow from the cardiovascular centers and a reciprocal increase in parasympathetic nerve activity.[8]

There is evidence that baroreceptors are dysfunctional in both experimental animals and humans with heart failure.[9] In animal models of heart failure, the sympathetic responses to increases or decreases in baroreceptor stimulation are blunted, suggesting decreased sensitivity of baroreceptors.[10] In patients with congestive heart failure, several observations likewise indicate a decrease in baroreceptor sensitivity.[8,9] In normal persons, reductions in arterial pressure caused by interventions such as nitroprusside infusion, head-up tilt, or lower body negative pressure reduce venous return, arterial pressure, and the volume of the heart, and thereby cause an increase in SNS outflow. In patients with heart failure, the SNS response to these maneuvers is blunted as indicated by diminished NE, vasoconstrictor, or heart rate responses.[11–13] Conversely, infusion of a vasopressor such as phenylephrine, which causes reflex SNS withdrawal and a slowing of heart rate in normal man, yields a blunted response in patients with heart failure.[8]

Baroreceptor sensitivity often is quantitated by measuring the relative changes in arterial blood pressure (mm Hg) and heart rate (R-R interval, ms) during the systemic infusion of phenylephrine to increase arterial pressure. Baroreceptor sensitivity is reflected by the slope of the line relating the R-R interval to arterial pressure, such that a decrease in sensitivity is indicated by a decrease in the slope of this line. Typically, the baroreceptor sensitivity in normal persons is approx-

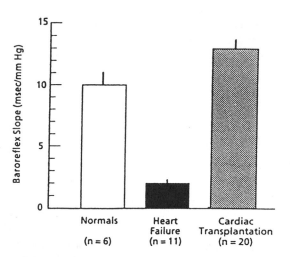

FIGURE 8.1. Arterial baroreflex slopes in normal persons, patients with congestive heart failure, and patients after cardiac transplantation. The arterial baroreflex slope is determined as the increase in R-R interval (ms) per increase in arterial blood pressure (mm Hg) during administration of a vasoconstrictor such as phenylephrine. The baroreflex slope is typically reduced in patients with congestive heart failure, reflecting reduced sensitivity of arterial baroreceptors. After cardiac transplantation, baroreceptor sensitivity is restored to normal, indicating that reduced baroreceptor sensitivity in heart failure is reversible. Reprinted with permission from ref. 14. Copyright by the American Heart Association.

imately a 10-ms increase in the R-R interval for each mm Hg rise in arterial pressure, and is markedly reduced to the range of 2 ms/mm Hg in patients with severe heart failure (Fig. 8.1). Interestingly, cardiac transplantation in man results in a normalization of baroreceptor function (Fig. 8.1) with a return of the baroreceptor slope to the normal range.[14] This suggests that baroreceptor dysfunction is not a primary abnormality inherent to congestive heart failure, but rather, a consequence of cardiac dysfunction. An important consequence of reduced baroreceptor sensitivity may be that SNS efferent activity is increased inappropriately relative to the level of cardiovascular performance. Such abnormal modulation of reflex sympathetic control likely contributes to the increased SNS activity that is characteristic of heart failure.

The cellular basis for baroreceptor dysfunction is not known, but may involve a number of factors such as mechanical alterations in the environment of the baroreceptor (e.g., vessel wall, myocardium), a resetting of baroreceptor reflex pathways, perhaps at the brain stem level, or alterations in the biochemical function of the baroreceptor, such as altered Na^+-K^+-ATPase activity.[9,10] In animals, baroreceptors can be isolated hemodynamically, and it can be shown that perfusion of a baroreceptor with digitalis to inhibit Na^+-K^+-ATPase or low K^+, which likewise inhibits

Na^+-K^+-ATPase, partially correct abnormal baroreceptor sensitivity.[10] This implies that increased Na^+-K^+-ATPase activity may be responsible for altered baroreceptor sensitivity in heart failure.

Abnormal baroreceptor function may be an important locus for therapeutic interventions. In patients with congestive heart failure, acute intravenous administration of a digitalis glycoside likewise results in normalization of baroreceptor sensitivity, as reflected by decreases in both forearm vascular resistance and sympathetic nerve activity to skeletal muscle.[15] Interestingly, acute administration of digitalis does not have this effect in normal persons. It is not known whether chronic administration of digitalis results in a similar, tonic withdrawal of SNS activity in patients with heart failure. However, if this were the case, it would provide a mechanism by which digitalis could produce long-term beneficial effects in patients, independent of a positive inotropic action.

Relatively little is known about the pharmacologic manipulation of baroreceptor sensitivity. Theoretically, it is possible that other agents might exert a digitalis-like effect on baroreceptor function in patients with heart failure, but lack some of the limiting characteristics of the digitalis glycosides (e.g., SNS activity). Likewise, the dose range for digitalis to cause sensitization of baroreceptors in patients with heart failure is not known. It is possible that this beneficial effect may occur at doses substantially lower than would be necessary to exert a positive inotropic effect. Since there is no established relationship between the dose of digitalis and the drug's positive inotropic effect or clinical benefit, it may be that lower doses of digitalis could be used without sacrificing clinical benefit.

Local Neurotransmitter Regulation

All of the effects of the SNS on cardiovascular end-organs are due to the interaction of the neurotransmitters, NE, and epinephrine, with α- and β-adrenergic receptors on the cell membrane of the target tissue. The primary neurotransmitter for sympathetic nerves is NE, which achieves substantial local concentrations in the area of the neuroeffector junction, estimated to be on the order of 10 μM in the vicinity of the receptor.[16] Circulating NE, which enters the circulation due to spillover from the neuroeffector junction, accounts for only approximately 10% of the total NE released from nerves (approximately 90% is taken up in the neuroeffector junction), and achieves plasma concentrations of only approximately 1 nM, which probably are not adequate to activate adrenergic receptors. However, under conditions of increased sympathetic nerve activity, such as in patients with severe heart failure or during strenuous exercise, plasma NE concentrations can

TABLE 8.1. Presynaptic receptors that may modulate the release of norepinepherine.

Inhibit norepinephrine release	Stimulate norepinephrine release
α_2-Adrenergic	Angiotensin II
Dopamine	β_2-Adrenergic
Muscarinic	
Opiate	
Prostaglandin	
Adenosine	
Serotonin	
Histamine	

be 5- to 10-fold higher,[17] and may contribute to the stimulation of adrenergic receptors.

Adrenergic nerves take up tyrosine, which is acted on by a series of enzymes (tyrosine hydroxylase, amino acid decarboxylase, and dobutamine β-hydroxylase) to yield NE.[18] NE is stored in vesicles in the nerve ending, where exocytotic release is triggered by a membrane depolarization–induced increase in the intracellular calcium concentration of the nerve. The amount of NE released in response to a nerve impulse can be modulated by a variety of hormones and substances that act on specific receptors located on the nerve ending[7] (Table 8.1). For instance, stimulation of presynaptic α_2-adrenergic receptors results in a decrease in NE release, whereas stimulation of angiotensin II receptors results in an increase in NE release.[19] Although these phenomena are clearly demonstrable in vitro, the importance of these mechanisms in vivo is not as certain. However, it can be shown that the nonselective α-adrenergic antagonist phentolamine, which inhibits the presynaptic α_2-adrenergic receptor, results in an increase in NE release from the forearm.[20] Likewise, the intracoronary infusion of phentolamine in man results in an increase in coronary sinus NE concentration (JD Parker, WS Colucci, *unpublished observations*). It has been suggested that one mechanism of action of the converting enzyme inhibitors may be to reduce the effect of angiotensin II at presynaptic nerve endings, thereby resulting in reduced NE release.

Most of the NE released from nerve ending is taken up by neuronal, and to a lesser extent, extraneuronal, tissues (e.g., endothelial cells, vascular smooth muscle cells), thereby resulting in resolution of the local concentration of neurotransmitter to the prestimulated level. NE taken up by neurons may be recycled into vesicles for future release, or metabolized to metabolites that are released into the circulation. NE taken up by extraneuronal cells is likewise metabolized to yield metabolites that are released to the interstitial space and may be recovered in the plasma.

The regulation of local NE concentration in the vicinity of the receptor is determined by several factors in addition to the level of electrical impulses, including (a) the amount of NE available in the nerve ending (which is determined by the relative rates of neurotransmitter synthesis, recycling, and release), (b) the rates of NE reuptake by neuronal and extraneuronal tissues, and (c) the presence of local modulating substances that act on the presynaptic neuron to regulate NE release.

Early work in patients with heart failure and in animal models found that the tissue concentration of NE was decreased in myocardium.[1,18] Likewise, the release of myocardial NE stores by tyrosine was decreased in patients with heart failure.[1] This depletion of cardiac NE may reflect a combination of factors, including (a) an increase in NE spillover,[6] (b) a defect in NE biosynthesis,[18] and/or, (c) a decrease in neuronal reuptake of NE.[21]

There has been substantial controversy regarding the relative roles of altered NE reuptake and release in heart failure. Working in dogs with right heart failure, Liang et al. found a chamber-specific decrease in NE reuptake in right ventricular myocardium, without an alteration in NE release, and associated with a decrease in the myocardial concentration of NE.[22] A number of investigators have now approached this issue in patients with heart failure. Rose et al. used a transient NE tracer method to assess cardiac NE spillover, reuptake, and interstitial concentration in patients with mild heart failure due to valvular heart disease.[21] In these patients there appeared to be decreases in both NE release and reuptake, and a substantially reduced tissue NE concentration. There also was a trend toward an increase in the interstitial concentration of NE.

Conflicting results were found by Hasking et al., who used a steady-state NE tracer approach to study patients with moderate congestive heart failure and elevated plasma NE concentrations.[6] These investigators found a marked increase in NE spillover from both heart and kidneys, but no evidence of altered neuronal reuptake (Fig. 8.2). Total plasma clearance of NE also was decreased by approximately 25% in patients with heart failure, presumably reflecting alterations in regional blood flow to tissues that metabolize NE. Thus, it was concluded that the increased plasma NE in patients with moderate congestive heart failure reflected both an increase in NE spillover from heart, kidney, and possibly other organs, and a modest decrease in clearance of NE from the circulation. Discrepancies in the findings of Rose et al.[21] and Hasking et al.[6] may reflect the substantial differences in the technique used and patient populations studied.

Recent work by Meredith et al.[23] has further evaluated this issue by studying the extraction of NE across the heart, as well as the release of dihydroxyphenylalaninè (DOPA) and dihydroxylphenylglycol (DHPG) in patients with and without congestive heart failure. Cardiac NE spillover and DOPA production were increased eightfold and twofold, respectively, whereas

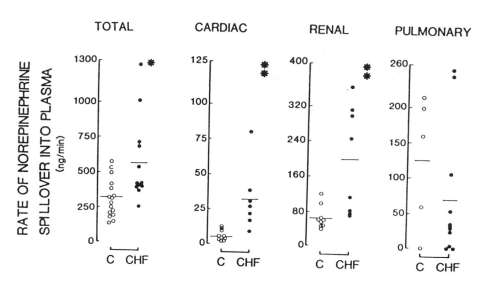

FIGURE 8.2. Total and regional norepinephrine spillover in patients with congestive heart failure and normal subjects. Reprinted with permission from ref. 6. Copyright by the American Heart Association.

cardiac extraction of NE was unchanged in patients with heart failure. The outward flux of DHPG, which reflects neuronal reuptake and intraneuronal metabolism of NE, was similar in normal persons and patients with heart failure, and was reduced to a comparable degree by desipramine, which blocks neuronal reuptake. These results led to the conclusion that increased NE release from the heart of patients with congestive heart failure is due to increased sympathetic nerve activity without a decrease in neuronal reuptake, and thus support the findings of Haskins et al.[6]

Postsynaptic Regulation of Adrenergic Responses

The effects of catecholamines are mediated entirely through their interaction with α- and β-adrenergic receptors located on various cardiovascular end-organs. It is now well established that end-organ responsiveness to adrenergic receptor stimulation can be modulated through changes in (a) receptor number, termed "upregulation" and "downregulation," (b) the expression or function of G-proteins that couple adrenergic receptors to the generation of second messengers, such as calcium and cyclic AMP, and (c) effector proteins, such as elements of the myocardial contractile apparatus, which are acted on by second messenger pathways.

There has been an intense investigation of the alterations in β-adrenergic receptor pathway expression and function in the myocardium of patients with congestive heart failure.[24,25] This attention reflects recognition of the central role of the β-adrenergic pathway in mediating the inotropic, chronotropic, and lusitropic effects of the sympathetic nervous system in the heart. Human myocardium expresses both β_1- and β_2-adrenergic receptors in a ratio of approximately 80:20.[26] Both subtypes of receptor are coupled to the stimulation of

adenylate cyclase and mediate similar contractile responses. In myocardium from patients with severe congestive heart failure, the contractile response to β-adrenergic stimulation is reduced, both in vitro[27] and in situ,[28] and in myocardium from such patients the total density of β-adrenergic receptors also is reduced, due primarily to a reduction in the β_1 receptor subpopulation.[26] Although there appears to be a substantial redundancy of β-adrenergic receptor number in the myocardium of several species, a phenomenon referred to as "spare receptors," existing evidence suggests that there are few or no spare receptors in man.[28] In this case, a decrease in β-adrenergic receptor density would result in a comparable decrease in the maximal amplitude of response. Thus, the attenuated physiologic response to β-adrenergic receptor stimulation in myocardium from patients with heart failure may be accounted for, in large part, by a downregulation of β-adrenergic receptors.

It also has been demonstrated that the functional activity of the G-protein, G_i, is increased in myocardium of patients with congestive heart failure.[29] This G-protein couples inhibitory receptors to adenylate cyclase, and thus might contribute to a reduced responsiveness of adenylate cyclase to stimulation. Surprisingly, the functional activity and expression of G_s, the stimulatory G-protein for adenylate cyclase that is coupled to β-adrenergic receptors, is not altered in myocardium of patients with congestive heart failure.[29] The mechanism by which the activity of G_i (as assessed by pertussis toxin-stimulated ribosylation) is increased in failing myocardium is not clear, since there does not appear to be increased expression of the protein as assessed by immunoblotting or of the mRNA as assessed by Northern blot analysis.

An alteration in G-protein function may contribute to the altered β-adrenergic responsiveness of failing myocardium. Such an alteration would result in a decrease in responsiveness out of proportion to the reduction in receptor density, a phenomenon referred to as uncoupling or desensitization. There is evidence that the relative roles of altered receptor density versus altered G-protein function may vary, depending on the underlying etiology of myocardial failure (i.e., ischemic vs. idiopathic).[30]

The third component of the β-adrenergic receptor pathway is the catalytic unit of adenylate cyclase, the protein responsible for the generation of cAMP. Although information regarding the expression and function of catalytic unit in failing myocardium is not available, it is theoretically possible that alterations in the catalytic unit may be involved in the altered physiologic responsiveness of the failing heart.

In vitro, exposure to NE causes both a decrease in β-adrenergic receptor density and an uncoupling from adenylate cyclase, and it is likely that exposure to increased NE levels is involved in the altered β-adrenergic responsiveness of failing human myocardium. There is some evidence to support this concept. For example, the density of myocardial β-adrenergic receptors is inversely related to the concentration of NE in coronary sinus blood,[24] which presumably is a reflection of the degree of NE spillover, and hence, the interstitial concentration of NE in the vicinity of the β-adrenergic receptor.

Altered β-adrenergic responsiveness contributes to the pathophysiology of heart failure by causing attenuation of the positive inotropic and chronotropic responses to β-adrenergic receptor stimulation. In vitro, myocardium obtained from patients with end-stage heart failure at the time of transplantation exhibits a normal contractile response to calcium, but a markedly attenuated response to β-adrenergic agonists.[24] In situ, the positive inotropic response to intracoronary infusion of the β-adrenergic agonist dobutamine is markedly depressed and bears an inverse relationship to the level of plasma NE[28] (Fig. 8.3).

β-Adrenergic receptor stimulation of the heart mediates two additional responses: an increase in heart rate (positive chronotropic response) and acceleration of the isovolumic phase of myocardial relaxation (positive lusitropic response). In patients with severe congestive heart failure, the chronotropic response to β-adrenergic receptor stimulation is markedly attenuated, as is the chronotropic response to exercise[17] (Fig. 8.4). Since heart rate is the predominant determinant of the increase in cardiac output that occurs with exercise, this may be a major way in which β-adrenergic receptor pathway dysfunction impacts the physiology of a patient with heart failure.

The isovolumic phase of left ventricular relaxation is prolonged in patients with severe congestive heart failure, and may contribute to elevated filling pressures and pulmonary congestion that are characteristic of this disorder.[31] Since β-adrenergic receptor stimulation is

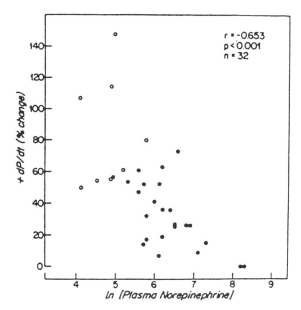

FIGURE 8.3. The positive inotropic response to an intracoronary infusion of dobutamine (25 μg/min) in patients with congestive heart failure (*solid circles*) and persons without congestive heart failure (*open circles*). The magnitude of positive inotropic response to β-adrenergic receptor stimulation with intracoronary dobutamine is inversely related to the resting plasma NE concentration at the time of study, suggesting that decreased β-adrenergic responsiveness of the heart in patients with heart failure is due, at least in part, to tonic elevation of sympathetic tone. Reproduced from *J Clin Invest.* 1988;81:1103, by copyright permission of American Society for Clinical Investigation.

known to accelerate left ventricular relaxation in normal tissue, it might be anticipated that this response would be attenuated in myocardium from patients with severe heart failure. Interestingly, it appears that the isovolumic relaxation response to β-adrenergic receptor stimulation is preserved, even in patients with end-stage congestive heart failure and attenuation of the inotropic response[31] (Fig. 8.5). This discrepancy between the inotropic and lusitropic responses to β-adrenergic receptor stimulation may be because they are mediated by different biochemical pathways: The inotropic response is mediated by cAMP-dependent phosphorylation of the calcium channel, whereas the lusitropic response involves cAMP-mediated activation of sarcoplasmic reticulum Ca^{2+}-ATPase.

Although attenuation of the β-adrenergic responsiveness of the failing heart may well contribute to reduced physiologic responsiveness and functional impairment, there is also reason to believe that a decrease in β-adrenergic responsiveness may exert a protective effect on the heart when it is exposed to excessive catecholamine stimulation. For example, by reducing the inotropic and chronotropic state of the heart, energy requirements might be reduced and the time for diastolic filling increased. In addition, reduced β-adrenergic respon-

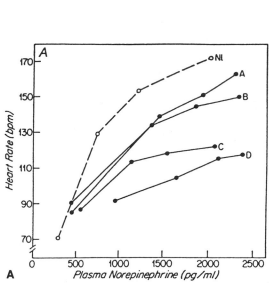

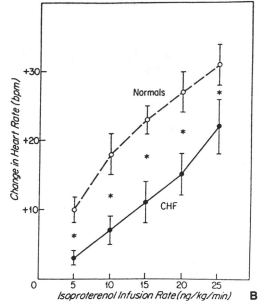

FIGURE 8.4. Relationship between the heart rate and plasma NE responses to exercise in normal persons (*dashed line*) and patients with mild, moderate, severe, and very severe congestive heart failure (**A–D**, respectively). **A**: Despite achieving comparable peak NE concentrations with exercise, the maximal heart rate response is reduced in patients with congestive heart failure, and is related to the severity of the clinical heart failure syndrome. **B**: Dose-response relationship for isoproterenol-stimulated heart rate increase in normal persons (*dashed line*) and patients with severe congestive heart failure (*solid line*). Taken together with the data in A, this observation suggests that chronotropic insufficiency in patients with congestive heart failure is due, at least in part, to desensitization of the β-adrenergic receptor pathway. Reprinted with permission from ref. 17. Copyright by the American Heart Association.

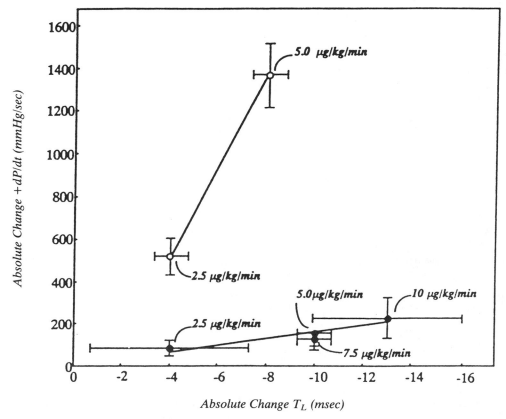

FIGURE 8.5. Relative changes in the positive inotropic (+dP/dt) and lusitropic (Tau, T_L) responses to intravenous infusion of the β-adrenergic agonist, dobutamine in normal persons (*open circles*), and patients with congestive heart failure (*filled circles*). Although the positive inotropic response to β-adrenergic receptor stimulation is markedly attenuated in the patients with heart failure, the positive lusitropic response is well maintained, possibly reflecting the differential second messenger coupling of these two physiologic responses. Reprinted with permission from ref. 31. Copyright by the American Heart Association.

BETA-RECEPTOR DENSITY

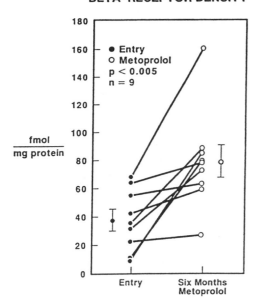

FIGURE 8.6. Myocardial β-adrenergic receptor density as assessed by radioligand binding in right ventricular endomyocardial biopsies obtained from patients with congestive heart failure before and after 6 months of therapy with the β-adrenergic antagonist, metoprolol. The data indicate a substantial upregulation of β-adrenergic receptor density, toward the expected normal levels. This correction in β-adrenergic receptor density was associated with a similar correction in myocardial inotropic responsiveness to a β-adrenergic agonist. Reprinted with permission from ref. 32. Copyright by the American Heart Association.

siveness might reduce the adverse electrophysiologic consequences of sympathetic stimulation. Interestingly, chronic administration of the β-adrenergic antagonist metoprolol to patients with severe congestive heart failure is associated with an increase in the density of myocardial β-adrenergic receptors and a restoration of cardiac responsiveness to β-adrenergic receptor stimulation[32] (Fig. 8.6). Other observations have suggested a similar upregulation of myocardial β-adrenergic receptors may occur during treatment with converting enzyme inhibitors.[33] Such improvement might reflect withdrawal of sympathetic tone due to improved cardiac performance and/or a decrease in peripheral NE release due to reduced angiotensin II levels.

Although most interest has focused on the β-adrenergic pathway, myocardial cells also express α_1-adrenergic receptors that, rather than coupling to adenylate cyclase, activate the phospholipase C/calcium/protein kinase C pathway, a pathway most often associated with vasoconstrictor responses in vascular smooth muscle. However, it can be shown that stimulation of α-adrenergic receptors also causes a posi-

tive inotropic effect in man, both in vitro[34] and in situ,[35] and there is some evidence that the α-adrenergic responsiveness of failing myocardium is reduced compared to that in nonfailing myocardium.[35]

It is now recognized that α-adrenergic receptors may be involved in regulating the growth of cardiac myocytes. In vitro, it can be shown that stimulation of α-adrenergic receptors results in hypertrophy of cardiac myocytes and is associated with changes in gene expression that are typical of the fetal or developing organism, and that are generally associated with pathological hypertrophy.[36] The role of the α-adrenergic receptor in contributing to the process of myocardial hypertrophy, an intermediate stage in the progression to myocardial failure, is an area of active research.

Summary

There are numerous alterations in sympathetic nervous system function in congestive heart failure. In most cases these alterations reflect an exaggeration of normal regulatory mechanisms that are involved in the maintenance of homeostatic cardiovascular function. Increased sympathetic nervous system outflow, likely reflecting both the normal response to impaired pump function and attenuation of baroreceptor sensitivity, contributes to the maintenance of adequate cardiac output, blood pressure, and the perfusion of vital organs. However, increased sympathetic nervous activity also may adversely affect hemodynamic function by increasing left ventricular afterload and preload. In addition, sympathetic activation may exert direct effects on myocardial cells, and thereby contribute to phenotypic and functional alterations involved in the progression of myocardial failure. Alterations in end-organ pathways further modify the overall impact of increased sympathetic nervous system activity by diminishing the responses to catecholamines. It is likely that many therapeutic agents currently in use for the treatment of heart failure act, to some degree, by affecting either sympathetic nervous system activity or end-organ responsiveness.[37] A better understanding of the role of the sympathetic nervous system in heart failure may lead to new therapeutic strategies for this disease.

References

1. Chidsey CA, Braunwald E. Sympathetic activity and neurotransmitter depletion in congestive heart failure. *Pharmacol Rev*. 1966;18;685–700.
2. Thomas JA, Marks BH. Plasma norepinephrine in congestive heart failure. *Am J Cardiol*. 1978;41:233–243.
3. Levine TB, Francis GS, Goldsmith SR, Simon AB, Cohn

JN. Activity of the sympathetic nervous system and renin-angiotensin system assessed by plasma hormone levels and their relation to hemodynamic abnormalities in congestive heart failure. *Am J Cardiol.* 1982;49:1659–1666.

4. Leimbach WN JR, Wallin BG, Victor RG, Aylward PE, Sundlof G, Mark AL. Direct evidence from intraneural recordings for increased central sympathetic outflow in patients with heart failure. *Circulation.* 1986;73:913–919.

5. Swedberg K, Viquerat C, Rouleau JL, et al. Comparison of myocardial catecholamine balance in chronic congestive heart failure and angina pectoris without failure. *J Clin Pharmacol.* 1984;54:783–786.

6. Hasking GJ, Esler MD, Jennings GL, Burton D, Johns JA, Korner PI. Norepinephrine spillover to plasma in patients with congestive heart failure: evidence of increased overall and cardiorenal sympathetic nervous activity. *Circulation.* 1986;73:615–621.

7. Langer SZ. Presynaptic regulation of the release of catecholamines. *Pharmacol Rev.* 1981;32:337–362.

8. Hirsch AT, Dzau VJ, Creager MA. Baroreceptor function in congestive heart failure: effect on neurohumoral activation and regional vascular resistance. *Circulation.* 1987;75:IV-36–IV-48.

9. Rea RF, Berg WJ. Abnormal baroreflex mechanisms in congestive heart failure. Recent insights. *Circulation.* 1990;81:2026–2027.

10. Wang W, Chen J-S, Zucker IH. Carotid sinus baroreceptor sensitivity in experimental heart failure. *Circulation.* 1990;81:1959–1966.

11. Olivari MT, Levine TB, Cohn JN. Abnormal neurohumoral response to nitroprusside infusion in congestive heart failure. *J Am Coll Cardiol.* 1983;2:411–417.

12. Levine TB, Francis GS, Goldsmith SR, Cohn JN. The neurohumoral and hemodynamic response to orthostatic tilt in patients with congestive heart failure. *Circulation.* 1983;67:1070–1075.

13. Kubo SH, Cody RJ. Circulatory autoregulation in chronic congestive heart failure: Responses to head-up tilt in 41 patients. *Am J Cardiol.* 1983;52:512–518.

14. Ellenbogen KA, Mohanty PK, Szentpetery S, Thames MD. Arterial baroreflex abnormalities in heart failure. Reversal after orthotopic cardiac transplantation. *Circulation.* 1989;79:51–58.

15. Ferguson DW, Abboud FM, Mark AL. Selective impairment of baroreflex-mediated vasoconstrictor responses in patients with ventricular dysfunction. *Circulation.* 1984;69:451–460.

16. Bevan JA, Su C. Variation of intra- and perisynaptic adrenergic transmitter concentrations with width of synaptic cleft in vascular tissue. *J Pharmacol Exp Ther.* 1974;190:30.

17. Colucci WS, Ribeiro JP, Rocco MB, et al. Impaired chronotropic response to exercise in patients with congestive heart failure. Role of postsynaptic β-adrenergic desensitization. *Circulation.* 1989;80:314–323.

18. Daly PA, Sole MJ. Myocardial catecholamines and the pathophysiology of heart failure. *Circulation.* 1990;82:I-35–I-43.

19. Isaacson JS, Reid IA. Importance of endogenous angiotensin II in the cardiovascular responses to sym-

pathetic stimulation in conscious rabbits. *Circ Res.* 1990;66:662–671.

20. Kubo SH, Rector TS, Heifetz SM, Cohn JN. α_2-Receptor-mediated vasoconstriction in patients with congestive heart failure. *Circulation.* 1989;80:1660–1667.

21. Rose CP, Burgess JH, Cousineau D. Tracer norepinephrine kinetics in coronary circulation of patients with heart failure secondary to chronic pressure and volume overload. *J Clin Invest.* 1985;76:1740–1747.

22. Liang C-S, Fan T-H, Sullebarger JT, Sakamoto S. Decreased adrenergic neuronal uptake activity in experimental right heart failure. A chamber-specific contributor to beta-adrenoceptor downregulation. *J Clin Invest.* 1989;84:1267–1275.

23. Meredith IT, Esler MD, Jennings GL, Eisenhofer G. Increased cardiac norepinephrine spillover in heart failure is due to Increased release and not reduced neuronal uptake. *Circulation.* 1991;84(suppl II):II-468. Abstract.

24. Bristow MR, Hershberger RE, Port JD, et al. β-Adrenergic pathways in nonfailing and failing human ventricular myocardium. *Circulation.* 1990;82:I-12–I-25.

25. Brodde O-E. β_1- and β_2-Adrenoceptors in the human heart: Properties, function, and alterations in chronic heart failure. *Pharmacol Rev.* 1991;43:203–242.

26. Bristow MR, Ginsburg R, Fowler M, et al. β_1 and β_2-adrenergic receptor subpopulations in normal and failing human ventricular myocardium: Coupling of both receptor subtypes to muscle contraction and selective β_1-receptor downregulation in heart failure. *Circ Res.* 1986;59:297–309.

27. Fowler MB, Laser JA, Hopkins GL, Minobe W, Bristow MR. Assessment of the β-adrenergic receptor pathway in the intact failing human heart: progressive receptor downregulation and subsensitivity to agonist response. *Circulation.* 1985;74:1290–1302.

28. Colucci WS, Denniss AR, Leatherman GF, et al. Intracoronary infusion of dobutamine to patients with and without severe congestive heart failure. Dose-response relationships, correlation with circulating catecholamines, and effect of phosphodiesterase inhibition. *J Clin Invest.* 1988;81:1103–1110.

29. Feldman AM, Cates AE, Veazey WB, et al. Increase of the 40,000-mol wt pertussis toxin substrate (G protein) in the failing human heart. *J Clin Invest.* 1988;82:189–197.

30. Bristow MR, Anderson FL, Port JD, et al. Differences in β-adrenergic neuroeffector mechanisms in ischemic versus idiopathic dilated cardiomyopathy. *Circulation.* 1991;84:1024–1039.

31. Parker JD, Landzberg JS, Bittl JA, Mirsky I, Colucci WS. Effects of β-adrenergic stimulation with dobutamine on isovolumic relaxation in the normal and failing human left ventricle. *Circulation.* 1991;84:1040–1048.

32. Heilbrunn SM, Shah P, Bristow MR, Valantine HA, Ginsburg R, Fowler MB. Increased β-receptor density and improved hemodynamic response to catecholamine stimulation during long-term metoprolol therapy in heart failure from dilated cardiomyopathy. *Circulation.* 1989;79:483–490.

33. Horn EM, Bilezikian JP. Mechanisms of abnormal transmembrane signaling of the β-adrenergic receptor in congestive heart failure. *Circulation.* 1990;82:I-26–I-34.

34. Benfey RG. Function of myocardial α-adrenoceptors. *Life Sci.* 1990;743–757.

35. Landzberg JS, Parker JD, Gauthier DF, Colucci WS Effects of myocardial α_1-adrenergic receptor stimulation and blockade on contractility in humans. *Circulation.* 1991;84:1608–1614.

36. Simpson PC. Norepinephrine-stimulated hypertrophy of cultured rat myocardial cells is an alpha-1 adrenergic response. *J Clin Invest.* 1983;72:732–738.

37. Bristow MR, Port JD, Hershberger RE, Gilbert EM, Feldman AM. The β-adrenergic receptor-adenylate cyclase complex as a target for therapeutic intervention in heart failure. *Eur Heart J.* 1989;10:45–54.

9
Nonadrenergic Hormonal Alterations in Congestive Heart Failure

Milton Packer

When cardiac output falls after an insult to the myocardium, several neurohormonal mechanisms are activated in an attempt to preserve circulatory homeostasis. These mechanisms include both endogenous vasoconstrictor systems (sympathetic nervous system, renin-angiotensin system, and vasopressin) that act to increase systemic blood pressure and expand intravasular volume, and endogenous vasodilator systems (atrial natriuretic peptide and prostaglandins) that limit the pressor, antinatriuretic, and antidiuretic effects of the vasoconstrictor systems.[1] The hemodynamic and metabolic abnormalities in heart failure result in large part from the complex interplay of these neurohormonal forces, which regulate systemic and regional blood flow as well as salt and water balance.

Among the neurohormonal systems activated in heart failure, some of the most important are those that modulate the interactions of the kidneys and the heart. The heart and the kidneys are the two organs principally designed to maintain the circulation. The heart pumps oxygen-containing blood to vital organs; the kidneys ensure that both the quantity of blood (its volume) and the quality of blood (its oxygen-containing capacity) are optimal. Although the essential elements of this concept have been recognized for several centuries, knowledge of the precise mechanisms by which the two organ systems communicate to achieve their common mission is still evolving. For many years, physicians believed that the heart and kidneys interacted primarily by utilizing hemodynamic signals (pressure and flow), largely because hemodynamic variables were the only ones that physiologists could measure. If the cardiac output decreased, renal perfusion pressures would fall, and this fall would elicit the retention of salt and water in an effort to restore cardiac output. Conversely, if renal function deteriorated, cardiac filling pressures would rise, and this increase would lead to an augmentation of cardiac performance (by the Frand-Starling mechanism) that might restore renal function. However, as techniques were developed to measure minute quantities of circulating substances, investigators have begun to recognize that the heart and kidneys communicate using a variety of signals. Not only are these organ systems linked hemodynamically, but they also are linked hormonally, and these hemodynamic-hormonal interactions control nearly every known aspect of cardiac and renal physiology.

This chapter focuses on the role of nonadrenergic hormonal mechanisms in heart failure, with a particular focus on the hormonal systems that mediate and modulate the functions of the kidneys and the heart.

Release of Hormones from the Kidney

The kidneys respond to circulatory stress by releasing two potent vasoactive factors—angiotensin II and prostaglandins—which are rapidly synthesized whenever renal blood flow is compromised or sympathetic nerve traffic to the kidneys in increased.[2-6] Once activated, these two hormonal signals are greatly amplified within the kidneys (both prostaglandins and angiotensin II stimulate the intrarenal release of each other[3,7]), and thus, high concentrations of both vasoactive substances are achieved within the renal cortex and medulla in both experimental and clinical heart failure.

Renin-Angiotensin System

Although the renin-angiotensin system traditionally has been regarded as a primary force supporting systemic blood pressure, its role is best understood by viewing its activation as an attempt to preserve renal function during states of circulatory stress.[8]

Regulation of the Renin-Angiotensin System

There is little activation of the renin-angiotensin system in normal individuals on a normal sodium diet, and thus, this system appears to play little physiologic role under normal conditions. Consequently, suppression of antiotensin formation in sodium-replete volunteers results in little change in blood pressure, renal blood flow, or glomerular filtration rate.[9,10] However, if individuals are sodium depleted, the intrarenal renin-angiotensin system is activated and exerts a vasoconstrictor effect that is largely confined to the efferent (postglomerular arteriole),[11,12] thereby increasing glomerular capillary hydraulic pressure and filtration fraction.[13–15] This microcirculatory response acts to preserve glomerular filtration, despite the threat posed by the restriction of salt; hence, renal function declines in salt-deplete states if the synthesis or actions of angiotensin II are experimentally or clinically inhibited.[14,16–19]

Intrarenal activation of the renin-angiotensin system plays a greater role in preserving glomerular filtration when renal perfusion pressure is impaired either by disease or by treatment.[14,16] Any change in cardiac performance that threatens renal blood flow is detected by sensory receptors in the renal arterioles; this baroreceptor stimulation leads to the release of renin from the kidneys, an effect that may be potentiated by a reduction in distal tabular sodium chloride transport and stimulation of the renal sympathetic nerves.[20] The subsequent formation of angiotensin II (AII) acts on the efferent arterioles to increase glomerular hydraulic filtration pressure (and to preserve renal function), despite the reduction in renal perfusion pressure.[21] Such an action may explain why patients with bilateral renal artery stenosis or congestive heart failure show a marked decline in renal function after converting-enzyme inhibition,[21–24] an effect that is exaggerated by sodium depletion and is ameliorated by the administration of salt.[24,25] Hence, renal hypoperfusion and sodium depletion act synergistically to determine the importance of the renin-angiotensin system during periods of circulatory stress.

The Renin-Angiotensin System in Heart Failure

Under normal conditions, if excessive activation of the renin-angiotensin occurs and results in an increase in systemic and atrial pressures, operation of arterial and atrial baroreceptors leads to the release of atrial natriuretic peptide as well as to a reduced stimulation of the renal sympathetic nerves, both of which act to reduce renin release. However, the function of atrial and arterial baroreceptors is markedly impaired in congestive heart failure, and thus, atrial distension does not suppress renal sympathetic activity in this disorder.[26] In addition, the ability of atrial distension to stimulate the release of atrial natriuretic peptide is impaired in chronic heart failure, as is the ability of the peptide to suppress renin release.[27,28] These derangements interfere with the capacity of the failing circulation to limit the

release of renin from the kidneys, particularly in the face of a persistent stimulus to such release (a low renal perfusion pressure). Consequently, most patients with heart failure demonstrate an excessive activation of the renin-angiotensin system at rest or during exercise.

Activation of the renin-angiotensin system subserves both beneficial and deleterious roles in patients with chronic heart failure. On the one hand, AII acts to support systemic perfusion pressures and to preserve glomerular filtration rate during states of renal hypoperfusion.[21] On the other hand, prolonged activation of the renin-angiotensin system may exert deleterious effects on ventricular function by a direct toxic effect on the heart, by causing direct systemic vasoconstriction and by facilitating the vasoconstrictor actions of the sympathetic nervous system as well as the release of vasopressin.[29,30] Furthermore, by stimulating the synthesis of aldosterone, angiotensin promotes the retention of salt and water by the kidney (which may further exacerbate loading conditions in the failing heart) and the depletion of potassium and magnesium (which may predispose to the occurrence of complex ventricular arrhythmias).[34]

Clinical Observations

The renin-angiotensin system is activated in patients with congestive heart failure in proportion to the severity of the disease.[32] In patients with mild symptoms, plasma renin activity is normal at rest but rises to high levels on exertion.[33] As symptoms become progressively more severe and renal perfusion pressure falls, plasma renin activity becomes elevated at rest, and the magnitude of the elevation parallels the degree of hemodynamic and functional impairment.[32] These observations may explain why plasma renin activity (or its marker, serum sodium concentration) provides important prognostic information in these patients.[34–36]

Several factors contribute to the activation of the renin-angiotensin system in chronic heart failure. In the early stages of the disease the increase in plasma renin activity is primarily due to stimulation of the renal sympathetic nerves and the use of diuretics,[37–39] whereas in the late stages the fall in renal perfusion pressure directly stimulates the release of renin from the kidney.[40] Interestingly, renal hypoperfusion acts not only to release renin but also to impair the clearance of free water (leading to dilutional hyponatremia); the development of hyponatremia is enhanced further by an increased intake of water, which results from the direct stimulation of the cerebral thirst center by AII.[41] these interactions explain why an inverse relation exists between plasma renin activity and serum sodium concentration in chronic heart failure[34,42] and why both hyponatremia and high levels of renin are markers of renal hypoperfusion.[40,43]

Drugs that interfere with the renin-angiotensin system (converting enzyme inhibitors, renin inhibitors, and AII antagonists) produce hemodynamic and clinical benefits in patients with heart failure,[44,45] but their efficacy in an individual patient cannot be predicted by conventional measurements of the activity of the renin-angiotensin system (e.g., the assessment of plasma renin activity).[46] This may be related to the fact that the range of "normal" values for plasma renin activity, established in hypertensive patients who were taking no medications and who were in sodium balance, are difficult to apply to patients with heart failure, who are commonly in a salt-retaining state despite treatment with diuretic drugs. To make matters more complicated, low levels of AII may exert a prolonged pressor effect that is reversed by long-term (but not short-term) angiotensin inhibition[47]; this may be related to the fact that renin and angiotensin may act as local tissue hormones, so that circulating levels may not reflect the concentration of these substances at active receptor sites.[48] Furthermore, converting enzyme inhibitors may act in a complex manner with hormonal systems other than the renin-angiotensin system (catecholamines, vasopressin, kinins, and prostaglandins), and these additional actions may contribute substantially to their clinical effects.

Renal Prostaglandin System

In response to the same circulatory stresses that lead to activation of the renin-angiotensin system, the kidneys release prostaglandins that serve to potentiate the beneficial and limit the deleterious actions of the renin-angiotensin system.

Regulation of the Renal Prostaglandin System

The kidneys release two types of prostaglandins that are important in the regulation of renal function: prostacyclin (PGI_2) and prostaglandin E_2. Both substances possess minimal vasodilator activity under basal conditions, but are potent vasodilators under conditions of prior vasoconstriction.[49-51] Hence, suppression of prostaglandin formation in sodium-replete individuals results in little change in blood pressure, renal blood flow, or glomerular filtration rate.[51-53] However, in the presence of sodium depletion or activation of the renin-angiotensin system, prostaglandins are synthesized within the kidneys[54-56] and exert a renal vasodilator action predominantly at the level of the afferent arteriole,[57,58] thereby increasing glomerular capillary hydraulic filtration pressure and filtration fraction.[49] This microcirculatory response acts to preserve glomerular filtration rate, despite the threat posed by the restriction of dietary salt; hence, renal function declines modestly in salt-deplete states if the formation of prostaglandins is inhibited.[54] Intrarenal prostaglandin synthesis plays a greater role in preserving glomerular filtration rate when renal perfusion pressure is impaired, either by disease or by treatment.[2,57,58] Such hypoperfusion may stimulate prostaglandin release directly or indirectly by the intrarenal activation of the renin-angiotensin system.[7,49,59] Consequently, glomerular filtration rate may decline markedly after cyclooxygenase inhibition when renal blood flow is anatomically or physiologically compromised,[6,57,60] an effect that is exaggerated by sodium depletion and can be ameliorated by the administration of salt.[61]

Thus, both prostaglandins and AII increase glomerular hydraulic filtration pressure and thereby act to preserve glomerular filtration rate—the prostaglandins by a dilating action on the afferent arteriole and AII by a constricting effect on the efferent arteriole. Yet, at nearly all other sites, the actions of renal prostaglandins oppose those of AII. Prostaglandins antagonize the actions of AII on systemic blood vessels and decrease loading conditions in the failing heart.[62] In addition, prostaglandins decrease total body sodium and water by several mechanisms: they directly inhibit sodium reabsorption in the renal tubules,[63] they antagonize the dipsogenic effects of AII,[64] and they oppose the actions of AII-mediated vasopressin release in the collecting duct.[65-67] Finally, prostaglandins may directly reduce the frequency and complexity of ventricular arrhythmias. Hence, the release of renal prostaglandins may neutralize many of the adverse effects that might be expected to accompany the activation of the renin-angiotensin system.

Clinical Observations

Renal hypoperfusion is a potent stimulus not only to the release of renin but also to the release of vasodilator prostaglandins from the kidney. Both hormones are released further in response to diuretic therapy and to stimulation of the renal sympathetic nerves, and once formed within the kidney, both prostaglandins and AII stimulate the intrarenal release of each other.[68,69] Hence, it is not surprising that patients with heart failure who show the highest plasma renin activity also show the highest circulating levels of prostacyclin and prostaglandin E_2[62] The physiologic marker of such activation is the presence of hyponatremia, since this marker identifies patients with heart failure who have the most compromised renal perfusion.[43]

The interaction between prostaglandins and AII in heart failure is potentiated by the administration of diuretics. Both hormones are released from the kidney during diuretic therapy but exert opposite effects on the systemic vasculature. This may explain why intravenous furosemide has been reported to cause vasodilation in some reports but vasoconstriction in others.[70,71] Both hormones also modify the natriuretic response to furosemide, which is potentiated and attenuated by converting enzyme inhibitors and cyclooxygenase inhibitors, respectively.

Finally, the importance of prostaglandins in limiting the actions of AII in heart failure may explain the effects of cyclooxygenase inhibitors in these patients. Indomethacin produces notable systemic vasoconstriction and hemodynamic deterioration in heart failure because of the unopposed action of AII and other systemic vasoconstrictor hormones.[62] Cyclooxygenase inhibition results in a marked reduction in renal blood flow in low-output states, unless the actions of AII are simultaneously blocked.[58] Indomethacin also may produce sodium and water retention in patients with heart failure. These adverse effects of prostaglandin inhibition are seen most likely in patients with hyponatremic heart failure, who have the highest circulating levels of prostaglandins and the most compromised renal perfusion.[43,62]

These observations suggest that in patients with severely compromised renal perfusion, the release of prostaglandins by the kidneys acts as an adaptive response that counteracts the deleterious effects of the renin-angiotensin system. Prostaglandins may not limit the response to AII in patients with less severe heart failure, however, whose renal blood flow is only modestly reduced. Furthermore, prostaglandins generally are regarded as sutocoids, and thus, their actions usually are confined to their organ of origin (the kidneys). Accordingly, for most patients with heart failure, atrial natriuretic peptide may function as the primary antagonist of the renin-angiotensin system. However, as the condition of the patient deteriorates and renal blood flow is progressively reduced, the intrarenal actions of the atrial peptides become attenuated, and renal prostaglandins become increasingly important as antagonists of the action of AII.

Release of Hormones from the Heart

As do the kidneys, the heart responds to circulatory stress by modulating the activity of two potent vasoactive factors: norepinephrine and atrial natriuretic peptide. These two hormonal signals in the heart are regulated by a common hemodynamic trigger (atrial distension), they oppose each other's actions, and their control mechanisms become progressively more deranged as the heart failure state advances.

Regulation of Atrial Natriuretic Peptide

Any change in cardiac performance that increases cardiac filling pressures is detected by stretch receptors in the right and left atria, leading to the release of atrial natriuretic peptides from the heart. Once released, atrial peptides exert potent direct vasodilator and natriuretic actions by virtue of their ability to increase intracellular cyclic guanesine monsphosphate (GMP); these effects unload the heart and reduce its energy consumption. In addition, atrial peptides antagonize the actions of most endogenous vasoconstrictor systems. Under experimental conditions, atrial natriuretic peptide inhibits the release of norepinephrine from nerve terminals as well as the vasoconstrictor actions of norepinephrine on systemic vessels; it also enhances baroreceptor sensitivity and thereby reduces central activation of the sympathetic nervous system. Atrial peptides suppress the formation of renin and oppose the systemic vasoconstrictor actions of AII as well as angiotensin's ability to stimulate thirst and the secretion of aldosterone and vasopressin. Atrial peptides inhibit the release of vasopressin as well as its vasoconstrictor effects on systemic blood vessels and its antidiuretic effects on the collecting duct. These observations suggest that atrial natriuretic peptides function as versatile neruohormonal antagonists.[72–75] Such antagonism not only ameliorates cardiac distension, but it also attenuates any adverse effect of endogenous vasoconstrictors on the kidneys.

Although atrial peptides exert important natriuretic and renin-suppressive effects in acute heart failure, the function of atrial stretch receptors becomes impaired and the content of atrial peptides becomes depleted when heart failure enters its chronic phase. As a result, although the circulating levels of atrial natriuretic peptide are increased markedly in heart failure, the slope of the atrial pressure/response curve is shifted, such that the circulating levels of atrial peptide are reduced at a given level of atrial pressure.[27] It is noteworthy that as the atrial content of natriuretic peptides becomes depleted in chronic heart failure, natriuretic peptides are synthesized by ventricular myocytes, and this source may contribute substantially to the circulating level of atrial peptides.[76] The localization of natriuretic peptides in the ventricular myocardium appears to represent regression to a more primitive evolutionary state, since natriuretic peptides normally are found in the ventricle only in nonmammalian species, but disappear from the ventricle in higher forms of life unless heart failure supervenes.[77]

Although atrial peptides exert potent natriuretic effects in acute heart failure, patients with chronic heart failure demonstrate marked sodium retention, despite the very high circulating levels of atrial peptides. This appears to be related to a marked attenuation of the ability of the released peptides to exert natriuretic effects and suppress neurohormonal activity.[28] This attenuation of the actions of atrial natriuretic factor may be related to a decline in the density of receptors for the peptide,[78,79] to a decline in renal blood flow,[80,81] or to the intrarenal antagonism of the actions of the peptide by the sympathetic nervous system and the renin-angiotensin system.[82] Regardless of the mechanism of attenuation, however, it is likely that atrial natriuretic peptide does not function as an important homeostatic hormone in most patients with chronic heart failure.

Clinical Observations

An elevation in the level of atrial natriuretic peptide in the circulation is one of the earliest hormonal markers of heart failure. The activity of this system is enhanced before the activation of other neurohormonal systems and increases progressively as the severity of heart failure becomes advanced.[83] This may explain why circulatory levels of atrial natriuretic peptide have prognostic significance in patients with chronic heart failure, with the highest levels seen in patients with the most unfavorable long-term outcome.[84]

Attempts have been made to increase circulating and tubular levels of atrial natriuretic peptide by the administration of agents that inhibit the activity of atriopeptidase, the enzyme responsible for the degradation of endogenous peptide. The administration of atriopeptidase inhibitors has produced favorable hemodynamic and natriuretic effects in patients with chronic heart failure,[85] but clinical experience with these drugs is limited. Conversely, a number of pharmacologic interventions that improve cardiac performance lead to a decrease in the circulating level of atrial natriuretic peptide, presumably as a consequence of a drug-induced decline in right and left atrial pressure.[86] This reduced release of atrial peptides is not necessarily accompanied by sodium retention, however. If therapy improves renal blood flow or decreases the activity of counteractive endogenous vasoconstrictor hormones, the reduced level of atrial peptides may be more effective in eliciting a natriuretic response than the higher levels seen before treatment.

Other Hormonal Derangements in Heart Failure

Endothelian-Derived Vasoconstrictors and Vasodilators

Many of the neurohormonal systems that are activated in patients with heart failure exert potent constrictor effects on peripheral blood vessels, but peripheral blood vessels (specifically, the endothelium) are capable of synthesizing and releasing their own vasoconstrictor and vasodilator factors in response to changes in pressure and flow and to alterations in the neurohormonal environment. The principal vasodilator substance produced by the endothelium is endothelium-derived relax-

ing factor (possibly mitric oxide), which induces relaxation by increasing levels of intracellular cyclic GMP in vascular smooth muscle. The principal vasoconstrictor produced by the endothelium is endothelin, which induces constriction possibly by activating the inositoltriphosphate pathway.

Under normal conditions, the vasoconstrictor effects of endothelin are counterbalanced by the vasodilator effects of endothelium-derived relaxing factor. However, in chronic heart failure, levels of endothelin are markedly elevated (in proportion to the severity of the disease),[87] and the release of endothelium-derived relaxing factor is markedly diminished.[88] Consequently, as in the case of circulating neurohormones, the balance between these locally active vasodilators is shifted in favor of vasoconstriction. This imbalance is restored toward normal after cardiac transplantation.[89]

Little is known about the effect of various pharmacologic interventions on the production of endothelial-derived vasoconstrictor and vasodilator factors. Nitrates mediate their vasodilator effects in part by increasing the release of endothelial-derived relaxing factor, and flosequinan may exert its vasodilator effects by interfering with the intracellular actions of endothelin. Pharmacologic agents that interfere with the production of endothelin or the interaction with its receptor are under development.

Vasopressin

Circulating levels of vasopressin are increased in patients with severe heart failure because of a nonosmotic stimulus to the release of the hormone consequent to the reduction in cardiac output and effective peripheral perfusion.[90–92] Hence, plasma vasopressin levels are elevated in heart failure in direct proportion to the hemodynamic and clinical severity of the heart failure state,[93,94] and vasopressin may contribute directly to the systemic vasoconstriction seen in this disorder.[95,96] Plasma vasopressin levels are increased in parallel to a rise in plasma renin activity,[92] in part because compromised end-organ perfusion and baroreceptor dysfunction are common stimuli to both vasopressin and renin release and in part because AII may directly stimulate the hypophyseal production of vasopressin.[97] Since hyponatremia is a marker of poor systemic perfusion, it is not surprising that both plasma renin activity and plasma vasopressin are markedly elevated in hyponatremic heart failure[90] and have been implicated in the pathogenesis of the abnormal water metabolism in this condition.[98] Given the prognostic importance of hyponatremia, it is likely that future work will demonstrate a close relation between elevated plasma levels of vasopressin and a poor long-term outcome in heart failure. There are no data, however, that suggest that vasopressin exerts a direct deleterious effect on survival in this disorder.

Tumor Necrosis Factor

Tumor necrosis factor is a pluripotent cytokine produced primarily by monocytes that has been shown experimentally to cause cachexia and anorexia.[99,100] Elevated circulating levels of tumor necrosis factor have been noted in patients with a variety of neoplastic, infectious, and collagen vascular disorders, many of which are characterized by severe weight loss and anorexia. Interestingly, circulating levels of cytokines (e.g., tumor necrosis factor) also are elevated in heart failure, particularly in patients with marked neurohormonal activation.[101] Cytokines may contribute to the development of the anorexia and cachexia, may exacerbate the production of cardiotoxic oxygen free radicals, and may explain the attenuated myocardial responsiveness to catecholamines and the diminished peripheral vascular responsiveness to endothelial-mediated vasodilators seen in this disorder.[102,103] All of these physiologic abnormalities are corrected after cardiac transplantation, as circulating levels of tumor necrosis factor decline.[104] Elevated levels of cytokines (and other markers of monocyte activation) bear an important relationship to survival in heart failure.[105] The role that cytokines may play in the progression of heart failure is an exciting area of future research.

References

1. Packer M. Neurohormonal interactions and adaptations in congestive heart failure. *Circulation.* 1988;77:721–730.
2. Jackson EK, Gerkens JF, Brash AR, Branch RA. Acute renal artery constriction increases renal prostaglandin I_2 biosynthesis and renin release in the conscious dog. *J Pharmacol Exp Ther.* 1982;222:410–413.
3. Freeman RH, Davis JO, Dietz JR, Villareal D, Seymour AA, Echtenkamp SF. Renal prostaglandins and the control of renin release. *Hypertension.* 1982;4(suppl II):106–112.
4. Vander AJ. Effects of catecholamines and renal nerves on renin secretion in anesthetized dogs. *Am J Physiol.* 1965;209:659–662.
5. Dunham EW, Zimmerman BG. Release of prostaglandin-like material from dog kidney during nerve stimulation. *Am J Physiol.* 1970;219:1279–1285.
6. Henrich WL, Anderson RJ, Bernes AS. The role of renal nerves and prostaglandins in control of renal hemodynamics and plasma renin activity during hypotensive hemorrhage in the dog. *J Clin Invest.* 1978;61:744–750.
7. Stahl RA, Paravincini M, Schollmeyer P. Angiotensin II stimulation of PGE_2 and 6–keto-PGF_{1a} formation by isolated human gloermuli. *Kidney Int.* 1984;26:30–34.
8. Packer M. Interaction of prostaglandins and angiotensin II in the modulation of renal function in congestive heart failure. *Circulation.* 1988;77(suppl I):64–73.
9. Hollenberg NK, Williams GH, Taub KJ, Ishikawa I, Brown C, Adams DF. Renal vascular response to interruption of the renin-angiotensin system in normal man. *Kidney Int.* 1977;12:285–293.
10. Faxon DP, Creager MA, Haperin JL, Bernard DB, Ryan TJ. Redistribution of regional blood flow following angiotensin-converting-enzyme inhibition. Comparison of normal subjects and patients with heart failure. *Am J Med.* 1984;76:104–110.
11. Edwards RM. Segmental effects of norepinephrine and angiotensin II on isolated renal microvessels. *Am J Physiol.* 1983;244:F526–F534.
12. Ichikawa J, Miele JF, Brenner BM. Reversal of renal cortical actions of angiotensin II by verapamil and manganese. *Kidney Int.* 1979;16:137–147.
13. Myers BD, Deen WM, Brenner BM. Effects of norepinephrine and angiotensin II on the determinants of glomerular ultrafiltration and proximal tubule fluid readsorption in the rat. *Circ Res.* 1975;37:101–110.
14. Hall JE, Guyton AC, Jackson TE, Coleman TG, Lohmeier TE, Trippodo NC. Control of glomerular filtration rate by renin angiotensin system. *Am J Physiol.* 1977;233:F366–F372.
15. Hall JE, Guyton AC, Smith MJ Jr, Coleman TG. Chronic blockade of angiotensin II formation during sodium deprivation. *Am J Physiol.* 1979;237:F424–F432.
16. Lohmeier TE, Cowley AW, Trippodo NC, Hall JE, Guyton AC. Effects of endogenous angiotensin II on renal sodium excretion and renal hemodynamics. *Am J Physiol.* 1977;233:F388–F395.
17. Kastner PR, Hall JE, Guyton AC. Control of glomerular filtration rate: role of intrarenally formed angiotensin II. *Am J Physiol.* 1984;246:F897–F906.
18. Murphy BF, Whitworth JA, Kincaid-Smith P. Renal insufficiency with combinations of angiotensin converting enzyme inhibitors and diuretics. *Br Med J.* 1984;288:844–845.
19. Pariente EA, Bataille C, Bercoff E, Lebrec D. Acute effects of captopril on systemic and renal hemodynamics and on renal function in cirrhotic patients with ascites. *Gastroenterology.* 1985;88:1255–1259.
20. Hirsch AT, Dzau VJ, Creager MA. Baroreceptor function in congestive heart failure: effect on neurohormonal activation and regional vascular resistance. *Circulation.* 1987;75(suppl IV):36–48.
21. Packer M, Lee WH, Kessler PD. Preservation of gloermular filtration rate in human heart failure by activation of the renin-angiotensin system. *Circulation.* 1986;74:766–774.
22. Hricik DE, Browning PJ, Kapelman R, Goorno WE, Madias NE, Dzau VJ. Captopril-induced functional renal insufficiency in patients with bilateral renal-artery stenosis or stenosis in a solitary kidney. *N Engl J Med.* 1983;308:373–376.
23. Curtiss JJ, Luke RG, Whelchel JD, Diethelm AG, Jones P, Dustan HP. Inhibition of angiotensin-converting enzyme in renal-transplant recipients with hypertension. *N Engl J Med.* 1983;308:377–381.
24. Packer M, Lee WH, Kessler PD. Functional renal insufficiency during long-term therapy with captopril and enalapril in severe chronic heart failure. *Ann Intern Med.* 1987;106:346–354.
25. Hricik DE. Captopril-induced renal insufficiency and the role of sodium balance. *Ann Intern Med.* 1985;103:222–223.
26. Zucker IH, Share L, Gilmore JP. Renal effects of left

atrial distension in dogs with chronic congestive heart failure. *Am J Physiol*. 1979;236:H554–H560.

27. Redfield MM, Edwards BS, McGoon MD, Heublein DM, Aarhus LL, Burnett JC Jr. Failure of atrial natriuretic factor to increase with volume expansion in acute and chronic congestive heart failure in the dog. *Circulation*. 1989;80:651–657.

28. Cody RJ, Atlas SA, Laragh JH, et al. Atrial natriuretic factor in normal subjects and heart failure patients: plasma levels and renal, hormonal, and hemodynamic responses to peptide infusion. *J Clin Invest*. 1986;78:1362–1374.

29. Tan LB, Jalil JE, Pick R, Janicki JS, Weber KT. Cardiac myocyte necrosis induced by angiotensin II. *Circ Res*. 1991;69:1185–1195.

30. Francis GS, Goldsmith SR, Olivari MT, Levine TB, Cohn JN. The neurohormonal axis in congestive heart failure. *Ann Intern Med*. 1984;101:370–377.

31. Packer M, Gottlieb SS, Kessler PD. Hormone-electrolyte interactions in the pathogenesis of lethal cardiac arrhymias in patients with congestive heart failure. The basis of a new physiologic approach to control of arrhythmia. *Am J Med*. 1986;80(4A):23–29.

32. Dzau VJ, Colucci WS, Hollenberg NK, Williams GH. Relation of renin-angiotensin-aldosterone system to clinical state in congestive heart failure. *Circulation*. 1981;63:645–651.

33. Kirlin PC, Grekin R, Das S, Ballor E, Johnson T, Pitt B. Neurohumoral activation during exercise in congestive heart failure. *Am J Med*. 1986;81:623–629.

34. Lee WH, Packer M. Prognostic importance of serum sodium concentration and its modification by converting-enzyme inhibition in patients with severe chronic heart failure. *Circulation*. 1986;73:257–267.

35. Rockman HA, Juneau C, Chatterjee K, Rouleau JL. Long-term predictors of sudden and low output death in chronic congestive heart failure secondary to coronary artery disease. *Am J Cardiol*. 1989;64:1344–1348.

36. Dargie HJ, Cleland JGF, Leckie BJ, Inglis CG, East BW, Ford I. Relation of arrhythmias and electrolyte abnormalities to survival in patients with severe chronic heart failure. *Circulation*. 1987;75 (suppl IV):98–107.

37. Dibner-Dunlap ME, Thames MD. Baroreflex control of renal sympathetic nerve activity is preserved in heart failure despite reduced arterial baroreceptor sensitivity. *Circ Res*. 1989;65:1526–1535.

38. Francis GS, Siegel RM, Goldsmith SR, Olivari MT, Levine TB, Cohn JN. Acute vasoconstrictor response to intravenous furosemide in patients with chronic congestive heart failure. *Ann Intern Med*. 1985;103:1–6.

39. Kubo SH, Clark M, Laragh JH, Borer JS, Cody RJ. Identification of normal neurohormonal activity in mild congestive heart failure and stimulating effect of upright posture and diuretics. *Am J Cardiol*. 1987;60:1322–1328.

40. Goldenberg IF, Levine TB, Olivari MT, Petein MA, Cohn JN. Markers of reduced renal blood flow in patients with congestive heart failure. *Circulation*. 1985;72(suppl III):III-284. Abstract.

41. Packer M, Medina M, Yushak M. Correction of dilutional hyponatremia in patients with severe chronic heart failure by converting-enzyme inhibition. *Ann Intern Med*. 1984;100:782–789.

42. Packer M, Medina N, Yushak M. Relationship between serum sodium concentration and the hemodynamic and clinical responses to converting-enzyme inhibition with captopril in severe heart failure. *J Am Coll Cardiol*. 1984;3:1035–1043.

43. Lilly LS, Dzau VJ, Williams GH, Rydstedt L, Hollenberg NK. Hyponatremia in congestive heart failure: implications for neurohormonal activation and response to orthostasis. *J Clin Endocrinol Metab*. 1984;59:924–930.

44. Packer M, Medina N, Yushak M, Meller J. Hemodynamic patterns of response during long-term captopril therapy for severe chronic heart failure. *Circulation*. 1983;68:803–812.

45. Neuberg GW, Kukin ML, Pinsky DJ, Medina N, Yushak M, Packer M. Hemodynamic effects of renin inhibition with enalkiren in severe chronic heart failure. *Am J Cardiol*. 1991;67:63–66.

46. Packer M, Medina N, Yushak M, Lee WH. Usefulness of plasma renin activity in predicting hemodynamic and clinical responses and survival during long-term converting-enzyme inhibition in severe chronic heart failure. Experience in 100 consecutive patients. *Br Heart J*. 1985;54:298–304.

47. Riegger AJC, Lever AF, Millar JA, Morton JJ, Slack B. Correction of renal hypertension in the rat by prolonged infusion of angiotensin II inhibitors. *Lancet*. 1977; 2:1317–1319.

48. Swales JD. Arterial wall or plasma renin in hypertension? *Clin Sci*. 1979;56:293–298.

49. Schor N, Ichikawa I, Brenner BM. Mechanisms of action of various hormones and vasoactive substances on glomerular ultrafiltration in the rat. *Kidney Int*. 1981; 20:442–451.

50. Chapnick BM, Paustian PW, Feigen LP. Influences of inhibitors of prostaglandin synthesis on renal vascular resistance and on renal vascular responses to vasopressor and vasodilator agents in the cat. *Circ Res*. 1977;40:348–354.

51. Terrago NA, Terragno A, McGiff JA. Contribution of prostaglandins to the renal circulation in conscious, anestehtized, and laparotomized dogs. *Circ Res*. 1977;40:590–595.

52. Blasingham MC, Shade RE, Share L, Nasjletti A. The effect of meclofenamate on renal blood flow in the unanesthesized dog: relation to renal prostaglandin and sodium balance. *J Pharmacol Exp Ther*. 1980;214:1–4.

53. Blasingham MC, Nasjletti A. Differential renal effects of cyclo-oxygenase inhibition on sodium-replete and sodium-deprived dog. *Am J Physiol*. 1980;239:F360–F365.

54. Muther RS, Potter DM, Bennett WM. Aspirin-induced depression of gloermular filtration rate in normal humans: role of sodium balance. *Ann Intern Med*. 1981;94:317–321.

55. DeForrest JH, Davis JO, Freeman RH, et al. Effects of indomethacin and meclofenamate on renin release and renal hemodynamic function during chronic sodium depletion in conscious dogs. *Circ Res*. 1980;47:99–107.

56. Stahl RA, Attallah AA, Bloch DL, Lee JB. Stimulation

of rabbit renal PGE$_2$ biosynthesis by dietary sodium restriction. *Am J Physiol*. 1979;237:F344–F349.

57. Echtenkamp SF, Davis JO, DeForrest JM, et al. Effects of indomethacin, renal denervation, and propranolol on plasma renin activity in conscious dogs with chronic thoracic caval constriction. *Circ Res*. 1981;49:492–500.

58. Oliver JA, Sciacca RR, Pinto J, Cannon PJ. Participation of prostaglandins in the control of renal blood flow during acute reduction of cardiac output in the dog. *J Clin Invest*. 1981;67:229–237.

59. Satoh S, Zimmerman BG. Influence of the renin-angiotensin system on the effect of prostaglandin synthesis inhibitors in the renal vasculature. *Circ Res*. 1977;40:348–354.

60. Walshe JJ, Venturo RC. Acute oliguric renal failure induced by indomethacin: possible mechanisms. *Ann Intern Med*. 1979;91:47–49.

61. DiBona GF. Prostaglandins and nonsterodial anti-inflammatory drugs. Effects on renal hemodynamics. *Am J Med*. 1986;80:12–21.

62. Dzau VJ, Packer M, Lilly JS, et al. Prostaglandins in heart failure: relation to activation of the renin-angiotensin system and hyponatremia. *N Engl J Med*. 1984;310:347–354.

63. Stokes JB, Kokko JP. Inhibition of sodium transport by prostaglandin E$_2$ across the isolated perfused rabbit collecting tubule. *J Clin Invest*. 1977;59:1099–1104.

64. Guaita DP, Chiaravigilio E. Effect of prostaglandin E$_1$ and its biosynthesis inhibitor indomethacin on drinking in the rat. *Pharamcol Biochem Behav*. 1980;13:787–792.

65. Anderson RJ, Berl T, McDonald KM, Schrier RW. Evidence for an in vivo antagnism between vasopressin and prostaglandin in the mammalian kidney. *J Clin Invest*. 1975;56:420–426.

66. Berl T, Raz A, Wald H, Horowitz J, Czaczkes W. Prostaglandin synthesis inhibition and the action of vasopressin: studies in man and rat. *Am J Physiol*. 1977; 232:F529–F537.

67. Fejes-Toth G, Magyar A, Walter J. Renal response to vasopressin after inhibition of prostaglandin synthesis. *Am J Physiol*. 1977;232:F416–F423.

68. Katayama S, Attallah AA, Stahl RAK, Bloch DL, Lee JB. Mechanism of furosemide-induced natriuresis by direct stimulation of renal prostaglandin E$_2$. *Am J Physiol*. 1984;247:F555–F561.

69. DeForrest JH, Davis JO, Freeman RH, et al. Effects of indomethacin and meclofenamate in renin release and renal hemodynamic function during chronic sodium depletion in conscious dogs. *Circ Res*. 1980;47:99–107.

70. Johnston GD, Hiatt WR, Nies AS, Payne NA, Murphy RC, Gerber JC. Factors modifying the early non-diuretic vascular effects of furosemide in man: the possible role of renal prostaglandins. *Circ Res*. 1983;53:630–635.

71. Francis GS, Siegel RM, Goldsmith SR, Olivari MT, Levine TB, Cohn JN. Acute vasoconstrictive response to intravenous furosemide in patients with chronic congestive heart failure. *Ann Intern Med*. 1985;103:1–6.

72. Laragh JH. Atrial natriuretic hormone, the renin-aldosterone axis, and blood pressure-electrolyte homeostasis. *N Engl J Med*. 1985;313:1330–1340.

73. Harris PJ, Thomas D, Morgan TO. Atrial natriuretic peptide inhibits angiotensin-stimulated proximal tubular sodium and water reabsorption. *Nature* 1987;326:697–701.

74. Lappe RW, Dinish JL, Bex F, Wendt RL. Effects of atrial natriuretic factor on drinking responses to central angiotensin II. *Pharmacol Biochem Behav*. 1986; 24:1573–1576.

75. Antunes-Rodrigures J, McCann SM, Rogers LC, Samson WK. Atrial natriuretic factors inhibits dehydration- and angiotensin II-induced water intake in the conscious, unrestrained rat. *Proc Natl Acad Sci USA*. 1985; 82:8720–8730.

76. Chapeau C, Gutowska J, Schiller PW, et al. Localization of immunoreactive synthetic atrial natriuretic factor (ANF) in the heart of various animal species. *J Histochem Cytochem*. 1985;33:541–550.

77. Nadal-Ginard B, Mahdavi V. Molecular basis of cardiac performance. Plasticity of the myocardium generated through protein isoform switches. *J Clin Invest*. 1989;84:1693–1700.

78. Schiffrin EL. Decreased density of binding sites for atrial natriuretic peptide on platelets of patients with severe congestive heart failure. *Clin Sci*. 1988;74:213–218.

79. Tsunoda K, Mendelsohn FA, Sexton PM, Chai SY, Hodsman GP, Johnston CI. Decreased atrial natriuretic peptide binding in renal medulla in rats with chronic heart failure. *Circ Res*. 1988;62:155–161.

80. Sosa RE, Volpe M, Marion DN, et al. Relationship between renal hemodynamic and natriuretic effects of atrial natriuretic factor. *Am J Physiol*. 1986;250:F520–F524.

81. Redfield MM, Edwards BS, Heublein DM, Burnett JC Jr. Restoration of renal response to atrial natriuretic factor in experimental low-output heart failure. *Am J Physiol*. 1989;257:R917–R923.

82. Petersson A, Hedner J, Hedner T. Renal interaction between sympathetic activity and ANP in rats with chronic ischaemic heart failure. *Acta Physiol Scand*. 1989; 135:487–492.

83. Francis GS, Benedict C, Johnstone DE, et al. Comparison of neuroendocrine activation in patients with left ventricular dysfunction with and without congestive heart failure. *Circulation*. 1990;82:1724–1729.

84. Gottlieb SS, Kukin ML, Ahern D, Packer M. Prognostic importance of atrial natriuretic peptide in patients with chronic heart failure. *J Am Coll Cardiol*. 1989;13:1534–1539.

85. Northridge DB, Jardine AG, Finlay IN, Archibald H, Dilly SG, Dargie HJ. Inhibition of the mtabolism of atrial natriuretic factor causes diuresis and natriuresis in chronic heart failure. *Am J Hypertension*. 1990;3:682–687.

86. Packer M, Nicod, P, Khandheria BR, et al. Randomized, multicenter, double-blind, placebo-controlled evaluation of amlodipine in patients with mild-to-moderate heart failure. *J Am Coll Cardiol*. 1991;17:274A.

87. Margulies KB, Hildebrand FL, Lerman A, Perrella MA, Burnett JC Jr. Increased endothelin in experimental heart failure. *Circulation*. 1990;82:2226–2230.

88. Kubo SH, Rector TS, Bank AJ, Williams RE, Heifetz SM, Endothelium- dependent vasodilation is attenuated

in patients with heart failure. *Circulation*. 1991;84:1589–1596.

89. Kubo SH, Rector TS, Bank AJ, et al. Heart transplantation reverses abnormalities in endothelium-dependent dilation of peripheral blood vessels in patients with heart failure. *Circulation*. 1991;84(suppl II):II-469.

90. Szatalowicz VL, Arnold PE, Chaimovitz C, Bichet D, Berl T, Schrier RW. Radioimmunoassay of plasma arginine vasopressin in hypoantremic patients with congestive heart failure. *N Engl J Med*. 1981;305:263–266.

91. Riegger GAJ, Leibau G, Hoehsiek K. Antidiuretic hormone in congestive heart failure. *Am J Med*. 1982;72:49–52.

92. Goldsmith SR, Francis GS, Cowley AW, Levine TB, Cohn JN. Increased plasma arginine vasopressin levels in patients with congestive heart failure. *J Am Coll Cardiol*. 1983;1:1385–1390.

93. Thrasher TN, Moore-Gillon M, Wade CE, Keil LC, Ramsay DJ. Inappropriate drinking and secretion of vasopressin after caval constriction in dogs. *Am J Physiol*. 1983;244:R850–R856.

94. Yamane Y. Plasma ADH level in patients with chronic congestive heart failure. *Jpn Circ J*. 1968;32:745–759.

95. Nicod P, Waeber B, Bussien J-P, et al. Acute hemodynamic effect of a vascular antagonist of vasopressin in patients with congestive heart failure. *Am J Cardiol*. 1985;55:1043–1047.

96. Creager MA, Faxon DP, Cutler SS, Kohlmann O, Ryan TJ, Gavras H. The contribution of vasopressin to vaso-

constriction in patients with congestive heart failure: comparison to the renin-angiotensin system and the sympathetic nervous system. *J Am Coll Cardiol*. 1986;7:758–765.

97. Uhlich E, Weber P, Eigler I, Groeschel-Stewart U. Angiotensin stimulates AVP-release in humans. *Klin Wocheschr*. 1975;53:177–180.

98. Packer M, Medina N, Yushak M. Correction of dilutional hyponatremia in severe chronic heart failure by converting-enzyme inhibition. *Ann Intern Med*. 1984;100:782–789.

99. Tracey KJ, Lowry SF, Cerami A. Cachectin: a hormone that triggers acute shock and chronic cachexia. *J Infect Dis*. 1988;157:413–420.

100. Oliff A. The role of tumor necrosis factor (cachectin) in cachexia. *Cell*. 1988;54:141–142.

101. Levine B, Kalman J, Mayer L, Fillit HM, Packer M. Elevated circulating levels of tumor necrosis factor in congestive heart failure. *N Engl J Med*. 1990;323:236–241.

102. Gulick T, Chung MK, Pieper SJ, Lange LG, Schreiner GF. Interleukin-1 and tumor necrosis factor inhibit cardiac myocyte β-adrenergic responsiveness. *Proc Natl Acad Sci USA*. 1989;86:6753–6757.

103. Kalman J. Levine B, Mayer L, Penn J, Kukin ML, Packer M. Prognostic importance of circulating neopterin in heart failure: evidence for monocyte activation in patients with cardiac cachexia. *Circulation*. 1990;82(suppl III):III-315. Abstract.

10
The Peripheral Circulation in Heart Failure

Alan T. Hirsch and Mark A. Creager

The development and progression of myocardial failure are heralded by the activation of circulating neurohormonal systems that modulate both vascular tone and renal retention of salt and water. In addition, the peripheral circulation undergoes local changes in response to heart failure that are fundamental to the pathophysiology of this disease state. The fractional distribution of blood flow to the kidneys, limbs, and splanchnic beds decreases, whereas blood flow to the heart and brain is preserved.[1,2] The diminished exercise capacity of limb muscles in patients with heart failure may be due, in part, to chronically diminished nutritive perfusion.[3,4] Renal hypoperfusion and altered intrarenal hemodynamics may contribute to sodium and water retention.[5,6] Previous chapters have focused on the mechanisms underlying systemic activation of the sympathetic nervous system, the renin-angiotensin system, as well as other circulatory neurohormones, such as arginine vasopressin and atrial natriuretic factor. In this chapter we examine the structural and functional changes that occur in the peripheral vasculature. Specifically, this chapter focuses on local vasodilator and vasoconstrictor mechanisms that are mediated by the endothelium, by tissue production of angiotensin II, and by adrenergic and vasopressinergic receptors.

Endothelial Mechanisms in Heart Failure

The response of large arteries and arterioles to both physiologic and pharmacologic stimuli is influenced by the presence of an intact endothelium. Vascular endothelial cells have been shown to synthesize endogenous vasodilators (e.g., endothelium-derived relaxing factor and prostacyclin) as well as vasoconstrictors (e.g., endothelin and vasoconstrictor prostanoids). Regulation of endothelium-derived vasodilation and constriction may be altered in heart failure and contribute to the vasoconstricted state. The limited data supporting this contention are reviewed below.

Endothelium-Dependent Relaxation

Furchgott and Zawadzki initially demonstrated that relaxation of vascular rings in response to acetylcholine was dependent on an intact endothelium; this relaxation was abolished by removal of the endothelium.[7] They found that this relaxation was due to the release of a diffusible substance. The subsequent chemical characterization of the endothelial-derived relaxant factor (EDRF) was made difficult by its short half-life. Biochemical evidence indicates that EDRF is nitric oxide, or a related nitroso compound derived from the metabolism of the amino acid, L-arginine.[8-10] This endogenous substance is a potent relaxant of vascular smooth muscle in both ex vivo and in vivo conditions.[11] EDRF elicits a vasodilator response in a manner analogous to other nitrovasodilators, by activating soluble guanylate cyclase and thereby increasing intracellular levels of cyclic guanosine monophosphate (GMP).

EDRF is released in response to a wide variety of stimuli. A number of endogenous vasoconstrictors, such as norepinephrine, vasopressin, thrombin, and endothelin, interact with specific receptors on the endothelial surface to induce the release of EDRF. In this way, EDRF modulates the direct vasoconstrictor effect of these endogenous substances. Aggregating platelets may release vasoactive substances (e.g., adenosine diphosphate and serotonin) that also can stimulate the release of EDRF production and thereby induce vasodilation. In the presence of an intact endothelium, these stimuli will induce vasodilation and inhibit further platelet activation. However, after endothelial cell injury, local serotonin and thrombin cause vasoconstriction and promote thrombosis.[12-14]

EDRF is the most potent endogenous vasodilator yet

identified and normally contributes to regulation of basal vascular tone. Pharmacologic inhibition of EDRF synthesis causes a significant increase in vascular resistance in both experimental animals and in humans. For example, L-N-mono-methyl-arginine (L-NMMA) inhibits the synthesis of EDRF by antagonizing the utilization of L-arginine by nitric oxide synthase. When L-NMMA is infused into the normotensive rabbit, blood pressure increases by 30 mm Hg.[15] When this antagonist of EDRF synthesis is infused into the brachial artery of healthy volunteers, forearm vascular resistance increases by 50%.[16] Thus, impaired release of EDRF may cause vasoconstriction. This mechanism has been postulated to underlie the pathophysiology of hypertension.[17–20] Decreases in the synthesis or release of EDRF in disease states might lead to elevations in vascular resistance since there will be less of this endogenous vasodilator to counterbalance vasoconstrictive neurohumoral stimuli. Also, deficiencies in EDRF production could be associated with changes in vascular structure and thrombosis because its antiplatelet and antimitogenic effects would be less.

Endothelial-Derived Relaxant Factor in Heart Failure

It remains uncertain whether abnormalities in the synthesis or action of EDRF contribute to vasoconstriction in heart failure. Studies have variably found attenuation as well as augmentation of endothelium-derived vasorelaxation. Vasodilator responses to acetylcholine, but not to nitroglycerin, are diminished in the pulmonary artery and the thoracic aorta of rats with stable compensated heart failure induced by coronary artery ligation, suggesting that endothelium-dependent relaxation is abnormal[21] (Fig. 10.1). Several groups of investigators have studied the role of endothelial-derived vasorelaxation on vascular function in experimental heart failure in canines subjected to rapid-ventricular pacing. In this model, heart failure develops gradually within 30 days after the onset of pacing. The findings among the various studies are not consistent. In one study, the sensitivity and maximal vasodilator response to the acute infusion of acetylcholine was decreased significantly in femoral arteries of dogs with heart failure; vascular responses to nitroglycerin and to norepinephrine were not altered.[22] These data suggest that endothelium-dependent vasodilation is abnormal. Alternatively, there may be increased endothelial secretion of a vasoconstrictor prostanoid, since indomethacin improved endothelium-dependent vasorelaxation in this study. Elsner et al. reported preliminary results of a study that examined the effect of inhibition of basal EDRF biosynthesis, by administration of L-NMMA. Inhibition of nitric oxide synthase caused a marked rise in mean arterial pressure in conscious healthy dogs but

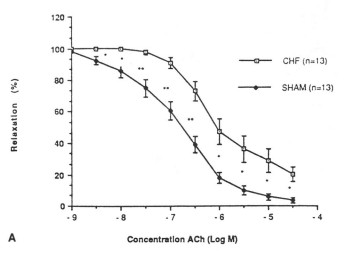

A

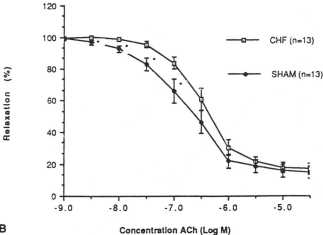

B

FIGURE 10.1. The effect of acetylcholine (ACh) on pulmonary artery (**A**) and thoracic aorta (**B**) relaxation in rats with congestive heart failure. The sensitivity to the endothelium-dependent vasodilator is reduced in heart failure rats compared to sham controls. Adapted with permission from ref. 21. Copyright 1991 by the American Heart Association.

not in dogs in whom heart failure was induced by rapid ventricular pacing.[23] This would suggest that basal release of EDRF is reduced in heart failure. In contrast, Hildebrand et al. reported that L-NMMA increased systemic vascular resistance more in dogs with heart failure than healthy dogs, suggesting that basal release of EDRF is increased in heart failure.[24] Also, Main et al. have found that endothelium-dependent vasodilation to norepinephrine and BHT 920, an α_2-adrenoceptor agonist, is enhanced in coronary arteries of dogs with pacing-induced heart failure.[25] Two reports suggest that endothelium-dependent vasodilation is abnormal in humans with heart failure. Treasure et al. reported that acetylcholine-mediated coronary vasodilation was diminished in a small study of eight patients with idiopathic dilated cardiomyopathy.[26] The maximal vasodilator re-

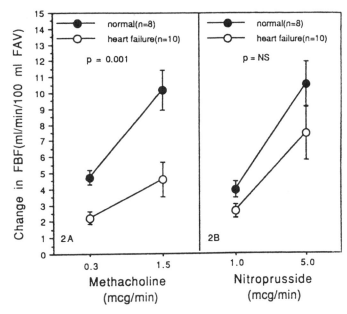

FIGURE 10.2. The vascular effects of intrabrachial infusion of an endothelium-dependent vasodilator (methacholine) and an endothelium-independent vasodilator (nitroprusside) in normal persons and in patients with heart failure. The methacholine dose-response was blunted in patients with heart failure (*lefthand panel*); in contrast, the nitroprusside dose-response was not significantly decreased in heart failure patients. Adapted with permission from ref. 27. Copyright 1991 by the American Heart Association.

sponse to adenosine, an endothelium-independent vasodilator, was similar in control and cardiomyopathic subjects. Kubo et al. evaluated the responsiveness of the forearm circulation to endothelium-dependent and endothelium-independent vasodilators[27] (Fig. 10.2). The increase in forearm blood flow during intrabrachial artery infusion of methacholine, an endothelium-dependent vasodilator, was blunted in patients with heart failure. In contrast, the forearm vascular responsiveness to the endothelium-independent vasodilator, nitroprusside, was similar in the patients with heart failure to the normal humans. These data suggest that the muscarinic release of EDRF is blunted in heart failure. The same authors recently have reported, in preliminary form, that endothelial dysfunction in patients with end-stage heart failure can be normalized by heart transplantation.[28]

Thus, available data are conflicting and there still is no consensus regarding endothelium-mediated vasodilation in heart failure. Furthermore, in Western society, many patients with heart failure have other coexisting diseases, such as atherosclerosis. It is well established that endothelium-dependent vasodilation is abnormal in atherosclerotic vessels.[29] Endothelial function is impaired in animals and humans with risk factors for atherosclerosis, such as hypercholesterolemia, hyper-

tension, and diabetes, even in vessels without overt atherosclerotic lesions. Therefore, it is conceivable that abnormalities in endothelium-dependent vasodilation in some patients with heart failure also reflect the presence of these other disease states, in addition to the effect of heart failure alone.

Prostaglandins

Endothelial cells synthesize the vasodilator prostaglandins E_2 and I_2 from arachidonic acid. Increased systemic levels of vasodilator prostaglandins have been observed in patients with heart failure, as reported by Dzau et al.[30] In their study of patients with severe left ventricular dysfunction, the prostaglandin metabolites of PGE_2 and PGI_2 were three- to sixfold higher than levels measured in normal humans. These investigators also noted that concentrations of these prostanoids were not increased in all patients, but that levels of the vasodilator prostaglandins correlated directly with the concentrations of angiotensin II and the plasma renin activity. Vasodilator prostaglandin levels were highest in patients with hyponatremia (serum sodium concentration less than 135 mEq/L); typically, these persons have high plasma concentrations of vasoconstrictor hormones. The mechanisms underlying increased prostaglandin levels in heart failure are not known. Local synthesis of vasoactive prostanoids is increased by hypoperfusion of regional vascular beds (e.g., the renal and coronary circulations).[31,32] Production of prostaglandins also can be stimulated directly by other vasoconstrictor hormones, such as angiotensin, vasopressin, and norepinephrine.[33–35]

The contribution of local vasodilator prostaglandins to vascular resistance has important clinical implications. Prostaglandin-synthetase inhibition in patients with heart failure causes a decline in cardiac output and an increase in pulmonary capillary wedge pressure, particularly in those subjects with the greatest activation of circulating vasoconstrictor hormones.[36] It appears that synthesis of prostaglandins by blood vessels counterbalances vasoconstrictor mechanisms in heart failure. Additionally, some pharmacologic agents produce their beneficial effects, in part, via increasing the production of endogenous vasodilator prostaglandins. Captopril has been shown to increase the plasma concentration of PGE_2-metabolite levels in hypertensive patients[37]; the antihypertensive effect of this angiotensin-converting enzyme (ACE) inhibitor is blunted by prior administration of indomethacin.[38] When captopril is administered to patients with heart failure, the plasma concentrations of PGE_2 metabolite and 6-keto-F_1 progressively increase.[39] The vasodilation induced by captopril, nitroglycerin, nitroprusside, and hydralazine is attenuated by pretreatment with indomethacin.[40–42]

Endothelium-Dependent Vasoconstriction

The endothelium also produces potent vasoconstrictor substances. The endothelial-derived vasoconstrictor, endothelin, was identified by Yanagisawa et al. in 1988.[43] Three subtypes of endothelin have been sequenced. Endothelin, a 21–amino acid peptide hormone, is the most potent endogenous vasoconstrictor substance identified to date. Endothelin is synthesized from its messenger RNA in endothelial cells as a pre-propeptide and is cleaved from proendothelin by an endogenous endopeptidase. Endothelin is then produced by an endothelin-specific converting enzyme, which is present in lung and in other endothelial cells.[44] Many of the same stimuli that increase release of EDRF including shear stress, epinephrine, thrombin, angiotensin II (AII), arginine vasopressin, and calcium ionophore also increase both transcription of the pre-proendothelin mRNA and endothelin release.[43,45-48]

Endothelin binds to specific receptors and activates two intracellular signal transduction systems via guanosine triphosphate (GTP)-binding proteins.[49] Endothelin stimulates phospholipase C (PLC) and opens voltage-dependent calcium channels. Activation of PLC degrades phosphoinositide to form inositol triphosphate (IP$_3$) and diacylglycerol (DG). IP$_3$ releases calcium from intracellular stores and DG sensitizes contractile proteins via protein kinase C.[49-52] Endothelin also stimulates phospholipase A$_2$ to produce several prostanoids.[49,51] It is presumed that the effects of endothelin are most prominent in adjacent vascular regions. In this manner endothelin would serve as an autocoid modulator of arteriolar resistance. Endothelin has been measured by radioimmunoassay in venous plasma of normal persons,[53] in patients with hypertension,[54] as well as other disease states[55,56]; thus, endothelin also may act as a circulating neurohormone and contribute to generalized arterial and venous vasoconstriction.

The cardiovascular effects of endothelin are complex and potentially profound. During exogenous infusion of endothelin there is an initial brief vasodilation followed by prolonged vasoconstriction.[57-61] In ex vivo studies, endothelin increases contractility in isolated heart preparations.[62-65] A dose-dependent chronotropic response also has been noted during endothelin perfusion in these isolated heart preparations.[66] The chronotropic and inotropic effects of this peptide are most prominent in immature ventricles and in atrial tissue. In vivo, endothelin infusion decreases cardiac output via direct cardiac and associated peripheral vascular effects.[67] Since endothelin has been shown to increase coronary vascular resistance, subendocardial myocardial ischemia and associated left ventricular dysfunction may occur.[67] An endothelin-induced increase in afterload may cause cardiac output to fall. Endothelin also may increase the release of endogenous atrial natriuretic factor, which could modulate the cardiac and vascular effects of endothelin.[68,69]

Endothelin in Heart Failure

A two- to threefold increase in plasma concentrations of endothelin has been observed in experimental heart failure induced by rapid ventricular pacing in the dog[70,71] (Fig. 10.3A). Similar elevations in plasma endothelin concentration occur in humans with stable or decompensated heart failure[72-76] (Fig. 10.3B). The significance of increased plasma endothelin concentration is not known, in part due to the lack of an appropriate inhibitor for use in physiologic investigation. The infusion of exogenous endothelin in normal animals increases systemic vascular resistance and reduces cardiac output.[60,61]

Plasma endothelin levels may be increased in heart failure by several mechanisms. Both AII and arginine vasopressin stimulate endothelin synthesis.[46,77] Also, endothelin clearance is decreased in heart failure. Infusion of endothelin into animals with heart failure induced by rapid ventricular pacing causes higher plasma concentrations than a comparable infusion in normal animals.[70] The relative increase in plasma endothelin concentration occurs out of proportion to the decrease in glomerular filtration.

Thus, the known elevation in endothelin in both experimental models of heart failure and in patients suggests that this vasoconstrictor may have important pathophysiologic effects. The ultimate role of endothelin in the pathophysiology of these disease states must await the availability of an inhibitor of the production of endothelin or an antagonist that blocks endothelin receptors.

Tissue Renin-Angiotensin System in Heart Failure

The role of the circulating renin-angiotensin system in the maintenance of cardiovascular homeostasis has been defined by use of specific antagonists. Anti-renin antibodies,[78,79] AII antagonists,[80] and inhibitors of ACE[81] have each been utilized in this context. Studies with these agents have demonstrated that acute hemodynamic responses correlate with pretreatment plasma renin-angiotensin system activity, and are most profound in individuals with high plasma renin activity and AII concentrations (see related chapter elsewhere in this book). In contrast, chronic responses to these agents are not predicted by plasma renin-angiotensin system activity. Indeed, ACE inhibition often is beneficial in pathophysiologic states in which plasma renin activity and AII levels are not elevated. ACE inhibition

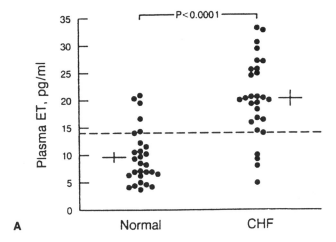

FIGURE 10.3A. Individual and mean plasma endothelin concentrations in control, sham, and experimental congestive heart failure (CHF) dogs induced by rapid ventricular pacing. Mean plasma endothelin concentrations were increased two- to threefold in dogs with experimental heart failure. Adapted with permission from ref. 70. Copyright 1990 by the American Physiological Society.

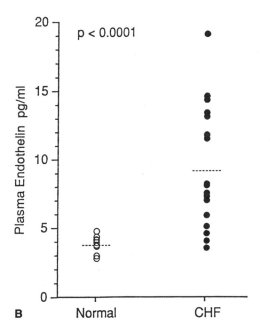

FIGURE 10.3B. Endothelin-1 levels in normal persons and patients with congestive heart failure. Peak endothelin-1 concentrations were significantly higher in the patients with heart failure. Adapted with permission from ref. 74. Copyright 1992 by the American Heart Association.

reduces blood pressure in normal-renin essential hypertension,[82] or in low-renin hypertension that occurs after bilateral nephrectomy.[83] These agents also are effective in heart failure patients with normal plasma activity.[84,85] Therefore, circulating AII may not account wholly for AII-mediated vasoconstriction in heart failure.

Endogenous renin-angiotensin systems have been demonstrated to exist in tissues that are important in cardiovascular regulation. The existence of tissue renin-angiotensin systems suggests that AII might be produced in target organs via local biochemical cascades. Renin substrate, renin-like enzymatic activity, and ACE each have been demonstrated at tissue sites by immunohistochemical and biochemical techniques.[86-89] Molecular biologic techniques have confirmed that both renin and angiotensinogen genes are expressed in many tissues associated with cardiovascular homeostasis (e.g., blood vessels, heart, kidney, brain, and adrenal tissues.[89,90] In addition, there is evidence for uptake of renin and angiotensinogen by the vessel wall.[91,92] The evidence supporting the existence and physiologic role of vascular, cardiac, and renal renin-angiotensin systems is reviewed below. The possibility that the tissue renin-angiotensin system might contribute to local AII production has important pathophysiologic and therapeutic implications. This section will review (a) the evidence that supports the presence of functional tissue renin-angiotensin systems, (b) the increasing body of data that suggests a role for these tissue renin-angiotensin system in the pathophysiology of heart failure, and (c) the pharmacologic implications of these local systems.

The Vascular Renin-Angiotensin System

The presence of renin, angiotensinogen, and AII in blood vessels has been reported by a number of laboratories.[93,94] The postulated distribution of the components of the renin-angiotensin system within the vessel wall is presented in Table 10.1. The vessel wall distribution of renin has been examined by use of anti–renin-specific antibody; intense staining has been noted throughout the thickness of the aorta, large and smaller arteries, as well as arterioles, particularly in endothelial and smooth muscle cells.[95] The isolated rat hindlimb artery is capable of generating AII from tetra-decapeptide renin-substrate in the absence of circulating renin.[92] Chronic oral captopril treatment decreases vascular AII release.[96] Furthermore AII is present in

TABLE 10.1. Postulated distribution of the renin-angiotensin system components in the blood vessel.

Localization	RAS component
Adventitia	Angiotensinogen
Media	Angiotensinogen
	Renin[a]
	Angiotensin-converting enzyme
Endothelium	Renin[a]
	Angiotensin-converting enzyme

[a] Renin may be synthesized in the blood vessel or taken up from the circulation.
RAS = Renin-angiotensin system.

rat plasma 48 hr after bilateral nephrectomy, when plasma renin activity is undetectable, suggesting a tissue source of this peptide.[97] Additionally, kinetic analysis of arteriovenous angiotensin I and AII differences in sheep and humans indicates that both angiotensin I and AII are synthesized in vascular tissues.[98,99]

The local synthesis of angiotensin II in the blood vessel wall has important physiologic implications. Local AII may contribute directly to regional blood flow regulation by activating vascular receptors in specific circulations (e.g., the kidney). AII also may alter vascular function by facilitating norepinephrine release from local noradrenergic nerve terminals.[100] These autocoid mechanisms may affect regional vascular tone even when circulating levels of AII are not increased.

Additional evidence to support the importance of local AII to arteriolar and conduit artery function is derived from experiments involving renin inhibition or angiotensin receptor blockade. Longnecker et al. demonstrated that topical administration of AII receptor antagonist saralasin to the microvasculature of the spontaneously hypertensive rat, which presumably elicits only local effects, resulted in selective vasodilation of third and fourth order arterioles.[101] Prolonged infusion of saralasin normalizes blood pressure in the chronic phase of two-kidney, one-clip hypertension.[102] This hypotensive response is not correlated with the pretreatment plasma renin activity. In the chronic hypertensive phase of this model, plasma renin activity is near normal, but vascular ACE activity is increased and is responsible for the increased vasoconstrictor response to angiotensin I infusion.[103] Unger et al. have observed a persistent hypotensive response after withdrawal of chronically administered ACE inhibitors in spontaneously hypertensive rats, despite the earlier return of plasma ACE activity to normal values,[104] suggesting that inhibition of plasma ACE activity is not essential to elicit a systemic hypotensive response. Sustained inhibition of vascular ACE activity has been observed in parallel to the blood pressure response in some of these studies and may underlie the antihypertensive effect.[105] In humans, the compliance and diameter of large (brachial and carotid) arteries is increased by ACE inhibition, even at doses that do not reduce blood pressure.[106,107] This latter observation suggests that local vascular renin-angiotensin system activity influences distensibility of these conduit vessels. Thus, multiple lines of evidence suggest that local vascular synthesis of AII exerts physiologically important responses.

The Renal Renin-angiotensin System

The juxtaglomerular apparatus is capable of releasing large amounts of renin into the circulation. In patients with heart failure, low renal perfusion pressure, decreased distal tubular sodium load, increased sympathetic activity, and diuretic administration all increase systemic levels of renin and AII. The presence of a locally active renin-angiotensin system in the kidney in sites other than the juxtaglomerular cells has been documented by molecular, biological, immunocytochemical, and biochemical techniques. Taugner et al. have demonstrated renin in afferent and efferent arterioles and in the proximal tubule by antirenin antiserum staining.[108,109] Cultured glomerular mesangial cells synthesize renin.[110] Angiotensinogen mRNA expression in the renal cortex has been demonstrated and in situ hybridization studies has shown that angiotensinogen mRNA is expressed principally in the proximal tubule[111,112]; renin mRNA is localized primarily to the juxtaglomerular cells.[113,114] Intrarenal ACE also has been demonstrated by the presence of the ACE mRNA.[115] In addition to the vasculature, ACE has been localized to the proximal tubule brush border by immunohistochemical and radioligand binding studies.[116,117] Since all the components are found in the proximal tubule, local synthesis of AII has been hypothesized.[114] Indeed, a recent micropuncture study demonstrated that proximal tubular fluid AII concentration is 1000-fold greater than that in the plasma.[118] Local AII production might be a major factor in regulation of basal renal hemodynamics and sodium reabsorption. In fact, this local system also is responsive to physiologic stimuli. Tissue-specific regulation has been demonstrated in response to sodium depletion and glucocorticoid and androgen administration.[112,119,120] Thus, intrarenal renin-angiotensin system thereby may be important in the regulation of sodium homeostasis and glomerular filtration.

The Renal Renin-Angiotensin System in Heart Failure

Experimental heart failure causes changes in the activity of the intrarenal renin-angiotensin system. In rats with chronic left ventricuar dysfunction after experimental myocardial infarction, the renal angiotensinogen mRNA level increases twofold as compared to sham-operated controls.[121] As described by Schunkert et al., the magnitude of increase correlates closely with the histopathologic size of the myocardial infarction, implying a relationship with the degree of ventricular dysfunction.[121] The effect of heart failure on the kidney renin-angiotensin system appears to be selective for this single component of the renin-angiotensin system, as renal renin and ACE activities are unchanged. Chronic ACE inhibition with enalapril normalizes renal angiotensinogen expression to that of sham-operated control rats, suggesting that angiotensin may have a positive feedback role on angiotensinogen expression in the kidney.

Little is known of the activity of the vascular renin-angiotensin system in heart failure. Conceptually, local vascular AII can cause constriction of large arteries and resistance vessels, resulting in increased systemic vascular resistance and reduced arterial compliance. Systemic administration of ACE inhibitors have regionally selective effects, suggesting a differential distribution of AII receptors. These drugs preferentially cause renal vasodilation but have less effect on limb or splanchnic vascular resistance in patients with heart failure.[122] Local infusion of ACE inhibitors cause limb and coronary vasodilation, indicating that local generation of AII may contribute to vascular resistance.[123,124] Additionally, ACE inhibition elicits venodilation.[125]

Vascular Adrenergic Mechanisms in Heart Failure

In patients with heart failure, sympathetic efferent activity is increased and plasma norepinephrine concentration often is elevated. The mechanisms underlying activation of the sympathetic nervous system are discussed in chapter 8. The effect of sympathetic nervous system activation on vascular tone is a consequence of the relative responsiveness of the adrenergic receptor pathways. Relatively little is known about potential abnormalities in the intracellular regulation of vascular smooth muscle cell adrenergic receptor pathways in heart failure. If changes in receptor density and/or coupling efficiency were to occur, sympathetic vascular responsiveness would be altered. Thus, this section will focus on vascular adrenergic receptor function in heart failure.

Adrenergic Receptor Pharmacology

There are two categories of α-adrenergic receptors, α_1 and α_2.[126] Three distinct subtypes of α_1 receptors have been identified.[127-130] Both α_{1a} and α_{1b} receptors modulate vascular smooth muscle tone. α_{1c} has been found to exist only in brain.[129,130] α_1 receptors activate phospholipase C to promote mobilization of Ca^{2+} and sensitization of contractile proteins via protein kinase C. Both the density and coupling of α_1-adrenergic receptors in vascular smooth muscle are affected by the adrenergic hormonal mileau. The density of α_1-adrenergic receptors on vascular smooth muscle is decreased in animals chronically exposed to high catecholamine levels.[131,132] In cultured rabbit aortic smooth muscle cells, norepinephrine decreases mRNA for the α_1-adrenergic receptor, decreases α_1-adrenergic receptor density, and uncouples the receptor from its intracellular second messenger pathways.[133,134] In rabbit aorta, norepinephrine decreases α-adrenergic receptor

sensitivity, but not receptor density.[135] α_2 receptors inhibit neural release of norepinephrine from the presynaptic nerve terminal. Postjunctional vascular α_2 receptors mediate vasoconstriction.[136] Three α_2 receptor subtypes have been identified,[137] but the selective function of these receptors is not known. α_2 receptors inhibit adenylate cyclase.[138] It is not established whether α_2 density or sensitivity in vascular smooth muscle is altered by norepinephrine, since this issue has not yet been investigated.

Three subtypes of β-adrenergic receptors have been identified.[139-141] β_1 receptors, when activated, increase cardiac contractility and heart rate and stimulate lipolysis. β_2 receptors are located in the heart and on blood vessels and bronchi. Activation of β_2 receptors causes vasodilation and bronchial dilation, and also increases cardiac contractility and heart rate. β_2 receptors also are present on lymphocytes and pancreatic islet cells. β_3 receptors recently have been isolated and described in adipose cells, liver, muscle, and ileum and may mediate adipose tissue thermogenesis, glycogen synthesis, and ileum relaxation.[140] β-adrenergic receptors are membrane-bound proteins that stimulate adenylate cyclase via GTP binding proteins. Adenylate cyclase hydrolyzes ATP to cyclic adenosine monophosphate (cAMP). cAMP has selective effects depending on the β-receptor subtype. In β_1 receptor cell types, an inotropic effect occurs when cyclic AMP binds to protein kinase A, ultimately resulting in an increase in intracellular calcium. In vascular smooth muscle, the increase in cAMP consequent to stimulation of β_2 receptors causes vasodilation; this results from sequestration of intracellular calcium by the sarcoplasmic reticulum, hyperpolarization of the cell due to increased potassium permeability; and effects on the myosin light chain, and/or activation of the electrogenic sodium pump.[142]

Both the density and coupling of β-adrenergic receptors can be regulated. Norepinephrine or isoproterenol desensitizes β-adrenergic receptors in cultures as rat myocardial cells and human fibroblasts.[143-145] In vivo, chronic administration of norepinephrine uncouples the β adrenoceptor from its second messengers.[146] The regulation of β receptors may be specific for each subtype and dependent on the level of specific agonists.[146-150]

Vascular Adrenergic Receptor Function in Heart Failure

Vascular α-adrenergic responsiveness has been studied in experimental models and in humans with heart failure. Two studies, performed in dogs with heart failure caused by rapid ventricular pacing, have yielded different findings. Wilson et al. found no difference in hindlimb vascular responsiveness to intraarterial norepinephrine between healthy and heart failure dogs.[151]

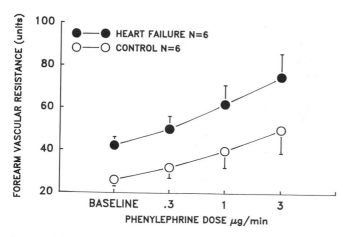

FIGURE 10.4. The effect of intraarterial phenylephrine on forearm vascular resistance in normal persons and patients with congestive heart failure. There was no significant difference in the dose-response curves to the α_1-adrenoceptor agonist between the two groups. Adapted with permission from ref. 153. Copyright 1990 by the American Physiological Society.

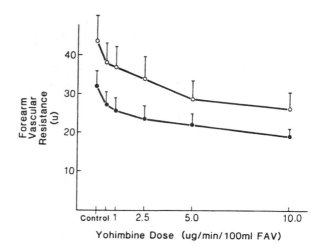

FIGURE 10.5. The effect of intraarterial yohimbine on forearm vascular resistance in normal persons and patients with congestive heart failure. There was no significant difference in the dose-response curves to this α_2-adrenoceptor antagonist between the two groups. Adapted with permission from ref. 154. Copyright 1989 by the American Heart Association.

In contrast, Forster et al. reported that the responses to the α-adrenergic agonists norepinephrine and phenylephrine were increased in the isolated pedal artery of dogs after the development of heart failure, and suggested that the increased responsiveness to these agonists was due to increased responsiveness of the α_1-adrenergic pathway.[152] In humans, Creager et al. found that intraarterial infusion of phenylephrine, a relatively selective α_1 receptor agonist, caused a dose-related increase in forearm vascular resistance that was similar in normal persons and patients with heart failure[153] (Fig. 10.4). Thus, this study did not find altered α-adrenergic vascular responsiveness in humans with congestive heart failure. Kubo and colleagues administered the highly specific α_2-adrenergic antagonist, yohimbine, into the brachial artery of patients with congestive heart failure and normal persons.[154] Yohimbine infusion decreased forearm vascular resistance comparably in the two groups, suggesting that the α_2-adrenergic vasoconstriction was not increased in the forearm vasculature of patients with heart failure (Fig. 10.5).

Changes in ventricular β-adrenoceptor number and sensitivity in animal models of patients with heart failure have been studied extensively and are reviewed elsewhere in this book.[146,147,155-157] Little information is available regarding peripheral vascular β receptors in heart failure. Forster and colleagues reported that β_2 receptor density is reduced in the hindlimb vessels of dogs with heart failure induced by rapid ventricular pacing. Yet, isoproterenol-induced hindlimb vasodilation was similar in the control dogs and the dogs with heart failure. Creager et al. examined β-adrenoceptor–mediated vasodilator function in the forearm resistance vessels of patients with congestive heart failure and normal

persons.[158] Intraarterial isoproterenol administration to normal persons and patients with heart failure increased forearm blood flow and decreased forearm vascular resistance comparably in each group. Thus, studies in one animal model of heart failure, and in humans, indicate that peripheral β_2-adrenoceptor–mediated vasodilation is not downregulated.

Vascular Vasopressin Receptors

Arginine vasopressin is a potent nonapeptide with dual vasopressor and antidiuretic properties. This peptide is synthesized by the hypothalamic magnocellular neurons of the supraoptic and paraventricular nuclei, and is released into the circulation by axonal terminals of the posterior pituitary gland. Vasopressin release is modulated in animals and humans by both osmotic and nonosmotic stimuli. Increases in plasma osmolality are sensed by hypothalamic osmoreceptors, and vasopressin is secreted into the circulation. Nonosmotic stimuli that increase vasopressin release include unloading of the cardiopulmonary and arterial baroreceptors, activation of chemoreceptors, and elevated concentration of AII. The effects of vasopressin are mediated by V_1 and V_2 receptors. Activation of the V_1 receptor causes vasoconstriction mediated by GTP binding proteins that activate phospholipase C and produce inositol triphosphate and diacylglycerol. Subsequently, intracellular calcium levels increase. The renal hydroosmotic effects of vasopressin are mediated by the V_2 receptor, which activates adenylate cyclase and increases intracellular cAMP. Hirsch et al. and others also have demonstrated that vasopressin can activate a vascular V_2 receptor and cause direct vasodilation of skeletal muscle.[159–161] In addition, vasopressin indirectly affects vascular tone. Vasopressin sensitizes baroreceptors and causes vasodilation by withdrawing sympathetic activity. Also, vasopressin may mediate vasodilation by increasing the synthesis and release of EDRF and vasodilator prostaglandins.[162,163] Thus, the peripheral vascular effects of vasopressin are complex, and include both vasoconstriction and vasodilation.

The vasoactive effects of vasopressin may be pertinent to the pathophysiology of heart failure. High plasma vasopressin concentrations have been demonstrated in some patients with heart failure.[164–168] The availability of a pharmacologic probe that specifically blocks the vasopressin receptors has permitted investigation of the pressor action of this peptide in pathophysiologic states. Mulinari and co-workers evaluated the role of elevated endogenous vasopressin levels by administering a vasopressin analogue with dual V_1/V_2 receptor blocking properties to rats with heart failure induced by surgically creating a large myocardial infarction.[169] In these animals, an 18% increase in cardiac output and a 4- to 10-fold increase in urine volume was observed during vasopressin receptor blockade. In dogs with low-output failure caused by tricuspid valve occlusion and pulmonary artery constriction, Stone et al. found that a vasopressin (V_1) receptor antagonist decreased systemic vascular resistance and increased peripheral blood flow.[170] Creager and co-workers have evaluated the role of endogenous vasopressin concentrations in clinical heart failure; in this study, baseline plasma vasopressin levels were increased in only 3 of 10 heart failure patients.[168] Subsequent administration of a V_1 receptor antagonist caused a decrease in systemic vascular resistance and increase in cardiac output only in those persons with the highest vasopressin concentrations. Nicod and associates evaluated the role of vasopressin blockade in an additional 10 patients with heart failure, similarly demonstrating that V_1 receptor blockade was effective only in the single patient with an elevated baseline plasma vasopressin level.[171] The relative role of local vascular V_1 and V_2 receptors in modulating the regional vasoconstrictor responses to this hormone in heart failure has not been evaluated.

Atrial Natriuretic Factor

Atrial natriuretic factor (ANF) is a vasorelaxant peptide hormone that is secreted from atrial myoctes into the circulation. Specific ANF receptors have been localized in vascular smooth muscle, endothelial cells, platelets, the adrenal glomerulosa, and renal epithelial and glomerular sites. Receptor binding and subsequent activation of particulate guanylate cyclase increases intracellular cGMP.[172,173] The effect is not dependent on the presence of normal endothelium.[173] ANF is a potent inhibitor of vascular smooth muscle contraction. Regional vascular beds have heterogeneous responses to ANF. Aortic and renal vascular strips are more sensitive to ANF than coronary, mesenteric, femoral, and carotid vessels.[174,175]

Plasma ANF levels are increased in patients with heart failure, and correlate with atrial filling pressures and disease severity.[176–179] It is possible that high circulating levels of ANF reduce receptor number or sensitivity in vascular smooth muscle. The vascular and renal responses to ANF are attenuated in both animal models and in patients with heart failure. The vasodepressor response to infusion of ANF is markedly blunted in rats with heart failure due to myocardial infarction.[180] Cody and co-workers have demonstrated that the hemodynamic effects of exogenous ANF decreased in patients with heart failure.[178] The forearm vascular responses to intrabrachial arterial ANF infusion in heart failure patients and normal persons recently was examined by Hirooka and co-workers.[181] ANF caused comparable increases in local venous plasma ANF and cGMP concentrations in heart failure patients and healthy persons; however, the direct vasodilator effect of ANF was markedly blunted in the heart failure patients. In contrast, the forearm vasodilator responses to the intra-arterial infusion of nitroglycerin, which causes vasodilation by activating soluble guanylate cyclase, was similar in healthy and heart failure patients. The mechanism(s) underlying altered vascular responsiveness to ANF in heart failure is not known, but might be due to changes in vascular smooth muscle ANF receptor density, uncoupling of intracellular signal transduction pathways, or increased local clearance of active ANF peptide.

Structural Contributions to Vascular Tone

In chronic heart failure, abnormalities in vascular structure may contribute to increased vascular resistance at rest and impair the vasodilator response to exercise or hormonal stimuli. Whereas there is no direct histopathologic evidence of altered vascular structure in humans with heart failure, physiologic evidence suggests that vascular remodeling does occur in this disease state. Structural abnormalities in resistance vessels have been surmised by experiments in which vascular tone is minimized by a maximal metabolic vasodilatory stimulus; the residual vascular resistance would then represent the "structural" contribution. The limb postocclusion peak hyperemic blood flow is blunted at rest in many patients with heart failure.[182,183] Also, during both static and dynamic exercise there is reduced limb vasodilation in individuals with heart failure compared to normal persons.[184] Zelis et al. have proposed that the blunted vasodilator capacity might be due to increased arteriolar sodium content and associated increased tissue edema and turgor.[185-188] Peak reactive hyperemia indeed can be improved by the administration of diuretics, but this treatment does not fully normalize this dilator response.[188] Mechanisms other than vascular wall salt and water retention may prevent maximal vasodilation. Physical conditioning may be one such mechanism that influences vascular structure. Sinoway demonstrated that the maximal hyperemic blood flow response was increased in the dominant forearm of tennis players, but not of persons who did not play tennis.[189] After a forearm physical training program peak reactive hyperemic blood flow increases.[190] Since patients with chronic heart failure usually are deconditioned, it is plausible that the abnormal vasodilator capacity observed in these patients might be reversed by therapy that improves exercise capacity. Both basal forearm vascular resistance as well as peak hyperemic blood flow normalize months after orthotopic heart transplantation, when physical activity has increased to normal levels.[191] Initially, vasodilator capacity remains blunted despite improvement in left ventricular function and reduction in neurohumoral stimuli, the improvement in peak forearm reactive hyperemia does not improve during the initial 2 to 3 weeks of recovery.

Structural changes in conductance vessels have been implied from studies that measure impedance or arterial compliance. Indirect measurements of compliance usually indicate that elasticity is reduced in conduit vessels of patients with heart failure. Pulse wave velocity correlates inversely with compliance and is increased in heart failure.[192] In addition, characteristic impedance is elevated in patients with heart failure.[193,194] Direct measurements of carotid artery compliance using high resolution ultrasonography have confirmed decreased distensibility in these individuals compared to healthy persons.[195] The structural changes contributing to altered compliance are not known. Nonetheless, decreased distensibility will increase the load on the heart during systole and further compromise cardiac function.

References

1. Leithe ME, Margorien RD, Hermiller JB, Unverferth DV, Leier CV. Relationship between central hemodynamics and regional blood flow in normal subjects and in patients with congestive heart failure. *Circulation.* 1984;69:57–64.
2. Zelis R, Flaim SF. Alterations in vasomotor tone in congestive heart failure. *Prog Cardiovasc Dis.* 1982;24:437–459.
3. Wiener DH, Maris J, Chance B, Wilson JR. Detection of skeletal muscle hypoperfusion during exercise using phosphorus-31 nuclear magnetic resonance spectroscopy. *J Am Coll Cardiol.* 1986;7:793–799.
4. Wilson JR, Wiener DH, Fink LI, Ferraro N. Vasodilatory behavior of skeletal muscle arterioles in patients with nonedematous chronic heart failure. *Circulation.* 1986;74:775–779.
5. Creager MA, Halperin AL, Bernard DB, et al. Acute regional circulatory and renal hemodynamic effects of converting-enzyme inhibition in patients with congestive heart failure. *Circulation.* 1981;64:483–489.
6. Cody RJ, Covit AB, Schaer GL, Laragh JH, Sealey JE, Feldschuh J. Sodium and water balance in chronic congestive heart failure. *J Clin Invest.* 1986;77:1441–1452.
7. Furchgott RF, Zawadzki JV. The obligatory role of endothelial cells in the relaxation of arterial smooth muscle by acetylcholine. *Nature.* 1980;288:373–376.
8. Ignarro LJ, Burns RE, Buga GM, Wood KS. Endothelium-derived relaxing factor from pulmonary artery and vein posesses pharmacologic and chemical properties identical to those of nitric oxide radical. *Circ Res.* 1987;61:866–879.
9. Palmer RMJ, Ferridge AG, Moncada S. Nitric oxide release accounts for the biological activity of endothelium-derived relaxing factor. *Nature.* 1987;327:524–526.
10. Myers PR, Guerra R, Harrison DG. Release of NO and EDRF from cultured bovine aortic endothelial cells. *Am J Physiol.* 1989;256:H1030–H1037.
11. Ignarro LJ. Biological action and properties of endothelium-derived nitric oxide formed and released from artery and vein. *Circ Res.* 1989;65:1–21.
12. Cohen RA, Zitnay KM, Haudenschild CC, Cunningham LD. Loss of selective endothelial cell vasoactive functions in pig coronary arteries caused by hypercholesterolemia. *Circ Res.* 1988;63:903–910.
13. DeMey JG, Vanhoutte PM. Heterogeneous behavior of the canine arterial and venous wall: Importance of the endothelium. *Circ Res.* 1982;51:439–447.
14. Shimokawa H, Vanhoutte PM. Impaired endothelium-dependent relaxation to aggregating platelets and related vasoactive substances in porcine coronary arteries in hypercholesterolemia and atherosclerosis. *Circ Res.* 1989;64:900–914.
15. Rees DD, Palmer RMJ, Moncada S. Role of endothelium-derived nitric oxide in the regulation of blood pressure. *Proc Natl Acad Sci USA.* 1989;86:3375–3378.
16. Vallance P, Collier J, Moncada S. Effects of endothelium-derived nitric oxide on peripheral arteriolar tone in man. *Lancet.* 1989;2:997–1000.
17. Luscher TF, Vanhoutte PM. Endothelium-dependent contractions to acetylcholine in the aorta of the spontaneously hypertensive rat. *Hypertension.* 1986;8:344–348.
18. Luscher TF, Vanhoutte PM, Raij L. Antihypertensive treatment normalizes decreased endothelium-dependent relaxations in rats with salt-induced hypertension. *Hypertension.* 1987;(suppl III):III193–III197.
19. Lockette W, Otsuka Y, Carretero OA. The loss of endothelium-dependent relaxation in hypertension. *Hypertension.* 1986;8:II61–II66.
20. Panza JA, Quyyumi AA, Brush JE Jr, Epstein SE. Abnormal endothelim-dependent vascular relaxation in

patients with essential hypertension. *N Engl J Med.* 1990;323:22–27.

21. Ontkean MT, Gay R, Greenberg B. Diminished endothelium-derived relaxing factor activity in an experimental model of chronic heart failure. *Circ Res.* 1991;69:1088–1096.

22. Kaiser L, Spickard RC, Olivier NB. Heart failure depresses endothelium-dependent responses in canine femoral artery. *Am J Physiol.* 1989;256:H962–H967.

23. Elsner D, Muntze A, Riegger AJR. The increase in total peripheral resistance by inhibition of EDRF-synthesis is attenuated in conscious dogs with heart failure. *Circulation.* 1990;III-591. Abstract.

24. Hildebrand FL Jr, Perrella MA, Burnett JD Jr. The role of endothelium-derived relaxing factor in experimental congestive heart failure. *J Am Coll Cardiol.* 1991; 17:281A. Abstract.

25. Main JS, Forster C, Armstrong PW. Inhibitory role of the coronary arterial endothelium to alpha-adrenergic stimulation in experimental heart failure. *Circ Res.* 1991;68:940–946.

26. Treasure CB, Vita JA, Cox DA, et al. Endothelium-dependent dilation of the coronary microvasculature is impaired in dilated cardiomyopathy. *Circulation.* 1990;81:772–779.

27. Kubo SH, Rector TS, Bank AJ, Williams RE, Heifetz SM. Endothelium-dependent vasodilation is attenuated in patients with heart failure. *Circulation.* 1991;84:1589–1596.

28. Kubo SH, Rector TS, Bank AJ, et al. Heart transplantation reverses abnormalities in endothelium dependent vasodilation of peripheral blood vessels in patients with heart failure. *Circulation.* 1991;84:II469.

29. Rubanyi GM. *Cardiovascular Significance of Endothelium-derived Vasoactive Factors.* Mount Kisco, NY: Futura Publishing, 1991.

30. Dzau VJ, Colucci WS, Hollenberg NK, Williams GH. Relation of the renin-angiotensin-aldosterone system to clinical state in congestive heart failure. *Circulation.* 1981;63:645–651.

31. Oliver JA, Sciacca R, Pinto J, Cannon PJ. Participation of the prostaglandins in the control of renal blood flow during acute reduction of cardiac output in the dog. *J Clin Invest.* 1981;67:229–237.

32. Friedman PL, Brown EJ Jr, Gunther S, et al. Coronary vasoconstrictor effect of indomethacin in patients with coronary artery disease. *N Engl J Med.* 1981;305:1171–1175.

33. Shebuski RJ, Aiken JW. Angiotensin II stimulation of renal prostaglandin synthesis elevated circulating prostacyclin in the dog. *J Cardiovasc Pharmacol.* 1980; 2:667–677.

34. Zusman RM, Keiser HR. Prostaglandin biosynthesis by rabbit renomedullary interstitial cells in culture: stimulation by angiotensin II, bradykinin and arginine vasopressin. *J Clin Invest.* 1977;60:215–223.

35. McGiff JC, Crawshaw K, Terragne NA, Malik KU, Lonigro AJ. Differential effect of noradrenaline and renal nerve stimulation on vascular resistance in the dog kidney and the release of a prostaglandin E-like substance. *Clin Sci.* 1972;42:223–233.

36. Dzau VJ, Packer M, Lilly LS, Swartz SL, Hollenberg NK, Williams GH. Prostaglandins in severe heart failure: Relation to renin-angiotensin system and hyponatremia. *N Engl J Med.* 1984;310:347–352.

37. Swartz SL, Williams GH. Angiotensin-converting enzyme inhibition and prostaglandins. *Am J Cardiol.* 1982;49:1405–1409.

38. Moore TJ, Crantz FR, Hollenbert NK, et al. Contribution of prostaglandins to the antihypertensive action of captopril in essential hypertension. *Hypertension.* 1981;3:168–173.

39. Dzau VJ, Creager MA. Prostaglandins in congestive heart failure. In: Robertson JIS, ed. *The Renin-Angiotensin System.* London: Gower Medical; 1986:912–918.

40. Lavin RI, Jaffe EA, Weksler BB, Tack-Goldman K. Nitroglycerin stimulates synthesis of prostacyclin by cultured human endothelial cells. *J Clin Invest.* 1981;67:762–769.

41. Morcillio E, Reid PR, Dubin N, Ghodgaonkar R, Pitt B. Myocardial prostaglandin E release by nitroglycerin and modification by indomethacin. *Am J Cardiol.* 1980;45:53–57.

42. Rubin IJ, Lazar JD. Influence of prostaglandin synthesis inhibitors on pulmonary vasodilatory effects of hydralazine in dogs with hypoxic pulmonary vasoconstriction. *J Clin Invest.* 1981;67:193–200.

43. Yanagisawa M, Kurihara S, Kimura S, et al. A novel potent vasoconstrictor peptide produced by vascular endothelial cells. *Nature.* 1988;332:411–415.

44. Wu-Wong JR, Budzik GP, Devine EM, Opgenorth TJ. Characterization of endothelin converting enzyme in rat lung. *Biochem Biophys Res Commun.* 1990;171:1291–1296.

45. Yanagisawa M, Masaki T. Endothelin, a novel endothelium-derived peptide: pharmacological activities, regulation and possible roles in cardiovascular control. *Biochem Pharm.* 1989;38:1877–1883.

46. Resink TJ, Hahn AWA, Scott-Burden T, Powell J, Weber E, Buhler FR. Inducible endothelin mRNA expression and peptide secretion in cultured human vascular smooth muscle cells. *Biochem Biophys Res Commun.* 1990;168:1303–1310.

47. Brenner BM, Troy JL, Ballerman BJ. Endothelium-dependent vascular responses: mediators and mechanisms. *J Clin Invest.* 1989;84:1373–1378.

48. Yoshizumi M, Kurihara H, Sugiyama T, et al. Hemodynamic shear stress stimulates endothelin production by cultured endothelial cells. *Biochem Biophys Res Commun.* 1989;161:859–864.

49. Masaki T, Kimura S, Yanagisawa M, Goto K. Molecular and cellular mechanism of endothelin regulation implications for vascular function. *Circulation.* 1991;84:1457–1468.

50. Marsden PA, Danthuluri NR, Brenner BM, Ballerman BM, Brock TA. Endothelin action on vascular smooth muscle involves inositol trisphosphate and calcium mobilization. *Biochem Biophys Res Commun.* 1989;158:86–93.

51. Resink TJ, Scott-Burden T, Buhler FR. Activation of phospholipase A2 by endothelin in cultured vascular

smooth muscle cells. *Biochem Biophys Res Commun.* 1989;158:279–286.

52. Simonson MS, Wann S, Mene P, et al. Endothelin stimulates phospholipase C, Na+/H+ exchange, c-fos expression and mitogenesis in rat mesangial cells. *J Clin Invest.* 1989;83:708–712.

53. Ando K, Hirata YU, Shichiri M, Emori T, Marumo F. Presence of immunoreactive endothelin in human plasma. *FEBS Lett.* 1989;245:164–166.

54. Saito Y, Nakao K, Mukoyama M, Imura H. Increased plasma endothelin level in patients with essential hypertension. *N Engl J Med.* 1989;322:205.

55. Ogburn PL, Thompson RL, Lerman A, Burnett JC Jr. Endothelin elevation in normal preganancy and preeclampsia. *Am J Obstet Gynecol.* 1990;164:274.

56. Lerman A, Hallet JW, Heublein DM, Burnett JC Jr. A role for endothelin as a marker of diffuse atherosclerosis in the human. *J Am Coll Cardiol.* 1991;17:370A. Abstract.

57. King AJ, Pfeffer JM, Pfeffer MA, Brenner BM. Systemic hemodynamic effects of endothelin in rats. *Am J Physiol.* 1990;258:H787–H792.

58. Knuepfer MM, Han SP, Trapani AJ, Fok KF, Westfall TC. Regional hemodynamic and baroreflex effects of endothelin in rats. *Am J Physiol.* 1989;257(*Heart Circ Physiol* 26):H918–H926.

59. Otsuka A, Mikami H, Katahira K, et al. Haemodynamic effect of endothelin, a novel potent vasoconstrictor in dogs. *Clin Exp Pharm Physiol.* 1990;17:351–360.

60. Miller WI, Redfield MM, Burnett JC Jr. Integrated cardiac, renal, and endocrine actions of endothelin. *J Clin Invest.* 1989;83:317–320.

61. Goetz KL, Wang BC, Madwed JB, Zhu JL, Leadley RJ Jr. Cardiovascular, renal and endocrine responses to intravenous endothelin in conscious dogs. *Am J Physiol.* 1988;255(*Heart Circ Physiol* 24):R1064–R1068.

62. Vigne P, Laxdunski M, Frelin C. The inotropic effect of endothelin-1 on rat atria involves hydrolysis of phosphatidylinositol. *FEBS Lett.* 1989;249:143–146.

63. Concas V, Laurent S, Brisac AM, Perret C, Safar M. Endothelin has potent direct inotropic and chronotropic effects in cultured heart cells. *J Hypertens.* 1989;7:S96–S97.

64. Hu JR, Hardorf RV, Lang RE. Endothelin has potent inotropic effects in rat atria. *Eur J Pharmacol.* 1988;158:275–278.

65. Lembeck F, Decrinis M, Pertl C, Amann R, Donner J. Effects of endothelin on the cardiovascular system and on smooth muscle preparations in different species. *Naunyn-Scmiedeberg's Arch Pharmacol.* 1989;340:744–751.

66. Ishikawa T, Yanagisawa M, Kimura S, Goto K, Masaki T. Positive chronotropic effects of endothelin, a novel endothelium-derived vasoconstrictor peptide. *Pfluger Arch.* 1988;413:108–110.

67. Kramer BK, Nishida M, Kelly RA, Smith TW. Endothelins: myocardial actions of a new class of cytokines. *Circulation.* 1992;85:350–356.

68. Stasch JP, Hirth-Kietrick C, Kazda S, Neuser D. Endothelin stimulates release of atrial natriuretic peptides in vitro and in vivo. *Life Sci..* 1989;45:869–875.

69. Schiebinger RJ, Gomez-Sanchez CE. Endothelin: a potent stimulus of atrial natriuretic peptide secretion by superfused rat atria and its dependency on calcium. *Endocrinology.* 1990;127:119–125.

70. Cavero PG, Miller WL, Heublein DM, Margulies KB, Burnett JC. Endothelin in experimental congestive heart failure in the anesthetized dog. *Am J Physiol.* 1990;259:F312–F317.

71. Margulies KB, Hildebrand FL Jr, Lerman A, Perrella MA, Burnett JC Jr. Increased endothelin in experimental heart failure. *Circulation.* 1990;82:2226–2230.

72. Robertston R, Susawa T, Sugiura M, et al. Circulating endothelin levels: modulation by heart failure in man. *Clin Res.* 1990;38:414A. Abstract.

73. Stewart DJ, Cernacek P, Costello KB, Rouleau JL. Elevated endothelin-1 in heart failure and loss of normal response to postural change. *Circulation.* 1992;85:510–517.

74. Cody RJ, Haas GJ, Binkley PF, Capers Q, Kelley R. Plasma endothelin correlates with the extent of pulmonary hypertension in patients with chronic congestive heart failure. *Circulation.* 1992;85:504–509.

75. Ray SG, McMurray J, Morton JJ. Endothelin and atrial natriuretic factor in acute myocardial infarction. *Circulation.* 1990;82(suppl III):III-279. Abstract.

76. Cernacek P, Stewart D. Immunoreactive endothelin in human plasma: marked elevations in patients in cardiogenic shock. *Biochem Biophys Res Commun.* 1989;161:562–567.

77. Emori T, Hirata Y, Ohta K, Shichiri M, Marumo F. Secretory mechanism of immunoreactive endothelin in cultured bovine endothelial cells. *Biochem Biophys Res Commun.* 1989;160:93–100.

78. Wakenlin GE. Antibodies to renin as proof of the pathogenesis of sustained renal hypetension. *Circulation.* 1958;17:653–657.

79. Dzau VJ, Copelman RI, Barger AC, Haber E. Renin-specific antibody for study of cardiovascular homeostasis. *Science.* 1980;207:1091–1093.

80. Pals DT, Masucci FD, Sipos F, Denning GS. A specific competitive antagonist of the vascular action of angiotensin II. *Circ Res.* 1971;29:664–647.

81. Ondetti MA, Rubin B, Cushman DW. Design of specific inhibitors of angiotensin converting enzyme: new class of orally active antihypertensive agents. *Science.* 1977; 196:441–444.

82. Brunner HR, Gavras H, Waeber B, et al. Oral angiotensin-converting enzyme inhibitor in long-term treatment of hypertensive patients. *Ann Intern Med.* 1979;90:19–23.

83. Wenting GJ, Blankestijn PJ, Pldermans D, et al. Blood pressure response of nephrectomized subjects and patients with essential hypertension to ramipril: indirect evidence that inhibition of tissue angiotensin converting enzyme is important. *Am J Cardiol.* 1987;59:92D–97D.

84. Kubo SH, Clark M, Laragh JH, Borer JS, Cody RJ. Identification of normal neurohormonal activity in mild congestive heart failure and stimulating effect of upright posture and diuretics. *Am J Cardiol.* 1987;60:1322–1328.

85. Creager MA, Faxon DP, Halperin SL, et al. Determi-

nants of clinical response and survival in patients with congestive heart failure treated with captopril. *Am Heart J.* 1982;104:1147–1153.

86. Dzau VJ, Re RN. Evidence for the existence of renin in the heart. *Circulation.* 1987;73(suppl I):I134–I136.

87. Philips MI, Stenstrom B. Angiotensin II in rat brain comigrates with authentic angiotensin II in high pressure liquid chromatography. *Circ Res.* 1985;56:212–219.

88. Deboben A, Inagami T, Ganten G. Tissue renin. In: Genest J, Kuchel O, Hamet P, eds. *Hypertension.* 2nd ed. New York: McGraw-Hill; 1983:194–209.

89. Field LS, McGowen RA, Dickensen DP, Gross KW. Tissue and gene specificity of mouse renin expression. *Hypertension.* 1984;6:597–603.

90. Lynch KR, Simnad VT, Ben-Ari ET, Maniatis T, Zinn K, Garrison JC. Localization of preangiotensinogen messenger RNA sequences in the rat brain. *Hypertension.* 1986;8:540–543.

91. Loudon M, Bing RF, Thurston H, Swales JD. Arterial wall uptake of renal renin and blood pressure control. *Hypertension.* 1983;5:629–634.

92. Oliver JA, Sciacca RR. Local generation of angiotensin II as a mechanism of regulation of peripheral vascular tone in the rat. *J Clin Invest.* 1984;4:1247–1251.

93. Dzau VJ, Gibbons GH. Autocrine-paracrine mechanisms of vascular myocytes in hypertension. *Am J Cardiol.* 1987; 60:991–1031.

94. Rosenthal JH, Pfeiffer B, Mecheilor ML, Pschort J, Jacob ICM, Dahlheim H. Investigations of components of the renin-angiotensin system in rat vascular tissue. *Hypertension.* 1984;6:383–390.

95. Molteni A, Dzau VJ, Fallon JT, Haber E. Monoclonal antibodies as probes of renin gene expression. *Circulation.* 1984;70(suppl II):II-196. Abstract.

96. Mizuno K, Nakamaru M, Higashimori K, Inagami T. Local generation and release of angiotensin II in peripheral vascular tissue. *Hypertension.* 1988;11:223–229.

97. Aguirela G, Schirar A, Baukai A, Gatt KJ. Circulating angiotensin II and adrenal receptors after nephrectomy. *Nature.* 1981;289:507–509.

98. Campbell DJ. The site of angiotensin production. *J Hypertens.* 1985;3:730–737.

99. Admiraal PJJ, Darkx FHM, Jan Danser AH, Pierman H, Schalenkamp MADH. Metabolism and production of angiotensin II in different vascular beds in subjects with hypertension. *Hypertension.* 1990;15:44–55.

100. Shepherd JT, Vanhoutte PM, George E. Brown memorial lecture: local modulation of adrenergic neurotransmission. *Circulation.* 1981;64:655–666.

101. Longnecker DJ, Durcus MI, Donovan KR, Miller ED, Peach MJ. Saralasin dilates arterioles in SHR but not WKY rats. *Hypertension.* 1984;1(suppl I):106–110.

102. Riegger AJG, Lever AF, Miller JA, Morton JJ, Slack B. Correction of renal hypertension in the rat by prolonged infusion of saralasin. *Lancet.* 1977;2:1317–1319.

103. Okamura T, Miyazcki M, Inagemi T, Toda N. Vascular renin-angiotensin system in two-kidney, one clip hypertensive rats. *Hypertension.* 1986;8:560–565.

104. Unger T, Ganten D, Lang RE, Scholkens VA. Is tissue converting inhibition a determinant of the antihyperten-

sive efficacy of converting enzyme inhibitors? Studies with two different compounds Hoe 398 and MD 421 in spontaneously hypertensive rats. *J Cardiovasc Pharmacol.* 1985;7:36–41.

105. Kaplan HR, Taylor DG, Olson SC, Andrews LK. Quinapril—a preclinical review of the pharmacology, pharmacokinetics, and toxicology. *Angiology.* 1989; 40:335–350.

106. Simon ACH, Levenson JA, Bouther JI, Safar ME. Comparison of oral MK 421 and propranolol in mild to moderate hypertension and their effects on arterial and venous vessels of the forearm. *Am J Cardiol.* 1984;53:781–783.

107. Dzau VJ, Safar MI. Large conduit arteries in hypertension: role of the vascular renin angiotensin system. *Circulation.* 1988;77:947–954.

108. Taugner R, Hackenthal E, Helmchen U, et al. The intrarenal renin-angiotensin system. An immunocytochemical study on the localization of renin, angiotensinogen, converting enzyme, and the angiotensins in the kidney of mouse and rat. *Klin Wochenschr.* 1982;60:1218–1222.

109. Taugner R, Hackenthal E, Rix E, Nibiling R, Poulsen K. Immunocytochemistry of the renin-angiotensin system: renin, angiotensinogen, angiotensin I, angiotensin II, and converting enzyme in the kidneys of mice, rats, and tree shrews. *Kidney Int.* 1982;22:S33–S43.

110. Dzau VJ, Kreisbert JI. Cultured glomerular mesangial cells contain renin: influence of calcium and isoproterenol. *J Cardiol Pharmacol.* 1986;8(suppl 10):S6–S10.

111. Dzau VJ, Ellison KE, Brody T, Ingelfinger J, Pratt RE. A comparative study of the distributions of renin and angiotensinogen messenger ribonucleic acids in rat and mouse tissues. *Endocrinology.* 1987;120:2334–2338.

112. Ingelfinger JR, Pratt RE, Ellison K, Dzau VJ. Sodium regulation of angiotensinogen mRNA expression in rat kidney cortex and medulla. *J Clin Invest.* 1986;78:1311–1315.

113. Ingelfinger JR, Fon EA, Ellison KE, Dzau VJ. Localization of the intratenal renin angiotensin system (RAS) by in situ hybridization of renin and angiotensinogen (Ang-n) mRNAs. *Kidney Int.* 1988;33:269. Abstract.

114. Ingelfinger JR, Zuo WM, Fon EA, Ellison KE, Dzau VJ. In situ hybridization evidence for angiotensinogen messenger RNA in the rat proximal tubule. *J Clin Invest.* 1990;85:417–423.

115. Soubrier F, Alhene-Gelas F, Hubert C, et al. Two putative active centers in human angiotensin I converting enzyme revealed by molecular cloning. *Proc Natl Acad Sci USA.* 1988;85:9386–9390.

116. Sakaguchi K, Chai SY, Jackson B, Johnston CI, Mendelsohn FAO. Inhibition of tissue angiotensin converting enzyme. Quantitation by autoradiography. *Hypertension.* 1988;11:230–238.

117. Ingelfinger JR, Anderson S, Hirsch AT, Dzau VJ, Brenner BM. Elevation of renal angiotensin converting enzyme (ACE) activity in nephrotic rats. American Society of Nephrology, Proceedings of 22nd Annual Meeting, Washington, DC, 1989;168A. Abstract.

118. Seikaly MG, Arant BS Jr, Seney FD Jr. Measurement of endogenous angiotensin levels in glomerular filtrate and

proximal tubule fluid. American Society of Nephrology, Proceedings of 22nd Annual Meeting, Washington, DC, 1989;171A. Abstract.

119. Campbell DJ, Habener JF. Angiotensinogen gene is expressed and differentially regulated in multiple tissues of the rat. *J Clin Invest.* 1986;78:31–39.

120. Ellison KE, Ingelfinger JR, Pivor M, Dzau VJ. Androgen regulation of rat renal angiotensinogen messenger RNA expression. *J Clin Invest.* 1989;83:1941–1945.

121. Schunkert H, Ingelfinger JR, Hirsch AT, et al. Evidence for tissue-specific activation of renal angiotensionogen mRNA expression in chronic stable experimental heart failure. *J Clin Invest.* 1992;90:1523-1529.

122. Creager MA, Halperin JL, Bernard DB, et al. Acute regional circulatory and renal hemodynamic effects of converting-enzyme inhibition in patients with congestive heart failure. *Circulation.* 1981;64:483–489.

123. Bank AJ, Kubo SH, Rector TS, Heifetz SM, Williams RE. Local forearm vasodilation with intra-arterial administration of enalaprilat in humans. *Clin Pharmacol Ther.* 1991;50:314–321.

124. Foult JM, Tavolaro O, Antony I, Nitenberg A. Direct myocardial and coronary effects of enalaprilat in patients with dilated cardiomyopathy: assessment by a bilateral intracoronary infusion technique. *Circulation.* 1988; 77:337–344.

125. Faxon DP, Halperin JL, Creager MA, Gavras H, Schick EC, Ryan TJ. Angiotensin inhibition in severe heart failure: acute central and limb hemodynamic effects of captopril with observations on sustained oral therapy. *Am Heart J.* 1981;191:548–556.

126. Hoffman BB, Lefkowitz RJ. Alpha-adrenergic receptor subtypes. *N Engl J Med.* 1980;302:1390–1396.

127. Cotecchia S, Schwinn DA, Randall RR, Lefkowitz RJ, Caron MG, Kobilka BK. Molecular cloning and expression of the cDNA for the hamster alpha1- adrenergic receptor. *Proc Natl Acad Sci USA.* 1988;85:7159–7163.

128. Schwinn DA, Lomasney JW, et al. Molecular cloning and expression of the cDNA for a novel alpha$_1$-adrenergic receptor subtype. *J Biol Chem.* 1990; 265:8183–8189.

129. Han C, Abel PW, Minneman KP. Alpha$_1$-adrenoceptor subtypes linked to different mechanisms for increasing intracellular Ca2+ in smooth muscle. *Nature.* 1987; 329:333–335.

130. Suzuki E, Tsujimoto G, Tamura K, Hashimoto K. Two pharmacologically distinct alpha1-adrenoceptor subtypes in the contraction of rabbit aorta: each subtype couples with a different Ca^{2+} signalling mechanism and plays a different physiological role. *Mol Pharmacol.* 1990; 38:725–736.

131. Colucci WS, Gimbrone MA Jr, Alexander RW. Regulation of the postsynaptic alpha-adrenergic receptor in rat mesenteric artery. Effects of chemical sympathectomy and epinephrine treatment. *Circ Res.* 1981;48:104–111.

132. Tsujimoto G, Honda K, Hoffman BB, Hashimoto K. Desensitization of postjunctional alpha 1- and alpha 2-adrenergic receptor-mediated vasopressor response in rat harboring pheochromocytoma. *Circ Res.* 1987;61:86–98.

133. Colucci WS, Alexander RW. Norepinephrine-induced alteration in the coupling of alpha$_1$-adrenergic receptor occupancy to calcium efflux in rabbit aortic smooth muscle cells. *Proc Natl Acad Sci USA.* 1986;83:1743–1746.

134. Izzo NJ Jr, Seidman CE, Collins S, Colucci WS. Alpha$_1$-adrenergic receptor mRNA level is regulated by norepinephrine in rabbit aortic smooth muscle cells. *Proc Natl Acad Sci USA.* 1990;87:6268–6271.

135. Lurie KG, Tsujimoto G, Hoffman BB. Desensitization of alpha-1 adrenergic receptor-mediated vascular smooth muscle contraction. *J Pharmacol Exp Ther.* 1985; 234:147–152.

136. Goldberg MR, Robertson D. Evidence for the existence of vascular alpha$_2$-adrenergic receptors in humans. *Hypertension.* 1984;6:551–556.

137. Lorenz W, Lomasney JW, Collins S, Regan JW, Caron MG, Lefkowitz RJ. Expression of three alpha$_2$-adrenergic receptor subtypes in rat tissues: Implications for alpha$_2$-receptor classification. *Mol Pharmacol.* 1990; 38:599–603.

138. Cotecchia S, Koblika BK, Daniel KW, et al. Multiple second messenger pathways of alpha-adrenergic receptor subtypes expressed in eukaryotic cells. *J Biol Chem.* 1990;265:63–69.

139. Ahlquist RP. A study of the adrenotropic receptors. *Am J Physiol.* 1948;153:586–600.

140. Emorine LJ, Marullo S, Briend-Sutrean M-M, et al. Molecular characterization of the human β_3-adrenergic receptor. *Science.* 1989;245:1118–1121.

141. Lefkowitz RJ, Stadel JM, Caron MG. Adenylate cyclase-coupled β-adrenergic receptors. *Annu Rev Biochem.* 1983;52:159–186.

142. Bulbring E, Tomita T. Catecholamine action on smooth muscle. *Pharmacol Rev.* 1987;39:49–96.

143. Hertel C, Perkins JP. Receptor-specific mechanisms of desensitization of β-adrenergic receptor function. *Mol Cell Endocrinol.* 1984;37:245.

144. Kassis S, Fishman PH. Different mechanisms of desensitization of adenylate cyclase by isoproterenol and prostaglandin E1 in human fibroblasts. *J Biol Chem.* 1982;257:5312–5318.

145. Strasser RH, Lefkowitz RJ. Homologous desensitization of β-adrenergic receptor coupled adenylate cyclase. *J Biol Chem.* 1985;260:4561–4564.

146. Vatner DE, Vatner SF, Nejima J, et al. Chronic norepinephrine elicits desensitization by uncoupling the β-receptor. *J Clin Invest.* 1989;84:1741–1748.

147. Vatner DE, Vatner SF, Fujii AM, Homcy CJ. Loss of high affinity cardiac β-adrenergic receptors in dogs with heart failure. *J Clin Invest.* 1985;76:2259–2264.

148. Brodde O-E, Daul A, Michel-Reher M, et al. Agonist-induced desensitization of α-adrenoceptor function in humans. *Circulation.* 1990;81:914–921.

149. Rothwell NJ, Stock MJ, Sudera DK. Changes in tissue blood flow and β-receptor density of skeletal muscle in rats treated with the β_2-adrenoreceptor agonist clenbuterol. *Br J Pharmacol.* 1987;90:601–607.

150. Colucci WS, Alexander RW, Williams GH, et al. Decreased lymphocyte a-adrenergic agonist pirbuterol. *N Engl J Med.* 1981;305:185–190.

151. Wilson JR, Lanoce V, Frey MJ, Ferraro N. Arterial

baroreceptor control of peripheral vascular resistance in experimental heart failure. *Am Heart J*. 1990;119:1122–1130.

152. Forster C, Carter SL, Armstrong PW. Alpha₁ adrenoceptor activity in arterial smooth muscle following congestive heart failure. *Can J Physiol Pharmacol*. 1989;67:110–115.

153. Creager MA, Hirsch AT, Dzau VJ, Nabel EG, Cutler SS, Colucci WS. Baroreflex regulation of regional blood flow in congestive heart failure. *Am J Physiol*. 1990; 258:H1409–H1414.

154. Kubo SH, Rector TS, Heifetz SM, Cohn JN. Alpha₂-receptor mediated vasoconstriction in patients with congestive heart failure. *Circulation*. 1989;80:1660–1667.

155. Gilson N, el Houda Bouanani N, Corsin A, Crozatier B. Left ventricular function and β-adrenoceptors in rabbit failing heart. *Am J Physiol*. 1990;258:H634–H641.

156. Fan T-H, Liang C-S, Kawashima S, Banerjee SP. Alterations in cardiac β-adrenoceptor responsiveness and adenylate cyclase system by congestive heart failure in dogs. *Eur J Pharmacol*. 1987;140:123–132.

157. Bristow MR, Hershberger RE, Port JD. β-adrenergic pathways in nonfailing and failing human ventricular myocardium. *Circulation*. 1990;82:1–12.

158. Creager MA, Quigg RJ, Ren CJ, Roddy MA, Colucci WS. Limb vascular responsiveness to β-adrenergic receptor stimulation in patients with congestive heart failure. *Circulation*. 1991;83:1873–1879.

159. Walker BR. Evidence for a vasodilatory effect of vasopressin in the conscious rat. *Am J Physiol*. 1986;251: H34–H39.

160. Liard J-F. Cardiovascular effects associated with antidiuretic activity of vasopressin after blockade of its vasoconstrictor action in dehydrated dogs. *Circ Res*. 1986;58:631–640.

161. Hirsch AT, Dzau VJ, Majzoub JA, Creager MA. Vasopressin-mediated forearm vasodilation in normal humans; evidence for a vascular vasopressin V2 receptor. *J Clin Invest*. 1989;84:418–426.

162. Zusman RM, Keiser HR. Prostaglandin biosynthesis by rabbit renomedullary interstitial cells in tissue culture. Stimulation by angiotensin II, bradykinin, and arginine vasopressin. *J Clin Invest*. 1977;60:215–233.

163. Katusic ZS, Shepherd JT, Vanhoutte PM. Vasopressin causes endothelium-dependent relaxations of the canine basilar artery. *Circ Res*. 1984;55:575–579.

164. Yamane Y. Plasma ADH level in patients with chronic congestive heart failure. *Jpn Circ J.*. 1968;32:745–759.

165. Szatalowicz VL, Arnold PE, Chaimovitz C, Bichet D, Berl T, Schrier RW. Radioimmunoassay of plasma arginine vasopressin in hyponatremic patients with congestive heart failure. *N Engl J Med*. 1981;305:263–266.

166. Riegger GAJ, Liebau G, Koehsiek K. Antidiuretic hormone in congestive heart failure. *Am J Med*. 1982;72:49–52.

167. Goldsmith SR, Francis GS, Cowley AW Jr, Levine TB, Cohn JN. Increased plasma arginine vasopressin levels in patients with congestive heart failure. *J Am Coll Cardiol*. 1983;1:1385–1390.

168. Creager MA, Faxon DP, Cutler SS, Kohlmann O, Ryan TJ, Gavras H. The contribution of vasopressin to vaso-constriction in patients with congestive heart failure: comparison to the renin-angiotensin system and the sympathetic nervous system. *J Am Coll Cardiol*. 1986;7:756–765.

169. Mulinari RA, Gavra I, Wang YX, Franco R, Gavras H. Effects of a vasopressin antagonist with combined antipressor and antidiuretic properties in rats with left ventricular dysfunction. *Circulation*. 1990;81:308–311.

170. Stone CK, Liang C, Imai N, Sakamoto S, Sladek CD, Hood WB. Short-term hemodynamic effects of vasopressin V1-receptor inhibition in chronic right-sided congestive heart failure. *Circulation*. 1988;78:1251–1259.

171. Nicod P, Waeber B, Bussein J-P, et al. Acute hemodynamic effect of a vascular antagonist of vasopressin in patients with congestive heart failure. *Am J Cardiol*. 1985;55:1043–1047.

172. Waldman SA, Rapoport RM, Murad F. Atrial natriuretic factor selectively activates particulate guanylate cyclase and elevates cyclic GMP in rat tissues. *J Biol Chem*. 1984;259:14332–14334.

173. Winquist RJ, Faison SA, Waldman SA, Schwartz K, Murad F, Rapoport RM. Atrial natriuretic factor elicits an endothelium-independent relaxation and activates particulate guanylate cyclase in vascular smooth muscle. *Proc Natl Acad Sci USA*. 1984;81:7661–7664.

174. Garcia R, Thibault G, Gutkowska J, Cantin M, Genest J. Changes of regional blood flow induced by atrial natriuretic factor (ANF) in conscious rats. *Life Sci*. 1985;36:1687–1692.

175. Ishihara T, Aisaka K, et al. Vasodilatory and diuretic actions of alpha-human atrial natriuretic polypeptide (alpha hANP). *Life Sci*. 1985;36:1205–1215.

176. Burnett JC Jr, Kao PC, Hu DC, et al. Atrial natriuretic peptide elevation in congestive heart failure in the human. *Science*. 1986;231:1145–1147.

177. Raine AEG, Erne P, Burgisser F, et al. Atrial natriuretic peptide and atrial pressure in patients with congestive heart failure. *N Engl J Med*. 1986;31:533–537.

178. Cody RJ, Atlas SA, Laragh JH, et al. Atrial natriuretic factor in normal subjects and heart failure patients. *J Clin Invest*. 1986;78:1362–1374.

179. Creager MA, Hirsch AT, Nabel EG, Cutler SS, Colucci WS, Dzau VJ. Responsiveness of atrial natriuretic factor to reduction in right atrial pressure in patients with chronic congestive heart failure. *J Am Coll Cardiol*. 1988;11:1191–1198.

180. Kohzuki M, Hodsman GP, Johnston CI. Attenuated response to atrial natriuretic peptide in rats with myocardial infarction. *Am J Physiol*. 1989;256:H533–H538.

181. Hirooka Y, Takeshita A, Imaizumi T, et al. Attenuated forearm vasodilatative response to intra-arterial atrial natriuretic peptide in patient with heart failure. *Circulation*. 1990;82: 147–153.

182. Zelis R, Mason DT, Braunwald E. A comparison of peripheral resistance vessels in normal subjects and in patients with congestive heart failure. *J Clin Invest*. 1968;47:960–970.

183. Creager MA, Quigg RJ, Ren CJ, Roddy M, Colucci WS. Limb vascular responsiveness to β-adrenergic receptor stimulation in patients with congestive heart failure. *Circulation*. 1991;83:1873–1879.

184. Longhurst J, Gifford W, Zelis R. Impaired forearm oxygen consumption during statis exercise in patients with congestive heart failure. *Circulation.* 1976;54:447–480.

185. Zelis R, Mason DT. Diminished forearm arteriolar dilator capacity produced by mineralocorticoid-induced salt retention in man. *Circulation.* 1970;41:589–592.

186. Zelis R, Delea CS, Coleman HN, Mason DT. Arterial sodium content in experimental congestive heart failure. *Circulation.* 1970;61:213–216.

187. Zelis R, Lee G, Mason DT. Influence of experimental edema on metabolically determined blood flow. *Circ Res.* 1974;34:482–490.

188. Sinoway L, Minotti J, Musch T, et al. Enhanced metabolic vasodilation secondary to diuretic therapy in decompensated congestive heart failure secondary to coronary artery disease. *Am J Cardiol.* 1987;60:107–111.

189. Sinoway LI, Musch TI, Minotti JR, Zelis R. Enhanced maximal metabolic vasodilation in the dominant forearms of tennis players. *J Appl Physiol.* 1986;61:1076–1079.

190. Sinoway LI, Shenberger J, Wilson J, McLaughlin D, Musch T, Zelis R. A 30-day forearm work protocol increases maximal forearm blood flow. *J Appl Physiol.* 1987;62:1063–1067.

191. Sinoway LI, Minotti JR, Davis D, et al. Delayed reversal of impaired vasodilation in congestive heart failure after heart transplantation. *Am J Cardiol.* 1988;61:1076–1079.

192. Arnold JMO, Marchiori GE, Imrie JR, Bunton GL, Pflugfelden PW, Kostuk WJ. Large artery function in patients with chronic heart failure. *Circulation.* 1991;84:2418–2425.

193. Finkelstein SM, Cohn JN, Collins VR, Carlyle PF, Shelly WJ. Vascular hemodynamic impedance in congestive heart failure. *Am J Cardiol.* 1985;55:423–427.

194. Repine CJ, Nichols WW, Conti CR. Aortic input impedance in heart failure. *Circulation.* 1978;58:460–469.

195. Lage S, Kopel L, Monachini M, Coleman S, Polak J, Creager MA. Compliant properties of the carotid artery in congestive heart failure. *Circulation.* 1991;84:II–56.

11
Renal Salt and Water Handling in Congestive Heart Failure

William T. Abraham and Robert W. Schrier

The kidneys are bestowed with the ability to regulate the composition and volume of body fluids within exquisitely fine limits. In 1909, Starling[1] wrote: "The kidney presents in the highest degree the phenomenon of 'sensibility,' the power of reacting to various stimuli in a direction which is appropriate for the survival of the organism; a power of adaptation which almost gives one the idea that its component parts must be endowed with intelligence." Homer Smith[2] rejected this exalted view of the kidney's innate wisdom and suggested that the kidney was "only a passive agent operating blindly and automatically according to the dictates of receptor-effector systems located elsewhere in the body; the integration of these receptor-effector systems constitutes the wisdom behind salt and water balance." Evidence that the kidney unquestionably responds to extrarenal stimuli has accumulated since 1957, the year Smith wrote his classic review on salt and water volume receptors.[2] In addition, as suggested by Starling, the kidney can be isolated from its extrarenal environment and yet be demonstrated to excrete a salt load that is added to its renal arterial perfusion circuit.[3] Thus, it is fair to state that both extrarenal and intrarenal mechanisms contribute to the kidney's ability to maintain the *milieu interieur*. Moreover, it is clear that the kidney plays the central role in body fluid composition and volume regulation in health and disease. This chapter explores the extrarenal and intrarenal mechanisms affecting renal salt and water handling in congestive heart failure (CHF).

The factors involved in renal salt and water handling in CHF can be classified broadly as belonging to either the afferent ("sensor") or efferent ("effector") limb of a volume regulatory system. Until recently, the nature of this volume regulatory system has escaped definitive delineation.

Afferent Mechanisms

The Concept of "Effective Blood Volume" or the Compartment Sensed

Undoubtedly, many circumstances exist in which total extracellular fluid (ECF), interstitial fluid (ISF), and intravascular (IV) volumes are expanded and yet avid renal sodium and water retention persists. Patients with advanced CHF have been found to have not only increased ECF volumes including interstitial edema but expanded total plasma and blood volumes.[4] In fact, this situation of avid renal sodium and water retention despite total body salt and water excess defines the edematous disorders, including CHF, cirrhosis, and the nephrotic syndrome. In these disease states, it is clear that the integrity of the kidney as the ultimate effector organ of body fluid regulation is intact. For instance, transplantation of the kidney from a cirrhotic patient with ascites and peripheral edema to a person with normal liver function totally reverses the renal sodium and water retention.[5] Moreover, the transplantation of a normal liver into the edematous cirrhotic patient also has been shown to abolish the renal sodium and water retention.[6] Thus, in such edematous disorders, the kidney must be responding to extrarenal signals from the afferent limb of a volume regulatory system. The exact pathogenesis of these extrarenal signals is not definitively known.

If the afferent volume receptors sensed primarily total blood volume, then the kidneys of edematous patients should increase their excretion of sodium and water as their total blood volume increases; yet as mentioned above, in patients with severe cardiac or liver disease this does not occur. Thus, there must be some body fluid compartment that is still "underfilled" even in the presence of expansion of total ECF and blood volume, which comprises the afferent limb of renal sodium and water retention in patients with edematous disorders. In 1948, John Peters at Yale coined the term "effective blood volume" as a reference to just such an underfilled body fluid compartment.[7] Thus, extrarenal signals must be initiated by this decrease in "effective blood volume," which enhances tubular sodium and water reabsorption by the otherwise normal kidney. In this regard, it is clear that renal sodium and water retention can occur in patients with cardiac failure before any diminution in glomerular filtration rate.

Borst and deVries[8] first suggested cardiac output as the primary modulator of renal sodium and water excretion. In this context, the level of cardiac output would constitute "effective blood volume." Although this concept is appealing, it is clear that profound renal sodium and water retention may occur in the presence of an increase in cardiac output. For example, a significant elevation in cardiac output may occur in the presence of avid renal sodium and water retention and expansion of ECF volume in association with cirrhosis, pregnancy, a large arteriovenous fistula (AV), and other causes of high output cardiac failure such as thyrotoxicosis and beriberi.[4]

Primacy of the Arterial Circulation in Volume Regulation

A series of investigations in experimental animals and man[9-19] has led to our proposal of a unifying hypothesis for body fluid volume regulation in health and disease.[4] This unifying hypothesis states that total ECF, ISF, or IV volumes are not primary determinants of renal sodium and water excretion. With this hypothesis, the venous component of IV volume is likewise excluded as the primary determinant of sodium and water excretion. It is acknowledged, however, that there are experimental and clinical circumstances in which selective rises in right and left or left atrial pressures stimulate the release of atrial natriuretic peptide (ANP)[20] and suppression of arginine vasopressin (AVP),[21] respectively, which may enhance sodium and water excretion. These events must, however, be subservient to more potent determinants of body fluid volume regulation since the patient with advanced left or right ventricular dysfunction or both exhibits avid sodium and water retention despite markedly elevated atrial pressures.

The proposed unifying hypothesis of body fluid regulation in health and disease states that the arterial circulation is the primary body fluid compartment that modulates renal sodium and water excretion.[4] In a 70-kg man, total body water approximates 42 L, of which only 0.7 L (1.7% of total body water) resides in the

TABLE 11.1. Body fluid distribution.

Compartment	Amount	Volumes in 70-kg man (liters)
Total body fluid	60% of body weight	42
Intracellular fluid	40% of body weight	28
Extracellular fluid	20% of body weight	14
Interstitial fluid	Two thirds of ECF	9.4
Plasma fluid	One third of ECF	4.6
Venous fluid	85% of plasma fluid	3.9
Arterial fluid	15% of plasma fluid	0.7

arterial circulation (Table 11.1). From a teleological viewpoint, it is attractive to propose that the primacy for regulation of renal sodium and water excretion, and thus body fluid volume homeostasis, is modulated by the smallest body fluid compartment, thus endowing the system with exquisite sensitivity to relatively small changes in body fluid volume, and resides in that fluid compartment that is responsible for the arterial perfusion of the body's vital organs and tissues.

Cardiac Output and Peripheral Arterial Resistance as the Determinants of "Effective Arterial Blood Volume"

According to this body fluid volume regulation hypothesis, there are two primary determinants of overfilling or underfilling of the arterial circulation, namely, cardiac output and peripheral arterial resistance. In this context, it is proposed that all renal sodium- and water-retaining states, which occur in the absence of intrinsic renal disease, are initiated by either a fall in cardiac output or peripheral arterial vasodilation. Thus, this hypothesis accounts for sodium and water retention in both low-output and high-output cardiac failure as well as in other edematous disorders.

Afferent Volume Receptors

The afferent volume receptors for such a volume regulatory system must reside in the arterial vascular tree, such as the high-pressure baroreceptors in the carotid sinus, aortic arch, and juxtaglomerular apparatus. As previously mentioned, the low-pressure volume receptors of the thorax (atria, right ventricle, and pulmonary vessels) must be of some importance to the volume regulatory system. However, there is considerable evidence that arterial receptors predominate over low-pressure receptors in volume control in mammals.[22-30]

Low-Pressure Volume Receptors

Various maneuvers that decrease central venous return, such as positive pressure breathing,[31] lower extremity tourniquets,[2,32] and prolonged standing,[33] are associated with decreased renal sodium excretion. Conversely, maneuvers that increase thoracic venous return, such as negative pressure breathing[34] and recumbency,[35] are associated with enhanced renal sodium excretion. Head-out water immersion, a technique that increases venous return to the heart, results in a significant increase in renal salt and water excretion independent of major changes in either glomerular filtration rate (GFR) or renal hemodynamics.[36] Moreover, in the dog, a direct correlation between renal sodium excretion and left atrial pressure has been demonstrated,[37,38] suggesting a role for an atrial receptor in volume regulation. As first suggested by Gauer and Henry,[34,39] physiologically important left atrial receptors have been shown to contribute to ECF volume regulation by exerting nonosmotic control over the antidiuretic hormone AVP.[21,37,39] In addition, changes in atrial stretch and transmural pressures have been shown to determine circulating plasma concentrations of the vasoactive and natriuretic hormone, ANP.[40–42]

High-Pressure Volume Receptors

Evidence for the presence of volume-sensitive receptors in the arterial circulation in humans originated from observations in patients with traumatic AV fistulae.[43] Closure of AV fistulae is associated with a decreased rate of emptying of the arterial blood into the venous circulation, as demonstrated by closure-induced increases in diastolic arterial pressure and decreases in cardiac output, and results in an immediate increase in renal sodium excretion without changes in either GFR or renal blood flow (RBF).[43] Further evidence implicating the "fullness" of the arterial vascular tree as a sensor in modulating renal sodium excretion can be found in denervation experiments. In these studies, pharmacologic or surgical interruption of sympathetic efferent neural pathways emanating from high-pressure areas inhibited the natriuretic response to volume expansion.[9,10,44–48] Moreover, reduction of pressure or stretch at the carotid sinus has been shown to activate the sympathetic nervous system and to promote renal sodium and water retention.[49,50] High-pressure baroreceptors also appear to be important factors in regulating the nonosmotic release of vasopressin and thus renal water excretion.[51,52]

Located in the afferent arterioles within the kidney, the juxtaglomerular apparatus is one of the most well defined of the high-pressure receptors implicated in body fluid volume regulation. The juxtaglomerular apparatus responds to decreased stretch or increased renal sympathetic tone with enhanced renal secretion of renin.[49] Thus, this baroreceptor is an important factor in the control of angiotensin II (AII) formation and aldosterone secretion and ultimately in renal sodium retention.

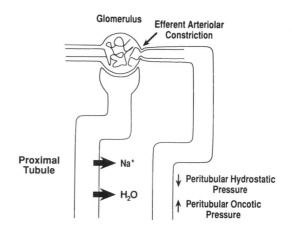

FIGURE 11.1. Efferent arteriolar constriction, mediated in CHF by increased renal sympathetic activity and AII concentrations, decreases net postglomerular Starling forces in a direction to enhance proximal tubular sodium and water reabsorption.

Efferent Mechanisms

Renal Hemodynamics

The GFR usually is normal in early or mild heart failure and is reduced only as cardiac performance becomes more severely impaired. Renal vascular resistance is increased with a concomitant decrease in RBF. In general, RBF decreases in proportion to the decrease in cardiac performance. Thus, the ratio of GFR to RBF, or the filtration fraction, usually is increased in patients with cardiac failure. This increased filtration fraction is a consequence of constriction of the efferent arterioles within the kidney. These changes in renal hemodynamics alter the hydrostatic and oncotic forces in the peritubular capillaries to favor increased proximal tubular reabsorption of sodium and water (Figure 11.1). The renal hemodynamic changes seen in CHF are mediated primarily by activation of various neurohormonal vasoconstrictor systems. In addition, neurohormonal activation directly influences enhanced sodium and water reabsorption in both the proximal and distal nephron in CHF, as discussed below.

The Neurohormonal Response to Cardiac Failure

Arterial underfilling secondary to a diminished cardiac output elicits a number of compensatory neurohormonal responses that act to maintain the integrity of the arterial circulation by promoting peripheral vasoconstriction as well as expansion of the ECF volume through renal sodium and water retention. The three major neurohormonal vasoconstrictor systems activated in response to cardiac failure are the sympathetic ner-

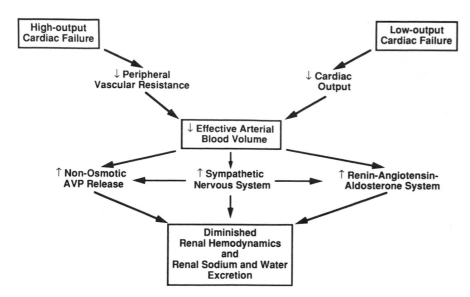

FIGURE 11.2. Proposed mechanism of renal sodium and water retention in high-output and low-output cardiac failure.

vous system, the renin-angiotensin-aldosterone system, and the nonosmotic release of vasopressin. Baroreceptor activation of the sympathetic nervous system appears to be the primary integrator of the hormonal vasoconstrictor systems involved in the volume control system, since the nonosmotic release of AVP involves sympathetic stimulation of the supraoptic and paraventricular nuclei in the hypothalamus[53] and activation of the renin-angiotensin-aldosterone system involves renal β-adrenergic stimulation.[54] Thus, in low-output cardiac failure, diminished integrity of the arterial circulation as determined by decreased cardiac output causes unloading of arterial baroreceptors in the carotid sinus and aortic arch. Peripheral vasodilation causes unloading of these arterial baroreceptors in the setting of high-output cardiac failure (Figure 11.2). This baroreceptor inactivation results in diminution of the tonic inhibitory effect of afferent vagal and glossopharyngeal pathways to the central nervous system and initiates an increase in sympathetic efferent adrenergic tone with subsequent activation of the other two major vasoconstrictor hormonal systems. Various counterregulatory, vasodilatory hormones also may be activated in CHF, including ANP and renal prostaglandins. Table 11.2 summarizes the renal effects of the various neurohormonal systems that are activated in CHF.

The Sympathetic Nervous System in Congestive Heart Failure

The sympathetic nervous system is activated early in patients with CHF. Evidence for this comes both from indirect and direct measurements of sympathetic nervous system activity in heart failure patients. Various studies have documented elevated peripheral venous plasma norepinephrine (NE) concentrations in patients with CHF.[55-59] Previous studies in advanced heart failure,

TABLE 11.2. Renal effects of neurohormonal activation in CHF.

Vasoconstrictor systems
Renal nerves
  Promote efferent greater than afferent arteriolar constriction
  Enhance sodium reabsorption in proximal tubule
  Stimulate renal renin release
Renin-angiotensin-aldosterone system
  Angiotensin II
    Promotes efferent greater than afferent arteriolar constriction
    Enhances sodium reabsorption in proximal tubule
    Stimulates adrenal aldosterone synthesis and release
  Aldosterone
    Enhances sodium reabsorption and potassium secretion in collecting duct
Arginine vasopressin
  Increases water reabsorption in cortical and medullary collecting duct
  Increases sodium chloride reabsorption in medullary ascending limb of Henle's loop

Vasodilator systems
Atrial natriuretic peptide
  Increases glomerular filtration rate
  Promotes diminished sodium reabsorption in collecting duct
  Suppresses renin activity
  Inhibits aldosterone synthesis and release
  Inhibits vasopressin release
Renal prostaglandins
  Promote renal vasodilation
  Decrease tubular sodium reabsorption in ascending limb of Henle's loop
  Inhibit vasopressin hydroosmotic action in collecting duct

using tritiated NE to determine NE kinetics, demonstrated that both increased NE secretion and decreased NE clearance contribute to the high venous plasma NE concentrations seen in these patients, suggesting that increased sympathetic activity is at least partially responsible for the elevated circulating plasma NE.[57,58] A more recent investigation of NE kinetics in earlier stages of heart failure demonstrated that the initial rise in plasma NE in CHF is due solely to increased NE secretion, providing evidence of increased sympathetic nervous activity early in the course of CHF.[59] Studies employing peroneal nerve microneurography to assess directly sympathetic nerve activity to muscle also demonstrate increased sympathetic activity in CHF patients. Using this technique, one group of investigators recorded sympathetic nerve activity to muscle while simultaneously measuring plasma NE concentrations in patients with CHF.[60] Sympathetic nerve activity was increased in these patients and strongly correlated with plasma NE levels.[60]

The peripheral effects of this increased sympathetic efferent discharge include (a) vasoconstriction of arterial resistance vessels with increased cardiac afterload, (b) splanchnic venoconstriction with central translocation of volume and increased cardiac preload, (c) positive chronotropic and inotropic effects on the heart, and, (d) increased renal neural traffic, which directly and indirectly enhances proximal tubular sodium reabsorption as well as stimulates renin release and thus activation of the renin-angiotensin-aldosterone system. Sympathetic activation, as measured by plasma NE concentration, correlates directly with the degree of left ventricular dysfunction in CHF.[55,56,61] Moreover, the plasma NE concentration correlates negatively with prognosis in CHF.[62] That is, high plasma NE levels are associated with poor prognosis in heart failure patients. This was demonstrated by Cohn and colleagues, who prospectively studied 106 patients with moderate or severe CHF and found that a single resting venous plasma NE level provided a better guide to prognosis than other commonly measured indices of cardiac performance.[62] Enhanced sympathetic activity may cause deleterious effects in CHF via several mechanisms, including increased ventricular pre- and afterload, downregulation of cardiac β-receptors, direct myocardial toxicity, stimulation of tachycardia and other arrhythmias, as well as through promoting renal sodium retention.

Effects of Increased Renal Sympathetic Activity in Congestive Heart Failure

Through renal vasoconstriction, stimulation of the renin-angiotensin-aldosterone system, and direct effects on the proximal convoluted tubule, enhanced renal sympathetic activity may contribute to the avid sodium and water retention of CHF. Indeed, intrarenal adrenergic blockade has been shown to cause a natriuresis in experimental animals and humans with CHF.[63-65] Moreover, in the rat, renal nerve stimulation has been demonstrated to produce approximately a 25% reduction in sodium excretion and urine volume.[66] The diminished renal sodium excretion that accom-

panies renal nerve stimulation may be mediated by at least two mechanisms. Studies performed in rats have demonstrated that norepinephrine-induced efferent arteriolar constriction alters peritubular hemodynamic forces in favor of increased tubular sodium reabsorption.[67] As previously mentioned, the increase in filtration fraction with a normal or only slightly reduced GFR that is often seen in CHF patients must be due to efferent arteriolar constriction. Constriction of the efferent arterioles in CHF has been confirmed by renal micropuncture studies performed in rats,[68] and is at least partially mediated by increased renal sympathetic activity and by AII. Thus, efferent arteriolar constriction in CHF tips the balance of hemodynamic forces in the peritubular capillaries in favor of enhanced proximal tubular sodium reabsorption.

In addition, renal nerves have been shown to exert a direct influence on sodium reabsorption in the proximal convoluted tubule.[66,69] Bello-Reuss et al. demonstrated this direct effect of renal nerve activation to enhance proximal tubular sodium reabsorption in whole-kidney and individual nephron studies in the rat.[66] In these animals, renal nerve stimulation produced an increase in the tubular fluid/plasma inulin concentration ratio in the late proximal tubule, an outcome of increased fractional sodium and water reabsorption in this segment of the nephron.[66] Hence, increased renal nerve activity may promote sodium retention by a mechanism independent of changes in renal hemodynamics. However, in dogs with denervated transplanted kidneys and chronic vena caval constriction, the sodium retention persists.[70] Moreover, renal denervation does not prevent ascites in the dog with chronic vena caval constriction.[71] Thus, renal nerves probably contribute to but do not fully account for the avid sodium retention of CHF.

The Renin-Angiotensin-Aldosterone System in Congestive Heart Failure

The renin-angiotensin-aldosterone system also is activated in CHF, as assessed by plasma renin activity (PRA).[56,72,73] Renin acts on angiotensinogen to produce angiotensin I, which is then converted by angiotensin-converting enzyme (ACE) to AII. In CHF, the resultant increased plasma concentration of AII exerts circulatory effects similar to sympathetic activation, including peripheral arterial and venous vascular constriction, renal vasoconstriction, and cardiac inotropism. AII also acts to promote the secretion of the sodium-retaining hormone aldosterone by the adrenal cortex and in positive-feedback stimulation of the sympathetic nervous system. Thus, in the kidney, activation of this hormonal system promotes sodium retention via several mechanisms as discussed below.

Activation of the renin-angiotensin-aldosterone system is associated with hyponatremia and an unfavorable prognosis in CHF.[74,75] The association of PRA and hyponatremia was first described by Dzau and others in a cohort of 15 CHF patients[74] These data demonstrated that normal or suppressed PRA is associated with a normal serum sodium level, whereas the highest PRA is associated with the lowest serum sodium concentrations.[74] This association of hyponatremia with renin-angiotensin-aldosterone system activation was later confirmed by Lee and Packer in a larger group of CHF patients.[75] Moreover, these investigators demonstrated the association of this hyponatremic, hyper-reninemic state with poor survival.[75] The mechanisms by which activation of the renin-angiotensin-aldosterone system might negatively impact on survival in CHF are primarily mediated by increased AII levels. As noted above, increased AII causes arteriolar and venous vasoconstriction, thus increasing ventricular pre- and afterload. AII stimulates nonosmotic AVP release, promoting renal water retention and increased thirst. AII also may act as a growth factor promoting myocardial hypertrophy, and thus ischemia. AII via several mechanisms augments renal sodium reabsorption.

Renal Effects of Increased Angiotensin II in Congestive Heart Failure

AII may contribute to the sodium and water retention of CHF through direct and indirect effects on proximal tubular sodium reabsorption and by stimulating the release of aldosterone from the adrenal gland. AII causes renal efferent vasoconstriction, resulting in decreased renal blood flow and an increased filtration fraction. As with renal nerve stimulation, this results in increased peritubular capillary oncotic pressure and reduced peritubular capillary hydrostatic pressure, which favors the reabsorption of sodium and water in the proximal tubule.[68,76] In addition, AII has been shown to have a direct effect on enhancing sodium reabsorption in the proximal tubule.[77] Finally, AII enhances aldosterone secretion by the adrenal gland, which promotes tubular sodium reabsorption in the distal tubule and collecting duct.

A role for renin-angiotensin-aldosterone system activation in the sodium retention of CHF is suggested by the finding that urinary sodium excretion inversely correlates with PRA and urinary aldosterone excretion in heart failure patients.[78] However, the administration of an ACE inhibitor during heart failure does not consistently increase urinary sodium excretion despite a consistent fall in plasma aldosterone concentration.[79] The simultaneous fall in blood pressure due to decreased circulating concentrations of AII, however, may activate hemodynamic and neurohormonal mechanisms that could obscure the natriuretic response

to lowered AII and aldosterone concentrations. Support for this hypothesis comes from a recent study performed by Hensen and associates in our laboratory.[80] We examined the effect of the specific aldosterone antagonist, spironolactone, on urinary sodium excretion in patients with mild to moderate CHF who were withdrawn from all medications before the study. Sodium was retained in all patients throughout the period prior to aldosterone antagonism. On an average sodium intake of 97 ± 8 mmol/day, the average sodium excretion before spironolactone was 78 ± 8 mmol/day. During therapy with spironolactone, all CHF patients exhibited a significant increase in urinary sodium excretion to an average of 131 ± 13 mmol/day. PRA and norepinephrine increased during the administration of spironolactone. Thus, this investigation demonstrates reversal of the sodium retention of CHF with the administration of an aldosterone antagonist, despite further activation of various antinatriuretic influences including stimulation of the renin-angiotensin and sympathetic nervous systems. These results indicate that the renin-angiotensin-aldosterone system is an important mediator of sodium retention in CHF.

The Nonosmotic Release of Vasopressin in Congestive Heart Failure

Plasma AVP is consistently elevated in patients with CHF and correlates in general with the clinical and hemodynamic severity of disease and with the serum sodium level.[12,19,81–83] Recently, through the use of a single intravenous bolus technique, we determined vasopressin clearance to be normal in six patients with mild to moderate heart failure (*unpublished observations*). Moreover, plasma AVP concentrations are inappropriately elevated in hypoosmotic patients with CHF, and these levels fail to suppress normally to acute water loading.[81,83] These data, taken together, suggest that there is enhanced release of AVP in heart failure and that nonosmotic mechanisms are responsible. As already suggested, baroreceptor activation of the sympathetic nervous system likely mediates the nonosmotic release of AVP in heart failure patients.[53]

Through its effects on vascular (V_1) and renal (V_2) receptors, AVP is a potent mediator of peripheral vasoconstriction and renal water retention, respectively. By analogy to norepinephrine, it can be speculated that both of these effects may be of some pathophysiologic importance in CHF. Numerous studies support a role for AVP in the altered hemodynamics of CHF. Experimental antagonists of the V_1 receptor of vasopressin have been used in patients with low-output cardiac failure.[84,85] Selective antagonism of these receptors in humans is associated with peripheral vasodilation and improved cardiac function in a subset of patients with severe CHF.[84,85] Conversely, small increases in plasma

AVP concentrations, within the basal range seen in CHF patients, increase peripheral vascular resistance and produce a corresponding fall in cardiac output in patients with cardiac failure.[86] These observations demonstrate a role for AVP in the peripheral vaso-constriction, and hence increased afterload, of CHF.

Renal Effects of Increased Arginine Vasopressin in Congestive Heart Failure

AVP, via stimulation of its V_2 receptor, enhances water reabsorption in the distal nephron, including the corti-cal and medullary collecting ducts. Two lines of evidence implicate nonosmotic AVP release in the abnormal water retention of CHF. First, in animal models of CHF, the absence of a pituitary source of AVP is asso-ciated with normal or near normal water excretion.[28,87] This observation was first made by Anderson and col-leagues in the dog during acute thoracic vena caval constriction.[28] In these animals, acute removal of the pituitary source of AVP by surgical hypophysectomy virtually abolished the defect in water excretion. Abnormal water excretion also occurs in the rat with an aortocaval fistula.[87] The impairment in water excretion seen in this high-output model of cardiac failure pre-sumably is the result of AVP release, since the defect is not demonstrable in rats with central diabetes insipidus.[87] The second line of evidence supporting a role for AVP in the water retention of CHF comes from studies using selective antagonists of the V_2 receptor of AVP in several animal models of cardiac failure.[88,89] Ishikawa and co-workers have assessed the antidiuretic effect of plasma AVP in a low-output model of cardiac failure secondary to vena caval constriction in the rat.[88] In these animals, plasma AVP concentrations were increased, and an antagonist of the antidiuretic effect of AVP reversed the defect in water excretion. Yared et al. also have shown a reversal of water retention using an antagonist to the antidiuretic effect of AVP in another model of heart failure, the rat coronary artery ligation model.[89] This effect of the nonosmotic release of AVP to cause water retention in CHF re-cently has been shown to be associated with increased transcription of messenger RNA for the AVP pre-prohormone in the rat hypothalamus.[90]

In a recent study by Bichet et al., the effect of the converting enzyme inhibitor, captopril, and the α_1-adrenergic blocker, prazosin, to reverse the abnormality in water retention in patients with Class III and IV CHF was examined.[19] The afterload reduction and in-creased cardiac output with either agent was associated with improved water excretion and suppression of AVP in response to an acute water load. A role of AII in modulating the effect of AVP in CHF seems unlikely, since captopril and prazosin had different effects on the renin-angiotensin system, yet their effects to improve

water excretion as plasma AVP was suppressed were comparable.[19] In this regard, it is important to note that in this study by Bichet and co-workers, the average de-crease in mean arterial pressure was 5 mm Hg, a decre-ment that is less than the 7% to 10% necessary to acti-vate the nonosmotic release of AVP.[91] Thus, these re-sults are compatible with the suggestion that a decrease in stroke volume and cardiac output, rather than a fall in mean arterial pressure, is the primary stimulus for the nonosmotic release of AVP in low-output cardiac failure. The association of improved cardiac output and water excretion during afterload reduction is compatible with an influence of ventricular receptors or barorecep-tors sensing pulse pressure in modulating AVP release.

Atrial Natriuretic Peptide in Congestive Heart Failure

ANP also is released in response to heart failure.[40–42] This circulating peptide hormone possesses natri-uretic,[92] vasorelaxant,[93] and renin-, aldosterone-, and possibly vasopressin-inhibiting properties.[94–96] These attributes suggest the possibility of an important coun-terregulatory role for ANP in cardiac failure. In fact, the significant vasodilatory action of elevated endo-genous ANP concentrations in CHF recently has been demonstrated during the infusion of a monoclonal ANP antibody in the rat.[97] In this coronary artery liga-tion model of CHF, infusion of a monoclonal antibody shown to specifically block endogenous ANP in vivo caused a significant rise in right atrial pressure, left ven-tricular end-diastolic pressure, and peripheral vascular resistance. Thus, ANP appears to attenuate to some de-gree the peripheral vasoconstriction of CHF. In human heart failure, ANP infusions result in decreased pul-monary arterial wedge pressure and decreased peripheral vascular resistance with an associated in-crease in cardiac output.[98]

Renal Effects of Increased Atrial Natriuretic Peptide in Congestive Heart Failure

In normal humans, ANP increases GFR with no change or only a modest fall in renal blood flow.[98,99] These changes in renal hemodynamics likely are mediated by afferent arteriolar vasodilation and constriction of the efferent arterioles, as demonstrated by micropuncture studies in the rat.[100,101] ANP infusions appear to be associated with diminished sodium reabsorption in the proximal tubule.[98,99] This effect of infused ANP may be a consequence of renal hemodynamic changes or as a result of a direct tubular effect. Against this latter possi-bility are recent enzymatic and binding studies of ANP in rat glomeruli and nephrons that demonstrate that the glomerulus and distal nephron are the important sites of renal ANP action, rather than the proximal

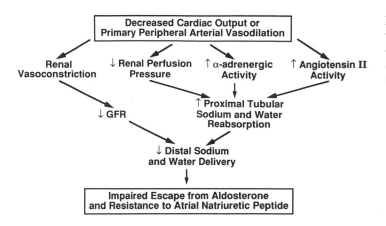

FIGURE 11.3. Factors that contribute to decreased distal tubular sodium and water delivery in CHF. Decreased distal sodium delivery is the postulated cause of impaired aldosterone escape and atrial natriuretic peptide resistance in CHF.

tubule.[102–104] Thus, in addition to increasing GFR and filtered sodium load as a mechanism of its natriuretic effect, ANP has been proposed as a specific inhibitor of sodium reabsorption in the collecting tubule.[102]

An important functional role for endogenous ANP in the renal sodium balance of CHF recently has been proposed by Lee and associates.[105] These investigators examined sodium excretion in two models of low-output cardiac failure in the dog, acute heart failure produced by rapid ventricular pacing, and a thoracic inferior vena caval constriction model. In the case of acute CHF produced by rapid ventricular pacing, cardiac output and arterial pressure were diminished while atrial pressures and plasma ANP concentrations were increased. Despite the arterial hypotension, sodium excretion was maintained. In addition, PRA and plasma aldosterone concentrations were not increased. Similar reductions in cardiac output and arterial pressure by thoracic inferior vena caval constriction were not associated with increased atrial pressures or plasma ANP. In these animals, PRA and plasma aldosterone were significantly increased. Moreover, avid sodium retention was observed in these animals with normal circulating, rather than elevated, ANP concentrations. Finally, dogs with thoracic inferior vena caval obstruction were administered exogenous ANP to achieve circulating levels comparable to that seen in the acute CHF animals. Exogenous administration of ANP to such levels prevented sodium retention, renal vasoconstriction, and activation of the renin-angiotensin-aldosterone system.[105] These results suggest that the high plasma ANP concentrations observed in CHF are important in attenuating the renal sodium retention.

However, despite such observations that suggest a natriuretic role for ANP in heart failure, the intravenous infusion of synthetic ANP to patients with low-output cardiac failure results in a much smaller increase in renal sodium excretion and less significant alterations in renal hemodynamics compared to normal persons.[98] The mechanism of this relative resistance to the natriuretic effect of ANP in CHF is uncertain.

Possible mechanisms include (a) downregulation of renal ANP receptors (b) secretion of inactive immunoreactive ANP (c) enhanced renal endopeptidase activity limiting the delivery of ANP to receptor sites and, (d) diminished sodium delivery to the distal renal tubule site of ANP action. This latter possibility is analogous to the impairment in aldosterone escape seen in CHF and may be mediated by neurohormonal vasoconstrictor activation.[4] Recently, it has been shown that human CHF is associated with downregulation of the platelet ANP receptor.[106] However, the functional significance of this finding remains unclear. Moreover, the first three mechanisms listed above should result in dissociation of plasma ANP and urinary cyclic guanosine monophosphate (cGMP), the second messenger for the natriuretic effect of ANP in vivo.[107,108] However, we have shown in CHF patients that urinary cGMP is increased and correlates with plasma ANP concentrations and hemodynamics.[109] Skorecki et al. have made similar observations in patients with cirrhosis.[110] These data support the hypothesis that the ANP resistance seen in patients with edematous disorders may be due to decreased sodium delivery to the distal tubule site of ANP action rather than a direct impairment of the ANP receptor-signal transduction system involving cGMP. In Figure 11.3 are the various factors that are activated in CHF and contribute to decreased distal sodium delivery.

Renal Prostaglandins in Congestive Heart Failure

In normal persons and in intact animals, renal prostaglandins do not regulate renal sodium excretion or renal hemodynamics to any significant degree.[111,112] In CHF patients, prostaglandin activity is increased and has been shown to correlate with the severity of disease as assessed by the degree of hyponatremia.[74] Moreover, it has been well documented that the administration of a cyclooxygenase inhibitor in heart failure patients may result in acute reversible renal failure, an effect

FIGURE 11.4. Glomerular and tubular sites of action of various neurohormonal systems which are activated in CHF. Renal nerves and angiotensin II (*AII*) influence sodium reabsorption in the proximal tubule. Aldosterone (*Aldo*) enhances sodium reabsorption and promotes potassium and hydrogen excretion in the cortical and medullary collecting duct. Arginine vasopressin (*AVP*) acts to increase water reabsorption in the cortical and medullary collecting duct. Atrial natriuretic peptide (*ANP*) promotes afferent arteriolar vasodilation and constriction of the efferent arterioles and inhibits sodium reabsorption in the collecting duct.

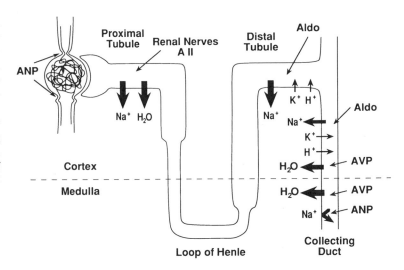

proposed to be due in part to inhibition of renal prostaglandins.[113] A recent investigation in patients with moderate CHF and a normal sodium intake demonstrated that the administration of acetylsalicylic acid in doses that decrease the synthesis of renal prostaglandin E_2 results in a significant reduction in urinary sodium excretion.[114] These observations suggest a possible role for vasodilating prostaglandins in CHF; however, their exact role in renal sodium handling in CHF remains to be elucidated.

Figure 11.4 reviews the renal sites of action of some of the neurohormonal systems activated in CHF.

Therapeutic Implications of Neurohormonal Activation in Congestive Heart Failure

Conventional medical therapy of CHF with dietary salt restriction, diuretics, and direct-acting vasodilators (e.g., nitrates, hydralazine), although shown to improve survival modestly in CHF,[115] may be limited by the development of drug tolerance. The emergence of diuretic resistance or vasodilator tolerance in patients with CHF may be due, in part, to further activation of vasoconstrictor mechanisms induced by these therapeutic agents. In fact, sodium depletion due to dietary salt restriction and the use of diuretics may activate all three of the aforementioned major neurohormonal vasoconstrictor systems.[116,117] Moreover in CHF patients, continuous vasodilator therapy with nitroglycerin results in the rapid development of drug tolerance and in weight gain occurring simultaneously with activation of the renin-angiotensin-aldosterone system.[118] Thus, it can be postulated that diuretic- or vasodilator-induced activation of neurohormonal vasoconstrictor mechanisms reverses the beneficial hemodynamic effects of these agents and stimulates renal sodium and water retention. A recent investigation that examined the interaction of continuous nitroglycerin administration and ACE in-

hibition in normal persons supports this hypothesis.[119] This study showed that the development of nitrate tolerance and the weight gain observed with chronic nitrate therapy was prevented by the simultaneous administration of either captopril or enalapril, suggesting that the development of drug tolerance and expansion of body fluid volume seen with chronic nitrate therapy is mediated by activation of the renin-angiotensin-aldosterone system.[119]

These findings suggest further that specific inhibition of neurohormonal vasoconstrictor mechanisms might be more beneficial than or of additive value to nonspecific vasodilator therapy in CHF. The proven beneficial effects of ACE inhibition on symptoms, hemodynamics, and survival in heart failure support the routine use of these agents in CHF.[120–122] Ongoing investigations of adrenergic-blocking agents and vasopressin antagonists in heart failure patients may lead to the broad application of such antihormonal therapy in CHF. The pharmacologic therapy of CHF is discussed in detail in Section IV of this volume.

Summary

Thus, the various neurohormonal systems activated in response to cardiac failure influence changes in renal hemodynamics and directly affect tubular sodium and water handling resulting in an avid salt- and water-retaining state. Vasoconstrictor neurohormonal activation appears to be mediated by ventricular and high-pressure baroreceptor stimulation of the sympathetic nervous system, leading to activation of the renin-angiotensin-aldosterone system and the nonosmotic release of vasopressin, in response to underfilling of the arterial circulation. Counterregulatory vasodilator and natriuretic hormones, such as ANP and prostaglandins, also are activated in heart failure. These hormones may serve to attenuate to some degree the antinatriuretic and antidiuretic effects of vasoconstrictor hormone activation.

References

1. Starling EH. The Fluids of the Body. In *The Herter Lectures*. Chicago: Keener; 1909:106.
2. Smith HW. Salt and water volume receptors: an exercise in physiologic apologetics. *Am J Med.* 1957;23:623–652.
3. Nizet A. Quantitative influence of non-hormonal blood factors on the control of sodium excretion by the isolated dog kidney. *Kidney Int.* 1972;1:27–37.
4. Schrier RW. Pathogenesis of sodium and water retention in high-output and low-output cardiac failure, cirrhosis, nephrotic syndrome, and pregnancy. *N Engl J Med.* 1988;319:1065–1072,1127–1134.
5. Koppel MH, Coburn JW, Mims MM, Goldstein H, Boyle JD, Rubini ME. Transplantation of cadaveric kidneys from patients with hepatorenal syndrome: evidence for the functional nature of renal failure in advanced liver disease. *N Engl J Med.* 1969;280:1367–1371.
6. Iwatsuki S, Popovtzer MM, Corman JL, et al. Recovery from hepatorenal syndrome after orthotopic liver transplantation. *N Engl J Med.* 1973;289:1155–1159.
7. Peters JP. The role of sodium in the production of edema. *N Engl J Med.* 1948;239:353–362.
8. Borst JGG, deVries LA. Three types of "natural" diuresis. *Lancet.* 1950;2:1–6.
9. Schrier RW, Humphreys MH. Factors involved in the antinatriuretic effects of acute constriction of the thoracic inferior and abdominal vena cava. *Circ Res.* 1971;29:479–489.
10. Schrier RW, Humphreys MH, Ufferman RC. Role of cardiac output and the autonomic nervous system in the antinatriuretic response to acute constriction of the thoracic superior vena cava. *Circ Res.* 1971;29:490–498.
11. Schrier RW, Berl T, Anderson RJ. Osmotic and non-osmotic control of vasopressin release. *Am J Physiol.* 1979;236:F321–F322.
12. Szatalowicz VL, Arnold PE, Chaimovitz C, Bichet D, Berl T, Schrier RW. Radioimmunoassay of plasma arginine vasopressin in hyponatremic patients with congestive heart failure. *N Engl J Med.* 1981;305:263–266.
13. Bichet DG, Szatalowicz VL, Chaimovitz C, Schrier RW. Role of vasopressin in abnormal water excretion in cirrhotic patients. *Ann Intern Med.* 1982;96:413–417.
14. Bichet DG, Van Putten VJ, Schrier RW. Potential role of the increased sympathetic activity in impaired sodium and water excretion in cirrhosis. *N Engl J Med.* 1982;307:1552–1557.
15. Bichet DG, Groves BM, Schrier RW. Mechanisms of improvement of water and sodium excretion by enhancement of central hemodynamics in decompensated cirrhotic patients. *Kidney Int.* 1983;24:788–794.
16. Nicholls KM, Shapiro MD, Van Putten VJ, et al. Elevated plasma norepinephrine concentrations in decompensated cirrhosis: association with increased secretion rates, normal clearance rates and suppressibility by central blood volume expansion. *Circ Res.* 1985;56:457–461.
17. Shapiro MD, Nicholls KM, Groves BM, et al. Interrelationship between cardiac output and vascular resistance as determinants of "effective arterial blood volume" in cirrhotic patients. *Kidney Int.* 1985;28:206–211.
18. Nicholls KM, Shapiro MD, Kluge R, Chung H-M, Bichet DG, Schrier RW. Sodium excretion in advanced cirrhosis: effect of expansion of central blood volume and suppression of plasma aldosterone. *Hepatology.* 1986;6:235–238.
19. Bichet DG, Kortas C, Mettauer B, et al. Modulation of plasma and platelet vasopressin by cardiac function in patients with heart failure. *Kidney Int.* 1986;29:1188–1196.
20. Bichet DG, Schrier RW. Cardiac failure, liver disease and nephrotic syndrome. In: Schrier RW, Gottschalk CW, eds. *Diseases of the Kidney.* 4th ed. Boston: Little, Brown; 1988:2703–2742.
21. de Torrente A, Robertson GL, McDonald KM, Schrier RW. Mechanism of diuretic response to increased left atrial pressure in the anesthetized dog. *Kidney Int.* 1975;8:355–361.
22. Goetz KL, Bond GC, Bloxham DD. Atrial receptors and renal function. *Physiol Rev.* 1975;55:157–205.
23. Zucker IH, Earle AM, Gilmore JP. The mechanism of adaptation of left atrial stretch receptors in dogs with chronic congestive heart failure. *J Clin Invest.* 1977;60:323–331.
24. Schrier RW, Lieberman RA, Ufferman RC. Mechanism of antidiuretic effect of beta adrenergic stimulation. *J Clin Invest.* 1972;51:97–111.
25. Schrier RW, Berl T. Mechanism of effect of alpha-adrenergic stimulation with norepinephrine on renal water excretion. *J Clin Invest.* 1973;52:502–511.
26. Berl T, Cadnapaphornchai P, Harbottle JA, Schrier RW. Mechanism of suppression of vasopressin during alpha-adrenergic stimulation with norepinephrine. *J Clin Invest.* 1974;53:219–227.
27. Berl T, Cadnapaphornchai P, Harbottle JA, Schrier RW. Mechanism of stimulation of vasopressin release during beta adrenergic stimulation with isoproterenol. *J Clin Invest.* 1974;53:857–867.
28. Anderson RJ, Cadnapaphornchai P, Harbottle JA, McDonald KM, Schrier RW. Mechanism of effect of thoracic inferior vena cava constriction on renal water excretion. *J Clin Invest.* 1974;54:1473–1479.
29. Anderson RJ, Pluss RG, Berns AS, et al. Mechanism of effect of hypoxia on renal water excretion. *J Clin Invest.* 1978;62:769–777.
30. Schrier RW, Berl T. Mechanism of antidiuretic effect of interruption of parasympathetic pathways. *J Clin Invest.* 1972;51:2613–2620.
31. Murdaugh HV Jr, Sieker HO, Manfredi F. Effect of altered intrathoracic pressure on renal hemodynamics, electrolyte excretion and water clearance. *J Clin Invest.* 1959;38:834–842.
32. Gauer OH, Henry JP. Circulating basis of fluid volume control. *Physiol Rev.* 1963;43:423–481.
33. Epstein FH, Goodyer AVN, Lawrason FD, Relman AS. Studies of the antidiuresis of quiet standing: the importance of changes in plasma volume and glomerular filtration rate. *J Clin Invest.* 1951;30:63–72.

34. Gauer OH, Henry JP, Sieker HO, Wendt WE. The effect of negative pressure breathing on urine flow. *J Clin Invest.* 1954;33:287–296.

35. Hulet WH, Smith HH. Postural natriuresis and urine osmotic concentration in hydropenic subjects. *Am J Med.* 1961;30:8–25.

36. Epstein M, Duncan DC, Fishman LM. Characterization of the natriuresis caused in normal man by immersion in water. *Clin Sci.* 1972;43:275–287.

37. Gillespie DJ, Sandberg RL, Koike TI. Dual effect of left atrial receptors on excretion of sodium and water in the dog. *Am J Physiol.* 1973;225:706–710.

38. Reinhardt HW, Kaczmarczyk G, Eisele R, Arnold B, Eigenheer F, Kuhl U. Left atrial pressure and sodium balance in conscious dogs on a low sodium intake. *Pflugers Arch.* 1977;370:59–66.

39. Henry JP, Gauer OH, Reeves JL. Evidence of the atrial location of receptors influencing urine flow. *Circ Res.* 1956;4:85–90.

40. Sato F, Kamoi K, Wakiya Y, et al. Relationship between plasma atrial natriuretic peptide levels and atrial pressure in man. *J Clin Endocrinol Metab.* 1986;63:823–627.

41. Raine AEG, Erne P, Bürgisser E, et al. Atrial natriuretic peptide and atrial pressure in patients with congestive heart failure. *N Engl J Med.* 1986;315:533–537.

42. Nakaoka H, Imataka K, Amano M, Fujii J, Ishibashi M, Yamaji T. Plasma levels of atrial natriuretic factor in patients with congestive heart failure. *N Engl J Med.* 1985;313:892–893.

43. Epstein FH, Post RS, McDowell M. Effects of an arteriovenous fistula on renal hemodynamics and electrolyte excretion. *J Clin Invest.* 1953;32:233–241.

44. Gilmore JP. Contribution of baroreceptors to the control of renal function. *Circ Res.* 1964;14:301–317.

45. Gilmore JP, Daggett WM. Response of chronic cardiac denervated dog to acute volume expansion. *Am J Physiol.* 1966;210:509–512.

46. Knox FG, Davis BB, Berliner RW. Effect of chronic cardiac denervation on renal response to saline infusion. *Am J Physiol.* 1967;213:174–178.

47. Pearce JW, Sonnenberg H. Effects of spinal section and renal denervation on the renal response to blood volume expansion. *Can J Physiol Pharmacol.* 1965;43:211–224.

48. Schedl HP, Bartter FC. An explanation for and experimental correction of the abnormal water diuresis in cirrhosis. *J Clin Invest.* 1967;46:1297–1308.

49. Davis JO. The control of renin release. *Am J Med.* 1973;55:333–350.

50. Guyton A, Scanlon CJ, Armstrong GG. Effects of pressoreceptor reflex and Cushing's reflex on urinary output. *Fed Proc.* 1952;11:61–62.

51. Anderson RJ, Cronin RE, McDonald KM, Schrier RW. Mechanism of portal hypertension-induced alterations in renal hemodynamics, renal water excretion, and renin secretion. *J Clin Invest.* 1976;58:964–970.

52. Schrier RW, Berl T, Anderson RJ, McDonald KM. Nonosmolar control of renal water excretion. In: Andreoli T, Grantham J, Rector F, eds. *Disturbances in Body Fluid Osmolality.* Bethesda, MD: American Physiological Society; 1977:149–178.

53. Sklar AH, Schrier RW. Central nervous system mediators of vasopressin release. *Physiol Rev.* 1983;63:1243–1280.

54. Berl T, Henrich WL, Erickson AL, Schrier RW. Prostaglandins in the beta adrenergic and baroreceptor-mediated secretion on renin. *Am J Physiol.* 1979; 235:F472–F477.

55. Thomas JA, Marks BH. Plasma norepinephrine in congestive heart failure. *Am J Cardiol.* 1978;41:233–243.

56. Levine TB, Francis GS, Goldsmith SR, Simon AB, Cohn JN. Activity of the sympathetic nervous system and renin-angiotensin system as assessed by plasma hormone levels and their relation to hemodynamic abnormalities in congestive heart failure. *Am J Cardiol.* 1982;49:1659–1666.

57. Davis D, Baily R, Zelis R. Abnormalities in systemic norepinephrine kinetics in human congestive heart failure. *Am J Physiol.* 1988;254:E760–E766.

58. Hasking JG, Esler MD, Jennings GL, Burton D, Korner PI. Norepinephrine spillover to plasma in patients with congestive heart failure: evidence of increased overall and cardiorenal sympathetic nervous activity. *Circulation.* 1986;73:615–621.

59. Abraham WT, Hensen J, Schrier RW. Elevated plasma noradrenaline concentrations in patients with low-output cardiac failure: dependence on increased noradrenaline secretion rates. *Clin Sci.* 1990;79:429–435.

60. Leimbach WN, Wallin BG, Victor RG, Aylward PE, Sundlöf G, Mark AL. Direct evidence from intraneural recordings for increased sympathetic outflow in patients with heart failure. *Circulation.* 1986;73:913–919.

61. Chidsey CA, Braunwald E, Morrow AG. Catecholamine excretion and cardiac stores of norepinephrine in congestive heart failure. *Am J Med.* 1965;39:442–451.

62. Cohn JN, Levine BT, Olivari MT. Plasma norepinephrine as a guide to prognosis in patients with chronic congestive heart failure. *N Engl J Med.* 1984;311:819–823.

63. Brod J, Fejfar Z, Fejfarová MH. The role of neurohumoral factors in the genesis of renal haemodynamic changes in heart failure. *Acta Med Scand.* 1954;148:273–290.

64. Gill JR Jr, Mason DT, Bartter FC. Adrenergic nervous system in sodium metabolism: effects of guanethidine and sodium-retaining steroids in normal man. *J Clin Invest.* 1964;43:177–184.

65. DiBona GF, Herman PJ, Sawin LL. Neural control of renal function in edema-forming states. *Am J Physiol.* 1988;254:R1017–R1024.

66. Bello-Reuss E, Trevino DL, Gottschalk CW. Effect of renal sympathetic nerve stimulation on proximal water and sodium reabsorption. *J Clin Invest.* 1976;57:1104–1107.

67. Meyers BD, Deen WM, Brenner BM. Effects of norepinephrine and angiotensin II on the determinants of glomerular ultrafiltration and proximal tubule fluid reabsorption in the rat. *Circ Res.* 1975;37:101–110.

68. Ichikawa I, Pfeffer J, Pfeffer MA, Hostetter TH, Brenner BM. Role of angiotensin II in the altered renal function of congestive heart failure. *Circ Res.* 1983;55:669–675.

69. DiBona GF. Neural control of renal tubular sodium reabsorption. *Am J Physiol.* 1977;233:F73–F81.

70. Carpenter CCJ, Davis JO, Holman JE, Ayers CR, Bahn RC. Studies on the response of the transplanted kidney and transplanted adrenal gland to thoracic inferior vena caval constriction. *J Clin Invest.* 1961;40:196–204.

71. Lifschitz MD, Schrier RW. Alterations in cardiac output with chronic constriction of thoracic inferior vena cava. *Am J Physiol.* 1973;225:1364–1370.

72. Francis GS, Goldsmith SR, Levine TB, Olivari MT, Cohn JN. The neurohumoral axis in congestive heart failure. *Ann Intern Med.* 1984;101:370–377.

73. Merrill AJ, Morrison JL, Brannon ES. Concentration of renin in renal venous blood in patients with chronic heart failure. *Am J Med.* 1946;1:468–472.

74. Dzau VJ, Packer M, Lilly LS, Swartz SL, Hollenberg NK, Williams GH. Prostaglandins in severe congestive heart failure: relation to activation of the renin-angiotensin system and hyponatremia. *N Engl J Med.* 1984;310:347–352.

75. Lee WH, Packer M. Prognostic importance of serum sodium concentration and its modification by converting-enzyme inhibition in patients with severe chronic heart failure. *Circulation.* 1986;73:257–267.

76. Ichikawa I, Brenner BM. Importance of efferent arteriolar vascular tone in regulation of proximal tubule fluid reabsorption and glomerulotubular balance in the rat. *J Clin Invest.* 1980;65:1192–1201.

77. Liu F-Y, Cogan MG. Angiotensin II: a potent regulator of acidification in the rat early proximal convoluted tubule. *J Clin Invest.* 1987;80:272–275.

78. Cody RJ, Covit AB, Schaer GL, Laragh JH, Sealy JE, Feldschuh J. Sodium and water balance in chronic congestive heart failure. *J Clin Invest.* 1986;77:1441–1452.

79. Pierpont GL, Francis GS, Cohn JN. Effect of captopril on renal function in patients with congestive heart failure. *Br Heart J.* 1981;46:522–527.

80. Hensen J, Abraham WT, Dürr J, Schrier RW. Aldosterone in congestive heart failure: analysis of determinants and role in sodium retention. *Am J Nephrol.* 1991;11:441–446.

81. Riegger GAJ, Liebau G, Koschiek K. Antidiuretic hormone in congestive heart failure. *Am J Med.* 1982;72:49–55.

82. Pruszczynski W, Vahanian A, Ardailou R, Acar J. Role of antidiuretic hormone in impaired water excretion of patients with congestive heart failure. *J Clin Endocrinol Metab.* 1984;58:599–603.

83. Goldsmith SR, Francis GS, Cowley AW Jr. Arginine vasopressin and the renal response to water loading in congestive heart failure. *Am J Cardiol.* 1986;58:295–299.

84. Nicod P, Biollaz J, Waeber B, et al. Hormonal, global and regional haemodynamic responses to a vascular antagonist of vasopressin in patients with congestive heart failure with and without hyponatraemia. *Br Heart J.* 1986;56:433–439.

85. Creager MA, Faxon DP, Cutler SS, Kohlmann O, Ryan TJ, Gavras H. Contribution of vasopressin to vasoconstriction in patients with congestive heart failure: comparison with the renin-angiotensin system and the sym-

pathetic nervous system. *J Am Col Cardiol.* 1986;7:758–765.

86. Goldsmith SR, Francis GS, Cowley AW, Goldenberg IF, Cohn JN. Hemodynamic effects of infused arginine vasopressin in congestive heart failure. *J Am Coll Cardiol.* 1986;779–783.

87. Handelman W, Lum G, Schrier RW. Impaired water excretion in high output cardiac failure in the rat. *Clin Res.* 1979;27:173A.

88. Ishikawa S, Saito T, Okada K, Tsutsui K, Kuzuya T. Effect of vasopressin antagonist on water excretion in inferior vena cava constriction. *Kidney Int.* 1986;30:49–55.

89. Yared A, Kon V, Brenner BM, Ichikawa I. Role for vasopressin in rats with congestive heart failure. *Kidney Int.* 1985;27:337.

90. Kim JK, Michel J-B, Soubrier F, Dürr J, Corvol P, Schrier RW. Arginine vasopressin gene expression in congestive heart failure. *Kidney Int.* 1988;33:270.

91. Dunn FL, Brennan TJ, Nelson AE, Robertson GL. The role of blood osmolality and volume in regulating vasopressin secretion in the rat. *J Clin Invest.* 1973;52:3212–3219.

92. Atlas SA, Kleinert HD, Camargo MJ, et al. Purification, sequencing, and synthesis of natriuretic and vasoactive rat atrial peptide. *Nature.* 1984;309:717–719.

93. Currie MG, Geller DM, Cole BR, et al. Bioactive cardiac substances: potent vasorelaxant activity in mammalian atria. *Science.* 1983;221:71–73.

94. Molina CR, Fowler MB, McCrory S, et al. Hemodynamic, renal, and endocrine effects of atrial natriuretic peptide in severe heart failure. *J Am Coll Cardiol.* 1988;12:175–186.

95. Atarashi K, Mulrow PJ, Franco-Saenz R, Snajdar R, Rapp J. Inhibition of aldosterone production by an atrial extract. *Science.* 1984;224:992–994.

96. Samson WK. Atrial natriuretic factor inhibits dehydration and hemorrhage-induced vasopressin release. *Neuroendocrinology.* 1985;40:277–279.

97. Drexler H, Hirth C, Stasch H-P, Lu W, Neuser D, Just H. Vasodilatory action of endogenous atrial natriuretic factor in a rat model of chronic heart failure as determined by monoclonal ANF antibody. *Circ Res.* 1990;66:1371–1380.

98. Cody RJ, Atlas SA, Laragh JH, et al. Atrial natriuretic factor in normal subjects and heart failure patients: plasma levels and renal, hormonal, and hemodynamic responses to peptide infusion. *J Clin Invest.* 1986;78:1362–1374.

99. Biollaz J, Nussberger J, Porchet M, et al. Four-hour infusion of synthetic atrial natriuretic peptide in normal volunteers. *Hypertension.* 1986;8:II96–II105.

100. Borenstein HB, Cupples WA, Sonnenberg H, Veress AT. The effect of natriuretic atrial extract on renal hemodynamics and urinary excretion in anesthetized rats. *J Physiol.* 1983;334:133–140.

101. Dunn BR, Ichikawa I, Pfeffer JM, Troy JL, Brenner BM. Renal and systemic hemodynamic effects of synthetic atrial natriuretic peptide in the anesthetized rat. *Circ Res.* 1986;237–246.

102. Kim JK, Summer SN, Dürr J, Schrier RW. Enzymatic and binding effects of atrial natriuretic factor in glomeruli and nephrons. *Kidney Int.* 1989;35:799–805.

103. Koseki C, Hayashi Y, Torikai S, Furuya M, Ohnuma N, Imai M. Localization of binding sites for alpha-rat atrial natriuretic polypeptide in rat kidney. *Am J Physiol.* 1986;250:F210–F216.

104. Healy DP, Fanestil DD. Localization of atrial natriuretic peptide binding sites within the rat kidney. *Am J Physiol.* 1986;250:F573–F578.

105. Lee ME, Miller WL, Edwards BS, Burnett JC Jr. Role of endogenous atrial natriuretic factor in acute congestive heart failure. *J Clin Invest.* 1989;84:1962–1966.

106. Schiffrin EL. Decreased density of binding sites for atrial natriuretic peptide on platelets of patients with severe congestive heart failure. *Clin Sci.* 1988;74:213–218.

107. Huang C-L, Ives HE, Cogan MG. In vivo evidence that cGMP is the second messenger for atrial natriuretic factor. *Proc Natl Acad Sci.* 1986;83:8015–8018.

108. Hamet PJ, Tremblay J, Pang SC, et al. Cyclic GMP as mediator and biological marker of atrial natriuretic factor. *J Hypertens.* 1986;4:S49–S56.

109. Abraham WT, Hensen J, Kim JK, et al. Atrial natriuretic peptide and urinary cyclic guanosine monophosphate in patients with chronic heart failure. *J Am Soc Nephrol.* 1992;2:1697–1703.

110. Skorecki KL, Leung W, Campbell P, et al. Role of atrial natriuretic peptide in the natriuretic response to central volume expansion induced by head-out water immersion in sodium-retaining cirrhotic subjects. *Am J Med.* 1988;85:375–382.

111. Swain JA, Heyndrickx GR, Boettcher DH, Vatner SF. Prostaglandin control of renal circulation in the unanesthetized dog and baboon. *Am J Physiol.* 1975;229:826–830.

112. Walker RM, Brown RS, Stoff JS. Role of renal prostaglandins during antidiuresis and water diuresis in man. *Kidney Int.* 1981;21:365–370.

113. Walshe JJ, Venuto RC. Acute oliguric renal failure induced by indomethacin: possible mechanism. *Ann Intern Med.* 1979;91:47–49.

114. Riegger GA, Kahles HW, Elsner D, Kromer EP, Kochsiek K. Effects of acetylsalicylic acid on renal function in patients with chronic heart failure. *Am J Med.* 1991;90:571–575.

115. Cohn JN, Archibald DG, Ziesche S, et al. Effect of vasodilator therapy on mortality in chronic congestive heart failure: results of a Veterans Administration Cooperative Study. *N Engl J Med.* 1986;314:1547–1552.

116. Francis GS, Siegel RM, Goldsmith SR, Olivari MT, Levine B, Cohn JN. Acute vasoconstrictor response to intravenous furosemide in patients with chronic congestive heart failure: activation of the neurohumoral axis. *Ann Intern Med.* 1985;103:1–6.

117. Bayliss J, Norell M, Canepa-Anson R, Sutton G, Poole-Wilson P. Untreated heart failure: clinical and neuroendocrine effects of introducing diuretics. *Br Heart J.* 1987;57:17–22.

118. Packer M, Lee WH, Kessler PD, Gottlieb SS, Medina N, Yushak M. Prevention and reversal of nitrate tolerance in patients with congestive heart failure. *N Engl J Med.* 1987;317:799–804.

119. Katz RJ, Levy WS, Buff L, Wasserman AG. Prevention of nitrate tolerance with angiotensin converting enzyme inhibitors. *Circulation.* 1991;83:1271–1277.

120. Captopril Multicenter Research Group. A placebo-controlled trial of captopril in refractory chronic congestive heart failure. *J Am Coll Cardiol.* 1983;2:755–763.

121. CONSENSUS Trial Study Group. Effects of enalapril on mortality in severe congestive heart failure: results of the North Scandinavian Enalapril Survival Study (CONSENSUS). *N Engl J Med.* 1987;316:1429–1435.

122. The SOLVD Investigators. Effect of enalapril on survival in patients with reduced left ventricular ejection fractions and congestive failure. *N Engl J Med.* 1991;325:293–302.

Part III
Differential Diagnosis of Congestive Heart Failure

12
Heart Failure Secondary to Coronary Artery Disease

Roger M. Mills, Jr., and Carl J. Pepine

In this chapter, we outline our approach to heart failure occurring as a consequence of coronary artery disease. Table 12.1 enumerates the common clinical syndromes of heart failure due to coronary artery disease, the three themes being (a) ischemia with reversible left ventricular (LV) dysfunction, either systolic or diastolic, leading to pulmonary congestion, (b) mechanical complications of infarction, and (c) irreversible myocardial scarring with impairment of LV systolic function leading to low forward cardiac output. The epidemiologic issues involved have been reviewed in prior chapters, but we emphasize again that heart failure represents a major public health problem with more than 400,000 new cases annually in the United States. In the U.S., coronary artery disease is the most common cause of heart failure. Once established, the prognosis with medical management is poor, with an average annual mortality of 30% to 40%.[1-3] In addition, patients who develop heart failure as a consequence of coronary artery disease have a significantly poorer prognosis than those whose heart failure results from nonischemic pathology. Franciosa and colleagues followed 182 patients with chronic LV failure, and reported 1- and 2-yr mortality rates of 46% and 69% in patients with coronary artery disease compared with 23% and 48% in patients with idiopathic dilated cardiomyopathy.[4] Similarly, in a study group of 201 patients with advanced heart failure, Likoff et al. found a 6-month mortality of 65% in patients with ischemic heart disease versus 40% in noncoronary heart failure patients.[5] This difference persists despite vasodilator therapy, as demonstrated by the Veterans Administration Cooperative Study data shown in Figure 12.1, comparing patients with heart failure due to coronary artery disease and noncoronary causes treated with vasodilators versus conventional therapy ("placebo").[6] Approximately onehalf of all deaths due to heart failure occur suddenly.[7] Despite advances in medical therapy, which may provide a modest reduction in deaths due to heart failure, the sudden death prob-

TABLE 12.1. Syndromes of heart failure with coronary artery disease.

Ischemia
Diastolic dysfunction—normal heart size
"Flash" pulmonary edema with multivessel CAD
Exertional dyspnea due to ischemia
Both systolic and diastolic dysfunction
Stunned and hibernating myocardium
Transient coronary occlusion during unstable
angina or PTCA
Anatomic disruption
Ischemic mitral regurgitation
Ventricular septal defect
Left ventricular aneurysm
Chronic scarring
Systolic dysfunction with cardiac enlargement
Ischemic cardiomyopathy

lem has not been reduced.[8,9] Also, about 35% of all patients with heart failure are hospitalized every year, representing a tremendous public health problem.[9]

The diagnostic approach to the patient with heart failure due to coronary artery disease should focus primarily on two important questions. First, can mechanical revascularization [e.g., percutaneous transluminal coronary angioplasty (PTCA), or coronary artery bypass grafting (CABG)] relieve reversible ischemia with clinical improvement? Second, can the function of the heart be improved by anatomic reconstruction, for instance, repair of an acquired ventricular septal defect, combined LV aneurysmectomy and revascularization, or repair or replacement of a damaged mitral valve?

With these questions in mind, we will develop the rationale for our approach by first reviewing our current understanding of coronary artery disease pathophysiology with a major emphasis on cardiac function. Although much basic and clinical investigation remains to be done, recent advances have improved our understanding of how variations in coronary flow act to pro-

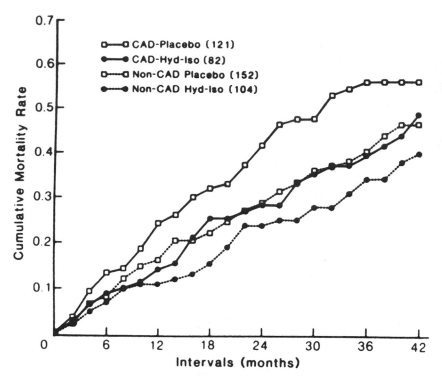

FIGURE 12.1. Cumulative mortality among patients with (n = 203) and without (n = 256) coronary artery disease (CAD) treated with placebo or hydralazine-isosorbide dinitrate (*Hyd-Iso*). Reprinted, with permission, of the *New England Journal of Medicine* (1986; 314;24).

duce acute and chronic hemodynamic dysfunction. Second, we discuss the acquisition of clinical data including the appropriate use of diagnostic tests including echocardiography, stress testing, ambulatory electrocardiographic monitoring, and the catheterization laboratory in the assessment of the heart failure patient with known or suspected coronary artery disease. Third, we attempt to integrate pathophysiologic and clinical data by reviewing the processes involved in decision making and choice of therapy.

Ischemia-Related Left Ventricular Dysfunction: Physiologic Principles

Coronary Blood Flow–Myocardial Oxygen Demand

Obstructive disease in the coronary arterial tree becomes clinically apparent as coronary artery disease by producing either reversible or irreversible myocardial oxygen supply-demand imbalance. Central to an appreciation of heart failure due to coronary artery disease is an understanding of the precise coupling of coronary blood flow to myocardial oxygen demand and the close association of the adequacy of this blood flow versus O_2 demand relationship with myocardial function. This coupling requires the ability to increase coronary blood flow markedly in response to augmentation in myocardial metabolic demand described as "coronary flow reserve."[10]

Coronary flow reserve in laboratory animal experiments can be measured directly using an open-chest preparation with a mechanical snare to produce variable degrees of stenosis in proximal vessels and an electromagnetic flow meter to measure distal flow. In this preparation, coronary flow at rest and after maximal coronary vasodilation can be compared during production of varying degrees of stenosis in the vessel. Using this technique and intracoronary injections of radiographic contrast as a vasodilator stimulus, Gould and associates[11] demonstrated that coronary flow in unobstructed vessels could increase four- to fivefold. Although resting blood flow did not fall until an 85% stenosis was imposed, this four- to fivefold coronary flow reserve was impaired by only 35% to 40% proximal stenosis. In further studies, these measurements appeared valid with either single or multiple coronary stenoses, and the investigators therefore proposed coronary flow reserve as a physiologic measurement that described the overall function of the artery as a unit.[11,12]

In human studies, coronary flow reserve has been measured using subselective intracoronary Doppler blood flow velocity catheters. Although the Doppler flow catheter directly measures flow velocity, if the studies are performed under conditions of prior nitroglycerin administration (e.g., maximal dilation of large coronary arteries), changes in coronary flow velocity are essentially proportional to changes in coronary flow volume. Using this technique, Wilson and colleagues demonstrated increases over resting flow velocity of 3.5-fold with intracoronary radiographic contrast material

FIGURE 12.2. Decreasing coronary flow reserve with progressive coronary obstruction.

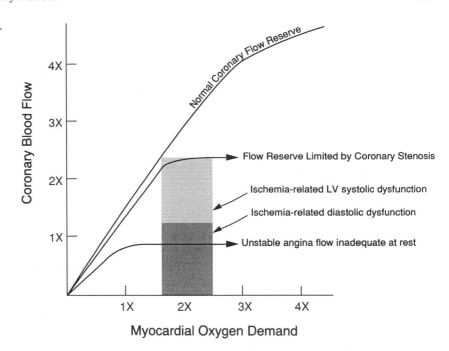

injections, 5-fold with dipyridamole,[13] and 5-fold with papaverine[14] in patients with angiographically normal coronary arteries. These studies convincingly demonstrate the existence of coronary flow reserve in humans, and indicate that the magnitude of coronary flow reserve, approximately fivefold, is similar to that seen in the laboratory preparations described above. Such increases in flow are not required during ordinary daily activities.

As the obstruction caused by coronary artery disease progresses, coronary flow reserve gradually declines to a level where ischemia ensues with only modest increases in myocardial oxygen need (Fig. 12.2). In the unstable coronary syndromes, the impairment of coronary blood flow that occurs may reduce myocardial perfusion below levels required to prevent ischemia during daily activities or even at rest. Under these circumstances flow reserve no longer exists.

Ischemia-Related Injury

In either situation, inadequate flow reserve in response to stress or impaired resting flow, myocardial hypoperfusion results in myocellular hypoxia. This leads to biochemical, electrical, and mechanical dysfunction because cardiac muscle metabolism is an obligate aerobic system with minimal anaerobic sources of energy. Jennings et al. have studied high energy phosphate metabolism in quick-frozen sections of the canine heart after coronary occlusion.[15] Their data show a shift from aerobic to anaerobic metabolism beginning within 8 to 10 s after coronary ligation. After 40 to 60 min, their studies demonstrate marked loss of high energy

phosphate and low tissue pH with characteristic ultrastructural changes, including cell swelling with mitochondrial and sarcolemma damage.

In addition to these metabolic changes, recent laboratory studies in the isolated perfused heart suggest that ischemia also leads to an increase in β-adrenergic receptors in the plasma membrane within as little as 15 min, leading to increased sensitivity to β-adrenergic stimulation in very early ischemia.[16]

The time course of these ischemia-related changes may vary with the mechanism of ischemia, as subtle differences between "supply ischemia" produced by transient balloon occlusion or arterial obstruction and "demand ischemia" produced by pacing tachycardia become evident. In addition, the phenomenon of "preconditioning" clearly plays a significant role in "supply ischemia." Preconditioning implies an increased tolerance to ischemia after repeated episodes and is discussed in greater detail below.

In human studies, diastolic function appears most sensitive to ischemia. Bonow and associates studied filling dynamics using radionuclide angiography in 26 patients with single vessel coronary disease and normal LV systolic function.[17] Comparison before and after PTCA showed improvement in filling rate from 2.5 ± 0.6 to 3.0 ± 0.6 end-diastolic volumes/s and a decrease in time to peak filling rate from 178 ± 30 to 162 ± 20 ms. These findings suggest that diastolic function may be measurably impaired, with regional asynchrony in relaxation associated with impaired global diastolic function, while regional and global systolic function remain normal. Piscione et al. studied LV function during balloon occlusion in 10 patients with normal LV function undergoing PTCA.[18] With high fidelity pressure records and LV angiography during the PTCA, these investigators demonstrated impairment of relaxation at 20 s after the onset of ischemia, associated with impairment of peak segmental shortening as well. They concluded that the severity of impairment of global filling dynamics during the early phase of acute ischemia was related to the magnitude of LV systolic and diastolic asynchrony. In summary, one of the earliest manifestations of cardiac ischemia that can be detected in patients is an alteration in diastolic function. In some situations, reversible alterations in diastolic function may be present without detectable impairment of systolic function.[19] More intense myocellular hypoxia leads to failure of contraction. Finally, as in the animal model, hypoxia results in irreversible ischemic injury to the structure of the myocyte.

Myocardial Stunning and Hibernation

Until recently, ischemia-related injury was thought of as an acute self-limited process with only two possible outcomes from the standpoint of LV function. Either prompt relief of ischemia completely restored mechanical function, or persistent ischemia led to cell necrosis with permanent loss of mechanical function through infarction and scar formation. There is now growing appreciation that ischemia-related LV dysfunction is much more complex (Figs. 12.3, 12.4). This conceptual expansion was necessary to explain continued cellular viability with ischemic contraction failure, which may later reverse under certain circumstances. Two different patterns of clinically important reversible ischemic dysfunction now have been described. When ischemic contraction failure or relaxation abnormalities of viable myocytes occur due to single or repetitive brief episodes of hypoperfusion followed by reperfusion as in acute myocardial infarction with reperfusion, the phenomenon is referred to as "myocardial stunning". When contractile failure occurs as a physiologic adaptation to chronic hypoperfusion, the descriptive term "hibernating myocardium" has been used.[20–25]

Myocardial stunning may occur after single prolonged or repetitive brief episodes of coronary hypoperfusion, as demonstrated by increased diastolic stiffness after repeated angioplasty balloon occlusion. Wijns and colleagues[26] studied the effect of 3 to 10 balloon inflations lasting from 15 to 75 s on diastolic performance and demonstrated decreased diastolic performance last-

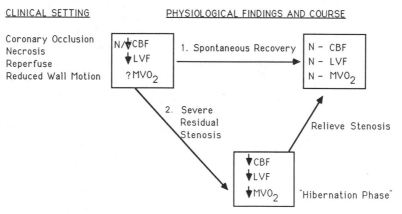

FIGURE 12.3. When a severe coronary stenosis reduces coronary flow without necrosis there may be a downregulation of myocardial function. The decrease in myocardial contractility reduces myocardial energy demands, hence no necrosis occurs. Thus, the physiological findings in the course of this clinical phenomenon would be reduced coronary blood flow, reduced LV function, and reduced myocardial oxygen demands. There are three possible consequences given these findings. The first, spontaneous recovery with which coronary blood flow may normalize due to collateral flow relief of coronary spasm, etc. This will result in return of LV myocardial oxygen requirements and function. The second possibility is to relieve the stenosis. Under these circumstances coronary blood flow normalizes immediately but LV function may recover immediately or its recovery may be delayed. If its recov- ery is delayed, the findings (basically, a normal coronary blood flow with reduced LV function and presumably myocardial oxygen demand) resemble those seen in myocardial stunning which occurs after myocardial infarction is reperfused. Thus, the hibernating myocardium may go through a delayed recovery phase, which we have termed a "stunned phase". With time spontaneous recovery should occur. A third possibility would be if the relationship between the reduced coronary blood flow and reduced myocardial oxygen demand is disturbed by further reduction in coronary blood flow for an increase in myocardial oxygen consumption, myocardial necrosis may ensue. Under these circumstances the necrosed myocardium may be reperfused, in which case coronary blood flow is normalized; this myocardial region also may go through a stunned phase before spontaneous recovery.

HIBERNATING MYOCARDIUM

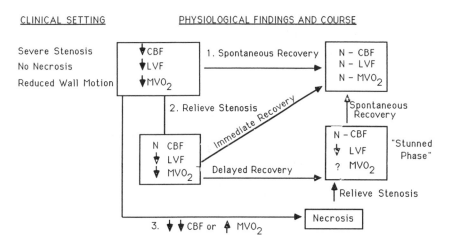

FIGURE 12.4. Stunned myocardium occurs in the clinical setting of severe acute onset coronary occlusion, which results in necrosis of myocardium in the region at risk. The occlusion is relieved when the myocardium is reperfused; however, reduced myocardial wall motion exists in the region at risk in the viable myocardium. Physiologically, coronary blood flow may be normal or slightly reduced in this stunned region, LV function is reduced, and myocardial consumption may be reduced. There are two possible consequences or courses to these findings. The first is spontaneous recovery, in which case coronary blood flow normalizes as LV function normalizes and myocardial oxygen consumption normalizes. However, in the course of a persistent severe residual coronary stenosis that persists after reperfusion there may be delayed recovery. Hence, the stunned myocardium may progress to a phase that is indistinguishable from the hibernating myocardium; that is, reduced coronary blood flow, reduced LV function and reduced oxygen consumption. Thus, stunned myocardium may go through a "hibernation phase." With time the hibernation phase may undergo delayed recovery as coronary blood flow is normalized and the stenosis is relieved.

ing up to 12 min after the last occlusion, whereas systolic function returned quickly to normal. Impairment of systolic function also may occur with repeated episodes of ischemia, as demonstrated by Nixon et al.[27] The stunned myocardium retains the ability to contract under positive inotropic stimulation or post-extrasystolic potentiation (PESP).[22] For example, after successful thrombolysis, ejection fraction (EF) may remain depressed shortly after treatment, but improves substantially 10 to 14 days later. Stack and associates[28] showed improvement in LV EF from $40 \pm 8\%$ to $48 \pm 6\%$ in 16 days after successful lytic therapy; Reduto et al.[29] also demonstrated a similar improvement from $46 \pm 14\%$ to $55 \pm 10\%$ in 10 days. Another characteristic of stunned myocardium is that given time, without other intervention, function will recover.

"Hibernating myocardium" describes persistent chronic LV contractile dysfunction that occurs as a response to decreases in coronary blood flow that is reversible by restoring coronary flow. The myocardium probably downregulates or depresses its mechanical function to match its reduced oxygen supply. Under some conditions, reduced flow may produce severe myocardial dysfunction without evidence of necrosis, which persists for days to weeks after the flow is corrected. Thus, there may be delayed recovery in hibernating myocardium

that resembles stunned myocardium. This new concept of "downregulation" of myocardial function is an attractive contrast to the prevailing view that the myocardium always commits suicide when its blood flow is reduced to a critical level for a long period.[30] Conceptually, hibernating myocardium implies that another equilibrium between myocardial oxygen supply and demand is established at a level that does not result in myocardial necrosis. Also, the usual signs (e.g., ST segment shifts) and symptoms (e.g., angina) of imbalance between myocardial oxygen supply and demand are not present.

Keller et al. have studied the effect of reduced coronary flow on myocardial metabolism in the isolated perfused rat heart using nuclear magnetic resonance (NMR) spectroscopy.[31] Their data indicate that modest coronary flow decreases produce significant reductions in contractile performance and myocardial oxygen consumption before any observable decrease in adenosine triphosphate (ATP) or myocardial pH occurs, and before significant lactate production begins. These balanced reductions in ventricular performance and oxygen consumption without the traditional metabolic markers of ischemia were felt to provide a model for hibernating myocardium. More dramatic reductions in coronary pressure and flow lead to decreases in ATP and pH with lactate production, and the impairment of contractility and the metabolic abnormalities observed returned to control values when coronary flow was restored. These data suggest that the reduction in myocardial contractility seen with low levels of hypoperfusion is not mediated by ADP, pH, or NADH, but may be directly related to reduced tissue oxygen delivery.

Further modifications and understanding of the metabolic bases of myocardial injury due to hypoperfusion has continued with recognition and investigation of the phenomenon of ischemic preconditioning. In contrast to expectations, repeated brief episodes of ischemia appear to offer some protection against ischemic injury. Deutsh and associates studied this phenomenon during PTCA in 12 patients with isolated left anterior descending coronary disease, and demonstrated lessened clinical, electrocardiographic, hemodynamic, and metabolic evidence of myocardial ischemia during a second balloon inflation, as compared to the first episode of ischemia.[32] Lactate extraction ratio fell from -0.11 ± 0.03 on the first inflation to -0.03 ± 0.02 during the second period. Although a variety of metabolic changes have been documented in the laboratory,[33] insights into the potential mechanism of ischemic preconditioning have come only recently, with the studies of Liu and associates, demonstrating that adenosine release may be intimately involved.[34] These laboratory studies involve examining the size of experimental infarctions produced by coronary occlusion with and without ischemic preconditioning and with and without an infusion of adenosine. Normalized myocardial infarct size averaged 39% of the area at risk in control animals, and approximately 8% of the area at risk with preconditioning. A 5-min infusion of adenosine into the isolated/perfused heart was as protective as 5 min of preconditioning, and the protection afforded by preconditioning disappeared when adenosine receptor blocking agents were given before preconditioning. These studies suggest that adenosine released during the preconditioning ischemic state is protective against recurrent episodes of ischemia.

Clinical demonstration that revascularization can restore function to viable ischemic hypocontractile myocardium provides validation of the importance of these new concepts. Topol and his associates evaluated the effect of surgical revascularization on systolic wall thickening using transesophageal echocardiography (TEE) in 20 patients at the time of surgery.[35] They found frequent improvement in regional myocardial function with the most marked improvement in segments showing the most severe preoperative impairment, and concluded that this may have been due to reversal of chronic ischemic dysfunction. Tillisch and associates studied 17 patients undergoing coronary bypass surgery.[36] Abnormal wall motion improved after revascularization in 35 of 41 myocardial segments showing preservation of glucose uptake on positron emission

tomography (PET) scanning. In contrast, 24 of 26 regions without glucose uptake failed to improve.

The benefits of mechanical revascularization are not confined to surgery. Cohen et al. identified 12 patients with severe wall motion abnormalities at rest who were felt to have potentially viable ischemic myocardium on the bases of persistent angina, PESP in the asynergic zone, or thallium-201 uptake in the asynergic zone.[37] After PTCA, global ejection fraction increased from 46 ± 20 to $62 \pm 19\%$ for this group. Carlson and associates also showed an improvement in LV EF from 43 ± 13 to $51 \pm 13\%$ in 22 patients after successful PTCA for unstable angina, again confirming the restoration of contractile function in previously ischemic tissue.[38] In summary, both laboratory and clinical evidence now supports the concept that myocardial ischemia leads to abnormalities of systolic and diastolic function that may be reversed by either surgical revascularization or PTCA. Parameters used in these studies to determine myocardial viability include a history of angina, PESP, thallium uptake, and PET scan evidence of metabolic activity. These approaches will be discussed in greater in the section on diagnostic methods to follow.

Recovery and Healing of Ischemia-Related Injury

We also now realize that the process of healing after myocardial infarction is very complex. Under most circumstances, prolonged periods of ischemia lead to myocyte necrosis and eventual replacement of muscle with fibrous tissue. The initial process involved in the regional shape distortion of the LV is infarct expansion. Infarct expansion describes the increase in ventricular size that occurs as a result of acute stretching, thinning and dilation of the injured myocardial segment. Erlebacher et al. studied 27 patients with acute anterior myocardial infarction with two-dimensional echocardiography, and localized early LV dilation to the infarct zone.[39] In follow-up, six of eight patients with infarct expansion were New York Heart Association Class II or worse, but only one of seven without infarct expansion had limiting symptoms. This documentation of early infarct expansion suggests that the anatomic stage is set for ventricular aneurysm formation within the first days after myocardial infarction. Expansion early after infarction and subsequent rupture are more common in Q-wave infarction than non–Q-wave infarction and in first infarctions compared with reinfarctions.[30] Early infarct expansion clearly has a critical role relative to the development of subsequent heart failure.

In association with infarct expansion, the process of "remodeling" has received considerable recent attention because of its important functional consequences.[40,41] The term "remodeling" implies global shape changes in the LV that occur over time in response to a regional injury. Remodeling of LV geometry begins early after an acute episode of irreversible myocardial injury (e.g., infarction) and continues well beyond the usually recognized convalescent phase. McKay et al. studied 30 patients with a first myocardial infarction acutely and 2 weeks later with direct LV angiography.[40] In patients showing ≥20% increase in LV end-diastolic volume at 2 weeks, the endocardial perimeter of the infarct segment increased 13%, and the noninfarct segments increased 19%. These findings suggest that early dilation is associated with later remodeling of the entire LV, including volume overload hypertrophy of the noninfarcted segments. This process is proportional to infarct size. Jeremy and colleagues studied 50 first myocardial infarction patients with serial radionuclide angiograms extending the follow-up period to 6 months.[41] Eleven patients showed LV dilation within 10 days, and 10 more showed dilation on the 6-month study. Eight of these 21 patients, all of whom had large anterior myocardial infarction, showed progressive dilation with a fall in ejection fraction from 35 ± 6 to $24 \pm 10\%$. Four of the 6 patients who died during follow-up had progressive dilation. Risk factors for progressive dilation included infarct size, early infarct expansion, a persistently occluded infarct related artery, and myocardial dysfunction secondary to ischemia.

In summary, infarct expansion occurs soon after acute myocardial infarction. LV remodeling follows closely, and is a corollary of infarct expansion, in that more dramatic remodeling is associated with more extensive initial infarction. Thus, the two processes are inextricably linked, and closely associated with the subsequent development of clinical heart failure.

The Open Artery Hypothesis

Clinical studies after thrombolytic therapy for myocardial infarction have suggested a significant improvement in long-term survival with restoration of coronary perfusion, even when reperfusion occurs beyond the time when cell death would have been expected to occur.[42] For instance, in patients who achieved reperfusion late after myocardial infarction, LV function did not improve, but mortality was reduced from 36% in patients with partial or no reperfusion to 5% in patients with complete restoration of flow. Similar clinical findings were evident with other thrombolytic agents, and in even later therapy, as reviewed by Braunwald.[42]

In a rat model,[43] with ligation of the left coronary artery, release of the ligature at 30 min resulted in salvage of the effected myocardium. However, no difference in infarct size was demonstrated between the animals with ligature release at 2 hr and those with permanent ligation. Despite similar infarct size, however, infarct expansion was significantly inhibited in the group reperfused at 2 hr, with fewer than 20% showing Gr III–IV expansion as against 60% in the permanent occlusion group.

These clinical and laboratory findings have led to the "open artery hypothesis," as formulated by Braunwald, who stated that "it may be important to achieve a patent infarct-related artery, even beyond the time period when that patency may be expected to salvage myocardium."[42] Clearly a significant benefit from the continued patency would be a reduction in infarct expansion or myocardial remodeling, effected by restoration of blood flow.

Vicious Cycles Associated with Ischemia and Heart Failure

Heart failure patients have a propensity for deterioration in a gradually worsening cycle. Impairment of systolic and diastolic function further compromises subendocardial perfusion as elevation of LV diastolic pressure diminishes the diastolic transcoronary pressure gradient for perfusion[44] (Fig. 12.5). When abnormal resistance to diastolic flow is imposed by epicardial coronary disease, this impairment of diastolic perfusion becomes even more important. The loss of diastolic perfusion time associated with tachycardia further compromises myocardial perfusion.[44,45,46,47] Atrial pacing in patients with coronary disease and normal LV function at rest can induce wall motion abnormalities and lactate production.[47] Ferro and associates have shown the importance of diastolic perfusion time as an index of myocardial oxygen supply in exercise stress and atrial pacing studies of the variability of ischemic threshold in patients with coronary artery disease as well as "Syndrome X."[48] Testing upright and supine, with and without therapy and pacing stress, diastolic perfusion time and ischemic threshold remained relatively constant. These observations, along with extensive laboratory studies reviewed by Crawford, suggest that heart rate–related limitation of subendocardial blood flow may be an important mechanism in the pathogenesis of exercise-induced ischemia.[49] The poorly perfused and poorly functioning ventricle under stress tends to enter into a negative feedback loop, exacerbating ischemia-related dysfunction (Fig. 12.6).

Acquisition of Clinical Data

In managing heart failure associated with coronary artery disease, clinical decisions are influenced by the following: (a) the amount of ischemic myocardium in relation to the function of the remaining nonischemic myocardium, (b) the potential reversibility of LV dys-

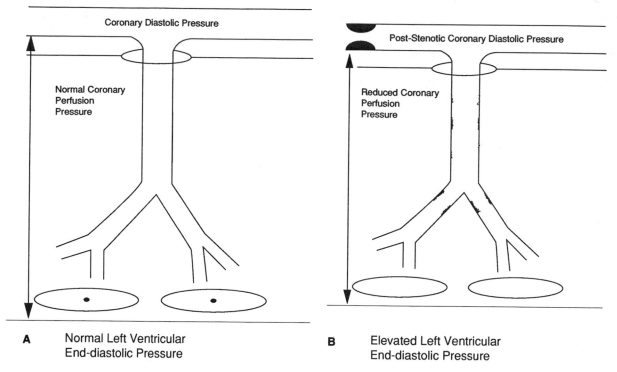

A   Normal Left Ventricular
        End-diastolic Pressure

B   Elevated Left Ventricular
        End-diastolic Pressure

FIGURE 12.5. Reduction in myocardial perfusion due to coronary stenosis and elevated LV diastolic pressure.

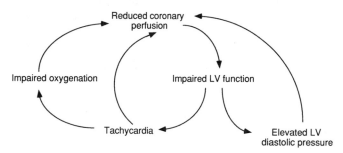

FIGURE 12.6. Negative feedback cycles in coronary disease with LV dysfunction.

function, and (c) whether the ischemic process is due to obstruction in the major epicardial conduit vessels or due to impairment of microvascular flow reserve without major vessel obstruction.[44]

Some of the multiple syndromes of heart failure seen with coronary artery disease are outlined in Table 12.1. Clinicians must be particularly alert to the combination of relatively well maintained chamber size with manifestations of congestion as a clue to potentially reversible ischemic states.[50,51]

Clinical Assessment

The potential for rapid deterioration in the patient with heart failure due to coronary artery disease justifies a thorough search for evidence of potentially reversible myocardial hypoperfusion. A meticulous history and physical examination remains the cornerstone of clinical assessment. The protean nature of anginal symptoms has been emphasized for the past 200 years. Nonetheless, the presence of an anginal equivalent (e.g., exercise intolerance due to dyspnea with reproducible symptoms of brief duration) remains an important clue to the possibility of reversible ischemia. Such a history may be the only definitive clue to potentially salvageable functional myocardium. The converse also is true. The absence of angina does not exclude asymptomatic "silent ischemia" as a cause of transiently worsening of LV dysfunction. Lack of a documented episode of myocardial infarction may be an important clue to potentially reversible systolic dysfunction, with "stunned" or "hibernating" myocardium. Diabetics, hypertensives, and the elderly have a high frequency of both asymptomatic ischemia and silent or unrecognized myocardial infarction.[52] In diabetic patients with coronary disease, the time from onset of 0.1 mV of ST segment depression to onset of angina during treadmill exercise testing is prolonged.[53] This impairment of angina perception led to an average increase of 86 s in onset of 0.1 mV ST segment depression to onset of angina in diabetic patients studied by Ranjadayalan and associates. These investigators suggested that repetitive asymptomatic ischemic episodes in these patients might predispose them to more frequent episodes of heart failure. A detailed history also may provide clues to important arrhythmias, neural factors altering cardiac perfusion, or other systemic diseases important to myocardial function (e.g., thyroid disease, anemia, etc.).

The physical examination should focus on bedside assessment of right heart filling pressure and LV function.[5,54,55] One can estimate the central venous pressure from examining of the right jugular vein as well as observing the V-wave systolic pulsations of tricuspid insufficiency. Careful precordial palpation, searching both supine and in the left lateral decubitus position for the sustained apical impulse of ventricular aneurysm, is important. Documentation of the presence or absence of diastolic filling sounds, increased intensity of the pulmonic second sound, and systolic murmurs of mitral and/or tricuspid insufficiency also are important in the patient with heart failure due to coronary artery disease. The examiner should search for clues to other associated cardiac diseases, such as aortic valve stenosis, which may be difficult to appreciate in low flow states. It is also important to look for systemic diseases such as hypertension, chronic obstructive pulmonary disease, thyrotoxicosis, anemia, etc. that may substantially alter myocardial oxygen supply/demand relationships.

Often overlooked, the standard resting 12-lead electrocardiogram (ECG) provides a number of useful diagnostic clues about heart failure in patients with known or suspected coronary artery disease. The rate and rhythm are most important, as uncontrolled tachycardia or atrial fibrillation may contribute to potentially reversible ischemic systolic dysfunction by raising myocardial oxygen requirements or decreasing diastolic perfusion time. The patterns of Q-wave myocardial infarction suggest specific problems, which are outlined in Table 12.2. In the absence of Q waves, the overall R-wave amplitude roughly reflects the amount of remaining viable myocardial tissue. Well maintained R-wave amplitudes and poor systolic function in the setting of coronary disease may suggest "myocardial stunning." On the other hand, Q waves with persistent ST segment elevations are highly specific for significant focal wall motion disorders (e.g., "ventricular aneurysm").[56]

TABLE 12.2. Specific heart failure syndromes with Q-wave infarction.

Q-waves	Syndromes
Leads II, III, AVF	Right ventricular infarction with high venous pressure low output
	Acute mitral regurgitation due to posterior papillary muscle ischemia
Leads V1-2-3	Cardiogenic shock due to extensive infarction
	Ventricular aneurysm
	Septal rupture

The standard anteroposterior (AP) x-ray film of the chest gives confirmatory estimates of heart size and pulmonary vascular congestion. A normal overall cardiac size without evidence of pulmonary vascular congestion suggests transient potentially reversible hypoperfusion with diastolic dysfunction perhaps precipitating heart failure.[57]

Noninvasive Laboratory Assessment

Echocardiography

Two-dimensional echocardiography and Doppler examination now play a central role in the evaluation of heart failure due to coronary artery disease. A quantitative echo examination is appropriate for all patients with suspected heart failure.[57] In the patient with coronary artery disease, the echo examination is particularly useful to help exclude important valvular disease, which may be inaudible in low-flow states, and to evaluate the functional state of the LV. The echocardiogram provides useful information concerning LV wall thickness, chamber sizes, global function, and aneurysm formation as well as mural thrombus. Focal wall motion disorders are generally evident with views obtained in multiple planes. An overall assessment of the functional state of the LV usually is possible in most patients. But it is important to emphasize that a technically limited echocardiographic examination, due to lung disease, pleural effusions, etc., should not be used for these assessments. In these cases, radionuclide angiography offers an alternative noninvasive method to evaluate ventricular function. Finally, evaluation of the blood flow filling patterns by Doppler echo or radionuclide angiography at rest and after exercise may provide objective data to support a diagnosis of diastolic dysfunction, particularly where diastolic dysfunction is increased by reversible ischemia.[58,59]

Stress Testing

In our clinical practice, we have found that many physicians underuse exercise tolerance testing in the assessment of known or suspected coronary artery disease with heart failure. Most of the difficulty arises from failure to separate diagnostic exercise testing from exercise testing for functional assessment. The diagnostic exercise test must be approached with a clearly stated clinical diagnosis and an objective assessment of the likelihood of that clinical diagnosis. The heart failure patient presents some unique problems relative to diagnostic exercise testing. The QRS-T pattern often is distorted at baseline and QRS prolongation and ST segment depression are not uncommon. Digitalis and diuretics often compound this distortion, so the baseline ECG often is limited for assessment of ischemia. The

With pharmacologic stress:

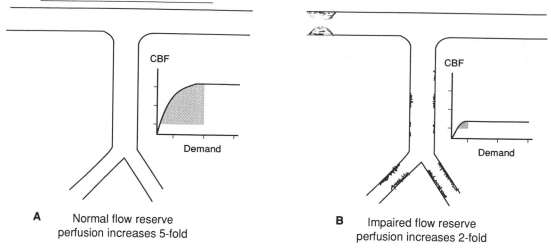

A Normal flow reserve
perfusion increases 5-fold

B Impaired flow reserve
perfusion increases 2-fold

with stress (increased demand)
A-counts = 2.5 X B-counts

At rest, flow is normal <u>after</u> redistribution
A-counts = B-counts

(CBF=coronary blood flow)

FIGURE 12.7. Pharmacologic stress and radionuclide imaging in coronary artery disease.

functional limits of heart failure result in marked reduction of exercise time and level attained by these patients.

By keeping these problems in mind, and understanding the interaction of pretest likelihood with the sensitivity and specificity of the test, the clinician can analyze the results of diagnostic exercise testing using standard Bayesian techniques to derive a posttest likelihood of coronary disease.[60,61]

Exercise Stress or Pharmacological Stress Combined with Myocardial Perfusion Imaging

In patients with heart failure due to known coronary artery disease, the potential benefits of mechanical revascularization require an attempt to demonstrate reversible versus irreversible ischemia in the distribution of each of the coronary lesions. Radioisotope imaging ([201]thallium or newer [99]technetium-labeled isonitriles) using exercise stress or pharmacologic stress offers the theoretical advantage of detecting ischemia and localizing the specific anatomic region of transient hypoperfusion as well as scar.[62,63] Unfortunately, this potential advantage often is confounded by technical limitations of the isotope tests. [201]Thallium is particularly limited as a perfusion agent in the presence of myocardial scarring, hypoperfusion of areas in the posterior septum, attenuation of emitted photons by overlying tissue (e.g., particularly breast shadows), and the somewhat subjective nature of most interpretations. Also, its long bio-

logical half-life limits the dose that can be used and an adequate time for redistribution must be permitted, prolonging the evaluation to 24 hr. Thallium imaging may be useful when attempting to understand the physiologic significance of lesions that appear angiographically to be of "borderline" significance. The "routine" use of thallium studies in the assessment of coronary disease is neither intellectually sound nor clinically useful and cannot be justified economically.

The use of either exercise or pharmacologic stressors (i.e., dipyridamole or adenosine) to enhance the detection of focal hypoperfusion is based on a set of physiologic assumptions outlined in Figure 12.7. Lesions in the major epicardial conductance vessels may not compromise resting blood flow, but may substantially impair coronary flow reserve. By maximally dilating the resistance vessels, regional inequalities in coronary reserve will become manifest as focal areas of hypoperfusion. Since this represents a nonphysiologic stress, one should search both for validation of the physiologic concepts and for some correlation of findings with other objective clinical events. The demonstration that dipyridamole-thallium scan abnormalities correlate with postoperative ischemic events in vascular surgery,[64] for instance, suggest that these studies may be valuable in selecting patients with silent myocardial ischemia for further evaluation. The absence of [201]thallium uptake in a myocardial region both at rest (redistribution) and during stress was thought to be good evidence that scar is present, but recent reports suggest that some non-redistribution [201]thallium defects may be viable myocardial regions.[30]

Stress Testing with Imaging of Myocardial Functional Imaging

When anatomic coronary disease has been demonstrated angiographically, with normal resting wall motion in the myocardium supplied by that vessel, demonstration of the physiologic significance of the lesion assumes considerable importance in the decision for revascularization. In this setting, the demonstration of reversible impairment of wall motion with exercise stress indicates that mechanical revascularization may well improve overall LV function. Both radionuclide ventriculography with exercise and two-dimensional echocardiography combined with exercise may demonstrate reversible wall motion disorders. With patients in whom technically satisfactory echo examinations are possible, the addition of echo examination may be extremely useful.[65]

In general, perfusion imaging techniques or demonstration of persistent metabolic activity will be required when assessing the potential effects of revascularization on myocardium that is hypokinetic under resting conditions. In contrast, imaging of mechanical function with stress provides useful data in assessing the functional significance of a coronary lesion supplying tissue that moves normally under resting conditions but may contribute to stress related heart failure.

Exercise Testing for Functional Evaluation

As a management tool, when the diagnosis of coronary artery disease has been angiographically confirmed, the exercise test is invaluable in the functional assessment of the patient. The information generated includes overall exercise capacity, and an evaluation of heart rate–blood pressure product required to evoke ischemia.[5,61,66,67] Furthermore, with the addition of relatively straightforward on-line measurements of O_2 consumption, the functional assessment during exercise can be expanded to include determination of maximum oxygen consumption. A substantial body of data, comprehensively reviewed by Jennings and Esler,[66] indicates that functional capacity in patients with heart failure does not correlate with resting hemodynamics or LVEF. For example, several studies have shown no correlation between overall functional capacity and pulmonary capillary wedge pressures at rest or during exercise.[67,68] As many as one fifth of patients with impaired systolic function do not show clinical heart failure,[69] and in many series as many as half the patients with clinical heart failure do not show impaired systolic function. Thus, the choice and assessment of interventions in heart failure due to coronary artery disease requires an initial assessment of functional

TABLE 12.3. Exercise tolerance testing in heart failure due to coronary artery disease.

Diagnostic testing	Management tool
Poor exercise tolerance limits usefullness Digitalis, diuretics both decrease sensitivity, specificity of ECG changes	Provides quantification of physical capacity (oxygen uptake) May help clarify role of inadequate flow reserve in pathogenesis of symptoms Quantitates pharmacologic control of heart rate and blood pressure during exercise May reassure patient about safety of moderate exercise Provides guidelines for exercise prescription

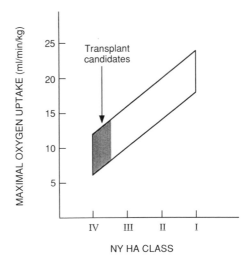

FIGURE 12.8. Comparison of assessment of heart failure using the New York Heart Association (*NYHA*) classification vs. functional assessment with maximal oxygen uptake.

capacity. Table 12.3 compares and contrasts standard exercise tolerance testing as a diagnostic procedure and as a management tool. Figure 12.8 compares the clinical versus functional approaches to the assessment of heart failure, using maximal oxygen uptake. We agree with Stevenson and Miller that functional assessment with determination of maximal oxygen uptake is mandatory for all but the most critically ill cardiac transplant candidates.[70]

Ambulatory Monitoring

Silent myocardial ischemia, particularly as a factor contributing to heart failure in the patient with coronary artery disease, remains a difficult and somewhat controversial problem. The primary clinical clue remains the association of relatively normal heart size and

TABLE 12.4. Ischemia detected by ambulatory monitoring and risk of untoward events: patients with stable angina or stable coronary artery disease.

Author	n	Follow-up duration (months)	% with detectable ischemia	Risk ratio Adverse outcome~	Death
Deedwania, 1990	107	23	44	2.7	2.9
Tzivoni, 1989	56	24	77	3.6	1.8
Aronow, 1988[a]	185	26	34	—	2.0
v. Arnim, 1988[b]	235	54	26	1.3	3.4
Rocco, 1988	86	12.5	57	13.6	>1.5[*c]
Dewood, 1986	59	36	44	4.9	3.7
Stern & Tzivoni, 1974	80	6–12	46	9.3	—
Totals (range)	563	(6–36)	(30–77)	(1.3–13.6)	(>1.5–3.7)

[a] Included elderly patients with angina or old myocardial infarction
[b] Included patients with coronary artery disease >75% stenosis
[c] Estimated by assuming that 1 death occurred in those without detectable ambulant ischemia
n = Number of patients; ~ = Adverse outcome included death and nonfatal myocardial infarction.
Adapted from Pepine CJ. *Circulation*. 1990;82:II-135-14

TABLE 12.5. Ischemia detected by ambulatory monitoring and risk of untoward events: patients with unstable angina.

Author	n	Follow-up duration (months)	% with detectable ischemia	Risk ratio Adverse outcome~	Death
Langer, 1989	135	In-hospital	66	2.5	3.7
Pozzati, 1988	88	12	55	2.1	2.7
v. Arnim, 1988	38	1	42	2.0	3.4
Nademanne, 1987	49	6	59	13.8	3.4
Gottlieb, 1987	70	24	53	3.2	9.0
Johnson, 1982	72	3	17	3.4	2.7
Totals (range)	492	(In-hospital to 24 months)	(17–66)	(2.0–13.8)	(2.7–9.0)

n = Number of patients; ~ = Adverse outcome included death and nonfatal myocardial infarction.
Adapted from Pepine CJ. *Circulation*. 1990;82:II-135-14

relatively normal systolic function with intermittent episodes of clinical heart failure. Ambulatory electrocardiographic monitoring offers potential insights into the timing and mechanisms responsible for silent or asymptomatic myocardial ischemia (e.g., tachycardia, etc.) and associated with evocative events (e.g., mental stress, environment, etc.). In addition, this technique has the potential for objectively documenting ischemic episodes for consideration of mechanical revascularization.[71] Forty-eight hours of ambulatory monitoring generally is recommended for patients in whom ischemia needs to be documented or clarified as day-to-day variability in the occurrence of ischemic episodes may be substantial. Individuals with stable or unstable ischemic syndromes manifesting intermittent ischemic-type ST segment depression on ambulatory ECG monitoring are at higher risk for subsequent cardiac events than individuals with similar coronary angiographic and exercise test findings who do not have ischemic-type ST depression (Tables 12.4, 12.5).[72] Unfortunately, only a small percentage of heart failure patients have baseline ST segment morphology that permits analysis for transient ischemia. However, patients with silent ischemia detected by exercise ECG abnormalities or thallium perfusion defects also are at high risk, and these procedures may be more suited for the patient with heart failure.[73,74]

PET Scanning

Ultimately, the issue of potentially reversible ischemic dysfunction must be addressed. Is there any objective evidence of potentially viable tissue that is inadequately perfused either at rest or with exercise? The objective of clinical assessment remains the demonstration of metabolic activity in myocardium known to be perfused by an obstructed vessel. This demonstration, along with the ability to construct a coronary flow reserve map of the myocardium, would provide invaluable information in planning therapeutic strategies. This is, in fact, the promise of PET technology.[36] PET scanning may become the ideal imaging modality for noninvasive assessment of coronary blood flow as well as viable myocardium. The potential for PET scanning, at present, unfortunately is limited by the need for an on-site cyclotron for generation of the imaging radiopharmaceuticals. However, as these technical challenges are met, imaging with PET scanning will allow comprehensive noninvasive assessment of LV metabolic function and perfusion.

Catheterization Laboratory Assessment

General Considerations in Cardiac Catheterization

Widespread use of technically simple methods of coronary angiography and revascularization procedures has caused many catheterization laboratories to limit their activities to relatively routine photographic procedures. However, in patients with severe congestive symptoms, a number of important considerations arise. The ability of the patient to tolerate radiographic contrast material and its attendant volume shifts must be considered.[75,76] Taliercio and associates showed that contrast nephropathy was independently associated with Class IV heart failure with low cardiac output. In that subgroup, 71% experienced contrast nephropathy defined as a ≥ 1 mg/dl rise in serum creatine after cardiac angiography.[75] As shown by Parfrey et al., patients with diabetes and preexisting renal insufficiency also are at risk of clinically important nephrotoxicity.[76] Patients with advanced, poorly compensated heart failure, diabetes, or renal insufficiency may benefit from a brief admission before catheterization in order to optimize their fluid status and renal function, including slight volume expansion and initiation of an active diuresis.[77]

The catheter study must not only carefully and accurately display coronary anatomy but also document its consequences in terms of ventricular function and mitral valve integrity. The cardiac catheterization study of heart failure patients must be carefully planned and the catheterization team should clinically evaluate each patient before his/her study.

Hemodynamic Issues in Heart Failure

Furthermore, the invasive cardiologist must be aware of the limitations of various techniques in assessing heart failure. For example, cardiac output determination by indicator dilution may be fraught with error and the assumptions made in equating pulmonary artery occlusion pressure, as recorded from the Swan-Ganz balloon flotation catheter, with true left atrial pressure may be invalid. Every attempt must be made to insure that hemodynamic measurements are accurate, reproducible, and truly representative of the heart failure patient's "best possible" hemodynamic state. Assessment of any transvalvular pressure gradients should be made with the realization that, in low output states, even relatively small gradients may reflect important valvular obstruction. If any question about the cardiac output determination arises, a carefully measured oxygen consumption should be done rather than relying only on indicator dilution techniques. Both techniques should be in agreement that a low output state is present. The specific areas of concern in catheterization assessment are dealt with in more detail below.

In patients with heart failure, a right and left heart catheterization, with accurate determination of cardiac output, is required to evaluate the feasibility of any type of surgical intervention. This includes biplane LV cineangiography, preferably before and after treatment with nitroglycerin,[78] and an inotropic agent if needed to provide maximum relief of ischemia-related dysfunction.[23,24] In addition, a sufficient amount of baseline information should be collected to evaluate the patient as a potential orthotopic heart transplant candidate. This requires left and right heart pressures to exclude definitely ventricular inflow or outflow obstruction. This may be done from a careful pullback tracing as the LV catheter is withdrawn to the aorta, provided that the patient is in a regular rhythm. When the latter is not present, simultaneous LV and ascending aortic pressure recordings, using equisensitive transducers, are required. Simultaneous recording of LV and pulmonary capillary wedge pressures also is needed. Blood samples for oxygen saturation from the pulmonary artery and systemic circulation should be obtained. A normal or high pulmonary arterial saturation in a patient with clinical heart failure may be a clue to unsuspected shunting or a high output heart failure state. A normal pulmonary artery (PA) oxygen saturation and cardiac output may suggest that transient ischemia is responsible for intermittent heart failure symptoms. A diminished arterial oxygen saturation may indicate that pulmonary problems have exacerbated myocardial dysfunction. Whenever the systemic arterial oxygen saturation is low, arterial blood gases should be sent for complete analysis with the patient breathing room air and repeated after several minutes of breathing with an FIO_2 of 100%.

Angiographic Considerations in Heart Failure

Biplane cine left ventriculography with a low osmolality, nonionic contrast agent is indicated. Regional wall motion disorders may be overlooked and cannot be evaluated completely with only single-plane ventriculography in the patient with coronary artery disease. Significant coronary lesions, in the distal right or circumflex artery distributions, require assessment of septal and lateral wall function. The left anterior oblique ventriculogram also will display the septum and angiographically demonstrate any left to right shunt through an acquired ventricular septal defect. In addition, the degree of mitral regurgitation often is better assessed angiographically with a slightly cranially angled left anterior oblique projection. This is because the left atrium, in this projection, does not overlie either the descending aorta or the thoracic spine. In this projection, the degree of opacification of the atrium is not obscured by the appearance of contrast in the descending aorta after two to three systoles. A high quality coronary angiographic examination also is mandatory. "Test" injections, of contrast agent, should be kept to a minimum and this is preferable to limiting the number of angiographic views filmed. Using 8 to 10 cc of contrast agent per injection, a satisfactory and complete examination of the left coronary can be obtained with five injections using single-plane technique. These include views with cranial and caudal angulations in the right anterior and left anterior oblique projections, and a lateral view. With two additional injections of the right coronary, the total amount of contrast used for the coronary artery examination should not exceed 100 ml. When contrast volume must be kept to the absolute minimum, use of biplane technique for both the LV angiography and coronary angiography will require a total volume of only 70 to 80 cc.

If the initial coronary artery injection reveals coronary artery disease, we recommend that the remainder of the examination be performed after administration of intracoronary nitroglycerin to dilate maximally the major epicardial vessels.[79]

Summary

The complete catheterization protocol must provide definitive answers for the following questions:

Do the coronary arteries, visualized by the angiogram, account for the arterial circulation to the entire heart? In other words, could there be a "flush" occluded vessel or an aberrant coronary artery?

Is the systolic LV dysfunction observed reversible or irreversible? Ventriculography and hemodynamic recordings after nitroglycerin and/or catecholamine treatment may be indicated to reverse ischemia-related dysfunction.

How much functioning myocardium is at risk from the coronary artery lesions that have been identified?

If the pulmonary vascular resistance is elevated to ≥ 5 Wood units, is this pulmonary hypertension reversible? The response to acute administration of a

vasodilator and an inotropic agent may restore the pulmonary resistance to the acceptable range. If a desirable response is not found, a Swan-Ganz catheter may be left in place for longer term monitoring during a continued infusion of catecholamine and/or vasodilators.

Information Management and Clinical Decision Making

After a complete diagnostic assessment of the patient with coronary artery disease and heart failure, one must structure the information obtained. A practical approach is outlined in Figure 12.9. The first step is to determine whether or not the coronary anatomy is suitable for mechanical revascularization. If so, is revascularization indicated on the basis of life-threatening anatomy, such as high grade left main coronary artery stenosis, or on the basis of objective evidence of reversible ischemia in the distribution of the lesions identified? Specific situations in which surgical revascularization has been shown to prolong survival also should be considered; for instance, the demonstration of significant coronary disease and impaired LV function in the patient who has experienced unstable angina.[80] In this setting, Luchi and his colleagues[80] in the Veterans Administration Cooperative Study group demonstrated that, in patients with progressive or unstable angina, LVEF was "strongly related" to mortality at 2 yr in medically treated patients. Patients with LVEF between 0.30 (the lower limit for acceptance into this study) and 0.59 enjoyed significantly improved survival with surgery.

After evaluating the coronary anatomy, one consid-

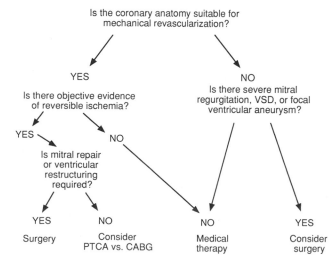

FIGURE 12.9. A practical approach to the management of heart failure due to coronary artery disease.

ers surgically correctable structural abnormalities of the LV, including severe mitral regurgitation, postinfarction ventricular septal defect, or ventricular aneurysm. In each of these pathologic conditions, the potential benefit from surgical intervention is related to the adequacy of residual LV function. Having dealt with the coronary arteries, attention should then focus on structural abnormalities of the LV that might be surgically corrected, including severe mitral regurgitation, postinfarction, ventricular septal defect, or ventricular aneurysm. In each of these pathologic conditions, the potential benefit from surgical intervention is related to the adequacy of residual LV function. If congestive heart failure is primarily related to the mechanical lesion, then repair, in general, will be associated with a favorable outcome. If, however, the mechanical lesion is merely a superimposed stress on an already badly scarred ventricle with markedly impaired EF, the risk of surgery rises dramatically and the benefit decreases.

The assessment of potential candidates for ventricular aneurysmectomy is difficult. Several studies show no long-term benefit from ventricular aneurysmectomy unless revascularization also is performed.[81–83] Faxon and associates reported The Coronary Artery Surgery Study (CASS) evaluation of the effect of surgery on the natural history of LV aneurysm.[81] The study included 1131 patients with angiographically documented aneurysm. Six hundred sixty-four patients comprised the medical group and 467 the surgical group, of whom 238 underwent LV resection, most with associated revascularization, and 229 had revascularization without resection. Survival rates for the medical and surgical patients with single- or double-vessel disease were similar. Despite an overall operative mortality of 7.9%, surgery was associated with significant improvement in 6-yr survival in patients with triple-vessel disease, 62% versus 47%. Improvement in survival with surgery was restricted to high-risk categories. LV resection did not appear to influence survival or overall symptoms of heart failure; however, some improvement was noted within the surgical group in patients who had LV resection as compared to revascularization alone.

Akins reported a series of 100 consecutive patients undergoing surgical aneurysmectomy.[82] In 93 patients who had anterior aneurysm, the overall survival rate at 38.5 months was 91.2% with associated bypass grafting versus 72% without associated revascularization.

In a series of 109 patients with heart failure due to postinfarction LV aneurysm, Louagie et al. found no difference in 5-yr survival between 49 patients undergoing surgical aneurysmectomy and 60 treated medically.[83] The surgical patients, however, had generally improved quality of life and functional class. The authors emphasized their conclusion that overall survival related to residual LV function, and their impression

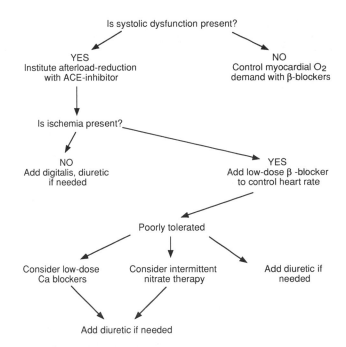

FIGURE 12.10. Algorithm for the medical management of heart failure due to coronary artery disease.

that left anterior descending revascularization and relief of ischemia was critical to improvement. They carefully evaluated residual segment contractile scores, using a computerized method of left ventriculographic analysis to exclude the noncontractile segment. The most important question for the cardiologist to attempt to answer is, "if the evident ventricular aneurysm is surgically removed, will the remaining LV myocardium be adequate to fill appropriately and generate a sufficient contraction to maintain stroke volume and cardiac output?" In the Montreal Heart series, described above, the best predictor of survival was contractile segment EF, with a "cutoff point" of 41%.[83] In this series right ventricular failure and cardiogenic shock also predicted poor outcome.

In the cyclosporin era, with 85% first-year survival after orthotopic cardiac transplantation, transplantation may offer a realistic alternative for many patients with irretrievably scarred ventricles and mechanical lesions.

If medical management is proposed for the patient with heart failure due to coronary artery disease, in addition to the algorithm shown in Figure 12.10, the physician must consider factors that may exacerbate the myocardial supply/demand mismatch associated with coronary disease. Patients with advanced LV dysfunction may show considerable physiologic reactions to psychological stress.[84,85] Other issues of importance include the possible exacerbating factors of weight, chronic pulmonary disease with hypoxemia, chronic renal insufficiency with inability to handle salt and water loads, endocrine disease particularly hypo- or hyperthyroidism, and the presence of significant hematologic disease, either anemia or polycythemia with thrombocytosis.

After carefully considering any possible noncardiac exacerbating factors, reversible disorders of cardiac rhythm, coronary vasomotion, or silent ischemia should be treated. Restoration of normal sinus rhythm, if possible, generally will be associated with improved hemodynamic function and better control of heart rate. The possibility of intermittent coronary obstruction due to platelet aggregation should be dealt with prophylactically by the administration of antiplatelet agents (e.g., aspirin). The possible benefits of a controlled exercise program should be considered. There is a sizeable body of evidence suggesting that cardiac rehabilitation is appropriate for coronary artery disease patients with moderately advanced heart failure.[86-88] Sullivan et al. have demonstrated that exercise training increases peak oxygen consumption and reduces blood lactate levels during submaximal exercise, without changes in cardiac output.[86,87] Coats and associates used a physician-blinded crossover trial to assess the effects of physical training in severe chronic heart failure, and demonstrated a beneficial effect of home exercise by increasing exercise tolerance, peak oxygen consumption, and symptoms.[88] Exercise time was prolonged by 18% to 20% with bicycle training, with no adverse experiences in the home setting. The training was associated with significant improvement in fatigue, breathlessness, and general well-being on a standardized questionnaire. The improvement in overall efficiency from a physical conditioning program may be sufficient to allow patients with moderately advanced LV dysfunction to return to satisfactory levels of activity.

In integrating the clinical, noninvasive, and catheterization data into an overall medical treatment plan tailored to the unique pathophysiology of heart failure that each patient with coronary artery disease manifests, several questions should be asked. Is diastolic ventricular dysfunction secondary to coronary flow reserve inadequacy that may be managed by control of heart rate (β-blockers, rate-controlling calcium antagonists), blood pressure, and LV end-diastolic pressure (nitrates, diuretics)? Or, is the problem systolic ventricular dysfunction secondary to scarring, where control of preload (diuretics, nitrates) and afterload (angiotensin-converting enzyme inhibitors, hydralazine) are of greater importance?

Repeat exercise tolerance testing after institution of a medical management program may give the clinician considerable insight into the adequacy of control of heart rate and blood pressure. Furthermore, repeat exercise testing may demonstrate persistent ischemia despite good medical therapy and thereby provide evidence favoring mechanical revascularization.

Summary

Multiple syndromes of heart failure may be seen in patients with coronary artery disease, reflecting the variety of coronary flow disturbances and myocardial responses to ischemia. The evaluation and treatment of heart failure on the basis of coronary disease requires clinical integration of data from many sources into a pathophysiologic conceptual framework.

In light of convincing evidence that both repeated episodes of ischemia and chronic hypoperfusion can produce prolonged systolic and diastolic dysfunction, and the poor prognosis of heart failure due to coronary artery disease, consideration of mechanical revascularization is critical in the management of congestive heart failure due to coronary artery disease. The clinician must aggressively seek evidence of myocardial viability with noninvasive or invasive studies and in uncertain situations must consider assessing the contractile response to revascularization with PTCA as a "therapeutic trial."

Structural defects resulting from ischemic injury, ventricular septal defect, ventricular aneurysm, or severe mitral regurgitation should be repaired if LV function is adequate and if the clinician is assured that the mechanical problem, not extensive irreversible scarring, is responsible for hemodynamic embarrassment.

In constructing a medical management program, the clinician must remember the variety of factors that follow a final common path to produce increased myocardial oxygen needs, ischemic increases in LV end-diastolic pressure, and overt clinical congestive heart failure. The clinical cardiologist must attempt, in the management of each individual patient, to decide where, when, and why heart failure occurs. Only in this framework can rational therapeutic steps be taken to control symptoms, prevent recurrences, and perhaps even prolong life.

References

1. Smith WM. Epidemiology of congestive heart failure. *Am J Cardiol.* 1985;55:3A–8A.

2. Bigger JT. Why patients with congestive heart failure die: arrhythmias and sudden cardiac death. *Circulation.* 1987;75:IV28–IV35.

3. Parmley WW. Pathophysiology and current therapy of congestive heart failure. *J Am Coll Cardiol.* 1989;13:771–785.

4. Franciosa JA, Wilen M, Ziesch S, Cohn JN. Survival in men with severe chronic left ventricular failure due to either coronary heart disease or idiopathic dilated cardiomyopathy. *Am J Cardiol.* 1983;51:831–836.

5. Likoff MJ, Chandler SL, Kay HR. Clinical determinants of mortality in chronic congestive heart failure secondary to idiopathic dilated or ischemic cardiomyopathy. *Am J Cardiol.* 1987;59:634–638.

6. Cohn JN, Archibald DG, Ziesche S, et al. Effect of vasodilator therapy on mortality in chronic congestive heart failure, results of Veterans Administration Cooperative Study. *N Engl J Med.* 1986;314:1547–1552.
7. Packer M. Sudden unexpected death in patients with congestive heart failure: a second frontier. *Circulation.* 1985;72:681–685.
8. Jaeschke R, Ruyatt GH. Medical therapy for chronic congestive heart failure. (editorial) *Ann Intern Med.* 1989;110:758–760.
9. The SOLVD Investigators. Effect of enalapril on survival in patients with reduced left ventricular ejection fractions and congestive heart failure. *N Engl J Med.* 1991; 325:293–302.
10. Winniford MD, Rossen JD, Marcus MC. Clinical importance of coronary flow reserve measurements in humans. *Modern Concepts Cardiovasc Dis.* 1989;58:25–35.
11. Gould KL, Lipscomb K, Hamilton GW. Physiologic bases for assessing critical coronary stenosis. *Am J Cardiol.* 1974;33:87–94.
12. Gould KL, Lipscomb K. Effects of coronary stenoses on coronary flow reserve and resistance. *Am J Cardiol.* 1974;34:48–55.
13. Wilson RF, Laughlin DE, Ackell PH, et al. Transluminal, subselective measurement of coronary artery blood flow velocity and vasodilator reserve in man. *Circulation.* 1985;72:82–92.
14. Wilson RF, White CW. Intracoronary papaverine: an ideal coronary vasodilator for studies of the coronary circulation in conscious humans. *Circulation.* 1986;73:444–451.
15. Jennings RB, Murry CE, Steenbergen C, Reimer KA. Development of cell injury in sustained acute ischemia. *Circulation.* 1990;82(suppl II):II.2–II.12.
16. Strasser RH, Marquetant R, Kubler W. Adrenergic receptors and sensitation of adenylyl cyclase in acute myocardial ischemia. *Circulation.* 1990;82(suppl II):II.23–II.37.
17. Bonow RO, Vitale DF, Bacharach SL, Frederick TM, Kent M, Green MV. A synchronous left ventricular regional function and impaired global diastolic filling in patients with coronary artery disease: reversal after coronary angioplasty. *Circulation.* 1985;71:297–307.
18. Piscione F, Hugenholtz RG, Serruys PW. Impaired left ventricular filling dynamics during percutaneous transluminal coronary angioplasty for coronary artery disease. *Am J Cardiol.* 1987;59:29–37.
19. Zile MR. Diastolic dysfunction: detection, consequences, and treatment. *Modern Concepts of Cardiovasc Dis.* 1989;58:67–72.
20. Braunwald E, Kloner RA. The stunned myocardium: prolonged, postischemic ventricular dysfunction. *Circulation.* 1982;66:1146–1149.
21. Zhao M, Zang H, Robinson TF, Factor SM, Sonnenblick EH, Eng C. Profound structural alterations of the extracellular collagen matrix in postischemic dysfunctional ("stunned") but viable myocardium. *J Am Coll Cardiol.* 1987;10:1322–1334.
22. Patel B, Kloner RA, Przyklenk K, Braunwald E. Postischemic myocardial "stunning." A clinically relevant phenomenon. *Ann Intern Med.* 1988;108:626–628.
23. Rahimtoola SH. The hibernating myocardium. *Am Heart J.* 1989;117:211–221.
24. Kloner RA, Przyklenk K, Patel B. Altered myocardial states: the stunned and hibernating myocardium. *Am J Med.* 1989;86(suppl 1A):14–22.
25. Bolli R. Mechanism of myocardial stunning. *Circulation.* 1990;82:723–738.
26. Wijns W, Serruys PW, Slager CJ, et al. Effect of coronary occlusion during percutaneous transluminal angioplasty in humans on left ventricular chamber stiffness and regional diastolic pressure-radius relations. *J Am Coll Cardiol.* 1986;7:455–463.
27. Nixon JV, Brown CN, Smitherman TC. Identification of transient and persistent segmental wall motion abnormalities in patients with unstable angina by two-dimensional echocardiography. *Circulation.* 1982;65:1497–1503.
28. Stack RS, Phillips HR III, Grierson DS, et al. Functional improvement of jeopardized myocardium following intracoronary streptokinase infusion in acute myocardial infarction. *J Clin Invest.* 1983;72:84–95.
29. Reduto LA, Freund GC, Gaetal JM, et al. Coronary artery reperfusion in acute myocardial infarction: beneficial effects of intracoronary streptokinase on left ventricular salvage and performance. *Am Heart J.* 1981;102:1168–1177.
30. Pepine CJ. New concepts in the pathophysiology of acute myocardial ischemia and infarction and their relevance to contemporary management. *Cardiovasc Clin.* 1989;20:3–18.
31. Keller AN, Cannon PJ, Wolny AC. Effective graded reductions of coronary pressure and flow on myocardial metabolism performance: a model of "hibernating myocardium." *J Am Coll Cardiol.* 1991;17:1661–1670.
32. Deutsh E, Berger M, Kussmaul WG, Hirshfeld JW Jr, Herrmann HC, Laskey WK. Adaptation to ischemia during percutaneous transluminal coronary angioplasty. *Circulation.* 1990;82:2044–2051.
33. Reimer KA, Murry CE, Jennings RB. Cardiac adaptation to ischemia. *Circulation.* 1990;82:2266–2268.
34. Liu GS, Thornton J, VanWinkle DM, Stanley AWH, Olsson RA, Downey JM. Protection against infarction afforded by preconditioning as mediated by A1 adenosine receptors in rabbit heart. *Circulation.* 1991;84:350–356.
35. Topol EJ, Weiss JL, Guzman PA, et al. Immediate improvement of dysfunctional myocardial segments after coronary revascularization: Detection by intraoperative transesophageal echocardiography. *J Am Coll Cardiol.* 1984;4:1123–1134.
36. Tillisch J, Brunken R, Marshall R, et al. Reversibility of cardiac wall motion abnormalities predicted by positron tomography. *N Engl J Med.* 1986;314:884–888.
37. Cohen M, Charney R, Hershman R, Fuster V, Gorlin R, Francis X. Reversal of chronic ischemic myocardial dysfunction after transluminal coronary angioplasty. *J Am Coll Cardiol.* 1988;12:1193–1198.
38. Carlson EB, Cowley MJ, Wolfgang TC, Vetrovec GW. Acute changes in global and regional rest left ventricular function after successful coronary angioplasty: comparative results in stable and unstable angina. *J Am Coll Cardiol.* 1989;13:1262–1269.
39. Erlebacher JA, Weiss JL, Weisfeldt ML, Buckley BH.

Early dilation of the infarcted segment in acute transmural myocardial infarction: role of infarct expansion in acute left ventricular enlargement. *J Am Coll Cardiol.* 1984;4:201–208.

40. McKay RG, Pfeffer MA, Pasternak RC, et al. Left ventricular remodeling after myocardial infarction: a corollary to infarct expansion. *Circulation.* 1986;74:693–702.

41. Jeremy RW, Alluran KC, Bautovitch G, Harris PJ. Patterns of left ventricular dilation during the six months after myocardial infarction. *J Am Coll Cardiol.* 1989;13:304–310.

42. Braunwald E. Myocardial reperfusion, limitation of infarct size, reduction of left ventricular dysfunction, and improved survival. *Circulation.* 1989;79:441–444.

43. Hochman JS, Choo H. Limitation of infarct expansion by reperfusion independent of myocardial salvage. *Circulation.* 1987;75:299–306.

44. Strauer BE. Functional dynamics of the left ventricle in hypertensive hypertrophy and failure. *Hypertension.* 1984;6:III 1141–1172.

45. Parker JO, Ledwich JR. West RO, Case RB. Reversible cardiac failure during angina pectoris. *Circulation.* 1969;39:745–757.

46. Dwyer EM Jr. Left ventricular pressure-volume alterations and regional disorders of contraction during myocardial ischemia induced by atrial pacing. *Circulation.* 1970;42:1111–1122.

47. Pasternak A, Gorlin R, Sonnenblick EH. Abnormalities of ventricular motion induced by atrial pacing in coronary artery disease. *Circulation.* 1972;45:1195–1205.

48. Ferro G, Spinelli L, Duillio L, Spadafora M, Guarnallia F, Condorelli M. Diastolic perfusion time at ischemic threshold in patients with stress-induced ischemia. *Circulation.* 1991;84:49–56.

49. Crawford MH. Exercise-induced myocardial ischemia importance of coronary blood flow. *Circulation.* 1991;84:424–425.

50. Dougherty AH, Naccerelli GV, Gray EL, Hicks CH, Godstein RA. Congestive heart failure with normal systolic function. *Am J Cardiol.* 1984;54:778–782.

51. Soufer R, Wohlgelernter D, Vita NA, et al. Intact systolic left ventricular function in clinical congestive heart failure. *Am J Cardiol.* 1985;55:1032–1036.

52. Kannel WB, Dannenberg AL, Abbott RD. Unrecognized myocardial infarction and hypertension: the Framingham study. *Am Heart J.* 1985;109:581–585.

53. Ranjadayalan K, Umachandran V, Ambepityia G, Kopelman PG, Mills PG, Timmis AD. Prolonged anginal perceptual threshold in diabetes: effect on exercise capacity and myocardial ischemia. *J Am Coll Cardiol.* 1990;16:1120–1124.

54. Mills RM, Kastor JA. Quantitative grading of cardiac palpation. *Arch Intern Med.* 1973;132:831–834.

55. Brill DM, Konstam MA, Vivino PG, et al. Importance of right ventricular systolic function as an independent predictor of mortality in patients with congestive heart failure. *Circulation.* 1989;80:II-649.

56. Mills RM, Young E, Gorlin R, Lesch M. Natural history of ST segment elevation after acute myocardial infarction. *Am J Cardiol.* 1975;35:609–614.

57. Kessler KM. Heart failure with normal systolic function. *Arch Intern Med.* 1988;148:2109–2111.

58. Robertson WS, Feigenbaum H, Armstrong WF, Dillon JC, O'Donnell J, McHenry PW. Exercise echocardiography: a clinically practical addition in the evaluation of coronary artery disease. *J Am Coll Cardiol.* 1983;2:1085–1091.

59. Kloner RA, Allen J, Zheng Y, Ruiz C. Myocardial stunning following exercise treadmill testing in man. *J Am Coll Cardiol.* 1990;15:203A. Abstract.

60. Sox HC, Blatt MA, Higgins MC, Marton KI. Differential diagnosis of heart failure secondary to coronary artery disease. In: *Medical decision making.* Boston: Butterworths; 1988:67–100.

61. Szlachcic J, Massie BM, Kramer BL, Topicn D, Tubau J. Correlates and prognostic implication of exercise capacity in chronic congestive heart failure. *Am J Cardiol.* 1985;55:1037–1042.

62. Legrand V, Mancini GBJ, Bates ER, Hodgson JMcB, Gross MD, Vogel RA. Comparative study of coronary flow reserve, coronary anatomy and results of radionuclide exercise tests in patients with coronary artery disease. *J Am Coll Cardiol.* 1986;8:1022–1032.

63. Kirkeede RL, Gould KL, Parsel L. Assessment of coronary stenoses by myocardial perfusion imaging during pharmacologic coronary vasodilation VII. Validation of coronary flow reserve as a single integrated functional measure of stenosis severity reflecting all its geometric dimensions. *J Am Coll Cardiol.* 1986;7:103–113.

64. Leppo J, Plaja J, Gionet M, Tumolo J, Paraskos JA, Cutler BC. Noninvasive evaluation of cardiac risk before elective vascular surgery. *J Am Coll Cardiol.* 1987;9:269–276.

65. Armstrong WF, O'Donnell J, Dillon JC, McHenry PL, Morris SN, Feigenbaum H. Complimentary value of 2-dimensional exercise echocardiography to routine treadmill exercise testing. *Ann Intern Med.* 1986;105:829–835.

66. Jennings GL, Esler MD. Circulatory regulation at rest and exercise and the functional assessment of patients with congestive heart failure. *Circulation.* 1990;81:II5–II13.

67. Franciosa JA. Why patients with heart failure die: hemodynamic and functional determinants of survival. *Circulation.* 1987;75:IV20–IV27.

68. Mancini DM, LeJentel TH, Factor S, Sonnenblick E. Central and peripheral components of cardiac failure. *Am J Med.* 1986;80(suppl 2B):2–12.

69. Marantz PR, Topin JN, Wasserthiel-Smoller S, et al. The relationship between left ventricular systolic function and congestive heart failure diagnosed by clinical criteria. *Circulation.* 1988;77:607–612.

70. Stevenson LW, Miller LW. Cardiac transplantation as therapy for heart failure. *Curr Prob Cardiol.* 1991;16:219–305.

71. Hoberg E, Kunze B, Rausch S, Konig J, Schafer H, Kubler W. Diagnostic value of ambulatory Holter monitoring for the detection of coronary artery disease in patients with variable threshold angina pectoris. *Am J Cardiol.* 1990;65:1078–1083.

72. Pepine CJ. Ambulant myocardial ischemia and its prognostic implications. (Editorial) *Circulation*. 1990;81:1136–1138.

73. Breitenbücher A, Pfisterer M, Hoffmann A, Burckhardt D. Long-term follow-up of patients with silent ischemia during exercise radionuclide angiography. *J Am Coll Cardiol*. 1990;15:999–1003.

74. Wolfe CL. Silent myocardial ischemia: its impact on prognosis. (Editorial) *J Am Coll Cardiol*. 1990;15:1004–1006.

75. Taliercio CP, Vlietstra RE, Fisher LD, Burnett JC. Risks for renal dysfunction with cardiac angiography. *Ann Intern Med*. 1986;104:501–504.

76. Parfrey PS, Griffiths SM, Barrett BJ, et al. Contrast material-induced renal failure in patients with diabetes mellitus, renal insufficiency, or both. *N Engl J Med*. 1989;320:143–149.

77. Brezis M, Epstein FH. A closer look at radio contrast-induced nephropathy. (Editorial) *N Engl J Med*. 1989;320:179–181.

78. Helfant RH, Pine R, Meister SG, Feldman MS, Trout RG, Banka VS. Nitroglycerin to unmask reversible asynergy: correlation with postcoronary bypass ventriculography. *Circulation*. 1974;50:108–113.

79. Feldman RL, Marx JD, Pepine CJ, Conti CR. Analysis of coronary responses to various doses of intracoronary nitroglycerin. *Circulation*. 1982;66:321–327.

80. Luchi RJ, Scott SM, Deupree RH, and the Principal Investigators and Their Associates of Veterans Administration Cooperative Study No. 28. Comparison of medical and surgical treatment for unstable angina pectoris. Results of a Veterans Administration Cooperative Study. *N Engl J Med*. 1987;316:977–984.

81. Faxon DP, Myers WO, McCabe CH, et al. The influence of surgery on the natural history of angiographically documented left ventricular aneurysm: the coronary artery surgery study. *Circulation*. 1986;74:110–118.

82. Akins CW. Resection of left ventricular aneurysm during hypothermic fibrillatory arrest without aortic occlusion. *J Thorac Cardiovasc Surg*. 1986;91:610–618.

83. Louagie Y, Alouini T, Lesperance J, Pelletier LC. Left ventricular aneurysm with predominating congestive heart failure. A comparative study of medical and surgical treatment. *J Thorac Cardiovasc Surg*. 1987;94:571–578.

84. Rozanski A, Krantz DS, Bairey CN. Ventricular responses to mental stress testing in patients with coronary artery disease. *Circulation*. 1991;83:II137–II144.

85. Mazzuero G, Temporelli PL, Tavazzi L. Influence of mental stress on ventricular pump function in postinfarction patients. *Circulation*. 1991;83:II145–II154.

86. Sullivan MJ, Higginbotham MB, Cobb FR. Exercise training in patients with severe left ventricular dysfunction: hemodynamic and metabolic effects. *Circulation*. 1988;78:506–515.

87. Sullivan MJ, Higginbotham MB, Cobb FR. Exercise training in patients with chronic heart failure delays ventilatory anaerobic threshold and improves submaximal exercise performance. *Circulation*. 1989;79:324–329.

88. Coats AJS, Adamopoulos S, Meyer TE, Conway J, Sleight P. Effects of physical training in chronic heart failure. *Lancet*. 1990;335:63–66.

13
The Cardiomyopathies

Jeffrey D. Hosenpud

The concept of primary myocardial disease was first suggested in the late 19th century by Krehl, who described several cases of "chronic myocarditis" in which autopsied hearts demonstrated myocardial degeneration, hypertrophy, and inflammation.[1] The term "primary myocardial disease" was coined by Josserand and Gallavardin at the beginning of this century.[2] But it was not until 1957 that the introduction of the term "cardiomyopathy," by Brigden, was used to describe myocardial disease of unknown etiology and in the absence of coronary disease.[3] Subsequently, in 1968 the terminology was specifically defined by the World Health Organization as myocardial disease excluding vascular, hypertension, and valvular disease. It was further broken down into "primary" and "secondary" cardiomyopathy depending on unknown or known etiologies, respectively.[4] This definition was refined further in 1980 by a combined task force of the World Health Organization and the International Society and Federation of Cardiology, which exchanged the term "secondary cardiomyopathy" for "specific heart muscle disease."[5] Despite these specific definitions, the term "cardiomyopathy" is used by most as defining primary myocardial disease, either of specific or unknown etiology. Unfortunately, it is used by many as a synonym for ventricular dysfunction of any cause (e.g., ischemic cardiomyopathy, valvular cardiomyopathy). For the purposes of this chapter, the term "cardiomyopathy" will be defined as diseases of the myocardium of either known or unknown etiology.

Traditionally, the cardiomyopathies have been grouped into anatomic/physiologic rather than etiologic groups (Fig. 13.1). These include dilated cardiomyopathy, hypertrophic cardiomyopathy, and restrictive cardiomyopathy. The dilated form is most common and the restrictive form least common. Although this classification does not take into account underlying etiologies, more often than not specific etiologies tend to fall into specific anatomic groupings. Furthermore,

this anatomic classification is helpful in the medical management of patients with cardiomyopathy, as will be described later. Finally, prognosis is linked more closely in most cases to anatomic/physiologic class rather than specific etiology.

Dilated Cardiomyopathy

Pathophysiology and Mechanisms of Disease

The primary myocardial defect in patients with dilated cardiomyopathy is an abnormality in contraction. As a result of reduction in myocardial contractility, the heart dilates out of proportion to the degree of hypertrophy, resulting in four-chamber enlargement with relatively thin cardiac walls.[6] This increase in radius to wall thickness increases myocardial wall stress[7] and decreases subendocardial coronary flow,[8] leading to further cardiac dysfunction. Figure 13.2 demonstrates a typical echocardiogram from a patient with dilated cardiomyopathy. On M mode (top), the left ventricle (LV) is markedly enlarged and systolic function is reduced. The two-dimensional echocardiogram (bottom) from the same patient demonstrates that all four chambers are enlarged.

In most cases of dilated cardiomyopathy, the mechanism(s) for the initial myocardial insult is unknown. Furthermore, it is unclear whether the defect is one of primary individual myocardial cell loss or cell dysfunction followed ultimately by myocardial cell loss and replacement with fibrous connective tissue. A host of molecular, biochemical, and cellular abnormalities have been described in patients with dilated cardiomyopathy. These include alterations in calcium handling by the sarcoplasmic reticulum,[9] a reduction β_1-receptor density,[10,11] alterations in Gs and Gi proteins,[12,13] alterations in cholinergic receptor density and function,[14] and expression of altered or fetal

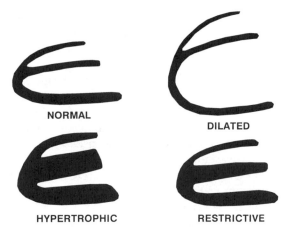

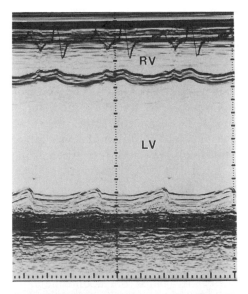

FIGURE 13.1. An anatomic classification of cardiomyopathy is depicted in this figure. In contrast with the normal ventricles, dilated cardiomyopathy has increased left and right ventricular chambers in relatively thin walls (increased radius/wall thickness ratio). Hypertrophic cardiomyopathy demonstrates thickened walls with the septal thickening usually predominating. Restrictive cardiomyopathy has relatively smaller ventricular cavities and relatively thickened walls, but not to the extent seen in hypertrophic cardiomyopathy.

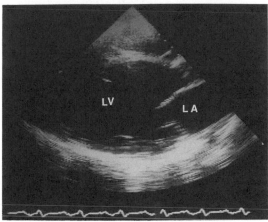

FIGURE 13.2. An M-mode (*top*) and two-dimensional (*bottom*) echocardiogram from a patient with dilated cardiomyopathy. Note the large chamber sizes and poor systolic contraction. LV = left ventricle; RV = right ventricle; LA = left atrium.

myosin subtypes.[15] It is not clear, however, whether many of these noted abnormalities are specific to dilated cardiomyopathy or are more general manifestations of cardiac dilatation and failure.

As noted previously, as early as the late 19th century it was hypothesized that cardiomyopathy was the result of chronic inflammatory disease.[1] After some 80 years, the concept that dilated cardiomyopathy may be the result of an acute, subacute, or chronic myocarditis again is receiving attention.[16] Although the inflammatory myocardial diseases are covered extensively elsewhere in this text, immune and infectious mechanisms of myocardial dysfunction as they relate to dilated cardiomyopathy will be briefly discussed here. The hypothesis put forth is that some myocardial insult, be it an acute viral infection or toxin, somehow alters the antigenicity of the myocardium resulting in it being mistaken for nonself and eliciting an autoimmune attack.[17] The problem with the hypothesis is that the pieces of the puzzle have been difficult to prove in a convincing way.

In terms of the initial insult, it has long been appreciated that Coxsackie group B virus was an important pathogen in acute viral myocarditis in patients and has provided an excellent model to study acute myocarditis in animals. Furthermore, in some murine strains, acute coxsackie myocarditis led to a more chronic myocarditis and cardiac dilation suggestive of dilated cardiomyopathy (DCM).[18] The difficulty linking Coxsackie virus to human DCM has been the inability to identify the virus in cardiac tissue. Serology is nonspecific,[19] viral cultures are rarely positive,[20] and electron microscopy for viral particles is difficult to interpret. With the recent growth of molecular biologic techniques, new methods for viral diagnosis have become available. Bowles and colleagues utilized invitro nucleic acid hybridization to study whether enterovirus RNA is present in the myocardium of patients with DCM.[21] Forty patients were studied: 21 with DCM and 19 controls with heart failure secondary to either coronary disease or congenital heart disease. Enterovirus RNA was detected in the myocardium of 6 of the 21 patients with DCM and only 1 of the controls. These and similar data by Kandolf and colleagues[22] are the first convincing evidence for enteroviral persistence in the myocardium of patients with DCM.

A number of studies have investigated the "immunologic milieu" in DCM. Limas and Limas found that

HLA-DR4 was represented in 40% of patients with DCM compared to 24% of controls.[23] Koike investigated cell-mediated immune function in 18 patients with DCM.[24] In these patients phytohemaglutinin (PHA)-mediated lymphocyte blastogenesis was reduced, the CD4 (helper lymphocytes) to CD8 (suppressor lymphocytes) ratio was higher, the PHA-mediated release of interleukin-2, a T-cell growth factor, was enhanced, and the number of activated lymphocytes (interleukin-2 receptor positive) was reduced when compared to controls. These data would suggest an inherited predisposition to immunologic disease.

Antimyocardial antibodies have been studied extensively over the past several years. However, a link between the presence of antibody and an alteration in cardiac function or metabolism has not been established. In previous studies by Schultheiss and colleagues, an antibody directed against the adenosine diphosphate–adenosine triphosphate (ADP-ATP) carrier protein of the mitochondrial membrane had been described in patients with DCM.[25] Subsequently, the group demonstrated the ability of this autoantibody to be transported intracellularly and alter myocardial metabolism.[26] In a more recent study, the investigators have isolated the ADP-ATP carrier from guinea pig hearts and immunized guinea pigs to this protein to produce specific antibodies and demonstrated that in those hearts from immunized animals, mean aortic pressure, stroke volume, stroke work, and external heart work were all significantly lower than in hearts from the control group.[27] Thus, it appears that this specific autoantibody can be related directly to an alteration in myocardial function and metabolism.

The regulation of β_1 receptors on myocardium in patients with heart failure has been well described.[10] The mechanism for this downregulation is felt to be a negative feedback related to chronically elevated levels of circulating catecholamines, presumably a nonspecific mechanism related to the degree of heart failure. Limas and colleagues demonstrated that a high percentage of patients with DCM, especially those that are HLA-DR4, had circulating anti-β_1 receptor autoantibodies.[28] An additional mechanism for modulating cell surface β receptors specific to DCM can therefore be hypothesized.

In addition to a direct cell-mediated or humoral response to the myocardium, a whole host of soluble cytokines are a part of the immunologic milieu. Our laboratory previously described a negative inotropic effect of interleukin-1 (IL-1) in an isolated rat heart preparation.[29] More recently we have demonstrated that IL-1 stimulates myocardial interstitial cells to produce a thus far undefined second compound (likely a small polypeptide) that inhibits myocardial cell RNA and protein synthesis in a cell culture system.[30] It is therefore evidence that the immune system could potentially affect myocardial function through a variety of pathways, including cell-mediated immunity, humoral immunity, and direct and indirect effects from soluble cytokines.

Mechanisms other than those involving immunologic abnormalities for DCM have been investigated. Based on their experimental data in the Syrian hamster, Factor and colleagues have postulated that some forms of DCM are secondary to small vessel disease and specifically to microvascular spasm.[31] This mechanism is presumed to play an important role in the DCM associated with pheochromocytoma.[32] In a recent study, Treasure and colleagues demonstrated that patients with DCM have impaired endothelial dependent coronary microvasculature dilation compared to controls.[33] van Hoeven and Factor reviewed endomyocardial biopsies from 145 patients with DCM and demonstrated small vessel thickening in 56% of these patients.[34] This, however, was not a specific finding as a significant proportion of patients with hypertension, diabetes, unexplained arrhythmias, and chest pain syndromes had similar changes.[34]

Direct myocardial toxicity is suggested for alcohol-induced cardiomyopathy[35] and clearly is present in anthracycline-induced DCM.[36,37] Although in the muscle bath, alcohol is a potent depressant of myocardial function, the effects and variability of alcohol on the myocardium in vivo are poorly understood. Although several mechanisms to be discussed later have been suggested for anthracycline cardiotoxicity, there is at least a dose-related effect of anthracyclines on cardiac function.

Finally, as will be discussed later, the association of DCM with several forms of muscular dystrophy is well described.[38,39] Caforio and colleagues demonstrated that in 35% of nonselected cases of both dilated and hypertrophic cardiomyopathy there was an abnormal reduction of skeletal motor unit potential duration. Furthermore, in nine patients who underwent skeletal muscle biopsies (five, DCM; four, HCM), all had abnormalities suggestive of a myogenic myopathy.[40] These data would suggest that some patients with cardiomyopathy may have a generalized muscle disease that manifests primarily in the heart. If this is true, the implications are that a primary (genetic) molecular defect in muscle metabolism may exist in patients with DCM as is present in the primary muscular dystrophies.

Clinical Features of Dilated Cardiomyopathy

Irrespective of underlying etiology, most patients with DCM present in similar fashion albeit in a continuum of heart failure. In general, patients present with progressive symptoms of exercise limitation that can span as short as days to months or years. Dyspnea with exertion, orthopnea, paroxysmal nocturnal dyspnea

TABLE 13.1. Hemodynamics in dilated cardiomyopathy.

Parameter	Series 1	Series 2	Series 3
Ejection fraction	.27	.30	.26
LV filling pressure (mm Hg)	20	20	22
Cardiac index (L/min/m²)	1.9	2.5	2.5
1-yr mortality	48%	35%	35%

Series 1: Adult, ref. #116; series 2: Adult, ref. #115; series 3: Pediatric, ref. #113.
LV = left ventricular.

(PND), and less commonly chest discomfort similar to typical angina can be presenting symptoms. Early in the course of the disease, left-sided symptoms seem to predominate and it is only later that evidence of right ventricular failure manifests. This is a curious feature as the myopathic process presumably involves both ventricles. Coexistent symptoms or even modes of presentation include the onset of ventricular or atrial arrhythmias and systemic embolization. Physical findings especially in the acute setting typically include traditional findings of heart failure including sinus tachycardia, elevated jugular venous pressure, pulmonary rales, a third and likely a fourth heart sound, mitral insufficiency, and in the most severe cases, hepatic congestion and peripheral edema.

In a study by Fuster and colleagues[41] of 104 patients with DCM, the mean time from initial symptoms to presentation to a physician was 1.3 years. At the time of diagnosis, 87% of patients had cardiomegaly, 80% had electrocardiographic abnormalities, a full 73% presented with overt heart failure, and 4% presented with evidence of systemic embolization. In a similar study of 68 patients with DCM by Schwarz and colleagues,[42] all had symptoms of congestive heart failure (CHF) (65% NYHA II, 35% NYHA III), 82% had cardiomegally, 97% had electrocardiogram (ECG) abnormalities, and 47% experienced episodes of chest pain.

Table 13.1 demonstrates a summary of several clinical series of patients with DCM. Typically the ejection fraction is reduced to approximately half normal; left, and when severe, right ventricular filling pressures are twice normal and cardiac index is reduced. This coupled with increased heart rate implies an even greater reduction of stroke volume. Differences between series likely reflect referral patterns in a given community and earlier or later stage of the disease process.

Differential Diagnosis of Dilated Cardiomyopathy

Table 13.2 lists some but not all of the etiologies and associations with DCM. Although the list is extensive, the vast majority of patients will have no obvious

TABLE 13.2. Reported causes and associations with dilated cardiomyopathy.

Idiopathic	Diabetes
Infectious	Beriberi
Viral Disease	Selenium Deficiency
Coxsackievirus	Kwashiorkor
Echovirus	Collagen vascular disease
Adenovirus	Lupus erythematosus
Arbovirus	Dermatomyositis
Bacterial	Polyarteritis nodosa
Diphtheria	Scleroderma
Tuberculosis	Neuromuscular disease
Leptospirosis	Duchenne's
Rickettsia	Fredreich's ataxia
Typhus	Limb girdle
Q fever	Neurofibromatosis
Protozoal	Myasthenia gravis
Chagastic	Toxins
Malarial	Alcohol
Leishmaniasis	Arsenic
Granulomatous disease	Cobalt
Idiopathic	Lead
Sarcoidosis	Carbon tetrachloride
Giant cell	Carbon monoxide
Wegner's	Catecholamines
Metabolic/endocrine	Amphetamines
Acromegally	Cocaine
Hypothyroidism	Anthracyclines
Pheochromocytoma	Cyclophosphamide

associated cause for their disease. Approximately 10% to 15% of patients will present with a clinical DCM and have evidence of a chronic myocarditis on endomyocardial biopsy.[17] This entity and other inflammatory diseases are discussed elsewhere in the text and are not discussed further here. The specific diseases that are expanded on here include alcohol-induced cardiomyopathy, diabetic cardiomyopathy, peripartum cardiomyopathy, and anthracycline-induced cardiomyopathy.

Alcohol-Induced Cardiomyopathy

The major difficulty with the diagnosis of alcohol-induced cardiomyopathy is that cardiomyopathy is an uncommon event and alcohol abuse is a common condition. Clinically, histologically and therapeutically, alcohol-induced cardiomyopathy, is not significantly different than idiopathic cardiomyopathy. The incidence of alcohol being identified as a significant risk factor in cardiomyopathy has been reported at between 20% and 30%.[41,42]

It is clear that high blood levels of alcohol produce mild negative inotropy.[43,44] Furthermore, several animal studies have investigated the effects of prolonged alcohol administration. In primates, chronic alcohol administration results in myocytolysis and fibrosis.[45] In dogs, cardiac fibrosis is produced and ultimately measurable myocardial dysfunction occurs.[46,47] In a hamster model, chronic alcohol administration resulted in a reduction in myocardial high energy phosphates.[48]

The specific mechanisms by which alcohol might produce myocardial dysfunction also have been investigated. Cellular events that have been described with chronic alcohol exposure include impaired sarcoplasmic reticular uptake of calcium,[49] inhibition of myosin ATPase,[50] elevation of intracellular Na^+ and water,[51] inhibition of the Na^+-K^+ ATPase,[52] and alterations in the incorporation of membrane fatty acids and phospholipids.[47,53]

The expression of alcohol-induced cardiomyopathy obviously is quite variable. There is evidence to suggest that excessive alcohol consumption is likely to be present for a minimum of 10 years before the onset of heart failure,[54-56] men are more susceptible than women,[57] and that concurrent smoking, hypertension, and malnutrition may be contributing factors. Furthermore, there appears to be a differential organ susceptibility to alcohol as those individuals who develop cardiomyopathy are unlikely to develop chronic cirrhosis.[58]

An interesting, likely unrelated phenomenon occurred in the 1960s where in a few areas of Europe and Canada, cobalt was added to beer as a foam-stabilizing agent. An acute and aggressive form of cardiomyopathy developed in heavy beer drinkers that was attributable to the cobalt.[59,60] When this element was no longer used, no further cases of this form of cardiomyopathy were reported.

There is some evidence to suggest that the abstinence of alcohol beneficially impacts prognosis in alcohol-induced cardiomyopathy. In one study of 64 patients, approximately one third discontinued excessive alcohol use. This subgroup had a 9% mortality rate over the subsequent 4 yr, contrasted with a 57% mortality rate in the remainder who continued drinking.[35] A second, although smaller study (31 patients), supported these findings.[61]

Diabetic Cardiomyopathy

Diabetic cardiomyopathy as a unique entity has been recognized only recently. First reported in 1972, Rubler and colleagues presented data on four patients with Kimmelsteil-Wilson disease and DCM in the absence of coronary, valvular, or other cardiomyopathic risk factors.[62] Supportive data have included retrospective analysis from the Framingham Study demonstrating a 2.4-fold higher incidence of developing heart failure in diabetics on insulin,[63] a higher than expected incidence of diabetes in a population of idiopathic DCM,[64] and animal data to be described below.

Animal data have been somewhat difficult to interpret. Drug-induced diabetic dogs, sheep, and primates demonstrate no evidence of systolic myocardial dysfunction,[65-67] although myocardial collagen was increased in one dog study.[68] In genetically diabetic mice, there is evidence of progressive myocardial damage and thickening of capillary basement membranes.[69] In drug-induced diabetic rats, hypertension is required to induce overt cardiomyopathy,[70,71] although lesser degrees of myocardial dysfunction have been demonstrated in the absence of hypertension.[72,73]

Potential pathogenetic mechanisms for diabetic cardiomyopathy have included increased vascular permeability resulting in increased glycosylation of collagen,[74] alterations in intracellular Ca^{2+} kinetics,[75] and microvascular damage[76] akin to diabetic retinopathy and nephropathy.

Clinical presentation of diabetic cardiomyopathy is not dissimilar from idiopathic DCM. In a series of 16 diabetics with cardiomyopathy, cardiac volumes, left ventricular filling pressures, and ventricular mass were increased in all patients and cardiac index reduced in approximately half.[64] These findings were confirmed in a small series that also demonstrated a decrease in myocardial compliance.[77] Several investigators have demonstrated that diabetics have abnormal cardiac function based on systolic time intervals.[78-80] Seneviratne noted that these abnormalities were present only in diabetic patients with evidence of other microangiopathy (retinopathy or nephropathy).[79]

Histopathologically, hearts from diabetic patients with DCM are similar to those from nondiabetic patients. Some investigators have reported in addition to the hypertrophy and interstitial fibrosis, an increase in interstitial PAS-positive material consistent with glycoprotein.[81] Other investigators have reported hyalin thickening of small vessels in the myocardium.[82] Factor and colleagues presented histopathologic data on patients with hypertension and diabetes, where interstitial fibrosis and myocytolysis were more pronounced than in patients with either diabetes or hypertension alone.[83] This added effect of hypertension on diabetic arteriopathy is consistent with other studies of retinopathy and nephropathy[84,85] and may lend additional credence to the diabetic-hypertensive rat model of cardiomyopathy.

Peripartum Cardiomyopathy

The syndrome of unexplained heart failure in women postpartum was detailed in the mid-1930s by a number of investigators,[86,87] but had been suggested even earlier. Initially described as occurring primarily in the postpartum period, it is clear now that the presentation of the disease can occur from as early as the end of the middle of the third trimester through several months after delivery. Most commonly, however, signs and symptoms of heart failure occur postpartum.[88]

The etiology of peripartum cardiomyopathy is unknown, although several factors have been associated with development of the disease. As the disease appears to be more common in less affluent populations, nutritional deficiencies during pregnancy have been postulated.[89,90] Other suggested associations have included toxemia of pregnancy,[90] immunologic factors including the development of antiheart antibodies,[91] genetic susceptibility,[92,93] and drug-induced hypersensitivity.[94]

A particularly interesting finding in a subset of patients with peripartum cardiomyopathy is that of chronic myocarditis. Melvin and colleagues first reported three patients who underwent endomyocardial biopsy soon after presenting with peripartum cardiomyopathy and had evidence of a chronic inflammatory process on histology.[95] A more recent series by Midei and colleagues suggested that 14 of 18 patients with peripartum cardiomyopathy had myocarditis.[96] The difficulty with these data is that a low grade inflammatory process can be present solely as a response to myocardial cell injury rather than the cause. It is of interest that of the 14 patients with "myocarditis" in the latter study, 6 patients had only "borderline" myocarditis manifest by a mild lymphocytic infiltrate.

Although the general clinical signs, symptoms, and histology (excepting patients with myocarditis) are no different from patients with idiopathic DCM, there appear to be certain factors, including race (with a much higher incidence in blacks), advanced maternal age, multiparae, and twin pregnancies.[88,97] In addition, one specific complication, embolic disease, is substantially more common in peripartum cardiomyopathy compared to other forms, likely because of the altered coagulative state during pregnancy.[97,98] There is no doubt that this entity is distinct from other forms of DCM based on three well documented phenomena. First, as previously stated, in most cases the timing of the onset of disease is closely related to the postpartum period.[88,97] Second, relatively speaking, the prognosis of peripartum cardiomyopathy is excellent compared to other forms of DCM, with a full third of patients recovering to normal function and another third stabilizing for prolonged periods of time.[99,100] Third, the disease appears to recur with subsequent pregnancies in a portion of patients, even in patients who have had complete recovery from their first episode.[92,100]

Anthracycline-Induced Cardiomyopathy

Anthracycline-induced cardiomyopathy, a form of toxin-induced cardiomyopathy, may affect anywhere from 5% to 20% of patients receiving the agent, depending on a variety of risk factors and total dose. It is a unique form of cardiomyopathy and as a result has provided several insights into toxin-induced cardiac disease and global cardiac function for the following reasons. First, as a toxin, it appears to affect individual cardiac cells while leaving others unaffected, based on electron microscopic studies.[101,102] The number of affected cells appears related to total dose. This is presumably a different phenomenon than in other forms of DCM where the insult or defect appears felt to affect cardiac tissue more diffusely. Second, there appears to be a threshold effect, where gross cardiac function remains normal until this threshold percentage of cells are affected and then cardiac function can deteriorate precipitously.[103] This would suggest a partial redundancy in the number of contractile units (myocytes) in the heart as is present in the functioning units of other organs (e.g., glomeruli).

Several hypotheses have been proposed to explain the cardiotoxic effect of anthracyclines. Oxygen free radicals, lipid peroxidation, altered arachidonic acid metabolism, a direct interaction with the calcium release protein from sarcoplasmic reticulum, and metabolite action on the calcium pump from sarcoplasmic reticulum all have been implicated in the cardiotoxicity effects.[104]

The clinical presentation of cardiomyopathy secondary to anthracycline toxicity is not dissimilar from DCM of other etiologies. It has been reported as early as a week after the last dose of doxorubicin but can present even years after chemotherapy.[105] It has been suggested that the severity and ultimate prognosis is least favorable when the latency period is shorter.[105] Most studies have suggested that cardiac toxicity is uncommon in cumulative doses of less than 450 mg/m² in the absence of other risk factors.[105] When risk factors are present, which include advancing age, mediastinal radiation, concomitant cardiotoxic chemotherapy, underlying cardiac disease, and large bolus therapy, cardiac toxicity has been noted at substantially lower total dosages.[105–109]

Although a variety of cardiovascular studies have been advocated to follow patients for cardiac toxicity, the most sensitive appears to be endomyocardial biopsy.[103] This is in part secondary to the threshold phenomenon described above. Most studies such as echocardiography, radionuclide angiography, and systolic time intervals rely on systolic cardiac function, which may not fall despite significant histologic evidence of toxicity.[110] It is conceivable that diastolic function might provide more sensitive data in following these patients.

Although specific pathologic findings are discussed in detail elsewhere in this text, a brief description of the histopathology in anthracycline cardiac toxicity is warranted. Most of the clinical work was performed by Billingham and colleagues at Stanford University. It became apparent to these investigators that standard light microscopy was inadequate to judge the severity and extent of cardiac toxicity. Low power electron microscopy therefore became the standard methodology.[101] Histopathologic findings include disruption of myofibrils and dissolution of the myofilaments, extensive vacuolization secondary to swelling of the sarcoplasmic reticulum, mitochondrial pleomorphism, and dissociation of the tight junctions.[101,102] These findings are then graded based on both number of cells affected and the severity of the changes.

Reduction in anthracycline cardiac toxicity has been accomplished first by a more careful monitoring of toxicity and understanding of risk factors. Once the total dose of doxorubicin exceeds 450 mg/m^2 (or lower if risk factors are present), histologic monitoring by endomyocardial biopsy is warranted before administering additional drug. A high grade biopsy should preclude additional anthracycline exposure irrespective of the left ventricular systolic function. Second, it appears that toxicity can be reduced by reducing peak levels of the drug. This has resulted in changing protocols from monthly large-dose infusions to weekly smaller dose infusions and even daily continuous intravenous administration. It has been noted that larger total doses can be achieved, efficacy is not impaired, and toxicity is lessened.[110]

Therapy

Therapy for DCM is directed primarily toward the treatment of CHF. This is extensively addressed elsewhere in the text. In brief, digitalis glycosides, diuretics, and vasodilators are the mainstays of therapy both from a symptomatic standpoint as well as for prognosis (vasodilator therapy). In the author's view, patients with DCM presenting with symptoms of left ventricular dysfunction should receive all three therapies instituted at doses appropriate for the patients' symptoms and their response to therapy. An angiotensin-converting enzyme (ACE) inhibitor probably is the vasodilator of choice because of the minimum side effect profile. For patients who present with DCM who are asymptomatic, approach to therapy is less well defined. Based on preliminary communications from ongoing studies (SOLVD), it is likely that the use of ACE inhibitors will be beneficial in this group.

Other complications of left ventricular dysfunction, including arrhythmia management and prevention of thromboembolism, likewise need to be addressed. The issue of arrhythmia management, especially that of ventricular arrhythmias, is a complicated one and is addressed extensively elsewhere. One might emphasize that conventional approaches to arrhythmia management as used in ischemic heart disease are less successful in DCM. If sudden death has occurred or sustained ventricular arrhythmias are documented, many clinicians will treat directly with amiodarone or if ap-

TABLE 13.3. Indications for anticoagulation.

| EF < .25 |
| Prior history of thrombosis |
| Venous insufficiency |
| Atrial fibrillation with EF < .40 |
| Peripartum cardiomyopathy |

EF = ejection fraction

propriate, consider an automatic implantable cardiovertor-defibrillator.[111]

The prevention of thromboembolism also is critical in patients with DCM. Again, based on the author's experience, patients should be anticoagulated with warfarin for any one of the following; (a) if the ejection fraction (EF) is less than 0.25, (b) if there is any history of thromboembolism, (c) if the patient is in atrial fibrillation (EF less than 0.40), or (d) if the underlying disease is peripartum cardiomyopathy, especially in the first few months after delivery (see Table 13.3). The addition of aspirin to those in atrial fibrillation with higher EFs also may be warranted.

Once a patient's symptoms progress to late NYHA functional class III or IV, despite intensive medical management, mortality is excessive and cardiac transplantation should be entertained.

Prognosis

In general, the prognosis of patients with DCM depends on cardiac function irrespective of underlying etiology. As previously discussed, exceptions include patients with peripartum cardiomyopathy where prognosis is more favorable, anthracycline cardiomyopathy with rapid onset where prognosis is poor, and alcoholic cardiomyopathy with continued alcohol consumption where likewise prognosis is worse than the group as a whole. Figure 13.3 demonstrates the actuarial survival from four patient series.[41,112–114] The differences in the two adult series are likely due to patients of differing severity of illness. Even in the better outcome group,

TABLE 13.4. Predictors of outcome in detailed cardiomyopathy.

| Ejection fraction |
| Functional class |
| Alcohol |
| Ventricular arrhythmias |
| Elevated filling pressures |
| Reduced cardiac output |
| Degree of ventricular hypertrophy |
| Degree of interstitial fibrosis |
| Intraventricular conduction abnormalities |
| Maximum oxygen consumption |
| Pediatric age group |

FIGURE 13.3. Survival in dilated cardiomyopathy. The actuarial survival from four series are presented (refs. 41, 112, 113, 114). One-year survival ranges from just below 90% to as low as 45%, depending on the series and underlying characteristics of the patients. Pediatric patients with the diagnosis of dilated cardiomyopathy appear to have the worst prognosis overall.

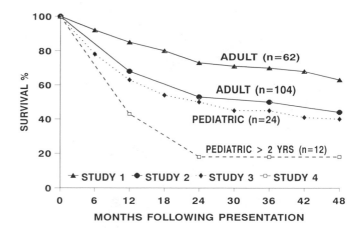

the 1- and 2-yr survivals are 83% and 72%, respectively. There appears to be an extremely poor prognosis in children who present after the age of 2 yr, although this series is quite small.

A variety of factors have been reported to influence prognosis in patients with DCM (Table 13.4). Most consistently, EF[42,115] and functional class[116] are powerful determinants. Other reported factors are filling pressures,[42,115,116] cardiac output,[115] age at both extremes,[41,114] ventricular arrhythmias,[115,116] atrial fibrillation,[115] ventricular conduction delay,[115] interstitial fibrosis,[115] and ventricular hypertrophy.[42,115]

Restrictive Cardiomyopathy

Pathophysiology

The primary myocardial defect in patients with restrictive cardiomyopathy is an abnormality of diastolic relaxation resulting in restricted ventricular filling, high filling pressures, and despite normal or near normal systolic function, a reduced stroke volume secondary to a reduction in total ventricular volume.[117] As a result, at any given diastolic volume diastolic pressure is increased compared to the normal heart (Fig. 13.4). In addition to the shift in the pressure/volume relationship to the left, the rate of rise in pressure for any given change in volume is greater in the restrictive myopathic heart.[118]

The characteristic left and right ventricular filling pressures are depicted in Figure 13.5. Initially after the ventricle empties, filling occurs rapidly but then plateaus early in diastole as the limits of ventricular compliance are reached. This "dip and plateau" configuration also is seen in constrictive pericarditis, making separation of these entities sometimes difficult.

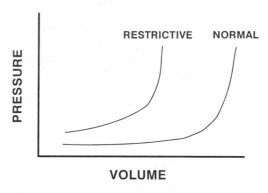

FIGURE 13.4. Theoretical ventricular pressure/volume relationships in ventricles with normal and restricted physiology. Not only is ventricular pressure greater for a given volume in the restricted heart, but the rate of pressure rise for a given increase in volume also is increased (reduced compliance).

More careful analysis of these filling characteristics have demonstrated that in constrictive pericarditis, the majority of filling of the ventricle occurs within the first half of diastole. In contrast in restrictive myopathy, approximately only half of the ventricular filling has occurred during this time.[119,120] An explanation for these differences is that in constriction, filling is relatively normal until the constraints of the pericardium are met, where as in restrictive disease, filling is abnormal throughout the diastolic period. In contrast to constrictive pericarditis, myocardial restriction usually results in differences in right and left ventricular filling pressures.[121] In addition, in severe restrictive disease, filling pressures even at the onset of diastole are elevated, suggesting that both ventricles empty incompletely.[122] This is in contrast to pericardial constriction where the initial diastolic pressure can be low.[123] In mild cases of restrictive cardiomyopathy or in patients who have been excessively volume depleted

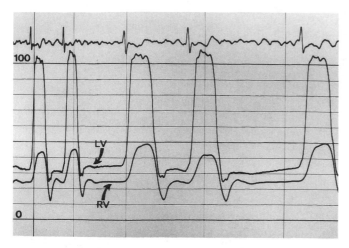

FIGURE 13.5. Left and right ventricular (*LV*, *RV*) pressure tracings in a patient with restrictive cardiomyopathy. Filling pressures are elevated in both chambers but not equalized. Note the early diastolic "dip" followed rapidly by a "plateau" in the pressure pulse. This "square root" sign also is seen in constrictive pericarditis. Reprinted, with permission, from Hosenpud JD. Restrictive cardiomyopathy. *Progress in cardiology*. 1989, Lea & Febiger.

with diuretic therapy, the restrictive physiology may be occult, requiring volume manipulation or exercise to become manifest.[122]

The mechanisms responsible for the reduction in ventricular compliance vary depending on the specific disease process. Potential mechanisms include an intrinsically abnormal myocardium, infiltration of the myocardium with nonmyocardial materials such as collagen or abnormal protein, endomyocardial disease, and space-occupying lesions (thrombus or tumor), reducing the total ventricular volumes. These different potential etiologies will be further delineated.

Differential Diagnosis and Specific Etiologies

Table 13.5 lists most of the reported causes of restrictive cardiomyopathy. Features of idiopathic restrictive cardiomyopathy, amyloidosis, and endocardial fibrosis will be expanded on, whereas other etiologies will be mentioned only briefly.

Idiopathic

It appears that as in DCM, no specific etiology for many patients with restrictive cardiomyopathy is found.[117,121,122,124] The histopathologic findings in these cases of primary or "idiopathic" restrictive cardiomyopathy are nonspecific and generally include myocardial cell hypertrophy and an increase in interstitial fibrosis. A primary defect in myocardial cell relaxation presumably is present. The clinical and hemodynamic findings of patients with idiopathic restrictive cardio-

TABLE 13.5. Reported causes of restrictive cardiomyopathy.

Primary (idiopathic)	Tumor infiltration
Amyloidosis	Storage diseases
Endocardial fibrosis	Anthracyclines
Eosinophilic heart disease	Radiation
Hemochromatosis	Cardiac transplant
Sarcoidosis	

Reprinted with permission from Hosenpud JD. Restrictive cardiomyopathy. *Progress in cardiology*. 1989, Lea & Febiger.

TABLE 13.6. Clinical and hemodynamic characteristics of 34 patients with primary restrictive cardiomyopathy.[a]

Age: mean: 39 yr; range: 1–77 yr	
Sex: 19 (56%) male; 15 (44%) female	
Symptomatology	
Chest pain	56%
Fatigue	50%
Dyspnea	61%
Clinical findings	
Jugular venous distension	62%
Rales	19%
S3	48%
S4	32%
Ascites	25%
Edema	32%
Hemodynamics	
Right atrial (mm Hg)	12 ± 6
Pulmonary wedge (mm Hg)	21 ± 7
Cardiac index (L/min/m²)	2.9 ± 1.0
LVEDVI (ml/m²)	67 ± 18
LV ejection fraction	$.68 \pm .10$

LVEDVI = left ventricular end-diastolic volume index.
[a]Compiled data from seven studies.[117,121,122,124–127] Results expressed as mean ± 1 SD.

myopathy are presented in Table 13.6, based on compiled data from seven series.[117,121,122,124–127] The mean age at presentation is similar to other forms of idiopathic cardiomyopathy with a very large age range. There is almost an equal distribution between males and females. Despite of one of the most frequent complaints being dyspnea, only a minority of patients have objective evidence of pulmonary interstitial or alveolar edema. Chest pain, which is atypical of angina, is the second most frequent complaint in these patients, followed by fatigue. Filling pressures are elevated as expected, but resting cardiac output tends to be normal. EFs are normal and, as expected, left ventricular end diastolic volumes tend to be small secondary to the restrictive process.

The characteristic gross anatomic findings in these patients are small left and right ventricles with normal or mildly increased ventricular wall thicknesses, and moderate to severely enlarged atria. Figure 13.6 presents

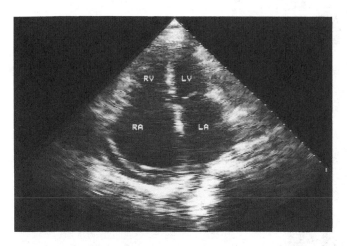

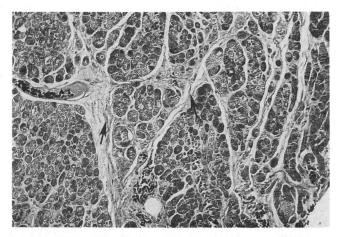

FIGURE 13.6. Echocardiogram from a patient with restrictive cardiomyopathy (apical four-chamber view). Note the small left (*LV*) and right (*RV*) chamber sizes and the relatively normal wall thicknesses. The left (*LA*) and right (*RA*) atria are markedly enlarged. Reprinted, with permission, from Hosenpud JD. Restrictive cardiomyopathy. *Progress in cardiology*. 1989, Lea & Febiger.

FIGURE 13.7. Endomyocardial biopsy (hematoxylin-eosin, ×255) from a patient with primary restrictive cardiomyopathy, showing extensive interstitial fibrosis (*arrows*) and relatively normal myocytes. Reprinted, with permission, from Hosenpud JD. Restrictive cardiomyopathy. *Progress in cardiology*. 1989, Lea & Febiger.

an echocardiographic apical four-chamber view from a patient with primary restrictive cardiomyopathy. Histopathologically, prominent interstitial fibrosis as seen in Figure 13.7 is a prominent finding.[117,122,128]

In contrast to patients with DCM who have an extremely high 1- and 2-yr mortality, as shown in Figure 13.8, patients with primary restrictive cardiomyopathy appear to have a better early prognosis (approximate 10% mortality at 1 yr). Ultimately, however, the prognosis is poor with only 10% of patients surviving at 10 yr.

Amyloidosis

A second frequently reported cause of restrictive cardiomyopathy is that associated with amyloid protein deposition into the myocardial interstitium. Amyloid is a generic term for the deposition of a variety of fibrous proteins arranged spatially in a beta-pleated sheet configuration. It is this spatial configuration that gives amyloid its characteristic staining properties in tissue. The two most common forms of amyloidosis are primary (including those associated with multiple myeloma) and secondary forms, which are associated with chronic inflammatory conditions.[129] A familial form of amyloidosis also has been described.[130] The protein found in primary amyloidosis consists of immunoglobulin light chains. In secondary amyloidosis, a variety of proteins associated with the acute phase response have been isolated.[129] The mechanism by which myocardial amyloid deposition produces its effects on diastolic function are unclear.

Table 13.7 presents data compiled from case reports

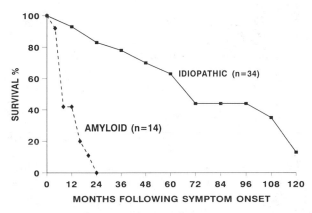

FIGURE 13.8. Actuarial survival data in primary restrictive cardiomyopathy compiled from several studies (refs. 6, 13, 18, 25, 39, 55, 60). Short and intermediate survival is reasonable, however, ultimate survival after onset of symptoms is approximately 10% at 10 yr. In contrast, actuarial survival of patients with amyloid heart disease from compiled data (refs. 17, 22, 30, 37, 38, 42, 63) is extremely poor. There essentially is no survival beyond 24 months from the onset of cardiac symptoms.

and small series of patients with amyloidosis where individual clinical and follow-up data were available.[120,131-136] Myeloma, plasmacytoma, or other plasma cell dyscrasias are present overall in 45% of cases of cardiac amyloidosis. Based on the age distribution for plasma cell diseases, one would expect and the data confirms an overall older group of patients in this

TABLE 13.7. Clinical characteristics of 14 patients with amyloid cardiomyopathy.[a]

Age: mean: 56 yr; range: 44–86 yr	
Sex: 50% male; 50% female	
Symptomatology	
Chest pain	0%
Fatigue	73%
Dyspnea	100%
Clinical findings	
Jugular venous distension	83%
Rales	58%
S3	91%
S4	50%
Ascites	55%
Edema	92%
Hemodynamics	
Right atrial (mm Hg)	14 ± 4
Pulmonary wedge (mm Hg)	20 ± 3
Cardiac index (L/min/m²)	2.1 ± 0.4
LVEDVI (ml/m²)	60 ± 14
LV ejection fraction	$.57 \pm .10$

LVEDVI = left ventricular end diastolic volume index.
[a] Compiled data from seven studies.[120,131–135]. Results expressed as mean $\pm$ 1 SD.

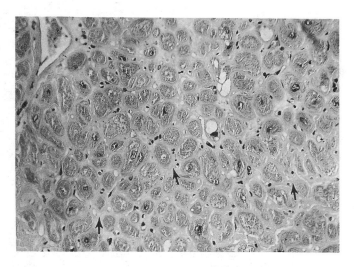

FIGURE 13.9. Endomyocardial biopsy (hematoxylin-eosin, ×250) from a patient with amyloid heart disease showing extensive deposits of amorphous material surrounding individual myocytes (*arrows*) within the interstitium. Reprinted, with permission, from Hosenpud JD. Restrictive cardiomyopathy. *Progress in cardiology*. 1989, Lea & Febiger.

form of restrictive cardiomyopathy compared to patients with primary disease. The remainder of cases of cardiac amyloidosis, with few exceptions, are manifestations of systemic disease and have amyloid deposition found in multiple other organs. Patients with amyloid heart disease tend to be more symptomatic, more often clinically in congestive heart failure, and have reduced cardiac indices in contrast to the normal cardiac outputs seen in primary restrictive cardiomyopathy.

The gross anatomic findings in amyloid heart disease are similar to those with primary restrictive cardiomyopathy with some notable differences. Both left and right ventricular wall thicknesses on echo tend to be increased symmetrically, and there is hypokinesis of the intraventricular septum. The AV valves also are involved and can appear thickened on echocardiography. Finally, a particular granular and speckled pattern of the myocardium has been described.[137–139] Unfortunately, this particular finding can be quite variable depending on gain settings and the particular machine used. Therefore, amyloid should not be ruled in or out based on the echo tissue characteristics. Figure 13.9 demonstrates histopathology from an endomyocardial biopsy on a patient with severe restrictive cardiomyopathy secondary to amyloid infiltration. The amyloid protein is deposited throughout the interstitium, surrounding individual myocytes, with larger deposition in the perivascular areas. If one views amyloid in tissue under polarized light, a characteristic green birefringance is present.

Reviewing again Figure 13.8, it is clear that the prognosis of patients with restrictive cardiomyopathy sec-

ondary to amyloidosis is extremely poor compared to those with idiopathic restrictive disease, in contrast to the relatively long survival of patients with no survival beyond 2 yr of symptoms. These prognostic data are supported further by a larger single study of patients with amyloid heart disease and CHF in whom median survival was 6 months.[140]

Endomyocardial fibrosis with or without eosinophilia was first described by Loeffler in 1930,[141] and is another frequently cited cause of restrictive cardiomyopathy. Since Loeffler's original two patients, more than 100 cases have been reported. It has been suggested that eosinophilic damage to the endocardium is the primary etiology in all cases of endomyocardial fibrosis, and that those patients without documented eosinophilia are presenting at a later stage of the disease.[142] The mechanism of injury appears to be a direct toxic effect of eosinophilic secretory products (granule basic proteins) on the myocardium.[143] The pattern of injury appears to progress through three stages: the necrotic stage, in which there is an eosinophilic endomyocarditis and arteritis, a mural thrombosis stage, during which platelets and thrombin are deposited along the damaged endothelium, and a fibrotic stage, where the endocardial thrombus and damaged endothelium are replaced by fibrous tissue.[144,145]

The resulting restrictive hemodynamic findings in patients with endomyocardial fibrosis may have different mechanisms depending on the stage of the disease process. During the thrombotic stage, in addition to the endomyocardial damage, ventricular thrombi may be so large that the remaining ventricular chamber volume is inadequate to sustain cardiac output. In the fibrotic stage, the thick endocardial peel presumably prevents normal diastolic relaxation.

The cardiovascular clinical findings in endomyocardial fibrosis are identical to those found in other forms of restrictive cardiomyopathy and include symptoms and signs of biventricular CHF.[146–149] The prognosis appears to be quite variable and probably depends on the underlying disease process. Although eosinophilia can be present for a prolonged period before the development of cardiac symptoms,[150] once cardiac symptoms develop, prognosis appears to be poor.[150–152] In studies where aggressive therapy is directed simultaneously to reducing the total eosinophil count, treating the CHF, and in some cases surgical endomyocardial stripping and valve replacement, the outcome may be modified.[144,146,148]

Other Causes

Other reported causes of restrictive cardiomyopathy have included sarcoidosis and other granulomatous diseases of the myocardium,[142,153] hemochromatosis,[154] cardiac tumors,[155,156] radiation,[157] anthracycline toxicity,[158] collagen vascular diseases,[159] genetic connective tissue diseases,[160] and coronary arteritis.[161] Most recently, it has been suggested that the cardiac allograft exhibits "restrictive" physiology.[162,163] Whether this is an intrinsic myocardial abnormality or an artifact of donor/recipient size matching and/or problems with recipient volume, regulation currently requires more investigation.

Restrictive Cardiomyopathy Versus Constrictive Pericarditis

Despite a large body of medical literature on the subject, differentiation between myocardial and pericardial disease frequently is difficult. Attempts to differentiate these entities have relied on subtle differences in physical findings, imaging techniques looking at both structural differences and subtle functional differences, and endomyocardial biopsy (Table 13.8). Even with careful noninvasive and less invasive studies, however, diagnostic thoracotomy sometimes is necessary.

Ramsey and colleagues in 1970 reported using coronary angiography and determining the relationship between the coronary arteries and the epicardium as a measure of pericardial thickening. In a small number of cases, they accurately distinguished pericardial constriction from myocardial disease and confirmed this at thoracotomy.[164] Chang and Grollman utilized both right ventricular wall motion as well as coronary

TABLE 13.8. Differentiation between constrictive pericarditis and restrictive cardiomyopathy.

Method	Constriction	Restriction
Physical exam		
A wave	Absent	Present (large)
Kussmaul's sign	Usually present	Absent
Pericardial knock	Can be present	Absent
AV valve murmurs	Usually absent	Usually present
Diagnostic studies		
Computerized tomography	Thickened pericardium	Normal pericardium
Magnetic resonance	Thickened pericardium	Normal pericardium
Coronary angiography	Coronaries displaced from epicardium	Normal anatomic relationship with epicardium
Echocardiography	Rapid early filling	Delayed filling
Left ventriculography	Rapid early filling	Delayed filling
Catheterization	Identical LV and RV filling pressures	Disparate LV and RV pressures at baseline or with volume changes
Endomyocardial biopsy	Normal histology	Myopathic or specific histology

Reprinted with permission from Hosenpud JD. Restrictive cardiomyopathy. *Progress in cardiology*. 1989, Lea & Febiger.
LV = left ventricular; RV = right ventricular.

angiography as previously described. They noted that in constrictive pericarditis although the right ventricular free wall had impaired motion, the crista supraventricularis moved normally. This was not the case in patients with amyloid heart disease.[165] Echocardiographic examination of the pericardium has yielded conflicting results presumably because transducer positioning and gain settings can substantially influence the reflected signal from the pericardium.[166] This does not appear to be a problem using either computerized tomographic (CT) imaging or magnetic resonance imaging (MRI). In three studies utilizing these modalities to assess pericardial thickness, differentiation between restrictive myocardial disease and constrictive pericarditis was uniformly successful.[167–169] The numbers of patients in these studies, however, were extremely small.

Attempts to make the myocardial/pericardial distinction using physiologic parameters have relied on relatively subtle differences in diastolic filling characteristics. Nye and colleagues noted that the right ventricular end-diastolic pressure was equal to or greater than one third of the systolic pressure in constriction and less than one third systolic pressure in restrictive disease.[170] Gould, in an early observation, noted the absence of the A wave on catheterization in patients with constriction and giant A waves in myopathic restriction.[171] Lewis and Gotsman demonstrated a reduction in the maximal rate of left ventricular pressure fall (negative dp/dt) in patients with constrictive pericarditis when compared to controls, however, these patients were not compared to patients with restrictive cardiomyopathy.[172] Tyberg and colleagues, using digitized left ventriculograms, demonstrated that patients with constrictive pericarditis had a premature plateau in diastolic filling, whereas patients with restriction had no plateau and the left ventricular filling rate was slower than normal during the first half of diastole.[120] A similar study by Janos et al. utilizing digitized M-mode echocardiography demonstrated that left ventricular filling was shortened in constriction and lengthened in restriction when compared to normals.[119]

In a recent study reported by Schoenfeld and colleagues,[173] a moderately sized population of patients with restrictive/constrictive physiology underwent endomyocardial biopsy in the hope of distinguishing cardiac from pericardial disease. In this study, there were no significant clinical or physiologic differences between those patients ultimately diagnosed with restriction versus those with constriction. Endomyocardial biopsy, however, yielded a specific myocardial diagnosis in 13 of the 19 patients with restriction, obviating the need for thoracotomy in these patients.[173]

It is clear from the above studies that differentiation between restrictive cardiomyopathy and constrictive pericarditis requires the compilation of data from a number of diagnostic studies. In most cases, the diagnosis should be achievable short of thoracotomy.

Therapy

Specific Therapy

In patients with primary restrictive cardiomyopathy, as no specific etiology is known, there obviously is no specific treatment. Although there is no evidence to suggest that the treatment of myeloma, plasma cell dyscrasias, or chronic inflammatory processes will alter the natural history of amyloid heart disease, one could hypothesize an arresting or stabilizing of the cardiac condition with control of the underlying disease. As discussed earlier, aggressive therapy of eosinophilic systemic disease may influence the endomyocardial damage[148]; once damage is present, aggressive surgical therapy may improve cardiac performance.[146] There have been isolated reports of aggressive total body iron removal influencing cardiac function in patients with hemochromatosis,[154] and corticosteroid therapy improving cardiac performance in patients with sarcoidosis and other granulomatous diseases of the myocardium.[153]

Generic Therapy

Generic therapy for restriction is extremely difficult once severe cardiovascular compromise is present. Diuretics are a mainstay of therapy but require cautious use. As the diastolic ventricular pressure/volume relationship in restrictive cardiomyopathy is quite steep, small changes in volume can produce large changes in filling pressures. The decrease in myocardial compliance requires higher filling pressures for adequate ventricular filling, so a reduction in filling pressures to alleviate symptoms of congestion may produce dramatic falls in cardiac output. Systolic performance in patients with restrictive cardiomyopathy usually is normal and may in some patients be at the upper range of normal. This finding limits the use of inotropic agents, and digitalis specifically may have a role only in rhythm control as many patients with restriction and atrial dilation will have atrial arrhythmias. In addition, patients with amyloid heart disease may have a supersensitivity to the toxic effects of digitalis.[140]

Vasodilator therapy, although a mainstay of therapy for most forms of heart failure, may have a very small role in restrictive disease. In restriction, stroke volume depends on high filling pressures and usually is fixed at peak pressures. As cardiac dilation is seldom present, this component of wall stress would not play a major role. The expected response in patients with restrictive cardiomyopathy to vasodilator therapy would be a reduction in preload, reducing filling, and stroke volume, and a potentially profound reduction in arterial pressure secondary to both arteriolar dilation and the fall in cardiac output. Furthermore, the beneficial effects of calcium channel blockers in hypertrophic cardiomyopathy have not been demonstrated with restrictive cardiomyopathy. As most calcium antagonists are vasodilators, the effects anticipated with vasodilator therapy also would be anticipated with calcium channel antagonists. In addition, both verapamil and diltiazam have direct suppressant effects on sinus node function resulting in a slowing of heart rate, and have negative inotropic properties.[174] In patients where stroke volume is fixed and cardiac output is heart-rate dependent, it is evident that calcium channel blocking agents have more potential deleterious than beneficial effects. Furthermore, in both the infiltrative diseases as well as those where the endomyocardium is primarily affected, one would expect the myocardial diastolic properties to be relatively normal.

Therapy for restrictive cardiomyopathy therefore is limited for all practical purposes to diuretic therapy for mild to moderate symptoms and cardiac transplantation for patients with severe disease.

Hypertrophic Cardiomyopathy

Pathophysiology and Mechanisms of Disease

Hypertrophic cardiomyopathy, initially described by Teare in 1958,[175] has since been surrounded by controversy and still is poorly understood. A reflection of

FIGURE 13.10. The presentation of hypertrophic cardiomyopathy is highly variable, even within the same family. One can present with hypertrophy primarily localized to the septum with or without obstruction, which when present occurs at the level of the anterior mitral leaflet or a more diffuse pattern of hypertrophic disease involving the entire left ventricle.

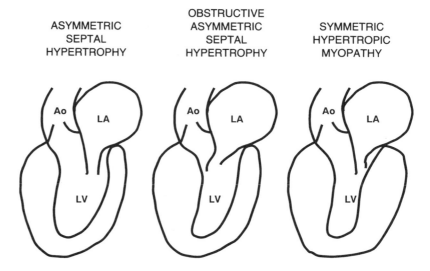

ASYMMETRIC SEPTAL HYPERTROPHY

OBSTRUCTIVE ASYMMETRIC SEPTAL HYPERTROPHY

SYMMETRIC HYPERTROPIC MYOPATHY

this are the several primarily descriptive names of the disease, including hypertrophic obstructive cardiomyopathy, idiopathic hypertrophic subaortic stenosis, asymmetric septal hypertrophy, and muscular subaortic stenosis, all related to the concept that outflow tract obstruction is a principal pathophysiologic mechanism. However, this aspect of the disease is controversial. In fact, most students of primary myocardial disease feel that although outflow tract obstruction may be present, the principal abnormality is that of impaired ventricular compliance, which is likely due to the inappropriate myocardial hypertrophy. Hence, hypertrophic cardiomyopathy, now the most commonly used terminology, is likely the most appropriate.

What is clear is that a distinctive pattern of hypertrophy involving the ventricular septum out of proportion to the other ventricular walls (asymmetric septal hypertrophy-ASH) is present in most patients. Microscopically, in the areas of hypertrophy the myocardial fibers are disorganized without evidence of the usual orientation parallel to the lines of stress. This has been referred to as myofibril disarray. In addition to the asymmetric septal hypertrophy, most patients will have evidence of a pressure gradient across the aortic outflow tract caused primarily by the mitral valve moving anteriorly during systole and abutting the septum, termed "systolic anterior motion" (SAM).[176] The specific controversies surrounding the measured pressure gradient are discussed later.

The disease appears to be inherited as an autosomal dominant one in between 50% and 75% of cases, with the remainder being sporadic.[177,178] As with other autosomal dominant diseases, penetrance and phenotype even within a given family can be quite variable. As previously stated, most patients manifest asymmetric septal hypertrophy and a measured gradient. Others, however (even within the same family), manifest a more concentric hypertrophy or ASH without "obstruction" (Figure 13.10). The etiology of the abnormal hypertrophy is unknown, although several theories have been proposed. The earliest of these was that hypertrophic cardiomyopathy was an abnormal response to hypertension.[179] It soon became clear, however, that hypertension was not present in most patients with the disorder. Hutchins and Bulkley suggested that the shape of the septum in hypertrophic cardiomyopathy is abnormal, resembling a catenoid, and that this shape promotes isometric contraction and hence the resulting hypertrophy.[180] Unfortunately this does not explain those cases where hypertrophy is more concentric. The finding of increased numbers of sympathetic nerve fibers in the septum,[181] the production of a similar syndrome in dogs using norepinephrine or nerve growth factor administration infusions,[182] have led some to suggest that hypertrophic cardiomyopathy is a developmental disorder of adrenergic nervous system regulation. Finally, Liew and colleagues have demonstrated abnormalities in myocardial nuclear proteins (nonhistone), suggesting abnormalities of regulation at the cellular and molecular levels.[183]

Figure 13.11 demonstrates the typical M-mode and two-dimensional echocardiographic findings from a patient with hypertrophic cardiomyopathy and an outflow tract gradient. As previously stated, the gradient is produced by the anterior leaflet of the mitral valve (MV) abutting the septum in late systole. It was assumed that the primary morbidity of this disease was based on this outflow tract "obstruction" similar to that of fixed aortic valvular disease. It was Criley who first suggested that the outflow tract gradients seen in patients with hypertrophic cardiomyopathy were due to the extremely powerful and rapid contraction of the ventricle and the resulting cavity obliteration.[184] This school proposed that the primary morbidity in hypertrophic cardiomyopathy was secondary to abnormal diastolic function and ventricular stiffness rather than obstruction.[185–187] Arguments for and against the importance of obstruction peppered the medical literature for the

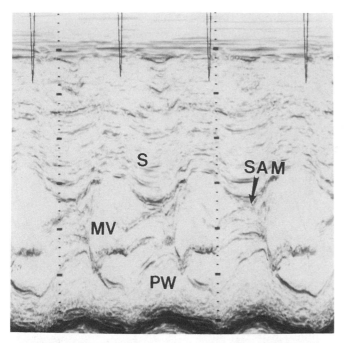

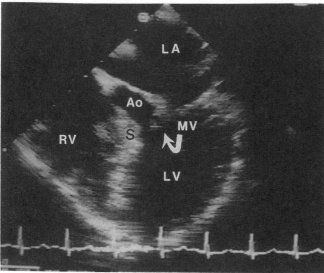

FIGURE 13.11. The typical M-mode (*top*) and transesophageal (*bottom*) echocardiograms seen in patients with hypertrophic cardiomyopathy. With the onset of systole, the mitral valve (*MV*) exhibits systolic anterior motion (*SAM*) and abuts the ventricular septum (*S*), causing an outflow tract gradient. LV = left ventricle; RV = right ventricle; PW = posterior wall; LA = left atrium; Ao = aorta.

the creation of a larger ventricular chamber allowing greater left ventricular filling, beta-blockers slowing heart rate and reducing contractility, thus allowing for improved diastolic function, and calcium antagonists both reducing contractility and possibly directly altering diastolic properties of the myocardium. Finally, there did not appear to be any difference in ultimate prognosis or symptoms between patients with or without an outflow tract gradient.[190,191]

Clinical Features of Hypertrophic Cardiomyopathy

Symptoms

The principal symptoms of patients with hypertrophic cardiomyopathy are dyspnea, chest pain, and syncope.[179,192-194] Exertional dyspnea certainly is the most common symptom and has been reported in upwards of 90% of patients with the disease.[195] The etiology of the dyspnea is likely secondary to high filling pressures, especially with exercise, secondary to the reduced myocardial compliance.[185-187] It is clear that this symptom (along with chest pain and syncope) does not correlate with the presence or amount of the outflow tract gradient.[196,197]

Angina is the next most frequent symptom and can occur in up to 75% of patients.[198] Moreover, myocardial infarction has been documented in 15% of patients at autopsy.[199] The infarction can, on rare occasion, involve the entire subendocardium resulting in complete shelling of the entire left ventricular subendocardium. The mechanism of the angina and myocardial necrosis is felt to be a combination of inadequate subendocardial coronary blood flow to meet the needs of the marked hypertrophy, direct subendocardial vascular compression due to high systolic and diastolic left ventricular cavity pressures, and abnormal regulation of the coronary microcirculation.[199-204]

Syncope or near syncope has been reported in up to 50% of patients with hypertrophic cardiomyopathy.[192-194] Although initially thought to be secondary to the outflow tract gradient through mechanisms similar to those seen in valvular aortic stenosis, it is clear now that there is no relationship between syncopal symptoms and the severity of outflow tract gradients.[192-194,197,205] Based on Holter monitor and treadmill exercise studies demonstrating frequent ventricular and atrial arrhythmias and overt ventricular tachycardia in up to 40% of patients, the syncope is most certainly arrhythmic in etiology in most cases.[206-209] Based on electrophysiologic studies, the propensity for ventricular tachyarrhythmias may be due to disordered electrophysiologic properties of the abnormally hypertrophied ventricle.[210] The mechanism for atrial arrhythmias may be solely the elevated ven-

next 15 years with proponents of the "obstruction school" citing the beneficial effects of septal myectomy, the reduction in gradients with beta blockers and calcium channel blockers as supportive evidence.[188,189] The opposing school countered with evidence suggesting that most of the ejection from the left ventricle occurred before the development of the gradient and the cavity obliteration seen in most patients.[184,190] The counter explanation for surgical improvement was

tricular filling pressures resulting in atrial stretch.[208,209] Other abnormalities including associated atrioventricular (A-V) bypass tracts have been reported.[211]

Finally, in a minority of patients and usually late in the disease, systolic ventricular function deteriorates and more characteristic symptoms of heart failure supervene. Signs and symptoms of both left and right ventricular dysfunction can occur, especially if patients lose sinus rhythm and atrioventricular synchrony.[192,196]

Overall, patients with hypertrophic cardiomyopathy are less symptomatic than patients with other forms of cardiomyopathy. A full 30% of patients will be asymptomatic, as evidenced by recent well publicized stories of athletes dying suddenly during a sporting event who subsequently were found to have hypertrophic cardiomyopathy. Another 50% of patients are NYHA functional class II; it is a rare patient who presents with functional class IV symptoms.[193,212]

Clinical Findings

Clinical findings in patients without resting or exercise outflow tract gradients can be entirely normal or may be confined to signs of elevated left ventricular filling pressures (fourth heart sound). In the more advanced stages, especially with loss of sinus rhythm and progressive ventricular dysfunction, signs of both systemic and pulmonary venous congestion can be present. In patients with a resting or provocable outflow tract gradient, the clinical examination can be diagnostic. Figure 13.12 demonstrates a representation of the carotid impulse from a patient with hypertrophic cardiomyopathy and contrasts this with a patient with valvular aortic stenosis (AS). In contrast to the patient with AS in whom

TABLE 13.9. Maneuvers differentiating aortic stenosis from hypertrophic cardiomyopathy.

Maneuver	AS	HCM
Decrease ventricular volume		
Valsalva	D	I
Upright posture	U	I
Amyl nitrate		
Increase contractility		
Post-PVC	I	I
Exercise	I	I
Increase ventricular volume		
Leg elevation	I	D
Pregnancy	I	D
Increase arterial pressure		
Handgrip	D	D
Phenylephrine	D	D

D = Decrease murmur intensity; I = increase murmur intensity; U = unchanged murmur intensity; PVC = premature ventricular contractions.

the carotid impulse is reduced in amplitude and delayed in timing, the carotid impulse in the patient with hypertrophic cardiomyopathy is rapid in upstroke, bifid, and followed by a prominent dicrotic notch. This "spike and dome" pulse tracing is secondary to the rapid ventricular emptying due to the enhanced contractility, followed by the abrupt reduction of flow secondary to the mitral valve anterior motion (SAM) occluding the outflow tract.

The jugular venous pressure is typical of patients with reduced ventricular compliance. So long as the patient remains in sinus rhythm, the a wave is large and usually the v wave is normal unless significant tricuspid regurgitation is present.

As the outflow tract gradient is dynamic, the murmur in patients with hypertrophic cardiomyopathy is quite characteristic and can be altered by a series of bedside maneuvers or pharmacologic interventions. Table 13.9 contrasts the murmur of hypertrophic cardiomyopathy with that of fixed AS. In general, the murmur is heard best along the left sternal border and usually does not radiate well into the carotid arteries. In contrast to valvular aortic stenosis, any maneuver that reduces preload and hence ventricular size accentuates the murmur due to an earlier abutment of the mitral valve against the septum and an increase in the outflow tract gradient. Conversely, any maneuver that increases ventricular size such as leg raising or squatting will reduce the intensity of the murmur. Similarly with AS, an increase in contractility or reduction in afterload (post-VPB (ventricular premature beat), amyl nitrate) will increase the intensity of the murmur. In contrast to AS, however, these latter maneuvers actually will decrease the pulse pressure as assessed by carotid or brachial palpation due to the earlier occurrence of SAM. Finally, in addition to the outflow tract murmur, many pa-

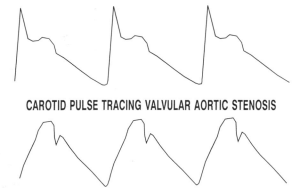

CAROTID PULSE TRACING HYPERTROPHIC CARDIOMYOPATHY

CAROTID PULSE TRACING VALVULAR AORTIC STENOSIS

FIGURE 13.12. The carotid impulse in patients with hypertrophic cardiomyopathy demonstrate a characteristic rapid initial upstroke followed by a "dip and plateau" resulting from the abrupt cessation of blood flow secondary to the anterior motion of the mitral valve. This contrasts the delayed upstroke and prominant dicrotic notch (especially with low cardiac output) seen in patients with native aortic stenosis.

tients, especially those with moderate to severe SAM of the mitral valve, will have coexistent mitral insufficiency of varying degrees.

Invasive and Noninvasive Studies

The electrocardiogram in patients with hypertrophic cardiomyopathy most often demonstrates left ventricular hypertrophy,[192] left atrial enlargement, and abnormal Q waves usually in the inferior and lateral leads.[213] As previously mentioned, holter monitoring demonstrates both atrial and ventricular arrhythmias.

The echocardiogram has become the primary diagnostic tool for confirming the diagnosis of hypertrophic cardiomyopathy. As previously discussed, the upper panel of Figure 13.11 demonstrates the typical M-mode echocardiogram from a patient with hypertrophic cardiomyopathy. The most striking feature is the markedly thickened intraventricular septum (S), but the posterior wall also is thickened compared to normal. The mitral valve (MV) moves anteriorly during systole (SAM), abutting the septum and "obstructing" the outflow tract. The lower panel demonstrates the similar findings on a transesophageal two-dimensional echocardiogram from a different patient. Other echocardiographic abnormalities described have included abnormalities in diastolic time intervals both by traditional echo as well as Doppler techniques.[214–219] Shaver and colleagues studying 84 patients with hypertrophic cardiomyopathy demonstrated abnormally prolonged isovolumic relaxation periods in 31 of the 84.[220]

The hemodynamic findings of patients with hypertrophic cardiomyopathy with outflow tract gradients are well described.[221–224] Figure 13.13 demonstrates a representation of left ventricular and aortic pressure tracings corresponding to the above clinical findings of the phenomenon first described by Brokenbrough and colleagues.[224] The systolic contraction immediately following a premature ventricular complex has augmented contractility, which results in higher intraventricular pressure. This augmentation of ventricular pressure results in an earlier anterior motion of the mitral valve, a larger outflow tract gradient, and a fall in aortic pressure compared to the normal beat. As described above, the same maneuvers used at the bedside to change loading conditions and volume of the ventricle alter a resting gradient or can provoke a gradient that was not present at rest.[222] With careful hemodynamic monitoring during left ventricular pullback, the gradient usually can be found within the left ventricular outflow tract before crossing the aortic valve. Other associated hemodynamic findings include elevations in both left and right ventricular filling pressures, a corresponding accentuation of the a wave in both ventricles, and in a minority of patients in the latter stages of the disease a reduction in cardiac output.[225]

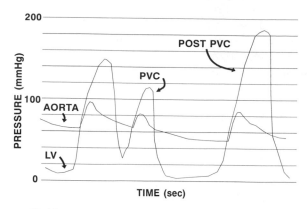

FIGURE 13.13. A representation of the aortic and left ventricular (LV) pressure tracing in a patient with hypertrophic cardiomyopathy. The "Brokenbrough" effect is produced by a premature ventricular contraction (PVC) causing postsystolic potentiation of the subsequent beat. The increase in contractility increases the intraventricular pressure, the outflow tract gradient increases, and pulse pressure actually falls.

Angiographic findings include the asymmetric septal hypertrophy, a small hypercontractile ventricle often with complete cavity obliteration (evidence against hemodynamically important "obstruction"), and hypertrophied papillary muscles. Mitral regurgitation can range from mild to severe. The shape of the ventricle in systole has been referred to as an inverted cone because of the massive hypertrophy and cavity obliteration that encroaches on the outflow tract.[221–225]

Therapy

Medical Management

As early as 1964, Harrison and colleagues reported the potential benefits of beta-blocking agents on the hemodynamics of patients with hypertrophic cardiomyopathy.[226] Since that time, several studies have demonstrated the efficacy of these agents both in reducing symptoms as well as improving hemodynamics. Most hemodynamic studies demonstrated a reduction in the outflow tract gradient with beta-blockade and suggested that improvement in symptoms was secondary to this reduction.[227,228] Other, more likely mechanisms include the reduction in contractility reducing myocardial oxygen demand both at rest and during exercise, the reduction of heart rate allowing for an increase in diastolic time and filling, and possibly a reduction in the amount of mitral regurgitation. Initial studies suggested that beta-blockade might improve diastolic function,[229,230] but subsequent careful studies of diastolic indicies have not supported this.[231,232] Finally, beta-blockers may impact the generation of ventricular arrhythmias, especially during exercise and stress when catecholamine levels are elevated. Although the initial response to beta-blockers in many patients is quite good, the long-term response has been less satisfactory, with many patients experiencing fatigue and depression especially if high doses of beta-blockers are required.

In contrast to beta-blockers, a large body of work has demonstrated the efficacy and sustained response of patients with hypertrophic cardiomyopathy to treatment with calcium channel blockers.[233–236] Although several of the calcium channel blockers have been demonstrated to be efficacious, most of the experience has been with verapamil. Rosing and colleagues demonstrated that verapamil improved exercise performance by an average of 45% in 19 patients with hypertrophic cardiomyopathy.[237] In this study there was no correlation between improvement in exercise and change in outflow tract gradient, which was reduced by an average of 35 mm Hg. Like the beta-blockers, calcium channel blockers exert their efficacy by a combination of factors including a reduction in contractility and a reduction in heart rate, but unlike the beta-blockers, there is reproducible evidence that calcium channel blockers improve diastolic function in this disease. Shaffer et al. demonstrated that verapamil improved two indices of diastolic function (peak filling rate and time to peak filling rate) and improved exercise performance in 10 children (ages 7 to 18 years) for an average treatment period of 1.8 yr.[238] The mechanisms responsible for improved relaxation potentially include an improvement in coronary flow resulting in reduced subendocardial ischemia, a possible improvement in ventricular synchrony, and an improvement in both preload and afterload.[239,240] There also is experimental evidence that abnormal cardiac hypertrophy results in altered calcium flux and an intracellular calcium overload state.[241] In experimentally induced calcium overload, verapamil improves relaxation in cultured myocardial cells.[242]

More recent studies have demonstrated a hemodynamically beneficial effect of the antiarrhythmic agent amiodarone.[243] The mechanisms responsible for this efficacy are unclear but may be due to the negative inotropic effects of this agent along with vascular dilation. There also may be the added benefit of suppression of ventricular arrhythmias. This agent has been demonstrated to improve symptoms of patients refractory to both beta-blockers and calcium channel blockers.[244]

In patients with elevated filling pressures, careful use of diuretic therapy is indicated. As with restrictive cardiomyopathy, one is hampered by the need to reduce resting filling pressures enough to eliminate symptoms of congestion but not enough to reduce ventricular filling. This is particularly difficult in patients who are in chronic atrial fibrillation, as atrial contraction in this disease can be responsible for as much as 50% of ventricular filling.

Arrhythmia management is a major concern in patients with hypertrophic cardiomyopathy. Patients may become severely symptomatic with loss of atrial synchrony as alluded to above. It is reasonable to attempt to convert atrial arrhythmias either electrically or pharmacologically and try to maintain sinus rhythm in patients who become symptomatic with loss of A-V synchrony. Amiodarone has been demonstrated to be beneficial in controlling both atrial and ventricular arrhythmias in patients with hypertrophic cardiomyopathy.

Finally, attempts to prevent comorbidity should be undertaken. In patients with intermittent or persistent atrial fibrillation, systemic anticoagulation is indicated and in patients with a systolic murmur consistent with SAM, endocarditis prophylaxis is required.

Surgical Management

The first report of surgical therapy for hypertrophic cardiomyopathy was presented by Morrow and Brockenbrough in 1961 in which a subaortic ventriculomyotomy was performed on two patients with a reduction in outflow tract gradient and clinical improvement.[245] Since that time, the procedure has been modified, and many patients refractory to medical management have undergone the procedure.[246] The overall operative mortality ranges from 0 to 26%, depending on the series, with additional late mortality.[247] Maron reported on 124 patients undergoing septal myotomy-myectomy at the National Institutes of Health with an operative mortality of 8%. Eighty-eight percent of patients showed clinical improvement in the first 6 months postoperation and this improvement persisted in 70% of the initial group.[188]

Figure 13.14 demonstrates the completed septal myotomy-myectomy procedure. The mechanisms by which improvement occurs after this operation are not clear. There is no doubt that the procedure reduces the resting outflow tract gradient.[188] It is also well documented that the clinical results of the operation do not correlate with the preoperative gradient or hemodynamics.[188] If reduction in the gradient is the principal mechanism for improvement, then the reduction in left ventricular pressures could be seen to reduce myocardial oxygen demand, improve coronary flow, and possibly improved diastolic function by reducing ischemia. Alternatively, septal myotomy-myectomy does increase the size of the ventricular chamber. This increase in size in and of itself may improve filling characteristics and increase stroke volume and cardiac output.

The current recommendations for septal myotomy-myectomy are that it be undertaken only for patients

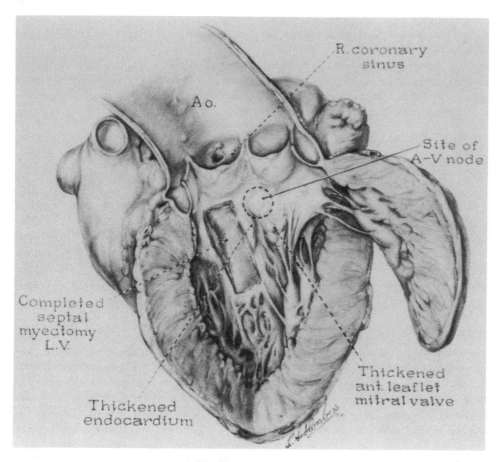

FIGURE 13.14. A completed septal myectomy is demonstrated. Reprinted, with permission, from Morrow AG, Hypertrophic subaortic stenosis. *J Thorac Cardiovasc Surg*. 1974;76:429.

who are refractory to medical management and who have an outflow tract gradient of at least 50 mm Hg. As there is no evidence that surgical therapy prolongs survival or has an impact on arrhythmias in these patients, symptoms alone must justify the surgical risks.

Prognosis

Figure 13.15 demonstrates the survival of four patient groups presented in three studies.[188,191,248] In a large cohort of patients from the United Kingdom in which 184 patients were adults at the time of diagnosis and 27 were children, the overall 10-yr actuarial survival was greater than 80% in the adults and less than 60 percent in the pediatric group.[191] In a large surgical series from the National Institutes of Health, the 10-yr actuarial survival was somewhat lower than the adult series, but above 70%.[188] However, in a meta-analysis of both surgical and medical approaches to this disease, Canedo and Frank compared 255 surgically treated and 184 medically treated patients with hypertrophic cardiomyopathy and could demonstrate no differences in outcome between groups.[247] In a selected series of 33 patients who had experienced cardiac arrest and were resuscitated successfully, their outcome was substantially poorer than the general adult experience, with a 10-yr actuarial survival of less than 65%.[248] Finally, an interesting study from Spirito and colleagues pointed out

the difficulty of determining the natural history of a disease using data from recognized referral centers for that disease. In a group of 25 outpatients with the diagnosis of hypertrophic cardiomyopathy and a mean follow-up period of 4.4 yr, there were no deaths nor evidence of clinical deterioration documented.[249] Therefore, the prognosis appears particularly good in the relatively asymptomatic patient with this disease.

Aside from mortality, there is a real incidence of morbid events in patients with hypertrophic cardiomyopathy. Approximately 5% of patients will develop endocarditis, another 5% to 10% will experience systemic emboli, approximately 10% to 15% eventually will develop atrial fibrillation, and around 5%–10% will have myocardial decompensation and symptoms of heart failure. Recognizing these comorbid events in this patient population and directing preventative therapy (antibiotic prophylaxis, anticoagulation) where available hopefully will impact the incidence of these complications.

Conclusions

The cardiomyopathies are a heterogeneous group of diseases with multiple associations but disease mechanisms that are largely unknown. The anatomic classification of cardiomyopathies, albeit primitive, allows for

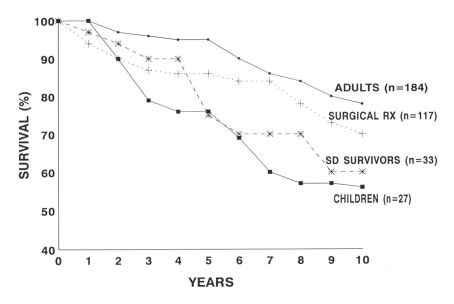

FIGURE 13.15. Survival in four groups of patients with hypertrophic cardiomyopathy is demonstrated (refs. 188, 192, 253). There appears to be no difference in survival in adult patients treated medically or surgically. High-risk groups appear to be children and those with a prior history of cardiac arrest.

some insight in etiology and association and definite insights into medical management and prognosis. Direct therapy currently is unavailable for most of the diseases and generic heart failure management certainly is limited. In those individuals where prognosis is poor, cardiac transplantation should be ultimately considered.

References

1. Krehl L. Beitrag zur Kentniss der idiopathischen Herzmuskelerkrankungen. *Dtsch Arch F Klin Med.* 1891; 48:414–431.
2. Josserand E, Gallavardin L. De l'asystole progressive des jeunes sujets par myocardite subaigue primitive. *Arch Gen Med.* 1901;6:684–704.
3. Brigden W. Uncommon myocardial diseases. The non-coronary cardiomyopathies. *Lancet.* 1957;2:1243–1249.
4. Fejfar Z. Accounts of international meetings: idiopathic cardiomegaly. *Bull WHO.* 1968;28:979–992.
5. WHO:ISFC Task Force. Report on the WHO/ISFC task force on the definition and classification of cardiomyopathies. *Br Heart J.* 1980;44:672–673.
6. Douglas PS, Morrow R, Ioli A, Reichek N. Left ventricular shape, afterload and survival in idiopathic dilated cardiomyopathy. *J Am Coll Cardiol.* 1989;13: 311–315.
7. Grossman W, Jones D, McLaurin LP. Wall stress and patterns of hypertrophy in the human left ventricle. *J Clin Invest.* 1975;56:56–64.
8. O'Keefe DD, Hoffman JIE, Cheitlin R, O'Neill, MJ, Allard JR, Shapkin E. Coronary blood flow in experimental canine left ventricular hypertrophy. *Circ Res.* 1978;43:43–51.
9. Limas CJ, Olivari MT, Goldenberg IF, Levine TB, Benditt DG, Simon A. Calcium uptake by cardiac sarcoplasmic reticulum in human dilated cardiomyopathy. *Cardiovasc Res.* 1987;21:601–605.

10. Bristow MR, Ginsburg R, Minobe W, et al. Decreased catecholamine sensitivity and beta-adrenergic-receptor density in failing human hearts. *N Engl J Med.* 1982;307:205–211.
11. Heilbrunn SM, Shah P, Bristow MR, Valentine HA, Ginsburg R, Fowler MB. Increased beta-receptor density and improved hemodynamic response to catecholamine stimulation during long-term metoprolol therapy in heart failure from dilated cardiomyopathy. *Circulation.* 1989;79:483–490.
12. Feldman AM, Cates AE, Veazey WB, et al. Increase of the 40,000-mol. wt. pertussis toxin substrate (G protein) in the failing human heart. *J Clin Invest.* 1988;82:189–197.
13. Bohm M, Gierschik P, Jakobs KH, et al. Increase of G_i alpha in human hearts with dilated but not ischemic cardiomyopathy. *Circulation.* 1990;82:1249–1265.
14. Bohm M, Ungerer M, Erdmann E. Beta adrenoceptors and M-cholinoceptors in myocardium of hearts with coronary artery disease or idiopathic dilated cardiomyopathy removed at cardiac transplantation. *Am J Cardiol.* 1990;66:880–882.
15. Walsh RA, Henkel R, Robbins J. Cardiac myocin heavy- and light-chain gene expression in hypertrophy and heart disease. *Heart Failure.* 1990–91;6:238–243.
16. Robinson JA, O'Connell JB. *Myocarditis: precursor of cardiomyopathy.* Lexington, MA: Collamore Press; 1983.
17. Hosenpud JD. Chronic idiopathic myocarditis: controversies in causes and therapy. *Cardiovasc Rev Rep.* 1988;9:31–37.
18. Reyes MP, Lerner AM. Coxsackievirus myocarditis-with special reference to acute and chronic effects. *Prog Cardiovasc Dis.* 1985;27:373–394.
19. Woodruff JF. Viral myocarditis. *Am J Pathol.* 1980; 101:427–479.
20. Daly K, Richardson PJ, Olsen EGJ, et al. Acute myocarditis—role of histological and virological ex-

amination in the diagnosis and assessment of immunosuppressive treatment. *Br Heart J.* 1984;51:30–35.

21. Bowles NE, Rose ML, Taylor P, et al. End-stage dilated cardiomyopathy; persistence of enterovirus RNA in myocardium at cardiac transplantation and lack of immune response. *Circulation.* 1989;80:1128–1136.

22. Kandolf R, Ameis D, Kirschner P, Canu A, Hofschneider PH. In situ detection of enteroviral genomes in myocardial cells by nucleic acid hybridization: an approach to the diagnosis of viral heart disease. *Proc Natl Acad Sci USA.* 1987;84:6272–6276.

23. Limas CJ, Limas C. HLA antigens in idiopathic dilated cardiomyopathy. *Br Heart J.* 1989;62:379–383.

24. Koike S. Immunological disorders in patients with dilated cardiomyopathy. *Jpn Heart J.* 1989;30:799–807.

25. Schultheiss HP, Schulze K, Kuhl U, Ulrich G, Klingenberg M. The ADP/ATP carrier as a mitochondrial autoantigen—facts and perspectives. *Ann NY Acad Sci.* 1986;488:44–64.

26. Schulze K, Becker BF, Schultheiss HP. Antibodies to the ADP/ATP carrier, an autoantigen in myocarditis and dilated cardiomyopathy, penetrate into myocardial cells and disturb energy metabolism in vivo. *Circ Res.* 1989;64:179–192.

27. Schulze K, Becker BF, Schauer R, Schultheiss HP. Antibodies to ADP/ATP Carrier-an autoantigen in myocarditis and dilated cardiomyopathy-impair cardiac function. *Circulation.* 1990;81:959–969.

28. Limas CJ, Limas C, Kubo SH, Olivari MT. Anti-beta receptor antibodies in human dilated cardiomyopathy and correlation with HLA-DR antigens. *Am J Cardiol.* 1990;65:483–487.

29. Hosenpud JD, Campbell SM, Mendelson DJ. Interleukin-1 induced myocardial depression in an isolated perfused beating heart preparation. *J Heart Transplant.* 1989;8:460–464.

30. Hosenpud JD, Campbell SM, Pan G. Indirect inhibition of myocyte RNA and protein synthesis by interleukin-1. *J Mol Cell Cardiol.* 1990;22:213–225.

31. Factor SM, Minase T, Cho S, Dominitz R, Sonnenblick EH. Microvascular spasm in the cardiomyopathic Syrian hamster: a preventable cause of focal myocardial necrosis. *Circulation.* 1982;66:342–354.

32. Leonard DA, Sonnenblick EH, LeJemtel TH. Endocrine cardiomyopathies. *Heart Failure.* 1985;July/August:179–186.

33. Treasure CB, Vita JA, Cox DA, et al. Endothelium-dependent dilation of the coronary microvasculature is impaired in dilated cardiomyopathy. *Circulation.* 1990;81:772–779.

34. van Hoeven KH, Factor SM. Endomyocardial biopsy diagnosis of small vessel disease: a clinicopathologic study. *Int J Cardiol.* 1990;26:103–110.

35. Demakis JG, Proskey A, Rahimtoola SH, et al. The natural course of alcoholic cardiomyopathy. *Ann Intern Med.* 1974;80:293–297.

36. Kantrowitz NE, Bristow MR. Cardiotoxicity of antitumor agents. *Prog Cardiovasc Dis.* 1984;27:195–200.

37. Bristow MR, Mason JW, Billingham ME, Daniels JR. Dose-effect and structure-function relationships in dox-

orubicin cardiomyopathy. *Am Heart J.* 1981;102:709–718.

38. Perloff JK, De Leon AC Jr, O'Doherty D. The cardiomyopathy of progressive muscular dystrophy. *Circulation.* 1966;33:625–648.

39. Alboliras ET, Shub C, Gomez MR, et al. Spectrum of cardiac involvement in Friedreich's ataxia: clinical, electrocardiographic and echocardiographic observations. *Am J Cardiol.* 1986;58:518–524.

40. Caforio ALP, Rossi B, Risaliti R, et al. Type 1 fiber abnormalities in skeletal muscle of patients with hypertrophic and dilated cardiomyopathy: evidence of subclinical myogenic myopathy. *J Am Coll Cardiol.* 1989;14:1464–1473.

41. Fuster V, Gersh BJ, Giuliani ER, Tajik AJ, Brandenburg RO, Frye RL. The natural history of idiopathic dilated cardiomyopathy. *Am J Cardiol.* 1981;47:525–531.

42. Schwarz F, Mall G, Zebe H, et al. Determinants of survival in patients with congestive cardiomyopathy: quantitative morphologic findings and left ventricular hemodynamics. *Circulation.* 1984;70:923–928.

43. Regan TJ, Levinson GE, Oldewurtel HA, Frank MJ, Weisse AB, Moschos CB. Ventricular function in noncardiacs with alcoholic fatty liver: role of ethanol in the production of cardiomyopathy. *J Clin Invest.* 1969;48:397–407.

44. Lang RM, Borow KM, Neumann A, Feldman T. Adverse cardiac effects of acute alcohol ingestion in young adults. *Ann Intern Med.* 1985;102:742–747.

45. Vasdev SC, Chakravarti RN, Subrahmanyam D, Jain AC, Wahi PL. Myocardial lesions induced by prolonged alcohol feeding in rhesus monkeys. *Cardiovasc Res.* 1975; 9:134–140.

46. Regan TJ, Khan MI, Ettinger PO, et al. Myocardial function and lipid metabolism in the chronic alcoholic animal. *J Clin Invest.* 1974;54:740–752.

47. Thomas G, Haider B, Oldewurtel HA, Lyons MM, Yeh CK, Regan TJ. Progression of myocardial abnormalities in experimental alcoholism. *Am J Cardiol.* 1980;46:233–241.

48. Wu S, White R, Wikman-Coffelt J, et al. The preventive effect of verapamil on ethanol-induced cardiac depression: phosphorous-31 nuclear magnetic resonance and high-pressure liquid chromatographic studies of hamsters. *Circulation.* 1987;75:1058–1064.

49. Segal LD, Rendig SV, Mason DT. Alcohol-induced cardiac hemodynamic and Ca^{2+} flux and dysfunctions are reversible. *J Mol Cell Cardiol.* 1981;13:443–455.

50. Sarma JSM, Ikeda S, Fischer R, Maruyama Y, Weishaar R, Bing RJ. Biochemical and contractile properties of heart muscle after prolonged alcohol administration. *J Mol Cell Cardiol.* 1976;8:951–972.

51. Polimeni, PI, Hoeschen O, Hoeschen LE. In vivo effects of ethanol on the rat myocardium: evidence for a reversible, non-specific increase of sarcolemmal permeability. *J Mol Cell Cardiol.* 1983;15:113–122.

52. Noren GR, Staley NA, Einzig S, Mikell FL, Asinger RW. Alcohol-induced congestive cardiomyopathy: an animal model. *Cardiovasc Res.* 1983;17:81–87.

53. Reitz RC, Helsabeck E, Mason DP. Effects of chronic alcohol ingestion on the fatty acid composition of the heart. *Lipids*. 1973;8:80–84.

54. Burch GE, Giles, TD. Alcoholic cardiomyopathy: concept of the disease and its treatment. *Am J Med*. 1971;50:141–145.

55. Koide T, Machida K, Nakanishi A, Ozeki K, Mashima S, Kono H. Cardiac abnormalities in chronic alcoholism. An evidence suggesting association of myocardial abnormality with chronic alcoholism in 107 Japanese patients admitted to a psychiatric ward. *Jpn Heart J*. 1972;13:418–427.

56. McDonald CD, Burch GE, Walsh JJ. Alcoholic cardiomyopathy managed with prolonged bed rest. *Ann Intern Med*. 1971;74:681–691.

57. Wu CF, Sudhakar M, Jaferi G, Ahmed SS, Regan TJ. Preclinical cardiomyopathy in chronic alcoholics: a sex difference. *Am Heart J*. 1976;91:281–286.

58. Lefkowitch JH, Fenoglio JJ Jr. Liver disease in alcoholic cardiomyopathy: evidence against cirrhosis. *Hum Pathol*. 1983;14:457–463.

59. Morin Y, Daniel P. Quebec beer-drinkers' cardiomyopathy: etiological considerations. *Can Med Assoc*. 1967;97:926–928.

60. Sullivan J, Parker M, Carson SB. Tissue cobalt content in "beer drinkers' myocardiopathy." *J Lab Clin Med*. 1968;71:893–896.

61. Shugoll GI, Bowen PJ, Moore JP, Lenkin ML. Follow-up observations and prognosis in primary myocardial disease. *Arch Intern Med*. 1972;129:67–72.

62. Rubler S, Dglugash J, Yuceoglu YZ, Kumral T, Branwood AW, Grishman A. New type of cardiomyopathy associated with diabetic glomerulosclerosis. *Am J Cardiol*. 1972;30:595–602.

63. Kannel WB, Hjortland M, Castelli WP. Role of diabetes in congestive heart failure: the Framingham study. *Am J Cardiol*. 1974;34:29–34.

64. Hamby RI, Zoneraich S, Sherman S. Diabetic cardiomyopathy. *JAMA*. 1974;229:1749–1754.

65. Regan TJ, Ettinger PO, Khan MI, et al. Altered myocardial function and metabolism in chronic diabetes mellitus without ischemia in dogs. *Circ Res*. 1974;35:222–237.

66. Lee JC, Downing SE. Coronary dynamics and myocardial metabolism in the diabetic newborn lamb. *Am J Physiol*. 1979;237:H118–H124.

67. Haider B, Yeh CK, Thomas G, Oldewurtel HA, Lyons MM, Regan TJ. Influence of diabetes on the myocardium and coronary arteries of rhesus monkeys fed an atherogenic diet. *Circ Res*. 1981;49:1278–1288.

68. Regan TJ, Wu CF, Yeh CK, Oldewurtel HA, Haider B. Myocardial composition and function in diabetes: the effects of chronic insulin use. *Circ Res*. 1981;49:1268–1277.

69. Giacomelli E, Wiener J. Primary myocardial disease in the diabetic mouse: an ultrastructural study. *Lab Invest*. 1979;40:460–473.

70. Rodrigues B, McNeill JH. Cardiac function in spontaneously hypertensive diabetic rats. *Am J Physiol*. 1986;20:H571–H580.

71. Rodgers RL. Depressor effect of diabetes in the spontaneously hypertensive rat: associated changes in heart performance. *Can J Physiol Pharmacol*. 1986;64:1177–1184.

72. Fein FS, Kornstein LB, Strobeck JE, Capasso JM, Sonnenblick EH. Altered myocardial mechanics in diabetic rats. *Circ Res*. 1980;47:922–933.

73. Heyliger CE, Pierce GN, Singal PK, Beamish RE, Dhalla NS. Cardiac alpha-and beta-adrenergic receptor alterations in diabetic cardiomyopathy. *Basic Res Cardiol*. 1982;77:610–618.

74. Brownlee M, Cerami A, Viassara H. Advanced glycosylation end products in tissue and the biochemical basis of diabetic complications. *N Engl J Med*. 1988;318:1315–1321.

75. Ganguly PK, Pierce GN, Dhalla KS, Dhalla NS. Defective cardiac sarcoplasmic reticular calcium transport in diabetic cardiomyopathy. *Am J Physiol*. 1983;244:E528–E535.

76. Factor SM, Minase T, Cho S, Fein F, Capasso JM, Sonnenblick EH. Coronary microvascular abnormalities in the hypertensive-diabetic rat. A primary cause of cardiomyopathy? *Am J Pathol*. 1984;116:9–20.

77. Regan TJ, Lyons MM, Ahmed SS, et al. Evidence for cardiomyopathy in familial diabetes mellitus. *J Clin Invest*. 1977;60:885–899.

78. Ahmed SS, Jaferi GA, Narang RM, Regan TJ. Preclinical abnormaility of left ventricular function in diabetes mellitus. *Am Heart J*. 1975;89:153–158.

79. Seneviratne BIB. Diabetic cardiomyopathy: The preclinical phase. *Br Med J*. 1977;1:1444–1446.

80. Sykes CA, Wright AD, Malins JM, Pentecost BL. Changes in systolic time intervals during treatment of diabetes mellitus. *Br Heart J*. 1977;39:255–259.

81. Blumenthal HT, Alex M, Goldenberg S. A study of lesions of the intramural coronary branches in diabetes mellitus. *Arch Pathol*. 1960;70:27–42.

82. Silver MD, Huckell VS, Lorber M. Basement membranes of small cardiac vessels in patients with diabetes and myxedema: preliminary observations. *Pathology*. 1977;9:213–220.

83. Factor SM, Minase T, Sonnenblick EH. Clinical and morphological features of human hypertensive-diabetic cardiomyopathy. *Am Heart J*. 1980;790:446–458.

84. Parving HH. Impact of blood pressure and antihypertensive treatment on incipient and overt nephropathy, retinopathy and endothelial permeability in diabetes mellitus. *Diabetes Care*. 1991;14:260–269.

85. Chase HP, Garg SK, Jackson WE, et al. Blood pressure and retinopathy in type I diabetes. *Ophthalmology*. 1990;97:155–159.

86. Hull E, Hafkesbring E. Toxic post-partal failure. *New Orleans Med Surg J*. 1937;89:556–557.

87. Gouley BA, McMillan TM, Bellet S. Idiopathic myocardial degeneration associated with pregnancy and especially the puerperium. *Am J Med Sci*. 1937;194:185–199.

88. Homans DC. Peripartum cardiomyopathy. *N Engl J Med*. 1985;312:1432–1437.

89. Metcalfe J. The maternal heart in the postpartum period. *Am J Cardiol*. 1963;12:439–440.

90. Demakis JG, Rahimtoola SH. Peripartum cardio-myopathy. *Circulation*. 1971;44:964–968.

91. Rand RJ, Jenkins DM, Scott DG. Maternal cardiomyopathy of pregnancy causing stillbirth. *Br J Obstet Gynaecol*. 1975;82:172–175.

92. Walsh JJ, Burch GE, Black WC, Ferrans VJ, Hibbs RG. Idiopathic myocardiopathy of the puerperium (post-partal heart disease). *Circulation*. 1965;32:19–31.

93. Pierce JA, Price BO, Joyce JW. Familial occurrence of postpartal heart failure. *Arch Intern Med*. 1963;111:651–655.

94. Brown AK, Doukas N, Riding WD, Jones EW. Cardiomyopathy and pregnancy. *Br Heart J*. 1967;29:387–393.

95. Melvin KR, Richardson PJ, Olsen EGJ, Daly K, Jackson G. Peripartum cardiomyopathy due to myocarditis. *N Engl J Med*. 1982;307:731–734.

96. Midei MG, DeMent SH, Feldman AM, Hutchins GM, Baughman KL. Peripartum myocarditis and cardio-myopathy. *Circulation*. 1990;81:922–928.

97. Julian DG, Szekely P. Peripartum cardiomyopathy. *Prog Cardiovasc Dis*. 1985;27:223–240.

98. Burch GE, McDonald CD, Walsh JJ. The effect of prolonged bed rest on postpartal cardiomyopathy. *Am Heart J*. 1971;81:186–201.

99. DeMakis JG, Rahimtoola SH, Sutton GC, et al. Natural course of peripartum cardiomyopathy. *Circulation*. 1971;44:1053–1061.

100. Meadows WR. Idiopathic myocardial failure in the last trimester of pregnancy and the puerperium. *Circulation*. 1957;15:903–914.

101. Billingham ME, Mason JW, Bristow MR, Daniels JR. Anthracycline cardiomyopathy monitored by morpho-logic changes. *Cancer Treat Rep*. 1978;62:865–872.

102. Ferrans VJ. Overview of cardiac pathology in relation to anthracycline cardiotoxicity. *Cancer Treat Rep*. 1978;62:955–961.

103. Mason JW, Bristow MR, Billingham ME, Daniels JR. Invasive and noninvasive methods of assessing adriamy-cin cardiotoxic effects in man: superiority of histopatho-logic assessment using endomyocardial biopsy. *Cancer Treat Rep*. 1978;62:857–864.

104. Olson RD, Mushlin PS. Doxorubicin cardiotoxicity: analysis of prevailing hypotheses. *FASEB J*. 1990;4:3076–3086.

105. Saltiel E, McGuire W. Doxorubicin (adriamycin) car-diomyopathy. *West J Med*. 1983;139:332–341.

106. Minow RA, Benjamin RS, Lee ET, Gottlieb JA. Adriamycin cardiomyopathy—risk factors. *Cancer*. 1977;39:1397–1402.

107. Billngham ME, Bristow MR, Glatstein E, Mason JW, Masek MA, Daniels JR. Adriamycin cardiotoxicity: endomyocardial biopsy evidence of enhancement by irradiation. *Am J Surg Pathol*. 1977;1:17–23.

108. Billingham ME. Endomyocardial changes in anthra-cycline-treated patients with and without irradiation. *Front Radiat Ther Oncol*. 1979;13:67–81.

109. Torti FM, Bristow MR, Howes AE, et al. Reduced cardiotoxicity of doxorubicin delivered on a weekly schedule. *Ann Intern Med*. 1983;99:745–756.

110. Bristow MR, Lopez MB, Mason JW, Billingham ME, Winchester MA. Efficacy and cost of cardiac monitoring in patients receiving doxorubicin. *Cancer*. 1982;50:32–41.

111. Neri R, Mestroni L, Salvi A, Pandullo C, Camerini F. Ventricular arrhythmias in dilated cardiomyopathy: efficacy of amiodarone. *Am Heart J*. 1987;113:707–715.

112. Figulla HR, Rahlf G, Nieger M, Luig H, Kreuzer H. Spontaneous hemodynamic improvement or stabilization and associated biopsy findings in patients with congestive cardiomyopathy. *Circulation*. 1985;71:1095–1104.

113. Taliercio CP, Seward JB, Driscoll DJ, Fisher LD, Gersh BJ, Tajik AJ. Idiopathic dilated cardiomyopathy in the young: clinical profile and natural history. *J Am Coll Cardiol*. 1985;6:1126–1131.

114. Griffin ML, Hernandez A, Martin TC, et al. Dilated car-diomyopathy in infants and children. *J Am Coll Cardiol*. 1988;11:139–144.

115. Unverferth DV, Magorien RD, Moeschberger ML, Bak-er PB, Fetters JK, Leier CV. Factors influencing the one-year mortality of dilated cardiomyopathy. *Am J Cardiol*. 1984;54:147–152.

116. Wilson JR, Schwartz JS, St John Sutton M, et al. Prog-nosis in severe heart failure: relation to hemodynamic measurements and ventricular ectopic activity. *J Am Coll Cardiol*. 1983;2:403–410.

117. Chew CYC, Ziady GM, Raphael MJ, Nellen M, Oakley CM. Primary restrictive cardiomyopathy non-tropical endomyocardial fibrosis and hypereosinophilic heart disease. *Br Heart J*. 1977;39:399–413.

118. Benotti JR, Grossman W. Restrictive cardiomyopathy. *Annu Rev Med*. 1984;35:113–125.

119. Janos GG, Arjunan K, Meyer RA, Engel P, Kaplan S. Differentiation of constrictive pericarditis and restrictive cardiomyopathy using digitized echocardiography. *J Am Coll Cardiol*. 1983;1(2):541–549.

120. Tyberg TI, Goodyer AVN, Hurst VW III, Alexander J, Langou RA. Left ventricular filling in differentiating re-strictive amyloid cardiomyopathy and constrictive peri-carditis. *Am J Cardiol*. 1981;47:791–796.

121. Benotti JR, Grossman W, Cohn PF. Clinical profile of restrictive cardiomyopathy. *Circulation*. 1980;61:1206–1212.

122. Hosenpud JD, Niles NR. Clinical hemodynamic and endomyocardial biopsy findings in idiopathic restrictive cardiomyopathy. *West J Med*. 1986;144:303–306.

123. Montgomery JF. Pericarditis. *West J Med*. 1975;127:295–308.

124. Siegel RJ, Shah PK, Fishbein MC. Idiopathic restrictive cardiomyopathy. *Circulation*. 1984;70:165–169.

125. Mehta AV, Ferrer PL, Pickoff AS, et al. M-mode echo-cardiographic findings in children with idiopathic restric-tive cardiomyopathy. *Pediatr Cardiol*. 1984;5:273–280.

126. Sapire DW, Casta A, Swischuk LE, Casta D. Massive dilatation of the atria and coronary sinus in a child with restrictive cardiomyopathy and persistence of the left superior vena cava. *Cathet Cardiovasc Diagn*. 1983;9:47–53.

127. Erath HG, Graham TP Jr, Smith CW, Boucek RJ Jr. Restrictive cardiomyopathy in an infant with massive

biatrial enlargement and normal ventricular size and pump function. *Cathet Cardiovasc Diagn.* 1978;4:289–296.

128. Arbustini E, Buonanno C, Trevi G, Pennelli N, Ferrans VJ, Thiene G. Cardiac ultrastructure in primary restrictive cardiomyopathy. *Chest.* 1983;84:236–238.

129. Glenner GG. Amyloid deposits and amyloidosis. *N Engl J Med.* 1980;302:1283–1292.

130. Olofsson BO, Bjerle P, Osterman G. Hemodynamic and angiocardiographic observations in familial amyloidosis with polyneuropathy. *Acta Med Scand.* 1982;212:77–81.

131. Maule WF, Martin RH. Primary cardiac amyloidosis: an angiocardiographic clue to early diagnosis. *Ann Intern Med.* 1983;98:177–180.

132. Kern MJ, Lorell BH, Grossman W. Cardiac amyloidosis masquerading as constrictive pericarditis. *Cathet Cardiovasc Diagn.* 1982;8:629–635.

133. Edhag O, Helmers C, Samnegard H, Sjogren A, Vallin H. Two cases of myocardial disease simulating constrictive pericarditis. *Scand J Thorac Cardiovasc Surg.* 1977;11:225–227.

134. Meaney E, Shabetai R, Bhargava V, et al. Cardiac amyloidosis, constrictive pericarditis in restrictive cardiomyopathy. *Am J Cardiol.* 1976;38:547–556.

135. Naggar CZ. Rapid amyloid infiltration of the heart. *Am J Cardiol.* 1986;80:276–278.

136. Garcia R, Alam M. Restrictive cardiomyopathy. *Henry Ford Hosp Med J.* 1986;34;168–173.

137. Child JS, Krivokapich J, Abbasi AS. Increased right ventricular wall thickness on echocardiography in amyloid infiltrative cardiomyopathy. *Am J Cardiol.* 1979;44:1391–1395.

138. Child JS, Levisman JA, Abbasi AS, MacAlpin RN. Echocardiographic manifestations of infiltrative cardiomyopathy. *Chest.* 1976;70:726–731.

139. Pierard L, Verheugt FWA, Meltzer RS, Roelandt J. Echocardiographic aspects of cardiac amyloidosis. *Acta Cardiol.* 1981;36:455–461.

140. Kyle RA, Greipp PR. Amyloidosis (AL): clinical and laboratory feature in 229 cases. *Mayo Clin Proc.* 1983;58:665–683.

141. Loeffler W. Endocarditis parietalis fibroplastica Mit Bluteosinophiline. *Schweiz Med Wchnscr.* 1930;66:817–820.

142. Roberts WC, Ferrans VJ. Pathologic anatomy of the cardiomyopathies. Idiopathic dilated and hypertrophic types, infiltrative types, and endomyocardial disease with and without eosinophilia. *Hum Pathol.* 1975;6:287–342.

143. Spry CJF, Tai P-C, Davies J. The cardiotoxicity of eosinophils. *Postgrad Med J.* 1983;59:147–151.

144. Fauci AS, Harley JB, Roberts WC, Ferrans VJ, Gralnick HR, Bjornson BH. The idiopathic hypereosinophilic syndrome. *Ann Intern Med.* 1982;97:78–92.

145. Olsen EGJ. Pathological aspects of endomyocardial fibrosis. *Postgrad Med J.* 1983;59:135–139.

146. Cherian G, Vijayaraghavan G, Krishnaswami S, et al. Endomyocardial fibrosis: report on the hemodynamic data in 29 patients and review of the results of surgery. *Am Heart J.* 1983;105:659–666.

147. Olsen EGJ, Spry CJF. Relation between eosinophilia and endomyocardial disease. *Prog Cardiovasc Dis.* 1985;27:241–254.

148. Parrillo JE, Borer JS, Henry WL, Wolff SM, Fauci AS. The cardiovascular manifestations of the hypereosinophilic syndrome. *Am J Med.* 1979;67:572–582.

149. Kudenchuk PJ, Hosenpud JD, Fletcher S. Eosinophilic endomyocardiopathy. *Clin Cardiol.* 1986;9:344–348.

150. Solley GO, Maldonado JE, Gleich GJ, et al. Endomyocardiopathy with eosinophilia. *Mayo Clin Proc.* 1976;51:697–708.

151. Benvenisti DS, Ultmann JE. Eosinophilic leukemia? Report of 5 cases and review of the literature. *Ann Intern Med.* 1969;71:732–736.

152. Chusid MJ, Dale DC, West BC, Wolff SM. The hypereosinophilic syndrome: analysis of 14 cases and review of the literature. *Medicine.* 1975;54:1–27.

153. Ratner SJ, Fenoglio JJ Jr, Ursell PC. Utility of endomyocardial biopsy in the diagnosis of cardiac sarcoidosis. *Chest.* 1986;90:528–533.

154. Cutler DJ, Isner JM, Bracey AW, et al. Hemochromatosis heart disease: an unemphasized cause of potentially reversible restrictive cardiomyopathy. *Am J Med.* 1980;69:923–928.

155. Kaplan A, Cohen J. Restrictive cardiomyopathy as the presenting feature of reticulum cell sarcoma. *Am Heart J.* 1969;77:307–314.

156. Landau E, Reisin LH. LV myxoma resembling restrictive cardiomyopathy. *Am Heart J.* 1986;112:1356.

157. Westerhof PW, van der Putte SCJ. Radiation pericarditis and myocardial fibrosis. *Eur J Cardiol.* 1976;4/2:213–218.

158. Mortensen SA, Olsen HS, Baandrup U. Chronic anthracycline cardiotoxicity: haemodynamic and histopathological manifestations suggesting a restrictive endomyocardial disease. *Br Heart J.* 1986;55:274–282.

159. Doherty NE, Siegel RJ. Cardiovascular manifestations of systemic lupus erythematosus. Am Heart J. 1985;110:1257–1265.

160. Navarro-Lopez F, Llorian A, Ferrer-Roca O, Betriu A, Sanz G. Restrictive cardiomyopathy in pseudoxanthoma elasticum. *Chest.* 1980;78:113–115.

161. Papapietro SE, Rogers LW, Hudson NL, Atkinson JB, Page DL. Intramyocardial coronary arteritis and restrictive cardiomyopathy. *Am Heart J.* 1987;114:175–178.

162. Humen DP, McKenzie FN, Kostuk WJ. Restricted myocardial compliance one year following cardiac transplantation. *J Heart Transplant.* 1984;3:341–345.

163. Young JB, Leon CA, Short D III, et al. Evolution of hemodynamics after orthotopic heart and heart-lung transplantation: early restrictive patterns persisting in an occult fashion. *J Heart Transplant.* 1987;6:34–43.

164. Ramsey HW, Sbar S, Elliott LP, Eliot RS. The differential diagnosis of restrictive myocardiopathy and chronic constrictive pericarditis without calcification. *Am J Cardiol.* 1970;25:635–638.

165. Chang LWM, Grollman JH Jr. Angiocardiographic differentiation of constrictive pericarditis and restrictive cardiomyopathy due to amyloidosis. *Am J Roentgenol.* 1978;130:451–453.

166. Anderson PAW. Diagnostic problem: constrictive peri-

carditis or restrictive cardiomyopathy? *Cathet Cardiovasc Diagn.* 1983;9:1–7.

167. Isner JM, Carter BL, Bankoff MS, et al. Differentiation of constrictive pericarditis from restrictive cardiomyopathy by computed tomographic imaging. *Am Heart J.* 1983;105:1019–1025.

168. Sechtem U, Higgins CB, Sommerhoff BA, Lipton MJ, Huycke EC. Magnetic resonance imaging of restrictive cardiomyopathy. *Am J Cardiol.* 1987;59:480–482.

169. Sechtem U, Tscholakoff D, Higgins CB. MRI of the abnormal pericardium. *AJR.* 1986;147:245–252.

170. Nye RE, Lovejoy FW, Yu PN. Clinical and hemodynamic studies of myocardial fibrosis. *Circulation.* 1957;16:332–338.

171. Gould L. Left atrial "a" waves in primary myocardial disease, constrictive pericarditis, and arteriosclerotic heart disease. *Am Heart J.* 1969;77:430–431.

172. Lewis BS, Gotsman MS. Maximal rate of fall of left ventricular pressure in cardiomyopathy and constrictive pericarditis. *S Afr Med J.* 1975;49:1287–1291.

173. Schoenfeld MH, Supple EW, Dec GW Jr, Fallon JT, Palacios IF. Restrictive cardiomyopathy versus constrictive pericarditis: role of endomyocardial biopsy in avoiding unnecessary thoracotomy. *Circulation.* 1987;75:1012–1017.

174. Braunwald E. Mechanism of action of calcium-channel-blocking agents. *N Engl J Med.* 1982;307:1618–1627.

175. Teare D. Asymmetrical hypertrophy of the heart in young patients. *Br Heart J.* 1958;20:1–8.

176. Maron BJ, Epstein SE. Hypertrophic Cardiomyopathy. *Am J Cardiol.* 1980;45:141–154.

177. Clark CE, Henry WL, Epstein SE. Familial prevalence and genetic transmission of idiopathic hypertrophic subaortic stenosis. *N Engl J Med.* 1973;289:709–714.

178. Maron BJ, Nichols PF, Pickle LW, Wesley YE, Mulvihill JJ. Patterns of inheritance in hypertrophic cardiomyopathy: assessment by M-mode and two-dimensional echocardiography. *Am J Cardiol.* 1984;53:1087–1094.

179. Brock R. Functional obstruction of the left ventricle (acquired aortic subvalvular stenosis). *Guy's Hosp Rep.* 1957;106:221–238.

180. Hutchins GM, Bulkley BH. Catenoid shape of the interventricular septum: possible cause of idiopathic hypertrophic subaortic stenosis. *Circulation.* 1978;58:392–397.

181. Pearse AGE. Histochemical and electron microscopy of obstructive cardiomyopathy. In Wolstenholme GEW, O'Connor M, eds. *Ciba Foundation Symposium on Cardiomyopathies.* London: Churchill Livingstone; 1964;132–164.

182. Witzke DJ, Kay MP. Hypertrophic cardiomyopathy induced by administration of nerve growth factor. *Circulation.* 1976;54(suppl 2):88. Abstract.

183. Liew C-C, Sole MJ, Silver MD, Wigle ED. Electrophoretic profiles of nonhistone nuclear proteins of human hearts with muscular subaortic stenosis. *Circ Res.* 1980;46:513–519.

184. Criley JM, Lewis KB, White RI Jr, Ross, RS. Pressure gradients without obstruction: a non concept of "hypertrophic subaortic stenosis." *Circulation.* 1965;32:881–887.

185. Stewart S, Mason DT, Braunwald E. Impaired rate of

left ventricular filling in idiopathic subaortic stenosis and valvular aortic stenosis. *Circulation.* 1968;37:8–14.

186. Sanderson JE, Gibson DG, Brown DJ, Goodwin JF. Left ventricular filling in hypertrophic cardiomyopathy: an angiographic study. *Br Heart J.* 1977;39:661–70.

187. Hanrath P, Mathey DG, Siegert R, Bleifeld W. Left ventricular relaxation and filling pattern in different forms of left ventricular hypertrophy: an echocardiographic study. *Am J Cardiol.* 1980;45:15–23.

188. Maron BJ, Merrill WH, Freier PA, Kent KM, Epstein SE, Morrow AG. Long-term clinical course and symptomatic status of patients after operation for hypertrophic subaortic stenosis. *Circulation.* 1978;57:1205–1213.

189. Epstein SE, Henry WL, Clark CE, et al. Asymmetric septal hypertrophy. *Ann Intern Med.* 1974;81:650–680.

190. Goodwin JF. An appreciation of hypertrophic cardiomyopathy. *Am J Med.* 1980;68:797–800.

191. McKenna W, Deanfield J, Faruqui A, England D, Oakley C, Goodwin J. Prognosis in hypertrophic cardiomyopathy: role of age and clinical, electrocardiographic and hemodynamic features. *Am J Cardiol.* 1981;47:532–538.

192. Braunwald E, Lambrew CT, Rockoff SD, Ross J Jr, Morrow AG. Idiopathic hypertrophic subaortic stenosis. I: a description of the disease based upon an analysis of 64 patients. *Circulation.* 1964;29, 30(suppl IV):3–119.

193. Swan DA, Bell B, Oakley CM, Goodwin J. Analysis of symptomatic course and prognosis and treatment of hypertrophic obstructive cardiomyopathy. *Br Heart J.* 1971;33:671–685.

194. Fiddler GI, Tajik AJ, Weidman WH, McGoon DC, Ritter DG, Giuliani ER. Idiopathic hypertrophic subaortic stenosis in the young. *Am J Cardiol.* 1978;42:793–799.

195. Nishimura RA, Giuliani ER, Brandenburg RO. Hypertrophic cardiomyopathy. *CVRR.* 1983;4:931–962.

196. Shah PM, Adelman AG, Wigle ED, et al. The natural (and unnatural) history of hypertrophic obstructive cardiomyopathy. *Circ Res.* 1974;34,35(suppl II):II-179–195.

197. Adelman AG, Wigle ED, Ranganathan N, et al. The clinical course in muscular subaortic stenosis. A retrospective and prospective study of 60 hemodynamically proved cases. *Ann Intern Med.* 1972;77:515–525.

198. Stewart S, Schreiner B. Coexisting idiopathic hypertrophic subaortic stenosis and coronary artery disease. Clinical implication and operative management. *J Thorac Cardiovasc Surg.* 1981;82:278–280.

199. Maron BJ, Epstein SE, Roberts WC. Hypertrophic cardiomyopathy and transmural myocardial infarction without significant atherosclerosis of the extramural coronary arteries. *Am J Cardiol.* 1979;43:1086–1112.

200. Pichard AD, Meller J, Teichholz LE, Lipnik S, Gorlin R, Herman MV. Septal perforator compression (narrowing) in idiopathic hypertrophic subaortic stenosis. *Am J Cardiol.* 1977;40:310–314.

201. Kostis JB, Moreyra AE, Natarajan N, Hosler M, Kuo PT, Conn HL Jr. The pathophysiology and diverse etiology of septal perforator compression. *Circulation.* 1979;59:913–919.

202. St John Sutton MG, Tajik AJ, Smith HC, Ritman EL. Angina in idiopathic hypertrophic subaortic stenosis: a

clinical correlate of regional left ventricular dysfunction; a videometric and echocardiographic study. *Circulation*. 1980;61:561–568.

203. Pitcher D, Wainwright R, Maisey M, Curry P, Sowton E. Assessment of chest pain in hypertrophic cardiomyopathy using exercise thallium-201 myocardial scintigraphy. *Br Heart J*. 1980;44:650–656.

204. Weiss MB, Ellis K, Sciacca RR, Johnson LL, Schmidt DH, Cannon PJ. Myocardial blood flow in congestive and hypertrophic cardiomyopathy: relationship to peak wall stress and mean velocity of circumferential fiber shortening. *Circulation*. 1976;54:484–494.

205. Hardarson T, de la Calzada CS, Curiel R, Goodwin JF. Prognosis and mortality of hypertrophic obstructive cardiomyopathy. *Lancet*. 1973;2:1462–1467.

206. Canedo MI, Frank MJ, Abdulla AM. Rhythm disturbances in hypertrophic cardiomyopathy: prevalence, relation to symptoms and management. *Am J Cardiol*. 1980;45:848–855.

207. Ingham RE, Rossen RM, Goodman DJ, Harrison DC. Treadmill arrhythmias in patients with idiopathic hypertrophic subaortic stenosis. *Chest*. 1975;68:759–764.

208. McKenna WJ, England D, Doi YL, Deanfield JE, Oakley C, Goodwin JF. Arrhythmia in hypertrophic cardiomyopathy. I. Influence on prognosis. *Br Heart J*. 1981;46:168–172.

209. Maron BJ, Savage DD, Wolfson JK, Epstein SE. Prognostic significance of 24-hour ambulatory electrocardiographic monitoring in patients with hypertrophic cardiomyopathy: a prospective study. *Am J Cardiol*. 1981;48:252–257.

210. Cosio FG, Moro C, Alonso M, de la Calzada CS, Llovet A. The Q-waves of hypertrophic cardiomyopathy. An electrophysiologic study. *N Engl J Med*. 1980;302:96–99.

211. Goodwin JF, Kirkler DM. Arrhythmia as a cause of sudden death in hypertrophic cardiomyopathy. *Lancet*. 1976;2:937–940.

212. Frank S, Braunwald E. Idiopathic hypertrophic subaortic stenosis: clinical analysis of 126 patients with emphasis on the natural history. *Circulation*. 1968;37:759–788.

213. Prescott R, Quinn JS, Littman D. Electrocardiographic changes in hypertrophic subaortic stenosis which stimulates myocardial infarction. *Am Heart J*. 1963;66:42–48.

214. St. John Sutton MG, Tajik AJ, Gibson DG, Brown DJ, Seward JB, Giuliani ER. Echocardiographic assessment of left ventricular filling and septal and posterior wall dynamics in idiopathic hypertrophic subaortic stenosis. *Circulation*. 1978;57:512–520.

215. Hanrath P, Mathey D, Siegert R, Blefield W. Left ventricular relaxation and filling pattern in different forms of left ventricular hypertrophy. An echocardiographic study. *Am J Cardiol*. 1980;45:15–23.

216. Sanderson JE, Traill TA, St John Sutton MG, Brown DJ, Gibson DG, Goodwin JF. Left ventricular relaxation and filling in hypertrophic cardiomyopathy. An echocardiographic study. *Br Heart J*. 1978;40:596–601.

217. Murgo JP, Alter BR, Dorethy JF, Altobelli SA, McGranaham GM Jr, Dunne TE. Dynamics of left ventricular ejection in obstructive and nonobstructive hypertrophic cardiomyopathy. *J Clin Invest*. 1980;66:1369–1382.

218. Stewart S, Mason DT, Braunwald E. Impaired rate of left ventricular filling in idiopathic hypertrophic subaortic stenosis and valvular aortic stenosis. *Circulation*. 1968;37:8–14.

219. Wigle ED, Marquis Y, Auger P. Muscular subaortic stenosis: initial left ventricular inflow tract pressure in the assessment of intraventricular pressure differences in man. *Circulation*. 1967;35:1110–1117.

220. Shaver JA, Salerni R, Curtiss EI, Follansbee WP. Clinical presentation and noninvasive evaluation of the patient with hypertrophic cardiomyopathy. *Cardiovasc Clin*. 1989;19:149–192.

221. Adelman AG, McLoughlin MJ, Marquis Y, Auger P, Wigle ED. Left ventricular cineangiographic observations in muscular subaortic stenosis. *Am J Cardiol*. 1969;24:689–697.

222. Whalen RE, Cohen AL, Sumner RG, Mc Intosh HD. Demonstration of the dynamic nature of idiopathic hypertrophic subaortic stenosis. *Am J Cardiol*. 1963;11:8–17.

223. Simon AR, Ross J Jr, Gault JH. Angiographic anatomy of the left ventricle and mitral valve in idiopathic hypertrophic subaortic stenosis. *Circulation*. 1967;36:852–867.

224. Glancy DL, O'Brien KP, Gold HK, Epstein SE. Atrial fibrillation in patients with idiopathic hypertrophic subaortic stenosis. *Br Heart J*. 1970;32:652–659.

225. Murgo JP. The hemodynamic evaluation in hypertrophic cardiomyopathy: systolic and diastolic dysfunction. *Cardiovasc Clin*. 1989;19:193–220.

226. Harrison DC, Braunwald E, Glick G, Mason DT, Chidsey CA, Ross J Jr. Effects of beta adrenergic blockade on the circulation, with particular reference to observations in patients with hypertrophic subaortic stenosis. *Circulation*. 1964;29:84–98.

227. Flamm MD, Harrison DC, Hancock EW. Muscular subaortic stenosis. Prevention of outflow obstruction with propranolol. *Circulation*. 1968;38:846–858.

228. Stenson RE, Flamm MD Jr, Harrison DC, Hancock EW. Hypertrophic subaortic stenosis. Clinical and hemodynamic effects of long-term propranolol therapy. *Am J Cardiol*. 1973;31:763–773.

229. de la Calzada CS, Ziady GM, Hardarson T, Curiel R, Goodwin JF. Effect of acute administration of propranolol on ventricular function in hypertrophic obstructive cardiomyopathy measured by non-invasive techniques. *Br Heart J*. 1976;38:798–803.

230. Swanton RH, Brooksby IAB, Jenkins BS, Webb-Peploe MM. Hemodynamic studies of beta blockade in hypertrophic obstructive cardiomyopathy. *Eur J Cardiol*. 1977;5:327–341.

231. Speiser KW, Krayenbuehl HP. Reappraisal of the effect of acute beta-blockade on left ventricular filling dynamics in hypertrophic obstructive cardiomyopathy. *Eur Heart J*. 1981;2:21–29.

232. Hess OM, Grimm J, Krayenbuehl HP. Diastolic function in hypertrophic cardiomyopathy: effects of propranolol and verapamil on diastolic stiffness. *Eur Heart J*. 1983;4(suppl F):47–56.

233. Kaltenbach M, Hopf R, Kober G, Bussman W-D, Keller M, Petersen Y. Treatment of hypertrophic obstructive

cardiomyopathy with verapamil. *Br Heart J*. 1979;42:35–42.

234. Rosing DR, Condit JR, Maron BJ, et al. Verapamil therapy: a new approach to the pharmacologic treatment of hypertrophic cardiomyopathy. III. Effects of long-term administration. *Am J Cardiol*. 1981;48:545–553.

235. Rosin DR, Idanpaan-Heikkla U, Maron BJ, Bonow RO, Epstein SE. Use of calcium channel blocking drugs in hypertrophic cardiomyopathy. *Am J Cardiol*. 1985;55:185B–195B.

236. Bonow RO, Dilsizian V, Rosing DR, Maron BJ, Bacharach SL, Green MV. Verapamil-induced improvement in left ventricular diastolic filling and increased exercise tolerance in patients with hypertrophic cardiomyopathy: short and long term effects. *Circulation*. 1985;72:853–864.

237. Rosing DR, Kent KM, Maron BJ, Epstein SE. Verapamil therapy: a new approach to the pharmacologic treatment of hypertrophic cardiomyopathy. II. Effects on exercise capacity and symptomatic status. *Circulation*. 1979;60:1208–1213.

238. Shaffer EM, Rocchini AP, Spicer RL, et al. Effects of verapamil on left ventricular diastolic filling in children with hypertrophic cardiomyopathy. *Am J Cardiol*. 1988;61:413–417.

239. Bonow RO, Vitale DF, Maron BJ, Bacharach SL, Frederick TM, Green MV. Regional left ventricular asynchrony and impaired global filling in hypertrophic cardiomyopathy: Effect of verapamil. *J Am Coll Cardiol*. 1987;9:1108–1116.

240. Bonow RO, Ostrow HG, Rosing DR, et al. Verapamil effects on left ventricular systolic and diastolic function in patients with hypertrophic cardiomyopathy: pressure-volume analysis with a non-imaging scintillation probe. *Circulation*. 1983;68:1062–1073.

241. Ito Y, Suko J, Chidsey CA. Intracellular calcium and myocardial contractility. V. Calcium uptake of sarcoplasmic reticulum fractions in hypertrophied and failing rabbit hearts. *J Mol Cell Cardiol*. 1974;6:237–247.

242. Lorell BH, Barry WH. Effects of verapamil on contraction and relaxation of cultured chick embryo ventricular cells during calcium overload. *J Am Coll Cardiol*. 1984;3:341–348.

243. Paulus WJ, Nellens P, Heyndrickx GR, Andries SE. Effects of long-term treatment with amiodarone on exercise hemodynamics and left ventricular relaxation in patients with hypertrophic cardiomyopathy. *Circulation*. 1986;74:544–554.

244. Leon MB, Rosing DR, Maron BJ, Bonow RO, Lesko LJ, Epstein SE. Amiodarone in patients with hypertrophic cardiomyopathy and refractory cardiac symptoms: an alternative to current medical therapy. *Circulation*. 1984;70(suppl II):II–18. Abstract.

245. Morrow AG, Brockenbrough EC. Surgical treatment of idiopathic hypertrophic subaortic stenosis: technic and hemodynamic results of subaortic ventriculomyotomy. *Ann Surg*. 1961;154:181–189.

246. Morrow AG. Hypertrophic subaortic stenosis. *J Thorac Cardiovasc Surg*. 1978;76:423–430.

247. Canedo MI, Frank MJ. Therapy of hypertrophic cardiomyopathy: medical or surgical? Clinical and pathophysiologic considerations. *Am J Cardiol*. 1981;48:383–388.

248. Cecchi F, Maron BJ, Epstein SE. Long-term outcome of patients with hypertrophic cardiomyopathy successfully resuscitated after cardiac arrest. *J Am Coll Cardiol*. 1989;13:1283–1288.

249. Spirito P, Chiarella F, Carratino L, Berisso MZ, Bellotti P, Vecchio C. Clinical course and prognosis of hypertrophic cardiomyopathy in an outpatient population. *N Engl J Med*. 1989;320:749–755.

14
Inflammatory Heart Disease

John B. O'Connell and Jay W. Mason

The application of transvenous endomyocardial biopsy to the evaluation of patients with unexplained heart failure has resulted in a rebirth of enthusiasm for the identification of inflammatory and immune mechanisms that result in myocardial injury. Although in most instances active viral myocarditis, the most commonly identified cause of immune-mediated injury, resolves spontaneously without sequelae, inflammation or other mediators occasionally may persist with progressive myocardial injury. A clinical syndrome indistinguishable from dilated cardiomyopathy (DCM) results.[1]

DCM is an important cause of cardiovascular morbidity precipitating premature death, functional limitation and providing the largest pool of patients requiring cardiac transplantation.[2] At present, medical treatment of DCM is palliative. The natural history of DCM will be altered only when the etiology of myocyte injury is clear and therapeutic modalities designed to reverse the cause rather than the effect of this disease are developed. Further understanding of the immunopathogenesis and treatment of active myocarditis and other forms of inflammatory heart disease in analogous animal models may be necessary before this goal has been reached.

In this chapter, new observations regarding the immunopathogenesis of myocarditis including analyses both in the animal model and observations made in the human disease are reviewed. The importance of endomyocardial biopsy in the diagnosis of myocarditis are emphasized and the controversies in treatment are delineated. Nonviral causes of myocarditis and of inflammatory heart muscle diseases in which the histopathology differs from the more commonly identified active lymphocytic myocarditis also are described.

Viral Myocarditis in the Animal Model

When Coxsackievirus B3 (CVB3), a common human cardiotropic virus, is injected into weanling mice, myocardial infection results.[3] Replicating virus can be detected in the myocardium for 7 to 9 days after inoculation. Evidence of congestive heart failure (CHF), however, is absent during this phase and the inflammatory infiltrate is sparse on histologic examination. In selected strains, progressive injury and persistent inflammation are detected after viral clearance.[4]

When Swiss ICR mice were sacrificed 6 months after infection with CVB3, some animals demonstrated persistent inflammation and hypertrophy with early evidence of CHF.[5] By 15 months after infection, progressive CHF ensues with mural thrombi and left ventricular dilatation in the absence of inflammatory infiltrate on histologic examination.[6] Therefore, viral infection triggers immune responses following viral clearance that result in progressive myocyte injury leading to a syndrome that is indistinguishable from human DCM. When Coxsackieviruses B1 or B4 were administered, left ventricular aneurysms commonly resulted.[7] With inoculation of encephalomyocarditis virus (EMC), a more rapidly progressive but immunologically similar disease results.[8]

When antithymocyte serum is administered during the acute infectious phase, viral clearance is unaffected.[9] However, the progressive inflammatory response is attenuated. These results imply that cell-mediated immune responses may be more important during the chronic phase than during the acute phase. Experimental analyses have demonstrated that the antigen driving these effector mechanisms either represents a neoantigen located on neighboring fibroblasts or auto-immune cytotoxic T-cell responses.[10,11] Antibodies also may play a role in the pathogenesis of this disease, with antibodies to the beta-receptor, myosin, and the adenosine diphosphate–adenosine triphosphate (ADP/ATP) carrier protein implicated in the myocyte injury and dysfunction.[12–14] Furthermore, administration of purified antigen (myosin) alone has reproduced some of the pathophysiologic and histologic characteristics of viral myocarditis.[15]

The immunologic response to viral infection is strain-specific, with some murine strains reacting more aggressively via humoral immune responses and antibodies and other strains responding more aggressively with T-cell effectors.[11] Some strains also are highly resistant to the effects of CVB3.[4] When pregnant females or animals fed large quantities of alcohol are infected with cardiotropic viruses, the injury is intensified.[16,17]

In an effort to draw comparisons and establish therapies for the human disease, prophylactic and therapeutic interventions have been applied to the animal model. Administration of the antiviral agent, ribavirin, shortly after the inoculation of virus dramatically attenuated the lymphocytic infiltrate and the myocyte necrosis.[18] Inactive virus vaccine has been administered in the EMC virus model and passive immunization with specific antiviral antibodies to EMC or CVB3 has been successful in prophylaxis.[19] Viral clearance is augmented by interferon administration with interferon alpha A/D interferon.[20]

Immunosuppression has been studied primarily by intervention concomitant with or soon after viral inoculation. Corticosteroids, nonsteroidal antiinflammatory drugs, and antimetabolites such as cyclophosphamide all have enhanced viral replication and mortality when initiated on the day of infection.[21–23]

A negligible effect occurred when administered after viral clearance. While antithymocyte serum attenuated the inflammatory reaction in some strains, in others viral-mediated myocyte damage was exacerbated.[9,24] The effect of cyclosporine is dependent on the murine strain analyzed. When BALB/c mice were infected with CVB3, cyclosporine administration at the time of infection enhanced mortality and attenuated the inflammatory infiltrate while the necrosis increased and viral replication was prolonged.[25] Conversely, in DBA/J mice, cyclosporine favorably affects the disease even when administration was initiated before or immediately after infection.[26]

While a great deal of evidence suggests that postinfectious immune response is the major cause of left ventricular dysfunction in certain murine models of myocarditis, direct myocardial damage by replicating virus may occur in mice as well as in humans. Therapeutic interventions directed against the immune response in the human disease could, in theory, worsen

this direct damage by weakening protective elements of the immune response as noted with immunosuppression in the murine model during the acute phase. However, documentation of deleterious effects of immunosuppression in the human disease has not been provided.

Further study of this latter possibility is needed. Nevertheless, therapeutic knowledge derived from the murine myocarditis model cannot be transferred directly to man, because the pathophysiology of myocarditis in humans is not clear.

Immunopathogenesis of the Human Disease

Defects in suppressor and natural killer cell functions were identified in patients with DCM and myocarditis but assay results were inconsistent.[27–29] Antibody-dependent cellular cytotoxicity also has been reported to be suppressed with active myocarditis.[30] Analysis of lymphocyte surface markers have been shown to be of little value in establishing the diagnosis.[31]

Antimyolemmal antibodies occur commonly in patients with DCM and myocarditis but the role of these antibodies in pathogenesis is unknown.[32] Cardiac-specific antibodies including those directed toward myosin, ADP/ATP carrier protein, and beta-receptors also have been identified.[12,14,33] The functional implications of these antibodies are speculative. To date, although clinical studies have identified the presence of antimyosin antibodies, their effect on cardiac function has not been reported. When sera from patients with DCM were analyzed for autoantibodies directed against the sera from ADP/ATP carrier protein, elevated titers were detected in 24 of 32 patients. In patients with coronary artery disease, hypertrophic cardiomyopathy, alcoholic cardiomyopathy, and normal controls had no detectable antibody binding. A statistically significant but weak relationship between antibody titer and ejection fraction below 40% in the patients with DCM was detected.[34] These investigators also have documented the impairment of energy metabolism in intact perfused hearts isolated from immunized and nonimmunized guinea pigs. Only immunized animals demonstrated a decreased phosphorylation potential of ATP as a result of a reduction of mitochondrial/cytosolic nucleotide transport. They also demonstrated that mean aortic pressure and stroke work were significantly lower in the immunized hearts compared to nonimmunized controls and the external heart work of the immunized hearts achieved only 20% of the performance level of control hearts.[35]

HLA D4 and DR1 were strongly associated with anti–beta-receptor antibodies detected by inhibition of radioligand binding of tritiated dihydroalprenolol.[12] These data suggest that cardiac beta-receptors and adenylate cyclase activity are modulated by circulating anti–beta-receptor antibodies that may be genetically controlled under the histocompatibility complex. Identification of these humoral antibodies that play a role in the immunopathogenesis of myocarditis and DCM may, in part, provide an explanation for reversibility of the disease because function is impaired by mechanisms other than direct cytotoxicity.

Immunohistochemistry of myocardial tissue has demonstrated a predominance of CD8+ or CD4+ lymphocytes.[36] Mononuclear cells can be cultured from endomyocardial biopsies in the presence of human recombinant interleukin-2 (IL-2) and the activated T cells specifically derived from these biopsies can be expanded in vitro for further analysis.[37] Major histocompatibility antigens are expressed more commonly in patients with active myocarditis than in control samples.[38] Perforin, the effector of cytotoxicity of CD8+ cells, can be demonstrated by immunohistologic biopsy examination.[39]

Endomyocardial biopsy also allows further analysis of the role of the virus in initiating this disease. Using the techniques of in situ hybridization and the sensitive polymerase chain reaction, enteroviral genomic fragments have been detected in the human myocardium both in patients with active myocarditis and those with DCM.[40–42] Although only 10% to 30% of biopsies with myocarditis demonstrate persistent enteroviral genomes, these analyses confirm the association of viral infection of the heart with active myocarditis. Whether these genomic fragments are capable of replicating has not been elucidated. These reports must be considered preliminary. The inconsistencies in immunohistochemical reports suggest that the multiple factors are operable in the immunopathogenesis of human myocarditis. However, the observation that viral genomic fragments are present in biopsy samples is strong support of an integral role of enterovirus in initiating this disease. A possible schema for the immunopathogenesis of myocarditis is presented in Figure 14.1.

Clinical Presentation of Human Myocarditis

Elevated antibody titers to cardiotropic viruses indicating previous infection are reported in more than 50% of normal adults.[43] Yet, DCM is much less common, occurring at a rate of 4 to 5 new cases per 100,000 population per year.[44] This large disparity can be explained if most cases of myocarditis are clinically silent and resolve without sequelae or despite cardiotropicity, the virus does not infect the myocardium. When patients are symptomatic during the acute phase of the illness, nonspecific complaints such as fever and symptoms of an antecedent enteroviral infection are

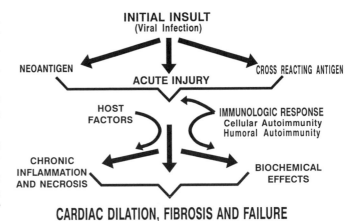

FIGURE 14.1. A possible schema for the immunopathogenesis of myocarditis.

common.[45] Specific cardiovascular manifestations include chest pain, dyspnea, palpitations, and syncope. Although unusual, sudden death has been reported as an initial manifestation of acute viral myocarditis. One noteworthy symptom is syncope due to AV block, which may require pacemaker implantation.[46] Cardiovascular collapse and cardiogenic shock also have been reported. An unusual presentation of active myocarditis is a syndrome that is indistinguishable from acute myocardial infarction.[47] CHF, without evidence of previous or ongoing infection, may represent the most common clinical presentation of this process.

On echocardiography, left ventricular dilatation with systolic dysfunction, increased wall thickness, and/or pericardial effusion may be identified.[48] These findings, however, do not help differentiate active myocarditis from other forms of myocardial disease.

Diagnosis of Myocarditis

At present, the diagnosis of active myocarditis is established when there is histologic evidence of inflammation in cardiac tissue. Until recently, this evidence was available only retrospectively through autopsy analysis. However, safe intravascular techniques for endomyocardial biopsy have made histologic analysis of myocardial tissue possible during life. After demonstration that active myocarditis can be identified histologically in patients with otherwise unexplained CHF,[49] several investigators reported their experience in detecting myocarditis[50–73] (Table 14.1). The wide variation in observed frequency could be explained by varying histologic criteria.[74]

Recognizing this problem, a panel of cardiovascular pathologists established a working definition of myocarditis, the "Dallas" criteria.[75] They defined "active" myocarditis as "an inflammatory infiltrate of the

TABLE 14.1. Incidence of biopsy-proven myocarditis in unexplained congestive heart failure.

Investigators	Year	Patients biopsied	Myocarditis (%)
Mason et al.[49]	1980	400	2
Noda[50]	1980	52	1
Baandrup and Olsen[51]	1981	201	4
Das et al.[52]	1981	12	8
Nippoldt et al.[53]	1982	34	12
Fenoglio et al.[54]	1983	135	25
Unverferth et al.[55]	1983	42	9
Parillo et al.[56]	1984	74	26
Zee-Cheng et al.[57]	1984	35	63
O'Connell et al.[58]	1984	68	7
Daly et al.[59]	1984	69	17
Regitz et al.[60]	1984	290	6
Rose et al.[61]	1984	76	0
Dec et al.[62]	1985	27	67
Salvi et al.[63]	1985	74	18
Mortensen et al.[64]	1985	65	18
Hosenpud et al.[65]	1985	38	16
Cassling et al.[66]	1985	80	2
Hammond et al.[67]	1987	52	19
Maisch et al.[68]	1988	123	8
Chow et al.[69]	1988	90	4
Leatherbury et al.[70]	1988	20	25
Hobbs et al.[71]	1989	148	21
Latham et al.[72]	1989	52	13
Vasiljevic et al.[73]	1990	85	12

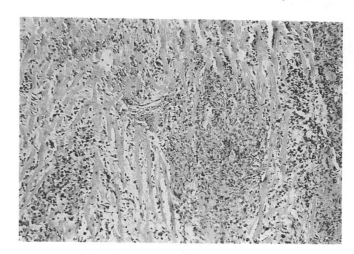

FIGURE 14.2. Photomicrograph of an endomyocardial biopsy fragment from a patient with unexplained congestive heart failure showing a dense lymphocytic infiltrate with myocyte necrosis characteristic of "active" myocarditis (hematoxylin and eosin, original magnification ×20).

myocardium with necrosis and/or degeneration of adjacent myocytes not typical of the ischemic damage associated with coronary artery disease" (Fig. 14.1). Using this convention or initial biopsy, the histologic diagnostic possibilities include active myocarditis with or without fibrosis (Fig. 14.2), borderline myocarditis, or no myocarditis. To confirm the clinical significance of these histologic categories, Dec and colleagues reported that in four of six patients whose initial biopsy demonstrated borderline myocarditis, repeat biopsy showed the diagnosis of active myocarditis.[76] In 22 patients in whom the initial biopsy showed either myocyte hypertrophy or interstitial fibrosis (no myocarditis), active myocarditis was not confirmed on repeat biopsy even when both ventricles were biopsied to minimize sampling error. Application of this working definition by the Pathology Panel of the Myocarditis Treatment Trial (see below) has yielded a very high rate of diagnostic agreement. The Dallas criteria have been widely applied and accepted as the standard against which other criteria are compared.

Radioisotopic imaging with the inflammation-avid radioisotope gallium-67 is quite sensitive but nonspecific in predicting active myocarditis in patients undergoing biopsy.[58] This imaging modality is expensive and cumbersome. Therefore, gallium scanning is not recommended as a screening test. Imaging with [111]indium-labeled antimyosin (Fab) fragments detects myocyte injury. The sensitivity of this technique for the diagnosis of active myocarditis is high with poor specificity.[77] The investigators propose that the lack of specificity was related to the sampling error of endomyocardial biopsy. A potentially more important problem is that this scanning technique cannot distinguish among the many causes for myocyte damage.

Unfortunately, only autopsy analyses, which cannot draw valid comparisons to endomyocardial biopsy in living patients, have been used to quantitate the degree of sampling error in myocarditis.[78–80] Biopsy studies in cardiac transplant rejection show a low false negative incidence when an adequate number of samples are obtained.[81] In addition, the study of Midei and colleagues[82] demonstrated a 78% incidence of myocarditis in peripartum CHF suggesting a very low false negative rate. While these two forms of inflammatory heart disease may not be representative, these studies are more convincing to us than autopsy reviews that necessarily examine a different stage of the disease.

When retrospective analyses of patients with active myocarditis were compared to patients in whom myocarditis was suspected but could not be proven histologically, clinical variables were not useful in predicting patients with active myocarditis. Heart failure presenting in the puerperium may be the exception in that patients with peripartum cardiomyopathy, if biopsied early, have an incidence of myocarditis three- to fourfold greater than other patients with unexplained CHF.[82,83] In more than 2000 patients logged into the Myocarditis Treatment Trial, 9% have active myocarditis on biopsy.

Before the application of endomyocardial biopsy, the proof of progression from active myocarditis to DCM was not available. Quigley and colleagues established the diagnosis of active myocarditis by biopsy in 23 patients and over long-term follow-up, DCM with histologic confirmation developed in 52%.[84] Endomyocardial biopsy, therefore, has been useful in confirming the relationship between myocarditis and DCM.

While histologic criteria currently provide the gold standard for diagnosing myocarditis, other diagnostic criteria undoubtedly will supercede histology in the future. If myocarditis is largely an infectious inflammatory or postinfectious immune-mediated disease, lymphocytic infiltration and myocyte necrosis may be present in only a proportion of cases. Myocyte damage or dysfunction might be induced by a variety of immunological insults that do not require a prominent cellular infiltrate.

Treatment

The initial treatment of active myocarditis is directed toward the clinical symptoms. Treatment of CHF should be initiated with diuretics, vasodilators, and digitalis glycosides. If bradyarrhythmias are present, a temporary pacemaker may be warranted. The inflamed endocardium is predisposed to development of mural thrombi and anticoagulation should be administered even if the left ventricular ejection fraction would not otherwise warrant this treatment.[85] In the murine model, forced physical exercise accentuates the myocyte necrosis and prolongs viral replication.[86,87] Although similar provocative studies have not been performed in man, it is wise to restrict physical activity until histologic resolution has been documented. When extreme degrees of hemodynamic compromise are present, inotropic support and mechanical circulatory assistance may be necessary.

Myocarditis may be complicated by life-threatening ventricular arrhythmias, and even may present with sudden death with minimal or no left ventricular dysfunction.[88] Since myocarditis may resolve spontaneously or respond to immunosuppression with reduction in the risk of arrhythmia recurrence, the decision to institute aggressive antiarrhythmic therapy, including electrophysiologic studies and possible defibrillator implantation, is very difficult. Both antiarrhythmic therapy and immunosuppressive therapy cause substantial morbidity. Thus, the decision to attempt prevention of life-threatening arrhythmias includes a choice between these two therapies, or use of both of them.

We recommended temporizing, if possible, with protracted inpatient monitoring until myocarditis resolves. At that point, an electrophysiologic study can be used to detect continued arrhythmia vulnerability. If, on the other hand, inflammation on biopsy persists, or LV dysfunction worsens, the need to treat the arrhythmia vulnerability is clear.

TABLE 14.2. Uncontrolled reports of immunosuppression in biopsy-proven myocarditis.

Investigator	Year	n	Improved	Therapy
Mason et al.[49]	1980	10	5	CS, AZA
Sekiguchi et al.[92]	1980	3	2	CS
Edwards et al.[93]	1982	4	2	CS
Fenoglio et al.[54]	1983	19	8	CS, AZA
Zee-Cheng et al.[57]	1984	11	5	CS, AZA, ATG
Daly et al.[59]	1984	9	7	CS, AZA
Vignola et al.[88]	1984	6	5	CS, AZA
Fenely et al.[94]	1984	2	2	CS, AZA
Dec et al.[62]	1985	9	4	CS, AZA
Mortensen et al.[64]	1985	12	8	CS, AZA, CYA
Hosenpud et al.[65]	1985	6	0	CS, AZA
Salvi et al.[95]	1989	14	8	CS, AZA
Chan et al.[96]	1990	13	6	CS, AZA
Total		118	62 (52%)	

CS = corticosteroids; AZA = azathioprine; ATG = antithymocyte globulin; CYA = cyclosporine; n = number of patients.

Immunosuppressive therapy has become a popular although unproven treatment. The use of corticosteroids predated endomyocardial biopsy. When children with suspected acute myocarditis were given adrenocorticotropic hormone (ACTH) or corticosteroid preparations, improvement was reported.[89,90] Patients with DCM in the absence of active inflammation who received corticosteroid therapy showed only short-lived improvement and the disadvantages of chronic corticosteroid therapy far outweighed its efficacy.[72,91] Several investigators have reported that immunosuppressive therapy results in improvement in patients with unexplained CHF or ventricular arrhythmias with biopsy-proven myocarditis (Table 14.2).[49,54,57,59,62,64,65,88,92–96] Administration of OKT3, a murine monoclonal antibody directed to the pan T cell CD3 antigen, also has been reported to result in improvement in active myocarditis.[97]

These data have serious shortcomings. The natural history of myocarditis is unknown; consequently, these uncontrolled nonrandomized studies do not verify efficacy of therapy. The specific immunosuppressive regimens were not consistent within or among the studies. Improvement was ill-defined and inconsistent. Additionally, most reports predated the Dallas criteria and consequently the standards used to establish the diagnosis of myocarditis were variable. The existent literature, therefore, cannot be interpreted because of lack of a meaningful clinical trial. Because of these deficiencies, the multicenter NIH-sponsored Myocarditis Treatment Trial was established.[98]

This clinical trial is designed to determine the efficacy of immunosuppressive therapy in active myocarditis and to elucidate the immunopathogenesis of the human disease. Patients with a radionuclide ejection fraction

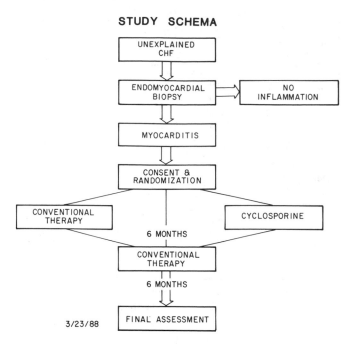

FIGURE 14.3. Study design of the Myocarditis Treatment Trial.

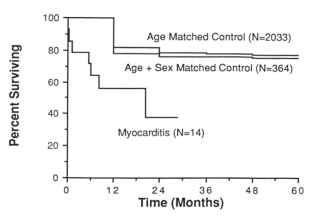

FIGURE 14.4. Comparison of survival in recipients with active myocarditis who undergo cardiac transplantation to sex- and age-matched and age-matched female controls. Reproduced with permission from O'Connell et al.[100]

below 45% who have unexplained CHF and evidence of biopsy-proven myocarditis are eligible for randomization to conventional therapy for CHF alone or conventional therapy with the addition of prednisone and cyclosporine (Fig. 14.3). After a 6-month period of randomized drug therapy, all patients are followed for another 6 months until final evaluation 1 yr after the initial randomization period.

At baseline, 12, 28, and 52 weeks after randomization, left ventricular ejection fraction (EF) by radionuclide angiography, exercise treadmill testing, endomyocardial biopsy, right heart catheterization and hemodynamic study, 12-lead electrocardiogram (ECG), 24-hr Holter monitor, and M-mode and two-dimensional echocardiography are performed to assess the serial changes and correlate the histology with the clinical and hemodynamic course. Within the clinical trial, a cellular immunology study is being conducted in which peripheral blood is studied for lymphocyte subset frequencies, natural killer cell activity, and antibody-dependent cellular cytotoxicity. Endomyocardial biopsy samples are studied for lymphocyte subpopulations and presence of enteroviral genomes. Immunofluorescence of endomyocardial biopsies and assessment of heart-specific antibodies in the peripheral blood have been incorporated into the clinical trial.

Enrollment of patients was initiated in October 1986 and it became readily apparent that enrollment would not meet the anticipated sample size. Enrollment was completed in October 1990 and final data analysis is pending. The results of the Myocarditis Treatment Trial should further elucidate the natural history of the disease, shed light on the immunopathogenesis of the disease and determine whether immunosuppressive therapy should be administered to patients with active myocarditis. If immunosuppressive therapy is not effective, endomyocardial biopsy should be restricted to cardiac transplantation centers where biopsy is necessary to survey for allograft rejection, to the occasional patient who with a form of cardiomyopathy in which a specific diagnosis can be made,[99] and oncology centers where cardiotoxicity of chemotherapeutic agents is monitored by histopathology.

Active myocarditis may not be responsive to medical management. Cardiac transplantation must then be considered. Because active myocarditis is characterized by humoral antibodies and cytotoxic lymphocytic effector cells directed toward human cardiac antigens, the pretransplantation immunologic milieu may predispose the allograft to aggressive early rejection. Retrospective analysis of the baseline characteristics and clinical outcome of 12 patients who had active myocarditis in their explanted heart demonstrated early rejection with a high mortality that achieved statistical significance when compared to age- and sex-matched controls[100] (Fig. 14.4). Beyond the early posttransplant period, the outcome was indistinguishable from the general transplant population. Before a patient with active myocarditis should be considered for cardiac transplantation, a period of hemodynamic support and perhaps a trial of immunosuppression should be considered to establish the need for transplantation. Prospective trials to determine whether pretransplant immunosuppression improves the outcome of the allograft should be considered.

Acquired Immunodeficiency Syndrome

The rapidly developing epidemic of acquired immunodeficiency syndrome (AIDS) has resulted in a flurry of information regarding the prevalence of myocarditis. Initially described in autopsy and necropsy studies, myocarditis may be found in up to 50% of patients dying with AIDS.[101,102] Although evidence of CHF occurs at a far lower frequency (10%), a wide range of pathogens including virus, protozoa, bacteria, fungi, and mycobacteria were present in myocardial sections. In one notable series, 45% of patients with AIDS had myocarditis at necropsy, 23% of whom had CHF and 15% had ventricular tachycardia.[103] Characteristic active lymphocytic myocarditis also has been reported.[104] More recently, identification of AIDS retrovirus genomic sequence in cardiac tissue has been confirmed.[105] Endomyocardial biopsy also has been useful in detecting lymphoma in an AIDS patient.[106] Careful prospective studies with immunosuppressive therapy have not been performed. However, the prevalence of AIDS has risen to the point that meaningful prospective clinical trials are now feasible.

Giant Cell Myocarditis

An aggressive form of active myocarditis is identified by the presence of giant cells in the endomyocardial biopsies.[107–109] At times this histologic abnormality has been noted with autoimmune diseases such as myasthenia gravis.[110] Brady- and tachyarrhythmias are common manifestations in patients with giant cell myocarditis. Although isolated reports have demonstrated a response to immunosuppression,[111] more commonly the disease is progressive and unresponsive. Giant cell myocarditis may recur in the allograft after transplantation.

Sarcoid Heart Disease

Another inflammatory heart disease that can be diagnosed by endomyocardial biopsy is sarcoid heart disease.[112,113] When systemic sarcoidosis is associated with cardiac symptoms, a high index of suspicion is present. However, periodically the diagnosis of sarcoid heart disease is made in the absence of extracardiac involvement.[114] Sarcoid heart disease is difficult to differentiate from giant cell myocarditis when extracardiac involvement is absent. Although controlled studies have not been performed, corticosteroids have been advocated. In a report of three patients undergoing transplantation, sarcoidosis did not recur in the allografts.[115]

Eosinophilic Heart Disease

When the eosinophil is the major cell infiltrating the myocardium, the diagnosis of eosinophilic myocarditis is established.[116] The eosinophil granule major basic protein has been detected in areas of acute necrotizing myocarditis, suggesting that the constituents of these granules are toxic to the heart.[117] Although endocardial thickening and restrictive myocardial disease may be detected, eosinophilic myocarditis may occur in the absence of pronounced peripheral eosinophilia with a clinical presentation characterized by systolic dysfunction comparable to DCM. In some reports, administration of corticosteroids has resulted in a prompt improvement in cardiac function or resolution of the histologic abnormalities.[118]

Lyme Carditis

Infection with the spirochete *Borrelia burgdorferi*, which is introduced by the bite of the tick Ixodes dammini, may result in Lyme disease characterized by erythema chronicum migrans, fever, myalgias, arthralgias, headache, lymphadenopathy, and fatigue.[119] The disease generally is responsive to tetracycline during the early phase but may progress to Lyme carditis. Lyme carditis is characteristically manifested by complete heart block, although left ventricular dysfunction may occur.[120,121] Endomyocardial biopsy may reveal active myocarditis. In at least one report a suspected spirochete was demonstrated in the biopsy specimen.[121] Treatment of active disease with corticosteroids has been successful in isolated case reports.[122]

Summary

Elucidation of the immune responses that adversely affect cardiac function provide new insight into the etiology of inflammatory heart disease and DCM. Further study of immune mechanisms may improve the diagnostic yield in patients with unexplained heart failure. A detailed understanding of mechanisms may result in development of therapies that effectively alter the natural history of this disease. The efficacy of conventional immunosuppressive therapy is being tested in the ongoing Myocarditis Treatment Trial.

References

1. O'Connell JB. Evidence linking viral myocarditis to dilated cardiomyopathy in humans. In: Robinson JA, O'Connell JB, eds. *Myocarditis: precursor of cardiomyopathy.* Lexington, MA: DC Heath and Co; 1983:93–108.
2. Kriett JM, Kaye MP. The registry of the international society for heart transplantation: seventh official report—1990. *J Heart Transplant.* 1990;9:323–330.
3. Woodruff JF. Viral myocarditis. *Am J Pathol.* 1980;101:427–479.
4. Herskowitz A, Wolfgram LJ, Rose NR, et al. Coxsackievirus B₃ murine myocarditis: a pathologic spectrum of myocarditis in genetically defined inbred strains. *J Am Coll Cardiol.* 1987;9:1311–1319.

5. Wilson FM, Miranda QR, Chason JL, et al. Residual pathologic changes following murine Coxsackie A and B myocarditis. *Am J Pathol*. 1969;55:253–269.

6. Reyes MP, Ho K-L, Smith F, et al. A mouse model of dilated-type cardiomyopathy due to Coxsackievirus B₃. *J Infect Dis*. 1981;144:232–236.

7. EL-Khatib, MR, Chason JL, Lerner AM. Ventricular aneurysms complicating Coxsackievirus group B, types 1 and 4 murine myocarditis. *Circulation*. 1979;59:412–416.

8. Matsumori A, Kawai C. An animal model of congestive (dilated) cardiomyopathy: dilatation and hypertrophy of the heart in the chronic stage in DBA/2 mice with myocarditis caused by encephalomyocarditis virus. *Circulation*. 1982;66:355–360.

9. Woodruff JF, Woodruff JJ. Involvement of T lymphocytes in the pathogenesis of Coxsackie virus B₃ heart disease. *J Immunol*. 1974;113:1726–1734.

10. Paque RE, Gauntt CJ, Nealon TJ, et al. Assessment of cell-mediated hypersensitivity against Coxsackievirus B3 viral-induced myocarditis utilizing hypertonic salt extracts of cardiac tissue. *J Immunol*. 1978;120:1672–1678.

11. Huber SA, Lodge PA. Coxsackievirus B-3 myocarditis: identification of different pathogenic mechanisms in DBA/2 and BALB/c mice. *Am J Pathol*. 1986;122:284–191.

12. Limas CJ, Goldenberg IF, Limas C. Autoantibodies against beta-adrenoceptors in human idiopathic dilated cardiomyopathy. *Circulation*. 1989;64:97–103.

13. Neu N, Craig SW, Rose NR, et al. Coxsackievirus induced myocarditis in mice: cardiac myosin autoantibodies do not cross-react with the virus. *Clin Exp Immunol*. 1987;69:566–574.

14. Schultheiss H-P. The significance of autoantibodies against the ADP/ATP carrier for the pathogenesis of myocarditis and dilated cardiomyopathy—clinical and experimental data. *Springer Semin Immunopathol*. 1989;11:15–30.

15. Neu N, Rose NR, Beisel, et al. Cardiac myosin induces myocarditis in genetically predisposed mice. *J Immunol*. 1987;139:3630–3636.

16. Modlin JF, Crumpacker CS. Coxsackievirus B infection in pregnant mice and transplacental infection of the fetus. *Infect Immun*. 1982;37:222–226.

17. Morin Y, Roy PE, Mohiuddin SM, et al. The influence of alcohol on viral and isoproterenol cardiomyopathy. *Cardiovasc Res*. 1969;3:363–368.

18. Matsumori A, Wang H, Abelmann WH, et al. Treatment of viral myocarditis with ribavirin in an animal preparation. *Circulation*. 1985;71:834–839.

19. Matsumori A, Crumpacker CS, Abelmann WH, et al. Virus vaccine and passive immunization for the prevention of viral myocarditis in mice. *Jpn Circ J*. 1987;51:1362–1364.

20. Matsumori A, Crumpacker CS, Abelmann WH. Prevention of viral myocarditis with recombinant human leukocyte interferon alpha A/D in a murine model. *J Am Coll Cardiol*. 1987;9:1320–1325.

21. Tomioka N, Kishimoto C, Matsumori A, et al. Effects of prednisolone on acute viral myocarditis in mice. *J Am Coll Cardiol*. 1986;7:868–872.

22. Costanzo-Nordin MR, Reap EA, O'Connell JB, et al. A nonsteroid anti-inflammatory drug exacerbates Coxsackie B3 murine myocarditis. *J Am Coll Cardiol*. 1985;6:1078–1082.

23. Kishimoto C, Thorp KA, Abelmann WH. Immunosuppression with high doses of cyclophosphamide reduces the severity of myocarditis but increases the mortality in murine Coxsackievirus B3 myocarditis. *Circulation*. 1990;82:982–989.

24. Khatib R, Khatib G, Chason JL, et al. Alterations in coxsackievirus B4 heart muscle disease in ICR swiss mice by anti-thymocyte serum. *J Gen Virol*. 1983;64:231–236.

25. O'Connell JB, Reap EA, Robinson JA. The effects of cyclosporine on acute murine Coxsackie B3 myocarditis. *Circulation*. 1986;73:353–359.

26. Estrin M, Herzum M, Buie C, et al. Immunosuppressives in murine myocarditis. *Eur Heart J*. 1987;8(suppl J):259–262.

27. Fowles RE, Bieber CP, Stinson EB. Defective in vitro suppressor cell function in idiopathic congestive cardiomyopathy. *Circulation*. 1979;59:483–491.

28. Anderson JL, Carlquist JF, Hammond EH. Deficient natural killer cell activity in patients with idiopathic dilated cardiomyopathy. *Lancet*. 1982;2:1124–1128.

29. Schervish E, O'Connell JB, Kowalczyk D. Suppressor cell function in dilated cardiomyopathy. *Eur Heart J*. 1987;8(suppl J): 141–143.

30. McManus BM, Switzer BL, Kendall TJ, et al. Markedly diminished natural killing and antibody-dependent cell-mediated cytotoxicity in patients with idiopathic dilated cardiomyopathy and biopsy-proven myocarditis. *Circulation*. 1989;80(suppl II):II-666. Abstract.

31. Deguchi H, Hayashi T, Kotaka M, et al. In situ analysis with monoclonal antibodies of lymphocyte subsets in myocardial biopsies from patients with dilated cardiomyopathy and idiopathic (viral) myocarditis. *Jpn Circ J*. 1987;51:13651372.

32. Maisch B, Deeg P, Liebau G, et al. Diagnostic relevance of humoral and cytotoxic immune reactions in primary and secondary dilated cardiomyopathy. *Am J Cardiol*. 1983;52:1072–1078.

33. Neumann DA, Burek CL, Baughman KL, et al. Circulating heart-reactive antibodies in patients with myocarditis or cardiomyopathy. *J Am Coll Cardiol*. 1990;16:839–846.

34. Schultheiss H-P, Schulze K, Kuhl U, Ulrich G, Klingenberg M. The ADP/ATP carrier as a mitochondrial autoantigen—facts and perspectives. *Ann NY Acad Sci*. 1986;488:44–64.

35. Schulze K, Becker B, Schauer R, Schultheiss H. Antibodies to ADP/ATP carrier—an autoantigen in myocarditis and dilated cardiomyopathy—impair cardiac function. *Circulation*. 1990;81:959–969.

36. McManus BM, Gauntt CJ, Casling RS. Immunopathologic basis of myocardial injury. *Cardovasc Clin*. 1987;18:231–252.

37. Kurnick JT, Leary C, Palacios IF, et al. Culture and characterization of lymphocytic infiltrates from endomyocardial biopsies of patients with idiopathic myocarditis. *Eur Heart J*. 1987;8(suppl J):135–139.

38. Herskowitz A, Ahmed-Ansari A, Neumann DA, et al.

Induction of major histocompatibility complex antigens within the myocardium of patients with active myocarditis: a nonhistologic marker of myocarditis. *J Am Coll Cardiol*. 1990;15:624–632.

39. Young LHY, Joag SV, Zheng L-M, et al. Perforin-mediated myocardial damage in acute myocarditis. *Lancet*. 1990;336:1019–1021.

40. Bowles NE, Richardson PJ, Olsen EGJ, et al. Detection of Coxsackie-B-virus-specific RNA sequences in myocardial biopsy samples from patients with myocarditis and dilated cardiomyopathy. *Lancet*. 1986;1:1120–1123.

41. Tracy S, Chapman NM, McManus BM, et al. A molecular and serologic evaluation of enteroviral involvement in human myocarditis. *J Mol Cell Cardiol*. 1990;22:403–414.

42. Jin O, Sole MJ, Butany JW, et al. Detection of enterovirus RNA in myocardial biopsies from patients with myocarditis and cardiomyopathy using gene amplification by polymerase chain reaction. *Circulation*. 1990;82:8–16.

43. Eggers HJ, Mertens T. Viruses and myocardium: notes of a virologist. *Eur Heart J*. 1987;8(suppl J):129–133.

44. Abelmann WH. Incidence of dilated cardiomyopathy. *Postgrad Med J*. 1985;61:1123–1124.

45. O'Connell JB, Robinson JA. Coxsackie viral myocarditis. *Postgrad Med J*. 1985;61:1127–1131.

46. Kawamura K, Kitaura Y, Morita H, et al. Viral and idiopathic myocarditis in Japan: a questionnaire survey. *Heart Vessel* 1985;(suppl 1):18–22.

47. Costanzo-Nordin MR, O'Connell JB, Subramanian R, et al. Myocarditis confirmed by biopsy presenting as acute myocardial infarction. *Br Heart J*. 1985;53:25–29.

48. Hosenpud JD. Cardiac structure and function in biopsy proven myocarditis: an echocardiographic substudy of the Myocarditis Treatment Trial. *J Am Coll Cardiol*. 1991;17:382A. Abstract.

49. Mason JW, Billingham ME, Ricci DR. Treatment of acute inflammatory myocarditis assisted by endomyocardial biopsy. *Am J Cardiol*. 1980;45:1037–1044.

50. Noda S. Histopathology of endomyocardial biopsies from patients with idiopathic cardiomyopathy: quantitative evaluation based on multivariate statistical analysis. *Jpn Circ J*. 1980;44:95–116.

51. Baandrup U, Olsen EGJ. Critical analysis of endomyocardial biopsies from patients suspected of having cardiomyopathy. I: Morphologic and morpometric aspects. *Br Heart J*. 1981;45:476–486.

52. Das JP, Rath B, Das S, et al. Study of endomyocardial biopsies in cardiomyopathy. *Indian Heart J*. 1981;33:18–26.

53. Nippoldt TB, Edwards WD, Holmes DR, et al. Right ventricular endomyocardial biopsy. *Mayo Clin Proc*. 1982;57:407–418.

54. Fenoglio JJ, Ursell PC, Kellogg CF, et al. Diagnosis and classification of myocarditis by endomyocardial biopsy. *N Engl J Med*. 1983;308:12–18.

55. Unverferth DV, Ketters JK, Unverferth BJ, et al. Human myocardial histologic characteristics in congestive heart failure. *Circulation*. 1983;68:1194–1200.

56. Parrillo JE, Aretz HT, Palacios I, et al. The results of transvenous endomyocardial biopsy can frequently be used to diagnose myocardial diseases in patients with idiopathic heart failure. *Circulation*. 1984;69:93–101.

57. Zee-Cheng C-S, Tsai CC, Palmer DC, et al. High incidence of myocarditis by endomyocardial biopsy in patients with idiopathic congestive cardiomyopathy. *J Am Coll Cardiol*. 1984;3:63–70.

58. O'Connell JB, Henkin RE, Robinson JA, et al. Gallium-67 imaging in patients with dilated cardiomyopathy and biopsy-proven myocarditis. *Circulation*. 1984;70:58–62.

59. Daly K, Richardson PJ, Olsen EGJ, et al. Acute myocarditis: role of histological and virological examination in the diagnosis and assessment of immunosuppressive treatment. *Br Heart J*. 1984;51:30–35.

60. Regitz V, Knoll P, Rudolph W. Clinical and hemodynamic findings in patients with histologically documented myocarditis. *Eur Heart J*. 1984;5(suppl I):65. Abstract.

61. Rose AG, Fraser RC, Beck W. Absence of evidence of myocarditis in endomyocardial biopsy specimens from patients with dilated (congestive) cardiomyopathy. *S Afr Med J*. 1984;66:871–874.

62. Dec GW, Palacios IG, Fallon JT, et al. Active myocarditis in the spectrum of acute dilated cardiomyopathies. *N Engl J Med*. 1985;312:885–890.

63. Salvi A, Silvestri F, Gori D, et al. La biopsia endomiocardica: un'esperienza relativa a 156 pazienti. *G Ital Cardiol*. 1985;17:251–259.

64. Mortensen SA, Baandrup U, Buch J, et al. Immunosuppressive therapy of biopsy proven myocarditis: experiences with corticosteroids and ciclosporin. *Int J Immunother*. 1985;1:35–45.

65. Hosenpud JD, McAnulty JA, Niles NR. Lack of objective improvement in ventricular systolic function in patients with myocarditis treated with azathioprine and prednisone. *J Am Coll Cardiol*. 1985;6:797–801.

66. Cassling RS, Linder J, Sears TD, et al. Quantitative evaluation of inflammation in biopsy specimens from idiopathically failing or irritable hearts: experience in 80 pediatric and adult patients. *Am Heart J*. 1985;110:713–720.

67. Hammond EH, Menlove RL, Anderson JL. Predictive value of immunofluorescence and electron microscopic evaluation of endomyocardial biopsies in the diagnosis and prognosis of myocarditis and idiopathic dilated cardiomyopathy. *Am Heart J*. 1987;114:1055–1065.

68. Maisch B, Bauer E, Hufnagel G, et al. The use of endomyocardial biopsy in heart failure. *Eur Heart J*. 1988;9(suppl H):59–71.

69. Chow LC, Dittrich HC, Shabetai R. Endomyocardial biopsy in patients with unexplained congestive heart failure. *Ann Intern Med*. 1988;109:535–539.

70. Leatherbury L, Chandra RS, Shapiro SR, et al. Value of endomyocardial biopsy in infants, children and adolescents with dilated or hypertrophic cardiomyopathy and myocarditis. *J Am Coll Cardiol*. 1988;12:1547–1554.

71. Hobbs RE, Pelegrin D, Ratliff NB, et al. Lymphocytic myocarditis and dilated cardiomyopathy: treatment with immunosuppressive agents. *Cleve Clin J Med*. 1989;56:628–635.

72. Latham RD, Mulrow JP, Virmani R, et al. Recently diagnosed idiopathic dilated cardiomyopathy: incidence

of myocarditis and efficacy of prednisone therapy. *Am Heart J*. 1989;117:876–882.

73. Vasiljevic JD, Kanjuh V, Seferovic P, et al. The incidence of myocarditis in endomyocardial biopsy samples from patients with congestive heart failure. *Am Heart J*. 1990;120:1370–1377.

74. Shanes JG, Ghali J, Billingham ME, et al. Interobserver variability in the pathologic interpretation of endomyocardial biopsy results. *Circulation*. 1987;75:401–405.

75. Aretz HT, Billingham ME, Edwards WD, et al. Myocarditis: a histopathologic definition and classification. *Am J Cardiovasc Pathol*. 1986;1:3–14.

76. Dec GW, Fallon JT, Southern JF, et al. "Borderline" myocarditis: an indication for repeat endomyocardial biopsy. *J Am Coll Cardiol*. 1990;15:283–289.

77. Dec GW, Palacios I, Yasuda T, et al. Antimyosin antibody cardiac imaging: its role in the diagnosis of myocarditis. *J Am Coll Cardiol*. 1990;16:97–104.

78. Chow LH, Radio SJ, Sears TD, et al. Insensitivity of right ventricular endomyocardial biopsy in the diagnosis of myocarditis. *J Am Coll Cardiol*. 1989;14:915–920.

79. Hauck AJ, Kearney DL, Edwards WD. Evaluation of postmortem endomyocardial biopsy specimens from 38 patients with lymphocytic myocarditis: implications for role of sampling error. *Mayo Clin Proc*. 1989;64:1235–1245.

80. Billingham ME. Acute myocarditis: is sampling error a contraindication for diagnostic biopsies? *J Am Coll Cardiol*. 1989;14:921–922.

81. Spiegelhalter DJ, Stovin TGI. An analysis of repeated biopsies following cardiac transplantation. *Stat Med*. 1983;2:33–40.

82. Midei MG, DeMent SH, Feldman AM, et al. Peripartum myocarditis and cardiomyopathy. *Circulation*. 1990;81:922–928.

83. O'Connell JB, Costanzo-Nordin MR, Subramanian R, et al. Peripartum cardiomyopathy: clinical, hemodynamic, histologic and prognostic characteristics. *J Am Coll Cardiol*. 1986;8:52–56.

84. Quigley PJ, Richardson PJ, Meany BT, et al. Long-term follow-up of acute myocarditis. correlation of ventricular function and outcome. *Eur Heart J*. 1987;8(suppl J):39–42.

85. Tomioka N, Kishimoto C, Matsumori A, et al. Mural thrombus in experimental viral myocarditis in mice: relation between thrombosis and congestive heart failure. *Cardiovasc Res*. 1986;20:665–671.

86. Tilles JG, Elson SH, Shaka JA, et al. Effects of exercise on Coxsackie A9 myocarditis in adult mice. *Proc Soc Exp Biol Med*. 1964;117:777–782.

87. Iback N-G, Fohlman J, Friman G. Exercise in Coxsackie B3 myocarditis: effects on heart lymphocyte subpopulations and the inflammatory reaction. *Am Heart J*. 1989;117:1298–1302.

88. Vignola PA, Aonuma K, Swaye PS, et al. Lymphocytic myocarditis presenting as unexplained ventricular arrhythmias: diagnosis with endomyocardial biopsy and response to immunosuppression. *J Am Coll Cardiol*. 1984;4:812–819.

89. Garrison RF, Swisher RC. Myocarditis of unknown etiology (Fiedler's) treated with ACTH. *J Pediatr*. 1953;42:591–599.

90. Ainger LE. Acute aseptic myocarditis corticosteroid therapy. *J Pediatr*. 1964;64:716–723.

91. Parrillo JE, Cunnion RE, Epstein SE, et al. A prospective randomized, controlled trial of prednisone for dilated cardiomyopathy. *N Engl J Med*. 1989;321:1061–1068.

92. Sekiguchi M, Hiroe M, Take M, et al. Clinical and histopathological profile of sarcoidosis of the heart and acute idiopathic myocarditis. II Myocarditis. *Jpn Circ J*. 1980;44:264–273.

93. Edwards WD, Holmes DR, Reeder GS. Diagnosis of active lymphocytic myocarditis by endomyocardial biopsy. *Mayo Clin Proc*. 1982;57:419–425.

94. Feneley MP, Gavaghan TP, Ralston M, et al. Diagnosis and management of acute myocarditis aided by serial myocardial biopsy. *Aust NZ J Med*. 1984;14:826–830.

95. Salvi A, Di Lenarda A, Dreas L, et al. Immunosuppressive treatment in myocarditis. *Int J Cardiol*. 1989;22:329–338.

96. Chain KT, Iwahara M, Benson LN, et al. Immunosuppressive therapy in the management of acute myocarditis in children: a clinical trial. *J Am Coll Cardiol*. 1991;17:458–460.

97. Gilbert EM, O'Connell JB, Hammond ME, et al. Treatment of myocarditis with OKT3 monoclonal antibody (letter). *Lancet*. 1988;1:759.

98. O'Connell JB, Mason JW. The applicability of results of streamlined trials in clinical practice: the Myocarditis Treatment Trial. *Stat Med*. 1990;9:193–197.

99. Mason JW, O'Connell JB. Clinical merit of endomyocardial biopsy. *Circulation*. 1989;79:971–979.

100. O'Connell JB, Dec GW, Goldenberg IF, et al. Results of heart transplantation for active lymphocytic myocarditis. *J Heart Transplant*. 1990;9:351–356.

101. Anderson DW, Virmani R, Reilly JM, et al. Prevalent myocarditis at necropsy in the acquired immunodeficiency syndrome. *J Am Coll Cardiol*. 1988;11:792–799.

102. Baroldi G, Corallo S, Moroni M, et al. Focal lymphocytic myocarditis in acquired immunodeficiency syndrome (AIDS): a correlative morphologic and clinical study in 26 consecutive fatal cases. *J Am Coll Cardiol*. 1988;12:463–469.

103. Reilly JM, Cunnion RE, Anderson DW, et al. Frequency of myocarditis, left ventricular dysfunction and ventricular tachycardia in the acquired immune deficiency syndrome. *Am J Cardiol*. 1988;62:789–793.

104. Levy WS, Varghese J, Anderson DW, et al. Myocarditis diagnosed by endomyocardial biopsy in human immunodeficiency virus infection with cardiac dysfunction. *Am J Cardiol*. 1988;62:658–659.

105. Grody WW, Cheng L, Lewis W. Infection of the heart by the human immunodeficiency virus. *Am J Cardiol*. 1990;66:203–206.

106. Andress JD, Polish LB, Clark DM, Hossack KF. Transvenous biopsy diagnosis of cardiac lymphoma in an AIDS patient. *Am Heart J*. 1989;118:421423.

107. Kean BH, Hoekenga MT. Giant cell myocarditis. *Am J Pathol*. 1952;28:1095–1105.

108. Davies MJ, Pomerance A, Teare RD. Idiopathic giant cell myocarditis-a distinctive clinico-pathological entity. *Br Heart J*. 1975;37:192–195.

109. Davidoff R, Palacios I, Southern J, et al. Giant cell versus lymphocytic myocarditis: a comparison of their clinical features and long-term outcomes. *Circulation*. 1991;83:953–961.

110. Burke JS, Medline NM, Katz A. Giant cell myocarditis and myositis. *Arch Pathol*. 1969;88:359–366.

111. McFalls EO, Hosenpud JD, McAnulty JH, et al. Granulomatous myocarditis: diagnosis by endomyocardial biopsy and response to corticosteroids in two patients. *Chest*. 1986;89:509–511.

112. Fleming HA. Sarcoid heart disease. *Br Heart J*. 1974;36:54–68.

113. Roberts WC, McAllister HA, Ferrans VJ. Sarcoidosis of the heart. *Am J Med*. 1977;63:86–108.

114. Lorell B, Alderman EL, Mason JW. Cardiac sarcoidosis. Diagnosis with endomyocardial biopsy and treatment with corticosteroids. *Am J Cardiol*. 1978;42:143–146.

115. Valantine HA, Taxelaar HD, Macoviak J, et al. Cardiac sarcoidosis: response to steroids and transplantation. *J Heart Transplant*. 1987;6:244–250.

116. Spry CJF, Tai P-C. The eosinophil in myocardial disease. *Eur Heart J*. 1987;8(suppl J):81–84.

117. DeMello DE, Liapis H, Jureidini S, et al. Cardiac localization of eosinophil-granule major basic protein in acute necrotizing myocarditis. *N Engl J Med*. 1990; 323:1542–1545.

118. Kim CH, Vlietstra RE, Edwards WD, et al. Steroid-responsive eosinophilic myocarditis: diagnosis by endomyocardial biopsy. *Am J Cardiol*. 1984;53:1472–1473.

119. Steere AC, Batsford WP, Weinberg M, et al. Lyme carditis: cardiac abnormalities of lyme disease. *Ann Intern Med*. 1980;93:8–16.

120. McAlister HF, Klementowicz PT, Andrews C, et al. Lyme carditis: an important cause of reversible heart block. *Ann Intern Med*. 1989;110:339–345.

121. Reznick JW, Braunstein DB, Walsh RL, et al. Lyme carditis: electrophysiologic and histopathologic study. *Am J Med*. 1986;81:923–927.

122. Olson LJ, Okafor EC, Clements IP. Cardiac involvement in Lyme disease: manifestations and management. *Mayo Clin Proc*. 1986;61:745–749.

15
Congestive Heart Failure as a Consequence of Valvular Heart Disease

Barry H. Greenberg

Congestive heart failure (CHF) is an extremely serious complication of valvular heart disease. Not only does it indicate that the valve lesion is severe but, in almost all instances, the onset of CHF has been related to an important deterioration in the subsequent clinical course. Thus, the prevention, prompt recognition, and effective treatment of CHF in patients with valvular disease are issues of utmost importance to the practicing physician.

This chapter examines the approach to patients who have CHF (or at risk for developing it) as a consequence of left heart valvular lesions. CHF due to right heart valve lesions is discussed in the chapter dealing with congenital abnormalities. After a brief overview of the pathophysiology of pressure and volume overload, the natural history and clinical manifestations of CHF in aortic and mitral valvular disease will be presented. Principles of diagnosis and management are discussed and the chapter concludes with a section on the therapeutic and preventive aspects of vasodilator therapy in patients with left heart valvular insufficiency.

Pathophysiology

CHF can develop in patients with valvular heart disease either as a direct result of excessive loading conditions that overwhelm the reserve capacity of normally functioning myocardium or it can be due to myocardial dysfunction that develops as a long-term consequence of these very loading conditions.[1] When the valve lesion develops acutely, the onset of CHF is almost always related to the deleterious effects of an abrupt increase in the volume or (less commonly) pressure load faced by the left ventricle (LV) or left atrium (LA). In chronic conditions, however, it may be quite difficult to distinguish between the effects of abnormal loading conditions and the onset of myocardial dysfunction as the cause of CHF in an individual patient.

Acute valvular insufficiency of either the aortic or mitral valve subjects the LV to a sudden increase in the volume of blood that it must process with each cardiac cycle. The pressure/volume relationship of the LV determines the increase in pressure that will occur in this situation. As a result of the structure of the myocardium itself and the constraining influence of the surrounding pericardium, the normal LV is relatively noncompliant. Thus, during the early stages of either aortic insufficiency (AI) or mitral regurgitation (MR), the LV has a limited capacity to accommodate an increased diastolic volume at normal levels of filling pressure. In MR, the problem is accentuated by the fact that during systole, the LV can eject blood into either the aorta or the left atrium. The impedance to flow in the atrium is considerably lower than in the systemic circulation. Thus, when the valve lesion is severe, direct regurgitation of blood from the LV to the LA during systole can cause dramatic increases in pressure in the upstream chamber.

Compensatory mechanisms to deal with volume overload that develops as a consequence of acute left heart valvular insufficiency are limited. An increase in LV volume will, to some extent, increase LV stroke volume. However, since sarcomere stretch is close to the maximal level under normal conditions (as far as systolic shortening is concerned),[2] this effect cannot compensate fully for the reduction in forward stroke volume caused by severe acute left heart regurgitant lesions. As cardiac output falls and congestive symptoms begin to develop, there is an increase in sympathetic tone. The resultant catecholamine stimulation has both positive inotropic and chronotropic effects on cardiac function. Alpha-adrenergic stimulation of vascular smooth muscle, however, also promotes vasoconstriction of resistance vessels. While this peripheral effect of catecholamine stimulation may serve to maintain arterial pressure in the face of low cardiac output, the increase in vascular resistance has the unwanted effect of increasing impedance to forward flow. In both AI and

MR, high levels of peripheral resistance tend to increase the severity of the regurgitant flow and hasten the development of CHF.

As a result of the limited capacity of the LV (and to some extent the LA) to compensate for the volume load imposed by a regurgitant lesion and the limits imposed by the pressure/volume relationship in the normal ventricle, individuals who develop acute left heart valvular regurgitation are vulnerable to developing high levels of filling pressure in the left-sided chambers. These pressures, in turn, are transmitted passively backward to the pulmonary circuit and result in an increase in the ambient pressure in the pulmonary capillary bed. Once these pressures begin to exceed levels of 18 to 20 mm Hg, signs and symptoms of pulmonary congestion begin to develop. Further increases in pulmonary capillary pressure lead to more extensive congestion and may result in the development of fulminant pulmonary edema. In general, the extent of CHF can be viewed as a direct indicator of the severity of acute left-sided valvular regurgitation.

In contrast to the acute situation, compensatory mechanisms play an important role in enabling the LV to adapt to chronic volume overload. Cardiac chamber dilatation is the most important of these adaptive changes. Dilatation of the LV and the pericardium allow a rightward shift of the pressure/volume relationship so that any given volume of blood can be accommodated at a lower pressure than in a normal-sized chamber.[3] In this way, volumes of regurgitant flow that would give rise to severe symptoms in the acute setting can be accommodated easily in a dilated LV. The increased volume in the LV also enables stroke volume to increase. Decreased aortic impedance and alterations in the geometry of the LV that permit more efficient external work also help to increase the LV stroke volume.[4,5] Through these mechanisms, cardiac output can be maintained in the normal range despite a regurgitant volume that can be upwards of 80% of the total LV stroke volume. Similarly, dilatation of the LA in the setting of chronic MR may allow that chamber to accommodate massive amounts of regurgitant flow with only minimal increases in pressure.

The increase in LV volumes that is characteristic of left heart valvular regurgitant lesions also serves as a stimulus for an increase in muscle mass. The LV hypertrophy that develops in this setting appears to be a compensatory mechanism that is designed to normalize wall stress.[6] Because the changes in LV chamber size and muscle mass tend to develop in parallel, the restructured chamber tends to resemble a magnified but otherwise normal appearing LV.

Overall, these changes in cardiac structure and function enable the heart to accommodate large amounts of blood volume in the LA and LV at relatively low pressure. They also enable the LV to deliver a substantially larger stroke volume than would be possible in the acute setting. In this way, cardiac performance can be maintained in the normal or near normal range for many years in the presence of severe AI or MR. Despite these adaptive changes, patients with chronic severe volume overload are at risk for developing CHF later in the course. The reason(s) for late decompensation in this setting is uncertain. Chronic myocardial ischemia due to a mismatch between myocardial oxygen supply and demand may be involved in this process.[7] It appears that failure of the LV hypertrophy to keep pace with prevailing loading conditions is an early indicator of impending problems.[8] When this occurs, wall stress is increased and the LV must operate in a situation where excessive afterload can begin to affect LV performance adversely.

Acute pressure overload of the heart due to valvular disease is quite uncommon. It can, however, occur in the setting of acute endocarditis (particularly, when the mitral valve is involved) and as a consequence of prosthetic valve dysfunction. Physiologic compensations for acute pressure load are limited. As with acute valvular regurgitation, increased sarcomere stretch and catecholamine-induced inotropic and chronotropic effects can help increase cardiac output. When loading conditions overwhelm the ability of the LA or LV to maintain blood flow through an acutely stenotic valve, forward flow is reduced and high levels of filling pressure develop. The severity of the valve lesion and the rapidity with which it develops are the main predictors of the ensuing clinical course.

The development of valve stenosis, however, usually is a leisurely process. For example, rheumatic mitral stenosis or congenital aortic stenosis (AS) due to a bicuspid valve may progress over a period of several decades before the clinical manifestations become apparent.[9–11] One important reason for the seemingly indolent course of AS is that as the aortic valve becomes progressively more stenotic over time, the gradual increase in pressure load imposed on the LV is a potent stimulus for the development of hypertrophy.[6] Unlike the situation in volume overload where eccentric hypertrophy predominates, pressure overload leads to the parallel replication of sarcomeres and to the development of concentric hypertrophy. The overall LV chamber size is not enlarged but the amount of muscle mass and the mass/volume ratio are both markedly increased.

The hypertrophy that develops in the setting of chronic pressure overload provides additional muscle mass for pushing blood through a stenotic valve orifice and serves the important function of helping to normalize wall stress. This can be exemplified in the situation of chronic AS where the LV must generate systolic pressures of 300 mm Hg or above in some circumstances. According to the Laplace relationship in which wall tension is directly related to chamber pressure, increases in pressure of this magnitude would cause an enormous increase in wall stress if they were unopposed. However, since wall tension varies inversely with wall thickness, the development of LV hypertrophy is a means of normalizing wall stress in the face of a pressure load.

Unfortunately, myocardial hypertrophy cannot indefinitely compensate for increases in pressure load. In addition, hypertrophied myocardium may not always function normally. In contrast to the situation that develops during chronic volume loading, the hypertrophic pressure-loaded ventricle tends to be "stiffer" or less compliant than normal. The pressure/volume relationship is shifted upward and to the left in this situation so that at any given diastolic volume, diastolic pressure will be increased. The increase in diastolic pressure, in turn, is transmitted backward into the LA and to the pulmonary circulation. Through this mechanism, abnormalities in diastolic function can be the cause of the signs and symptoms of CHF.

Systolic function also may be compromised either as a result of intrinsic abnormalities in hypertrophic myocardium or due to myocardial ischemia. The latter may develop as a result of either supply-demand mismatch, limited myocardial oxygen reserve in a grossly hypertrophied ventricle, or the concurrence of coronary artery disease. In any event, once the ventricle starts to fail in this setting, the downward spiral can be rapid. Paradoxically, during the decompensated phase of pressure overload, evidence of LV dilatation may become apparent for the first time. However, the increase in chamber radius leads to a further increase in the level of systolic wall stress that is imposed on the failing LV and this factor contributes to the progressive deterioration in performance.

Aortic Valve Disease

Aortic Insufficiency

Acute AI is a medical emergency and the development of CHF in this setting requires immediate action. The causes of acute AI are limited. In most instances, aortic valve endocarditis, aortic root dissection, or trauma are involved. Spontaneous rupture of a normal or myxomatous valve or rheumatologic disorders such as ankylosing spondylitis also can cause acute AI. Since the underlying disease often is life-threatening, the early diagnosis and treatment of the cause of acute AI is essential. As indicated in the section on pathophysiology, the relative noncompliance of the LV limits the capacity of the chamber to accommodate regurgitant flow at acceptable levels of filling pressure. As the volume load in the chamber increases, the ventricle begins to ascend onto the steep upward portion of the pressure/volume

relationship. Signs and symptoms of pulmonary congestion develop as the increase in LV diastolic pressure is transmitted through the LA and into the pulmonary vasculature. It is important to note that once the steep ascending portion of the pressure-volume curve has been reached, diastolic pressures may increase quite rapidly with only small increases in volume. Thus, the amount of volume overload in the LV that gives rise to mild CHF may not be much less than that which gives rise to fulminant pulmonary edema. For this reason, the appearance of mild CHF, rather than being reassuring, should be viewed with the utmost concern since it is an early harbinger of extreme instability.

Unlike the situation in chronic AI where the manifestations of the valve lesion are readily apparent and roughly correlated with the severity of regurgitant flow, the physical findings of acute AI may be quite subtle.[12] The differences in physical findings between acute and chronic AI are outlined in Table 15.1. Peripheral evidence of increased total LV stroke volume (such as increased systolic blood pressure, bounding peripheral pulses, and head bob) is absent in acute AI since the diastolic volume of the LV is limited. Furthermore, the reduction in cardiac output caused by regurgitant flow leads to peripheral vasoconstriction and this also serves to diminish the peripheral manifestations. Even the characteristic diastolic murmur may be difficult to detect in the acute setting. This is particularly true when regurgitant flow leads to rapid diastolic filling of the LV and the pressure gradient that drives blood from the aorta to LV is diminished. However, the new onset of a third heart sound usually is a good indication that there is a significant amount of regurgitation present; the development of pulmonary congestion always should be a warning that the lesion is hemodynamically important.

Patients who survive the acute stage of AI with medical therapy alone and those in whom the valve lesion progresses slowly (and often silently) will develop compensatory changes that enable them to tolerate massive amounts of regurgitation for many years with little or no symptoms.[13] In these patients, the usual clinical signs of AI generally are present. The peripheral manifestations are due to the large initial stroke volume that is ejected into the aorta and subsequent regurgitation of up to 80% to 90% of that blood back into the LV during diastole. In general, the more pronounced the peripheral manifestations and the wider the pulse pressure, the more severe the valve lesion.

Patients with mild degrees of AI rarely deteriorate to the point where they develop signs and symptoms of CHF unless there is an associated worsening of the underlying valve function. Even when more severe degrees of AI are present, the adaptive mechanisms available to the LV are successful and patients can tolerate severely regurgitant valves for many years.[13] A recent study of 50 patients with moderate to severe AI evalu-

TABLE 15.1. Signs and symptoms of acute and chronic aortic insufficiency.

	Acute	Chronic
Congestive heart failure	Early and sudden	Late and insidious
Arterial pulse		
Rate/min	Increased	Normal
Rate of rise	Not increased	Increased
Systolic pressure	Normal to decreased	Increased
Diastolic pressure	Normal to decreased	Decreased
Pulse pressure	Near normal	Increased
Contour of peak	Single	Bisferiens
Pulsus alternans	Common	Uncommon
Left ventricular impulse	Near normal to moderately displaced, not hyperdynamic	Displaced, hyperdynamic
Auscultation		
First heart sound	Soft to absent	Normal
Aortic component of the second sound	Soft	Normal or decreased
Pulmonic component of the second sound	Normal or increased	Normal
Fourth heart sound	Consistently absent	Usually absent
Third heart sound	Common	Uncommon
Aortic systolic murmur	Grade 3 or less	Grade 3 or more
Aortic regurgitant murmur	Short, medium pitched	Long, high pitched
Austin Flint	Mid-diastolic	Presystolic, mid-diastolic, or both
Peripheral arterial auscultatory signs	Absent	Present
Electrocardiogram	Normal LV voltage with minor repolarization abnormalities	Increased LV voltage with major repolarization abnormalities
Chest roentgenogram		
Left ventricle	Normal to moderately increased	Markedly increased
Aortic root and arch	Usually normal	Prominent
Pulmonary venous vascularity	Increased	Normal

Reproduced, with permission, from Morganroth et al. *Annals of Internal Medicine* 1977;87:228.

ated the rate of progression to aortic valve replacement for either the onset of CHF and/or the development of LV dysfunction.[14] Patients enrolled in this survey were clinically stable and had preserved LV ejection fractions at the time of entry. All were at risk for future deterioration based on the presence of LV dilatation. The life table analysis for progression to aortic valve replacement is shown in Figure 15.1. The overall rate of progression in this trial was in the range of 4% per annum.

The above study also sought to determine if patients at increased risk for progression to aortic valve replacement could be identified. Factors that had a positive association with the future risk of deterioration were an LV end-diastolic volume ≥ 150 cc/m^2, an LV end-systolic volume ≥ 60 cc/m^2, an LV ejection during exercise of <0.50, and LV end-systolic wall stress that exceeded 86 dynes/cm^2 (which was the mean value in the group). Despite the fact that these variables defined a subgroup of patients with severe AI who were at relatively high risk for future deterioration, it is important to note that in most instances less than 50% had required aortic valve replacement within 3 years. Thus, although high-risk patients can be identified based on these variables, prophylactic surgery seems unnecessary

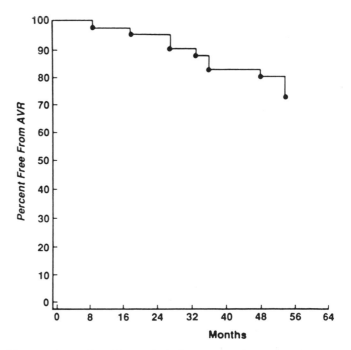

FIGURE 15.1. Life table analysis for progression to aortic valve replacement (*AVR*) in 50 patients with chronic stable aortic insufficiency. Reproduced, with permission, from Siemienczuk et al. *Annals of Internal Medicine* 1989;110:587–592.

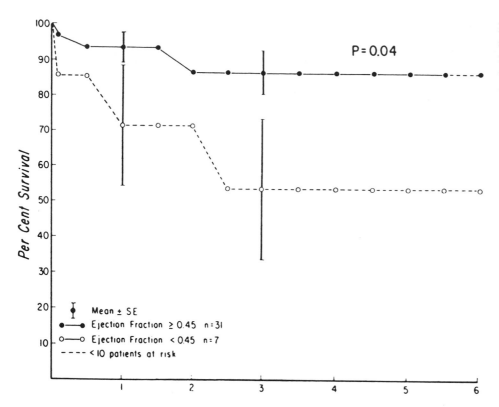

FIGURE 15.2. Actuarially determined survival after aortic valve replacement for aortic insufficiency. Reproduced, with permission, from *American Heart Journal* 1981;101:300.

since such a high proportion will remain clinically stable over an extended period of time.

Once LV dysfunction occurs in the setting of chronic aortic insufficiency, the long-term prognosis is less favorable than in patients with normal LV function.[15,16] As shown in Figure 15.2, survival of patients undergoing aortic valve replacement for aortic insufficiency was significantly less in patients with an LV ejection fraction (EF) <0.45 than in those patients with a higher EF. Recovery of normal LV function and complete regression of LV dilatation also is less likely in patients who have evidence of LV dysfunction at the time of surgical intervention. It does appear, however, that there is a period of time soon after LV dysfunction develops that the process is reversible. If patients with LV dysfunction are operated on within this "window," the LV is able to recover and the long-term outlook appears to be similar to that of patients who had no evidence of LV dysfunction at the time of surgery.[17,18]

Aortic Stenosis

Even more than chronic AI, AS tends to be an insidious disease that develops silently over many years. If the disease is not picked up on a routine physical examination during the asymptomatic period, the first manifestation may be one of the triad of angina, syncope, or CHF. The appearance of any of these conditions in the patient with AS marks a distinct turning point in the natural history of the disease and if surgical correction is not undertaken at this time, survival is substantially diminished.[19,20] CHF is a particularly ominous development and its occurrence is an indication that either all of the compensatory mechanisms for dealing with the pressure load have been exhausted and cardiac function is beginning to deteriorate as a result of "afterload mismatch," or that intrinsic myocardial abnormalities have begun to develop. As mentioned previously, it often is difficult to distinguish between the two circumstances in an individual patient. Nonetheless, the onset of symptoms in patients with AS is a strong indication for surgical intervention (see section below).

In AS, increases in LV end-diastolic pressure that develop as a consequence of changes in the diastolic properties of the LV result in an increase in LA pressure and volume. The increased wall stress in the LA in turn predisposes the patient with AS to the development of atrial fibrillation. The consequences of this rhythm disturbance may be catastrophic. The reason for this is that the LV is stiffer in patients with AS than in normal persons. In this setting, a forceful atrial contraction is needed to complete diastolic emptying of the LA and to maintain filling of the LV. It is estimated that the atrial contribution to LV stroke volume is close to 50% in patients with AS whereas it is in the range of 15% to 20% in normal persons.[21] When the atrial kick is lost in atrial fibrillation (and diastolic filling is compromised by the rapid heart rate), patients with AS may develop the rapid onset of CHF or cardiogenic shock.

The classical physical findings in AS include a low volume, slowly rising carotid pulse, a sustained apical impulse, a single second heart, a prominent S4, and a systolic ejection murmur. Although the predictive accuracy for any individual finding may not be high, a constellation of findings in the appropriate clinical setting should be sufficient to direct the clinician's attention toward the diagnosis of AS. In the author's experience, the physical findings that are of the greatest value in detecting or excluding the presence of hemodynamically significant AS are the following: a slow rising, low volume carotid pulse, a late peaking systolic ejection murmur (which may be accompanied by a thrill over the aortic region), and the presence of only a single component to the second heart sound. With regard to the latter finding, it is essential to note that many elderly or obese patients may have only a single audible component to S^2 so that the specificity of this finding in identifying patients with hemodynamically important AS will be quite low. Its value, though, is in the fact that the presence of a normally split second heart sound is strong evidence against the presence of hemodynamically significant AS.

Mitral Valve Disease

Mitral Regurgitation

As with acute AI, the development of acute MR is considered to be a medical emergency. Since management decisions are strongly influenced by the cause of the valve lesion, it is essential to determine the etiology of acute MR. The most common causes include such disparate diseases as acute myocardial infarction, infectious endocarditis, and spontaneous rupture of normal or myxomatous chordae tendineae. Whatever the cause, however, the heart is poorly prepared to handle the resultant volume overload imposed on the LV and LA. The compensatory mechanisms are the same as for acute AI and they include increased sarcomere stretch and (as CHF develops) catecholamine-induced increases in myocardial inotropy and chronotropy. When these compensatory mechanisms are exhausted, signs and symptoms of CHF begin to develop.

A characteristic of MR is the development of a large v wave in the LA or pulmonary artery wedge pressure tracing. It is due to the rapid filling of the LA during early systole as both venous return and regurgitant flow enter the chamber simultaneously. In acute MR, the amplitude of the v wave is a good indicator of the severity of the valve lesion. In chronic MR, however, LA dilatation dampens the increase in pressure due to regurgitant flow. In this setting, the height of the v wave is related less closely to the severity of the disease.

In chronic MR, patients often are able to tolerate the increase in LV and LA loading conditions for many years with few symptoms. However, CHF can develop later in the course as a result of excessive volume load that eventually overcomes the compensatory changes in LV structure and function (described above) or, more commonly, due to the onset of LV dysfunction. The issue is somewhat more complicated in MR than in AI since the changes in cardiac structure and function that are stimulated by the mitral valve lesion actually may lead to worsening valvular incompetence. The reason for this is that normal functioning of the mitral valve is strongly dependent on the structural and functional integrity of the subvalvular apparatus.[22] This anatomical unit is composed of the mitral valve annulus, the chordae tendineae, the papillary muscles, and the subjacent LV myocardium. As MR progresses, alterations in the geometry or function of these components can lead to greater incompetence of the valve and worsening MR. Thus, an important factor in the natural history of the disease is that MR tends to beget further MR. An extreme example of the effects of abnormalities in the subvalvular apparatus on mitral valve competence can be seen in patients with advanced CHF who develop secondary MR as a consequence of LV dilatation and dysfunction. In such patients it may be difficult (or even impossible) to determine whether hemodynamically important MR is the cause or an effect of severe LV dysfunction unless an antecedent history of the clinical course is available.

Mitral Stenosis

Acquired mitral stenosis (MS) is almost always rheumatic in origin and with this disease narrowing of the mitral orifice tends to be slowly progressive over a period of years. The anatomical changes in valve structure lead to a gradual decrease in transvalvular flow and to an increase in the transvalvular pressure gradient. Signs and symptoms of CHF tend to develop only after the lesion has been present for many years.[9,10] Increases in LA and pulmonary capillary pressures result in the transudation of fluid from the intra- to the extravascular lung spaces. The increases in hydrostatic pressure, however, develop slowly and this allows time for compensatory changes in the lymphatic drainage of the lung to develop. Lymphatic hypertrophy is an extremely effective means of reducing the amount of lung water and it helps explain why signs and symptoms of pulmonary congestion may be absent from some patients with long-standing MS despite the fact that LA pressures may be in excess of 30 to 35 mm Hg.

As MS progresses, there is a passive increase in pulmonary artery pressure due to the increase in LA pressure. In some patients, there also is an active component in the pulmonary vascular bed that contributes to the development of pulmonary hypertension. Whatever the cause, the resultant increase in right ventricular after-load can lead to right heart failure.[23] When the right ventricle begins to fail, the time course of clinical deterioration accelerates considerably. As right ventricular stroke volume goes down, the amount of blood pushed through the pulmonary circulation to the LA is reduced and LA pressure actually may be reduced in this setting. Although pulmonary congestion may be reduced as a consequence of the development of right heart failure, there often is a significant drop in cardiac output since high levels of filling pressures in the LA are required at this stage of the disease to push blood across the stenotic mitral valve. The onset of right ventricular failure also leads to the development of systemic congestion.

Once symptoms begin in patients with MS, the clinical course is slowly but relentlessly downhill. From information available from the presurgical era, we know that functional class III patients have a 5-yr survival of only 62% whereas functional class IV patients have a 5-yr survival of 15%.[10] Two conditions, in particular, have been associated with the onset of CHF in patients with MS. The onset of atrial fibrillation often marks a turning point in the clinical course of the disease. The atrial kick is an important mechanism for pushing blood across a stenotic mitral valve.[21] When it is lost, LA pressures can be expected to increase rapidly and cardiac output is likely to fall. The problem is accentuated by the increase in heart rate, which usually occurs since this produces a selective decrease in the diastolic filling period. Pregnancy is another condition that may bring about a precipitous decline in the course of a patient with MS. The reason for this is that cardiac output can be expected to increase by 30% to 50% by the 20th to 24th week of pregnancy. With a relatively fixed obstruction at the level of the mitral valve, this flow increase brings about an increase in the transvalvular gradient and LA pressure. As a result, it is not uncommon for patients with MS to develop the onset of pulmonary congestive symptoms or even pulmonary edema for the first time during this period.

Diagnosis and Management

As described in the above sections, the onset of CHF in a patient with a left heart valve disease tends to obscure the physical findings that are generally associated with the particular lesion. This is mainly due to a reduction in cardiac output, which reduces the intensity of the characteristic murmurs. Patients who present with "silent" AS or MS are an example of this phenomenon. Other factors such as arterial vasoconstriction (which may dampen the peripheral manifestations of AI) or right ventricular enlargement (which obscures the murmur and opening snap of MS by moving the mitral area

away from the chest wall) also are involved. Thus, although physical findings can lead the clinician to consider the possibility that an important valvular abnormality is present, it must be remembered that the sensitivity of the physical examination often is diminished when CHF is present. It remains essential, then, for the practicing clinician always to keep in mind the possibility that CHF could be on the basis of a valve lesion and that the clinical manifestations of hemodynamically important valvular heart disease may be quite subtle in this setting.

The chest x ray is a valuable test for alerting the physician to the presence of a valvular lesion in the patient with CHF. Unusual patterns of chamber enlargement (such as a small LV and large LA in MS) and the appearance of valvular calcification are helpful in this regard. The presence of aortic root dilatation in a patient with CHF should raise the possibility of hemodynamically significant AI. Viewed from the opposite perspective, the presence of the usual roentgenographic changes associated with CHF in a patient with a known valvular lesion is an indication that the disease has entered a new and more serious stage. Thus, a chest x ray should be a standard part of the routine examination of patients with valvular heart disease.

Ultrasound examination of the heart has proved to be an extremely useful means of screening and confirming the presence of left heart valvular lesions in patients with CHF. By this technique, LV function can be estimated. LV size and wall thickness can be measured reliably and the relative size of the other cardiac chambers can be assessed. Most importantly, the mitral and aortic valves can be visualized. Abnormal flow patterns due to either stenotic or regurgitant valve lesions can be detected and the severity of the valve disease can be quantified by a combined Doppler-echographic study. Radioisotope angiography is another noninvasive method that can be used in patients with valvular lesions to evaluate LV size and function. This technique also has been used to give an estimate of the amount of left heart valvular regurgitation.[24]

Cardiac catheterization remains an extremely useful way to evaluate patients with CHF and a known or suspected left heart valvular lesion. The precise measurements of intracardiac and intravascular pressures combined with assessment of cardiac output that are available with this technique can provide definitive information regarding the severity of a valve lesion. Catheterization is of greatest value when the status of the patient based on physical examination and noninvasive testing remains ambiguous or there are inconsistencies in the information that has been obtained.[25] The procedure often is performed before corrective valve surgery (or valvuloplasty) since it can confirm noninvasive results, provide essential anatomical information to the surgeon (or valvuloplasty operator), and be used to evaluate the coronary circulation when there is a question of coronary artery disease being present.

In general, the approach to the medical therapy of patients with CHF as a consequence of a left heart valvular lesion is similar to that in a patient with this syndrome in the absence of any valve disease. Since the standard approach to the treatment of CHF is discussed at length elsewhere in this text, it will not be repeated here. There are, however, a few peculiarities of the management of CHF in patients with valve lesions that deserve comment. Diuretic therapy in patients with and without valvular disease is an effective means of treating volume overload and the excessive fluid retention that occurs in CHF. Patients with either MS or AS, however, can be extremely sensitive to a reduction in volume. They are prone to experience a reduction in cardiac output when diuresis reduces LA or LV filling pressures below a critical level. Consequently, a degree of caution always is indicated when initiating diuretic therapy in such patients. Similarly, AS and MS patients tend to be exceedingly sensitive to the hemodynamic perturbations caused by atrial fibrillation. The prevention (by antiarrhythmic drugs) and prompt treatment of this condition can avoid many problems when a stenotic left heart valvular lesion is present.

As mentioned earlier in the chapter, CHF can develop either as a consequence of abnormal loading conditions that overwhelm normally functioning myocardium or it can be due to the occurrence of myocardial dysfunction. When abnormal loading conditions are the cause, surgical correction of the valve lesion will be a highly effective treatment of CHF. This is almost always the case in acute left heart valvular regurgitation and in most cases of chronic valvular regurgitation in which heart failure is of brief duration. When systolic performance of the left ventricle deteriorates due to the chronic effects of volume overload, the likelihood of a favorable long-term outcome is less certain.[15,26,27] This is particularly true in patients with MR. In this setting, surgical correction of the valve lesion actually may lead to a further reduction in left ventricular systolic performance. The reason for this is that when the valve lesion is present, the LV can empty a substantial quantity of blood into the LA. Impedance to regurgitant flow tends to be quite low and, as a result, the load that opposes LV systole is reduced. When the valve lesion is corrected, however, the low impedance sink is closed off and the LV is obliged to direct all of its systolic flow into the relatively high impedance systemic circulation. In cases where there is underlying myocardial damage, the sudden imposition of increased loading conditions can cause a further worsening of LV systolic performance.

As alluded to earlier in the chapter, the onset of CHF in a patient with AS is an extremely ominous sign. Although CHF is a risk factor for surgical mortality, surgical correction is strongly indicated in most cases.

Medical therapy is of limited value in this setting and there is good evidence that LV function may return to normal levels when the valve lesion is corrected even in patients with low LV EF before surgery.[28,29] The situation in AS is somewhat the obverse of that in MR, where the patient faces increased LV afterload after surgery. In AS, afterload is reduced by removal of a stenotic valve and impedance to LV emptying is reduced.

Surgical correction of MS can be expected to yield good results as far as relief of congestive symptoms are concerned, provided that it is undertaken before there are fixed changes in the pulmonary vasculature or before right ventricular dysfunction develops. However, late survival in patients with MS after valve replacement is substantially diminished.[30] Fortunately, many patients with MS will be candidates for mitral valve commissurotomy as opposed to valve replacement. The results of this procedure are excellent and the problems associated with a valve prosthesis can be avoided by this approach.[31]

Despite the great success of valve replacement surgery for all of the left heart valvular lesions, it must be remembered that the operation substitutes one disease for another. Surgery itself may damage myocardium and this factor may lead to the late development of CHF. Furthermore, most prosthetic valves are inherently stenotic. While this may be of little consequence in most patients, there are some in whom valve replacement offers little in the way of relief from valve stenosis.[32] Finally, prosthetic heart valves may deteriorate over time and this factor may again place the patient at risk for developing CHF due to the occurrence of prosthetic valve stenosis or regurgitation.

Vasodilator Therapy of Left Heart Valvular Regurgitation

In either AI or MR, the distribution of total LV stroke volume between forward and regurgitant flows is determined in large part by the relative impedance to flow in the two directions. When AI is present, blood in the aorta is either propelled through the systemic circulation or (during diastole) emptied back into the LV. MR enables LV stroke volume to be divided between forward flow into the aorta and regurgitation back into the LA. In both situations, the distribution of flow is sensitive to manipulations that alter the impedance to flow in the systemic circulation. If aortic impedance is increased, as it is during hand-grip exercise, then regurgitant flow will be enhanced. Conversely, interventions that reduce aortic impedance can favorably redistribute flow. As shown schematically in Figure 15.3, this is what occurs when arterial dilating agents are given to patients with left heart valvular regurgitation.

There is extensive documentation in the medical lit-

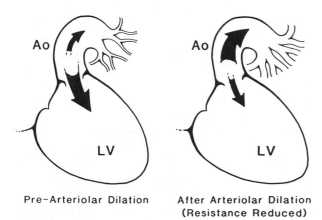

Pre-Arteriolar Dilation   After Arteriolar Dilation
                                  (Resistance Reduced)

FIGURE 15.3. Distribution of stroke volume in aortic insufficiency. By decreasing impedance to forward flow arteriolar dilation can increase cardiac output and reduce regurgitant flow. Reproduced, with permission, from *Cardiology Clinics* 1991;9:255–270.

erature that the acute administration of arterial dilating agents to patients with either AI or MR will improve cardiac function.[33–35] A summary of the hemodynamic effects of hydralazine in patients with AI is given in Figure 15.4. Similar findings have been observed when this drug is given to patients with MI. An example of the effects of the acute administration of hydralazine on the characteristic v wave in MI is shown in Figure 15.5. In this case, the reduction in the amplitude of the regurgitant v wave is, more or less, a direct reflection of

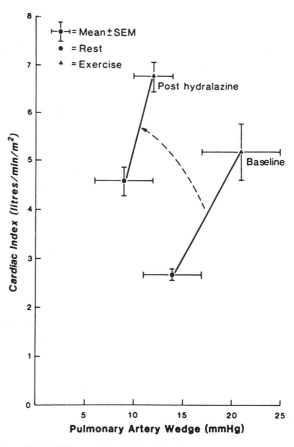

FIGURE 15.4. Effects of oral hydralazine on rest and exercise hemodynamic variables in 10 patients with chronic severe aortic insufficiency. Reproduced, with permission, from *Cardiology Clinics* 1991;9:255–270.

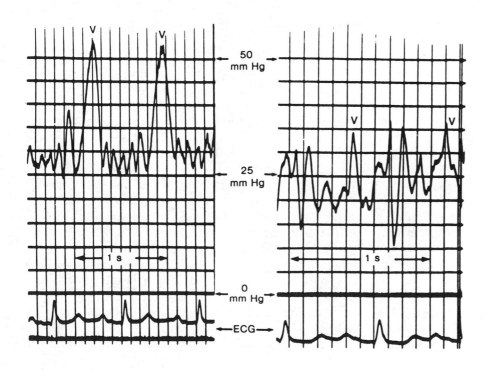

FIGURE 15.5. Effects of hydralazine on v waves due to MR. The tracing is from the pulmonary artery wedge position. Reproduced, with permission, from *JAMA* 1981;246. Copyright 1981 by the American Medical Association.

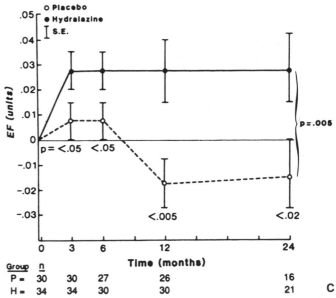

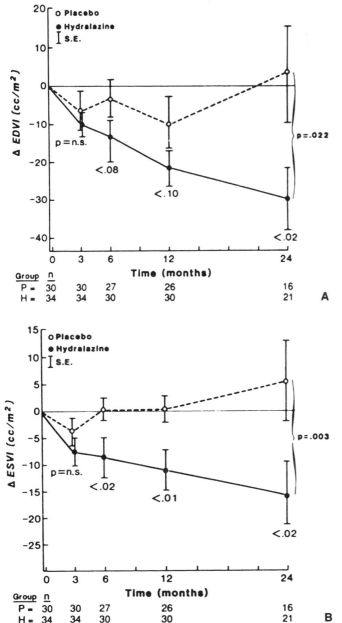

FIGURE 15.6. Effects of long-term vasodilator therapy in patients with chronic aortic insufficiency. **A** depicts changes in left ventricular end-diastolic volume index (*EDVI*) over time. **B** and **C** depict changes in end-systolic volume index (*ESVI*) and ejection fraction (*EF*), respectively. Reproduced, with permission, from *Circulation* 1988;78:92–103. Copyright by the American Heart Association.

the reduction in regurgitant flow that can be obtained with arterial dilator therapy.

The hemodynamic studies noted above suggest that arterial dilator therapy should have beneficial effects on the clinical course of patients with left heart valvular regurgitation. There are few long-term studies available, however, in symptomatic patients and much of the data is not controlled. Nonetheless, the results seem to indicate that this form of therapy is of value in patients with CHF secondary to either AI or MI.[36,37]

Another possible role for the use of arterial dilator therapy in patients with left heart valvular regurgitation is to prevent progression of LV dilatation and hypertrophy and the ultimate development of LV dysfunction. This issue was evaluated recently in a double-blinded,

placebo-controlled trial of hydralazine in patients with chronic AI.[38] In this study, clinically stable patients with minimal or no symptoms and a normal resting LV EF were enrolled. All patients were judged to have AI of at least moderate severity and to have evidence of LV enlargement at the time of entry into the trial. Patients were then randomized to receive either placebo or hydralazine over a 2-yr period. The primary endpoint of the trial was a change in LV end-diastolic volume between the two treatment groups during this time.

The results of this trial are summarized in Figure 15.6. Over a 2-yr period, patients in the placebo group demonstrated little change in LV volumes. Patients randomized to hydralazine showed a step-wise reduction in both end-diastolic and end-systolic volumes and these changes were significantly different from those seen in the placebo control group. Small, but highly significant, differences in LV EF in favor of the hydralazine group also were seen.

Since LV enlargement is an extremely strong risk factor for the future development of CHF or LV dysfunction,[14] the observation that long-term arterial dilator therapy can reduce ventricular size suggests that this approach can be used to delay or prevent the deterioration in LV performance due to chronic volume overload. In general, patients with more severe AI, as indicated by LV volumes greater than 150 cc/m², are the most likely to respond favorably.[39]

Conclusion

This chapter has provided an overview of the pathophysiological mechanisms involved in the development of CHF in patients with left heart valvular lesions and has summarized aspects of the clinical presentation and management of CHF that are unique to this setting. Since the development of CHF has such a profoundly negative effect on the clinical course of patients with a hemodynamically significant valve lesion, early recognition and treatment are imperative. Prevention of structural and functional changes in the myocardium, as with vasodilator therapy, is an important goal in the management of patients with valvular lesions. As more becomes known about the cellular and molecular basis of myocardial dysfunction, it is likely that novel strategies for preventive therapy will become available for more patients with valve lesions.

Acknowledgment. The author wishes to express his gratitude for the conscientious and diligent administrative and secretarial support that has been provided by Ms. Marita Schmit.

References

1. Gunther S, Grossman W. Determinants of ventricular function in pressure-overload hypertrophy in man. *Circulation.* 1979;59:679–688.
2. Sonnenblick EH, Ross J Jr, Covell JW et al. Ultrastructure of the heart in systole and diastole: changes in sarcomere length. *Cir. Res.* 1967;21:423–431.
3. McCullagh WN, Covell JW, Ross J Jr. Left ventricular dilatation and diastolic compliance changes during chronic volume overloading. *Circulation.* 1972;45:943–951.
4. Ross J Jr, McCullagh WH. Nature of enhanced performance of the dilated left ventricle in the dog during chronic volume overloading. *Circ Res.* 1972;30:549–556.
5. Urschel CW, Covell JW, Connenblick GH, et al. Myocardial mechanics in aortic and mitral valvular regurgitation:

the concept of instantaneous impedance as a determinant of the performance of the intact heart. *J Clin Invest.* 1968;47:867–883.
6. Grossman W, Jones D, McLauren LP. Wall stress and patterns of hypertrophy in the human left ventricle. *J Clin Invest.* 1975;56:56–64.
7. Pichard AD, Smith H, Holt J, et al. Coronary vascular reserve in left ventricular hypertrophy secondary to chronic aortic regurgitation. *Am J Cardiol.* 1983;51:315–320.
8. Greenberg B, Massie B, Thomas D, et al. Association between the exercise ejection fraction response and systolic wall stress in patients with chronic aortic insufficiency. *Circulation.* 1985;71:458–465.
9. Rowe JC, Bland F, Sprague HB, et al. Course of mitral stenosis without surgery: ten and twenty year perspectives. *Ann Intern Med.* 1960;52:741–749.
10. Oleson KH. The natural history of 271 patients with mitral stenosis under medical treatment. *Br Heart J.* 1962;24:349–357.
11. Campbell M. The natural history of congenital aortic stenosis. *Br Heart J.* 1968;30:514–526.
12. Morganroth J, Perloff JK, Zeldis SM, et al. Acute severe aortic regurgitation: pathophysiology, clinical recognition, and management. *Ann Intern Med.* 1977;87:223–232.
13. Bland EJ, Wheeler EO. Severe aortic regurgitation in young people. *N Engl J Med.* 1957;256:667–672.
14. Siemienczuk D, Greenberg B, Morris C, et al. Chronic aortic insufficiency: factors associated with progression to aortic valve replacement. *Ann Intern Med.* 1989;110:587–592.
15. Greves J, Rahimtoola S, McAnulty JH, et al. Preoperative criteria predictive of late survival following valve replacement for severe aortic regurgitation. *Am Heart J.* 1981;101:300.
16. Bonow RO, Picone AL, McIntosh CL, et al. Survival and functional results after valve replacement for aortic regurgitation from 1976 to 1983: impact of preoperative left ventricular function. *Circulation.* 1985;72:1244–1256.
17. Bonow RO, Rosing DR, Maron BJ, et al. Reversal of left ventricular dysfunction after aortic valve replacement for chronic aortic regurgitation: influence of duration of preoperative left ventricular dysfunction. *Circulation.* 1984;70:570–579.
18. Carabello BA, Usher BW, Hendrix GH, et al. Predictors of outcome in patients with aortic regurgitation and left ventricular dysfunction: a change in the measuring stick. *J Am Coll Cardiol.* 1987;10:991–997.
19. Frank S, Johnson A, Ross J Jr. Natural history of valvular aortic stenosis. *Br Heart J.* 1973;35:41–46.
20. Rapaport E. Natural history of aortic and mitral valve disease. *Am J Cardiol.* 1975;35:221–229.
21. Stott DK, Marpole DGF, Bristow JD, et al. The role of left atrial transport in aortic and mitral stenosis. *Circulation.* 1970;41:1031–1041.
22. Perloff JK, Roberts WC. The mitral apparatus: functional anatomy of mitral regurgitation. *Circulation.* 1972;46:227–239.
23. Grose R, Strain J, Yipintosoi T. Right ventricular function in valvular heart disease in relation to pulmonary artery pressure. *J Am Coll Cardiol.* 1983;2:225–232.
24. Bough E, Glandsmen EJ, North DL, Shulman RS. Gated

radionuclide angiographic evaluation of valve regurgitation. *Am J Cardiol.* 1980;46:423–428.

25. Hosenpud J, Greenberg B. The preoperative evaluation in patients with endocarditis: is cardiac catheterization necessary? *Chest.* 1983;84:690–694.

26. Henry WL, Bonow RO, Borer JS, et al. Observations on the optimum time for operative intervention for aortic regurgitation. *Circulation.* 1980;61:471–483.

27. Samuels DA, Curfman GD, Freidlich AL, et al. Valve replacement for aortic regurgitation: long-term follow-up with factors influencing the results. *Circulation.* 1979;60:647–654.

28. Schwartz F, Flameng W, Thormann J, et al. Recovering from myocardial failure after aortic valve replacement. *J Thorac Cardiovasc Surg.* 1978;75:854–864.

29. Smith W, McAnulty JH, Rahimtoola SH. Severe aortic stenosis with impaired left ventricular function and clinical heart failure: results of valve replacement. *Circulation.* 1978;58:258–264.

30. Tepley J, Grunkmeier G, Sutherland HD, et al. The ultimate prognosis after valve replacement: an assessment at 20 years. *Ann Thorac Surg.* 1981;32:111–119.

31. Vega JL, Fleitas M, Martinez R, et al. Open mitral commissurotomy. *Ann Thorac Surg.* 1981;31:266–270.

32. Rahimtoola SH. The problem of valve prosthesis-patient mismatch. *Circulation.* 1978;58:20–24.

33. Greenberg BH, DeMots H, Murphy E, et al. Beneficial effects of hydralazine on rest and exercise hemodynamics in patients with chronic severe aortic insufficiency. *Circulation.* 1980;62:49–55.

34. Greenberg BH, DeMots H, Murphy E, et al. Mechanisms for improved cardiac performance with arterial dilators in aortic insufficiency. *Circulation.* 1987;63:263–268.

35. Greenberg BH, Massie BM, Brundage BH, et al. Beneficial effects of hydralazine in severe mitral regurgitation. *Circulation.* 1978;58:273–279.

36. Greenberg BH, Rahimtoola SH. Long-term vasodilator therapy in aortic insufficiency: evidence for regression of left ventricular dilatation and hypertrophy and improvement in systolic pump function. *Ann Intern Med.* 1980;93:440–442.

37. Greenberg BH, DeMots H, Murphy E, Rahimtoola SH. Effects of arterial dilatation on cardiac performance during rest and exercise in patients with mitral regurgitation. *Circulation.* 1982;65:181–185.

38. Greenberg B, Massie B, Bristow JD, et al. Long-term vasodilator therapy of chronic aortic insufficiency. A randomized double-blinded, placebo-controlled clinical trial. *Circulation.* 1988;78:92–103.

39. Greenberg B, Massie B, Bristow JD, et al. Factors influencing the response to long-term arterial dilator therapy for aortic insufficiency. *Circulation.* 1987;76(suppl IV):516.

16
Heart Failure Secondary to Congenital Heart Disease

Mark J. Morton

The management of patients with congenital heart disease that results in congestive heart failure needs to be examined from several aspects: (a) age group, (b) rhythm, (c) volume overload, pressure overload, or cardiac muscle disease, (d) surgical sequelae, (e) pulmonary vascular disease, and (f) the consequences of chronic hypoxemia. Unlike many of the disorders in adults with acquired heart disease for which the development of congestive heart failure is necessary to warrant the risk of surgery, most congenital heart defects are corrected or palliated before the development of congestive heart failure (CHF). Thus, for many defects, prevention through surgery is the most effective management of heart failure. When CHF supervenes late in the course of the disease, the opportunity for intervention, short of transplantation, may be primarily medical.

Fetus

Fetal CHF is recognized as hydrops by the obstetrician or ultrasonographer. The fetus develops massive fluid accumulation in serous cavities (pericardial, pleural, abdominal) and soft tissue. The uterus rapidly increases in size by examination and is large for dates. Ultrasound identifies the fetus as the source of the abnormal growth. Before the availability of anti–D gamma globulin, Rhesus incompatibility with resultant fetal hemolysis and anemia was the cause of approximately 80% of hydrops fetalis. Now, most of cases of hydrops are nonimmune. The etiologies of nonimmune hydrops are diverse but at least 20% are cardiovascular (Table 16.1).[1]

The mortality ranges from 50% to 98% for fetuses with hydrops. Thus, early identification of fetuses doomed to expire can allow pregnancy termination. Conversely, otherwise well fetuses with readily correctable problems might be approached surgically, (e.g.,

urinary tract obstruction or with chemical cardioversion of fetal tachyarrhythmias). The possibility of fetal cardiac corrective surgery recently has been explored.

Fetal tachyarrhythmias that can be diagnosed easily by fetal echocardiography have been the most amenable abnormalities to treatment in utero. The variety of sustained fetal arrhythmias encountered is shown in Table 16.2.[2]

TABLE 16.1. Causes of nonimmune hydrops.

Cardiovascular (arrhythmia)	21 (6)
Chromosomal	16
Malformation syndromes	11
Twin-twin transfusion	10
Pulmonary	8
Hematologic	6
Infection	4
Urinary	3
Gastrointestinal	3
Miscellaneous	6
Unknown	16
	110

Modified from Holzgreve et al.[1] with permission.

TABLE 16.2. Fetal arrhythmias.

SVT	15
VT	2
2° AV block	2
Complete heart block	8
Flutter	3
Fibrillation	2
Sinus bradycardia	2

SVT = supraventricular tachycardia; VT = ventricular tachycardia; 2° AV = second degree atrioventricular. From Kleinman et al.[2] with permission.

TABLE 16.3. Maternal drug therapy for fetal arrhythmias.

	Digoxin	Verapamil	Propranolol	Procainamide	Quinidine
Loading dose	1–2.5 mg po	5–10 mg iv	.5 mg q5 min iv	12 mg kg iv	—
	0.75–2.0 mg iv				
Maintenance dose	0.25–0.75 mg po	80–120 mg q8h po	20–160 mg q6–8h po	6 mg/kg q4h po	250–500 mg q6h
cord/maternal ratio	0.6–1.0	0.3–0.4	0.1–0.3	0.8–1.3	0.2–0.9

Modified from Kleinman et al.[2] with permission.

The vulnerability of the fetus to tachyarrhythmias has physiologic bases.[3] As the fetal myocardium matures, calcium release and uptake shifts from sarcolemma to sarcoplasmic reticulum with the development of that organelle. Thus, the immature myocardium may be less able to relax at elevated heart rates because of the lack of development of the sarcoplasmic reticulum. Fetal muscle also is stiffer than neonatal or adult heart muscle. This may be due to the relative lack of fibril in the immature myocyte. The fetus has a reversed E/A ratio on Doppler evaluation of mitral or tricuspid flow, indicating increased importance of atrial booster pump function. Thus, fetal tachycardia may cause incomplete ventricular filling even at elevated pressures because of poor myocardial relaxation and loss of atrial booster pump function.

Transplacental antiarrhythmic therapy frequently is employed to convert supraventricular tachycardia (SVT) or to control the rate in atrial flutter or fibrillation. Commonly used drugs and their cord/maternal serum concentration ratios are shown in Table 16.3.[2]

In Kleinman's series[2] of 16 patients with SVT, 15 were controlled medically with digoxin alone (6), digoxin and verapamil (7), or digoxin and propranolol (2). The decision to treat fetal arrhythmias is based on evidence of fetal distress (hydrops) and knowledge that premature delivery may have considerable complications. Thus, Kleinman recommends delivery only for failure of in utero rhythm management.

Neonate

The transition from intrauterine life to a terrestrial existence is accompanied by a cardiovascular revolution.[3] Oxygen consumption is doubled because of the need for movement, respiration, digestion, and thermal regulation. This increase in oxygen consumption is effected by doubling of left ventricular (LV) output and a 50% increase in right ventricular output as well as near complete saturation of the arterial blood. The fetal circulation is characterized by four shunts and high pulmonary vascular resistance, which keeps pulmonary blood flow at only 10% of combined ventricular output before birth. The shunts exist at the atrium (foramen ovale), great vessels (ductus arteriosus), umbilical artery

TABLE 16.4. Causes of CHF in infants with congenital heart disease.

Preterm	Term	1–2 Weeks
Patent ductus arteriosus	Hypoplastic left heart	Large VSD
	Coarctation of aorta	AV canal
	Severe aortic stenosis	Transposition of the great vessels
	Arrhythmia	Truncus arteriosus
		Total anomalous pulmonary venous return with obstruction

VSD = ventricular septal defect; AV = atrioventricular; CHF = congestive heart failure.

(placenta), and umbilical vein (ductus venosus). The two fetal ventricles pump in parallel with right ventricular stroke volume 50% to 100% greater than LV stroke volume and with nearly equal atrial and arterial pressures. With the onset of neonatal respiration, pulmonary vascular resistance falls and pulmonary venous return raises left atrial pressure with respect to right atrial pressure, closing the foramen. Ligation of the cord eliminates the placental and ductus venosus shunts. The ductus arteriosus closes in response to elevated oxygen levels, eliminating any left to right shunt by 48 hr. Pulmonary artery pressure falls while aortic pressure increases. Thus, by 48 hr, the fetal circulation has acquired the characteristics it will retain for the rest of life. However, if anatomic abnormalities exist, the circulation may not be able to adapt and CHF may ensue. The neonatal period has by far the greatest incidence of CHF in the pediatric population.

The common causes of CHF are listed in Table 16.4 for premature infants, term infants, and infants 1 to 2 weeks of age.[4]

The persistence of fetal circulation in the premature infant (right to left shunting at the foramen ovale and patency of the ductus arteriosus) usually is associated with important pulmonary disease. The pulmonary disease prevents the normal drop in pulmonary vascular resistance with birth but the pulmonary disease may be aggravated by overperfusion of the lungs through the ductus arteriosus. The indications for ductal closure by surgery, catheter device, or prostaglandin inhibition are controversial and under active investigation. The man-

TABLE 16.5. Recognition of CHF in infants.

Poor feeding
Respiratory distress, rales, wheezing
Tachycardia
Hepatomegaly
Gallop
Sweating
Pale, ashen color
Decreased urine output
Cardiomegaly, CHF on chest x ray

CHF = congestive heart failure.

ifestations of heart failure in infants are listed in Table 16.5.[4]

Severe obstruction to flow through the left heart and aorta becomes manifest as heart failure soon after birth because of the separation of the parallel circulation of the fetus into series circulation with the closure of the fetal shunts. Thus, with hypoplastic left heart syndrome, severe mitral stenosis, severe aortic stenosis, or coarctation of the aorta, the right ventricle supplies blood to the body through the ductus arteriosus in utero. After birth, with closure of the ductus, systemic blood flow is reduced and pulmonary venous return has nowhere to go in the left heart if the left heart cannot fill or empty properly. The blood then builds up in the lungs and causes pulmonary edema. These infants are critically ill and need prompt diagnosis and, where possible, prompt surgical repair or palliation.

Paroxysmal supraventricular tachycardia also may cause CHF in infants. Whether the mechanism is dual atrioventricular (AV) nodal pathways or Wolff-Parkinson-White syndrome, the rapid ventricular response may be poorly tolerated. Attention should be directed toward conversion of the rhythm to sinus, maintenance of sinus rhythm, and delineation of any underlying cardiac abnormalities or precipitating events.

The progressive decline in pulmonary vascular resistance after birth invites increasing pulmonary blood flow when unrestricted communication between the high pressure left ventricle or aorta and the right heart or pulmonary artery exists. While the systemic ventricle normally doubles its output at birth, pulmonary blood flow may exceed systemic blood flow fourfold with large defects. In this setting, the systemic ventricle will be swamped with pulmonary venous return and CHF due to massive volume overload may ensue. It is important to recognize that these infants may appear well at birth when the pulmonary vascular resistance is still relatively high and the defect may not be detected. In addition, the rapid fall in pulmonary vascular resistance may be retarded by the high flows and pressures in the pulmonary artery pushing the threshold for clinical presentation out to 1 to 2 weeks after birth. The lesions most commonly responsible for CHF due to large left to right shunts are large ventricular septal defect (VSD) and abnormalities of the atrial ventricular canal. Transposition of the great vessels with a large VSD and truncus arteriosus also may produce CHF with a progressive fall in pulmonary vascular resistance, but cyanosis usually is the presenting sign. Total anomalous pulmonary venous return also is associated with cyanosis but may develop pulmonary edema. Here, the mechanism for elevated pulmonary capillary pressure is not high flow and systemic ventricular failure but rather obstruction to pulmonary venous return. Of note, atrial septal defect, regardless of size, rarely results in CHF. Unlike left to right shunting at the ventricular or great vessel level, left to right shunting at the atrial level depends on diastolic rather than systolic or arterial pressure differences. Thus, blood will shunt left to right only to the extent that the right ventricle is larger and more compliant than the left. Right ventricular diastolic pressure cannot exceed left ventricular pressure and thus right ventricular failure is rare until late in the natural history of this lesion.

Other less common causes of CHF include congenital anomalies of the coronary arteries and obstruction to pulmonary venous return at the left atrial level (cor triatriatum). The coronary artery anomalies usually present with evidence for myocardial ischemia or infarction and most frequently are associated with anomalous origin of the left coronary or left anterior descending coronary arteries from the pulmonary artery.

The management of infants with CHF should be considered a medical emergency. Attention is directed quickly to stabilization of respiratory, acid-base, and hemodynamic variables, followed immediately by anatomic definition of the underlying cardiovascular abnormalities by echocardiography. Surgical therapy when appropriate is then undertaken urgently with or without additional information from cardiac catheterization and angiography. The general approach to infants with CHF is shown in Table 16.6.[5] The general approach is not significantly different from other age groups or from discussions elsewhere in this book regarding adult patients except for manipulation of the ductus and caution regarding the use of vasodilators. Relaxation of ductal constriction by prostaglandin E_1 in the presence of hypoplastic left heart syndrome allows the right ventricle to continue its fetal role of supplying systemic blood flow, thus improving systemic perfusion and reducing pulmonary venous return. With severe juxtaductal coarctation, ductal constriction aggravates the obstruction by eliminating the remaining channel for antegrade flow. Relaxation of the ductus with prostaglandin E_1 will greatly reduce left ventricular afterload and improve CHF as well as systemic perfusion. Conversely, premature infants with respiratory failure and CHF may benefit from ductal constriction with prostaglandin inhibition produced by indomethacin.

TABLE 16.6. General measures to treat heart failure in infancy.

Maximize oxygen supply/demand
  Supplemental oxygen or ventilation
  Rest
  Controlled temperature environment
  Treat infection
Reduce pulmonary venous pressure
  Reduce sodium and water intake
  Diuretic
  Ventilation
  Dialysis
Increase contractility
  Digitalis
  Catecholamines
  Correct acid base abnormalities
Pharmacology manipulation of ductus arteriosus
  Dilate with prostaglandin E_1 for severe coarctation or hypoplastic left heart
  Constrict with indomethacin in premature infants

TABLE 16.7. Dosage regimens for digoxin.

Age and weight	Dose and route[a] of acute digitalization	Maintenance
Premature infants < 1.5 kg	10–20 μg/kg iv TDD: $\frac{1}{2}$, $\frac{1}{4}$ of dose q8h	4 μg/kg/day iv (may increase to 4 μg/kg q12h at age 1 month)
1.5–2.5 kg	Same as above	4 μg/kg q12h iv
Full-term newborn infants	30 μg/kg iv, TDD	4–5 μg/kg q12h iv
Older infants (1–12 mo)	35 μg/kg iv, TDD	5–10 μg/kg q12h iv

[a] Oral dose is approximately 20% greater than intravenous dose.
TDD = total digitalizing dose.
Reproduced, with permission, from George and Friedman.[5]

TABLE 16.8. Dosage regimens for diuretics.

Drug	Site of action	Intravenous	Dose oral
Chlorothiazide	Distal tubule		< 6 mo: 20–30 mg/kg/day q8–12h > 6 mo: 10–20 mg/kg/day q12h (max = 2g/day)
Hydrochlorothiazide	Distal tubule		2–3 mg/kg/day q8–12h (max = 200 mg/day)
Ethacrynic acid	Loop of Henle (ascending limb)	0.5–1.0 mg/kg/dose q8–12h	Not recommended for neonates and infants in oral form
Furosemide	Loop of Henle (ascending limb)	1 mg/kg/dose q8–12h (max = 6 mg/kg/dose)	1–2 mg/kg/dose q12h (max = 6 mg/kg/dose)
Spironolactone	Collecting tubule		1.5–3.5 mg/kg/day q6–8h

Reproduced, with permission, from George and Friedman.[5]

As with adult patients, vasodilator therapy either for afterload reduction or preload reduction is effective therapy for severe cardiac dysfunction caused by ischemia, cardiomyopathy, postoperative state, or severe aortic or mitral valve regurgitation.[6] However, the high prevalence of CHF caused by left to right shunts in this age group suggests that a secure anatomic diagnosis should be made before empiric use of vasodilator therapy is begun. The pulmonary vasculature may be variably sensitive to vasodilators commonly used. Thus, attempts to unload the systemic ventricle by systemic vasodilation may be confounded by increased left to right shunting due to simultaneous reduction in pulmonary vascular resistance.

Digitalis and diuretics remain the cornerstone of pharmacologic therapy and the doses used are reviewed in Tables 16.7 and 16.8.[5] Digoxin is the glycoside of choice and furosemide the most commonly used diuretic. Catecholamines are useful for chronotropic and inotropic stimulation and when necessary peripheral vasoconstriction. The doses and properties of frequently used catecholamines are noted in Table 16.9.[5]

Child-Adolescent

The initial occurrence of CHF in a child with congenital heart disease is uncommon in the absence of prior corrective or palliative surgery.[7] Thus, the initial occurrence of CHF in this age group should cause a physician to suspect acquired heart disease. Nevertheless, several congenital defects may present with CHF in childhood or adolescence. Postoperative patients may present in this age group with CHF due to the progression of uncorrected abnormalities or due to late postoperative complications.

Unoperated Patients

Causes of CHF in unoperated children and adolescents are shown in Table 16.10.

Eisenmenger's Syndrome

Progressive pulmonary vascular obstruction occurs with high pressure or flow in the pulmonary circuit. This re-

TABLE 16.9. Dosage regimens for inotropic agents.

Drug	Dose	Comments
Epinephrine	0.05–1.0 μg/kg/min iv	May cause hypertension and cardiac arrhythmias, inactivated in alkaline solution
Isoproterenol hydrochloride	0.05–0.5 μg/kg/min iv	May decrease coronary blood flow; results in peripheral and pulmonary vasodilation
Norepinephrine bitartrate	0.05–0.5 μg/kg/min iv	Causes significant vasodilation
Dobutamine hydrochloride	2–10 μg/kg/min iv (max = 40 μg/kg/min)	No direct effect on renal perfusion, little or no peripheral vasodilation or tachycardia
Dopamine hydrochloride	2–20 μg/kg/min iv (max = 50 μg/kg/min)	
	2–5 μg/kg/min	Significant renal vasodilation
	5–8 μg/kg/min	Inotropic ± heart rate acceleration
	8 μg/kg/min	Significant heart rate acceleration
	10 μg/kg/min	± Vasoconsriction
	15–20 μg/kg/min	Significant vasoconstriction

ᵃ Above dose/effect relations are speculative in neonates.
Reproduced, with permission, from George and Friedman.[5]

TABLE 16.10. Causes of CHF in children and adolescents (unoperated).

Eisenmenger's syndrome
Ebstein's anomaly
Aortic insufficiency with VSD
Tricuspid insufficiency with CTGA
Mitral regurgitation with tricuspid atresia
AV valve regurgitation with single ventricle
Myocardial dysfunction due to severe cyanosis
Arrhythmia
Endocarditis

CHF = congestive heart failure; VSD = ventricular spetal defect; CTGA = corrected transposition of the great arteries; AV = atrioventricular.

sults from left to right shunting because of atrial, ventricular, or great vessel communication. With severely elevated pulmonary vascular resistance, pulmonary artery pressures equal systemic and right to left shunting occurs, resulting in cyanosis and Eisenmenger's syndrome. Because of long-standing right ventricular systolic and in some cases diastolic overloading, right ventricular failure may occur in childhood. This usually is associated with severe right ventricular systolic dysfunction, pulmonary insufficiency, and tricuspid insufficiency. The tricuspid valve is particularly vulnerable. The three-leaflet arrangement and the tendency for both the right ventricular cavity and tricuspid annulus to dilate with episodes of CHF may pull the leaflets apart, preventing effective coaptation and allowing severe tricuspid regurgitation. However, "easy come, easy go": the converse also is true. If the CHF can be treated effectively, the tricuspid regurgitation may diminish markedly. The initial episode of CHF may be heralded by atrial flutter, fibrillation, or tachycardia.

Ebstein's Anomaly

Downward displacement of the tricuspid valve in Ebstein's anomaly is associated with tricuspid insufficiency and varying amounts of dysfunction of the remainder of the right ventricle. As right atrial pressure rises with respect to left atrial pressure, cyanosis may occur because of a patent foramen ovale or less commonly atrial septal defect. As with Eisenmenger's syndrome, CHF may be precipitated by an atrial arrhythmia, usually atrial fibrillation or flutter. However, Kent bundles are quite frequent in Ebstein's anomaly and paroxysmal supraventricular tachycardia utilizing the Kent bundle and AV node may be the mechanism.

Aortic Insufficiency

A congenitally abnormal aortic valve usually does not cause CHF in this age group but the valve can be rendered incompetent by a ventricular septal defect. A ventricular septal defect located in the supracristal region undermines support for the right coronary leaflet and may allow it to prolapse into the VSD, thus producing progressive and severe aortic insufficiency.

Congenitally Corrected Transposition of the Great Arteries

Although children with congenitally corrected transposition of the great arteries may be unrecognized and indeed may live a normal life span, some will develop left-sided CHF in childhood or adolescence. Although a natural correction mimicking the Senning or Mustard procedures for transposition of the great arteries, this lesion is not without its difficulties. The problems relating to disturbances of the conduction system result in atrial ventricular block and in the relegation of the right ventricle to systemic duties. Neither the right ventricle nor the tricuspid valve is ideally suited for long-term function at systemic pressures. Thus, as with the Eisenmenger's syndrome, the right ventricle, exposed to systemic pressures, may dilate and result in tricuspid insufficiency and eventually CHF.

Mitral Regurgitation

The mitral valve is more resistant to pressure and volume overload than the tricuspid valve, but it is not immune to these effects. Thus, mitral valve insufficiency may occur in tricuspid atresia because of the increased volume of the ventricle in dilatation of the mitral annulus. Annular dilation and ventricular enlargement combine to prevent effective leaflet coaptation; this results in mitral regurgitation by mechanisms similar to those involving tricuspid insufficiency. In a similar manner, the single AV valve of single ventricle will face high flow and have a ventricle dilated by increased volumes and accordingly be susceptible to regurgitation.

Severe Cyanosis

With complex congenital heart disease, it often is difficult to determine what the mechanisms are that lead to ventricular dysfunction. Both pressure and volume loading frequently are present for long duration. Nevertheless, it seems likely that reduced oxygen delivery to the myocardium contributes significantly to the subendocardial ischemia, necrosis, and fibrosis that ultimately result in ventricular dysfunction and heart failure in complex congenital heart disease.

Endocarditis

Infection of the heart and great vessels in patients with congenital heart disease is most common in locations with high velocity jets and turbulence. Thus, restrictive ventricular septal defects, restrictive patent ductus arteriosus, aortic valve disease, aortic coarctation, left-side AV valve regurgitation, moderate to severe pulmonary stenosis, and truncal valve regurgitation all are at high risk for infection. CHF usually occurs because of destruction of the left side atrioventricular valve or semilunar valve with resultant left heart failure. However, pulmonary embolization and tricuspid valve destruction with endocarditis involving a small VSD also can present with severe right heart failure.

Operated Patients

Causes of CHF in surgically treated children and adolescents are shown in Table 16.11. The list of operations for congenital heart disease is daunting and most can have CHF as an unnatural or natural occurrence

TABLE 16.11. Causes of CHF in children and adolescents (operated).

Myocardial dysfunction
Perioperative ischemic injury
Ventriculotomy
Preoperative myocardial disease
Coronary artery injury
Volume overload
Valvular regurgitation
Persistent VSD
Large bronchial collaterals
Large systemic to pulmonary shunt
Prosthetic dysfunction
Prosthetic valve dysfunction
Conduit obstruction
Patient-prosthesis mismatch
Pulmonary hypertension
Status post-Fontan
Arrhythmias
Endocarditis

CHF = congestive heart failure; VSD = ventricular septal defect.

after the procedure. Nevertheless, patients with heart failure can be divided into major groups of dysfunction for recognition and management.

Myocardial Dysfunction

Myocardial necrosis, scarring, and dysfunction occur after surgery because of intraoperative injury (ischemia or incision) or excessive postoperative loading conditions. Advances in myocardial preservation have greatly reduced intraoperative myocardial damage. It is now possible to arrest the myocardium physiologically for extended periods of time. The greatest limitation in vivo is obtaining adequate cooling of both ventricles in the face of complicated anatomy. Right ventriculotomy is still necessary for resection of infundibular stenosis in tetralogy but most simple ventricular septal defects are now repaired through the tricuspid valve. Coronary artery laceration is uncommon but remains a concern.

Unfortunately, myocardial dysfunction may be present before surgery due to the combined assaults of pressure and volume overload and cyanosis. Unsatisfactory results have pressed cardiologists and surgeons to intervene as soon as technically feasible to effect definitive repair of congenital defects. Because of this practice, the number of patients with postoperative myocardial dysfunction has dropped dramatically and short- and long-term prognosis have improved accordingly.

Volume Overload

Volume overload occurs after surgery for many reasons. Surgeons create systemic to pulmonary shunts to palliate hypoperfused lungs that cannot be treated definitively. Even the perfect size anastomosis necessarily increases the work of the systemic ventricle and eventually it may fail. Shunts that are too large may result in CHF as early as the perioperative period or take years to do their damage. Uncorrected, an excessively large shunt also may damage the pulmonary vasculature and result in severe pulmonary hypertension. Systemic-pulmonary shunts also may be difficult to close or obliterate during definitive surgery. For example, the Pott's shunt between the left pulmonary artery and the aorta is notoriously difficult to close during surgery and persistent left to right shunting through this defect may result in significant left ventricular volume overload and CHF. Naturally occurring collaterals from the bronchial arteries may be too numerous or difficult to locate at the time of definitive surgery. While providing necessary pulmonary blood flow before correction, with the rerouting of systemic venous return to the lungs, persistent collateral blood flow results in pulmonary over-perfusion and systemic ventricular volume overload and may result in CHF. Collaterals unapproachable at definitive surgery subsequently may be embolized by the interventionists.

All four valves may leak after surgery and result in or contribute to CHF. Generally, tricuspid and pulmonary regurgitation are tolerated better than mitral and aortic regurgitation. However, right ventricular pressure overload due to pulmonary valve, pulmonary artery, or pulmonary arteriolar constriction frequently is present to some degree and the volume overload will be less well tolerated in this setting. Unsuccessful repair of the valve in Ebstein's anomaly may result in recurrent right heart failure even with normal pulmonary artery pressures. Late right heart failure after tetralogy repair usually is multifactorial, including myocardial dysfunction from presurgical pressure overload, ventriculotomy, patch aneurysm, and pulmonary insufficiency. Nevertheless, carefully selected patients may respond well to pulmonary valve replacement. Mitral or left-side AV valve regurgitation may be associated with failed repair of a cleft mitral valve, transposition after atrial baffling, or with congenitally "corrected" transposition, single ventricle, or tricuspid atresia after Fontan repair. Aortic insufficiency may follow surgical or balloon valvotomy, VSD repair, or an incompetent truncal valve.

Persistent VSD may cause CHF after an operation to relieve pulmonary valve, subvalvular, or artery stenosis or atresia. Whereas the pulmonary circuit was protected before surgery, after surgery a large left to right shunt may occur, causing left ventricular volume overload and congestive heart failure.

Prosthetic Dysfunction

Prosthetic dysfunction results when biological or artificial valves or conduits fail or are outgrown. It must be recognized that insertion of prosthetic material into a patient represents a new disease whose natural history may or may not be known.[8] For example, there was tremendous enthusiasm for porcine prosthetic valves in the 1970s. The major attraction for children was the lack of need for anticoagulation as opposed to a mechanical valve. However, children and young adults proved to have accelerated calcification and degeneration of these prostheses whether placed in anatomic valve positions or conduit. These prostheses are now avoided in this age group. Enthusiasm has now shifted to the use of cryopreserved homografts, which are implanted in the aortic position, pulmonary position, or conduits between the right ventricle and pulmonary artery. The durability of these valves is certainly greater than for glutaraldehyde-preserved tissue, but the ultimate fate of these devices in patients remains to be determined.

Mechanical prostheses require warfarin anticoagulation to reduce the incidence of thromboembolic complications. Despite anticoagulation, and related to poor anticoagulation, these prostheses may develop thrombotic obstruction. The prostheses in the tricuspid position are most vulnerable with the mitral intermediate and aortic position least susceptible. Material failure of mechanical prostheses currently implanted is uncommon. A number of Bjork-Shiley convexo-concave valves remain in patients especially in the mitral position, which may be susceptible to strut fracture and acute sudden insufficiency or poppet embolization.

Conduit obstruction may occur because of the development of pseudointimal proliferation, thrombosis of the conduit or associated valve, or fibrocalcific degeneration of an associated bioprosthesis.

Bioprosthesis dysfunction usually is associated with fibrocalcific degeneration of the leaflets. This process results in mixed stenosis and regurgitation of the valve. Occasionally, a leaflet will tear and the manifestation of dysfunction may be severe regurgitation.

Patient prosthesis mismatch occurs as a natural consequence of growth when a child must have a heart valve or conduit placed that may be too small for that individual after puberty. Unfortunately, a hypoplastic annulus or great vessel also may require that a small prosthesis be placed in even fully grown young adults.

The Fontan Procedure

The Fontan procedure connects the right atrium directly to the pulmonary arteries or through an outflow chamber to the pulmonary valve for patients with single ventricle or tricuspid atresia. Without an effective pulmonary ventricle, mean right atrial and pulmonary artery pressures are the same. Thus, right atrial pressure must be greater than left atrial pressure to drive blood through the lungs both at rest and during exercise. Obviously, left ventricular end-diastolic pressure must be normal, the mitral valve competent, and pulmonary vascular resistance low for this operation to be successful. Even then, many patients have systemic congestion with ascites and pleural liquid after the procedure. This problem usually can be managed successfully by the judicious use of diuretics and afterload reduction.

Endocarditis

Endocarditis remains a threat for any prosthetic valve with an incidence of approximately 1% per year. Small residual VSDs and mild aortic and mitral insufficiency also are fertile grounds for endocarditis in the postsurgical patient and may result in leaflet destruction and CHF.

Arrhythmias

Arrhythmias are precipitating causes of CHF in patients with borderline ventricular systolic function, stiff ventricles dependent on atrial booster pump function, and with the Fontan procedure. Patients with atrial baffling procedures (Mustard, Senning) and the Fontan procedure also are at increased risk for atrial arrhythmias. Thus, atrial flutter in a patient with transposition who has had previous Mustard repair may be tolerated poorly because of systemic ventricular dysfunction. Likewise, atrial tachycardia in a patient with tetralogy repair with moderate residual outflow tract obstruction and insufficiency may develop right heart failure. Last, the Fontan patient needs both atrial ventricular synchrony for booster pump function in the systemic ventricle and right atrial booster pump function to enhance pulmonary blood flow. Atrial arrhythmias are a major cause of CHF in these patients. Congenital or acquired complete heart block also may become a manifest problem in this age group. While the bradycardia and lack of atrial ventricular synchrony may be tolerated well for years, the concurrent insults of ventricular dysfunction, prosthetic heart valve, or other postsurgical changes may promote CHF. Restoration of atrial ventricular synchrony with heart rate responsive to a normally innervated atrium or to patient activity may be indicated.

Pulmonary Hypertension

Pulmonary hypertension due to either pulmonary arteriolar changes associated with volume overload or multiple pulmonary arterial stenoses may remain after otherwise successful corrective surgery. In this setting, the competence of the pulmonary and tricuspid valves as well as pulmonary ventricular function are critical. Unless all of the components of the right heart are intact, right heart failure may ensue.

The recognition of CHF in children and adolescents makes full use of the history, physical examination, laboratory data base, and echocardiography (Table

TABLE 16.12. Recognition of CHF in children and adolescents.

Weight loss (anorexia)
Weight gain (edema, ascites)
Dyspnea
Reduced exercise tolerance
Tachycardia
Tachypnea
Elevated venous pressure
Gallop
Rales
Hepatomegaly, ascites, edema
Cardiomegaly, pulmonary congestion on chest x ray
Dysrhythmias on electrocardiogram
Abnormal anatomy and function on echo

CHF = congestive heart failure.

TABLE 16.13. Management of CHF in children and adolescents with congenital heart disease.

1. Obtain complete records of previous anatomic studies or operations
2. Obtain complete current anatomic-functional data with echo and if necessary catheterization
3. Repair surgically correctable lesions
4. Reoperate on incomplete or failed repairs, failed or outgrown prostheses
5. Correct arrhythmias
6. Optimize preload and afterload
7. Exclude or treat endocarditis

CHF = congestive heart failure.

16.12). Usually, the diagnosis of CHF can be made securely at the bedside, with confirmation of left heart failure by the chest x ray and with a mechanism established from the past history and the current echocardiographic findings. Occasionally, cardiac catheterization may be necessary for further delineation of abnormalities or for therapy. The importance of a carefully performed echocardiogram cannot be overemphasized.

The management of CHF in children and adolescents with congenital heart disease is shown in Table 16.13. Management begins with a thorough understanding of the underlying anatomy (natural and surgical), physiology, and function of the cardiovascular system. Most of these patients will have had multiple interactions with the medical system, including prior surgery. It is imperative that old records documenting prior findings at catheterization, surgery, and echocardiography be available and be understood. Current anatomy, physiology, and function must be meticulously determined. Usually, this can be accomplished with echocardiography. Where necessary, catheterization is used to measure pressures, flows, and resistances or to visualize pathoanatomy with contrast angiography. Where surgical therapy has the possibility of improved survival or reduced morbidity, it should be applied judiciously. For

TABLE 16.14. Digitalis and diuretic therapy in children and adolescents with CHF.

Digoxin
Digitalizing dose:
  0.04 mg/kg iv, 0.05 mg/kg po (max 1 mg)
  50% stat, 25% q3–12h depending on urgency
Maintenance:
  0.01–0.02 mg/kg (max 0.25 mg/day), 50% bid

Furosemide
Acute 1 mg/kg iv
Chronic 2–5 mg/kg/day in 1–2 doses po

Ethacrynic acid
Acute 1 mg/kg iv
Chronic 2–3 mg/kg/day in 1–2 doses

Hydrochlorothiazide
2–5 mg/kg/day po

Spironolactone
1–3 mg/kg/day po

CHF = congestive heart failure.
Modified from Artman et al.[7] with permission.

TABLE 16.15. Vasodilator treatment of CHF in children and adolescents with congenital heart disease.

Acute
Nitroprusside 0.5–8 μg/kg/min iv
Hydralazine 0.5–1 mg/kg iv

Chronic
Hydralazine 0.5–5 mg/kg/day po in 3 divided doses
Captopril 0.5–6 mg/kg/day po in 2–4 divided doses

CHF = congestive heart failure.
Modified from Artman et al.[7] with permission.

failed conduits or prostheses, reoperation usually is the only option. When increased pulmonary vascular resistance, ventricular dysfunction, arrhythmia, or endocarditis are present, initial medical management usually is indicated.

Drug therapy for children and adolescents with congenital heart disease and CHF is shown in Tables 16.14 and 16.15.[7] While digitalis and diuretics remain the mainstay of therapy for ventricular dysfunction, afterload reduction must be considered integral therapy when Eisenmenger's syndrome or severe pulmonary hypertension without a shunt are not present. Patients with systemic ventricular dysfunction or left-side regurgitant lesions should be considered early for treatment with afterload reducing agents. Although large randomized trials in this population do not exist to justify this approach, extrapolation from trials in adults with CHF seems warranted. Considering the ease with which therapy with angiotensin-converting enzyme (ACE) inhibitors can be carried out, the burden of proof might be on those who recommend against such empiric treatment.

The goal of diuretic therapy should be to obtain the lowest possible filling pressure or preload that does not decrease cardiac output. Without intravascular pressure measurement, this requires careful integration of the patient's weight, jugular venous pressure, free fluid, and blood urea nitrogen. Similarly, afterload reduction with ACE inhibitor therapy can be taken to the maximum doses until hypotension or azotemia occur. If azotemia remains a problem at high doses of diuretics and ACE inhibitors, hydralazine and lower doses of ACE inhibitors may be useful. Critically ill patients may require inotropic and vasodilator support with dobutamine and nitroprusside.

Adult

Adults with congenital heart disease are a rapidly increasing patient population.[9] This has occurred because of the increasing survival of patients with congenital heart disease palliated or corrected earlier in life. Although extracardiac defects such as patent ductus and coarctation were approached in 1930s and 1940s, intracardiac repair awaited the advent of the heart/lung machine in the 1950s. Ventricular septal defect and tetralogy were first repaired in 1955 and transposition in 1959. The first Fontan procedure was performed in 1971. Thus, many young adults are emerging with operated congenital heart disease. Adults with inoperable or deferred surgery also exist, and at the UCLA Adult Congenital Heart Disease Clinic occur in numbers equal to those who have had previous surgery.[10] Thus, the spectrum of adults with congenital heart disease is broad.

The mechanisms for development of CHF in adults with congenital heart disease are similar to those for children and adolescents. In addition, adults have had more time to develop other degenerative diseases that contribute to the development of CHF. These include diabetes, hypertension, coronary artery disease, and renal insufficiency. Pulmonary vascular obstructive disease frequently runs its final course in the fourth and fifth decades. Dystrophic fibrosis and calcification of congenitally abnormal aortic valves progresses rapidly in some young adults, bringing either important aortic stenosis or insufficiency or their combination to the clinical threshold. Previously asymptomatic patients with atrial septal defect may be pushed into CHF by the development of mitral regurgitation. Finally, adults have access to cardiotoxic drugs including alcohol, cocaine, and tobacco, which may aggravate myocardial, coronary, or vascular disease.

The management of adult patients with congenital heart disease and CHF follows the guidelines listed in Table 16.13. The following cases are illustrative of typical patients and their problems.

TABLE 16.16. Causes of CHF in adults with congenital heart disease (unoperated).

Eisenmenger's syndrome
Fibrocalcific degeneration of abnormal aortic valve
Systemic ventricular dysfunction and/or tricuspid regurgitation in CTGA
Atrial septal defect with mitral regurgitation due to myxomatous mitral valve
Congenital mitral regurgitation
Arrhythmia
Endocarditis
Other degenerative disease (CAD, hypertension, etc.)
Drug, alcohol abuse

CHF = congestive heart failure; CTGA = corrected transposition of the great arteries; CAD = coronary artery disease.

TABLE 16.17. Causes of CHF in adults with congenital heart disease (operated)

Myocardial dysfunction
Valvular regurgitation
Persistent left to right shunt
Pulmonary vascular disease
Prosthetic dysfunction
Status post-Fontan
Arrhythmia
Endocarditis
Other degenerative disease (CAD, hypertension, etc.)
Drug, alcohol abuse

CHF = congestive heart failure; CAD = coronary artery disease.

Case Studies

Twenty-Two-Year-Old Man, Status Post-Mustard Operation for Transposition

This young man recently moved to our area. He had balloon septostomy and then atrial septectomy soon after birth for transposition of the great vessels. The Mustard procedure was performed at age 3 yr. Over the last several years, he has had multiple admissions to hospitals for CHF, atrial tachyarrhythmias, and hemoptysis. He has been unemployed and essentially homeless. He binged alcohol and smoked. Recent evaluation at our institution by echocardiography and right heart catheterization showed severe systemic ventricular dysfunction, moderate to severe systemic atrioventricular valve regurgitation, and hemodynamics consistent with CHF. The atrial arrhythmias were identified as atrial flutter and paroxysmal supraventricular tachycardia. Inpatient treatment with intravenous nitroprusside, Lasix, and digitalis was begun. The etiology of hemoptysis was not clear, but was thought to be related to severe CHF. He responded well to treatment of CHF and was discharged on digitalis, furosemide, and captopril. He was readmitted with hemoptysis, but his heart failure was under good control. An aortogram showed a large bronchial collateral to the right lung (previously documented site of bleeding), and this was embolized with cessation of bleeding.

As an outpatient, he was counseled regarding the importance of taking his medications and refraining from the use of alcohol and tobacco. On this regimen, he responded dramatically, with normalization of his jugular venous pressure, resolution of his S3 gallop, and improvement to functional Class II status. Recently, while visiting relatives, he again binged alcohol and was treated in a local emergency room for atrial tachycardia and CHF. He definitely has been able to associate his clinical deterioration with the use of alcohol and with medical noncompliance. With abstinence and reinstitution of his medications, he has been restabilized.

This young man has complications of his congenital heart disease and its surgical treatment. He has systemic ventricular dysfunction and atrioventricular valve regurgitation related to the anatomic unsuitability of the morphologic right ventricle and tricuspid valve for systemic pressures. He has atrial arrhythmias associated with his Mustard repair. The ventricular dysfunction, atrioventricular valve regurgitation, and arrhythmias, however, all were exacerbated by alcohol and medical noncompliance. On medication and off alcohol, he improved from functional Class IV with multiple emergency room and hospital visits to functional Class II. When originally seen, we thought his prognosis was bleak, with transplantation the only possible long-term solution, but contraindicated because of his lifestyle. Currently, he may have many more years of service from his heart.

Twenty-Six-Year-Old Man, Status Postrepair of Tetralogy

A Blalock shunt was placed soon after birth to improve pulmonary blood flow for this cyanotic infant with tetralogy. Definitive repair was performed at age 5 yr. Ventricular septal defect closure, infundibular resection, and outflow tract patch, including the pulmonary valve annulus, were performed. Peripheral pulmonary stenoses were present in both arteries, however, and moderate pulmonary hypertension was present postoperatively. He did well as a child, nevertheless. Because of right heart failure and fatigue, he was reevaluated when he was a teenager. This showed normal left ventricular function, moderate pulmonary hypertension due to multiple pulmonary stenoses, severe pulmonary regurgitation, and tricuspid regurgitation with right ventricular dilatation and dysfunction. Pulmonary valve replacement with a homograft and tricuspid annuloplasty were performed, with improvement in symptoms. At age 21, he had fatigue, malaise, low-grade fever, and the return of CHF. Reevaluation revealed the cause to be streptococcus viridans endocarditis. This was treated successfully with antibiotics. No significant valve dysfunction was present, but mild CHF requiring digitalis and diuretics remained. Atrial arrhythmias became a recurrent problem, clearly exacerbating his symptoms of CHF. He was able, however, to work 30 to 40 hours per week as a computer operator. One year ago, he had progressive weakness and fatigue associated with palpitations. He was exhausted at work. Increased diuretics did not help. He was referred back for evaluation. He appeared ill, with irregularly irregular pulse of 80 to 90 bpm. His chest was clear, jugular venous pressure 10 cm, and pulmonary systolic and diastolic murmurs were present, but unchanged. Mild hepatomegaly and edema were present. Repeat echocardiographic evaluation showed normal left ventricular function, satisfactory pulmonary valve prosthetic function, moderate right ventricular dysfunction, and mild tricuspid insufficiency. Electrocardiogram showed atrial fibrillation. It was felt that the atrial fibrillation with loss of atrial booster pump function had tipped this delicately balanced patient with moderate pulmonary hypertension, pulmonary valve homograft, right ventricular dysfunction, and tricuspid insufficiency into right heart failure. Accordingly, he was anticoagulated with warfarin and cardioverted 3 weeks later to sinus rhythm. Quinidine was added to the regimen because of the seriousness of his clinical deterioration in atrial fibrillation. He responded slowly over the next 6 weeks with a decrease in his diuretic requirement, and returned to work half time. Quinidine therapy was complicated by loose stools, but was tolerable.

Although most patients with tetralogy repair are functional Class I or II, some have significant right ventricular dysfunction and arrhythmias. This patient is delicately balanced, and atrial fibrillation, even at normal heart rate, is enough to cause clinical deterioration. Since deterioration of the homograft also could contribute to right heart failure, this possibility needed to be considered as well. Eventually, right heart failure will return and be unresponsive to medical manipulation. Because of the peripheral pulmonary stenoses, heart transplantation will not be suitable. Heart-lung transplantation may be the only recourse.

Thirty-Three-Year-Old Man with Congenitally Corrected Transposition

We first saw this patient 3 years ago. As an infant, he had a loud murmur thought to be consistent with pulmonary stenosis. Surgery was performed and corrected transposition found unexpectedly. Pulmonary valve commissurotomy was performed, but some residual pulmonary subpulmonic stenosis remained. Follow-up catheterization in 1979 showed pulmonary ventricular pressure of 90 mm Hg, but the pulmonary arteries could not be en-

tered. Systemic ventricular function was reduced. He was lost to follow-up. He worked as a truck driver and delivery person. He was married and had three children. Several months before evaluation, he developed exertional dyspnea, fatigue, and could not keep up with his work. He was evaluated by a physician. The chest x ray showed CHF, and echocardiography confirmed the previous anatomy and showed severe systemic ventricular dysfunction associated with moderate systemic atrioventricular valve regurgitation and aortic insufficiency. The pulmonary ventricular outflow tract gradient was mild to moderate. The patient was referred to our Adult Congenital Heart Clinic. Therapy was begun with digoxin, hydrochlorothiazide, and captopril. He responded well and returned to early functional Class II status and worked full time.

One year ago, he had multiple respiratory infections over the winter, associated with his children's illnesses. Pulmonary infiltrates were intermittently identified. Several courses of antibiotics were given. Multiple blood cultures were negative. His clinical condition deteriorated with increasing dyspnea, fatigue, edema, hepatomegaly, and increasingly abnormal liver function tests. He was admitted to the hospital for evaluation. Right heart catheterization was performed with some difficulty in the Catheterization Laboratory. It should be noted that the continuity of the atrioventricular and semilunar valves of the pulmonary ventricle requires the catheter to double back on itself to cross into the pulmonary artery. Combined with severe atrioventricular valve regurgitation, the catheter could not be maintained in the pulmonary artery for long-term monitoring. Severe CHF with cardiac index of 1.5 L/min/m^2 was confirmed. Intensive intravenous therapy with dobutamine, nitroprusside, Lasix, and amrinone was instituted and a diuresis effected. Repeat echocardiography confirmed severe systemic ventricular dysfunction. Repeat right heart catheterization 1 week later showed improvement in his output and filling pressures, with the pulmonary vascular resistance less than 2 Wood units. The patient's status was still tenuous, however, and he was "drip-dependent." He was referred for consideration of heart transplantation and was accepted. He was listed, and transplantation performed within a month, although he remained in the hospital on intensive medical treatment until then.

This man had exhausted the reserve of his morphologic right ventricle, which was functioning as his systemic ventricle, by the fourth decade of his life. Because he had congenitally corrected transposition of the great arteries, he was never exposed to cyanosis, and his only previous surgery was a brief pump run for pulmonary valve commissurotomy. We thus conclude that the morphologic right ventricle may not be well suited for long-term service as the systemic ventricle. In this case, the pulmonary circuit was never overperfused, and thus pulmonary vascular resistance was low enough to allow cardiac transplantation without lung transplantation. For many patients with end-stage congenital heart disease, pulmonary vascular disease also will be present, and heart-lung transplantation will be the only possible operation. For some, for example, those who have ventricular septal defect with Eisenmenger's syndrome, ventricular function may be relatively preserved, and ventricular septal defect closure with single lung transplantation considered.

Conclusion

The management of patients with congenital heart disease and CHF has long been the responsibility of the pediatrician, neonatologist, and pediatric cardiologist. As noted above, prompt therapy and diagnosis accompanied by sophisticated surgical correction or palliation has improved the outcome for many children with congenital heart disease and CHF. Now, many of these patients are in the adult age group. A strong argument can be made for interdisciplinary care of these complicated patients, many of whom are defining the natural history for a new disease. The opportunities for life-prolonging surgical therapy are less in the adult with congenital heart disease and these opportunities cannot be missed. Strategies for early and effective medical management of ventricular dysfunction and valvular regurgitation need to be devised and implemented. Finally, this aging population will produce many patients with end-stage heart or heart and pulmonary disease. Unfortunately, many will not have adequate insurance coverage. Both the timing and funding of transplantation in these patients will be a thorny issue.

References

1. Holzgreve W, Holzgreve B, Curry CR. Nonimmune hydrops fetalis: diagnosis and management. *Semin Perinatol*. 1985;9:52–67.
2. Kleinman CS, Copel JA, Weinstein EM, Santulli Jr TV, Hobbins JC. In utero diagnosis and treatment of fetal supraventricular tachycardia. *Semin Perinatol*. 1985;5: 113–129.
3. Thornburg KL, MJ Morton. Development of the cardiovascular system. In: Thorburn GD, Harding R, eds. Textbook of fetal physiology. Oxford: Oxford University Press; 1992.
4. Friedman WF. Congenital heart disease in infancy and childhood. In: Braunwald E, ed. *Heart disease*. Philadelphia: Saunders; 1985:896–975.
5. George BL, Friedman WF. Treatment of cardiac failure in infants. *Comprehen Ther*. 1986;12:8–14.
6. Friedman WF, George BL. Treatment of congestive heart failure by altering loading conditions of the heart. *J Pediatr*. 1985;106:697–706.
7. Artman M, MD Parrish, TP Graham Jr. Congestive heart failure in childhood and adolescence: recognition and management. *Am Heart J*. 1983;105:471–480.
8. Haas G, Laks H, Perloff JK. The selection, use, and long-term effects of prosthetic materials. In: Perloff JK, Child JS, eds. *Congenital heart disease in adults*. Philadelphia: Saunders; 1991:213–223.
9. Perloff JK. A brief historical perspective. In: Perloff JK, Child JS, eds. *Congenital heart disease in adults*. Philadelphia: Saunders; 1991:3–17.
10. Perloff JK. The UCLA adult congenital heart disease program. *Am J Cardiol*. 1986;57:1190–1192.

17
Right Heart Failure

Marvin A. Konstam and James E. Udelson

Right heart failure may result from dysfunctional right ventricular (RV) myocardium, excessive load imposed on the right ventricle during systole and/or diastole, or obstruction to RV inflow. The clinical expression of right heart failure is similar regardless of cause, and is mediated via a combination of elevated systemic venous pressure and depressed cardiac output, with resulting sodium and water retention. The primary manifestations are edema, fatigue, and breathlessness. In addition, the failed right ventricle may adversely influence left ventricular (LV) performance through ventricular interaction, and thus may promote signs and symptoms of left heart failure.

In this chapter, we first review the pathophysiology and clinical manifestations of right heart failure; second, we review assessment of RV function; third, we describe the various specific causes of right heart failure; fourth, we discuss the physiology and clinical implications of ventricular interdependence; fifth, we discuss the manner in which RV performance may relate to the clinical expression of left heart failure; sixth, we review therapy for right heart failure.

Pathogenesis and Clinical Manifestations of Right Heart Failure

Right heart failure may be separated into diastolic failure, defined as abnormal elevation in right heart filling pressure, and systolic failure, defined as abnormally low RV forward output. In the absence of a perturbation in the serial nature of left and right heart output, as with intracardiac shunt, depression of right heart forward flow is a necessary accompaniment of a primary reduction in left heart output. This interaction is mediated through an increase in RV afterload and/or relative reduction in right heart inflow.

Load-Dependence of Right Ventricular Function

RV volume and systolic function are exquisitely sensitive to changes in load. The thin RV free wall, normally no more than 4 mm thick,[1] renders the right ventricle more compliant during both diastole and systole than is the left ventricle.[2-6] That is, increases in diastolic pressure or in systolic pressure are accompanied by relatively large increments in diastolic volume and in end-systolic volume, respectively. This difference implies that the magnitude of change in stroke volume is greater in relation to change in systolic pressure for the right ventricle than for the left ventricle (Fig. 17.1A). In contrast, increases in diastolic distending pressure effect less augmentation in stroke work—that is, shallower Starling curve—for the RV than for the LV (Fig. 17.1B). The relation between RV afterload and systolic function may be expressed quantitatively through the RV end-systolic pressure/volume relation[5,6-8] (Fig. 17.2). The slope of this relation represents RV chamber elastance, or the ability to sustain contractile performance in response to changes in systolic load. It has been found to increase in response to inotropic stimulation.[5] The ventricular systolic pressure-volume slope is shallower for the RV than for the LV, because for the thin-walled RV a given change in pressure translates into a greater change in wall stress than for the thick-walled LV.[6]

A clinically relevant corollary of these observations is that, relative to the LV, the RV is less suited to accommodate to pressure overload, but more suited to accommodate to volume overload. The sensitivity of RV volume to changes in pressure during diastole is responsible for the ability of the RV to accommodate substantial increases in preload with relatively small increases in systemic venous pressure. However, the sensitivity of RV end-systolic volume to changes in end-systolic pressure is responsible for the fact that re-

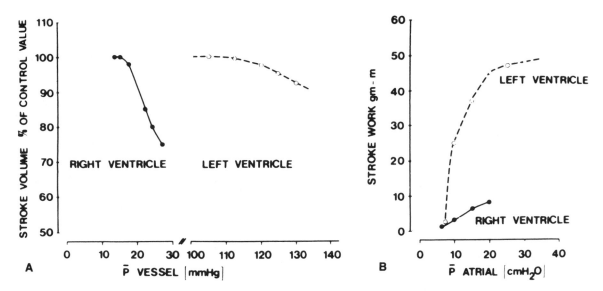

FIGURE 17.1. Effects of increasing afterload and preload on RV and LV function. The data in the left panel were obtained by constricting the main pulmonary artery or aorta in dogs. The right panel demonstrates the effect of increasing preload.

Reprinted, with permission, from McFadden ER Jr, Braunwald E. Corpulmonale and pulmonary thromboembolism In: Braunwald E, ed. *Heart disease. A textbook of cardiovascular medicine.* Philadelphia: Saunders; 1988.

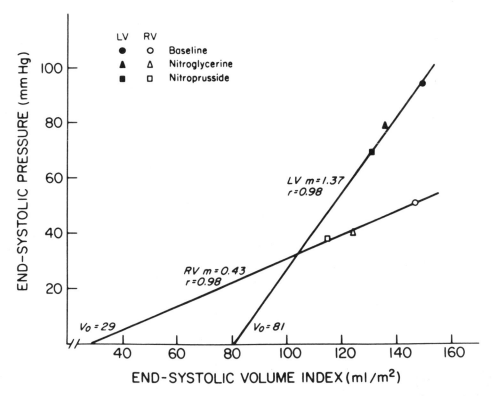

FIGURE 17.2. Comparison of LV and RV end-systolic pressure/volume relations (group mean data with linear regression lines) derived from 10 patients with biventricular failure due to healed myocardial infarction or DCM. Pulmonary or systemic arterial end-systolic (*dicrotic notch*) pressures are plotted against radionuclide-derived RV or LV end-systolic volumes, respectively, at baseline and during infusion of nitroglycerin and nitroprusside. The shallower slope of the RV relation in-

dicates lesser RV systolic stiffness compared with the LV. That is, identical changes in systolic pressure effect greater changes in systolic performance for the RV than for the LV. Reprinted, with permission, from Konstam MA, Levine HJ. Effects of afterload and preload on right ventricular systolic performance. In: Konstam MA, Isner JM, eds. *The right ventricle.* Boston, Dordrecht, Lancaster: Kluwer; 1988.

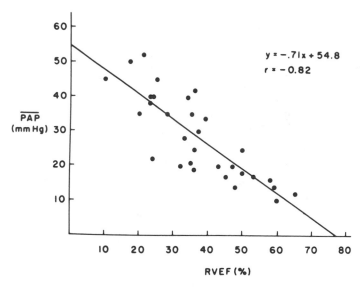

$$y = -.71x + 54.8$$
$$r = -0.82$$

FIGURE 17.3. Relation between right ventricular ejection fraction (*RVEF*) and mean pulmonary artery pressure (*PAP*) patients with diagnoses of coronary artery disease or valvular heart disease. Reprinted, with permission, from Korr et al. *Am J Cardiol.* 1982;49:71–77.

duction in RV ejection fraction (EF) and clinical findings of right heart failure more commonly are manifestations of abnormal afterload, due to left heart failure or pulmonary vascular pathology, than to intrinsic pathology of the RV myocardium[9–14] (Fig. 17.3). Conversely, RV EF may be maintained in the normal range despite moderate myocardial derangement, as long as it is ejecting into a low resistance circulation. Canine studies indicate that in the setting of acute pulmonary hypertension, inadequacy of RV coronary flow to meet the increased metabolic demand contributes to reduction in RV systolic performance.[15]

The development of RV hypertrophy in response to chronic pressure overload results in reduction in wall stress for any given intracavitary pressure. As hypertrophy progresses, the mechanical characteristics of the RV become more similar to those of the LV, retaining systolic function in the face of heightened pulmonary artery (PA) pressure, but requiring higher filling pressure to maintain preload and forward flow. In patients with pulmonary hypertension the degree to which RV hypertrophy develops and serves to maintain systolic function depends, in part, on the rapidity and age of onset of the hemodynamic stimulus. With progressive hypertrophy, RV systolic function may deteriorate, possibly due to intrinsic myocardial contractile dysfunction associated with cardiac hypertrophy. This occurrence is controversial, with some, but not all, studies of experimentally induced RV hypertrophy showing reduction of intrinsic contractility.[16–20] These studies have documented intrinsic contractile derangement during the early stages of pressure-overload hypertrophy, as

indicated by reduction in the maximum unloaded velocity and in the maximum rate of tension development of isolated myocardium. However, in time, these abnormalities generally have been observed to revert toward normal. Alternatively, a limitation in coronary flow reserve has been documented in animal models and in patients with RV myocardial hypertrophy and may result in ischemic contractile dysfunction.[21,22]

Depending on the rate and extent of progression of RV pressure overload, of any etiology, RV hypertrophy may be inadequate to maintain a normal level of systolic stress. As RV systolic stress becomes excessive, perhaps compounded by intrinsic RV myocardial contractile dysfunction, ejection performance declines. Under these conditions, the RV generally distends during diastole, in part representing a compensatory mechanism, by which preload is recruited to maintain stroke volume. RV distension is accelerated by the advent of tricuspid regurgitation (TR), which tends to thwart the compensatory Starling mechanism. Thus, in a variety of circumstances, RV pressure overload and volume overload coexist.

Clinical Findings in Right Heart Failure

In clinical practice, systolic and diastolic right heart failure, regardless of cause, often coincide. The clinical expression of right heart failure depends on a combination of elevated systemic venous pressure and depressed cardiac output. Clinical findings depend on the chronicity of hemodynamics derangement. Acute right heart failure, as due to RV infarction, is characterized by signs and symptoms of depressed cardiac output and elevated jugular venous pressure, often with prominent V-wave and Y descent. Other findings that may be present include RV S3 gallop, a murmur of TR, and Kussmul's sign.[23–26] Edema has not had time to develop. Acute severe pulmonary embolism presents a similar picture.[27–29] Additional signs of chronic pulmonary hypertension with RV hypertrophy—RV heave, RV S4 gallop, prominent jugular venous a wave—may or may not be present, since hypertrophy has not had time to develop, and the normal thin-walled RV is limited in the level of PA pressure that it can generate.[30,31]

With chronic right heart failure of any cause, edema becomes a prominent feature.[32] In addition to peripheral edema and ascites, edema of the visceral organs contributes to alteration in hepatic, renal, and intestinal function. Pleural effusions develop because of impediment to parietal pleural drainage. Other clinical signs depend on the etiology of right heart failure. For example, pulmonary vascular disease or recurrent pulmonary emboli are associated with signs of pulmonary hypertension and RV hypertrophy: RV heave, loud pulmonic component of the second heart sound, and RV S4 gallop.[27–29]

Neurohormonal Changes and Accumulation of Extravascular Fluid

Edema of peripheral tissues and systemic organs, a prominent feature of chronic right heart failure,[32] generally requires both elevation of central venous pressure and a stimulus for renal sodium and water retention. Since detectable edema requires an increase of approximately 5 L of extracellular fluid in an adult,[33] hemodynamic derangement must be prolonged before edema becomes apparent. Additional factors may accelerate the development of edema. Normally, competent venous valves and muscular activity in anatomically dependent zones tend to mitigate against transudation of intravascular fluid to the extravascular compartment. Potential factors that may provoke or accentuate tissue edema include incompetence of peripheral venous valves, muscular inactivity, and reduced plasma oncotic pressure.

In patients with right heart failure, the development of edema is supported by renal sodium retention provoked by reduced forward cardiac output and perturbation of neuroendocrine activity.[34] These mechanisms are described in detail elsewhere in this volume. In brief, reduction in cardiac output directly reduces glomerular filtration rate, thus diminishing tubular sodium delivery. Activation of the renin-angiotensin-aldosterone axis stimulates sodium-potassium exchange.[35,36] In the setting of right heart failure, increased renin secretion, leading to enhanced vasoconstriction and sodium retention, is accentuated by augmented adrenergic activity.[36] The latter is supported by impairment of baroreceptor function.[37]

Experimentally induced right heart failure has been found to diminish RV norepinephrine uptake-1 carrier density and norepinephrine uptake activity[38] (Fig. 17.4). This abnormality appears to be related directly to a regional perturbation of cardiac function, perhaps due to altered myocardial stress, since it was not evident within LV myocardium in a model with isolated right heart failure.[38] Reduced norepinephrine uptake may, in part, be responsible for excess exposure of myocardial beta-receptors to circulating and neuronally released norepinephrine, thereby yielding reduced norepinephrine sensitivity.

An increase in right atrial (RA) pressure stimulates release of atrial natriuretic factor (ANF), and patients with heart failure have been found to have a 2- to 10-fold increase in circulating levels of ANF, compared with normals.[39-42] However, in patients with heart failure, end-organ responsiveness to ANF is severely reduced.[43] This feature accounts for further reduction in glomerular filtration rate, through glomerular afferent arteriolar constriction, and may accelerate tubular sodium resorption.

Thus, manifestations of right heart failure are not

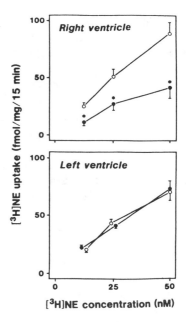

FIGURE 17.4. Specific ³H uptake activity (representing tissue [³H]norepinephrine [NE] uptake), at three concentrations of [³H]NE, using fresh tissue slices taken from the right and left ventricular free walls of sham-operated dogs (*open circles*) and dogs with experimentally induced right heart failure (*closed circles*). In dogs with right heart failure, there is reduction in NE uptake within RV, but not LV, myocardium. * = significant difference from sham-operated group. Reprinted, with permission, from Liang CS, et al. *J Clin Invest.* 1989;84:1267–1275.

merely the direct effect of altered RV hemodynamics. Rather, the right heart interfaces with, and contributes to, a perturbed neurohormonal milieu. A vicious cycle is established, with altered RV systolic and diastolic performance leading to vascular, renal, and neuroendocrine abnormalities, leading to further right heart dysfunction due to progressively abnormal RV loading conditions.

In patients with heart failure, excess pleural fluid is most common when elevations of pulmonary venous pressure and central venous pressure coincide. Pleural fluid is drained by parietal pleural lymphatic vessels that empty into the systemic veins, as well as via visceral pleural communication to the pulmonary venous system.[44-46] Therefore, in the presence of left heart failure or right heart failure in isolation, one drainage route is likely to compensate for failure of the alternate route. In studies of patients with chronic cor pulmonale and elevated RA pressure, in the absence of left heart failure, pleural effusions have not been observed frequently.[47] However, pleural effusion has been ascribed to systemic venous hypertension without pulmonary venous hypertension in the setting of acute RV myocardial infarction.[25,48] It is likely that in patients with chronic right heart failure, without left heart failure, alternative pleural drainage routes, which are not operative acutely, ultimately are recruited.

Clinical findings published in the 1940s tended to support the view that pleural effusions due to heart failure occurred predominantly on the right.[49–51] However, more recent post-mortem and clinical studies have indicated that between 70% and 90% of patients with heart failure and pleural effusions manifest bilateral pleural fluid.[52,53] In the few patients with unilateral effusions, the ratio of right-sided to left-sided effusions is approximately 2:1. Differences between the findings of older versus newer literature have been attributed to implementation of potent diuretics.[53] In patients in whom pleural effusions occur in association with primary pericardial disease, the pleural fluid has been observed to be predominantly left-sided.[54] It has been speculated that this finding may be related directly to the presence of pericardial inflamation.[54] Pleural effusions due to heart failure are predominantly transudative, being primarily the product of abnormal hydrostatic forces. In some studies, diuresis has been observed to transform the chemical composition of pleural fluid to that of a "pseudoexudate,"[55] although others have found this occurrence to be unusual.[56]

In patients with heart failure, failure of systemic organs predominantly results from a combination of increased venous pressure and reduced arterial perfusion. Tissue ischemia tends to accelerate formation of interstitial edema through capillary membrane injury. In turn, edema contributes to tissue ischemia through an increase in interstitial pressure, thus impeding blood flow. A vicious cycle is established that may be exacerbated acutely by an abrupt increase in venous pressure and/or abrupt reduction in perfusion pressure. These events may lead to chronic renal dysfunction, sometimes with superimposed acute tubular necrosis. Similarly, severe right heart failure frequently is associated with chronic hepatic dysfunction due to a combination of edema, ischemia, and impediment to venous drainage, with chronic elevation in serum transaminase as well as alkaline phosphatase and bilirubin. The latter often is predominantly indirect, indicating a deficiency in conjugation. Acute severe liver injury is common and may or may not be preceded by abrupt overt elevation in systemic venous pressure. Severe elevation in serum transaminase may occur and may be associated with a cholestatic picture. It is not uncommon that these findings are confused with acute viral hepatitis or chronic primary liver disease, until it is appreciated that central venous pressure is elevated. Furthermore, since venous pressure may fluctuate, and since abrupt reduction of hepatic arterial perfusion, rather than abrupt increase in hepatic venous pressure, may be the direct stimulus to liver necrosis, systemic venous pressure may not be elevated severely at the time when hepatic injury is clinically recognized.

Anorexia, malabsorption, and reduced responsiveness to oral medications have been attributed to intestinal edema in patients with right heart failure. However, cachexia in heart failure is likely to be multifactorial, resulting from a combination of anorexia, malabsorption, relatively increased metabolic demand, and possibly humoral factors.[57–61] Recently, patients with heart failure and cachexia have been found to have increased circulating levels of tumor necrosis factor, which may play a causative role in this syndrome.[62]

Assessment of Right Ventricular Function

RV systolic function may be assessed by use of any modality with the capability of estimating relative changes in RV volume: contrast ventriculography,[63–67] radionuclide ventriculography,[68–73] echocardiography,[74–79] magnetic resonance imaging,[80] cine-computerized tomography, high-frequency indicator dilution,[81–83] or impedance volumetrics.[84]

Employing any of these techniques, quantitation of ventricular function is technically more difficult and less exact for the RV than for the LV. The RV is characterized by coarse trabeculations and geometric complexity, with discrete inflow and outflow portions. The RV body, or inflow region, normally is concave around the interventricular septum. Contraction resembles the movement of a rounded bellows, the walls of which approach each other in a parallel manner during systole. The RV often changes its shape and its motion patterns substantially in the setting of pressure and/or volume overload.[85–93] Paradoxical septal motion consists of septal movement toward the RV during systole, rather than its normal pattern toward the center of the LV cavity. In patients with volume overload, the curvature of the interventricular septum is displaced toward the LV at end-diastole, concave toward the RV due to the increased diastolic load. At end-systole, the ventricles return toward a more normal configuration, resulting in motion of the septum toward the RV. For all of these reasons, the RV is poorly amenable to geometric modeling for the purpose of volume measurement. Despite these difficulties, numerous studies have employed these modalities to estimate relative change in RV volume through the cardiac cycle, and thus to measure RV EF.

Most studies investigating RV function have found the range of normal EFs to be lower than that of the LV. The lower limit of RV EF generally has been found to be in the range of 40% to 45%. This finding indicates that normal end-diastolic and end-systolic volumes are larger for the RV than for the LV, with the upper limit of normal for RV end-diastolic volume estimated as 120 ml/m^2.[94]

Although considerable attention has been given to the role of diastolic dysfunction of LV myocardium in the pathogenesis of heart failure, few studies have addressed the clinical assessment of RV diastolic performance.[95] The relative neglect of RV diastolic performance is due in part to difficulty in accurate measurement of RV volume throughout the cardiac cycle, for reasons cited above. In addition, whereas temporal indices of LV isovolumic pressure decline are used to assess ventricular relaxation, analogous indices may not be appropriate for analysis of RV relaxation, since the RV isovolumic relaxation period is brief, making mathematical modeling imprecise. Altered RV compliance, due to intrinsic myocardial disease or extrinsic compression, may be assessed by examination of RV pressure/volume relations, which may be approximated using radionuclide[8] or other techniques.

Etiologies of Right Ventricular Failure

Table 17.1 presents a differential diagnosis of right heart failure, broadly subdivided into primary myocardial dysfunction, pressure overload, and volume overload. As mentioned above, these pathophysiologic states often coexist. The most common cause of RV pressure overload, left heart failure, is discussed further in a later section. In additional, RV failure may be simulated by disorders that impede inflow into the RV. These disorders include tricuspid stenosis, cardiac tamponade, pericardial constriction, and restrictive myopathy. Although this category is discussed here in detail, restrictive myopathies are covered under Cardiomyopathy.

Right Ventricular Myocardial Dysfunction

Right Ventricular Myocardial Infarction

The clinical syndrome of RV myocardial infarction was first described in the 1970s as a syndrome involving diminished cardiac output with clear lungs and jugular venous distension.[23,25,96] Since those initial descriptions, the described clinical spectrum of RV involvement in myocardial infarction has broadened considerably.[97–99] Pathologically, infarction involving the RV most often is an accompaniment of infarction involving the posterior free wall of the LV and the posterior portion of the ventricular septum.[96] The extent of involvement of the RV free wall is variable, and does not necessarily correlate with the degree of hemodynamic perturbation. Profoundly abnormal hemodynamics may be observed in the presence of an anatomically small extent of RV involvement with infarction. Less common pathologically is involvement of the anterolateral RV free wall with anterior infarctions.[99] These

TABLE 17.1. Differential diagnosis of right heart failure.

RV myocardial dysfunction
RV myocardial infarction
Dilated cardiomyopathy
RV dysplasia

Primary RV pressure overload
Left ventricular failure
Mitral valve disease
Atrial myxoma
Pulmonary veno-occlusive disease
Cor pulmonale
   Obstructive lung disease
   Primary pulmonary hypertension
   Pulmonary emboli
Pulmonic stenosis
   Supravalvular
   Valvular
   Subvalvular
Ventricular septal defect
Aortopulmonary communication

Primary RV volume overload
Pulmonic regurgitation
Tricuspid regurgitation
Atrial septal defect
Partial anomalous pulmonary venous return

Impediment to RV inflow
Tricuspid stenosis
Cardiac tamponade
Pericardial constriction
Restrictive cardiomyopathy

infarctions tend to be antero-septal, extensive, and associated with moderate to severe reduction in LV EF.[99] Hemodynamically relevant RV infarction almost always signifies evidence of right coronary occlusion proximal to the RV free wall branches.[100]

Elevation of jugular venous pressure in a patient with an electrocardiographic inferior infarction usually indicates RV infarction. Right precordial leads often document RV infarction, with ST segment elevation in leads V3R and V4R.[98] Radionuclide ventriculography or echocardiography may demonstrate RV dilatation, with regional and global RV functional abnormalities.[101] Hemodynamic measurements in the setting of acute RV infarction most commonly reveals elevation of RA and RV diastolic pressure, which often are equilibrated with PA diastolic and PA wedge pressures, a pattern similar to pericardial constriction.[23,35,96] The RA pressure wave form often resembles an "M'" or a "W," with Y descent deeper than X descent. In some patients, however, these findings are not seen, and low pressures may be observed in both the right atrium and the pulmonary wedge position. In such patients, the hemodynamic abnormalities may be brought out by volume loading.[102] The constellation of hemodynamic findings seen in RV infarction appears to require the presence of an intact pericardium. In animal models of RV infarction, the hemodynamic abnormalities improve markedly after pericardiotomy.[103]

The outcome of patients sustaining a myocardial infarction with RV involvement appears to depend on the extent of LV infarction, as the presence or absence of hemodynamic or noninvasive evidence of RV dysfunction in acute myocardial infarction does not influence the long-term prognosis.[104] Serial noninvasive studies of patients with RV myocardial infarction document the common occurrence of improvement in RV performance over the weeks to months that follow an RV infarct.[101,105] Occasionally, patients with large RV myocardial infarction will manifest a syndrome of chronic severe right heart failure with TR.

Cardiomyopathy, Myocardial Infiltration, and Metabolic Disease

In most cases of dilated cardiomyopathy (DCM), right heart failure results, at least in part, from left heart involvement with resulting excessive RV afterload. However, the RV myocardium may be involved in the cardiomyopathic process, to an extent that may be less than, similar to, or greater than involvement of the LV. In some such cases, the clinical manifestations of myocardial involvement will be predominantly those of right heart failure.

There have been reports of cardiomyopathy predominantly involving the RV.[106] A quantitative histologic analysis performed in patients dying of DCM demonstrated that the cell diameter of myocytes in the RV free wall often was as enlarged as those in the LV free wall, and the myocyte cell diameter in both locations was significantly greater than that in control myocytes.[107] Furthermore, the percent volume fibrosis in the RV free wall was greater than that of controls. While these data do not prove primary involvement of the RV myocardium (i.e., these changes may have occurred from long-standing excess in afterload), they suggest that in some patients with cardiomyopathy, the RV may be importantly involved histologically.

Cardiac amyloidosis most often presents with clinical manifestations of biventricular failure. Left-sided involvement is commonly heralded by a restrictive cardiomyopathy with abnormal diastolic compliance characteristics. Prominent manifestations relating to right-sided failure often are seen. Edema and ascites may be exacerbated by concomitant nephrotic syndrome. In a histologic study of 54 necropsy patients with cardiac amyloidosis, most patients had amyloid deposits involving the myocardium of both ventricles, as well as gross involvement of the tricuspid leaflets in more than 80% of patients and gross involvement of pulmonic leaflets in more than 50% of patients.[108] Thus, amyloid deposition is an infiltrative cardiomyopathy that may importantly involve the RV di-

rectly. Evidence of RV failure in patients with cardiac amyloidosis, whether from direct involvement from amyloid deposition or as a consequence of severe derangement in LV hemodynamics, carries a grim prognosis, with a greater than 70% mortality within 6 months.[109] There is to this date no proven treatment regimen to reverse the infiltrative abnormalities of cardiac amyloidosis.

Primary or secondary hemochromatosis may involve the heart, and particularly the RV, with iron deposition and toxic damage to myocytes.[110] Clinically, hemachromatosis may appear as either a restricted or a dilated cardiomyopathy.[110] Once heart disease secondary to iron deposition is clinically manifest, the course of the disease often is progressive and refractory to therapy. In some cases, however, a degree of reversal of the hemodynamic derangement and improvement in ventricular function may be seen with repeated phlebotomy or after treatment with the iron-chelating agent deferoxamine.[111,112]

While sarcoidosis of the heart is associated most often with abnormalities of the cardiac conduction system, myocardial involvement and clinical evidence of heart failure also are seen.[113] RV myocardial involvement by the granulomatous process was observed in almost half of the specimens in a necropsy study of patients with clinically manifest cardiac sarcoidosis.[113] Sudden death, syncope, paroxysmal arrhythmias, and heart failure are the common clinical syndromes of cardiac sarcoidosis. Survival is variable; in some cases the initial clinical presentation of cardiac involvement is sudden death.[113] In contrast, survival over 10 years has been reported.[114,115] Treatment can be problematic, as arrhythmias may be refractory to conventional pharmacologic management. Symptoms associated with conduction system abnormalities are treated with permanent pacing. The use of steroids is controversial. While there may be improvement in conduction abnormalities, arrhythmias, and ventricular function by steroid-induced reduction in the inflammatory granulomatous burden,[116] some evidence exists that this approach may facilitate ventricular aneurysm formation.[113]

Within the spectrum of hypereosinophilic syndromes, there exist several types that involve the heart. Loffler's original description of endomyocardial fibrosis involved two patients who, at autopsy, were found to have extensive fibrous thickening of the mural endocardium of both the RV and LV.[117] Loffler referred to this as "endocarditis parietalis fibroplastica." Among patients with the variant known as endomyocardial fibrosis, the mural endocardial fibrosis and overlying thrombosis usually is limited to the inflow tracts of both ventricles with frequent involvement of the ventricular aspect of the posterior mitral and tricuspid leaflets. Among patients described as having cardiac involvement with the hypereosinophilic syndrome at the National Institutes of Health, RV mural endocardial thickening was noted in 13 of 16 autopsied patients.[117] Most schemes now classify the spectrum of endomyocardial disease and eosinophilia into two varieties.[118] The "temperate region" syndrome is characterized by endomyocardial disease, which is also accompanied by a systemic illness and eosinophilia. In this type, almost 100% of the patients have biventricular endomyocardial involvement. Cardiomegaly and mitral regurgitation often are present, although heart failure may or may not be manifest. A beneficial effect on clinical symptoms and survival has been seen with medical therapy consisting of steroids and cytotoxic drugs (particularly hydroxyurea) early in the course of the disease, as well as surgical therapy for the fibrotic endomyocardial disease with restrictive physiology.[117,118]

The second type of endomyocardial disease with eosinophilia, referred to as the "tropical" variety, may be a late manifestation of what was initially a temperate region variant. The tropical syndrome tends to have no systemic illness, may or may not have eosinophilia, and demonstrates biventricular endomyocardial involvement in approximately 75% of patients. Isolated involvement of the RV is found in this syndrome in 20% of cases.[118] Generally, patients with this type of endomyocardial disease demonstrate a progressive downhill course, although prolonged survival has been reported.[119] Predominant right heart involvement seems to be associated with more prolonged survival. Surgical endocardiectomy with associated valve replacement or repair offers symptomatic relief, although operative mortality is high with this complex operation.[120,121]

Carcinoid syndrome is an endocrinopathy that in its more severe forms often will have important right heart involvement. Among 21 patients with clinically important carcinoid heart disease studied at necropsy, 12 had gross RV mural endocardial involvement with carcinoid plaques.[122] In all 21 patients, both the tricuspid and the pulmonic valve were involved. In more than 70% of patients, all of the involvement with carcinoid plaques was limited to the right side of the heart. Such carcinoid plaques are composed of an unusual type of fibrous tissue devoid of elastic fibrils within which are contained smooth muscle cells and mucopolysaccharide. Most often, these plaques are located on the downstream aspect of the valve, which results in a distinct physiologic abnormality for each valve involved.[122] TR is far more common than tricuspid stenosis. In contrast, pulmonic stenosis is the predominant lesion resulting from involvement of the pulmonic valve. In selected cases, percutaneous tricuspid and/or pulmonic balloon valvuloplasty may be a useful palliative treatment. The prognosis in patients with carcinoid heart disease is generally related to the extent of the primary carcinoid tumor rather than the extent of cardiac involvement.

Signs and symptoms of RV failure may be noted in patients with massive obesity. Although abnormal RV performance may be due to pulmonary hypertension, resulting from hypoventilation or chronic pulmonary emboli, gross and histologic myocardial abnormalities have been described.[123] All 12 patients in one autopsy study of patients with massive obesity had dilated RVs, many of which demonstrated evidence of cellular hypertrophy. Three of the 12 patients demonstrated clear-cut fatty infiltration within the RV myocardium by both gross observation and by microscopy.

Right Ventricular Dysplasia

RV dysplasia comprises a spectrum of RV morphologic abnormalities, with clinical manifestations ranging from little or no derangement of RV performance to severe right heart failure.[124] The functional abnormalities range from subtle areas of hypokinesis[125] to severe generalized hypokinesis of a parchment-thin RV, referred to as Uhl's anomaly.[126] RV dysplasia may be associated with ventricular or supraventricular arrhythmias. Characteristically, ventricular tachycardia in arrhythmogenic RV dysplasia has a left bundle branch morphology with right axis deviation, indicating its origin from the RV. In patients with RV dysplasia, symptoms depend on the extent and functional importance of RV myocardial involvement, as well as on the presence and rate of the tachyarrhythmia. The natural history of this condition is not known. RV dysplasia must be distinguished from Ebstein's anomaly, atrial septal defect (ASD), partial anomalous pulmonary venous return, congenital absence of the left pericardium, RV infarction, or primary or secondary TR. In patients with ventricular arrhythmias, antiarrhythmic therapy has met with varying success, although fatal dysrhythmias are relatively uncommon. When antiarrhythmic therapy is not efficacious, surgical therapy has been advocated. The RV is dissected from its LV attachments and reattached such that a scar forms around the suture line and does not allow the arrhythmic focus to spread to the LV.[127]

Right Ventricular Pressure Overload States

Cor Pulmonale

Cor pulmonale refers to the combination of pressure overload, hypertrophy, and dilatation of the RV in the face of pulmonary hypertension. The latter may result from lung disease, such as chronic obstructive pulmonary disease, or from a primary abnormality in the pulmonary vasculature (i.e., primary pulmonary hypertension).

In contrast to conventional thought, normal pulmonary vessels have been found experimentally to be intrinsically stiffer than systemic vessels. The ability of the

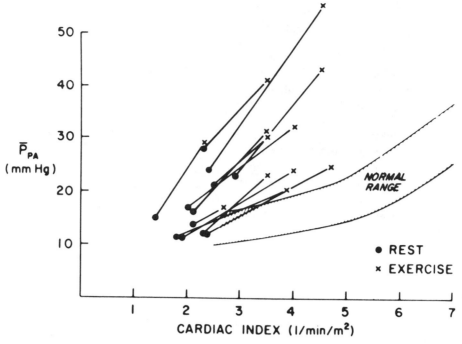

FIGURE 17.5. Relationship of resting and exercise cardiac index vs. mean pulmonary artery pressure (P$_{PA}$) in 12 patients with chronic obstructive pulmonary disease. Normal range represents values taken from 75 normal subjects. Reprinted, with permission, from Mahler et al. *Am Rev Respir Dis.* 1984;130:722–729.

pulmonary vascular bed to accept increases in cardiac output (and thus flow), without important increments in pressure and RV afterload, predominantly relates to the ability of the pulmonary vasculature to recruit portions of the vasculature that are underperfused at rest. This large amount of vascular reserve explains why substantial reductions in the size of the pulmonary vascular bed must occur before clinically relevant pulmonary hypertension develops. Even so, other factors must be involved in the pathophysiolgy of pulmonary hypertension due to chronic lung disease, beyond reduction in the size of the vascular bed. For example, in emphysema, despite reduction in the number of alveolar vessels due to pulmonary parenchymal destruction, it is unusual for cor pulmonale to be present until late in the course of the disease. Additional factors contributing to pulmonary hypertension in patients with obstructive lung disease include hypoxia, hypoxemia, and acidosis, resulting in pulmonary vasoconstriction, and polycythemia, resulting in hyperviscosity.

In the presence of these abnormalities of the pulmonary vascular bed, the pulmonary vasculature cannot accept increases in cardiac output during stress without substantial increases in PA pressure[128] (Fig. 17.5). The resulting reduction in RV systolic function is associated with limitation in cardiac output response to exercise.

Cor pulmonale is relatively common in patients with chronic bronchitis, in whom the disease is characterized by chronic productive cough, frequent respiratory infections, hypoxemia and hypercapnea at rest, and elevated hematocrit. Diffusion capacity is relatively maintained, since anatomic destruction of alveolae is not a prominent feature. Hypoxic vasoconstriction results from extensive ventilation-perfusion mismatching. Pulmonary hypertension at rest may be marked, and worsened further with modest degrees of exertion, resulting in overt right heart failure. The degree of reduction in RV EF correlates with the magnitude of pulmonary hypertension, which is, in turn, related to the degree of hypoxemia and hypercapnea.

In contrast, in patients with emphysema, cough and sputum production are not prominent, and hyperventilation generally can maintain arterial oxygen tension in a relatively normal range, despite a widened alveolar-arterial oxygen gradient. Thus, pulmonary hypertension in general is less prominent despite variable degrees of pulmonary vascular destruction. Signs and symptoms of right heart failure and noninvasive evidence of abnormalities in RV ejection performance are relatively late events.

Mitral Stenosis

Pulmonary hypertension in patients with mitral stenosis (MS) is multifactorial, resulting from a combination of elevated left atrial pressure, reactive pulmonary vasoconstriction, potentially reversible pulmonary arteriolar medial hypertrophy, and fixed obliterative pulmonary vascular changes.

In patients with mild mitral stenosis, PA pressure usually is normal or only slightly elevated at rest, resting RV systolic performance is normal, and symptoms of right heart failure are absent. However, PA pressure may rise markedly during exercise, causing excessive RV afterload and reduced RV systolic function.[11,12,129,130] As the severity of the valvular abnormality worsens, PA pressure may become elevated at rest and occasionally may exceed systemic pressure. Under such conditions, signs and symptoms of right heart failure frequently accompany reduction in resting RV EF. The magnitude of the change in EF with exercise is related to the degree of elevation in PA pressure.[131]

In patients with MS, once a substantial degree of precapillary obstructive change occurs within the pulmonary circulation, clinical findings of reduced cardiac output and right heart failure predominate. On the one hand, these vascular changes tend to mitigate against transudation of fluid into the pulmonary extravascular space. On the other hand, RV afterload becomes excessive, resulting in RV systolic failure, RV dilatation, TR, and manifestations of systemic venous hypertension.

Improvement in RV function after correction of MS results directly from alleviation of mitral valve obstruction and from regression of pulmonary vascular medial hypertrophy. Remodeling of RV architecture with diminished RV dilatation, in combination with diminished PA pressure, results in improvement in forward cardiac output due to both augmented RV ejection performance with the relief of afterload, as well as reduction in TR.

Pulmonic Stenosis

Most cases of pulmonic stenosis are due to congenital abnormalities of the pulmonic valve, either with fusion and variable thickening of the normal tricuspid leaflet or, much less commonly, a bicuspid valve. In addition, patients with Noonan's syndrome may demonstrate dysplastic changes of the pulmonic valve. Secondary hypertrophy of the RV infundibulum may occur with advancing age in adults with valvular pulmonic stenosis and contribute to RV systolic pressure overload.

Mild to moderate pulmonic stenosis may remain asymptomatic throughout life. However, in patients with more severe stenosis, symptoms such as dyspnea and fatigue, particularly with exercise, may occur and are due to the inability of the RV to augment cardiac output with increased demand.[132] With severe outflow obstruction, RV hypertrophy may not suffice to maintain normal wall stress. Reduction in forward output

will be exacerbated by TR, and signs and symptoms of right heart failure will appear. Exertional syncope or lightheadedness may occur, although sudden death is rare.[133] Angina pectoris may occur due to the increased demand on the RV in concert with an inability of RV vasodilator reserve to increase coronary perfusion maximally.

Noninvasive studies are able to document the severity of the valvular obstruction and consequent preservation or impairment of RV function. When a QR complex is present in lead V1 of the electrocardiogram, the pressure gradient across the pulmonic valve generally exceeds 80 mm Hg. Doppler interrogation of the RV outflow tract and proximal PA can quantify the gradient based on the flow velocity across the valve.[134] This technique is useful for serial assessment of asymptomatic patients, as well as determining the degree of postoperative improvement and potential onset of pulmonic regurgitation.

Pulmonic valvuloplasty now appears to be the initial treatment of choice for patients with right heart failure due to valvular pulmonic stenosis.[135] The degree to which RV hemodynamics and function return to normal is related to the relative contribution of afterload mismatch and of intrinsic myocardial dysfunction to the original hemodynamic syndrome. In some patients, RV end-diastolic pressure may remain elevated after relief of outflow tract obstruction, presumably due to a degree of interstitial fibrosis that had occurred on the basis of the long-standing pressure overload. In patients with a significant contribution of subvalvular stenosis, relief of the valvular obstruction may not improve symptoms and, in fact, may worsen obstruction at the infundibular level. The treatment of choice for such patients is surgical relief of both the valvular abnormality and the infundibular obstruction.

Right Ventricular Volume Overload States

Tricuspid Regurgitation

By far the most common etiology of TR is derangement of valve function due to (a) excessive RV systolic pressure and/or (b) dilatation of the RV with secondary enlargement of the tricuspid annulus. Rheumatic heart disease may directly affect the tricuspid valve, almost always in combination with anatomic or clinical involvement of at least two other valves. Other nonrheumatic etiologies that may be associated with TR include infective endocarditis, particularly in intravenous drug abusers, Ebstein's anomaly, Marfan's syndrome, and carcinoid syndrome. Cardiac tumors, in particular right atrial myxoma, may be associated with functional TR.

TR is common in patients with major RV infarction,[136] and may substantially exacerbate the clinical syndrome, contributing to reduction in forward flow and to RV dilatation with severe elevation in central venous pressure. In RV infarction, valve dysfunction may be due to RV distension alone. Alternatively, the papillary apparatus may be dysfunctional due to ischemic injury.

In the absence of pulmonary hypertension, TR usually causes no clinical symptoms. In the setting of pulmonary hypertension, TR exacerbates the clinical expression of right heart failure. In patients with heart failure of any etiology, functional TR may result in an effective descending limb of the Starling curve. As the RV distends, TR worsens and forward output decreases. In severe TR, the physical exam reflects "ventricularization" of the RA pressure wave form, with a prominent V wave in the jugular venous profile. The murmur of TR usually increases during inspiration, a finding known as Rivero-Carvello's sign. Echocardiography can aid in the grading of TR, and Doppler interrogation of the TR jet allows estimation of the PA peak systolic pressure.[137]

Specific surgical correction of a regurgitant tricuspid valve usually is not needed; rather, both medical and surgical therapy is directed at the underlying cause of RV pressure overload. However, when significant primary abnormality of the tricuspid valve exists and/or when pulmonary hypertension cannot be fully reversed, surgical palliation of TR may be performed by insertion of a Carpentier ring,[138] which diminishes annular dilatation and improves valvular coaptation.

Atrial Septal Defect

An atrial level left to right shunt is characterized by chronic RV volume overload. The magnitude of shunt flow is related primarily to the relative compliance of the RV and LV. The RV chamber, already capable of accommodating volume flow due to its chamber compliance characteristics, can increase its capacity further through dilatation as well as some degree of hypertrophy to maintain normal levels of wall stress, despite higher chamber radius. In the absence of pulmonary vascular obstructive changes, most patients with atrial septal defects (ASDs) remain asymptomatic throughout life. Symptoms may intervene in later life due to gradual elevation in PA pressure, in association with increasing left to right shunting, as LV compliance diminishes. Pulmonary hypertension transforms an ASD from a condition of pure RV volume overload to one of combined pressure and volume overload.

In patients with ASDs, signs and symptoms of right heart failure may result directly from left-sided abnormalities, in the absence of RV failure, since left atrial pressure is transmitted directly into the systemic venous circulation via the interatrial shunt. In this setting mitral regurgitation may manifest elevated jugular venous pressure, with a prominent regurgitant pressure wave, in the absence of TR.

A minority of patients develop pulmonary vascular obstructive disease, resulting in pulmonary hypertension, reduced RV compliance, reversal of shunt flow, reduction in pulmonary flow, and cyanosis (Eisenmenger's syndrome). The right to left flow reduces the degree of right heart failure by reducing the degree of RV volume load that would otherwise coincide with the worsening pressure load. In this circumstance, surgical closure is no longer feasible, since it would result in abrupt worsening of right heart failure. In contrast, there have been several reports regarding patients with pulmonary hypertension who have had modest clinical improvement after the induction of right to left shunting by balloon septostomy. Although this procedure produces or worsens cyanosis, it relieves RV volume overload and augments forward flow.

In one study, RV systolic function was found to be reduced in a group of patients with ASDs and normalized after surgical repair.[139] However, in another study,[140] RV EF was found to be higher in patients with ASDs than in patients with comparable elevations in PA pressure but without left to right shunt. In the latter study, after surgical repair, RV volume normalized, but EF decreased. Thus, RV volume overload tends to increase EF, although under these circumstances, EF overestimates the intrinsic level of RV contractility and may mask myocardial dysfunction.

Ventricular Interdependence: Effect of Right Heart Failure on the Left Heart

The potential exists for direct interaction between the two ventricles through direct transseptal pressure transmission and/or alteration in intrapericardial pressure.[94,141–147] A distended right heart may aggravate or possibly induce left heart failure via direct ventricular interaction. Abnormally elevated RV systolic or diastolic load has been shown to induce perturbations in septal geometry and in the mechanics of septal contribution to LV filling and ejection.[85–93] Under most circumstances changes in intrapericardial pressure match changes in RA pressure.[148] Elevations in RA pressure therefore reduce LV transmural (or distending) pressure at any given level of LV intracavitary pressure. Alternatively, for transmural pressure to be maintained, intracavitary pressure must rise. During diastole, transmural pressure determines the degree of LV filling, whereas an increase in intracavitary pressure is the stimulus for pulmonary venous hypertension and transudation of fluid into the pulmonary interstitium. Thus, RV and right atrial (RA) distension may adversely alter observed LV compliance characteristics; that is, the relation between intracavitary pressure and volume.

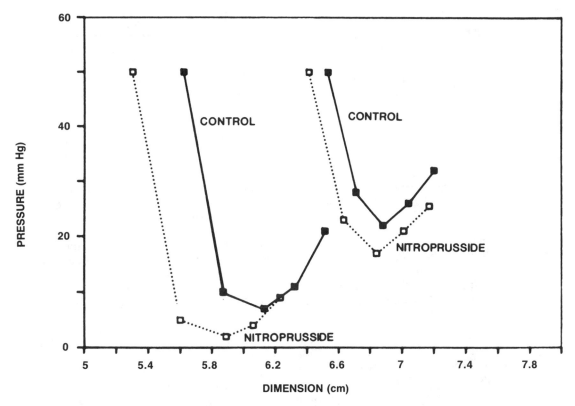

FIGURE 17.6. The average LV diastolic pressure/dimension relations before and after nitroprusside. Panel on left represents data from patients with normal right atrial pressure (n=5), in whom nitroprusside caused LV dimension and pressure to decrease along a constant pressure/volume relation. Panel on right represents data from patients with elevated right atrial pressure (n=5), in whom nitroprusside caused a reduction in intracavitary pressure out of proportion to the change in chamber size (i.e., a downward shift in the diastolic pressure/volume relation), suggesting an effect related to pericardial constraint and/or ventricular interaction. Reprinted, with permission, from Carroll JD et al. *Circulation*. 1986;74:815–825. Copyright by the American Heart Association.

In contrast to changes in intrinsic distensibility of LV myocardium, which are associated with changes in the slope of the LV diastolic pressure/volume relation, increased LV chamber stiffness due to ventricular interaction is characterized by a parallel shift in the LV compliance curve.[141–143,147] In addition, increased RA pressure may reduce LV compliance due to myocardial vascular engorgement ("erectile effect"), resulting from an increase in coronary venous pressure.[149] These effects may cause reduction in LV filling, with attendant decrease in stroke volume via the Starling mechanism, and/or an increase in the stimulus to develop pulmonary edema.

Acute severe right heart dilatation, such as occurs with RV myocardial infarction, may present a hemodynamic picture that is similar to pericardial constriction with near-equalization of RA and PA wedge pressures, prominent atrial Y descent, and "dip and plateau" of ventricular pressure contours during diastole.[25] These findings suggest intrapericardial constraint on left heart filling, imposed by the distended right heart. If these direct interventricular forces were not in effect, cardiac output would be sustained as long as LV intracavitary pressure were maintained in a physiologic range. However, since increased intrapericardial pressure renders LV intracavitary pressure an underestimate of transmural distending pressure, there is an apparent downward displacement of the LV Starling curve, and supranormal PA wedge pressure is needed to sustain a normal LV stroke volume.

In patients with right heart failure, withdrawal of RV constraint on LV filling appears to contribute to vasodilator-induced augmentation of stroke volume and reduction in pulmonary venous pressure.[146,147] In the presence of right heart failure, nitroprusside induces a parallel downward shift in the LV pressure-volume or pressure-dimension curve[147] (Fig. 17.6). Presumably, this shift results from a change in the relation between LV intracavitary pressure and transmural distending pressure, as nitroprusside reduces RA, and therefore intrapericardial pressure, through venodilatation. Similarly, the effect of acute angiotensin-converting enzyme (ACE) inhibition on the rate of LV diastolic filling is related to the state of the RV. We observed that enalaprilat has no effect on LV peak filling rate in patients with isolated LV failure. However, enalaprilat augments LV

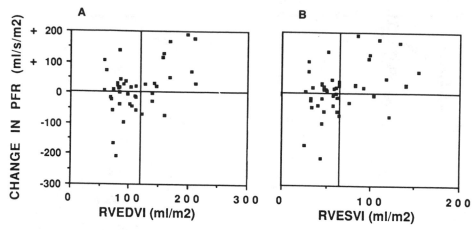

FIGURE 17.7. Relationship of enalaprilat-induced change in LV peak filling rate (*PFR*) vs. baseline RV end-diastolic volume index (*RVEDVI*) (**A**) and vs. baseline RV end-systolic volume index (*RVESVI*) (**B**). Vertical lines mark the upper limits of normal for RV volumes. Enalaprilat had no consis- tent effect on peak filling rate in patients with normal RV volumes, but increased peak filling rate in most patients with enlarged RV volumes. Reprinted, with permission, from Konstam et al. *Circulation*. 1990;81(suppl III):III-115–III-122. Copyright by the American Heart Association.

peak filling rate in patients with LV systolic dysfunction and RV dilation, presumably reflecting withdrawal of RV constraint to LV filling[94] (Fig. 17.7).

Thus, it appears reasonable to presume that right heart failure may induce or exacerbate left heart failure through direct ventricular interaction and that the manner and magnitude of response to therapeutic intervention may be influenced by this interaction.

Role of the Right Heart in Left Heart Failure

The maintenance or loss of normal right heart performance has been linked to the clinical expression of left heart failure in a number of respects. In a population of patients with depressed LV systolic performance, RV EF has been observed to be correlated positively with functional capacity[150] (Fig. 17.8) and with survival.[151,152] In addition, the state of RV systolic function is linked to the nature of symptomatology in patients with left heart failure. The relationship of RV performance to clinical manifestations and outcomes in the setting of left heart failure is multifactorial.

As discussed above, RV systolic performance is strongly influenced by systolic load. During vasodilator administration in patients with left heart failure, a linear relation exists between the fractional or absolute reductions in PA dicrotic notch pressure and RV end-systolic volume.[6,7,10] This close association between RV systolic performance and afterload is likely to be a major mediator of the relation between RV EF and functional capacity. As left heart failure progresses, RV afterload is augmented and RV stroke volume and EF decrease. As RV systolic failure ensues, RV dilatation

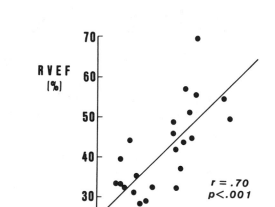

FIGURE 17.8. The correlation between resting right ventricular ejection fraction (*RVEF*) and maximum oxygen consumption (MVO$_2$) in 25 patients with congestive heart failure due to LV systolic dysfunction. Reprinted, with permission, from Baker BJ et al. *Am J Cardiol*. 1984;54:596–599.

must occur in order to maintain forward stroke volume. This defense mechanism is thwarted by the development of TR, which may establish a vicious cycle of progressive right heart failure, cardiac output reduction, salt and water retention, left heart failure, and further increments in RV afterload.

We have compared the ventricular mechanisms for augmentation of cardiac output during cycle exercise in patients with symptomatic versus asymptomatic LV systolic dysfunction.[153] In asymptomatic patients, despite exhaustion of contractile reserve, stroke volume increases during exercise through augmentation of LV end-diastolic volume (i.e., recruitment of preload reserve). In contrast, in patients with symptomatic heart failure, preload reserve appears to be exhausted, with no detectable change in LV end-diastolic volume during exercise, and increases in cardiac output being totally dependent on tachycardia. Right heart failure may relate to these phenomena in at least two ways. First, the failing RV may not be capable of augmenting PA perfusion pressure during exercise sufficiently to increase LV preload. Second, as discussed above, the failed RV may directly impede left heart filling through ventricular interdependence. Thus, in a number of respects, RV performance is likely to impact directly on functional capacity.

In a large cohort of patients with LV systolic dysfunction and heart failure, a multivariate analysis indicated that the strongest identifiable correlate of rapid onset pulmonary edema without associated overt myocardial ischemia was RV EF.[154] Compared to the remainder of the population, patients with rapid onset pulmonary edema manifested substantially higher RV EFs, with many patients having hypercontractile RVs. These observations may be explained on the basis of variation in the manner in which the RV responds to left heart failure. As discussed above, in most patients with left heart failure, the thin-walled, compliant RV succumbs to increased afterload, fails to maintain normal pump function, and dilates during diastole. It is limited in the degree to which it may augment PA pressure, and therefore sustain an increase in pulmonary capillary pressure, in the face of an expanded intravascular volume. Instead, under such conditions, the failed RV distends further during systole and diastole and may fail to maintain its forward stroke volume. However, it contributes to a buffering of intravascular volume, thus mitigating against abrupt changes in pulmonary capillary pressure. It appears likely that in some patients with left heart failure, the RV hypertrophies before dilating, and is capable of maintaining systolic performance in the face of augmented afterload. In response to increased intravascular volume the RV might move up a relatively steep Starling curve and augment PA pressure sufficiently to sustain a substantial augmentation of pulmonary capillary pressure. A hypertrophied, hypercontractile RV tends to maintain forward output but is associated with a reduced capacity to buffer acute changes in intravascular volume and may predispose the patient to rapid-onset pulmonary edema. The precise determinants of RV hypertrophy remain to be elucidated.

Thus, in a variety of ways, the maintenance or failure of RV performance is closely linked to various aspects of the clinical expression of left heart failure, beyond manifestations of right heart failure, per se. It is likely that in some respects, RV performance and clinical symptomatology are coincident by-products of altered RV load produced by left heart failure. In other respects, primary variability in RV performance may directly influence the clinical presentation.

Therapy

In this section, we review physiologic and practical aspects of the treatment of right heart failure. Treatment for right heart failure is directed largely at (a) optimizing RV loading conditions and (b) minimizing the peripheral effects of right heart failure. Most therapeutic modalities strive toward both of these goals in concert. Efforts to optimize load differ somewhat, depending on the primary pathologic stimulus to abnormal load. Additionally, we discuss the role of inotropic agents.

Optimizing Right Ventricular Preload

Optimization of RV preload generally represents the most appropriate primary intervention in patients with right heart failure. The direction of change to be instituted depends on the clinical circumstance and the predominant clinical manifestation of right heart failure, namely low output or systemic venous hypertension. In patients with severe acute right heart failure, as due to acute RV infarction, or postoperative RV dysfunction, volume loading should be instituted to increase RV filling pressure,[25,155] thus forcing the RV to ascend its relatively shallow Starling curve. However, two cautions to this approach should be stated. First, excessive RV dilation may worsen functional TR, thus establishing an effective descending Starling curve limb and reducing forward output. Second, in the setting of acute RV dilation, PA wedge pressure may not adequately reflect true LV filling pressure. This caveat is a result of ventricular interdependence and pericardial restraint on left heart filling. Otherwise stated, as the right heart distends and RA pressure increases, intrapericardial pressure increases as well, and LV transmural, or distending, pressure diverges from intracavitary pressure.[148] Thus, even in the absence of primary LV systolic dysfunction, forward output will be less than anticipated for a given level of PA wedge pressure. For these reasons, as volume loading is instituted, its effect on forward output must be tracked. Since in the setting of right heart distension with TR thermodilution cardiac output measurements may be spurious, it may be helpful to monitor an alternative indicator of forward output, such as mixed venous oxygen saturation.

Maintenance of atrial contribution to RV filling represents an important means for optimizing RV preload in the setting of acute right heart failure. Significant clinical deterioration may occur with the onset of atrial fibrillation or initiation of ventricular pacing for bradyarrhythmias. Thus, in these circumstances, consideration should be given to emergent cardioversion or institution of dual chamber pacing.[156]

In patients with chronic right heart failure, diuretics act to reverse sodium and water retention, reduce central venous pressure, and relieve edema.[157,158] Diuretics also may improve forward output by relieving RV distension, thus reducing the degree of functional TR. In addition to loop diuretics, spironolactone often is effective in reducing the edema associated with right heart failure since a hyper-renin hyper-aldosterone state is almost universal in patients with right heart failure, and contributes substantially to sodium retention.

Nitrates have been found to exert salutary hemodynamic effects and to improve exercise performance in patients with various forms of heart failure, including patients with cor pulmonale and primary right heart failure.[159-165] Nitrates exert venodilator effect, acting to recruit venous capacitance, thus reducing systemic venous hypertension. In addition, nitrates have been found to augment exercise capacity in patients with heart failure, an effect that may be mediated via arterial dilation with reduction in LV afterload.[160] Alternatively, to the extent that RV distension impedes left heart filling through ventricular interdependence, a reduction in RV diastolic pressure may contribute to the effect of nitrates on functional capacity.[147]

Reduction of Right Ventricular Systolic Load

As discussed above, the most effective way to augment RV systolic performance is reduction of afterload.[7,164,166,167] Thus, any intervention that reduces RV systolic load will tend to augment forward output and presumably improve functional capacity. In patients with left heart failure, this effect is best achieved by reducing left heart filling pressure and pulmonary venous pressure. Thus, systemic arteriolar dilators, which augment LV stroke volume and reduce the stimulus for augmenting LV preload, serve secondarily to reduce RV afterload and augment RV systolic performance. In addition, most systemic arteriolar dilators also act as pulmonary vasodilators, thus reducing the additional afterload imposed on the RV by pulmonary vasoconstriction. This group of agents includes α-adrenergic antagonists, calcium channel antagonists, ACE inhibitors, and direct-acting vasodilators, including nitrates. Thus, in addition to impacting directly on RV diastolic failure, through venodilation, nitrates influence RV systolic failure through reduction in pulmonary venous pressure and in pulmonary vascular resistance.

Despite the fact that angiotensin II has little, if any, direct effect on systemic venous tone, ACE inhibitors may benefit patients with systolic and/or diastolic right heart failure via a variety of mechanisms.[167] For reasons cited above, RV afterload may be reduced. In addition,

reduction in plasma aldosterone reduces the stimulus to renal sodium retention.

Reduction of Right Ventricular Afterload in Cor Pulmonale

Efforts to minimize RV afterload require special additional considerations in the setting of right heart failure due to pulmonary vascular pathology. These considerations differ depending on whether obstruction to pulmonary blood flow results from hypoxic vasoconstriction, thromboembolism, or primary vascular pathology, as in the case of primary pulmonary hypertension.

In most cases of cor pulmonale related to chronic obstructive pulmonary disease (COPD), reversible vasoconstriction due to hypoxia plays a role. Under such circumstances efforts should be directed primarily toward maximizing oxygenation. In patients with COPD, use of supplemental oxygen has been found to improve hemodynamics, functional status, and survival.[163,168-171] The latter effect appears to be related to reversibility of pulmonary hypertension.[170]

In patients with COPD, bronchodilators may improve RV function and reduce signs and symptoms of right heart failure through a number of mechanisms. Both β-adrenergic agonists and phosphodiesterase inhibitors potentially exert their clinical effects through a combination of bronchodilation, direct pulmonary vasodilation, and inotropic action. In patients with COPD, terbutaline has been found to reduce pulmonary vascular resistance, increase cardiac output, and improve RV EF, without significant change in arterial oxygen tension.[172,173] PA pressure tends to remain unchanged. Theophylline has been found to reduce PA pressure and vascular resistance and to increase RV EF.[173-177]

Several classes of direct and indirect vasodilators have been employed, with variable success in patients with COPD and pulmonary vascular disease. The likelihood of clinical efficacy probably is related to the degree to which active vasoconstriction contributes to pulmonary hypertension. In patients with COPD, several studies have documented augmentation of cardiac output by hydralazine.[178-181] However, benefit in terms of other hemodynamic functional parameters has been variable, with some investigators finding an increase in pulmonary arterial pressure and worsening of hypoxia and dyspnea,[179] possibly related to an adverse change in ventilation/perfusion relationships. Calcium channel antagonists have been found to blunt hypoxic pulmonary vasoconstriction,[182] increase cardiac output, and reduce pulmonary vascular resistance and PA pressure.[183] However, some investigators have identified a worsening of hypoxemia with administration of calcium channel blockers, which has been attributed to augmented blood flow to poorly ventilated areas of lung.[184] In a rat model, the ACE inhibitor, captopril, has been found to reduce the degree to which hypoxia induces pulmonary vascular pathology and RV hypertrophy.[185] In patients with COPD, the hemodynamic benefits of ACE inhibitors have been found to be minor,[186,187] although long-term clinical data are lacking.

In the setting of right heart failure due to fixed pulmonary vascular disease, as due to primary pulmonary hypertension, Eisenmenger's syndrome, or long-standing mitral valve disease, a variety of vasodilators have been advocated. Although individual patients have been reported to manifest hemodynamic efficacy, in general, vasodilator therapy is considerably less rewarding than in the setting of left heart failure and must be undertaken with caution.[188,189] In such patients, the reflex systemic vasoconstriction associated with reduced cardiac output is more responsive to vasodilators than is the morphologically altered pulmonary circulation. Therefore, all available vasodilators have the potential for inducing abrupt severe hypotension in patients with fixed pulmonary vascular disease. Systemic vasodilation may initiate a vicious cycle, with reduced coronary perfusion pressure, diminished RV contractile function, and further hypotension. If vasodilator therapy is to be attempted, it should be initiated under careful hemodynamic monitoring to confirm hemodynamic benefit and facilitate rapid drug withdrawal with necessary countermeasures, including volume expansion and/or administration of α-adrenergic agonists, in the event of hypotension.

Inotropic Agents

The role of inotropic agents in right heart failure has received considerable debate and has not been definitively clarified. In patients with left heart failure, the effect of amrinone on RV systolic performance has been found to be entirely explainable on the basis of reduced RV afterload due to a combination of improved LV performance and pulmonary vasodilation[190] (Fig. 17.9). In contrast, dobutamine has been found to augment RV contractility significantly in patients with COPD, as shown by end-systolic pressure-volume analysis.[10] In patients with LV failure, the effect of dobutamine on RV systolic performance has been found to be greater than that of milrinone, for a given reduction in RV afterload, suggesting that some of dobutamine's hemodynamic effects may be due to augmented RV contractility.[191]

In the clinical setting, it is difficult to sort out the degree to which improvement in RV systolic performance results from augmentation of RV contractility, as opposed to direct and/or indirect effects on RV load. For example, both β-adrenergic agents and amrinone have a vasodilator effect on the pulmonary circulation.[192] Digoxin and the selective β-1 agonist dobutamine have little or no direct pulmonary vasodilator

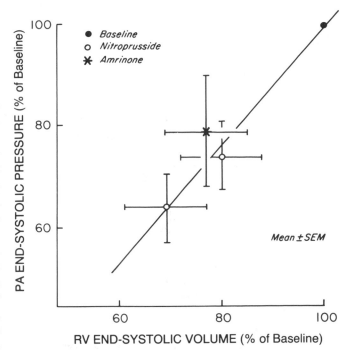

END-SYSTOLIC PRESSURE-VOLUME RELATION:
AMRINONE vs NITROPRUSSIDE

FIGURE 17.9. Relations between pulmonary artery (*PA*) end-systolic pressure vs. radionuclide-derived right ventricular (*RV*) end-systolic volume (group means) in nine patients with LV systolic dysfunction related to healed myocardial infarction or DCM. The effect of amrinone on RV systolic performance is explainable predominantly on the basis of reduced RV afterload. There is a lack of demonstrable shift of the amrinone pressure-volume point from the regression line formed by data derived at baseline and during nitroprusside infusion. Reprinted, with permission, from Konstam et al. *Circulation.* 1986;74:359–366. Copyright by the American Heart Association.

effect. However, in patients with left heart failure, LV inotropic effect results in reflex withdrawal of vasoconstrictor stimuli, resulting in reduction of pulmonary, as well as systemic, vascular resistance. Therefore, even in the absence of direct pulmonary vasodilator effect, inotropic agents may reduce RV systolic load. When these effects are present, it is likely that they predominate in determining the RV systolic functional response.

The clinical role of digitalis glycosides in patients with cor pulmonale has received considerable debate.[193–198] Several studies have documented some hemodynamic improvement in such patients, consisting of augmented cardiac output, stroke volume, and stroke work, with reduction in RV filling pressure.[194,195] However, digitalis glycosides may increase pulmonary vascular resistance by direct vasoconstrictor effects.[196,197] The net hemodynamic benefit of these agents appears to be less than that of other classes of agents. For example, the benefit of digitalis has been found to be less than that of oxygen.[198] For this reason and because of the relatively high incidence of adverse effects, digitalis generally is not recommended for the management of cor pulmonale in the absence of concomitant supraventricular arrhythmia or LV failure.

Treatment of Postoperative Right Ventricular Failure

After cardiopulmonary bypass, right heart failure is common and results from ischemic injury to the RV and/or pulmonary vascular injury. RV dysfunction may result from antecedent RV infarction or from acute RV ischemic insult due to inadequate RV myocardial protection, particularly in the setting of right coronary arterial occlusive disease. RV failure may be provoked or exacerbated by preexisting pulmonary vascular disease, as induced by chronic valvular or congenital heart disease. In addition, acute RV failure may complicate cardiac transplantation,[199] particularly in the setting of pulmonary vascular obstructive disease combined with an inadequately sized donor heart.

In patients with postoperative RV failure, attention should be directed first toward optimizing oxygenation and acid-base status to minimize pulmonary vasoconstriction, maintaining adequate volume status to optimize RV preload, and maintaining atrial contribution to RV filling (see above).[200,201] The potent pulmonary vasodilators prostacyclin and prostaglandin E_1 may be valuable,[202-204] although their effects may be limited by concomitant systemic vasodilation. Both β-adrenergic agents and amrinone may exert substantial clinical benefit through combined inotropic and pulmonary vasodilator effects.[192,205,206] If these various measures prove inadequate to sustain forward output, urgent consideration should be given to mechanical support of the RV. Such support may take the form of PA balloon counterpulsation[207-209] or, preferably, a mechanical assist pump.[199,210,211] Such devices may be life-sustaining until RV mechanical function recovers.

References

1. Suzuki J, Sakamoto T, Takenaka K, et al. Assessment of the thickness of the right ventricular free wall by magnetic resonance imaging in patients with hypertrophic cardiomyopathy. *Br Heart J*. 1988;60:440–445.
2. Laks MM, Garner D, Swan HJC. Volumes and compliances measured simultaneously in the right and left ventricles of the dog. *Circ Res*. 1967;20:565.
3. Abel FL, Waldhausen JA. Effects of alterations in pulmonary vascular resistance on right ventricular function. *J Thorac Cardiovasc Surg*. 1967;54:886.
4. Sarnoff SJ, Berglund D. Ventricular function. I. Starling's law of the heart studied by means of simultaneous right and left ventricular function curves in the dog. *Circulation*. 1954;9:706.
5. Maughan WL, Shoukas AA, Sagawa K, Weisfeldt ML. Instantaneous pressure-volume relationship of the canine right ventricle. *Circ Res*. 1979;44:309–315.
6. Konstam MA, Cohen SR, Salem DN, et al. Comparison of left and right ventricular end-systolic pressure-volume relations in congestive heart failure. *J Am Coll Cardiol*. 1985;5:1326–1334.
7. Konstam MA, Salem DN, Isner JM, et al. Vasodilator effect on right ventricular function in congestive heart failure and pulmonary hypertension: end-systolic pressure-volume relationship. *Am J Cardiol*. 1984; 54:132–6.
8. Friedman BJ, Lozner EC, Curfman GD, Herzberg D, Rolett EL. Characterization of the human right ventricular pressure-volume relation: effect of dobutamine and right coronary artery stenosis. *J Am Coll Cardiol*. 1984,4:999–1005.
9. Iskandrian AS, Hakki AH, Ren BF, et al. Correlation among right ventricular preload, afterload and ejection fraction in mitral valve disease: radionuclide, echocardiographic and hemodynamic evaluation. *J Am Coll Cardiol*. 1984,6:1403–1411.
10. Brent BN, Berger HJ, Matthay RA, Mahler D, Pytlik L, Zaret BL. Physiologic correlates of right ventricular ejection fraction in chronic obstructive pulmonary disease: a combined radionuclide and hemodynamic study. *Am J Cardiol*. 1982;50:255–262.
11. Wroblewski E, James F, Spann JF, Bove AA. Right ventricular performance in mitral stenosis. *Am J Cardiol*. 1981;47:51–55.
12. Winzelberg GC, Boucher CA, Pohost GM, et al. Right ventricular function in aortic and mitral valve disease. *Chest*. 1981;79:520–528.
13. Korr KS, Gandsman EJ, Winkler ML, Shulman RS, Bough EW. Hemodynamic correlates of right ventricular ejection fraction measured with gated radionuclide angiography. *Am J Cardiol*. 1982;49:71–77.
14. Konstam MA, Weiland DS, Conlon TP, et al. Hemodynamic correlates of left ventricular versus right ventricular radionuclide volumetric responses to vasodilator therapy in congestive heart failure secondary to ischemic or dilated cardiomyopathy. *Am J Cardiol*. 1987;59:1131–1137.
15. Vlahakes GJ, Turley K, Hoffman JIE. The pathophysiology of failure in acute right ventricular hypertension: hemodynamic and biochemical correlations. *Circulation*. 1981;63:87–95.
16. Spann JF, Buccino RA, Sonnenblick EH, Braunwald E. Contractile state of cardiac muscle obtained from cats with experimentally produced ventricular hypertrophy and heart failure. *Circ Res*. 1967;21:341–354.
17. Kaufmann RL, Homburger H, Wirth H. Disorder in excitation-contraction coupling of cardiac muscle from cats with experimentally produced right ventricular hypertrophy. *Circ Res*. 1971;28:346–357.
18. Bing OHL, Matsushita S, Fanburg BL, Levine HJ. Mechanical properties of rat cardiac muscle during experimental hypertrophy. *Circ Res*. 1973;28:234–245.
19. Williams JF, Potter RD. Normal contractile state of hypertrophied myocardium after pulmonary artery constriction in the cat. *J Clin Invest*. 1974;54:1266–1272.
20. Cooper G, Tomanek RJ, Ehrhardt JC, Marcus ML.

Chronic progressive pressure overload of the cat right ventricle. *Circ Res*. 1981;48:488–497.

21. Murray PA, Vatner SF. Reduction of maximum coronary vascular response to exercise in dogs with severe right ventricular hypertrophy. *J Clin Invest*. 1981;67:1314–1323.

22. Doty D, Wright C. Eastham C, Marcus M. Coronary reselve in atrial septal defect. *Circulation*. 1980;62:(suppl III): III-115.

23. Cohn JN, Gwha NH, Broder MI, Limas CJ. Right ventricular infarction. Clinical and hemodynamic features. *Am J Cardiol*. 1974,33:209–214.

24. Sharpe DN, Botvinick EH, Shames DM, et al. The noninvasive diagnosis of right ventricular infarction. *Circulation*. 1978;57:483–490.

25. Lorell B, Leinbach RC, Pohost GM, et al. Right ventricular infarction. *Am J Cardiol*. 1979;43:465–471.

26. Dell'Italia LJ, Starling MR, Orourke RA. Physical examination for exclusion of hemodynamically important right ventricular infarction. *Ann Intern Med*. 1983;99:608–611.

27. Dalen JE, Haffajee CI, Alpert JS 3d, Howe JP, Ockene IS, Paraskos JA. Pulmonary embolism, pulmonary hemorrhage and pulmonary infarction. *N Engl J Med*. 1977;296:1431–1435.

28. Sharma GV, Schoolman M, Cella G, Dalen JE, Sasahara AA. Pulmonary embolism. Part I. *Circulation*. 1983;67:245–247.

29. Sharma GV, Schoolman M, Cella G, Dalen JE, Sasahara AA. Pulmonary embolism. Part II. *Circulation*. 1983;67:474–477.

30. Dalen JE, Haynes FW, Hoppin FG, Evans GL, Bhardwaj P, Dexter L. Cardiovascular responses to experimental pulmonary embolism. *Am J Cardiol*. 1967;20:3–9.

31. Dobell AR. Capability of the right ventricle. *Can J Cardiol*. 1988;4:12–16.

32. Jaenike JR, Waterhouse C. The nature and distribution of cardiac edema. *Lab Clin Med*. 1958;52:384–393.

33. Braunwald E: Clinical manifestatins of heart failure. In: Braunwald E, ed. *Heart disease*. Philadelphia: Saunders; 1988.

34. Davis JO. The mechanism of salt and water retention in cardiac failure. *Hosp Pract*. 1970;5:63–76.

35. Davis JO, Freeman RH. Mechanisms regulating renin release. *Physiol Rev*. 1976;56:1–56.

36. Zanchetti A, Stella A. Neural control of renin release. *Clin Sci Mol Med*. 1975;48:215s–223s.

37. Ferguson DW, Abboud FM, Mark AL. Selective impairment of baroreflex-mediated vasoconstrictor responses in patients with ventricular dysfunction. *Circulation*. 1984;69:451–460.

38. Liang CS, Fan TH, Sullebarger JT, Sakamoto S. Decreased adrenergic neuronal uptake activity in experimental right heart failure. A chamber specific contributor to beta-adrenoceptor downregulation. *J Clin Invest*. 1989;84:1267–1275.

39. Cody RJ, Atlas SA, Laragh JH, et al. Atrial natriuretic factor in normal subjects and heart failure patients. *J Clin Invest*. 1986;78:1362–1374.

40. Raine AEG, Erne P, Burgisser E, et al. Atrial natriuretic peptide and atrial pressure in patients with congestive heart failure. *N Engl J Med*. 1986;315:533–537.

41. Creager MA, Hirsch AT, Nabel EG, Cutler SS, Colucci WS, Dzau VJ. Responsiveness of atrial natriuretic factor to reduction in right atrial pressure in patients with chronic congestive heart failure. *J Am Coll Cardiol*. 1988;11:1191–1198.

42. Keller N, Sykulski R, Thamsborg G, Storm T, Larsen J. Changes in atrial natriuretic factor during preload reduction with nitroglycerin in patients with congestive heart failure. *Clin Physiol*. 1988;8:57–64.

43. Koepke JP, DiBona GF. Blunted natriuresis to atrial natriuretic peptide in chronic sodium-retaining disorders. *Am J Physiol*. 1987;252:F865–F871.

44. Remetz MS, Cleman MW, Cabin HS. Pulmonary and pleural complications of cardiac disease. *Clin Chest Med*. 1989;10:545–592.

45. Wiener-Kronish JP, Berthiaume Y, Albertine KH. Pleural effusions and pulmonary edema. *Clin Chest Med*. 1985;6:509–519.

46. Wiener-Kronish JP, Matthay MA, Callen PW, Filly RA, Gamsu G. Relationship of pleural effusions to pulmonary hemodynamics in patients with congestive heart failure. *Am Rev Respir Dis*. 1985;132:1253–1256.

47. Wiener-Kronish JP, Goldstein R, Matthay RA, et al. Lack of association of pleural effusion with chronic pulmonary arterial and right atrial hypertension. *Chest*. 1987 Dec;92:967–970.

48. Isner JM. Right ventricular myocardial infarction. In: Konstam MA, Isner JM, eds. *The right ventricle*. Boston, Dordrecht, Lancaster: Kluwer; 1988.

49. White PD, August S, Michael CR. Hydrothorax in congestive heart failure. *Am J Med Sci*. 1947;214:243–247.

50. McPeak EM, Levine SA. The preponderance of right hydrothorax in congestive heart failure. *Ann Intern Med*. 1946;25:916–927.

51. Bedford DE, Lovibond JL. Hydrothorax in heart failure. *Br Heart J*. 1941;3:93–111.

52. Race GA, Scheifley CH, Edwards JE. Hydrothorax in congestive heart failure. *Am J Med*. 1957;22:83–90.

53. Weiss JM, Spodick DH. Laterality of pleural effusions in chronic congestive heart failure. *Am J Cardiol*. 1984;53:951.

54. Weiss JM, Spodick DH. Association of left pleural effusion with pericardial disease. *N Engl J Med*. 1983,308:696–697.

55. Chakko SC, Caldwell SH, Sforza PP. Treatment of congestive heart failure. Its effect on pleural fluid chemistry. *Chest*. 1989;95:798–802.

56. Shinto RA, Light RW. Effects of diuresis on the characteristics of pleural fluid in patients with congestive heart failure. *Am J Med*. 1990;88:230–234.

57. Pittman JG, Cohen P. The pathogenisis of cardiac cachexia. *N Engl J Med*. 1964;271:403–409,453–460.

58. Resnick H Jr, Friedman B. Studies on the mechanism of the increased oxygen consumption in patients with cardiac disease. *J Clin Invest*. 1935;14:551–562.

59. Berkowitz D, Croll MN, Likoff W. Malabsorption as a compilcation of congestive heart failure. *Am J Cardiol*. 1963;11:43–47.

60. Estes NAM, Levine HJ. Cardiac cachexia. *Med Grand Rounds*. 1982;1:188–200.

61. Carr JG, Stevenson LW, Walden JA, Heber D. Prevalence and hemodynamic correlates of malnutrition in severe congestive heart failure secondary to ischemic or idiopathic dilated cardiomyopathy. *Am J Cardiol*. 1989;63:709–713.

62. Levine B, Kalman J, Mayer L, Fillit HM, Packer M. Elevated circulating levels of tumor necrosis factor in severe chronic heart failure. *N Engl J Med*. 1990;323:236–241.

63. Arcilla R, Tsai P, Thilenius 0, Ranniger K. Angiographic method for volume estimation of right and left ventricles. *Chest*. 1971;60:446.

64. Ferlinz J, Gorlin R, Cohn PF, Herman MV. Right ventricular performance in patients with coronary artery disease. *Circulation*. 1975;52:608–615.

65. Fisher EA, DuBrow IW, Hastreiter AR. Right ventricular volume in congenital heart disease. *Am J Cardiol*. 1975,36:67–75.

66. Gentzler RD, Briselli MF, Gault JH. Angiographic estimation of right ventricular volume in man. *Circulation*. 1974;50:324–330.

67. Graham TP, Jarmakani JM, Atwood GF, Canent RV. Right ventricular volume determinations in children: normal values and observations with volume or pressure overload. *Circulation*. 1973;47:144–153.

68. Steele P, Kirch D, LeFree M, Battock D. Measurement of right and left ventricular ejection fractions by radionuclide angiocardiography in coronary artery disease. *Chest*. 1976;70:51.

69. Berger HJ, Matthay RA, Loke J, Marshall RC, Gottschalk A, Zaret BL. Cardiac performance with quantitative radionuclide angiocardiography: right ventricular ejection fraction with reference to findings in chronic obstructive pulmonary disease. *Am J Cardiol*. 1978;41:897–905.

70. Reduto LA, Berger HJ, Cohen LS, Gottschalk A, Zaret BL. Sequential radionuclide assessment of left and right ventricular performance after acute transmural myocardial infarction. *Ann Intern Med*. 1978;89:441–448.

71. Tobinick E, Schelbert HR, Henning H, et al. Right ventricular ejection fraction in patients with acute anterior and inferior myocardial infarction assessed by radionuclide angiography. *Circulation*. 1978;57:1078–1084.

72. Maddahi J, Berman DS, Matsuoka DT, et al. A new technique for assessing right ventricular ejection fraction using rapid multiple-gated equilibrium cardiac blood pool scintigraphy. *Circulation*. 1979;60:581–589.

73. Konstam MA, Kahn PC, Curran BH, Idoine J, Wynne J, Holman BL. Accuracy of equilibrium (gated) radionuclide ejection fraction measurement in the pressure or volume overloaded right ventricle. *Chest*. 1984;86:681–687.

74. Bommer W, Weinert L, Neumann A, et al. Determination of right atrial and right ventricular size by two dimensional echocardiography. *Circulation*. 1979;60:91.

75. Panidis IP, Ren J, Kotler MN, et al. Two dimensional echocardiographic estimation of right ventricular ejection fraction in patients with coronary artery disease. *J Am Coll Cardiol*. 1983;2:911.

76. Silverman NH, Hudson S. Evaluation of right ventricular volume and ejection fraction in chirdren by two dimensional echoardiography. *Pediatr Cardiol*. 1983;4:197.

77. Levine RA, Gibson TC, Aretz T, et al. Echocardiographic measurement of right ventricular volume. *Circulation*. 1984;69:497.

78. Kaul S, Tei C, Hopkins JM, Shah PM. Assessment of right ventricular function using two dimensional echocardioraphy. *Am Heart J*. 1984;107:526.

79. Starling MR, Crawford MH, Sorensen SG, O'Rourke, RA. A new two dimensional echocardiographic technique for evaluating right ventricular size and performance in patients with obstructive lung disease. *Circulation*. 1982;66:612.

80. Byrd BF, Schiller NB, Botvinick EH, Higgins CB. Normal cardiac dimensions by magnetic resonance imaging. *Am J Cardiol*. 1985;55:1440–1442.

81. Dhainaut J, Brunet F, Monsallier JF, et al. Bedside evaluation of right ventricular performance using a rapid computerized thermodilution method. *Crit Care Med*. 1987;15:148–152.

82. Morrison DA, Stovall R, Sensecqua J, Friefeld G. Thermodilution measurement of the right ventricular ejection fraction. *Cathet Cardiovasc Diag*. 1987;13:167–173.

83. Voelker W, Gruber HP, Ickrath O, Unterberg R, Karsch KR. Determination of right ventricular ejection fraction by thermodilution technique—a comparison to biplane cineventriculography. *Intens Care Med*. 1988;14:461–466.

84. McKay RG, Spears JR, Aroesty JM, et al. Instantaneous measurement of left and right ventricular stroke volume and pressure-volume relationships with an impedance catheter. *Circulation*. 1984;69:703–710.

85. Diamond MA, Dillon JC, Haine CL, et al. Echocardiographic features of atrial septal defect. *Circulation*. 1971;43:129–135.

86. Tajik AJ, Gau GT, Ritter DG, et al. Echocardiographic pattern of right ventricular diastolic volume overload in children. *Circulation*. 1972;46:36–43.

87. Meyer RA, Schwartz DC, Benzing G, et al. Ventricular septum in right ventricular volume overload. *Am J Cardiol*. 1972;30:349–353.

88. Kerber RE. Dippel WF, Abbound FM. Abnormal motion of the interventricular septum in right ventricular volume overload. *Circulation*. 1973;48:86–96.

89. Hagen AD, Francis GS, Sahn DJ, et al. Ultrasound evaluation of systolic anterior septal motion in patients with and without right ventricular volume overload. *Circulation*. 1974;50:248–254.

90. Pearlman AS, Clark CE, Henry WL, et al. Determinants of ventricular septal motion. Influence of relative right and left ventricular size. *Circulation*. 1976;54:83–91.

91. Visner MS, Arentzen CE, O'Connor MJ, Larson EV, Anderson RW. Alterations in left ventricular three-dimensional dynamic geometry and systolic function during acute right ventricular hypertension in the conscious dog. *Circulation*. 1983;67:353–365.

92. Badke FR. Left ventricular dimensions and function dur-

ing exercise in dogs with chronic right ventricular pressure overload. *Am J Cardiol.* 1984;53:1187–1193.

93. Feneley M, Gavaghan T. Paradoxical and pseudoparadoxical interventricular septal motion in patients with right ventricular volume overload. *Circulation.* 1986; 74:230–238.

94. Konstam MA, Kronenberg MW, Udelson JE, et al. Effect of acute angiotensin converting enzyme inhibition on left ventricular filling in patients with congestive heart failure: relation to right ventricular volumes. *Circulation.* 1990;81(suppl III):III-115–III-122.

95. Coma-Canella I, Lopez-Sendon J. Ventricular compliance in ischemic right ventricular dysfunction. *Am J Cardiol.* 1980;45:555–561.

96. Isner JM, Roberts WC. Right ventricular infarction complicating left ventricular infarction secondary to coronary heart disease. Frequency, location, associated findings and signficance from analysis of 236 necropsy patients with acute or healed myocardial iinfarction. *Am J Cardiol.* 1978;42:885–894.

97. Ratliff NB, Hackel DB. Combined right and left ventricular infarction: pathogenesis and clinicopathologic correlations. *Am J Cardiol.* 1980;45:217–221.

98. Chou TC, Fowler NO, Gabel M, Van Der Bel, Kahn J, Feltner J. Electrocardiographic and hemodynamic changes in experimental right ventricular infarction. *Circulation.* 1983;67:1258–1267.

99. Cabin HS, Clubb S, Wackers FJ, Zaret BL. Right ventricular myocardial infarction with anterior wall left ventricular infarction: an autopsy study. *Am Heart J.* 1987;113:16–23.

100. Weinshel AJ, Isner JM, Salem DN, Konstam MA. The coronary anatomy of right ventricular myocardial infarction: relationship between the site of right coronary occlusion and origin of the right ventricular free wall branches. *Circulation.* 1983;68:III-351.

101. Shah PK, Maddahi J, Berman DS, Pichler M, Swan HJ. Scintigraphically detected predominant right ventricular dysfunction in acute myocardial infarction: clinical and hemodynamic correlates and implications for therapy and prognosis. *J Am Coll Cardiol.* 1985;6:1264–1272.

102. Lopez-Sendon J, Coma-Canella I, Gamello C. Sensitivity and specificity of hemodynamic criteria in the diagnosis of right ventricular infarction. *Circulation.* 1981;64:515–525.

103. Goldstein JA, Vlahakes GJ, Verrier ED, et al. The role of right ventricular systolic dysfunction and elevated intrapericardial pressure in the genesis of low output in experimental right ventricular infarction. *Circulation.* 1982;65:513–522.

104. Haines DE, Beller GA, Watson DD, et al. A prospective clinical, scintigraphic, angiographic and functional evaluation of patients after inferior myocardial infarction with and without right ventricular dysfunction. *J Am Coll Cardiol.* 1985;6:995.

105. Dellitalia LJ, Starling MR, Crawford MH, Boros BL, Chaudhuri TK, O'Rourke RA. Right ventricular infarction identification by hemodynamic measurements before and after volume loading and correlation with non-invasive techniques. *J Am Coll Cardiol.* 1984;4:931.

106. Ibsen HHW, Baandrup U, Simonsen EE. Familial right

107. Unverferth DV, Baker PB, Swift SE, et al. Extent of myocardial fibrosis and cellular hypertrophy in dilated cardiomyopathy. *Am J Cardiol.* 1986;57:816–820.

108. Roberts WC, Waller BF. Cardiac amyloidosis causing cardiac dysfunction: analysis of 54 necropsy patients. *Am J Cardiol.* 1983;52:137–146.

109. Johnson RA, Palacios I. Nondilated cardiomyopathies. In Stollerman G, et al., eds. *Advances in internal medicine.* Chicago: Year Book Medical Publishers; 1984.

110. Buja LM, Roberts WC. Iron In the heart. Etiology and significance. *Am J Med.* 1971;51:209–221.

111. Cutler DJ, Isner JM, Bracey AW, et al. Hemachromatosis heart disease. An unemphasized cause of potentially reversible restrictive cardiomyopathy. *Am J Med.* 1980;69:923.

112. Short EM, Winkle RE, Billingham ME. Myocardial involvement in idiopathic hemachromatosis. Morphologic and clinical improvement following venesection. *Am J Med.* 1981;70:1275.

113. Roberts WC, McAllister HA, Ferrans VJ. Sarcoidosis of the heart. *Am J Med.* 1977;63:86–108.

114. Fleming HH. Sarcoid heart disease. *Br Med J.* 1986;292,1095.

115. Koide T, Itoyzma S, Kato K, Kato A, Murao S. Cardiac sarcoidosis with 12-year survival. *Jpn Heart J.* 1982;23:263.

116. Ishikawa T, Kondoh H, Nagakaw S, Koiwaya Y, Tanaka K. Steroid therapy in cardiac sarcoidosis: increased left ventricular contractility concomitant with electrocardiographic improvement after prednisolone. *Chest.* 1984;85:445.

117. Fauci AS, Harley JB, Roberts WC, Ferrans VJ, Gralnick HR, Bjornson BH. The idiopathic hypereosinophilic syndrome. *Ann Intern Med.* 1982;97:78–92.

118. Olsen EGJ, Spry CJF. Relation between eosinophilia and endomyocardial disease. *Prog Cardiovasc Dis.* 1985;27:241.

119. Davies JNP, Coles RM. Some considerations regarding obscure disease affecting the mural endocardium. *Am Heart J.* 1960;59:606.

120. Cherian G, Vijayaraghavan G, Krishnaswami S, et al. Endomyocardial fibrosis: report on the hemodynamic data in 29 patients and review of the results of surgery. *Am Heart J.* 1983;105:659.

121. Metras D, Coulibaly AO, Ouattara Ka. The surgical treatment of endomyocardial fibrosis: results in 55 patients. *Circulation.* 1985;72:II-274.

122. Ross EM, Roberts WC. The carcinoid syndrome: comparison of 21 necropsy subjects with carcinoid heart disease to 15 necropsy subjects without carcinoid heart disease. *Am J Med.* 1985;79:339–354.

123. Warnes CA, Roberts WC. The heart in massive (more than 300 pounds or 136 kilograms) obesity: analysis of 12 patients studied at necropsy. *Am J Cardiol.* 1984;54:1087–1091.

124. Marcus FI, Fontaine GH, Guiraudon G, et al. Right ventricular dysplasia—a report of 24 adult cases. *Circulation.* 1982;65:384.

125. Robertson JH, Brady GH, German LD, Gallagher JJ,

Kisslo J. Comparison of two-dimensional echocardiographic and angiographic findings in arrhythmogenic right ventricular dysplasia. *Am J Cardiol.* 1985;55:1506.

126. Diggelmann U, Baur HR. Familial Uhl's anomaly in the adult. *Am J Cardiol.* 1984;53:1402.

127. Guiraudon GM, Klein GJ, Gulamhusein SS, et al. Total disconnection of the right ventricular free wall: surgical treatment of right ventricular tachycardia associated with right ventricular dysplasia. *Circulation.* 1983;67:464.

128. Mahler DA, Brent BN, Like J, Zaret BL, Matthay RA. Right ventricular performance and central circulatory hemodynamics during upright exercise in patients with chronic obstructive pulmonary disease. *Am Rev Respir Dis.* 1984;130:722–729.

129. Cohen M, Horowitz SF, Machac J, Mindich BP, Fuster V. Response of the right ventricle to exercise in isolated mitral stenosis. *Am J Cardiol.* 1985;55:1054–1058.

130. Grose R, Strain J, Yipinatosoi T. Right ventricular function in valvular heart disease: relation to pulmonary artery pressure. *J Am Coll Cardiol.* 1983;2:225–232.

131. Johnston DL, Kostuk WJ. Left and right ventricular function during symptom-limited exercise in patients with isolated mitral stenosis. *Chest.* 1986;89:186.

132. Krabill KA, Wang Y, Einzig S, Moller JH. Rest and exercise hemodynamics in pulmonary stenosis: comparison of children and adults. *Am J Cardiol.* 1985;56:360.

133. Johnson LW, Grossman W, Dalen JE, Dexter L. Pulmonic stenosis in the adult: long-term follow-up results. *N Engl J Med.* 1972;287:1159.

134. Johnson GL, Kwan IL, Handshoe S, Noonan JA, De Maria. Accuracy of combined two-dimensional echocardiography and continuous wave recordings in the estimation of pressure gradient in right ventricular outlet obstruction. *J Am Coll Cardiol.* 1984;3:1013.

135. Locke J, Keane J, Ferllows K. The use of catheter intervention procedures for congenital heart disease. *J Am Coll Cardiol.* 1986;7:1420.

136. McAllister RG, Friesinger GC, Sinclair-Smith BC. Tricuspid regurgitation following inferior myocardial infarction. *Arch Inter Med.* 1976;136:905.

137. Yock PG, Popp RL. Non-invasive estimation of right ventricular systolic pressure by Doppler ultrasound in patients with tricuspid regurgitation. *Circulation.* 1984; 70:657.

138. Carpentier A, Deloche A, Dauptain A. A new reconstructive operation for correction of tricuspid and mitral insufficiency. *J Thorac Cardiovasc Surg.* 1971;61:1.

139. Liberthson RR, Boucher CA, Strauss HW, Dinsmore RE, McKusick KA, Pohost GM. Right ventricular function in adult atrial septal defect: preoperative and postoperative assessment and clinical implications. *Am J Cardiol.* 1981;47:56–60.

140. Konstam MA, Idoine J, Wynne J, et al. Right ventricular function in pulmonary hypertensive adults with and without atrial septal defects. *Am J Cardiol.* 1983;51:1144–1148.

141. Ludbrook PA, Byrne JD, McKnight RC. Influence of right ventricular hemodynamics on left ventricular diastolic pressure-volume relations in man. *Circulation.* 1979;59:21–31.

142. Ross J. Acute displacement of the diastolic pressure-volume curve of the left ventricle: role of the pericardium and the right ventricle. *Circulation.* 1979;59:32–37.

143. Lorell BH, Palacios I, Daggett WM, Jacobs ML, Fowler BN, Newell JB. Right ventricular distension and left ventricular compliance. *Am J Physiol.* 1981;240:H87–89.

144. Lavine SJ, Tami L, Jawad I. Pattern of left ventricular diastolic filling associated with right ventricular enlargement. *Am J Cardiol.* 1988;62:444–448.

145. Smith ER, Tyberg JV. Ventricular interdependence. In: Konstam MA, Isner JM, eds. *The right ventricle.* Boston, Dordrecht, Lancaster; Kluwer; 1988.

146. Dittrich HC, Chow LC, Nicod PH. Early improvement in left ventricular diastolic function after relief of chronic right ventricular pressure overload. *Circulation.* 1989;80:823–830.

147. Carroll JD, Land RM, Neumann AL, Borow KM, Rajfer SI. The differential effects of positive inotropic and vasodilator therapy on diastolic properties in patients with congestive cardiomyopathy. *Circulation.* 1986;74:815–825.

148. Tyberg JV, Taichman GC, Smith ER, Douglas MWS, Smiseth OA, Keon WJ. The relation between pericardial pressure and right atrial pressure: an intraoperative study. *Circulation.* 1986;73:428–432.

149. Watanabe J, Levine MJ, Bellotto F, Johnson RG, Grossman W. Effects of coronary venous pressure on left ventricular diastolic distensibility. *Circ Res.* 1990;67:923–932.

150. Baker BJ, Wilen MM, Boyd CM, Dinh H, Franciosa JA. Relation of right ventricular ejection fraction to exercise capacity in chronic left ventricular failure. *Am J Cardiol.* 1984,54:596–599.

151. Polak JF, Holman BL, Wynne J, Colucci WS. Right ventricular ejection fraction: an indicator of increased mortality in patients with congestive heart failure associated with coronary artery disease. *J Am Coll Cardiol.* 1983;2:217–224.

152. Brill DM, Konstam MA, Vivino PG, et al. Importance of right ventricular systolic function as an independent predictor of mortality in patients with congestive heart failure. *Circulation.* 1989;80:II-649.

153. Konstam MA, Kronenberg MW, Udelson JE, et al. Preload reserve: a determinant of clinical status in patients with left ventricular systolic dysfunction. *J Am Coll Cardiol.* 1991;17:89A.

154. Brill DM, Konstam MA, Vivino PG, et al. Rapid-onset pulmonary edema in patients with left ventricular systolic dysfunction: a syndrome related to right ventricular ejection fraction. *J Am Coll Cardio.* 1989;13:179A.

155. Goldstein JA, Vlahakes GJ, Verrier ED, et al. Volume loading improves low cardiac output in experimental right ventricular infarction. *J Am Coll Cardiol.* 1978;2:270-278.

156. Isner JM, Fisher GP, DelNegro AA, Borer JS. Right ventriuclar infarction with hemodynamic decompensation due to transient loss of active atrial augmentation: successful treatment with atrial pacing. *Am Heart J.* 1981;102:792-794.

157. Taylor SH: Diuretics in cardiovascular therapy. Perusing

the past, practicing in the present, preparing for the future. *Z Kardiol*. 1985;74(suppl 2):2–12.

158. Heinemann HO. Right-sided heart failure and the use of diuretics. *Am J Med*. 1978;64:367–370.

159. Franciosa JA, Nordstrom LA, Cohn JN. Nitrate therapy for congestive heart failure. *JAMA* 1978;240:443–446.

160. Leier CV, Huss P, Magorien RD, Unverferth DV. Improved exercise capacity and differing arterial and venous tolerance during chronic isosorbide dinitrate therapy for congestive heart failure. *Circulation*. 1983;67:817–822.

161. Armstrong PW. Pharmacokinetic-hemodynamic studies of transdermal nitroglycerin in congestive heart failure. *J Am Coll Cardiol*. 1987;9:420–425.

162. Packer M, Halperin JL, Brooks KM, Rothlauf EB, Lee WH. Nitroglycerin therapy in the management of pulmonary hypertensive disorders. *Am J Med*. 1984;76:67–75.

163. Morrison D, Caldwell J, Lakshminaryan S, Ritchie JL, Kennedy JW. The acute effects of low flow oxygen and isosorbide dinitrate on left and right ventricular ejection fractions in chronic obstructive pulmonary disease. *J Am Coll Cardiol*. 1983;2:652–660.

164. Brent BN, Berger HJ, Matthay RA, Mahler D, Pytlik L, Zaret BL. Contrasting acute effects of vasodilators (nitroglycerin, nitroprusside, and hydralazine) on right ventricular performance in patients with chronic obstructive pulmonary disease and pulmonary hypertension: a combined radionuclide-hemodynamic study. *Am J Cardiol*. 1983;51:1682–1689.

165. Banahy DT, Tobis JM, Aronow WS, Chetty K, Glauser F. Effects of isosorbide dinitrate on pulmonary hypertension in chronic obstructive pulmonary disease. *Clin Pharm Ther*. 1979;25:541–548.

166. Geggel RL, Dozor AJ, Fyler DC, Reid LM. Effect of vasodilators at rest and during exercise in young adults with cystic fibrosis and chronic cor pulmonale. *Am Rev Respir Dis*. 1985;131:531–536.

167. Zielinski J, Hawrylkiewicz I, Gorecka D, Gluskowski J, Koscinska M. Captopril effects on pulmonary and systemic hemodynamics in chronic cor pulmonale. *Chest*. 1986;90:562–565.

168. Wilson RH, Hoseth W, Dempsey ME. The effects of breathing of 99.6% oxygen on pulmonary vascular resistance and cardiac output in patients with pulmonary emphysema and chronic hypoxia. *Ann Intern Med*. 1955;42:629–637.

169. Abraham AS, Cole RB, Bishop JM. Reversal of pulmonary hypertension by prolonged oxygen administration in patients with chronic bronchitis. *Circ Res*. 1968;23:147–157.

170. Ashutosh K, Mead G, Dunsky M. Early effects of oxygen administration on prognosis in chronic obstructive pulmonary disease and cor pulmonale. *Am Rev Respir Dis*. 1983;127:399–404.

171. Stark RD, Finnegan P, Bishop JM. Daily requirement of oxygen to reverse pulmonary hypertension in patients with chronic bronchitis. *Br Med J*. 1972;3:724–728.

172. Brent BN, Mahler DA, Berger HJ, Matthay RA, Pytlik L, Zaret BL. Augmentation of right ventricular performance in chronic obstructive pulmonary disease by terbutaline: a combined radionuclide and hemodynamic study. *Am J Cardiol*. 1982;50:313–319.

173. Teule GJ, Majid PA. Hemodynamic effects of terbutaline in chronic obstructive airways disease. *Thorax*. 1980;35:536–542.

174. Rutherford JD, Vatner SF, Braunwald E. Effects of mechanisms of action of aminophylline on cardiac function and regional blood flow distribution in conscious dogs. *Circulation*. 1981;63:378–387.

175. Parker JO, Ashekian PB, DiGiorgi S, West RO. Hemodynamic effects of ammophylline in chronic obstructive pulmonary disease. *Circulation*. 1967;35:365–372.

176. Matthay RA, Berger HJ, Toke J, Gottschalk A, Zaret BL. Effects of aminophylline upon right and left ventricular performance in chronic obstructive pulmonary disease. Noninvasive assessment by radionuclide angiocardiography. *Am J Med*. 1978;65:903–910.

177. Matthay RA, Berger HJ, Davies R, Toke J, Gottschalk A, Zaret BL. Improvement in cardiac performance by oral long-acting theophylline in chronic obstructive pulmonary disease. *Am Heart J*. 1982;104:1022–1026.

178. Keller Ca, Shepard JW, Chun DS, Dolan GF, Vasquez P, Minh VD. Effects of hydralazine on hemodynamics, ventilation, and gas exchange in patients with chronic obstructive pulmonary disease and pulmonary hypertension. *Am Rev Respir Dis*. 1984;130:606–611.

179. Tuxen DV, Powles ACP, Mathur PN, Pugsley SO, Campbell EJM. Detrimental effects of hydralazine in patients with chronic air-flow obstruction and pumlonary hypertension. *Am Rev Respir Dis*. 1984;129:388–395.

180. Dal Nogare AR, Rubin L. The effects of hydralazine on exercise capacity in pulmonary hypertension secondary to chronic obstructive pulmonary disease. *Am Rev Respir Dis*. 1986;133:385–389.

181. Rubin LJ, Peter RH. Hemodynamics at rest and during exercise after oral hydralazine in patients with cor pulmonale. *Am J Cardiol*. 1981;47:116–122.

182. Simmoneau G, Escourrou P, Puroux P, Lockhart A. Inhibition of hypoxic pulmonary vasoconstriction by nifedipine. *N Engl J Med*. 1981;304:1582–1585.

183. Sturani C, Bassein L, Schiavani M, Gunella G. Oral nifedipine in chronic cor pulmonale secondary to severe chronic obstructive pulmonary disease (COPD). *Chest*. 1983;84:135–142.

184. Melot C, Hallemans R, Naeije R, Mols P, Lejeune P. Deleterious effect of nifedipine on pulmonary gas exchange in chronic obstructive pulmonary disease. *Am Rev Respir Dis*. 1984;130:612–616.

185. Zakheim RM, Mattioli L, Molteni A, Nullis KB, Bartley J. Prevention of pulmonary vascular changes of chronic alveolar hypoxia by inhibition of angiotensin I converting enzyme in the rat. *Lab Invest*. 1975;33:57–61.

186. Bertoli L, LoCicero S, Busnardo I, Rizzato G, Montanari G. Effects of captopril on hemodynamics and blood gases in chronic obstructive lung disease with pulmonary hypertension. *Respiration*. 1986;49:251–256.

187. Boschetti E, Tantucci C, Cocchieri M, Fornari G, Grassi V, Sorbini CA. Acute effects of captopril in hypoxic pul-

monary hypertension. Comparison with transient oxygen administration. *Respiration*. 1985;48:296–302.

188. Packer M, Greenberg B, Massie B, Dash H. Deleterious effects of hydralazine in patients with pulmonary hypertension. *N Engl J Med*. 1982;306:1326–1332.

189. Packer M. Vasodilator therpy for primary pulmonary hypertension. Limitations and hazards. *Ann Intern Med*. 1985;103:258–270.

190. Konstam MA, Cohen SR, Salem DN, Das D, Aronovitz M, Brockway B. Amrinone effect on right ventricular function: predominance of afterload reduction. *Circulation*. 1986;74:359–66.

191. Eichhorn EJ, Konstam MA, Weiland DS, et al. Differential effects of milrinone and dobutamine on right ventricular preload, afterload, and systolic performance in congestive heart failure secondary to ischemic or idiopathic dilated cardiomyopathy. *Am J Cardiol*. 1987;60:1329–1333.

192. Hill NS, Rounds S. Amrinone dilates pulmonary vessels and blunts hypoxic vasoconstriction in isolated rat lungs. *Proc Soc Exp Biol Med*. 1983;173:205–212.

193. Green LH, Smith TW. The use of digitalis in patients with pulmonary disease. *Ann Intern Med*. 1977;87:419–465.

194. Ferrer MI, Harvey RM, Cathcart RT, Webster CA, Richards DW, Cournand A. Some effects of digoxin upon the heart and circulation in man. Digoxin in cor pulmonale. *Circulation*. 1950;1:161–186.

195. Jezek V, Schrijen F. Haemodynamic effect of deslanoside at rest and during exercise in patients with chronic bronchitis. *Br Heart J*. 1973;35:2–8.

196. Kim YS, Aviado DM. Digitalis and the pulmonary circulation. *Am Heart J*. 1961;62:680–686.

197. Linde LM, Goldberg SJ, Gaal P, Momma K, Masato T, Sarna G. Pulmonary and systemic hemodynamic effects of cardiac glycosides. *Am Heart J*. 1968;76:356–364.

198. Berglund E, Widimsky J, Malmberg R. Lack of effect of digitalis in patients with pulmonary disease with and without heart failure. *Am J Cardiol*. 1963;11:477–482.

199. Fonger JD, Borkon AM, Baumgartner WA, Achuff SC, Augustine S, Reitz BA. Acute right ventricular failure following heart transplantation: improvement with prostaglandin E₁ and right ventricular assist. *Heart Transplant*. 1986;5:317–321.

200. Spence PA, Weisel RD, Salerno TA. Right ventricular

201. Payne DD, Cleveland RJ. Perioperative right heart dysfunction. In Konstam MA, Isner JM, eds. *The right ventricle*. Boston, Dordrecht, Lancaster: Kluwer; 1988.

202. Esmore DS, Spratt PM, Branch JM, et al. Right ventricular assist and prostacyclin infusion for allograft failure in the presence of high pulmonary vascular resistance. *J Heart Transplant*. 1990;9:136–141.

203. DAmbra MN, LaRaia PJ, Philbin DM, Watkins WD, Hilgenberg AD, Buckley MJ. Prostaglandin E₁. A new therapy for refractory right heart failure and pulmonary hypertension after mitral valve replacement. *J Thorac Cardiovasc Surg*. 1985;89:567–572.

204. Armitage JM, Hardesty RL, Griffith BP. Prostaglandin E₁: an effective treatment of right heart failure after orthotopic heart transplantation. *J Heart Transplant*. 1987;6:348–351.

205. Deeb GM, Bolling SF, Guynn TP, Nicklas JM. Amrinone versus conventional therapy in pulmonary hypertensive patients awaiting cardiac transplantation. *Ann Thorac Surg*. 1989;48:665–669.

206. Hess W, Arnold B, Veit S. The haemodynamic effects of amrinone in patients with mitral stenosis and pulmonary hypertension. *Eur Heart J*. 1986;7:800-807.

207. Jett GK, Siwek LG, Picone AL, Applebaume RE, Jones J. Pulmonary artery balloon counterpulsation for right ventricular failure. *J Thorac Cardiovasc Surg*. 1983;86:364–372.

208. Flege JB Jr, Wright CB, Reisinger TJ. Successful balloon counterpulsation for right ventricular failure. *Ann Thorac Surg*. 1984;37:167–168.

209. Symbas PN, McKeown PP, Santora AH, Vlasis SE. Pulmonary artery counterpulsation for treatment of intraoperative right ventriuclar failure. *Ann Thorac Surg*. 1985;39:437–440.

210. Dembitsky WP, Daily PO, Raney AA, Moores WY, Yoyo CI. Temporary extracorporeal support of the right ventricle. *J Thorac Cardiovasc Surg*. 1986;91:518–525.

211. O'Neill MJ Jr, Pierce WS, Wisman CB, Osbakken MD, Parr GV, Waldhausen JA. Successful management of right ventricular failure with the ventricular assist pump following aortic valve replacement and coronary artery bypass grafting. *J Thorac Cardiovasc Surg*. 1984;87:106–111.

failure. Pathophysiology and treatment. *Surg Clin North Am*. 1985;65:689–697.

18
Other Causes and Contributing Factors to Congestive Heart Failure

Constantine A. Hassapoyannes, William P. Nelson, and Christie B. Hopkins

The onset of symptoms of congestive heart failure (CHF) reflects the inability of the heart as a pump to meet the metabolic requirements of the body at all levels of activity despite the recruitment of numerous compensatory mechanisms. When cardiac reserve is already diminished, any further insult to the contractile status of the myocardium may decompensate previously controlled heart failure. Similarly, conditions that transiently or permanently increase cardiac work or interfere with the adaptive mechanisms governing cardiac work may lead to rapid deterioration of an already impaired ventricular function. This chapter deals first with factors contributing to CHF, then with exogenous causes, and finally with specific disease processes that independently affect the myocardium.

Factors Contributing to Congestive Heart Failure

High Output States

Anemia

Chronic anemia is associated with high cardiac output when hemoglobin equals 7 g% or less.[1] A distinguishing feature of all high output states is the reduced total peripheral resistance resulting from decreased systemic arteriolar tone and, in the case of anemia, also from lowered blood viscosity (Fig. 18.1). According to Guyton,[2] cardiac output in the normal heart is determined primarily by the systemic venous return, which in turn is proportional to the pressure gradient between small systemic veins (mean systemic pressure) and the right atrium. In anemia, arteriolar dilatation, due to tissue hypoxia and production of lactate or other vasodilatory metabolites, increases the rate at which blood is delivered from the arterial to the venous side of the cir-

culation, thus augmenting the mean systemic pressure and the systemic venous return. The prompt reversal of the high output state with orthostatic stress or use of pressor agents underscores the importance of vasodilation as a pathophysiologic mechanism.[3] Further, Fowler and Holmes quantitated the effect of low blood viscosity in the canine model after induction of the same degree of anemia by exchange transfusion of either low or high molecular weight dextran.[4] These investigators observed a greater increase in cardiac output (93% vs. 53%) with low compared to high molecular weight dextran, which was attributed to the lower blood viscosity in the former group. However, the fact that the cardiac output rose even when blood was exchanged with high molecular weight dextran indicates that the effects of anemia per se and altered blood viscosity are additive and independent of each other. Although the rise in cardiac output exceeds that in stroke volume,[3] the heart rate increase is insignificant in chronic as opposed to acute or subacute anemia. Finally, even though the presence of a circulating noncatecholamine inotrope has been suggested,[5] it is unlikely that an increase in intrinsic contractility contributes significantly to the high output state.[2]

Despite a high venous return/cardiac output, the arterial pressure decreases in anemia in response to a number of events including generalized vasodilation, reduced blood viscosity, and a reduced total blood volume.[3] Stroke work usually remains unchanged[3] since the increase in stroke volume is countered by the decrease in systemic vascular resistance and left ventricular end-systolic wall stress.[5] In terms of myocardial energetics, this change acts favorably on the heart, which is an effective volume pump rather than pressure pump.[6] In fact, Sarnoff et al.[7] have shown that for the same stroke work, switching from pressure work to flow work reduces myocardial oxygen consumption, although this has not been validated in the anemic

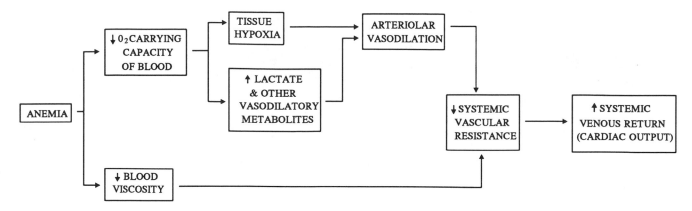

FIGURE 18.1. Diagram of pathophysiologic mechanisms effecting high output state in anemia.

state. However, in severe anemia myocardial oxygen consumption has been shown to increase,[8] possibly in response to very high cardiac output.

The ventricular myocardium responds to increased venous return and end-diastolic wall stress with replication of sarcomeres in series resulting in chamber enlargement and normalization of end-diastolic pressure. In turn, chamber enlargement and increased radius augment peak systolic wall stress resulting in replication of sarcomeres in parallel and wall thickening.[9] Thus, in chronic anemia as in chronic volume overload, the left ventricle undergoes eccentric hypertrophy. In chronic anemic states (hemoglobin 5 ± 1 g%), Olivetti et al. observed ventricular hypertrophy (50% heart weight increase) that occurred with greater increases in wall area than in wall thickness, suggesting an eccentric pattern.[10] Furthermore, myocardial growth was accompanied by a 60% lengthening of the capillary network which, in combination with an increase in capillary diameter, resulted in a 65% expansion of capillary luminal volume in the left heart; this may prevent the potential of ischemic injury. Thus, the heart can adapt itself appropriately to the hyperkinetic circulation of even moderately severe anemia for years without evidence of functional impairment. Conversely, anemic patients with hematocrit >20% exhibiting signs or symptoms of heart failure or ischemic heart disease almost invariably have underlying organic heart disease.

In patients with left ventricular (LV) dysfunction, the decrease in systemic vascular resistance due to anemia would be expected to enhance LV emptying by reducing the afterload. However, the overall impact of a reduction in the oxygen-carrying capacity of blood is usually deleterious since the impaired LV may have little or no reserve to meet an increase in metabolic requirements. The fact that anemia is a stimulus for development of eccentric hypertrophy also would exert an adverse effect in chronic heart failure when cardiac enlargement is already an issue. Finally, lowered oxygen-carrying capacity due to anemia would be expected to

clinically manifest more easily in patients with heart failure than in those with normal cardiac function since an increase in tissue oxygen extraction is an important compensatory mechanism in a setting of reduced cardiac output. A decrease in oxygen-carrying capacity would limit the effectiveness of this means of prevserving tissue oxygenation. Noteably, at hemoglobin levels <4 g%, patients may develop LV dysfunction, CHF, or overt pulmonary edema in the absence of intrinsic heart disease.

Fever

Endogenous increase in body temperature (e.g., infection or hyperthyroidism) augments cellular metabolism and, therefore, oxygen demand and production of metabolites, which act in concert to effect systemic vasodilation and an increase in systemic venous return/cardiac output. Furthermore, to preserve thermal homeostasis the body dissipates excess heat by means of selective cutaneous vasodilation and increase in blood flow. Normally, the body can efficiently dissipate excess heat as evidenced by the fact that during pyrexia the arteriovenous oxygen gradient remains unchanged or decreases; this indicates that the increase in cardiac output is equal to or exceeds the rise in oxygen requirements due to the hypermetabolic state.[11] In low-output CHF, however, pyrexia may cause the myocardium to decompensate due to either inability to sustain high output and dissipate heat, or to an increase in its own metabolic rate and an unfavorable myocardial oxygen supply/demand ratio.

Arteriovenous Fistulas

Arteriovenous fistulas (Table 18.1) are congenital or acquired (Fig. 18.2). Congenital fistulas are localized or diffuse, single or multiple, and may occur independently or as a manifestation of Osler-Weber-Rendu disease (hereditary hemorrhagic telangiectasia). The size of the communication determines the flow through the shunt

TABLE 18.1. Arteriovenous communications.

Congenital
Hemangiomas
    Capillary[a]
        Nevus flammeus ("portwine stain")
        Nevus vasculosus ("strawberry" hemangiomas)
    Cavernous
        Skin, bone, brain, kidneys, hepar, lungs
Hereditary hemorrhagic telangiectasia
(Osler-Weber-Rendu disease)

Acquired
Traumatic
    Stab or through-and-through gunshot wounds
Iatrogenic
    After diagnostic procedures (e.g., percutaneous femoral artery
        catheterization)
    After surgery (e.g., nephrectomy, thyroidectomy, laminectomy,
        cholecystectomy)
Infectious
    Syphilitic, mycotic
Artificial
    Hemodialysis
Tumors [e.g., nephroblastoma (Wilm's tumor)]

Ateriovenous shunting during hyperactivity of highly vascular tissues
Skin [e.g., dermatitis exfoliativa (erythroderma)]
Thyroid gland
    Severe thyrotoxicosis
Uterus
    Pregnancy
Bone
    Osteitis deformans (Paget's disease)
    Fibrous dysplasia (McCune-Albright syndrome)

[a]Capillary hemangiomas are highly unlikely to have hemodynamic repercussions.

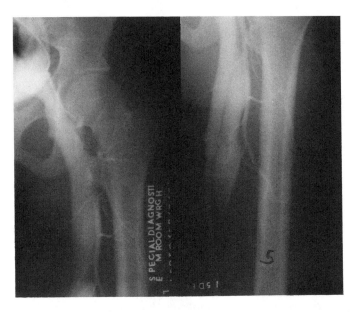

FIGURE 18.2. Left femoral arteriovenous fistula due to a pitchfork wound.

and reduction in systemic vascular resistance. Accordingly, a very small fistula may be merely of aesthetic consequence (e.g., a strawberry hemangioma), whereas an intrahepatic fistula in Osler-Weber-Rendu disease may lower the systemic vascular resistance enough to produce high output state.[12]

Hepatic hemangioendotheliomas[13] or Wilms' tumor[14]

of the kidney may lead to massive arteriovenous communication with high cardiac output and heart failure in infancy or childhood. Iatrogenic fistula of interest to cardiologists is one that follows percutaneous femoral artery catheterization, while a rare form of acquired fistula results from spontaneous rupture of an aortic aneurysm into the inferior vena cava with rapid development of heart failure.[15]

Manual compression of fistulas leads to reversal of the hyperkinetic circulation, which includes slowing of the heart rate (Branham's sign), increase of the arterial pressure, and decrease of the venous pressure (Fig. 18.3). In its rapidity, this response resembles the acute reversal of the high output state of chronic anemia effected by orthostasis or use of pressor agents and suggests reflex or chemical mediation as a common pathogenetic mechanism.[16] The presence and degree of

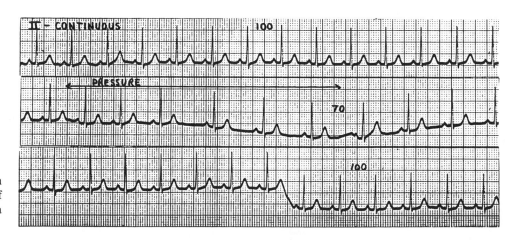

FIGURE 18.3. Continuous rhythm strip depicting the effect of manual compression of a fistula on heart rate.

underlying heart disease as well as the size of the arteriovenous communication and rapidity of onset are instrumental in the development of heart failure, an example being the onset of high output heart failure in hemodialyzed patients upon surgical shunt construction.

Observations in the canine model suggest that, when myocardial impairment is present, closure of a fistula results in little, if any, improvement in cardiac function.[17] Although clinical data to this effect are lacking, comparison can be made to patients with aortic insufficiency, which bears hemodynamic similarity to arteriovenous fistulas. Once severe ventricular diastolic dysfunction is established, mortality remains high and chances of symptomatic improvement are low after valve repair.[18] This has been attributed to repair-induced sudden reduction in preload and, therefore, loss of the ability to utilize the Starling mechanism, which is necessary to maintain cardiac output at a time when the cardiac function is depressed.

Vitamin B_1 Deficiency

Marked vasodilation is a central feature, and mediates the hyperkinetic state of cardiac beri-beri ("wet beri-beri"). The cause of the vasodilation is not known, but autonomic system dysfunction is possible since energy metabolism of the nervous system depends mostly on carbohydrates.[19] The hemodynamic response to vasodilation includes reflex tachycardia,[20] rapid circulation time, and widened pulse pressure, which indicates high cardiac output.[21] The quietening of the circulation after vasopressin injection and the stormy response to subcutaneous adrenaline confirm the role of vasodilation.[22] In contrast to chronic anemia, the hyperkinetic state of beri-beri also is characterized by blood volume expansion due to sodium and water retention by the kidneys.[20] Heart failure may develop suddenly with fulminant course leading to a fatal issue.[23]

Chronic Tachycardia

In the normal heart, when the rate increases acutely, the stroke volume decreases while the cardiac output rises because the increase in heart rate is greater than the corresponding decrease in stroke volume. However, upon reaching a peak at a critical heart rate, 120 to 138 beats/min during right atrial pacing in conscious instrumented dogs,[24] the cardiac output starts declining. This can be explained easily by the inadequate ventricular filling due to reduced duration of diastole which, at shorter cardiac cycles, decreases more than, and in favor of, systole. Given that increasing heart rate per se augments the myocardial oxygen requirements and further, that rate increases above a critical value are accompanied by a decline in cardiac output, the repercussions of tachycardia on cardiac efficiency seem obvious. Until recently, however, controversy had existed whether chronic (incessant) tachycardia could independently affect the myocardium and result in cardiac failure.

In dogs, rapid ventricular pacing for 3 weeks resulted in low output cardiac failure characterized by biventricular dilatation and impaired LV contractility.[25] Although it is now established that chronic supraventricular tachycardia can induce cardiomyopathy leading to marked cardiac dysfunction,[26–28] the precise requisite rate and duration are not known. While the exact pathophysiologic mechanism has not been identified, experimental studies suggest that the continuing rate burden results in a depletion of myocardial stores of creatine, creatine phosphate, and adenosine triphosphate.[27] Reported cases have most often had accessory atrioventricular pathways as the substrate for chronic reentrant supraventricular tachycardia. In these cases, antiarrhythmic therapy, utilizing multiple drugs, did not result in satisfactory suppression. Surgical incision or catheter ablation of the accessory pathway removed the arrhythmia substrate, with lasting effect. Depressed ejection fraction increased significantly, often returning to normal, while symptomatic improvement paralleled the objective change in cardiac performance.

Diet and Compliance

Diet

The major nutritional factors potentiating or contributing to CHF are cardiac cachexia and sodium/water imbalance.

Cardiac Cachexia

Heymsfield et al.[29] have noted two groups of cardiac patients likely to develop cardiac cachexia. First, about one third of their outpatients with class III or IV heart failure manifested mildly to moderately severe loss of lean body mass ("classic" cachexia). Second, after heart surgery, about 1 in every 15 patients was unable to resume normal eating habits (nosocomial cachexia). Reduced mid-arm muscle circumference, recessed temples, parchment-like skin, and low serum albumin level indicate undernutrition, which may otherwise go unnoticed due to normal body weight, secondary to edema.

Pathophysiologic mechanisms leading to cardiac cachexia involve anorexia, malabsorption, hypermetabolism, and impaired delivery of nutrients to, or clearance of, metabolites from the peripheral tissues.[29–31] It is unclear, however, which of the above is the leading or primary noxious factor. Two concepts have been proposed, the first of which suggests impaired delivery of nutrients to the periphery and the resultant tissue hypoxia as central in the cascade of cardiac cachexia. Tissue hypoxia leads to dyspnea, which may cause anorexia, whereas intestinal and hepatic or pancreatic hypoxia cause fat and nitrogen malabsorption by limiting active transport of nutrients across the intestinal villous membrane and reducing synthesis of bile salts or pancreatic enzymes, respectively.[29] Anorexia and malabsorption are in a sense adaptive abnormalities in that they reduce the energy requirements associated with ingestion of meals and active transport of nutrients. Resting hypermetabolism occurs in response to enhanced respiratory and cardiac muscle work and does not constitute an adaptive response. Instead, it magnifies further the reduction in net available energy.[30,31] In this model, the nutritional status can be improved only by enhancing cardiac output. In fact, increasing food intake without prior improvement of cardiac output would further compromise ventricular function.[29]

In the second model, the cascade of cachexia originates from anorexia, malabsorption, and hypermetabolism. In turn, the reduced supply of nutrients to the myocardium further depresses cardiac function. Based on this concept, hyperalimentation would ameliorate both the cardiac cachexia and the cardiac function.[29–32]

Sodium and Water Imbalance

The low cardiac output in CHF results in reduced renal perfusion. Consequently, several renal mechanisms are activated to enhance sodium and water retention and expand effective systemic blood volume.[33,34] Changes include enhanced activity of the renin-angiotensin-aldosterone system, altered intrarenal blood flow, and enhanced sodium reabsorption in the proximal tubule. In addition, reduced medullary blood flow decreases the kidney's ability to excrete water. Hence, total body sodium and total body water are increased in CHF.

For the average patient with CHF, moderate restriction of dietary sodium usually suffices, with a daily allowance of 2 g sodium.[33] More rigid salt restriction may render the diet unpalatable leading to undernourished state and/or poor compliance with the overall therapeutic regimen. At times, a more liberal salt intake is necessary, as in patients with a salt-losing nephropathy. Administration of angiotensin-converting enzyme (ACE) inhibitors may result in symptomatic hypotension, functional renal insufficiency, and hyperkalemia.[35] Increased dietary intake of salt and/or reduction in diuretic dosage can reverse these changes. Moderate water restriction, to about 1500 cc daily, is generally recommended.[33,34]

Compliance and Patient Behavior

A common cause of worsening CHF in treated patients is their failure to take their medications properly. Vinson et al.[36] reported that about one half of elderly patients with CHF require readmission within 90 days of initial discharge, usually for recurrence of symptoms.

Almost half of these readmissions were judged preventable: the causative factors included noncompliance with medications (15%) or diet (18%), inadequate discharge planning (15%), inadequate follow-up (20%), failure of the social support system (21%), and failure to seek medical attention promptly when symptoms recurred (20%). Further, in working-class urban minorities, a study observed that two thirds of readmissions for heart failure were due to noncompliance with medicines and/or diet.[37]

Hypertension

Systemic arterial hypertension (discussed as a primary cause elsewhere in this chapter) may contribute to or precipitate heart failure in the case of clinically latent LV dysfunction. Hypertension may adversely affect the myocardial oxygen supply/demand ratio in several ways: by increasing LV end-systolic wall stress (afterload) and myocardial oxygen demand; by increasing LV diastolic (mean left atrial) pressure and, thus, decreasing the diastolic pressure time index (DPTI, the area under the diastolic aortic pressure curve minus mean left atrial pressure times heart rate), which is an index of diastolic perfusion of the endocardium;[38] and by prolonging the isovolumic relaxation interval[39] by an average of 50 ms, which may increase further the extravascular resistance to coronary flow in early diastole.[6] In regard to pump function, acute elevation of the aortic pressure (afterload) in the animal model[40] shifts the cardiac function (Frank-Starling) curve downward and rightward; the maximum stroke volume decreases[40] and the end-diastolic volume rises.[41] These changes do not necessarily reflect a reduction in intrinsic contractility; an increase in afterload pressure, by definition, shifts the end-systolic point of the pressure-volume loop up along the line of the end-systolic pressure/volume relation and can alone decrease the stroke volume (Fig. 18.4). In fact, the intrinsic contractility may acutely increase, as suggested by the steeper slope of the end-systolic pressure/volume relation,[42] possibly due to enhanced adrenergic tone. In LV dysfunction (Panel B), when the slope of the end-systolic pressure/volume relation is decreased, a similar increase in afterload may cause a significantly greater decrease in stroke volume, prompting forward failure, and an increase in LV end-diastolic pressure, which may lead rapidly to pulmonary edema.

Drugs

A wide spectrum of drugs has the potential of precipitating or intensifying CHF. These agents are presented in Table 18.2, categorized by their effect(s) on the determinants of cardiac performance; that is, heart rhythm, inotropic status, preload, and afterload. For

A

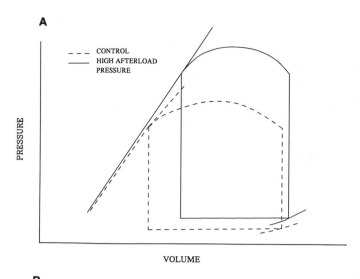

B

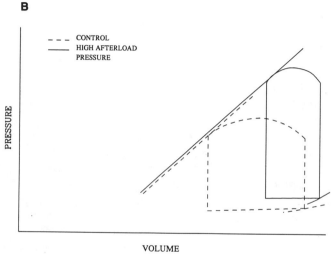

Figure 18.4. Pressure-volume loops and end-systolic pressure/volume relations in the normal (**A**) and failing ventricle (**B**), at normal and high afterload pressures. Note the greater reduction in stroke volume in the failing ventricle when afterload is increased.

completeness, direct cardiotoxins (see chapter 13) also are included.

The net effect of a pharmacologic agent on cardiac function can vary depending on the prevailing clinical conditions such as inotropic status, heart rhythm, neurohumoral milieu and presence of significant coronary artery disease, and their interaction. For instance, the in vitro negative inotropic effect of nifedipine usually is countered, in vivo, by reflex sympathetic hyperactivity in response to decreased systemic vascular resistance; however, under conditions of reduced inotropy and maximal sympathetic stimulation, the direct effect may be unmasked, prompting overt heart failure. The significance of the sympathetic tone as an independent variable also can be found in the xamoterol experience. This β_1-selective partial agonist exhibits β_1-adreno-

TABLE 18.2. Pharmacologic agents causing or contributing to CHF.

Mechanism	Agent
Inappropriate heart rhythm	
Bradycardia	β-adrenergic blockers; calcium channel blockers: verapamil, diltiazem; centrally acting α_2-adrenergic agonists: methyldopa, clonidine; adrenergic neuron blockers: reserpine
Tachycardia	Xanthines; sympathomimetic amines: epinephrine, isuprel, dobutamine, ephedrine
Arrhythmias	Antiarrhythmics (particularly encainide, flecainide); xanthines; digoxin; lithium carbonate; tricyclic antidepressants; phenothiazines
Negative inotropism	β-adrenergic blockers; calcium channel blockers (predominantly first generation); antiarrhythmics: disopyramide, encainide, flecainide, quinidine, procainamide; general anesthetics
Altered preload	
Salt and water retention	Vasodilators: diazoxide, hydralazine, minoxidil; nonsteroidal anti-inflammatory agents; corticosteroids; adrenergic neuron blockers: guanethidine, reserpine; centrally acting α_2-adrenergic agonists: methydopa; androgens; estrogens; salicylates (high dose); lithium carbonate; volume expanders: mannitol, albumin; high sodium–containing agents: carbenicillin disodium
Excess salt and water loss	Diuretics
Elevated afterload	Sympathomimetic amines: nasal decongestants (phenylephrine, ephedrine, mephentermine, propylhexedrine), norepinephine, dopamine, metaraminol
Cardiotoxicity	Antineoplastic agents: anthracyclines[a] [doxorubicin (adriamycin), daunorubicin], cyclophosphamide, 5-fluorouracil; cyclosporin A; methysergide; antimalarials or amebicidals: chloroquine, emetine; lithium carbonate; tricyclic antidepressants; phenothiazines

[a] Cumulative dose-dependent toxicity.

receptor antagonism at high levels of sympathetic tone, which may explain the detrimental effect in class III and IV heart failure.[43]

Perhaps in no other clinical syndrome does the burden of accurately assessing risks and benefits of pharmacologic intervention fall more heavily on the physician; a fine example of the intricacies encountered can be found in the decision to treat the so-called potentially malignant arrhythmias on a substrate of ventricular dysfunction. For, although it is true that more than one third of deaths in heart failure are sudden, it also may be argued that arrhythmia suppression does not necessarily imply improved survival. In fact, in the Cardiac Arrhythmia Suppression Trial the mortality was 100% or higher in the flecainide and encainide-treated groups compared to the placebo group, even though the patients were given these drugs only after demonstration of short-term arrhythmia suppression. The dilemma to treat or not is compounded further by the facts that heart failure occurred or worsened at a high frequency in the Cardiac Arrhythmia Pilot Study[44] and that a proarrhythmic effect is more likely in patients with low ejection fraction (EF). Finally, in the context of a discussion on CHF it is appropriate to stress that negative inotropism is not pharmacologically unique to class IC agents but, rather, a natural sequela of the intended action in most antiarrhythmics.[45-47]

Obesity

Obesity may be a lifelong problem or, more commonly, one of adulthood. Adipocytes (fat cells) are differentiated from precursor cells, preadipocytes. Excess caloric intake initially leads to an increase in size (hypertrophy) of existing fat cells until a maximum mass per cell, approximately 1 μg, is reached when new adipocytes are being formed (hyperplasia). In contrast, a negative energy balance may alter the size but not the number of existing adipocytes. Defining obesity on the basis of "weight tables" provided by insurance companies is rather arbitrary and requires judgment. For instance, a heavily muscled individual may weigh more than published norms, but not be obese. However, obesity usually is present when fat makes up a greater than a normal fraction of total body weight, approximately 15% and 20% in the average young man and woman, respectively.

Although studies on the relationship of obesity and risk of coronary artery disease are divergent, follow-up data from the Framingham Study indicate obesity as an independent cardiac risk factor. Further, the National Health and Nutrition Examination Surveys documented a strong correlation between obesity and other cardiovascular risk factors; the prevalence of both hypertension and diabetes mellitus is 2.9 times higher for overweight than lean persons, and the incidence of hypercholesteremia is 2.1 times higher in young overweight compared to nonoverweight individuals.[48]

As body fat accumulates, cardiac output increases to meet the oxygen needs of the excess adipose tissue. The rise in cardiac output is achieved by increases in stroke volume, while the resting heart rate remains unchanged.[49] In addition, both the total blood volume and the central blood volume, that is, the volume distributed between the right atrium and aortic valve, increase.[50] Due to an increase in ventricular end-diastolic volume and pressure, and in order to normalize end-diastolic wall stress, the ventricular mass (not the wall thickness) expands and the cavity dilates by addition of sarcomeres in series. Upon reaching the point when the end-systolic radius increases, the end-systolic wall stress starts rising. Then, to prevent further elevation in end-systolic wall stress, the LV wall thickens by addition of sarcomeres in parallel. Therefore, the additive effect of obesity is ventricular dilation and wall thickening (eccentric hypertrophy).[51] As a rule of thumb, LV hypertrophy can be anticipated in over 50% of patients who are more than 50% overweight.[49,51] Despite these adaptations, the left atrial emptying index,[52] a marker of ventricular diastolic compliance and function, and the end-systolic pressure/volume ratio, a load-independent index of inotropic status, are reduced even in mild obesity and in the absence of other cardiomyopathic processes.[53]

Comparison is made between the lean hypertensive patient who develops concentric LV hypertrophy and the obese normotensive patient who manifests eccentric hypertrophy. Both exhibit an equivalent, approximately 40%, increase in LV stroke work due, in the lean hypertensive, to increased afterload and in the obese normotensive, to augmented stroke volume. In a patient who is obese and hypertensive, the increase in stroke work may exceed 60%.[49,51]

Weight reduction correlates significantly with a decrease in mean arterial pressure and LV mass.[54] Total and central blood volume also decrease. Further, weight loss is accompanied by a decrease in plasma norepinephrine level, which suggests that a reduction in adrenergic tone may be a factor in lowering blood pressure, plasma renin activity of at least 50%, and aldosterone levels irrespective of sodium intake.[50] These favorable hemodynamic and humoral responses to weight reduction afford, in reverse fashion, insight to the role of obesity in CHF.

Pulmonary Disease

Pulmonary disease can affect the cardiac function by several mechanisms, including increased work of breathing, altered afterload, hypoxemia, hypercapnia, and accompanying metabolic and electrolytic imbalance, and cardiac effects of drugs used to treat respiratory abnormalities.

The work of normal quiet breathing equals 2% to 3% of the total body energy expenditure and is used completely for inspiration, since expiration is a passive process driven by the elastic recoil.[55] In heavy breathing, however, substantial muscle effort is needed to overcome airway and tissue resistance and under certain conditions such as asthma, the expiratory work can exceed that of inspiration. During heavy exertion a 25-fold increase in breathing work can occur along with a parallel rise in total body energy expenditure.

The inspiratory work has three components: compliance work required for lung expansion against elastic forces, tissue resistance work needed to overcome lung and chest wall viscosity, and airway resistance work.[55] Compliance work equals the change in lung volume times the average pleural pressure needed to cause the expansion. During quiet normal breathing, tissue and airway resistance constitute less than one third of the total work of breathing. Ratios of these components to the total work of breathing are altered during heavy breathing or in various disease states. For instance, diffuse pulmonary fibrosis increases both the compliance and the tissue resistance work. In addition, pulmonary disease can augment the work of breathing to the point that it absorbs one fourth or more of the total body energy, in which case the work of breathing alone could cause death through exhaustion.

Markedly negative intrathoracic pressure swings, as seen with reduced chest compliance, severe obstructive disease, or high tissue viscosity, can increase the LV transmural pressure (ventricular pressure relative to atmosphere minus pericardial pressure), a major determinant of wall stress (afterload), and impair cardiac performance. For instance, the increase in afterload effected by the Mueller maneuver has been shown to prompt LV wall motion abnormalities in patients with coronary artery disease.[56] Further, an acute asthmatic attack alone is sufficient to precipitate acute pulmonary edema.[57] Conversely, increases in intrathoracic pressure by means of mechanical ventilation, with or without positive end-expiratory pressure and with or without gating to the cardiac cycle, decrease the afterload inasmuch as negative intrathoracic pressure augments it. In the normal heart, where systemic venous return is the major determinant of cardiac output, an increase in intrathoracic pressure decreases the cardiac performance. In heart failure, however, when output is primarily dependent on pump performance and less sensitive to altered preload, increases in intrathoracic pressure may augment cardiac output and decrease myocardial oxygen consumption.[58]

The effect of acute and chronic hypoxemia on LV function can be significant. In a canine model of acute hypoxemia, Walley et al.[59] observed that when arterial blood oxygen saturation was decreased from 95% to 64%, coronary blood flow increased, thus maintaining normal myocardial oxygen delivery. However, at oxygen saturation below 64%, there was no further increase in coronary blood flow but instead, the myocar-

dial oxygen extraction started to rise. Subsequently, there was a fall in the LV pressure-volume area, a measure of the external cardiac work, and a decrease in the end-systolic pressure/volume relation, suggesting depressed contractility. Wexler et al.[60] showed that 2-min hypoxemia resulted in decreased diastolic distensibility (hypoxemic contracture). Further, the chronicity of hypoxemia may result in irreversible myocardial impairment. In assessing LV function of patients after correction of Fallot's tetralogy, Hausdorf et al.[61] noted that the severity of preoperative hypoxemia was an important risk factor for late dysfunction.

Arrhythmias complicating chronic pulmonary disease, cor pulmonale, and sleep apnea[62] are well documented, and the underlying mechanisms are complex including hypoxemia, hypercapnia, acid-base imbalance, electrolytic abnormalities, and cardiac effects of xanthines and β-adrenoreceptor agonists. Little is known about the arrhythmogenic effect of an acute asthmatic attack. In 13 asthmatic children with presumed normal cardiac function before a fatal crisis, Drislane et al.[63] noted the presence of myocardial contraction band necrosis in four, two of whom had not received sympathomimetics. This finding raised the possibility of an adrenergic surge-mediated arrhythmic death. However, Molfino et al.[64] observed no serious cardiac arrhythmias in 10 patients resuscitated from near-fatal asthma.

Of the various pharmacologic agents used in pulmonary disease, three classes have important cardiovascular effects.

β-Adrenergic Agonists

The earlier used, nonselective β-adrenergic agonists such as epinephrine and isuprel, have now been largely superseded by more specific β_2-agonists including terbutaline, albuterol, isoetharine, and bitolterol. For patients with heart failure, the advantages of these agents, particularly when given in aerosol form, include less tachycardia, fewer arrhythmias,[65] and less cardiac work. When given systemically, β-adrenergic agonists may enhance cardiac function but this effect often is transient.[66,67] In fact, there have been reports where systemic use of β-adrenergic agonists during pregnancy induced heart failure.[68–70]

Steroids

Preexisting heart failure may deteriorate with systemic corticosteroids due to sodium retention and volume expansion, hypokalemia, and rarely, hypertension. In contrast, inhaled corticosteroids (beclomethasone, fluocinonide, and triamcinolone) have no significant side effects and their use may afford reduction of oral steroid dosage.

Methylxanthines

These agents exert a positive inotropic and chronotropic effect, part of which is mediated by the release of catecholamines. In addition, they dilate the resistance vessels including the coronary arteries, and increase coronary blood flow. Since the cardiac work also increases, however, the outstanding question is whether the rise in oxygen supply exceeds that in demand. Patients with heart failure are at increased risk of theophylline toxicity due to the drug's half-life prolongation. Also, theophylline-related multifocal atrial tachycardia may rapidly lead to hemodynamic compromise owing to decreased ventricular filling.

Environmental Factors

Heat and Humidity

To preserve normothermia, the rates of heat production and heat loss from the body must be in equilibrium. At normal ambient temperature, heat dissipation is regulated largely by changes in cutaneous blood flow; from the skin surface, heat is lost by means of radiation and conduction (convection). With increases in thermal load (e.g., fever, physical exertion) or with rising ambient temperature, the cutaneous vasodilation needed to dissipate heat effects a marked decrease in systemic vascular resistance. This, in turn, results in an increase in systemic venous pressure and venous return/cardiac output, reflex tachycardia, and widened pulse pressure. Unfortunately, when the ambient temperature exceeds the body temperature not only is heat absorbed from the environment, but the increased cutaneous blood flow enhances the absorption of heat by the body. In addition, radiation and conduction are, obviously, no more effective and excess body heat can be lost only by evaporation of sweat. For evaporative heat loss to occur, the water vapor saturation of the surrounding air, relative humidity (RH), must be less than 100%; the lower the RH, the more rapid the evaporation will be. Thus, heat imparts a volume overload onto the myocardium while high humidity potentiates and prolongs this burden by delaying heat dissipation.

Burch and his colleagues pioneered research on the effect of climatic factors in the cardiac patient.[71] In one study, they examined the effect of heat at two levels of humidity (41% and 75% RH) in 23, predominantly (90%) female patients with functional class II or III CHF secondary to hypertensive, rheumatic, or ischemic heart disease.[72] This earlier work did not include invasive hemodynamic monitoring. Sixty-five percent and 78% of patients developed overt, albeit unspecified, heart failure upon exposure to a hot-dry (90°F, 41% RH) and hot-humid (90°F, 75% RH) environment, respectively. Further, the cardiac and respiratory rates increased significantly only in hot-humid environment. These data emphasize that a hot-humid environment is more unfavorable to the cardiovascular system than a hot-dry one and underscore the need for a controlled climate in patients with significant myocardial dysfunction.

Cold

Exposure to cold causes reflex cutaneous vasoconstriction in order to minimize body heat loss. This results in an increased systemic vascular resistance and arterial pressure, with little change in heart rate.[73] The increase in stroke work imparted to the myocardium may precipitate failure in the presence of ventricular dysfunction. Furthermore, reflex coronary vasoconstriction may occur in conjunction with the cutaneous vascular response, while focal coronary artery spasm can be provoked by the cold pressor test.[74] In patients with a history of angina pectoris and intolerance to cold, exercise in a cold environment resulted in symptoms and electrocardiographic changes of ischemia in a 30% shorter time interval than exercise in normal temperature.[75]

In conclusion, the hemodynamic response to altered ambient temperature is dimorphic; that is, an increase in cardiac work results from a rise in total peripheral resistance at low temperature (pressure work) and a rise in cardiac output when the temperature is high (flow work).

Electrolyte Abnormalities

Electrolyte disorders in CHF can cause two major problems: serious ventricular arrhythmias and decreased contractility.

Arrhythmias

The patient with organic or structural heart disease is at higher risk for sudden cardiac death and serious ventricular arrhythmias.[76,77] In general, the degree of risk parallels the extent of cardiac disease.

Hypokalemia

The importance of diuretic-induced hypokalemia in hypertension is controversial.[78,79] In the patient with heart failure, hypokalemia plays an important role in ventricular ectopy and sudden cardiac death.[80,81] Patients with CHF have reduced total body potassium even in the absence of diuretic therapy.[82,83] Indeed, intracellular hypokalemia may be secondary to hypomagnesemia. Since magnesium acts on sodium-potassium adenosine triphosphatase, it follows that hypomagnesemia may decrease intracellular potassium even when serum potassium is normal. The potassium-sparing diuretics, such as spironolactone, appear to be effective in restoring potassium balance since they spare magnesium as well as potassium.[84] In the patient with CHF, particularly when treated with digitalis, serum potassium levels should be maintained, ideally at $\geq$4.5 mEq/L and certainly above 4 mEq/L.

Hypomagnesemia

Magnesium is the second most abundant intracellular cation that is involved in the metabolism of adenosine triphosphate, membrane transport systems (sodium-potassium pump), muscle contraction, and countless other enzymatic processes. Magnesium decreases AV nodal conduction, which might explain its efficacy in suppressing supraventricular arrhythmias, and reduces the amplitude of cesium-induced afterdepolarizations in the animal model, which may underlie its effectiveness in torsade de pointes.

In a recent study of 199 patients with CHF, Gottlieb and colleagues found 38 patients with hypomagnesemia.[85] This group, compared to patients with normomagnesemia, exhibited more frequent ventricular tachycardia and a lower 1-yr survival rate (45% vs. 71%). Dyckner[86] notes that both hypokalemia and hypomagnesemia are important in patients with CHF, especially those receiving diuretics or digitalis. However, the association between hypomagnesemia and ventricular arrhythmias is not universally agreed on, partly because of the difficulty in establishing a cause and effect relationship between the two conditions. This is compounded by the lack of a universal standard for magnesium deficiency and inherent problems in assessing magnesium balance due to a poor correlation between serum magnesium and its concentration in muscle, red blood cells, or the myocardium.

In conclusion, even though the serum level is the most readily available method for magnesium measurement, the above limitations should always be borne in mind. Finally, correction of serum potassium to normal level does not necessarily imply intracellular normokalemia. In fact, since potassium and magnesium depletion often occur concurrently, magnesium supplements are necessary for intracellular potassium stores to be repleted.

Decreased Contractility

Hypocalcemia

CHF can be precipitated by hypocalcemia[87] and a cardiomyopathy apparently due to hypocalcemia (6 mg%) alone occasionally is recognized.[88,89] Patients on chronic dialysis with heart failure and hypocalcemia have an unrecognized element of hypocalcemic cardiomyopathy.[90] Correction of serum calcium may result in substantial clinical improvement.[87]

Exogenous Causes of Congestive Heart Failure

Carbon Monoxide

Carbon monoxide is an odorless, colorless, tasteless gas produced by incomplete combustion of organic matter. It binds to hemoglobin by displacing oxygen and therefore disrupts the oxygen transport system. With an affinity for hemoglobin 220 times that of oxygen, even in minute concentrations, carbon monoxide results in high carboxyhemoglobin levels.[91] Since the oxygen concentration in the atmosphere is approximately 21% by volume, exposure to 0.1% carbon monoxide in air would effect 50% carboxyhemoglobinemia, which constitutes severe and life-threatening poisoning.[92] In addition, carbon monoxide shifts the oxyhemoglobin dissociation curve to the left, thereby reducing further the oxygen availability to the tissues, and exerts a direct toxic effect by binding to cellular cytochrome. The last two effects may explain why, despite a similar oxygen-carrying capacity, an anemic patient with hemoglobin of 8 g% and a person with 50% carboxyhemoglobin manifest dissimilar symptoms, the former being relatively asymptomatic, the latter nearing collapse.

Cigarette smoke is a major environmental source of carbon monoxide. The fraction of carboxyhemoglobin to total hemoglobin is less than 2% in nonsmokers, 3% to 8% in chronic smokers, and 10% to 15% immediately after smoking a cigarette.[93] These levels of carboxyhemoglobin can be hazardous both in the presence and absence of cardiac disease. In nonsmokers with ischemic heart disease, an induced carboxylhemoglobinemia of 6% decreased the exercise tolerance, aggravated the anginal symptoms,[93] and enhanced the incidence and complexity of ventricular arrhythmias.[94] Further, myocardial infarction has been reported in a patient with normal coronary arteries after carbon monoxide poisoning due to smoke inhalation.[95] These data suggest that in patients with existing cardiac dysfunction, exposure to carbon monoxide may further impair the myocardium.[96]

Radiation

Although the heart is considered resistant to ionizing irradiation, mediastinal radiotherapy may have important cardiac sequelae[97] including pericarditis with effusion, tamponade, and constriction; coronary microvascular injury and thrombosis; accelerated narrowing of epicardial coronary arteries; acute and chronic involvement of the myocardium (fibrosis); and endocardial fibrosis. Burns et al.[98] observed a slightly decreased LV ejection fraction in 57% of pediatric patients after mediastinal irradiation for Hodgkin's disease. In a study of 21 women after mediastinal irradiation, Ikaheimo et al.[99] showed LV dysfunction to occur transiently; by 6 months, the cardiac function had normalized, but one third of the patients still manifested small pericardial effusion.

There are no data on the effect of radiation on patients with preexisting heart failure. However, in keeping with the above observations, the effect would be expected to be mild. Further, with current mediastinal radiotherapy techniques, irradiation of the heart is likely to be negligible.

Electrical Shock

The hazard of electrical shock is ubiquitous[100,101] in the home, at the workplace, and in nature. The awesome force of a lightning strike causes several hundred deaths yearly, and another 1500 fatalities result from high voltage electricity. It is estimated that the electromotive force of a lightning discharge ranges between millions and one billion volts; hence, a direct strike is always fatal. An indirect strike or splash results when a lightning bolt hits a tree or other object and is then reflected to a person nearby. Depending on skin resistance, the intensity of the direct current traversing through the body may vary from 50,000 to 200,000 amperes. The most frequent cause of death in lightning strike is cardiac, the massive electrical discharge being analogous to the effect of a direct current cardioverter. Flow of electrical current through the heart prompts myocardial contraction, often followed by a period of asystole and, usually, a return to sinus rhythm. However, should asystole persist so as to cause serious hypoxemia or respiratory center paralysis, ventricular fibrillation and death may ensue. Thus, due to protracted depression of the respiratory center, sustained resuscitative efforts may be necessary. Reports of individuals who survived lightning strike with minor or no sequelae abound. However, myocardial infarction and late onset severe LV dysfunction can occur.[102] The electrocardiographic findings include transient, diffuse ST-T abnormalities that may persist for weeks or months.

Electrical injuries in the home or workplace are related to alternating current, which causes tetanic muscle contraction, thus "locking" the victim onto the electrical source. The risk for cardiac arrhythmias and ventricular asystole or apnea is high and correlates with the intensity of the voltage of the alternating current source, although even the low household voltage (110 volts) can be fatal. Discharge from a high tension source (1000 volts or more) can result in widespread focal myocardial necrosis and myocardial fiber rupture.[103] In addition, contraction band necrosis involving the tunica media of the coronary arteries can occur, implying protracted coronary artery spasm, which may lead to a fatal myocardial infarction.

Cocaine

Cocaine usage can be traced in the Andes for untold years. However, its current recreational use in the United States has reached epidemic proportions. Of 30 million Americans who have tried it at least once, 6 million are regular, and 1 million are compulsive users.[104] Reports of myocardial ischemia, acute myocardial infarction, and sudden death due to cocaine abuse abound. Angiography performed after acute myocardial infarction documented normal coronary anatomy in 20% of cases, occlusive thrombus in 30%, and significant stenoses in the remaining 50%.[105–108] In young men who presented with chest pain after cocaine use and in whom myocardial infarction was ruled out, the coronary arteries were normal and neither diffuse vasoconstriction nor local spasm could be provoked by ergonovine;[109] however, endomyocardial biopsy revealed considerable wall thickening of intramural coronary arteries in 64% of patients, indicating small vessel coronary artery disease.

Cocaine is a local anesthetic that inhibits the reuptake of norepinephrine and dopamine at the presynaptic sympathetic nerve terminal and thus increases the postsynaptic concentration of these agents. In addition, cocaine stimulates catecholamine release from the adrenal medulla and its effects on heart rate and arterial blood pressure are dose-dependent. Kuhn et al.[110] investigated the effect of graded doses of cocaine on the coronary and the systemic circulation in the canine model. At a dose of 2 mg/kg there was a significant increase in coronary vascular resistance and an approximately 20% reduction in the diameter of the left anterior descending coronary artery. Cocaine-induced coronary vasoconstriction was mediated by α-adrenergic receptors and was prevented by pretreatment with an α-adrenergic antagonist, but not by a β-adrenergic antagonist. Further, the coronary vasoconstriction was diffuse without focal spasm and without electrocardiographic or biochemical (lactate production) evidence of ischemia. Lange and colleagues[111] quantified the degree of vasoconstriction in human epicardial coronary arteries at the time of diagnostic angiography; intranasally administered cocaine produced an 8% to 12% reduction in luminal diameter of the left anterior descending artery with a corresponding decrease in coronary sinus blood flow. In distinction from the effects on the coronary vasculature, the systemic hemodynamic response to cocaine is mediated by both α- and β-adrenoceptors.[110]

There is convincing evidence that, apart from adrenoreceptor-mediated vasoconstriction, cocaine exerts a direct effect on vascular smooth muscle. The fact that cocaine augments tension in human umbilical arteries in vitro, even though these arteries are devoid of sympathetic innervation, indicates a direct effect, possibly through enhancement of calcium flux across the cell membrane.[112] In addition to direct and indirect effects resulting in coronary vasoconstriction, there is evidence that cocaine increases thromboxane production and platelet aggregation, and cases have been reported of transient depression of myocardial contractility.[113]

Specific Diseases Causing Congestive Heart Failure

Several diseases can lead to, or exacerbate, CHF. These disorders may affect the myocardium, the specialized conduction system, or the loading conditions of the heart. Some of these disorders and their mechanisms of action are discussed briefly in this section.

Hypertension

Hypertension is a frequent cause of CHF in the United States. Cardiac dysfunction occurs six times more frequently in hypertensive versus normotensive individuals.[114] LV hypertrophy, echocardiographically defined as 110 g/M^2 or greater for women and 134 g/M^2 or greater for men,[115] conveys a six- to eightfold increase in risk of cardiac death due to either pump failure or coronary artery disease[116] and also enhances risk for sudden cardiac death.

The cardiac muscle fiber loses mitotic activity soon after birth, and myocardial cell enlargement becomes the principal process by which the heart enlarges. Ventricular wall thickness increases by addition of sarcomeres in series and parallel.[117] This results in less tension per sarcomere, but also augments the myocardial energetic requirements. Thus, the ability of the mitochondria to increase proportionately to energy demand may determine whether the muscle shortening velocity will be decreased, normal, or increased.[118] Similar to limited growth of mitochondrial mass in hypertrophy, there is restricted proliferation of capillaries that does not keep pace with contractile protein synthesis during the process of hypertrophy. This may result in hypoxia, which serves as a stimulus for collagen synthesis.[119] Wilkman-Coffelt et al.[118] defined hypertrophy as physiological when it is accompanied by a normal or augmented contractility. In this case, the maximum rate at which myosin hydrolyzes adenosine triphosphate (ATP) and the maximum velocity of muscle shortening are either normal or elevated. Pathological hypertrophy is defined as the situation in which contractility is depressed and both the rate of myosin ATPase activity and velocity of muscle shortening are decreased.

In patients with pressure overload, Grossman et al.[120] found that LV peak systolic and end-diastolic pressures were increased as compared to controls, whereas the wall stress remained normal throughout the cardiac cycle. However, with volume overload, the systolic wall stress did not differ from control, but the diastolic wall stress was high, supporting the contention that hypertrophy develops to normalize systolic, but not diastolic, wall stress. Based on these observations, the authors[120] postulated that when increased afterload is the primary stimulus, the myocardium hypertrophies through replication of sarcomeres in parallel (concentric hypertrophy, increased wall thickness/radius ratio), which normalizes the systolic wall stress and that, when the primary stimulus is volume overload (increased end-diastolic wall stress), the myocardium first undergoes replication of sarcomeres in series with ventricular cavity enlargement. Then, the enlarged cavity leads to an increase in end-systolic radius and wall stress, thereby promoting replication of sarcomeres in parallel (eccentric hypertrophy, normal wall thickness/radius ratio).

Pathophysiologically, the myocardial response to hypertension varies widely from minor increase in LV mass to LV hypertrophy with or without systolic and/or diastolic dysfunction. The early cardiac response to hypertension consists of a hyperdynamic state, characterized by increased contractility due to enhanced adrenergic tone,[121] as seen after isoproterenol administration in normotensives.[122] This initial upward and leftward shift of the cardiac function curve may subside upon development of sufficient wall thickness to normalize systolic wall stress. With progressively increasing LV wall thickness, the cavity dimensions and compliance decrease, resulting in prolonged relaxation time index (minimum LV dimension to mitral valve opening),[123] reduced filling rates,[124] vigorous atrial contraction, and gradual atrial enlargement (diastolic dysfunction stage). At this stage, symptoms and signs of backward failure including dyspnea of effort, paroxysmal nocturnal dyspnea, S$_4$ gallop, pulmonary vascular plethora, and rales may appear, although systolic LV function remains characteristically normal or supranormal. In our institution, serving a population with a high prevalence of hypertension, it is not infrequent to encounter patients presenting in florid pulmonary edema despite the presence of an ejection fraction of 70% or more. In later stages of hypertensive hypertrophic cardiomyopathy and in association with severe, sustained, and often poorly treated hypertension, resting LV systolic function declines.[125] This stage, often referred to as "burned-out" hypertension, usually is associated with cavity dilatation, which further increases systolic wall stress, thereby perpetuating a vicious cycle.

Connective Tissue Diseases

Since vasculitis is a common histologic characteristic, cardiac involvement is inevitable in all collagen vascular

TABLE 18.3. Cardiac manifestations in connective tissue disorders.

	Systemic lupus erythematosus	Scleroderma	Dermatomyositis/ polymyositis	Rheumatoid arthritis	Polyarteritis nodosa
Clinical expressivity	50%[a]	5–15%[a]	Up to 50%	3%	50–65%[b]
Incidence at nercropsy	>80%	80–95%	Up to 75%	30%	>50%
Cardinal histologic lesion	Diffuse vasculitis	Marked fibrosis	Fibrosis	Nodular[c] granulomas	Necrotizing vasculitis
Pericarditis	>80%; in 50% clinical	30%, subclinical	Rare	In 50% of patients with granulomas	Rare
Endocarditis	>30%, verrucous	Uncommon	Common	10%	Uncommon
Myocarditis	10–40%	Uncommon	Common	20%	Uncommon
Incidence of atherosclerosis compared to controls	Higher	Not different	Not different	Less common	Not different
Atrioventricular conduction defects	Rare	10–20%	Common	Rare	Rare
Hypertension, pulmonary, and systemic	Common	Very common	Rare	Rare	Very common

[a] Clinical cardiac disease is in part associated to systemic disease.
[b] In most cases, congestive heart failure is secondary to hypertension and renal failure.
[c] Vasculitis is central in the development of the rheumatoid nodule.

diseases (Table 18.3). In earlier years, subclinical cardiac disease could be recognized only at necropsy, but newer sophisticated techniques allow ante mortem diagnosis in most cases. The prevalence of clinical cardiac disease varies from very common, as in systemic lupus erythematosus, to rare, as in rheumatoid arthritis. Finally, the commonly occurring CHF in polyarteritis nodosa is in most cases secondary to severe hypertension and renal failure rather than primary cardiomyopathy due to necrotizing vasculitis.

Systemic Lupus Erythematosus

Multifaceted cardiac involvement is common in systemic lupus erythematosus (SLE) and includes pericarditis (most common) with or without effusion; myocarditis or cardiomyopathy, occasionally with conduction system defect; LV hypertrophy secondary to renal hypertension; myocardial infarction secondary to atherosclerosis rather than coronary arteritis; and nonbacterial verrucous endocarditis (Libman-Sacks).[126]

Myocardial involvement in SLE is well established.[127] Myocarditis manifests with tachycardia, mild dyspnea, or overt heart failure and nonspecific T-wave changes, and P-R prolongation on the electrocardiogram (Fig. 18.5). Diffuse foci of myocardial necrosis due to arteritis can globally depress LV function,[127] while thrombotic occlusion of a major coronary artery branch is bound to cause segmental wall motion abnormalities. Nihoyannopoulos et al.[128] found a high sensitivity and specificity of high level anticardiolipin antibodies in predicting cardiac abnormalities, not only in SLE, but also in other lupus-like syndromes. Strikingly, all their patients with thrombotic coronary artery lesions had increased anticardiolipin antibodies. These data support the theory that cardiac involvement is mediated by antiphospholipid antibodies, possibly via a primary stimulation of vascular endothelium by immunologic factors,[129] and perhaps similar immunologic mechanisms may underlie the enhanced atherogenesis[130] and increased incidence of myocardial infarction among patients with SLE.

Polymyositis (Dermatomyositis)

Polymyositis is a disease of unknown etiology primarily affecting striated muscle[131] and various connective tissues. When skin involvement is present, the disease is called dermatomyositis.[132] Diffuse cardiac involvement is common and includes conduction system abnormalities (fibrosis of sinoatrial node, AV node, bundle of His and bundle branches), and cardiomyopathy with scattered areas of fibrosis, pericarditis, and endomyocardial fibrosis.[133]

Although survival studies in polymyositis relate death to pneumonitis, autopsies in patients with this syndrome suggest higher frequency of cardiac involvement.[134] Cardiomyopathy presents with cardiac failure or arrhythmias in the form of complete heart block or ventricular tachycardia and may result in syncope, cardiac arrest, or death.

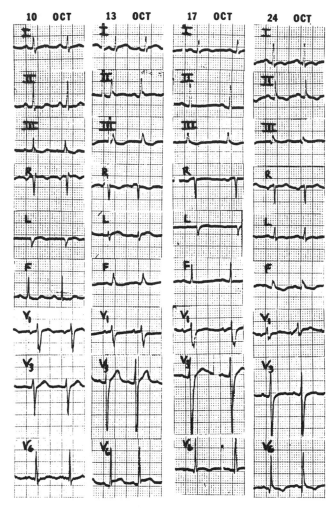

FIGURE 18.5. The electrocardiogram of a young woman with SLE and acute pericarditis.

Scleroderma (Progressive Systemic Sclerosis)

Scleroderma is an uncommon disease. It is characterized by generalized involvement, through an unknown mechanism, of small arteries and microvessels and is manifest by increased fibrosis and vascular obliteration of skin and visceral connective tissue. Endothelial cell changes, vasomotor and permeability changes, platelet activation, and perivascular mononuclear cell infiltrates are present in target tissues before fibrosis becomes prominent.[135]

Atherosclerosis of major coronary arteries occurs as frequently in patients with systemic sclerosis as in controls, but intimal sclerosis of small coronary arteries with ischemic wall infarctions and fibrosis is much more common in scleroderma.[135] Pericardial effusion, usually asymptomatic, can be large enough to cause tamponade and occurs even in the absence of uremia. Studies employing diverse diagnostic procedures including [201]Thallium scintigraphy, echocardiography, electrocardiography, 24-hr Holter monitoring, and rest and exercise nuclear ventriculography have shown the prevalence of cardiac involvement in diffuse systemic sclerosis to vary from 80% to 95% even in the absence of cardiovascular symptoms,[136,137] presumably reflecting small vessel disease.

Scleroderma heart disease manifests itself as pericarditis and CHF. Primary heart failure usually appears late in the disease and needs be differentiated from failure secondary to hypertension from renal disease. Mortality in scleroderma patients with overt heart failure is 100% by 7 yrs.[138]

Sickle Cell Anemia

Cardiovascular adaptation to steady-state sickle cell anemia includes marked reduction in systemic vascular resistance, increase in venous return and LV filling, and a 70% to 100% rise in cardiac output. For the same hemoglobin level, cardiac output is higher in sickle cell anemia compared to other anemias.[139] Anemia and arterial oxygen desaturation due to chronic pulmonary disease reduce the blood oxygen-carrying capacity, but this is balanced by the high cardiac output needed to maintain adequate oxygen delivery. Studies employing echocardiographic evaluation of patients with homozygous sickle cell disease and comparison to normal controls suggest a cardiac appearance consistent with the volume overload effects of chronic anemia[140,141] and no evidence of distinct sickle cell cardiomyopathy or cardiac dysfunction. However, in chronic blood transfusion cases with inadequate chelation treatment, cardiac hemosiderosis may impair contractility. After periodic transfusion of packed red blood cells in children with homozygous sickle cell anemia in order to maintain a hemoglobin concentration of greater than or equal to 10 g% and the proportion of hemoglobin S to 20% or less, Lester et al.[142] observed normalization of left heart chambers' size and significant decrease in heart rate, LV mass, and cardiac output. During vasoocclusive sickle cell crises, there is marked elevation in cardiac output and further reduction in systemic vascular resistance compared to steady-state values to which there is gradual return; in turn, steady-state values are different from those of normal persons.[143] The mechanism by which a minor insult, such as cold weather, results in crisis is unclear. Extracorpuscular changes have been causally associated with crises, with the sickled erythrocyte not being primarily responsible. This is supported by changes in polymorph adhesiveness and chemotaxis, and in plasma and platelet prostanoid levels. Singer et al.[143] suggested that inflammatory factors may act to arrest sickled erythrocytes in areas of constricted microvasculature and divert blood flow via "shunts" into alternate vascular beds resulting in focal hypoxia and infarction.

Pulmonary infarction (probably the result of thrombosis rather than embolism) and pneumonia are common, although pulmonary hypertension and cor pulmonale are rare in sickle cell anemia. The volume overload in sickle cell disease usually is well tolerated by the myocardium, so that development of CHF in children or young adults usually suggests underlying cardiac or other organ pathology. Given that even in the resting state the myocardium extracts approximately 75% of the delivered oxygen, myocardial infarction is rare, although necrosis of papillary muscles may occur due to their unfavorable location, and blood supply by terminal coronary rami with scant collateral vasculature.

Vitamin B₁ Deficiency

Vitamin B₁ (thiamine) is a precursor of thiamine pyrophosphate, a coenzyme required for oxidative decarboxylation of α-ketoacids to aldehydes. These reactions are an important source for high energy generation. Moreover, thiamine may have a role in facilitating peripheral nerve conduction, since the initiation of nerve impulses is associated with hydrolysis of thiamine pyrophosphate or thiamine triphosphate.[144] Advanced thiamine deficiency predominantly affects the cardiovascular system ("wet beri-beri") and/or the nervous system, both central and peripheral ("dry beri-beri").

Beri-beri was studied extensively in Java by Wenckebach.[145] The disease used to be common in the Far East among people subsisting on polished rice. Milling removes the husk where most of vitamin B₁ is found, but boiling before husking disperses thiamine throughout the grain. Use of enriched flour in white bread has virtually eradicated the disease in the West, but beri-beri occasionally is seen in alcoholics and diet faddists. Sporadic cases of wet beri-beri have been reported in Japanese teenagers[146] subsisting on thiamine deficient and carbohydrate-rich diets who were not alcohol users. Even among alcoholics with CHF and documented thiamine deficiency, beri-beri is rare. In a recent study from South Africa, the possibility of thiamine and vitamin B₆ deficiency was explored in 73 black alcoholic patients with cardiac failure. One third and one fifth of patients were found to have thiamine and vitamin B₆ deficiency respectively, but beri-beri heart disease was confirmed in only one patient.[147]

Secondary thiamine deficiency may arise under conditions of increased demand as in hyperthyroidism, pregnancy, fever, high ambient temperature, and strenuous exertion; decreased absorption as in protracted diarrhea; or decreased utilization as in advanced liver disease.

The pathophysiologic hallmarks of cardiac beri-beri are marked peripheral vasodilation and blood volume expansion (see High Output States). Although the circulation time is shortened, fluid retention gradually leads to biventricular enlargement with significantly elevated venous pressure often resulting in anasarca, hepatomegaly with ascites, and pleuro-pericardial effusion. "Dry beri-beri" presents with unpleasant paresthesiae in the feet and calves, painful cramps, a feeling of walking on cotton-wool, unsteady gait especially in the dark, sensorimotor deficits, and loss of deep tendon reflexes. Several biochemical values, such as increased pyruvate and lactate, low transketolase, and thiamine levels, are characteristic of thiamine deficiency, but not pathognomonic of beri-beri.[147] However, a rise in circulating erythrocyte transketolase activity after treatment or upon addition of thiamine diphosphate to the patient's blood in vitro indicates clinical avitaminosis.[15]

Polycythemia

Polycythemia vera (primary) is classified as a myeloproliferative disorder where erythropoietin is not the stimulus for increased red cell production. Secondary polycythemia develops in response to hypoxia,[148] as in cyanotic congenital heart disease and chronic obstructive pulmonary disease. Blood viscosity increases exponentially as a function of hematocrit[149] and, in turn, augments the systemic vascular resistance and cardiac work. The cardiac output also rises due to blood volume expansion.

Hypervolemia, hyperviscosity, thrombocytosis, and defective platelet function are responsible for most clinical manifestations. Intermittent claudication, headaches due to cerebral hypoperfusion, mild arterial hypertension, and angina pectoris are common. Paradoxically, bleeding and thrombosis both can occur. Bleeding results from thrombopathy and hypervolemia-induced venous and capillary distention, whereas thrombosis is caused by thrombocytosis, hyperviscosity, and increased platelet aggregation. Cerebrovascular, coronary, and abdominal vascular thrombosis (one third of fatalities)[150] or hemorrhage are the most common complications and the disease leads rapidly to death within 6 to 18 months if left untreated.

Venesection results in dramatic decreases in blood viscosity. In polycythemia vera, the increased oxygen delivery to the body due to high cardiac output and arterial oxygen content permits liberal phlebotomy.[151] In secondary polycythemia, however, the disadvantages relating to hemodynamic overload and risk of thrombosis first must be weighed against the advantage of enhanced oxygen delivery before considering venesection or erythropheresis as a therapeutic modality.

Hypophosphatemia and Other Electrolyte Abnormalities

Hypophosphatemia is defined as serum phosphate of less than 0.8 mmol/L. The three mechanisms leading to hypophosphatemia are decreased intake or intestinal

TABLE 18.4. Frequent causes of hypophosphatemia.

Diabetic ketoacidosis
Chronic alcoholism and alcoholic withdrawal
Hyperosmolar nonketotic coma
Phosphate-deficient hyperalimentation
Recovery from severe burns
Phosphate-binding antacids
Chronic renal failure
Renal transplantation
Hyperparathyroidism (all types)
Recovery from hypothermia
Lymphomas
Tumor phosphaturia
Fanconi's syndrome
Respiratory alkalosis
Malabsorption syndromes

absorption, increased loss, and transcellular shifts. As noted in Table 18.4, many clinical conditions are associated with hypophosphatemia[152] that may result in intracellular ATP depletion and dysfunction of many organ systems. Cardiac depletion of ATP leads to decreased myocardial contractility,[153] due to impaired actin-myosin interaction, as well as decreased function of the various ion exchange pumps in the cell wall and sarcolemmal membranes. These changes can be reversed with phosphate repletion.

Clinical hypokalemia has little effect on ventricular function. O'Regan et al.[153] found no abnormality of myocardial performance attributable to chronic hypokalemia. In the patient with CHF, the primary risk from hypokalemia is the potential exacerbation of cardiac arrhythmias.

Summary

This chapter dealt with factors that precipitate or potentiate existing heart failure as well as with systemic disease processes or noxious agents that can directly or indirectly, transiently or irreversibly, impair pump function. With the exception of conditions that affect the myocardial integrity through an inflammatory process (vasculitides), decreased oxygen availability (carbon monoxide poisoning, cocaine use), or altered cellular metabolism (hypophosphatemia, hypomagnesemia and hypokalemia), most of these factors augment the workload of the LV.

The increase in external cardiac work results from a rise in cardiac output (flow work), afterload pressure or impedance (pressure work), or both. Conditions that raise the cardiac output usually are well tolerated with few or no cardiac symptoms or pathoanatomic residuals, reflecting the heart's efficiency as a volume pump. In contrast, the myocardial response to pressure overload is not always predictable and may vary from physiological to pathological hypertrophy, the latter leading inexorably to irreversible dilation. This less favorable outcome is due to the fact that although hypertrophy can successfully normalize the systolic wall stress (afterload), it can also, by itself, enhance the myocardial energy requirements. Finally, the heart's endurance under a wide range of hemodynamic and metabolic conditions may be related to the autoregulatory capacity of the coronary circulation, the ability to use lactate as a nutrient, and the high rate of oxygen extraction even at rest.

The clinical response to the factors discussed in this chapter is determined to a great extent by the etiology and extent of LV dysfunction and to the presence and severity of coronary artery disease. Recognition of such factors and their interplay with existing cardiac abnormalities should be of help in managing patients with CHF.

Acknowledgment. We would like to thank Mya D. Kline for her technical support.

References

1. Graettinger JS, Parsons RL, Campbell JA. A correlation of clinical and hemodynamic studies in patients with mild and severe anemia with and without congestive heart failure. *Ann Intern Med.* 1963;58:617–626.
2. Guyton AC. Cardiac output, venous return and their regulation. In: Guyton AC, ed. *Textbook of medical physiology.* Philadelphia: Saunders; 1986:272–286.
3. Duke M, Abelmann WH. The hemodynamic response to chronic anemia. *Circulation.* 1969;39:503–514.
4. Fowler HO, Holmes JC. Blood viscosity and cardiac output in acute experimental anemia. *J Appl Physiol.* 1975;39:453–456.
5. Florenzano F, Diaz G, Regonesi C, Escobar E. Left ventricular function in chronic anemia: evidence of non-catecholamine positive inotropic factor in the serum. *Am J Cardiol.* 1984;54:638–645.
6. Berne RM, Rubio R. Coronary circulation. In: *Handbook of physiology. The cardiovascular system.* Bethesda, MD: American Physiological Society; 1979:873–952.
7. Sarnoff SJ, Braunwald E, Welch GH Jr, Case RB, Stainsby WN, Macruz R. Hemodynamic determinants of oxygen consumption of the heart with special reference to the tension-time index. *Am J Physiol.* 1958;192(1):148–156.
8. Bing RJ. Coronary circulation in health and disease as studied by coronary sinus catheterization. *Bull NY Acad Med.* 1951;27:413–421.
9. Grossman W, Jones D, McLaurin LP. Wall stress and patterns of hypertrophy in the human left ventricle. *J Clin Invest.* 1975;56:56–64.
10. Olivetti G, Lagransta C, Quaini F, et al. Capillary growth in anemia-induced ventricular wall remodeling in the rat heart. *Circ Res.* 1989;65(5):1182–1192.
11. Burch GE, DePasquale N, Hyman A, Degraff AC. In-

fluence of tropical weather on cardiac output, work, and power of right and left ventriculars of man resting in hospital. *Arch Intern Med.* 1959;104:553–60.

12. Burckhardt D, Staider GA, Ludin H, Bianchi L. Hyperdynamic circulatory state due to Osler-Weber-Rendu disease with intrahepatic arteriovenous fistulae. *Am Heart J.* 1973;85:797–800.

13. Zavota L, Bini F, Carano N, Agnetti A, Squuarcia U. Hepatic hemangiomatosis with congestive cardiac failure and development into a cholestatic hepatopathy. *Pediatr Med Chir.* 1984;6:621–624.

14. Sanyal SK, Saldivar V, Coburn TP, Wrenn EL Jr, Kumar M. Hyperdynamic heart failure due to A-V fistula associated with Wilms' tumor. *Pediatrics.* 1976;57:564–568.

15. Grossman W, Braunwald E. High cardiac output states. In: Braunwald E, ed. *Heart disease: A textbook of cardiovascular medicine.* Philadelphia: Saunders; 1988:778–792.

16. Stead EA, Warren JV. Cardiac output in man. *Arch Intern Med.* 1947;80:237–248.

17. Pinsky WW, Lewis RM, Hartley CJ, Entman ML. Permanent changes of ventricular contractility and compliance in chronic overload. *Am J Physiol.* 1979;237:H575–583.

18. Hirshfield JW Jr, Epstein SE, Roberts AV, Glancy DL, Morrow AG. Indices predicting long-term survival after valve replacement in patients with aortic regurgitation and patients with aortic stenosis. *Circulation.* 1974;50:1190–1199.

19. Waterlow JC, Eddy TP. Nutrition and nutritional disorders. In: Scott RB, ed. *Price's textbook of the practice of medicine.* Oxford: Oxford University Press; 1978:451–475.

20. Wood P. Hyperkinetic circulatory states. In: Wood P, ed. *Paul Wood's diseases of the heart and circulation.* London: Eyre and Spottiswoode, 1968:1039–1055.

21. Weiss S, Wilkins RW. The nature of the cardiovascular disturbances in vitamin deficiency states. *Trans Assoc Am Phys.* 1936;51:341–343.

22. Wenckebach KF. St. Cyres lecture on heart and circulation in a tropical avitaminosis (beri-beri). *Lancet.* 1928;ii:265–268.

23. Hashimoto H. Acute pernicious form of beri-beri and its treatment by intravenous administration of vitamin B_1, with special reference to electrocardiographic changes. *Am Heart J.* 1937;13:580–588.

24. Noble MIM, Trenchard D, Guz A. Effect of changing heart rate on cardiovascular function in conscious dogs. *Circ Res.* 1966;19:206–213.

25. Wilson JR, Douglas P, Hickey WF, et al. Experimental congestive heart failure produced by rapid ventricular pacing in the dog: cardiac effects. *Circulation.* 1987;75:857–867.

26. Gillette P, Smith R, Gasron A, et al. Chronic supraventricular tachycardia. *JAMA.* 1985;253:391–392.

27. Packer DL, Bardy GH, Worley SJ, et al. Tachycardia-induced cardiomyopathy: a reversible form of left ventricular dysfunction. *Am J Cardiol.* 1986;57:563–570.

28. Cruz FE, Cheriex EC, Smeets JL, et al. Reversibility of tachycardia-induced cardiomyopathy after cure of incessant supraventricular tachycardia. *J Am Coll Cardiol.* 1990;16:739–744.

29. Heymsfield SB, Smith J, Redd S, Whitworth HB Jr. Nutritional support in cardiac failure. *Surg Clin North Am.* 1981;61(3):635–652.

30. Pittman JG, Cohen P. The pathogenesis of cardiac cachexia (part 1). *N Engl J Med.* 1964;271:403–409.

31. Pittman JG, Cohen P. The pathogenesis of cardiac cachexia (part 2). *N Engl J Med.* 1964;271:453–460.

32. Heymsfield SB, Casper K. Congestive heart failure: clinical management by use of nasoenteric feeding. *Am J Clin Nutr.* 1989;50(3):539–544.

33. Skorecki KL, Brenner BM. Body fluid homeostasis in congestive heart failure and cirrhosis with ascites. *Am J Med.* 1982;72:323–38.

34. Cohn JN. Current therapy of the failing heart. *Circulation.* 1988;78(5 pt 1):1099–1107.

35. Packer M, Kessler PD, Gottlieb SS. Adverse effects of converting enzyme inhibition in patients with severe congestive heart failure: pathophysiology and management. *Postgrad Med J.* 1986;62(suppl 1):179–182.

36. Vinson JM, Rich MW, Sperry JC, Shah AS, McNamara T. Early readmission of elderly patients with congestive heart failure. *J Am Geriatr Soc.* 1990;38:1290–1295.

37. Ghali JK, Kadakia S, Cooper R, Ferlinz J. Precipitating factors leading to decompensation of heart failure. *Arch Intern Med.* 1988;148:2013–2016.

38. Buckberg GD, Rixler DE, Archie JP, Hoffman JIE. Experimental subendocardial ischemia in dogs with normal coronary arteries. *Circ Res.* 1977;30:67–81.

39. Hanrath P, Methey DG, Siegert R, Bleifeld W. Left ventricular relaxation and filling pattern in different forms of left ventricular hypertrophy: an echocardiographic study. *Am J Cardiol.* 1980;45:15–23.

40. Friberg P, Hallbäck-Nordlander M, Lundin S. Left ventricular hypertrophy improves cardiac function in spontaneously hypertensive rats. *Clin Sci.* 1981;(suppl)61:109s–111s.

41. Smiseth OA, Scott-Douglas NW, Thompson CR, Smith ER, Tyberg JV. Nonuniformity of pericardial surface pressure in dogs. *Circulation.* 1987;75:1229–1236.

42. Crozatier B, Caillet D, Bical O. Left ventricular adaptation to sustained pressure overload in the conscious dog. *Circ Res.* 1984;54:21–29.

43. The xamoterol in severe heart failure study group. Xamoterol in severe heart failure. *Lancet.* 1990;336:1–6.

44. Greene HL, Richardson DW, Hallstrom AP, et al. Congestive heart failure after acute myocardial infarction in patients receiving antiarrhythmic agents for ventricular premature complexes (Cardiac Arrhythmia Pilot Study). *Am J Cardiol.* 1989;63:393–398.

45. Podrid PJ, Schoenberger A, Lown B. Congestive cardiac failure caused by oral disopyramide. *N Engl J Med.* 1980;302:614–617.

46. Josephson MA, Ikeda N, Singh BN. Effects of flecainide on ventricular function: clinical and experimental correlation. *Am J Cardiol.* 1984;53(5):95B–100B.

47. Gottlieb SS, Kukin ML, Medina N, Yushak M, Packer M. Comparative hemodynamic effects of procainamide, tocainide, and ecainide in severe chronic heart failure. *Circulation.* 1990;81:860–864.

48. National institutes of health consensus development panel on the health implications of obesity. Health Implications of Obesity. *Ann Intern Med.* 1985;103:147–151.

49. Messerli FH, Sundgaard-Riise, Eeisin ED, et al. Dimorphic cardiac adaptation to obesity and arterial hypertension. *Ann Intern Med.* 1983;99:757–761.

50. Reisin E, Frohlich ED, Messerli FH, et al. Cardiovascular changes after weight reduction in obesity hypertension. *Ann Intern Med.* 1983;98:315–319.

51. Lavie CJ, Messerli FH. Cardiovascular adaptation to obesity and hypertension. *Chest.* 1986;90:275–279.

52. Lavie CJ, Amodeo C, Ventura HO, Messerli FH. Left atrial abnormalities indicating diastolic ventricular dysfunction in cardiomyopathy of obesity. *Chest.* 1987;92:1042–1046.

53. Garavaglia GE, Messerli FH, Nunez BD, Schmieder RE, Grossman E. Myocardial contractility and left ventricular function in obese patients with essential hypertension. *Am J Cardiol.* 1988;62:594–597.

54. MacMahon SW, Wilcken DEL, MacDonald GJ. The effect of weight reduction on left ventricular mass. *N Engl J Med.* 1986;314:334–338.

55. Guyton AC. Pulmonary Ventilation. In: Guyton AC, ed. *Textbook of medical physiology.* Philadelphia: Saunders; 1986:466–479.

56. Scharf SM, Bianco JA, Tow DE, Brown R. The effects of large negative intrathoracic pressure on left ventricular function in patients with coronary artery disease. *Circulation.* 1981;63:871–875.

57. Stalcup SA, Mellius RB. Mechanical forces producing pulmonary edema in acute asthma. *N Engl J Med.* 1977;297:592–595.

58. Hassapoyannes CA, Harper JF, Stuck LM, Hornung CA, Abel FL. Effects of systole-specific pericardial pressure increases on coronary flow. *J Appl Physiol.* 1991;71(1):104–111.

59. Walley KR, Becker CJ, Hogan RA, Teplinsky K, Wood LD. Progressive hypoxemia limits left ventricular oxygen consumption and contractility. *Circ Res.* 1988;63:849–859.

60. Wexler LS, Weinberg EO, Ingwall JS, Apstein CS. Acute alterations in diastolic left ventricular chamber distensibility: mechanistic differences between hypoxemia and ischemia in isolated perfused rabbit and rat hearts. *Circ Res.* 1986;59:515–528.

61. Hausdorf G, Hinrichs C, Nienaber CA, Schark C, Keck EW. Left ventricular contractile state after surgical correction of tetralogy of Fallot: risk factors for late left ventricular dysfunction. *Pediatr Cardiol.* 1990;11:61–68.

62. Shepard JW. Cardiopulmonary consequences of obstructive sleep apnea. *Mayo Clin Proc.* 1990;65:1250–1259.

63. Drislane FW, Samuels MA, Kozakewich H, Schoen FJ, Strunk RC. Myocardial contraction band lesions in patient with fatal asthma: possible neuroendocrine mechanisms. *Am Rev Respir Dis.* 1987;135:498–501.

64. Molfino NA, Nannini LJ, Martelli AN, Slutsky AS. Respiratory arrest in near-fatal asthma. *N Engl J Med.* 1991;324:285–288.

65. McFadden ER, Ingram RH. Relationship between diseases of the heart and lungs. In: Braunwald E, ed. *Heart disease.* Philadelphia: Saunders; 1988:1879.

66. Mifune J, Kuramoto K, Ueda K, et al. Hemodynamic effects of salbutamol an oral long-acting beta stimulant, in patients with congestive heart failure. *Am Heart J.* 1982;104:1011–1015.

67. Andersson KE. Some new positive inotropic agents. *Acta Med Scand.* 1986;707(suppl):65–73.

68. Tan SL, Lui PS, Salmon YM. Cardiac failure associated with the use of salbutamol for inhibition of premature labor. *Asia Oceania J Obstet Gynaecol.* 1987;13:147–149.

69. Jacobs MM, Knight AB, Arias F. Maternal pulmonary edema resulting from beta-mimetic and glucocorticoid therapy. *Obstet Gynecol.* 1980;56:56–59.

70. Carpenter RJ, Decuir P. Cardiovascular collapse associated with oral terbutaline tocolytic therapy. *Am J Obstet Gynecol.* 1984;148:821–823.

71. Burch GE, Giles TD. The burden of a hot and humid environment on the heart. *Mod Concepts Cardiovasc Dis.* 1970;39:115–120.

72. Ansari A, Burch GE. Influence of hot environments on the cardiovascular system. *Arch Intern Med.* 1969;123:371–378.

73. Epstein SE, Stampfer M, Beiser GD, Goldstein RE, Braunwald E. Effects of a reduction in enviromental temperature on the circulatory response to exercise in man. Implications concerning angina pectoris. *N Engl J Med.* 1969;280:7–11.

74. Raizner AE, Chahin RA, Ishimori T, et al. Provocation of coronary artery spasm by the cold pressor test. *Circulation.* 1980;62:925–932.

75. Juneau M, Johnstone M, Dempsey E, Waters DD. Exercise-induced myocardial ischemia in a cold environment. *Circulation.* 1989;79:1015–1020.

76. Chakko CS, Gheorghiade M. Ventricular arrhythmias in severe heart failure: incidence, significance and effectiveness of antiarrhythmic therapy. *Am Heart J.* 1985;109:497–504.

77. Packer M. Sudden unexpected death in patients with congestive heart failure: a second frontier. *Circulation.* 1985;72:681–685.

78. Freis ED. Critique of the clinical importance of diuretic-induced hypokalemia and elevated cholesterol level. *Arch Intern Med.* 1989;149:2640–2648.

79. Kaplan NM. How bad are diuretic-induced hypokalemia and hypercholesterolemia? *Arch Intern Med.* 1989;149:2649.

80. Podrid PJ, Fuchs T, Candinas R. Role of the sympathetic nervous system in the genesis of ventricular arrhythmia. *Circulation.* 1990;82(suppl 1):I103–113.

81. Hollifield JW. Electrolyte disarry and cardiovascular disease. *Am J Cardiol.* 1989;63:21–6B.

82. White RJ, Chamberlain Da, Hamer J, McAlister J, Hawkins LA. Potassium depletion in severe heart disease. *Br Med J.* 1969;2:606–610.

83. Cort JH, Mathews HL. Potassium deficiency in congestive heart failure: three cases with hyponatremia including results of potassium replacement in one case. *Lancet.* 1954;1:1202–1206.

84. Ryan MP. Magnesium and potassium sparing diuretics. *Magnesium*. 1986;5:282–292.

85. Gottlieb SS, Baruch L, Kukin ML, Bernstein JL, Fisher ML, Packer M. Prognostic importance of the serum magnesium concentration in patients with congestive heart failure. *J Am Coll Cardiol*. 1990;16:827–831.

86. Dyckner T. Relation of cardiovascular disease to potassium and magnesium deficiencies. *Am J Cardiol*. 1990;65:44K–46K.

87. Connor TB, Rosen BL, Blaustein MP, Applefeld M, Doyle A. Hypocalcemia precipitating congestive heart failure. *N Engl J Med*. 1982;307:869–872.

88. Rimailho A, Bouchard P, Schaison G, Richard C, Auzepy P. Improvement of hypocalcemic cardiomyopathy by correction of serum calcium level. *Am Heart J*. 1985;109:611–613.

89. Bashour R, Basha HS, Cheng TO. Hypocalcemic cardiomyopathy. *Chest*. 1980;78:663–665.

90. Feldman AM, Fivush B, Zahka KG, Oyuyang P, Baughman KL. Congestive cardiomyopathy in patients on continuous ambulatory peritoneal dialysis. *Am J Kidney Dis*. 1988;11:76–79.

91. Winter PM, Miller JN. Carbon monoxide poisoning. *JAMA*. 1976;236:1502–1504.

92. Ilano AL, Raffin TA. Management of carbon monoxide poisoning. *Chest*. 1990;97:165–169.

93. Adams KF, Koch G, Chatterjee B, et al. Acute elevation of blood carboxyhemoglobin to 6% impairs exercise performance and aggravates symptoms in patients with ischemic heart disease. *J Am Coll Cardiol*. 1988;12:900–901.

94. Sheps DS, Herbst MC, Hinderliter AL, et al. Production of arrhythmias by elevated carboxyhemoglobin in patients with coronary artery disease. *Ann Intern Med*. 1990;113:343–351.

95. Marius-Nunez AL. Myocardial infarction with normal coronary arteries after acute exposure to carbon monoxide. *Chest*. 1990;97:491–494.

96. Kjeldsen K, Thomsen JK, Astrup P. Effects of carbon monoxide on myocardium. *Circ Res*. 1974;34:339–348.

97. Selwyn AP. The cardiovascular system and radiation. *Lancet*. 1983;2(8342):152–154.

98. Burns RJ, Bar-Shlomo BZ, Druck MN, et al. Detection of radiation cardiomyopathy by gated radionuclide angiography. *Am J Med*. 1983;74:297–302.

99. Ikaheimo MJ, Niemela KO, Linnaluoto MM, Jakobsson MJT, Takkunen JT, Taskinen PJ. Early cardiac changes related to radiation therapy. *Am J Cardiol*. 1985;56:943–946.

100. Taussig HB. "Death" from lightning—and the possibility of living again. *Ann Intern Med*. 1968;68:1345–1353.

101. Hiestand D, Colice G. Lightning-strike injury. *J Intens Care Med*. 1988;3:303–314.

102. Kleiner J, Wilkin J. Cardiac effects of lightning stroke. *JAMA*. 1978;240:2757–2759.

103. James T, Riddick L, Embry J. Cardiac abnormalities demonstrated postmortem in four cases of accidental electrocution and their potential significance relative to non-fatal electrical injuries of the heart. *Am Heart J*. 1990;120:143–157.

104. Amin M, Gabelman G, Karpel J, Buttrick P. Acute myocardial infarction and chest pain syndromes after cocaine use. *Am J Cardiol*. 1990;66:1434–1437.

105. Rezkalla SH, Hale S, Kloner RA. Cocaine-induced heart diseases. *Am Heart J*. 1990;120(suppl):1403–1408.

106. Smith HWB, Liberman HA, Brody SL, Battey LL, Donohue BD, Morris DC. Acute myocardial infarction temporally related to cocaine use. *Ann Intern Med*. 1987;107:13–18.

107. Kossowsky WA, Lyon AF, Chou SY. Acute non–Q wave cocaine-related myocardial infarction. *Chest*. 1989;96:617–622.

108. Isner JM, Estes NA, Thompson PD, et al. Acute cardiac events temporally related to cocaine abuse. *N Engl J Med*. 1986;315:1438–1443.

109. Majid PA, Patel B, Kim HS, Zimmerman JL, Dellinger RP. An angiographic and histologic study of cocaine-induced chest pain. *Am J Cardiol*. 1989;64:811–814.

110. Kuhn FE, Johnson MN, Gillis RA, Visner MS, Schaer GL. Effect of cocaine on the coronary circulation and systemic hemodynamics in dogs. *J Am Coll Cardiol*. 1990;16:1481–1491.

111. Lange RA, Cigarroa RG, Yancy CW, Willard JE, Popma JJ. Cocaine-induced coronary-artery vasoconstriction. *N Engl J Med*. 1989;321:1557–1606.

112. Isner JM, Chokshi SK. Cardiovascular complications of cocaine. *Curr Probl Cardiol*. 1991;16:95–123.

113. Fraker TD, Temesy-Armos PN, Brewster PS, Wilkerson RD. Mechanism of cocaine-induced myocardial depression in dogs. *Circulation*. 1990;81:1012–1016.

114. Kannel WB, Castelli WP, McNamara PM, Mckee PA, Feinleib M. Role of blood pressure in the development of congestive heart failure. *N Engl J Med*. 1972;287:781–788.

115. Kaplan NM. Systemic hypertension: mechanisms and diagnosis. In: Braunwald E, ed. *Heart disease. A textbook of cardiovascular medicine*. Philadelphia: Saunders; 1988:819–861.

116. Kannel WB. Prevalence and natural history of electrocardiographic left ventricular hypertrophy. *Am J Med*. 1983;75(suppl 3A):4–12.

117. Laks MM, Morady F, Garner D, Swan HJ. Temporal changes in canine right ventricular volume, mass, cell size and sarcomere length after binding the pulmonary artery. *Cardiovasc Res*. 1974;8:106–111.

118. Wilkman-Coffelt J, Parmley WW, Mason DT. The cardiac hypertrophy process. Analysis of factors determining pathological versus physiological development. *Circ Res*. 1979;45(6):697–707.

119. Honig CR, Bourdeau-Martini J. Extravascular component of oxygen transport in normal and hypertrophied hearts with special reference to oxygen therapy. *Circ Res*. 1974;35(suppl II):97–103.

120. Grossman W, Jones D, McLaurin LP. Wall stress and patterns of hypertrophy in the human left ventricle. *J Clin Invest*. 1975;56:56–64.

121. Frohlich ED, Pfeffer MA. Adrenergic mechanisms in human hypertension and spontaneously hypertensive rats. *Clin Sci Mol Med*. 1975;48:2255–2385.

122. Tarazi RC, Ibrahim MM, Dustan HP, Ferrario CM. Cardiac factors in hypertension. *Circ Res.* 1974;34:1213–1221.

123. Hanrath P, Methey DG, Siegert R, Bleifeld W. Left ventricular relaxation and filling pattern in different forms of left ventricular hypertrophy: an echocardiographic study. *Am J Cardiol.* 1980;45:15–23.

124. Inouye I, Massie B, Loge D, et al. Abnormal left ventricular filling: an early finding in mild to moderate systemic hypertension. *Am J Cardiol.* 1984;53:120–126.

125. Devereux RB, Savage DD, Sachs I, Laragh JH. Effect of blood pressure control on left ventricular hypertrophy and function in hypertension. *Circulation.* 62(suppl 3):III-36.

126. O'Rourke RA. Antiphospholipid antibodies. A marker of lupus carditis? *Circulation.* 1990;82:636–638.

127. Borenstein DG, Fye WB, Arnet FC, Stevens MB. The myocarditis of systemic lupus erythematosus: association with myositis. *Ann Intern Med.* 1978;89:619–624.

128. Nihoyannopoulos P, Gomez PM, Joshi J, Loizou S, Walport MJ, Oakley CM. Cardiac abnormalities in systemic lupus erythematosus. Association with raised anticardiolipin antibodies. *Circulation.* 1990;82:369–375.

129. Bidaui AK, Roberts JL, Schwartz MM, Lewis EJ. Immunopathology of cardiac lesions in fatal systemic lupus erythematosus. *Am J Med.* 1980;69:849–858.

130. Hang LM, Izui S, Dixon FJ. A model of acute lupus and coronary vascular disease with myocardial infarction. *J Exp Med.* 1981;154:216–221.

131. Hochberg MC, Feldman D, Stevens MB. Adult onset polymyositis/dermatomyositis: an analysis of clinical and laboratory features and survival in 76 patients with a review of the literature. *Semin Arthritis Rheum.* 1968;15:168–185.

132. Tymms KE, Webb J. Dermatopolymyositis and other connective tissue disorders: a review of 105 cases. *J Rheumatol.* 1985;12:1140–1146.

133. Rossi MA. Endomyocardial fibrosis in dermatomyositis. *Int J Cardiol.* 1990;28(1):119–122.

134. Haupt HM, Hutchins GM. The heart and conduction system in polymyositis-dermatomyositis: a clinicopathologic study of 16 autopsied patients. *Am J Cardiol.* 1982;50:998–1106.

135. LeRoy EC. Systemic sclerosis (scleroderma). In: Wyngaarden JB, Smith Jr LH, eds. *Cecil's textbook of medicine.* Philadelphia: Saunders; 1988:2018–2024.

136. Follansbee WP. The cardiovascular manifestation of systemic sclerosis (scleroderma). In: O'Rourke RA, ed. *Current problems in cardiology.* Chicago: Year Book Medical Publishers; 1986;11(5):241–298.

137. Gustafsson R, Mannting F, Kazzam E, Waldenström A, Hälgren R. Cold-induced reversible myocardial ischemia in systemic sclerosis. *Lancet.* 1989;2:475–480.

138. Medsger TA Jr, Masi AT. Survival with scleroderma. II. A life-table analysis of clinical and demographic factors in 358 male U.S. veteran patients. *J Chron Dis.* 1973;26:647–652.

139. Varat MA, Adolph RJ, Fowler NO. Cardiovascular effects of anemia. *Am Heart J.* 1972;83:415.

140. Estrade G, Poitrineau O, Bernasconi F, Garnier D, Donatien Y. Left ventricular function and sickle cell anemia. *Arch Mal Coeur.* 1989;82(12):1975–1988.

141. Lester LA, Sodt PC, Hutcheon N, Arcilla RA. Cardiac abnormalities in children with sickle cell anemia. *Chest.* 1990;98(5):1169–1174.

142. Lester LA, Sodt PC, Hutcheon N, Arcilla RA. Cardiovascular effects of hypertransfusion therapy in children with sickle cell anemia. *Pediatr Cardiol.* 1990;11(3):131–139.

143. Singer M, Boghossian S, Bevan DH, Bennett ED. Hemodynamic changes during sickle cell crisis. *Am J Cardiol.* 1989;64:1211–1213.

144. Rivlin RS. Disorders of vitamin metabolism deficiencies, metabolic abnormalities, and excesses. In: Wyngaarden JB, Smith Jr LH, eds. *Cecil's textbook of medicine.* Philadelphia: Saunders; 1988:1228–1241.

145. Wenckebach KF. St. Cyres lecture on heart and circulation in a tropical avitaminoisis (beri-beri). *Lancet.* 1928;ii:265–268.

146. Kawai C, Wakabayashi A, Matsumura T, Yui Y. Reappearance of beri-beri heart disease in Japan; a study of 23 cases. *Am J Med.* 1980;69:383–386.

147. Tobias SL, Van der Westhuyzen J, Davis RD, Atkinson PM. Alcohol intakes and deficiencies in thiamine and vitamin B_6 in black patients with cardiac failure. *S Afr Med J.* 1989;76(7):299–302.

148. Polycythemia due to hypoxemia: advantage or disadvantage? *Lancet.* 1989;2(8653):20–22.

149. Castle WB, Jaandle AJH. Blood viscosity and blood volume: opposing influences upon oxygen transport in polycythemia. *Semin Hematol.* 1966;33:193–198.

150. Berk PD. Erthrocytosis and polycythemia. In: Wyngaarden JB, Smith Jr LH, ed. *Cecil's textbook of medicine.* Philadelphia: Saunders; 1988:975–984.

151. Chetty KG, Brown SE, Light RW. Improved exercise tolerance of the polycythemic lung following phlebotomy. *Am J Med.* 1983;74:415–420.

152. O'Connor LR, Wheeler WS, Bethune JE. Effect of hypophosphatemia on myocardial performance in man. *N Engl J Med.* 1977;297:901–903.

153. O'Regan S, Heitz F, Davignon A. Echocardiographic assessment of left ventricular function in patients with hypokalemia. *Miner Electrolyte Metab.* 1985;11:1–4.

19
The Pathology of Congestive Heart Failure

Margaret E. Billingham

"Heart failure may be defined as the pathophysiologic state in which an abnormality of cardiac function is responsible for failure of the heart to pump blood at a rate commensurate with the requirements of the metabolizing tissues. Heart failure occurs as the consequence of many forms of heart disease afflicting at least 4 million Americans of all ages."[1] Heart failure also occurs with the failure of compensatory mechanisms such as myocardial hypertrophy, which may accompany dilatation of the ventricular chambers. Heart failure can be divided into left and right heart failure, although if the heart failure becomes chronic then left heart failure can result in right heart failure, so that both can occur concomitantly. Heart failure may be due to failure of myocardial contraction or it may be due to an excessive hemodynamic burden. The heart will compensate for this physiologically, but also pathologically with myocyte hypertrophy with or without ventricular dilatation. The rate of onset of heart failure also will influence the clinical and pathological manifestations. For example, the right ventricle may dilate rapidly and the systemic venous pressure may rise to high levels immediately after an acute pulmonary embolus, without change in the myocytes themselves and therefore without compensatory hypertrophy. This chapter describes the pathomorphology of heart failure in the common conditions that cause heart failure (excluding congenital heart disease). Many of the significant morphologic changes encountered in congestive heart failure (CHF) are distant from the heart and are produced by the effect of hypoxia and congestion due to the failing circulation upon other organs and tissues. The pathology of the effect of CHF on the most important organs, the lungs, liver, and spleen, also are described. Apart from the general manifestations of heart failure, the specific pathology of conditions causing cardiac failure are described.

The Pathology of Left- and Right-Sided Heart Failure

Left-Sided Heart Failure

Left-sided heart failure[2] may be caused by hypertension, ischemic heart disease, aortic and mitral valve disease (rheumatic heart disease and calcific aortic stenosis), and other specific heart muscle diseases. Grossly, left-sided heart failure due to systolic pump failure results in massive dilatation of the left ventricle, which also may result in dilatation of the left atrium. The dilated ventricle may result in stretching of the papillary muscles to the point where they become thin and band-like (Fig. 19.1). If the heart failure has been present for a moderate amount of time, there also will be compensatory hypertrophy of the heart muscle, and although the ventricle is dilated, this may result in some increase in the width of the left ventricular (LV) wall. The atrial ventricular ring will become dilated as a result of the ventricular dilatation. Sometimes the aortic valve ring also is increased in size. As the LV failure becomes chronic, patchy fibrosis may be seen on the endocardial surface of the LV and also within the walls of the ventricle extending to the subepicardial surface. In long-standing chronic LV failure, gray striations of fibrosis may be seen on the epicardial surface of the heart. Chronic ventricular dilatation also may result in the formation of mural thrombi because of the poor ventricular contraction, the stasis of blood, and the substrate of fibrosis, which is conducive to the formation of thrombi. Depending on the cause of the LV failure, the left atrium also may dilate and the endocardium becomes thicker. Only with a LV restrictive disorder or mitral stenosis (occasionally atrial myxoma or atrial ball thrombus occluding the mitral valve) will dilatation confined only to the left atrium occur. Chronic cardiac in-

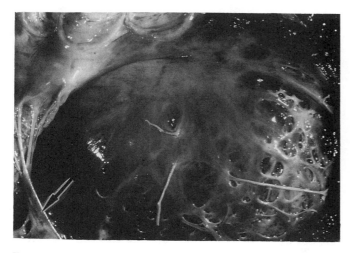

FIGURE 19.1. Left-sided heart failure showing dilated LV with flattened trabeculae and band-like papillary muscle (*arrows*).

sufficiency will result from extensive myocardial disease. Mechanical dysfunction of the cardiac valves, particular aortic and mitral defects, and tricuspid valvular defects may precipitate heart failure without being accompanied by significant myocardial disease.

Left-sided failure due to diastolic pump failure such as hypertrophic cardiomyopathy, endomyocardial fibrosis (EMF), and other restrictive and constrictive cardiac conditions will result in a normal-sized ventricle, but abnormally dilated left atrium because of damming up of blood from entering a ventricle that is unable to expand in diastole. Even in long-standing heart failure due to diastolic pump failure, due to restrictive or constrictive disease, myocyte hypertrophy and fibrosis will not occur as the myocardium is protected from dilatation.

Chronic long-standing LV failure will result in pathologic manifestations remote from the heart. The organs most affected by left ventricular failure are the lungs, kidneys, and sometimes the brain.

Lungs

LV failure due to volume overload results in back flow and pressure into the left atrium, which in turn results in damming of the blood flow from the pulmonary veins. Because of the progressive obstruction of blood within the pulmonary circulation, there is an increase in the pressure in the pulmonary veins and this is ultimately transmitted to the capillaries. Pulmonary congestion and edema result with a perivascular transudate due to leaking of the capillaries. Sections of the lung at this time will show perivascular clear spaces due to the transudate and this may progress into the alveolar septae, which become edematous and congested with edema fluid and blood. Edema fluid containing proteinaceous material and red blood cells may accumulate

in the alveolar spaces (pulmonary edema). Alveolar capillaries distended with blood will become tortuous and may rupture, causing intraalveolar hemorrhage. In chronic cases, the transudate may accumulate in the pleural spaces and result in pleural effusions. Pulmonary pathology at this time will show the features of hemosiderin-laden macrophages due to breakdown and phagocytosis of red blood cells within the alveoli the so-called heart failure cells. If the heart failure develops slowly and is progressive, in time the alveolar septae will become thickened by fibrosis and together with hemosiderin may cause "brown induration." Features of pulmonary hypertension also will manifest themselves by the thickening of the walls of the pulmonary arteries, sclerotic plaques within the larger vessels, and tortuosity of the small vessels. Sections of the kidney in chronic heart failure will show marked congestion of the vessels within the kidney; this also applies to the brain. Progression of the left-sided heart failure eventually will translate into a rise in pulmonary pressure and right sided heart failure, which will be dealt with next.

Right-Sided Heart Failure

As mentioned above, right-sided heart failure[2] often is a consequence of left-sided failure, because any increase in pressure in the pulmonary circulation due to left-sided failure is translated into an increased burden in the right side of the heart. The causes of right-sided failure therefore must include all those causes of left-sided failure, including congenital left to right shunts. Isolated right-sided failure will occur in cor pulmonale; in this case, the right ventricle (RV) will respond to the increase resistance in the pulmonary circulation. Right heart failure may be acute or chronic. Acute right heart failure may occur as a result of a massive pulmonary embolus (see Fig. 19.2) or showers of microemboli causing a rapid rise in pulmonary vascular resistance. Acute right heart failure also may occur at the time of cardiac transplantation if the nonhypertrophied normal RV is placed in series with pulmonary hypertension from a previous heart failure situation. Acute right heart failure results in acute, rapid dilatation of the RV.

In acute right heart failure, the accumulation of blood in the failing RV will manifest itself with acute right atrial failure and dilatation. In acute RV dilatation, myocyte morphology may be within normal limits, however, in time marked RV hypertrophy may occur also with some thickening of width of the RV free wall. Long-standing RV heart failure also will result in endocardial and intramyocardial fibrosis. The tricuspid valve ring may become dilated and the papillary muscles thinned and flattened. The right atrium also will become dilated and fibrosis becomes evident if right heart failure is long-standing. Chronic right heart failure also may result in mural thrombi both in the ventricle or in

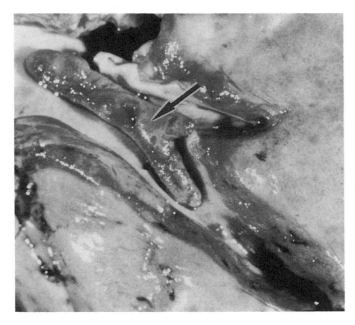

FIGURE 19.2. Large, organized pulmonary embolus [*arrow* (from deep vein thrombosis in the leg)] obstructing a branch of the pulmonary artery.

congestion, the central veins become widened by fibrous thickening and the fibrosis may extend into the lobules, resulting in a pattern similar to cirrhosis of the liver, which is termed "cardiac cirrhosis." In severe acute congestion, the liver cells may become atrophic because of the congestive hypoxia related to the stagnant flow in the central lobular sinusoids. If the congestion develops rapidly, rupture of the sinusoids may occur with central hemorrhagic necrosis of the liver lobules. Congestion of the portal system, of course, will lead to congestion of the spleen.

Pathologic Changes in the Spleen in Right-Sided Heart Failure

In chronic right-sided failure, the spleen will become large and tense with a cyanotic color. The cut surface will exude blood and this will result in reduction of tension with collapse of the organ and wrinkling of the surface capsule. In chronic congestion, the spleen parenchyma becomes more fibrotic but retains its shape, and does not have the soft consistency of a normal spleen.

the right atrial appendage. The pulmonary outflow tract may become dilated and endocardial fibrosis may be seen. As in the case of left heart failure, right heart failure also will result in pathologic manifestations in other organs remote from the heart, but mainly the liver and spleen because of damming up of the blood in those organs.

Pathologic Changes in the Liver in Right-Sided Heart Failure

Acute and chronic passive congestion from right-sided heart failure will occur in the liver. Both the size and the weight of the liver will increase and the liver surface will become smooth because of the stretched capsule. The cut surface of the liver will show marked congestion with oozing of blood. Microscopically, there will be prominent central veins with red accentuation of the centers of the liver lobule surrounded by a paler area. This results in the so-called nutmeg appearance of the liver seen grossly. With long-standing chronic passive

Ultrastructural Changes Relating to Heart Failure

A study comparing the ultrastructural changes in endomyocardial biopsies obtained at cardiac catheterization in patients with CHF compared with patients without CHF but with abnormal cardiac conditions fails to show ultrastructure differences that could distinguish patients in heart failure.[3] We compared the ultrastructural changes of these 13 heart failure patients (pulmonary artery wedge pressure >18 mm Hg) who ranged in age from 19 to 62 years (average 43 years) with the ultrastructural changes in 13 age-matched patients with heart disease who were not in heart failure (see Table 19.1). Seven of the patients in heart failure had a duration of symptoms from 2 to 5 yr and one had symptoms for more than 5 yr. Three of the non–heart failure patients had had other cardiac symptoms from 2 to 5 yr. The changes looked for and compared in the two groups were abnormalities and myocyte contraction, mitochondrial morphology, nuclear structure, sarcotubular swelling, myofibrillar loss, and myocyte edema.

TABLE 19.1. Ultrastructural comparison of myocardium from patients in heart failure with that of patients with heart disease but not in heart failure.

	No. of patients	Mean age (yrs)	PAW	Sarcotubular swelling	Myocyte degeneration	Myocyte edema	Vascular edema
Heart failure	13	43	33	10/13	7/13	1/13	0/13
No heart failure	13	43	7	4/13	3/13	4/13	0/13
Normal hearts	13	21	—	0/13	0/13	0/13	0/13

In the interstitium the degree of fibrosis, interstitial exudate, and vascular swelling (capillaries) were compared. Those patients with the most changes were listed in Table 19.1. It can be seen that, except for an increase in sarcotubular swelling ($p > .004$), both groups had morphologic changes because of their underlying heart disease, but it was not possible to distinguish morphologically which patients were actually in heart failure. The duration of symptoms had no effect on these results. There were, however, significant differences in the morphologic changes as can be expected from biopsies from eight normal disease-free young adults (organ transplant donors) (see Table 19.1).

Heart Failure Secondary to Ischemic Heart Disease

The most common pathologic abnormality of the heart that gives rise to the clinical syndrome of heart failure is disease of the myocardium, so that if the myocardium is damaged by acute infarction or ischemia heart failure may ensue. In diminishing the blood supply to the heart, coronary atherosclerosis becomes manifest in four major forms: acute myocardial infarction, angina pectoris, sudden death, and heart failure. There is some overlap and angina may precede a myocardial infarct by some days or even by months. Ischemia or angina is the clinical entity of chest pain due to the demand of myocardial oxygen exceeding the supply. The major cause of angina is a severe degree of coronary atherosclerosis; however, anemia, aortic valve disease, hypertrophic cardiomyopathy, hyperthyroidism, or hypertension without significant coronary atherosclerosis also can lead to angina. Post-mortem studies of patients with angina have found that 90% of them have at least one major coronary artery occlusion and coronary angiography in life has shown a similar relationship of old occlusions and severe stenosis causing angina. Progression of the vascular lesions with increasing frequency and severity of symptoms is seen, although a proportion of these cases remains static. In some cases, patients will develop angina after acute myocardial infarction, as in the Framingham study.[4] The same study shows that 25% of men with angina will have an acute infarction within 5 yr. Occasionally at autopsy, severe stenosis is found in a coronary artery where there had been no history of angina during life. On the other hand, coronary angiography has revealed some patients with typical angina, but apparently normal coronary arteries; this may be due to spasm of small arteries or disease of the small branches of the coronary arteries. It is usually estimated that 15% of the overall mortality of ischemic heart disease is due directly to chronic left heart failure.[5] It is also considered that the loss of 25% of the

LV muscle results in rises of LV filling pressure, which in effect will mean cardiac failure.[6]

The Pathology of Coronary Artery Atherosclerosis

Coronary atherosclerosis is a diffuse intimal thickening occurring with age in many people, but which can become more severe in others. Mild concentric intimal proliferation may occur with a normal aging process. Atherosclerosis usually is an asymmetric plaque-like lesion containing fibrosis, but also lipid-rich, macrophages, cholesterol crystals, and differing amounts of fibrosis and sometimes calcification. These asymmetric plaques actually occlude the lumen and in the worst cases may occlude altogether, resulting in a slit-like eccentric channel. The composition of the atherosclerotic lesions varies with the amounts of lipid material and fibrous tissue. In advanced cases the elastica of the intima usually is damaged and there is myointimal migration from the media with smooth muscle extending into the intima. Plaques can be complicated by hemorrhage into them, creating a false lumen that effectively will block off the main lumen (Fig. 19.3). Ruptures and fissures occurring in the plaques are common and may lead to the final occlusion of the vessel. If the lumen is occluded by thrombus or atherosclerosis and the patient recovers, recanalization of the lumen can occur, resulting in small central channels. If occlusion of the coronary artery lumen occurs gradually, it is not unusual to find small vessels forming a collateral circulation into the myocardium. As has been mentioned, calcification may occur not only in the grumous plaques of atherosclerosis, but also may occur in the walls of the vessels

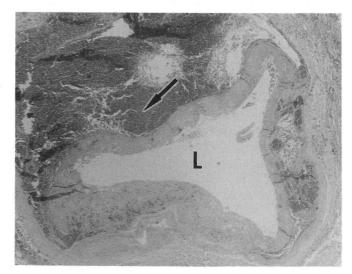

FIGURE 19.3. Transverse section of the left anterior descending coronary artery showing hemorrhage (*arrow*) creating a false lumen, which compromises the lumen of the artery (*L*).

TABLE 19.2. Myocardial infarction: sequence of changes.

Time	Gross changes	Microscopic changes	Histochemistry
0–2 hr	—	Separation of myocytes	↓ Dehydrogenase, oxidase phosphorylase, glycogen potassium ↑ Calcium and sodium
12 hr	Early pallor	Eosinophilia, pyknotic nuclei; contraction bands	
18–24 hr	Pallor	Myocyte shrinkage and changes as above	
24–72 hr	Pallor and hyperemia	Loss of nuclei, many neutrophils	
5 days	Hyperemic border	Granulation tissue and resorption	
2–3 wks	Hyperemic border	Cellular replacement with early fibrosis	
3 months	Scar	Mature scar	

forming a stiff pipe-like structure. There is a good correlation between the presence of wall calcification in coronary arteries and the absence of actual stenosis.

Myocardial Infarction

Heart failure due to coronary artery disease can be due to occlusion of the coronary arteries as described above with infarction of the myocardium. If this occurs suddenly and is large enough, then cardiogenic shock may ensue. If smaller infarcts occur over time and replacement fibrosis occurs, then the myocardium eventually may be compromised sufficiently to cause heart failure as described before. Acute ischemic necrosis of an area of myocardium will result in myocardial infarction. Most myocardial infarctions are localized in the left ventricle and are either (a) a transmural lesion extending from endocardium into the subepicardial area or (b) a subendocardial infarct confined to the inner third of the LV wall. The transmural variety of infarct is more common than the subendocardial lesions. Infarcts can occur in the interventricular septum and occasionally in the RV in about 20% of transmural infarcts of the inferoposterior wall and posterior portion of the septum related to right coronary artery atherosclerosis. According to Buja,[2] the left anterior descending coronary artery accounts for 40% to 50% of anterior wall and anterior two thirds of the interventricular septal infarcts. The right coronary artery accounts for 30% to 40% of the posterior inferior wall of the LV and posterior one third of the interventricular septum.[2] The left circumflex coronary artery accounts for 15% to 20% of infarcts of the lateral wall of the LV. The gross appearance of a myocardial infarction depends on the length of time from the initial infarction. Immediately after infarction, a slightly paler area may be present or it may be possible to see a hemorrhagic area in the region of the infarct. Some special stains can be used: for example, triphenyl-tetrosodium chloride, which highlights

the infarcted area by leaving it unstained and paler than the surrounding myocardium. After 48 hr a hyperemic rim may be seen around the paler infarcted area (see Fig. 19.5). Over the course of 3 months after the infarction, the area becomes replaced with patchy fibrosis and scar, following an ingrowth of granulation tissue. If the infarct extends to the epicardium, fibrinous pericarditis over the area of the infarct also may be seen. The histologic progression of a myocardial infarct allows more accurate dating than the gross appearance. These changes have been described well before[7] and are outlined in Table 19.2. For medicolegal and other reasons, there is great emphasis on the accurate dating of myocardial infarcts, but this is outside the realm of this chapter. Subendocardial infarcts have a similar light and gross appearance as the transmural, but usually become more visible grossly earlier than the transmural infarcts.

Clinical Sequelae of Myocardial Infarcts

Arrhythmias have been reported in up to 90% of carefully monitored patients having myocardial infarcts and they often result in early deaths. The clinical picture, however, often is dominated by the onset of pump failure manifested by CHF; CHF is present in most patients having significant myocardial infarctions. Acute failure may result in pulmonary edema and drop in blood pressure. If the infarct is greater than 40% of the LV, then a profound drop in cardiac output will result in cardiogenic shock.[8]

Complications of Myocardial Infarction Resulting in Heart Failure

Myocardial Rupture

Myocardial rupture may occur between 3 and 5 days after myocardial infarction. At this time, the infarcted myocardium is at its "softest," being filled with enzyme-secreting neutrophils digesting the necrotic myocardium. A sudden rise in blood pressure at this time, such as coughing or straining at stool, may result in myocardial rupture. Most infarcts undergoing external rupture are in the anterior wall of the LV. Rupture is said to be more common in women and to be associated with hypertension. Spontaneous rupture of an acute myocardial infarction generally is fatal. Rupture also can occur through the interventricular septum, but this is not thought to be as common as external wall rupture.

Ventricular Aneurysm

Ventricular aneurysm results in a localized bulging of the free wall of the ventricle over the area of infarction. Aneurysms may occur from 2 weeks to 2 yr after an episode of infarction and results in an akinetic area of the ventricle. Occasionally, calcification occurs in the wall of the aneurysm. Often the aneurysms become filled with mural thrombi. In some cases, surgical resection of the aneurysm is possible, resulting in improvement of function. The aneurysm wall consists mainly of fibrosis with islands of hypertrophied myocardium. Ventricular pseudoaneurysms may occur in ruptured myocardial infarctions that are contained by the pericardium, which becomes organized into a large fibrous sac communicating with the ventricle by a narrow aperture. The wall of the sac, however, is not derived from the myocardium; hence the designation of false aneurysm. The lesion is quite rare. Rupture of the sac may occur.

Papillary Muscle Rupture

Myocardial infarction including the LV papillary muscles occasionally may result in rupture of the papillary muscle so that mitral incompetence results, which also leads to heart failure.

Other Conditions of the Coronary Arteries Causing Occlusion

Occasionally, coronary artery emboli can be seen occluding or partially occluding the lumen of a vessel. The usual emboli are either calcific from surgery (from the removal of a calcific aortic valve), or they may be septic (Fig. 19.4), for example, from an endocarditis of the aortic or mitral valves, and occasionally they may be due to tumor, although this is rare. Ulcerated atheromatous plaques in the region of the coronary ostia also may lead to embolic atheromatous material. Mural thrombi within the LV also may cause embolic phenomenon.

Coronary arteritis due to systemic polyarteritis nodosa or Wegener's granulomatosis rarely involves the myocardium. Coronary arteritis for whatever cause may

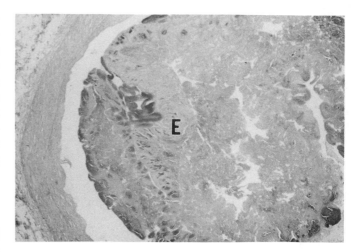

FIGURE 19.4. Transverse section of coronary artery almost occluded by a septic embolus (*E*).

result in thrombotic occlusion of the lumen; however, this also is rare.

Coronary arteries can develop true congenital aneurysms, but it is more common to have generalized dilatation of the coronary arteries occurring in old age. Localized atherosclerotic aneurysms also have been described. Micotic embolic aneurysms will occur after septic emboli. Aneurysms may result in thrombotic occlusion or rupture and, in both cases, may result in myocardial infarction. Some drugs have been associated with dissection of coronary arteries (e.g., ritalin) and in others dissection can emanate from damage to the endothelium by coronary angiography or by fissures in a plaque. Dissection of the coronary arteries due to Marfan's syndrome also has been recorded.

Primary Cardiomyopathies

Cardiomyopathy is a condition affecting primarily the myocardium unassociated with significant narrowing of the extramural coronary arteries, systemic hypertension, anatomic valvular disease, congenital malformation of the heart and vessels, extrinsic pulmonary parenchymal, or vascular disease. In other words, the diagnosis depends on the exclusion of other common types of heart disease. The diagnosis often is made by exclusion of the usual causes of cardiac failure. The incidence of this form of cardiac disease in the general population is not well known, in part due to the confusion in the terminology and classification of these disorders. It has been proposed recently by the task force on cardiomyopathies and the World Health Organization and the Scientific Council on Cardiomyopathies and the International Society and Federation of Cardiology that the nomenclature of this disease entity be

TABLE 19.3. Pathologic classification of cardiomyopathy.

Primary cardiomyopathy (idiopathic)
Dilated (congestive)
Hypertrophic
   With subaortic stenosis (IHSS or Hocm)
   Without subaortic stenosis
Obliterative type

IHSS = Idiopathic hypertrophic subaortic stenosis.
Hocm = Hypertrophic obstructive cardiomyopathy.

made more specific and less ambiguous. According to the new classification, the term "cardiomyopathy" should be used only to describe the group previously known as "primary cardiomyopathy" or "heart muscle disease of unknown cause" and that "secondary cardiomyopathy" should be replaced by the term "specific heart muscle disease." For example, a disease entity in which a viral agent is the proposed etiologic factor should be referred to as "viral heart muscle disease," not "viral cardiomyopathy." It is well known that many clinicians use the term "cardiomyopathy" to mean end-stage cardiac disease for whatever cause, for example, "ischemic cardiomyopathy." This should be called "end-stage ischemic heart disease" and the term "cardiomyopathy" should be used only when referring to idiopathic cardiomyopathy. There have been many classifications for the various cardiomyopathies; the following is a pathological classification of cardiomyopathies, which is generally accepted at this time (Table 19.3).

Dilated (Congestive) Cardiomyopathy

Cardiomyopathy may present with arrhythmias in a previously, apparently healthy young individual or it may present insidiously as the onset of LV failure manifested by shortness of breath on exertion and then at rest, and finally, with pulmonary edema and evidence of right-sided CHF. In many cases a history of malaise and flu-like syndromes may be elicited by the patient weeks before the development of heart failure. The physical findings are described elsewhere in this book.

Gross Pathology of Dilated Congestive Cardiomyopathy

The heart usually is markedly enlarged and, in some cases, will weigh 800 to 1000 g. The heart also is global in shape (see Fig. 19.6) with four-chamber dilatation, particularly the LV. The apex of the heart is rounded rather than triangular, as in the normal heart. The surface of the heart usually is smooth and glistening without evidence of pericarditis; however, streaks of gray fibrosis may be seen through the pericardium (see Fig. 19.6). The coronary arteries are by definition quite normal without atherosclerosis. In many patients with car-

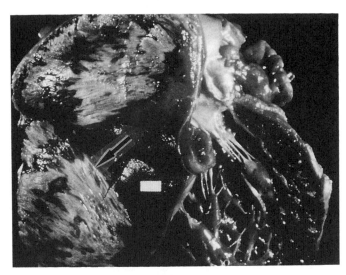

FIGURE 19.5. Gross pathology of interventricular myocardial infarct (the septum is sectioned) to show the paler areas of the infarct surrounded by darker hemorrhagic areas (*arrow*).

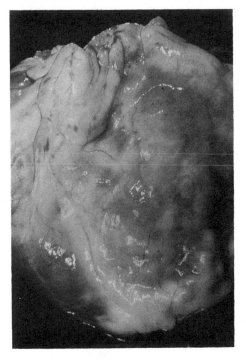

FIGURE 19.6. Gross pathology of a large (800-g) DCM heart with a rounded, globular shape. Note fibrosis seen through glistening epicardium.

diomyopathy minimal intimal proliferation with plaques sometimes may be seen in the proximal portions of the major coronary arteries. It must be stressed that these small lesions do not and could not result in ischemic heart disease or heart failure. These lesions result in 10% or less compromise of the coronary lumens. On opening the heart, the rounded dilated ventricles

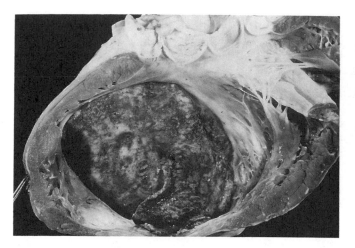

FIGURE 19.7. Dilated LV opened to show massive mural thrombus lining the interventricular wall.

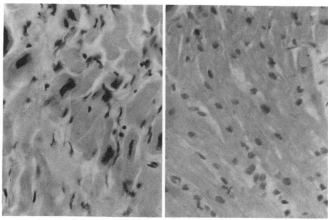

FIGURE 19.8. Photomicrograph showing hypertrophy and large, hyperchromatic nuclei of idiopathic cardiomyopathy in the left panel compared with nuclei of normal myocardium in the right panel.

are evident (see Fig. 19.1). Because of the dilatation, the endocardial surface of the ventricles may be flattened with concomitant stretching and flattening of the papillary muscles. Depending on the length of time for the developing cardiomyopathy, streaks of fibrosis may be seen in the subendocardium or there may be thicker and more extensive areas of endocardial fibrosis resulting from an earlier mural thrombosis on the endocardium or it may itself result in the formation of a mural thrombus over the fibrotic plaque. Mural thrombus is seen in approximately 50% of end-stage cardiomyopathies (see Fig. 19.7). The atrial ventricular ring will be dilated from normal because of the generalized dilatation of the ventricles in cardiomyopathies, however; the valve morphology for all cardiac valves should be within normal limits.

Microscopic Features of Idiopathic Cardiomyopathy

The microscopic features of idiopathic cardiomyopathy (Fig. 19.8) include a definite increase in both fine and coarse interstitial fibrosis. This can be so extensive that when the heart muscle is cut into it has a firm gritty or grizzly effect. Heart muscle hypertrophy is always present compared with normal, even though there may be marked dilatation of the ventricles. The myocyte nuclei show large bizarre-shaped patterns. The nuclei are much bigger than normal and the nuclear form factor (bizarre shapes) also is quite different (see Table 19.4). The other striking feature is the myofibrillar attenuation and loss. This means actual loss of contractile elements within the myocytes, leaving "ghost cells" that are almost empty (see Fig. 19.9). Partial myofibrillar loss also is seen at an electron microscopic level; however, these changes should be viewed with caution and total

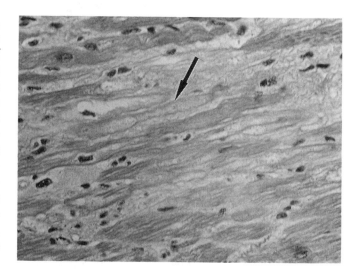

FIGURE 19.9. Section of myocardium from a DCM showing myofibrillar loss and "ghost cells" (arrow).

myofibrillar loss is preferred to make the diagnosis. The etiology of cardiomyopathy is uncertain, but a viral etiology has long been suspected. It is interesting therefore that in all cases of end-stage cardiomyopathy, small focal areas of inactive lymphocytes (not causing myocyte damage) can be found in 83% of cases.[9] It has been suggested that the fibrosis in cardiomyopathy is due to a vascular attenuation of small vessels as described in the cardiomyopathic hamster model.[10] More recent studies, however, do not show a reduction in small vessels within the myocardium.[11] Dilated cardiomyopathy (DCM) is a systolic pump failure with increasing dilatation of the ventricles due to insufficient working myocardium. Electron micrographs of a failing end-stage dilated cardiomyopathy show a high percen-

TABLE 19.4. Morphometrics of idiopathic dilated cardiomyopathy compared with normal control myocardium.

				Controls				
Case	Measured myocyte width (μm)	Sarcomere length (μm)	Corrected myocyte width (μm)	Nuclear area (μm²)	Measured nuclear form factor	Corrected nuclear form factor	Nucleolar area (μm²)	Mitochondrial area (μm²)
1	17.2 ± 5.4	1.18 ± 0.52	20.3	31.0 ± 10.1	0.50 ± 0.13	0.43	2.29 ± 0.85	0.36 ± 0.15
2	21.4 ± 5.3	1.34 ± 0.19	28.7	59.2 ± 20.4	0.38 ± 0.08	0.29	2.03 ± 0.94	0.31 ± 0.19
3	18.7 ± 3.2	0.94 ± 0.39	17.6	40.2 ± 14.0	0.31 ± 0.08	0.34	2.83 ± 1.15	0.40 ± 0.20
4	16.9 ± 3.2	1.21 ± 0.29	20.4	54.7 ± 16.5	0.47 ± 0.18	0.39	2.73 ± 0.97	0.39 ± 0.25
5	18.1 ± 3.7	1.17 ± 0.51	21.2	53.6 ± 17.2	0.47 ± 0.11	0.41	2.77 ± 1.07	0.32 ± 0.16
6	14.3 ± 5.9	1.37 ± 0.21	19.6	43.4 ± 16.5	0.47 ± 0.09	0.35	2.13 ± 1.11	0.35 ± 0.17
7	15.8 ± 4.1	1.14 ± 0.36	18.0	36.3 ± 9.7	0.34 ± 0.08	0.30	2.15 ± 1.10	0.39 ± 0.20
8	16.3 ± 5.4	1.35 ± 0.36	22.0	47.4 ± 30.0	0.47 ± 0.11	0.36	2.27 ± 0.85	0.36 ± 0.15
9	13.9 ± 3.2	1.20 ± 1.24	16.6	47.5 ± 13.2	0.42 ± 0.10	0.36	1.74 ± 0.59	0.39 ± 0.20
10	15.3 ± 3.9	1.24 ± 0.28	19.0	36.7 ± 9.9	0.45 ± 0.14	0.37	1.70 ± 0.52	0.22 ± 0.10
Mean	16.8 ± 2.2	1.22 ± 0.13	20.3 ± 3.4	45.0 ± 9.2	0.43 ± 0.06	0.36 ± 0.04	2.26 ± 0.40	0.35 ± 0.05
				Idiopathic DCM				
Case	Myocyte width (μm)	Sarcomere length (μm)		Nuclear area (μm²)	Nuclear form factor		Nucleolar area (μm²)	Mitochondrial area (μm²)
1	27.2 ± 6.9	1.04 ± 0.40		78.3 ± 25.9	0.23 ± 0.09		3.15 ± 2.32	0.24 ± 0.12
2	30.0 ± 9.4	1.29 ± 0.36		113.0 ± 72.3	0.21 ± 0.08		2.70 ± 2.22	0.23 ± 0.15
3	20.6 ± 4.0	1.34 ± 0.82		51.5 ± 17.5	0.40 ± 0.15		2.11 ± 1.04	0.32 ± 0.15
4	29.0 ± 4.7	1.10 ± 0.55		90.0 ± 33.5	0.35 ± 0.09		1.80 ± 0.85	0.32 ± 0.19
5	37.1 ± 5.6	1.08 ± 0.41		95.1 ± 52.6	0.23 ± 0.11		1.84 ± 1.31	0.30 ± 0.18
6	31.1 ± 10.3	0.86 ± 0.46		111.9 ± 88.0	0.22 ± 0.09		5.16 ± 3.10	0.29 ± 0.21
7	37.2 ± 7.8	1.04 ± 0.39		129.7 ± 69.9	0.20 ± 0.08		2.11 ± 1.36	0.31 ± 0.16
8	19.2 ± 4.8	0.84 ± 0.25		45.0 ± 14.0	0.28 ± 0.09		1.64 ± 1.26	0.33 ± 0.17
9	21.9 ± 4.9	1.27 ± 0.41		72.7 ± 34.0	0.23 ± 0.07		2.78 ± 1.46	0.38 ± 0.25
10	39.3 ± 6.0	1.01 ± 0.53		99.4 ± 28.4	0.49 ± 0.13		2.99 ± 2.63	0.23 ± 0.13
Mean	29.3 ± 7.2	1.09 ± 0.17		88.7 ± 27.1	0.28 ± 0.09		2.63 ± 1.04	0.30 ± 0.05

Note: All data are means plus or minus SD.
Modified from Rowan R, Masek MA, Billingham ME. Ultrastructural morphometric analysis of endomyocardial biopsies. *Am J Cardiovasc Path.* 1988; 2(2): 140.

tage of myofibrils without any contractile elements (Fig. 19.10). There has been some suggestion in the past of a "mitochondriosis"; however, although occasionally seen, this is not borne out in most cases of DCM.

Dilated Cardiomyopathy with Specific Associations

Peripartum Cardiomyopathy or Postpartum Cardiomyopathy

Peripartum or postpartum cardiomyopathy manifests itself during pregnancy or within 3 months after the puerperium. The myocardial changes gross light and electron microscopic exactly similar to that in patients with idiopathic DCM occurring in nonpuerperal states. The question has to be raised that since the morphology is identical, is this a fortuitous development of cardiomyopathy brought on by the stress of childbirth, or would it have occurred in any case.

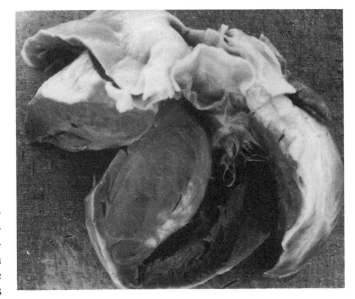

FIGURE 19.10. Hypertrophic cardiomyopathy showing widened interventricular septum with fibrosis on the outflow tract and reduced LV size.

Alcoholic Cardiomyopathy

Much has been written about the changes in alcoholic cardiomyopathy.[11,12] A large study by Alexander described very accurately the changes in alcoholic cardiomyopathy in more than 200 patients as obtained by needle biopsies of the LV.[13] These changes, however, were not compared with those of idiopathic cardiomyopathy, which appear to be the same morphologically with the exception of an increase in intracellular lipid and sarcotubular reticulum swelling.[14] It is said that alcoholic cardiomyopathy is reversible; however, the changes in idiopathic cardiomyopathy are not reversible and there may be an acute toxic change from alcoholism that is reversible, but the end stage change is similar both grossly, light microscopically, and electron microscopically to that of idiopathic DCM. There is no good correlation, to our knowledge, between alcoholic cardiomyopathy and liver cirrhosis, which is known to occur in chronic alcoholism. In any case, if this heart failure is due to chronic alcohol intake and strictly adhering to the WHO guidelines, this should not be called a cardiomyopathy, but rather alcoholic-specific heart muscle disease.

Familial Cardiomyopathy

Familial cardiomyopathy also is thought to be idiopathic grossly however, the changes are a little different from the usual idiopathic cardiomyopathy in that the hearts do not attain the same large size as those of idiopathic cardiomyopathy. Although the heart fails as a systolic pump failure, the myocardium does not contain the same degree of damage with regard to fibrosis and myofibrillar loss as is seen in end-stage idiopathic cardiomyopathy.[15,16] There are most likely several kinds of familial cardiomyopathy and some including mitochondrial changes have been described.[17] In our own institution, we have described abnormalities of the mitochondria (thumb-print mitochondria) observed in 10 cases of siblings who came to cardiac transplantation for end-stage cardiomyopathy.[18] Other changes due to carnitine deficiency also have been described. It does seem that familial cardiomyopathy is a subset of idiopathic cardiomyopathy, but that it is not entirely the same morphologically.

Hypertrophic Cardiomyopathy

Hypertrophic cardiomyopathy is an idiopathic cardiomyopathy; however, the congenital nature of the disease is supported by numerous reported cases of hypertrophic cardiomyopathy in infants and childhood and the occasional association with other congenital abnormalities and Friedrich's ataxia. Some of the ultrastructural changes seen are reminiscent of the early stages of myocardial embryogenesis. Familial incidence is common and the inheritance is that of an autosomal dominant.

In hypertrophic cardiomyopathy, the interventricular septum is by definition wider and thicker than the LV free wall and the LV cavity is thereby reduced in size (see Fig. 19.10). The heart may attain a large size, but is not so large as those hearts seen in end-stage DCM. Grossly, the heart may look like concentric hypertrophy, however, the difference between the size of the interventricular septum and the LV free wall will allow distinction. In this case, the clinical signs are those of diastolic pump failure. In some cases, the extensive interventricular septum impinges on the aortic outflow tract from the LV. Because of the increased hemodynamics in this area, there is often a thickened area of endocardium, just below the aortic valve (see Fig. 19.10). If this condition becomes severe, the aortic outflow is narrowed markedly and sudden death may occur with the same presenting features as those in aortic stenosis. Due to the obstructive element in hypertrophic cardiomyopathy, which may or may not be present, the terms "idiopathic subaortic stenosis" and "obstructive" cardiomyopathy may be used, but are dwindling in usage and importance, reflecting the realization that hypertrophic cardiomyopathy essentially is a disease of heart muscle rather than an outflow tract obstruction. The understanding of the importance of the diastolic dysfunction manifested by impaired relaxation represents an advance in knowledge of this disease. The reduction in the cavetry volume of the LV may result in apposition and slackness of the mitral valve cordae, so that mitral valve incompetence may ensue; these patients have been known to present with mitral valve murmurs. Treatment includes myomectomy of the outflow tract. Sections through the interventricular septum will reveal a pathognomic change of myocyte hypertrophy and disarray in the central of the interventricular septum within the bulbospiral muscle (see Fig. 19.11). In addition, small vessels in this area show marked thickening of the wall and are quite different from those normally seen in the myocardium. There also is an increase in fibrosis in the septum. Although areas of disarray can be seen in other parts of the heart, the disarray is pathognomic when it is in the center of the interventricular septum if that is wider than the LV free wall. These changes of disarray also are seen in electron microscopy, both between the myocytes themselves and a disarray of myofibrils within the myocytes, and these have been described previously.[19]

Obliterative (Restrictive) Cardiomyopathy

The obliterative type of cardiomyopathy results also in a diastolic pump failure rather than a systolic pump failure. Endomyocardial disease or fibrosis is a disease of unknown etiology characterized by severe focal en-

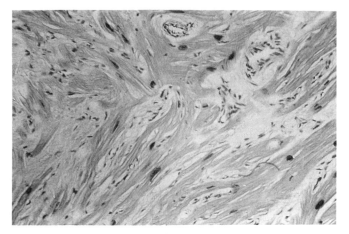

FIGURE 19.11. Section through the interventricular septum in hypertrophic cardiomyopathy showing the hypertrophy, fibrosis, and marked myocyte disarray.

docardial fibrosis of one or both ventricles with underlying subendocardial fibrosis with or without associated eosinophilia. The original description of this disease included an endocarditis with eosinophilia (Loeffer's fibroplastic endocarditis), which on healing resulted in the endocardial fibrosis (see Fig. 19.12). Fibrosis is predominantly in the inflow tracts of the ventricles and apices of the heart. Mural thrombi often overlie the fibrous plaques. The disease is prevalent in Africans and has been called "Uganda" disease in the past. Clinically, this disease represents a restrictive pattern of heart function and diastolic pump failure.

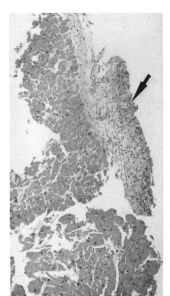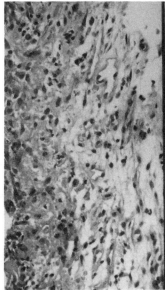

FIGURE 19.12. Section showing Loeffler's endocarditis (*arrow*, *left panel*) and higher power of the endocarditis with the eosinophilia.

Fibroelastosis

Fibroelastosis is more prevalent in infants and young children; they rarely survive more than 1 yr. The disease is congenital and the etiology is not clear. The pathology of endomyocardial fibroelastosis differs from that of EMF in that the thickened endocardium usually will line the entire LV, but also may include the RV. The thickened endocardium contains elastic fibers throughout the width of the thickened endocardium. In the case of EMF, the thickened endocardium consists mainly of fibrosis with the elastic tissue remaining in a thin band next to the myocardium.

Specific Heart Muscle Disease (Secondary Cardiomyopathies)

Specific heart muscle disease is all those cardiac conditions not termed idiopathic cardiomyopathy.

Inflammatory Myocarditis

Severe myocarditis is known to cause symptoms simulating idiopathic DCM. The myocarditis may result in a four-chamber dilatation, although at first the heart may remain within normal limits. Myocarditis, an inflammatory process affecting the myocardium, may be caused by any viral, bacterial, reckettsial, mycotic, or parasitic organism. In Europe and in the United States, however, most cases of acute myocarditis are thought to be caused by a viral infection. Evidence of myocarditis has been reported in up to 10% of routine autopsies. Myocarditis affects persons of all ages and in all areas of the world. Because it is often difficult to prove the viral etiology of cases of myocarditis, such cases are often referred to as idiopathic myocarditis. Although the most common causes are microbiologic infections, myocarditis also may be induced by hypersensitivity reactions, radiation therapy, and chemical and physical agents or drugs that cause myocyte necrosis, with secondary inflammatory changes.

Bacterial Myocarditis

Bacterial myocarditis is relatively rare in comparison with the idiopathic or viral myocarditis. It is often encountered as a complication of bacteremia or infective endocarditis. Diphtheritic myocarditis is not seen commonly these days and the damage is thought to be due to exotoxin of the bacteria. Young infants with severe bacterial pneumonia and septicemia sometimes will have a bacterial myocarditis. In this case, the pathology shows a florid "wall-to-wall" infiltrate that is predominantly mixed; that is, of neutrophils and monocytes together with areas of myocyte damage. Bacterial

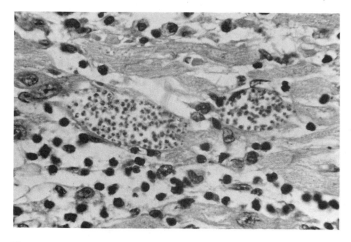

FIGURE 19.13. Section showing encysted *Toxoplasma gondii* with myocytes in an immunosuppressed patient.

myocarditis also may be seen in immunosuppressed patients and drug addicts who use the intravenous approach and it may result from a preceding endocarditis. Syphilis and *Borrelia recurrientis* are rare causes of bacterial endocarditis.

Protozoal Myocarditis

Infections also may cause myocarditis, the most common being Chagas' disease in some parts of the world, caused by *Trypanosoma Cruzi*. It is said that up to half of the population in endemic areas of South America are infected. Ten percent of these patients die in the acute phase.[2] This is an interesting infection because the acute phase is followed by a latent period of 10 to 20 yr when the chronic phase becomes manifest. The chronic phase is one of end-stage DCM; however, often there also is an aneurysmal dilatation at the apex of the LV described. *Toxoplasma gondii* is seen in immunosuppressed patients, particularly in the cardiac transplant cohort and also in those infected with the acquired immunodeficiency syndrome (AIDS) virus (see Fig. 19.13). The inflammatory infiltrate in toxoplasma usually is fairly focal and not diffuse. The organisms are seen only if they are still in the encysted form within the myocardium; however, the encysted form does not evoke an inflammatory reaction. Other parasites such as trichinosis may affect heart muscle as well as skeletal muscle. Trichinosis larvae (the trichinella spiralis) never encyst in the myocardium and the myocarditis that has been described with this condition is thought to be a nonspecific inflammatory manifestation of the larval invasion and a reaction to the death of the parasite or a hypersensitivity response.[2]

Tinea Echinococcus embryos also may invade the myocardium by the coronary and lymphatic circulations. The myocardial dysfunction often is due to the cyst size or if the cyst ruptures to anaphylaxis.

Viral Myocarditis

The Coxsackie-B enterovirus is especially cardiotropic in man. The echovirus group of enteroviruses also can cause acute myopericarditis. Even when a causative organism is isolated it is sometimes not known whether this is due to direct invasion of the virus with tissue damage or whether it is a toxic allergic or hypersensitivity response. Viral particles have never been seen unequivocally in the myocardium, except for cytomegalovirus in the immunocompromised host. Coxsackie-B virus causing myocarditis appears more commonly in young people and children where the acute disease is often symptomatic; it affects males twice as often as females.[2] The acute myocarditis often is preceded by an acute illness of upper respiratory tract infection accompanied by myalgias and fever. Many other viruses also are known to cause acute myocarditis such as influenza virus, infectious mononucleosis, measles, and other childhood viral illnesses as well as hepatitis and *Psittacosis*. It is thought that rubella virus contracted during the first trimester of pregnancy may result in cardiac as well as other congenital defects. Idiopathic myocarditis refers to cases of myocarditis that occur without an obvious cause in previously healthy individuals. Giant cell myocarditis usually is more common in adults and affects men more frequently than women. Myocardial failure is intractable and death usually ensues within a short time. The etiology of giant cell myocarditis is not known. There have not been many reports of survival once the diagnosis has been made; cardiac transplantation would seem to offer the only treatment at present.

Morphology of Myocarditis

In some cases of acute myocarditis, the heart is not increased in size significantly, but in most patients, particularly those dying of acute myocarditis, there is enlargement of the heart with four-chamber dilatation similar to that seen in idiopathic cardiomyopathy. In acute myocarditis, the heart muscle may be flabby with yellow streaks due to the inflammatory infiltrate. In the case of giant cell myocarditis, a serpiginous outline of yellow myocyte necrosis may be seen. In other cases, edema is more evident and the myocardium is somewhat stiff due to the interstitial edema and florid inflammatory infiltrate. It is a widely held concept that acute myocarditis may, in some patients, progress to a burnt-out phase, which is thought to be idiopathic cardiomyopathy of the dilated type. There is a good deal of circumstantial evidence to suggest this; however, actual proof is still lacking at this time.

Microscopic changes of acute myocarditis are variable; however, there always is an inflammatory infiltrate associated with interstitial edema. The Dallas criteria definition for acute myocarditis is defined "as a process characterized by inflammatory infiltrate of the myocardium with necrosis and/or degeneration of adjacent myocytes that is not typical of ischemic damage associated with coronary artery disease."[20] The more acute the disease, the more the numbers of polymorphonuclear leukocytes are present. In cases thought to be predominantly viral in origin, the infiltrate is mainly mononuclear. The inflammatory infiltrate causing death usually is a florid one extending from the endocardium to the epicardium and, sometimes, the pericardium. More recently, with the use of the endomyocardial biopsy, focal forms of acute myocarditis have been described and some autopsy descriptions also have included the focal type of myocarditis. Where drug or other hypersensitivity is thought to be involved, the number of eosinophils is markedly increased. In giant cell myocarditis (Fiedlers' myocarditis), the inflammatory infiltrate is confined within serpiginous borders and includes large areas of myocyte necrosis and giant cells. Recently, viral genomes have been isolated from idiopathic cardiomyopathy, suggesting progression from acute myocarditis; however, recent control studies in noncardiomyopathic hearts also have isolated viral genomes so the etiology of both idiopathic myocarditis and cardiomyopathy still is not entirely solved.[21–23]

Myocarditis and Collagen Diseases

Acute myocarditis may occur in rheumatic fever, rheumatoid arthritis, and lupus erythematosus. In polyarteritis nodosa there is a necrotizing vasculitis as well as an adjacent myocarditis. Microscopic changes in heart muscle have been reported in dermatomyocytis and scleroderma. In these cases, there is fibrous tissue replacement of the myocardium without a significant inflammatory component. Acute rheumatic disease has been described in many previous publications and textbooks. Grossly, in acute rheumatic carditis, the heart is enlarged, globular and frequently has a fibrinous pericarditis. On opening the heart, there is ventricular hypertrophy and dilatation, particularly of the LV. The most striking abnormality usually is on the valves of the left side of the heart, which are thickened and opaque and may display vegetations on their apposing surfaces. Microscopically, lesions may be found in any part of the heart. The specific lesion is the Aschoff body, which is seen mainly in the interstitial connective tissue adjacent to small vessels, but also is seen in the pericardium, interventricular septum, and in the posterior papillary muscle. The Aschoff body is a granulomatous focus found in the early part of the disease and is thought to be pathognomic. The Aschoff body is characterized by degenerative collagen and multinuclear cells with basophilic cytoplasm and the caterpillar (longitudinal) or owl-eye (transverse) appearance of the nuclei. These also are known as Anitschkow cells. In acute rheumatic disease, there often is also an acute valvulitis and mural

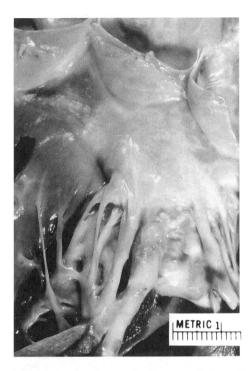

FIGURE 19.14. Chronic rheumatic disease of the mitral valve showing shortened, fused, and thickened chordae tendinae.

endocarditis also may be present. The conducting system sometimes is affected. If the patient survives the acute damage, chronic rheumatic disease is mainly a disease of the valves causing thickening, opaqueness, and shortening of the cordae with fibrosis (see Fig. 19.14). This results in rheumatic and aortic valvular heart disease. Although the etiology of rheumatic fever is not clear, it may represent an immune reaction induced by Group A, betahemolytic streptococcus. Rheumatic heart disease results from sensitization to streptococcal antigens and thus usually follows 1 to 4 weeks after streptococcal infection. The cellular zone contains Anitschkow cells and occasionally, multinucleated giant cells. Although any of the four cardiac valves may be affected (Fig. 19.15), the mitral valve is affected in nearly 50% of cases. Chronic healed mitral valvulitis in rheumatic heart disease consists of a markedly thickened leaflet that has fused and are cord-like and shortened cordae tendineae (see Fig. 19.14). The left atrium is greatly dilated and shows fibrous thickening of the endocardium.

Hypersensitivity Disease

Myocarditis has been associated with a number of drugs. With the increase in the use and abuse of new drugs, there has been an increase in toxic manifestations in the heart and adverse reactions to drugs are an increasingly important problem. Drugs may cause either a hypersensitivity or a true toxic myocarditis, and

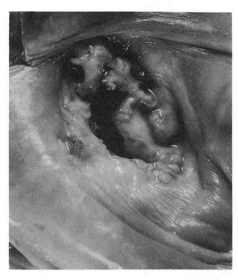

FIGURE 19.15. Chronic, incompetent, rheumatic heart valve with aortic valve deformity, fibrosis, and calcification.

TABLE 19.5. Drugs known to cause toxic myocarditis.

| Anthracyclines |
| Arsenicals |
| Lithium carbonate |
| Catecholamines |
| Quinidine |
| Cyclophosphamide |
| Fluorouracil |
| Phenothiazines |
| Theophylline |
| Barbiturates |

those thought to be responsible for each are listed in Table 19.5.

Hypersensitivity Allergic Myocarditis

Drugs known to cause hypersensitivity myocarditis are listed in Table 19.6. These lesions are not dose- or time-dependent and may occur at any time during delivery of the drug. When the drug is stopped the lesions regress. There may be other systemic signs or hypersensitivity such as rashes or fever. Morphologically, hypersensitivity myocarditis is manifested by an interstitial inflammatory infiltrate that contains a predominant number of eosinophils and atypical lymphocytes. The infiltrate is prominent in the ventricles; however, it may be both focal or diffuse. Myocyte damage is minimal in hypersensitivity disease. Some drugs will cause granulomatous infiltrates (e.g., isoniazide). Although hypersensitivity vasculitis involving arterioles and venules may be seen, necrotizing arteritis is not present. Hypersensitivity myocarditis also may be seen in allergies, particularly asthma.

TABLE 19.6. Some drugs causing hypersensitivity myocarditis.

| Penicillin |
| Tetracyclines |
| Phenylbutazone |
| Tetanus toxoid |
| Horse serum |
| Sulphonamides |
| Streptomycin |
| Isoniazid |
| Diphtheria toxin |
| Amphotericin B |

Drug-Induced Toxic Myocarditis

Drugs known to cause toxic myocarditis are shown in Table 19.5. Toxic myocarditis is dose related and the effects are cumulative, becoming worse as the drug dosage is increased. The inflammatory infiltrate surrounding damaged myocytes are predominantly acute mixed infiltrate including neutrophils as well as lymphocytes and histiocytes. Toxic myocarditis also includes an acute necrotizing vasculitis with hemorrhage, for example, as seen in cyclophasphamide-induced myocarditis. In older lesions, focal scarring may occur around the vessels. Because of the toxic vasculitis, microthrombi may be seen in small vessels and even aneurysmal dilatation has been described. Toxic myocarditis may result in multiple focal scars of the myocardium. Catecholamine cardiotoxicity is produced by sympathetic catecholamines, particularly norepinephrine. These lesions produce patchy intramyocardial hemorrhage, edema, and very focal myocyte necrosis, often with a small mixed cellular infiltrate including neutrophils. Early catecholamine injury shows hypereosinophilia. Later these small lesions are replaced by granulation tissue and scars. Similar lesions are seen in patients with brain tumors because raised intracranial pressure may cause catecholamine release. These small focal lesions of myocyte damage also are seen when patients are treated with high-dose pressor agents.

Myocarditis Due to Physical Agents, Poisons, and Drugs

Myocarditis may be seen in response to cardiac trauma, as in car accidents. Irradiation of the heart muscle causes an acute inflammatory reaction with damage to small vessels and many poisons and drugs will cause both toxic and hypersensitivity myocarditis.

Collagen Diseases

Collagen diseases may affect the myocardium. The most common are rheumatic fever; however, rheumatoid arthritis and systemic lupus erythematosus also may affect the myocardium and the cardiac valves. Scleroderma (progressive systemic sclerosis) may cause myocardial fibrosis without involvement of the coronary arteries. In scleroderma cardiac disease, however, usually is secondary to systemic hypertension from renal involvement or to cor pulmonale from the vascular involvement of the lung. Myocardial involvement in dermatomyositis is very rare.

Endocrine Disorders

CHF can occur as a result of thyrotoxicosis, although the light microscopic changes in the heart are somewhat nonspecific. CHF and cardiomegaly also can occur in patients with acromegaly. Patients with Cushings' syndrome or with hyperaldosteronism usually have systemic hypertension and electrolyte imbalance. Focal acute myocarditis has been observed with patients with pheochromocytoma and this is most likely due to the norepinephrine release described above.

Neurologic Disorders

Thirty percent of patients with Friedrich's ataxia, progressive muscular dystrophy, and myotonic muscular dystrophy may present with heart failure (see Fig. 19.16). The pathologic changes include myocardial fibrosis and, in some cases, the small vessels are thickened by fibrointimal proliferation. Fabry's disease is an X-linked disorder that may produce a DCM with heart failure. Pompe's disease may cause a pseudohypertrophic type of cardiomyopathy or even a restrictive pattern (e.g., Gaucher's disease). These diseases have been described elsewhere.

Anthracycline Cardiotoxicity

Anthracycline cardiotoxicity has two phases; an acute myocarditis, pericarditis syndrome, which is extremely rare, but that may cause death within 48 hr of an intravenous bolus of anthracyclines. Much more common, however, is the "cardiomyopathy" that becomes prevalent in some patients who have had high doses of anthracycline (usually 500 mg/m^2 or more). Chronic anthracycline change will result in a heart with four-chamber dilatation, however, usually it does not attain the same size as in idiopathic cardiomyopathy. The chronic changes in anthracycline cardiotoxicity have been described elsewhere.[24,25] Morphologically, two types of myocyte damage are recognized: the myocyte showing complete myofibrillar loss and the other type of cell with dilated sarcotubular reticulum often coalescing and causing vacuolization of the cells. Both of these cells are graded equally in the anthracycline grading system, which has been described.[24] Patients who have had previous mediastinal irradiation are more prone to cardiotoxicity at lower cumulative doses.

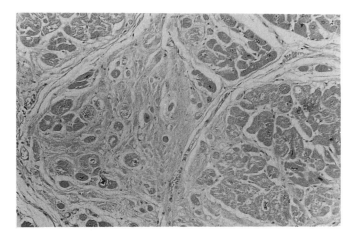

FIGURE 19.16. Section of myocardium in a patient with progressive muscular dystrophy showing myocyte loss and replacement fibrosis.

Infiltrative Disorders

Sarcoidosis

Sarcoidosis may involve the heart and circulation in several ways. It may produce cor pulmonale through pulmonary involvement or it may produce myocardial involvement leading to arrhythmias or heart failure and sudden death. Sarcoidosis is a disease, the etiology of which is unknown. Myocardial involvement is said to occur in 15% to 20% of patients. Sarcoidosis of the heart usually manifests itself by discrete noncaseating granulomas throughout the myocardium, but not usually involving the pericardium (see Fig. 19.17). Sarcoidosis often is accompanied by marked interstitial fibrosis with compensatory hypertrophy and can cause heart failure.

Amyloidosis

The heart may be affected in generalized forms of amyloidosis in chronic sepsis, rheumatoid arthritis, and

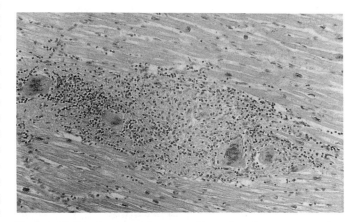

FIGURE 19.17. Section of myocardium showing noncaseating granulomas of sarcoidosis containing giant cells.

other predisposing diseases. The heart is involved in approximately 25% of cases (this has consisted mostly of small amounts of amyloid in myocardial arteries with minimal perimyocytic deposits). The heart is involved with amyloidosis in about 15% of cases of multiple myelomatosis. In addition, the heart is involved in primary amyloidosis with no recognized predisposing condition, particularly in men over the age of 60 years. Grossly, the heart is markedly enlarged with thick rigid walls and may weigh more than 1000 g. Multiple small translucent nodules may be seen through the endocardium. Microscopically, amyloid deposition appears as filamentous waxy bands surrounding myocytes and "hugging" the sarcolemma as opposed to fibrosis, which is mainly within the interstitium. In advanced cases, large masses of amyloid material may replace the myofibers. Nodular masses of amyloid in heart valves also may occur. The coronary arteries also may be involved with amyloid within the media.

Hemosiderosis

The accumulation of excessive amounts of iron pigment in the heart from prolonged hemolysis or repeated transfusions may occur. In hemochromatosis, the heart usually is enlarged and may be dilated. Brown pigmentation also may be visible. Microscopically, hemosiderin appears as brown granular material within the myocytes and sometimes in the interstitium. Iron stains show these deposits to consist of siderin granules, which are also quite striking on electron microscopy. The study by Buja and Roberts[26] confirmed earlier observations that the pigmentation is greatest in the epicardial third of the ventricular walls and least in the middle third. Other storage diseases such as oxalosis, gout and ochronosis and alcaptonuria have been described within the heart.

Heart Failure due to Pericardial Disease

Pericardial Effusion

Pericardial effusion, particularly if it occurs rapidly, may simulate CHF because there is enlargement of the cardiac silhouette, increase in venous pressure, increase in liver size, tenderness, and peripheral edema. An accumulation of blood in the pericardial sac (hemopericardium) usually is secondary to rupture of an acute myocardial infarction or dissection of the aorta or from penetrating wounds, endomyocardial biopsy, or pacemaker perforation. Intrapericardial hemorrhage or fluid may cause cardiac tamponade. Cardiac tamponade increases the pressure around the heart to the point where there is a diastolic pump failure and the ventri-

cles cannot enlarge to take in sufficient blood to pump to the systemic or coronary circulation and the heart fails.

Pericarditis

Inflammation of the pericardium/pericarditis may be due to infections as previously described: viral, bacterial, fungal, and others or it may be due to metabolic disorders such as uremia. Accumulation of pericardial fluid also may be due to neoplastic disease or postmyocardial infarction. Idiopathic pericarditis also can occur and usually is thought to be due to a viral origin, particularly the Coxsackie virus. The term "acute pericarditis" refers to a serous, fibrinous, or serofibrinous inflammation with an exudate of effusion within the pericardial sac. The presence of fibrin will give a shaggy appearance to the pericardium. Microscopically, the subserosal inflammation consists of fibrin, neutrophils, and mononuclear leukocytes. A suppurative effusion will contain bacteria or fungi. Effusions due to neoplasms often contain malignant cells or blood and tuberculosis may result in a caseous exudate. When the volume of pericardial effusion is massive or when the accumulation is rapid, diastolic filling is impaired and cardiac tamponade occurs, causing heart failure. Chronic pericarditis occurs after healing of any of the previous entities causing a chronic constrictive pericarditis characterized by encasement of the heart within dense fibrous tissue, sometimes with calcification. Heart failure ensuing from constrictive pericarditis requires pericardiectomy to relieve the symptoms.

Cardiac Tumors Causing Heart Failure

Primary neoplasms of the heart are very rare (an incidence of 0.02%). Tumors of the heart may result in heart failure by large metastases blocking an outflow tract (Fig. 19.18) or if the tumors are large enough, such as fibroma of the LV, they may cause diastolic failure. Tumors also may contribute to pleural effusions and constrictive pericarditis, as described above (Fig. 19.19). In common with tumors elsewhere in the body, tumors of the heart and pericardium may be classified as benign or malignant.

Benign Tumors
Myxomas

A myxoma is an exophytic tumor that may fill the cardiac chamber or prolapse through one of the atrioventricular (A-V) valves. Usually they are single, but they may be multiple, occupying multiple chambers. Ninety-five percent involve the atria with a 3 to 4 times

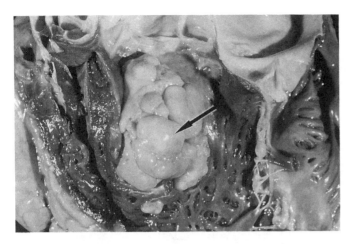

FIGURE 19.18. Metastases of osteosarcoma obstructing the subpulmonic outflow tract (*arrow*).

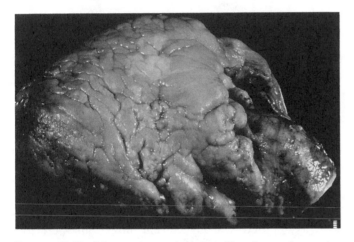

FIGURE 19.19. Metastatic carcinoma infiltrating and encasing the pericardial sac causing constrictive pericarditis.

increased predilection for the left atrium. Cardiac myxomas may result in left heart failure and cor pulmonale if the myxoma is large enough in the left atrium. These tumors usually are attached by one pedicle to the interatrial septum. Microscopically, the tumors contain islands of gland-like vascular spaces in a background of mucopolysaccharide. For this reason, the tumors feel "slimy" on the cut surface. They may, depending on the rapidity of growth, contain patchy hemorrhage and calcification as well as hemosiderin-laden macrophages.

Rhabdomyomas

Rhabdomyomas may be intramyocardial or project into a ventricular cavity. They occur in young children and are associated with tuberous sclerosis. Rhabdomyomas are circumscribed, but they are not encapsulated and usually occur in infancy and early childhood. Microscopically, the rhabdomyomas contain irregular vacuolization of cell cytoplasm, producing so-called spider cells.

Lipomas

The most common sites of lipomas are the LV and the right atrium. The tumors are circumscribed cecile polypoid or intramuscular and often are quite symptomless unless they become very large. Microscopically, they are composed of mature fat cells.

Fibromas

Fibromas occur more often in the interventricular septum or the anterior wall of the LV. These tumors are nonencapsulated and consist of interlacing bundles of fibrous tissues of varying cellularity. They may attain very large sizes and cause heart failure by their size.

Hemangiomas, Lymphangiomas, and Mesotheliomas

Hemangiomas, lymphangiomas, and Mesotheliomas also may occur in the heart. Teratomas are exceedingly rare. Tumors of the heart valves have been described, such as fibromas, myxomas, hematomas, and papillary tumors. One variety is polypoid or flat and occurs in children; the other is papillary and occurs in adults.

Malignant Tumors of the Heart

Sarcomas

Sarcomas comprise either smooth or skeletal muscle and appear to be the most common cardiac primary malignant tumors. Fibrosarcomas, fibromyxosarcomas, and rhabdomyosarcomas are exceedingly rare.

Malignant Vascular Tumors

Malignant vascular tumors (angiosarcomas, Kaposi's sarcoma, malignant hemangioendothelioma, and malignant hemangiopericytomas) have been reported.

Primary Lymphomas

Involvement by primary lymphomas of the heart is rare; they may be diffuse, nodular, or rarely present as an endocardial polypoid growth.

Rare Examples

Rare examples of primary cardiac neoplasms include granular cell myoblastomas, neurogenic sarcomas, ganglioneuromas, and malignant mesenchymoma.

Metastatic Heart Disease

Secondary deposits from malignant neoplastic cells are the most common tumors seen in the heart, outnumbering primary benign or malignant cardiac lesions at least 30-fold. Of all the patients with disseminated malignant

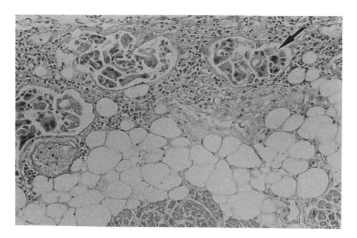

FIGURE 19.20. Lymphatic channels filled with metastasizing breast carcinoma (*arrow*) in the epicardium of the heart.

disease, up to 15% have cardiac lesions. Metastases reach the heart by direct spread (lung and breast), lymphatics (see Fig. 19.20), and the blood stream. The most common primary sites of origin are carcinomas of the lung, breast, large bowel, and stomach, followed by malignant lymphomas. Fifty percent of melanomas will metastarize to the heart (see Fig. 19.21). While metastases often are asymptomatic, patients may present with cardiac failure, arrhythmias, or pericarditis.

Heart Failure Due to Cardiac Allograft Rejection

Cardiac transplantation now is an accepted form of treatment for end-stage heart disease, as has been described elsewhere. Heart failure in the transplant recipient may occur at various stages.

Immediate Heart Failure

On rare occasions the donor heart will fail to function satisfactorily before the patient has left the operating room after cardiac allograft transplantation. This can be due to a number of surgical problems: either a prolonged ischemic time if the heart has been procured distantly or by actual trauma to the heart if the donor was an accident victim. Hemorrhage into the heart from either of these causes may prevent inadequate contraction. If the recipient has severe pulmonary hypertension, the normal RV of the donor may become discolored and fail to contract adequately because it is unable to overcome the increased pulmonary resistance.

Hyperacute Rejection

Hyperacute rejection also is very rare since it results from inaccurate cross-matching of the blood and major

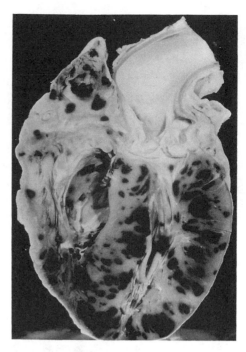

FIGURE 19.21. Longitudinal section of the heart showing metastases of malignant melanoma.

histocompatibility difference of the donor and recipient. Usually the heart dilates, becomes darker in color, and begins to fibrillate or does not contract well before the patient leaves the operating room. Histopathologic changes of hyperacute rejection consist of a marked interstitial hemorrhage seen diffusely throughout the heart as opposed to a myocardial infarction where the hemorrhage is confined to the watershed of a particular vessel. There may be evidence of interstitial edema as well. If the heart is kept going for a while, neutrophils also will become evident in the interstitium. Small vessels often contain "sludging" of red cells, which may block the capillaries, and fibrin thrombi may form.

Acute Rejection

During the first year after cardiac transplantation, particularly the first 3 months, the most common changes are those of acute rejection affecting the myocardium. There are now several different grading systems for acute rejection, but the most generally accepted at this time is that of the International Society for Heart Transplantation.[28] Mild acute rejection is characterized by perivascular and sometimes an endocardial infiltrate of large activated mononuclear cells with prominent nucleolar and pyroninophilic cytoplasm. These cells usually are perivascular in position in Grade 1A and do not cause any myocyte damage. Grade 1B consists of lymphoid cells that have disseminated in the interstitium, but do not cause myocyte damage. The infiltrating mononuclear cells are T cells; depending on the immunosuppressive treatment, they have a preponderance of cytotoxic suppressor T cells, although a few helper T cells also may be present. Patients usually do not go into heart failure with mild acute rejection.

Moderate Acute Rejection

The mononuclear lymphocytic infiltrate still may be perivascular, but also extends into the interstitium causing damage to the adjacent myocytes. The lymphocytes may overlap or actually indent myocytes, causing cell death. Sometimes the myocyte necrosis is quite focal (Grade 2); this usually will not cause heart failure. The amount of infiltrate and its distribution may not be sufficient to cause heart failure, although this will ensue if the patient is not treated with augmentation of immunosuppression. Grade 3B, which is "borderline severe," is an extension of the previous grade with a more extensive infiltrate, more myocyte damage with hemorrhage, and vasculitis in some cases. In severe acute rejection, Grade 4, the diagnosis of severe acute rejection usually is not made until there is a marked increase in interstitial inflammatory infiltrate with obvious myocyte damage. As the rejection becomes more severe, the inflammatory infiltrate becomes mixed, including some neutrophils and eosinophils as well as lymphocytes. At this stage, small vessels become involved with vasculitis and hemorrhage is prominent. Edema is frequently obvious in severe acute rejection. In the same way that heart failure occurs in acute myocarditis, heart failure will ensue in acute rejection.

Acute Vascular (Humoral) Rejection

Recently investigators have observed clinical examples of patients with hemodynamic and echocardiographic and clinical evidence of graft dysfunction without the usual cellular infiltrate described above. The tissue demonstrates evidence of endothelial cell injury of small vessels, which may later proceed to vasculitis and infiltration of vessels by lymphocytes. The interstitium may become edematous, but lacks the features of cellular rejection. Cases of mixed cellular and humoral rejection have been reported. In addition to the light microscopic findings described above, humoral rejection requires immunofluorescent evidence of vascular injury.[29] This is characterized by deposition of immunoglobulins (IgG or IgM, complement $-C_3'$ and/or C1Q and fibrinogen) in a linear staining pattern within the interstitium, suggesting sections of vessel walls. Some of these changes, however, are known not to be entirely specific and can occur with ischemia or other damage to the myocardium. There is some question of whether vascular rejection will increase the risk for the development of coronary graft disease. These findings are still under investigation.

The Pathology of Long-Term Survivors of Cardiac Transplantation Causing Heart Failure

Accelerated graft coronary disease in long-term survivors is a condition sometimes referred to as "chronic rejection." This has been described previously.[30–32] The coronary circulation in the transplanted allograft is subject to the development of a rapidly progressive form of concentric intimal proliferation extending along the entire length of the coronary vessels and including the small branches. Myocardial infarcts can result from this condition, even though angiographic changes of the major epicardial coronaries apparently are not yet totally occluded. These changes can occur as rapidly as 3 months after cardiac transplantation. Pathologic findings take the form of concentric intimal proliferation, which is unlike naturally occurring atherosclerosis because it is not focal or asymmetric as a rule.[32] Also, the internal elastic lamina frequently is intact and not fragmented. Although occasional plaques with cholesterol clefts can be seen, it is not clear whether these are legacies of the donor heart or whether they occur after many years in the transplanted heart. The concentric intimal proliferation may result in silent myocardial infarcts. The infarcts may be small and stellate if the small vessels and branches are occluded. If the infarcts are sufficiently big and sufficient myocardium is damaged, then left heart failure will ensue as in myocardial infarction from other causes.

Conclusions

As can be seen, all the various lesions presented ultimately can result in signs and symptoms of heart failure. If many contractile elements are primarily involved, the principal characteristics of myocardial dysfunction will be systolic in nature. Alternatively, if the lesion is infiltrative or obstructive, or if fewer contractile elements are replaced with noncontractile fibrosis (e.g., endocardial fibrosis), diastolic pump dysfunction will predominate. Often, however, the pathophysiologic states coexist in the most common causes of CHF.

References

1. Braunwald E. Historical overview and pathophysiologic considerations. In: Braunwald E, Mock MB, Watson J, eds. *Congestive heart failure.* Grune & Stratton; New York: 1982:3–9.
2. Buja LM. The heart. In: Robbins SC, Kumar V, eds. Basic pathology. 4th ed. Philadelphia: Saunders; 1987.
3. Billingham ME, Bristow MR, Mason JW, Joseph LJ. Endomyocardial biopsy: In: Braunwald E, Mock MB, Watson J, ed. *Congestive heart failure.* New York: Grune & Stratton; 1982:237–251.

4. Kannel WB, Feinlieb M. Natural history of angina pectoris in the Framingham study. *Am J Cardiol.* 1972;29:154.

5. Titus JL. Pathology of coronary heart disease. *Cardiovasc Clin.* 1969;1:9.

6. Hood WB. Pathophysiology of ischemic heart disease. *Prog Cardiovasc Dis.* 1971;14:197.

7. Bigger JT Jr, Dresdale RJ, Heissenbuttel RH, et al. Ventricular arrythmias in ischemic heart disease: mechanism, prevalence, significance, and management. *Prog Cardiovasc Dis.* 1977;19:255.

8. Page DL, Caulfield JB, Kastor JA, et al. Myocardial changes associated with cardiogenic shock. *N Engl J Med.* 1971;285:133.

9. Tazelaar HD, Billingham ME. Leukocytic infiltrates in idiopathic dilated cardiomyopathy: a source of confusion with active myocarditis. *Am J Surg Pathol.* 1986;10:405–412.

10. Factor SM, Minase T, Okun E, et al. Coronary microvascular spasm in the cardiomyopathic Syrian hamster: primary cause of focal cell necrosis? *Circulation.* 1980;62:111.

11. Alexander CS. Idiopathic heart disease II: electron microscopy examination of myocardial biopsy speciments in alcoholic heart disease. *Am J Med.* 1966;41:229.

12. Alexander CS. Idiopathic heart disease. *Am J Med.* 1966;41:213.

13. Alexander CS. Cobalt-beer cardiomyopathy. *Am J Med.* 1972;53:395.

14. Kouvaras G, Coikkincz D. Effects of alcohol on the heart: current views. *Angiology.* 1986;37:592.

15. Keren A, Billingham ME, Popp RL. Mildly dilated congestive cardiomyopathy: use of prospective diagnostic criteria and description of the clinical course without heart transplantation. *Circulation.* 1990;81:506–517.

16. Keren A, Billingham ME, Popp R. Features of dilated congestive cardiomyopathy compared with idiopathic restrictive cardiomyopathy and typical dilated cardiomyopathy. *J Am Soc of Echocardiogr.* 1988;1:78–87.

17. Silver MM, Silver MD. Cardiomyopathies. In: Churchill Livingstone; Silver MD, ed. *Cardiovascular pathology.* 2nd ed. New York: 1991.

18. Urie PM, Billingham ME. Ultrastructural features of familial cardiomyopathy. *Am J Cardiol.* 1988;62:325–327.

19. Maron BJ. Myocardial disorganization in hypertrophic cardiomyopathy. Another point of view. *Br Heart J.* 1983;50:1.

20. Aretz HT, Billingham ME, Edwards WD, et al. Myocarditis: a histopathologic definition and classification. *Am J Cardiovasc Pathol.* 1986;1:3–4.

21. Schultheiss HP, Kuhl U, Schulze K, et al. Biomolecular changes in dilated cardiomyopathy. In: Baroldi G, Camerini F, Goodwin JF, eds. *Advances in cardiomyopathies.* Berlin: Springer-Verlag; 1990.

22. Archard LC, Bowles NE, Cunningham L, et al. Enterovirus RNA sequences in hearts with dilated cardiomyopathy: a pathogenetic link between virus infection and dilated cardiomyopathy. In: Baroldi G, Camerini F, Goodwin JF, eds. *Advances in cardiomyopathies.* Berlin: Springer-Verlag; 1990.

23. Weiss LM, Movahed LA, Billingham ME, Cleary ML. Detection of Coxsackievirus B3 RNA in myocardial tissues by the polymerase chain reaction. *Am J Pathol.* 1991;138:497–503.

24. Billingham ME. Endomyocardial changes in anthracycline-treated patients with and without irradiation. (Ed. Jerome Vaeth) In: Vaeth J, ed. *Frontiers of radiation therapy and oncology.* Basel: Karger; 1979;13:67–81.

25. Billingham ME, Bristow M. Evaluation of anthracycline cardiotoxicity: predictive ability and functional correlation of endomyocardial biopsy. *Cancer Treat Symp.* 1984;3:71–76.

26. Buja LM, Roberts WC. Iron in the heart: etiology and clinical significance. *Am J Med.* 1971;51:209.

27. Pomerance A. Papillary tumors of the heart valves. *J Pathol Bact.* 1961;81:135.

28. Billingham ME, Cary NRB, Hammond ME, et al. A working formulation for the standardization of nomenclature in the diagnosis of heart and lung rejection: heart rejection study group. *J Heart Transplant.* 1990;9:587–592.

29. Hammond EH, Yowell RL, Nunoda S, et al. Vascular (humoral) rejection in heart transplantation: pathologic observations and clinical implications. *J Heart Transplant.* 1989;8:430–443.

30. Billingham ME. Cardiac transplant atherosclerosis. *Transplant Proc.* 1987;4(5):19–25.

31. Pucci AM, Forbes C, Billingham ME: Pathologic features in long-term cardiac allografts. *J Heart Transplant.* 1990;9(4):339–345.

32. Billingham ME. Graft coronary disease: the lesions and the patients. *Transplant Proc.* 1989;21:3665–3666.

33. Billingham ME. Histopathology of graft coronary disease. *J Heart Lung Transplant.* 1992;11:S38–S44.

Part IV
Pharmacologic Therapy of Congestive Heart Failure

20
Clinical Pharmacokinetics in Congestive Heart Failure

Alan S. Nies

Pharmacokinetics is the study of drug movement in the body from the time of dosing to the time at which all of the drug has been eliminated. Knowledge of pharmacokinetics is key to the design of dosing regimens for optimizing a drug's therapeutic effect. Drug movement across short distances, such as from the lumen of the gastrointestinal tract into the intestinal mucosa or across a cell membrane in the body, is not dependent on blood flow. Intuitively, the circulation must be an important determinant of a drug's movement over longer distances. However, only in the past two decades has there been an attempt to model and quantify the effect of changes in circulatory function on various pharmacokinetic parameters.[1-4] It is now known that all aspects of pharmacokinetics (i.e., absorption, distribution, and elimination) are critically dependent on the circulation. Changes produced by heart failure that would be expected to influence these pharmacokinetic parameters include a) reduced blood flow to sites of drug absorption such as skin, subcutaneous tissue, or intestine, b) interstitial edema at sites of absorption in the intestine or skin, c) delayed gastric emptying due to increased sympathetic and reduced parasympathetic tone, d) reduced blood flow to tissues that normally store drug in the body, such as fat and muscle, e) reduced blood flow to the liver; f) hepatocellular damage due to hypoxia or congestion, and g) reduced blood flow to the kidney with resulting changes in renal function.[5-7] Data exist for some model compounds regarding the influence of an altered circulation on pharmacokinetic variables, and from these data certain generalizations can be made to guide therapy with drugs for which data do not yet exist. This chapter starts with the basics. A description of the important aspects of pharmacokinetics as they relate to the circulation is followed by information on specific drugs that are important for the treatment of patients with congestive heart failure.

Pharmacokinetic Principles

Absorption

To produce systemic effects, drugs must be delivered into the central circulation (see Table 20.1). When a drug is given directly into the vascular space, all of the drug administered is available to produce its effect. For other routes of administration, the drug must pass a variety of barriers before it is able to gain access to the circulation. This absorption process will delay delivery of drug to its site of action and in some circumstances, will reduce the total quantity of drug reaching the circulation. At a minimum, a single cell layer, the capillary endothelium, must be traversed even when a drug is administered intramuscularly. Much more complex is absorption after oral administration where several cell layers must be crossed before the drug reaches the portal circulation, after which the drug must make it through the liver before it reaches the systemic circulation. Many β-adrenergic receptor antagonists, calcium channel blockers, antiarrhythmic agents, and nitrates are substantially metabolized by the liver before they reach the systemic circulation. This "presystemic" or "first pass" elimination accounts for the much larger oral dose required to produce the same effect as an intravenous dose. "Bioavailability" is the term that quantifies the amount of a dose that actually reaches the systemic circulation and varies from zero (none of the drug reaches the circulation) to 1 (100% of the dose reaches the systemic circulation). A reduction of bioavailability after oral administration of a drug indicates either poor absorption or presystemic elimination.[8]

Most drugs are absorbed from their site of administration by passive diffusion with the driving force for absorption being the concentration of drug in contact with the absorbing surface. Thus, the rate of absorption

TABLE 20.1. Influence of heart failure on pharmacokinetic factors influencing the plasma concentration of drugs.

	Effects of heart failure	Consequences	Examples
Absorption			
Oral	Delayed but extent not usually affected	Steady-state concentration unaffected but peak concentration reduced and delayed	Furosemide and bumetanide delivered later and in lower concentration to tubular fluid
Percutaneous	May be reduced	Reduced blood concentration	Nitroglycerin levels reduced
V_D	May be reduced if large	Increased plasma concentration after a loading dose, but concentration at steady state is unaffected; shortens $t_{1/2}$	Lidocaine and procainamide loading doses must be reduced
Hepatic blood flow	Reduced	Reduced clearance and increased concentration at steady state of high clearance drugs that are administered parenterally. Steady-state concentration of orally administered drugs is unaffected	Lidocaine maintenance infusion rate must be reduced
Hepatic metabolic capacity	May be reduced by ischemia and/or congestion	Reduced clearance and increased concentration at steady state of drugs that undergo Phase I metabolism (oxidation, reduction, dealkylation). This affects low clearance drugs given by any route and high clearance drugs given orally. Phase II metabolism (conjugation) usually unaffected. Increased $t_{1/2}$ (see also V_D)	Theophylline and quinidine maintenance doses may need to be reduced. Plasma concentration of these drugs should be used to guide dosing
Renal function	May be reduced	Reduced clearance and increased concentration at steady state of drugs cleared mainly by the kidney. Increased $t_{1/2}$ (see also V_D)	Procainamide, digoxin, enalapril, and lisinopril maintenance doses may need to be reduced in proportion to the reduction in creatinine clearance. For procainamide, the concentration of both the parent drug and its active metabolite (acecainide) must be monitored

V_D = apparent volume of distribution.

can be manipulated by controlling the dissolution of drug from the dosage form. This principle has been useful for designing drug preparations that delay and prolong absorption after oral, intramuscular, subcutaneous, or percutaneous sites of administration. In this way drugs that have short durations of action can be used for chronic therapy with relatively infrequent dosing. Depot preparations for intramuscular use (penicillin, progesterone) slowly release drug, which then is dissolved in tissue fluids and absorbed into the circulation, sustaining an effect over days or weeks. Long-acting oral preparations (e.g., calcium channel blockers, procainamide, theophylline) release drug slowly from the dosage form. For these oral preparations, the duration of sustained absorption is limited to 12 to 24 hr by the transit time of the gastrointestinal tract. Percutaneous absorption is achieving increasing use for a few, highly potent, lipid-soluble drugs. The duration of absorption is limited by the ability to incorporate sufficient drug into the patch that is applied to the skin. The absorption of percutaneous clonidine is sustained over a week; nitroglycerin is administered daily. The advantages of these sustained release preparations are that they are more convenient and thus have the ability to enhance compliance, and they produce a relatively constant blood level so that toxicity associated with the peaks and inefficacy associated with troughs of blood concentration are avoided. With preparations other than oral, drug can reach the systemic circulation without having to pass through the liver and be subjected to hepatic presystemic metabolism. This can improve the bioavailability for a drug, such as nitroglycerin, that is essentially metabolized completely by the liver after oral administration. However, presystemic metabolism may not be avoided entirely since skin also may metabolize nitroglycerin before it reaches the circulation during percutaneous absorption. A disadvantage is that interindividual variation in absorption is increased with the sustained release preparations, and with oral dosage forms, sustained release preparations are more likely to be affected by changes in gastrointestinal motility such that increases in motility can reduce the total quantity of drug absorbed. Another disadvantage that is unrelated to pharmacokinetics is the increased potential for the development of tolerance to the drug's effect when blood levels are sustained relatively constant over long periods of time. This has been of particular interest with the use of percutaneous nitroglycerin, which is discussed elsewhere in this book.

Factors other than drug concentration are important for absorption, particularly in disease states such as congestive heart failure (CHF).[5] Resistance of the absorbing surface to diffusion is a function of the area available for absorption as well its permeability to the drug. Blood flow to the absorption site also is important to remove drug and thereby maximize the concentration gradient across the absorbing surface.[9] For drugs that dissolve readily from the dosage form and diffuse rapidly across cells, blood flow to the site of absorption may be rate limiting. For most drugs, however, the rate of drug delivery from the dosage preparation or the resistance of the absorbing surface to diffusion is the rate limiting step in absorption such that alterations in blood flow become less important. In CHF, edema and a reduction of blood flow at the absorbing site have the potential to reduce bioavailability and/or alter the time course of drug absorption.[10] After oral dosing, most drugs are absorbed across the mucosa of the small intestine so that a delay in gastric emptying can retard absorption. This most commonly delays and decreases the height of the peak concentration in the blood. In heart failure the sympathetic nervous system is activated and the parasympathetic nervous system is depressed. In the gastrointestinal tract these consequences of heart failure reduce peristaltic activity and delay gastric emptying. Thus, several features of heart failure including edema formation, a reduction of blood flow, and a delay in gastric emptying would be predicted to reduce the rate and/or extent (i.e., the bioavailability) of absorption of some drugs.[11] It is important to recognize the consequences of a reduction in the rate or extent of drug absorption. For drugs such as digoxin and theophylline that are administered chronically and for which the target blood levels must remain within a certain range for therapeutic effect, a delay in the rate without a decrease in the extent of absorption is of little or no importance. In fact, a delay in absorption will result in a more constant blood concentration than would be achieved if the dose were absorbed rapidly. However, the rate of absorption can be important if the circulating drug concentration must reach a threshold level or if the rate of drug delivery to the site of action is a critical determinant of the drug's effect. This is the case for furosemide, which has a renal response that is determined by the rate as well as the extent of drug reaching the tubular fluid.[12] A reduction in the rate of oral absorption is one mechanism accounting for the resistance to the diuretic effect of oral furosemide in patients with heart failure.

In contrast to the relative unimportance of a reduc-

tion in rate of absorption for most drugs, a reduction in extent of absorption (bioavailability) will be of importance for all drugs affected since the steady-state concentration of the drug in the plasma will be reduced. The limited amount of data available in CHF indicates that the extent of drug absorption by the gastrointestinal tract usually is affected only minimally and unpredictably. However, the rate of drug absorption from the gut often is delayed, probably as a consequence of a delay in gastric emptying, although edema of the gut wall and a diminished blood flow also could play a role. With transdermal nitroglycerin, there is some evidence that bioavailability is variably reduced in patients with severe CHF, probably as a consequence of subcutaneous edema and reduced dermal blood flow.

Distribution

Once absorbed into the blood, drugs are distributed throughout the body, initially to the well perfused tissues, including the vasculature, heart, and brain, and then to the less well perfused tissues including fat and skeletal muscle. The extent of uptake into tissues depends on the ability of the tissues to bind or partition the drug relative to the binding or partitioning in the plasma. The pharmacokinetic term that describes the distribution of drugs is called the "apparent volume of distribution," often abbreviated as V_D. V_D is defined as the volume that would be required to contain an amount of drug at the concentration achieved in plasma, and therefore is a constant that describes the ratio of the amount of drug in the body (Amt) to the resulting plasma concentration (C_p):

$$V_D = \frac{Amt}{C_p} \qquad (1)$$

Depending on the rate of drug entry into the circulation, the body often behaves as if it were composed of two or more compartments that each have their own V_D. Drug is introduced initially to a smaller V_D (often designated as the "central compartment") and only more gradually is distributed to a larger V_D (often called the "peripheral compartment"). Thus, immediately after an intravenous bolus of a drug such as lidocaine, the drug concentration in the blood is high, but the drug rapidly disappears from the central compartment as it is distributed to the peripheral compartment. The drug concentration then falls more gradually as drug is eliminated from the body. The two phases have been called the initial "distribution phase" followed by the "elimination phase." The most important phase for chronic drug therapy is the elimination phase, during which drug is in equilibrium between the blood and the tissues of the body, and the concentration of drug in the blood therefore bears a consistent relationship to drug at the site of action. The V_D describing this apparent volume of the peripheral compartment therefore is the most clinically relevant value for most drugs and is the V_D listed in tables describing drug pharmacokinetics. Whether the drug concentration in plasma during the distribution phase is predictive of drug effects is dependent on the individual drug. For many drugs such as lidocaine that quickly reach their site of action, plasma concentrations achieved during the distribution phase are associated with therapeutic or toxic effects on the well perfused tissues such as the heart and brain. On the other hand, for a few drugs like digoxin, the plasma concentrations during the distribution phase are not predictive of drug effects. Only after 4 to 8 hr after a dose is there sufficient time for equilibrium to occur such that digoxin in the blood reflects drug at the site of action. A common error in the interpretation of digoxin concentrations in plasma is to ascribe meaning to the high values obtained when blood is sampled within 4 to 6 hr after a dose of digoxin.[13] Although concentrations of 4 to 10 ng/ml may be present at this time, they have no predictive value since they are not in equilibrium with digoxin at its site of action.

The V_D is an apparent volume that is rarely related to an actual volume, and it is a common mistake to attempt to label the V_D as plasma volume, extracellular water, or some other actual fluid space. For drugs that are bound to tissues, the V_D can be much larger than any real volume contained in any fluid space in the body. For instance, digoxin has a V_D of the peripheral compartment of 7 L/kg in normal individuals. Thus, an intravenous dose of 0.5 mg digoxin will be distributed in a peripheral compartment that has an apparent volume of about 500 L in a 70-kg patient, resulting in a plasma concentration of 1 μg/L or 1 ng/ml. A large V_D is the quantitative expression of the fact that drug in the body is present in the tissues at a higher concentration than in the blood. Even drugs that have a V_D similar to a body fluid compartment are rarely distributed everywhere at the same concentration.

The physiological determinants of the V_D are the relative affinities of the tissues and the plasma for the drug and the state of the circulation.[2,5,14] Binding of drug to plasma proteins acts to retain drug in the plasma since it limits the amount of unbound drug that can distribute to the tissues. Displacement of drug from plasma proteins will increase its V_D since there is an increase in the fraction of drug that is unbound, which will leave the central compartment. Drug binding to plasma proteins can be affected by diseases and other drugs. Uremia can reduce the binding of some drugs to plasma albumin since retained acidic metabolites can compete for binding sites. Nephrotic syndrome and hepatic disease can reduce the albumin concentration and thereby reduce the binding of drugs to plasma proteins. CHF usually is not associated with changes in binding to plasma proteins unless it is also accompanied

by renal or hepatic failure. However, the state of the circulation itself is apparently an important determinant of the V_D. This is probably related to the fact that drug is not as readily delivered to the tissues when the circulation is impaired.[15] During heart failure, intense peripheral vasoconstriction restricts access of drug to poorly perfused tissues that make up the peripheral compartment of the V_D. Thus, drugs that are extensively distributed out of the plasma, and therefore have a large V_D, may have a contraction of the V_D in patients with heart failure. This is perhaps counterintuitive on first glance since the edema present in patients with heart failure might suggest that the V_D should be increased. However, this is a fallacy based on the thinking of the V_D as a real volume. One model compound for which the V_D has been shown to be increased is aminopyrine, a substance that actually does seem to distribute only in body water.[16] For most drugs the following rule generally holds: If the V_D is large (1 L/kg or more) then the V_D may be reduced in patients with heart failure; for drugs with small V_D (<1 L/kg), there is little or no change in V_D with heart failure. Lidocaine is the best studied example of a drug that has a reduced V_D of the central and peripheral compartments by about 50% in patients with heart failure.[17]

The size of a loading dose is determined by the volume of distribution of the drug. The concept is that sufficient drug must be given such that after the distribution phase, the plasma concentration is in the desired range ($C_{desired}$). Generally, the V_D of the peripheral compartment is the constant used to calculate a loading dose (LD) delivered into the circulation by rearranging Equation (1):

$$LD = V_D \times C_{desired} \qquad (2)$$

For many drugs the calculated LD must be administered slowly to allow time for distribution so that the very high concentrations resulting from the initial distribution into the small V_D of the central compartment are avoided. In the presence of heart failure, LDs of some drugs must be reduced to account for the reduced V_D in this condition. For lidocaine, therefore, the loading boluses in a patient with heart failure should be about half the standard doses because the V_D for lidocaine is reduced by half in such patients.

Elimination

Most drugs are eliminated from the body by the liver, the kidney, or both organs. For a few drugs elimination occurs in the lung, the blood, or in other tissues. For most drugs the elimination rates are directly proportional to the concentration of drug in the plasma, a process mathematically described as "first order elimination." The most useful concept for describing the variables that are physiologically important for drug elimination is "drug clearance." Drug clearance usually is defined as the volume of fluid (blood or plasma) completely cleared of drug in a unit of time, and thus clearance has units of flow. Clearance was a concept originally used by renal physiologists to describe renal function. Creatinine clearance is the volume of plasma that is completely cleared of creatinine per minute and is calculated as the urinary elimination rate of creatinine divided by the plasma creatinine concentration. By analogy, drug clearance (Cl) can be considered as the rate of drug elimination (R_e) normalized to the plasma concentration (C_p)[4]:

$$Cl = \frac{R_e}{C_p} \quad (3)$$

The total body drug clearance is the sum of all the individual organ clearances, that is, renal clearance plus hepatic clearance plus lung clearance plus clearance by all other means.

Physiologically, clearance is equal to the product of blood flow (Q) to the eliminating organ and the extraction ratio (E), which is the fraction of the drug in the blood removed during a single passage through the organ:

$$Cl = Q \times E \quad (4)$$

Clearance is thus an index of the efficiency of drug removal from the blood and is *not* influenced by the distribution of drug in the body. Equation (4) implies that hepatic drug clearance (Cl_H) would be related directly to hepatic blood flow. However, this is not the case because the extraction ratio is not a constant. Hepatic extraction of drug from the blood is a function of a) hepatic blood flow, b) the inherent ability of the liver to irreversibly remove drug from the blood, and c) the binding of drug to the plasma proteins and the cellular components of blood.[2,3] A number of models of hepatic elimination have been proposed.[4] The most useful is the "well stirred model," which assumes that drug available to the eliminating processes of the liver is in equilibrium with hepatic venous blood.[1] Based on this model, the following relationship can be derived:

$$Cl_H = Q[E] = Q\left[\frac{f_B Cl_{int}^u}{Q + f_B Cl_{int}^u}\right] = Q\left[\frac{Cl_{int}}{Q + Cl_{int}}\right] \quad (5)$$

where f_B is the free (unbound) fraction of drug in the blood and Cl_{int}^u is the "intrinsic hepatic clearance," an index of the ability of the liver to remove unbound drug from liver water by metabolizing enzymes and transport processes. Since binding of drug to plasma proteins is not changed by heart failure, $f_B Cl_{int}^u$ can be combined into a single term, Cl_{int} which represents the ability of the liver to remove drug from blood rather than from liver water. Although Equation (5) appears formidable, it is useful for predicting the changes in hepatic drug clearance that occur when hepatic blood flow is impaired in CHF. It is instructive to consider two drug types that represent the limits of this equation. First consider a drug with a very high intrinsic hepatic clearance. In this case Cl_{int} is much larger than hepatic blood flow, and so the extraction ratio [$Cl_{int}/(Q + Cl_{int})$] is very high and approaches 1. Thus, hepatic drug clearance [Equation (5)] approaches hepatic blood flow. Drugs that have this type of Cl_{int} are called "high clearance drugs" and include lidocaine, propranolol, nifedipine, diltiazem, and verapamil. When given intravenously, their clearance is dependent on hepatic blood flow. Because of the very high hepatic extraction, such drugs are subject to a high first pass hepatic extraction and consequently have poor oral bioavailability. Contrast this with the situation when Cl_{int} is much less than hepatic blood flow. In this case the extraction ratio approaches [Cl_{int}/Q], and hepatic drug clearance therefore approaches Cl_{int} and is independent of hepatic blood flow. Such drugs are called "low clearance drugs" and include warfarin, theophylline, quinidine, and mexiletine. Thus, the model predicts that the hepatic clearance of drugs with a high hepatic extraction ratio and hence a high hepatic clearance are very sensitive to changes in hepatic blood flow, whereas the clearance of drugs with a low extraction ratio and consequently a low hepatic clearance are insensitive to changes in blood flow. This is because the extraction of these low clearance drugs is inversely proportional to hepatic blood flow so that as blood flow is reduced, the extraction ratio increases nearly proportionally and clearance, which is the product of blood flow and extraction, is therefore little changed. This is illustrated graphically in Figure 20.1. In the top portion (A) is illustrated the hepatic clearance (solid line) and hepatic extraction ratio (dashed line) versus hepatic blood flow for a high clearance drug that has a hepatic extraction of 0.9 at a normal liver blood flow of 1500 ml/min. Cl_{int} is assumed to remain constant as hepatic blood flow changes. As hepatic blood flow varies from 400 ml/min to 2000 ml/min, the actual hepatic clearance for the high clearance drug varies almost proportionally, and the extraction ratio remains relatively constant. In the bottom portion of Figure 20.1 (B) the effect of changes in hepatic blood flow on the actual hepatic clearance (solid line) and extraction ratio (dashed line) is depicted for a low clearance drug that has a hepatic extraction ratio of 0.1 at a normal liver blood flow of 1500 ml/min. Here the hepatic clearance remains relatively constant as liver blood flow changes because the extraction of the low clearance drug is increased as hepatic blood flow is reduced.[2,3]

A similar series of arguments can be applied to changes in hepatic function related to high and low clearance drugs. In the model, changes in hepatic function are reflected by changes in Cl_{int}. Thus, the hepatic clearance of low clearance drugs is influenced primarily

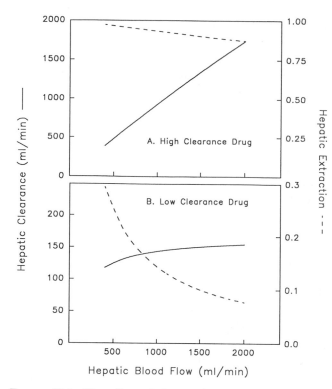

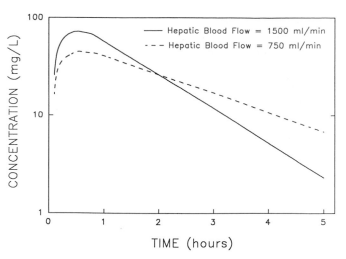

FIGURE 20.1. The effect of changes in hepatic blood flow on the actual hepatic clearance (*solid line*) and extraction ratio (*dashed line*) of two drugs that are metabolized entirely by the liver. A high clearance drug (E = 0.9 at a liver blood flow of 1500 ml/min) is shown in the top of the figure and a low clearance drug (E = 0.1 at a liver blood flow of 0.1 ml/min) is shown on the bottom. Liver blood flow is varied over the range of 400 to 2000 ml/min. Modified, with permission, from Wilkinson GR, Shand DG. *Clin Pharmacol Ther.* 1975; 18:377–390.

FIGURE 20.2. The effect of a change in hepatic blood flow on the plasma concentration–time profile of a high clearance drug (E = 0.9 at a liver blood flow of 1500 ml/min) that is metabolized entirely by the liver and is administered orally at time zero. The curve with a normal liver blood flow is depicted by the solid line, and the curve with a liver blood flow of half normal (750 ml/min) is depicted by the dashed line. When liver blood flow is reduced, the peak plasma concentration is reduced, indicating an increased hepatic presystemic elimination. However, once in the circulation the drug is eliminated less rapidly because the hepatic blood flow is reduced. As a result of these two effects of a reduction in hepatic blood flow, the average plasma concentration (i.e., the area under the curve) is unchanged. Modified, with permission, from Wilkinson GR, Shand DG. *Clin Pharmacol Ther.* 1975; 8:377–390.

by changes in hepatic function and is relatively independent of changes in blood flow and vice versa for high clearance drugs. Severe CHF can produce hepatocellular damage from hypoperfusion or congestion, which will result in a reduction of Cl_{int}. Therefore, since heart failure can reduce hepatic function as well as hepatic blood flow, the hepatic clearance of both high clearance and low clearance drugs can be affected, but for different reasons.

A powerful prediction from the model that is not intuitively obvious is that the average plasma concentration of an orally administered drug that is eliminated solely by hepatic metabolism is not affected by changes in hepatic blood flow, even if the drug is a high clearance drug. This is because a change in hepatic blood flow will alter the extraction of drug not only on the first pass through the liver but also on each subsequent pass, and these influences cancel each other. As shown in Figure 20.2, a reduction in hepatic blood flow will increase the first-pass hepatic extraction (E) of a high clearance drug [Equation (5)], reducing the amount of

an oral dose reaching the systemic circulation and thereby reducing the peak plasma concentration achieved after the dose. However, this reduced amount of drug is then cleared less well because of the decrease in hepatic blood flow [Equation (5)], which, if V_D is unchanged, will prolong the drug's half-life. This reduction in hepatic clearance exactly counters the reduced amount escaping hepatic extraction on the first pass resulting in no change in average plasma concentration. Mathematically, the apparent clearance of a hepatically metabolized drug administered orally (Cl_O) is the hepatic clearance (Cl_H) divided by the fraction of the dose escaping first pass hepatic extraction (1-E). By substituting in Equation (5) and solving for Cl_O, one derives the surprising fact that:

$$Cl_O = Cl_{int} \qquad (6)$$

indicating that the apparent clearance for a drug given orally is independent of hepatic blood flow and only dependent on the Cl_{int}, which is the functional capacity of the liver to remove drug from blood. Clinically, Equation (6) suggests that if heart failure produces changes in steady-state blood levels for any given oral dosing regimen of a drug that is solely eliminated by hepatic metabolism, then there must be a reduction in hepatocellular function. It is only for intravenous infusions of high clearance drugs, such as lidocaine, that hepatic blood flow has a significant effect on steady-state blood levels.

Renal clearance of drugs is much simpler and more predictable than hepatic drug clearance. Fortunately, drug clearance by the kidney is proportional to glomerular filtration rate even if the drug is cleared by tubular secretion and/or reabsorption rather than by filtration. Thus, by estimating or measuring creatinine clearance one can determine the effect of renal dysfunction on renal drug clearance and dosage adjustments can be made accordingly.[8]

Half-life

The most commonly used pharmacokinetic term is "drug half-life" ($t_{1/2}$), which is the time required to reduce the plasma concentration of drug by half. Half-life often is used to characterize drug elimination. However, it frequently is not appreciated that $t_{1/2}$ is actually a hybrid term that is dependent on two independent variables, drug clearance (Cl) and V_D:

$$t_{1/2} = \frac{0.693 V_D}{Cl} \tag{7}$$

Thus, at any given clearance more time will be required (i.e., a longer $t_{1/2}$) to clear the body of drug if there is a large V_D than if the V_D is smaller. If clearance is reduced, $t_{1/2}$ will be prolonged as long as V_D isn't changed. Thus, a change in $t_{1/2}$ cannot be used as an index of efficiency of drug elimination unless the apparent volume of distribution is unchanged. Cardiac failure can reduce the clearance as well as the volume of distribution of some drugs, and therefore $t_{1/2}$ is a particularly poor index of changes in drug elimination in this disease state. The best example is that of lidocaine, which has a reduction of both clearance and V_D of about 50% in some patients with heart failure. However, because of the relationship in equation (7), $t_{1/2}$ may not be changed. Nonetheless, the loading doses and maintenance doses of lidocaine (see below) must be reduced to avoid toxicity. If only $t_{1/2}$ is measured, there will be no clue to the major changes in kinetics that have occurred in this illness.

Half-life is important for the time course of drug elimination and accumulation. If drug administration ceases, only half the drug leaves the body in one $t_{1/2}$, half the remaining drug is eliminated in the second half life, and so forth. Thus, if 100% is present at time zero, 50% will be present after one $t_{1/2}$, 25% after two $t_{1/2}$, 12.5% after three $t_{1/2}$, 6.25% after four $t_{1/2}$, and 3.125% after five $t_{1/2}$. In theory, an infinite time is needed to rid the body of all drug; in practice, three to five $t_{1/2}$ are needed to effectively eliminate drug.

When drugs are given as a continuous infusion or as repeated intermittent doses, drug accumulates in the body until a steady state is achieved. The rate of drug accumulation depends on drug $t_{1/2}$ and is the mirror image of the rate of drug elimination discussed above. Thus, accumulation to half of the ultimate steady-state level occurs in one $t_{1/2}$, but it takes three $t_{1/2}$ to achieve 87.5% of steady state and five $t_{1/2}$ to reach 96.875% of steady state. For practical purposes, steady state is achieved when 90% of the ultimate accumulation occurs. For drugs with a long $t_{1/2}$ accumulation occurs slowly, and a LD may be necessary to achieve therapeutic effects quickly. However, regardless of whether a loading dose is given, the final steady state achieved is independent of the loading dose or the $t_{1/2}$ and is determined solely by the maintenance dose and the drug clearance (see below). The concept of accumulation applies equally well to a continuous infusion or to intermittent doses. As smaller doses are given more frequently the variation in peaks and troughs diminishes, but the average blood level reached at steady state is independent of dose frequency and is determined only by the dose per unit time and the clearance.

Half-life also describes the time course of changes in drug concentration when the dose or infusion rate is changed. Using the same reasoning as discussed above, three to five $t_{1/2}$ will be required to achieve a new steady state. Thus, the consequences of changing doses or infusion rates are delayed, and this delay is dependent on the $t_{1/2}$.

Maintenance Doses

When the amount of drug administered and absorbed over a period of time (dose/time, D/t) is the same as the amount of drug eliminated during the same time (elimination rate, R_e), steady state has been achieved. From the definition of clearance in Equation (3) it can be readily appreciated that both the dose/time and the elimination rate are equal to drug clearance times the steady-state plasma concentration (C_{ss}):

$$R_e = \frac{D}{t} = Cl \times C_{ss} \tag{8}$$

Thus, drug clearance and the dose/time are the sole determinants of the concentration of drug in the blood and the amount of drug in the body at steady state. Importantly, the steady-state concentration is independent of the V_D or the $t_{1/2}$. For drugs given intravenously, hepatic clearance is dependent on both hepatic blood flow and hepatic function, which therefore influence the steady state concentration. For drugs given orally, the hepatic portion of drug clearance is independent of hepatic blood flow and only dependent on the liver's metabolic capacity [Equation (5)]. Equation (8) can be used to calculate the dose required to achieve a given plasma concentration of the drug if clearance is known. As an example, the clearance of lidocaine in an average adult without heart failure or hepatic disease is about 800 ml/min. Thus, to achieve a therapeutic plasma concentration of 3 mg/L will require an infusion of 2.4 mg/min. In a patient with heart failure and reduced hepatic blood flow, lidocaine clearance may be reduced to 400 ml/min, and thus an infusion rate of 1.2 mg/min will be all that is necessary to achieve the same therapeutic level of 3 mg/L.

Effect of Heart Failure on Pharmacokinetics of Specific Drugs[9]

Antiarrhythmic Drugs[18]

Quinidine

Much of the early data on quinidine kinetics in heart failure are confusing because of nonspecific assay methodology. Oral absorption can be delayed in some patients with heart failure, and the V_D (normally 2.7 L/kg) may be reduced such that quinidine concentrations peak later and are higher after an oral dose in patients with heart failure.[19,20] Quinidine is largely metabolized by the liver as a low clearance drug (normally 4.7 ml/min/kg). However, if heart failure is severe enough to cause hepatocellular dysfunction, the clearance of quinidine will be reduced so that higher blood levels will result from usual oral doses.[21,22] Quinidine's $t_{1/2}$ (normally 6–7 hr), however, is not changed in most patients with heart failure because of an equivalent reduction in V_D and clearance. However, an occasional patient with very severe heart failure and hepatic dysfunction with markedly depressed hepatic quinidine clearance will have a prolonged $t_{1/2}$.[23]

Quinidine has pharmacokinetic drug interactions with a number of drugs. Its metabolism can be induced by several common enzyme inducers including phenobarbital,[24] phenytoin,[24] and rifampin,[25] resulting in an increase in hepatic clearance as a consequence of an increase in Cl_{int}. Quinidine plasma concentration therefore will decrease as a result of this interaction and may fall below the therapeutic range. Cimetidine,[26] verapamil,[27] and amiodarone[28] can reduce the metabolism of quinidine and thereby reduce its clearance resulting in an increase in steady-state quinidine levels. Quinidine and verapamil also produce additive effects on the vasculature and the combination can result in severe hypotension.[29] Importantly, quinidine can reduce the clearance of digoxin[30] and to a lesser extent digitoxin,[31] increasing the blood levels of these glycosides. Finally, quinidine can block the enzyme that accounts for the rapid metabolism of encainide and propafenone in 93% of the population who are exten-

sive metabolizers of these drugs.[32,33] The consequences of this interaction are complex since both encainide and propafenone have active metabolites, and whether dosage adjustments are required is not clear.

Procainamide

Procainamide is normally well absorbed from the gastrointestinal tract, but in the presence of severe heart failure absorption may be delayed and/or incomplete. The V_D of procainamide (normally 1.9 L/kg) has been found to be reduced in some patients with heart failure,[34] but this has not been a universal finding.[35] Procainamide is metabolized to an active metabolite N-acetylprocainamide (NAPA, acecainide) that has class III antiarrhythmic activity. The metabolism rate is genetically determined with about half of the American population being fast and half slow acetylators. In all patients with normal renal function, 60% to 80% of procainamide and essentially all of the acetylated metabolite is excreted in the urine. Hepatic clearance of procainamide is low and not affected much by liver blood flow. The major determinant of the drug's clearance therefore is the renal function.[36] When renal function is diminished, the acetylated metabolite accumulates more than the parent drug, and this can be the case in heart failure–induced renal dysfunction.[37] Thus, for optimum patient management, the blood concentrations of both procainamide and acecainide should be monitored. In the absence of renal dysfunction, patients with heart failure do not have any consistent changes in procainamide clearance and therefore require drug doses similar to patients without heart failure to maintain therapeutic concentrations of the drug in the blood.[35]

Cimetidine,[26] ranitidine,[26] trimethoprim,[38] and amiodarone[28] can reduce the renal clearance of procainamide and its active metabolite NAPA, resulting in increased plasma concentration of both at any given dose of procainamide.

Disopyramide

Disopyramide is contraindicated in patients with heart failure because of its potent negative inotropic effects.[39–41] Therefore, there are not many studies of its kinetics in this situation. Oral absorption of disopyramide is not changed by heart failure. The clearance of disopyramide (normally 1.2 ml/min/kg) is about 55% renal with the remainder being hepatic metabolism. Clearance can be reduced in heart failure, and $t_{1/2}$ (normally 6 hr) can be prolonged, especially if there is renal dysfunction.[42] The V_D of disopyramide is relatively small (normally 0.6 L/kg) and is unchanged in heart failure.

The most important interactions with disopyramide are with other negatively inotropic drugs such as β-adrenergic receptor antagonists that can add to the cardiac depression produced by disopyramide. A few pharmacokinetic interactions with potential clinical importance have been reported including a reduction of disopyramide clearance with hepatic P450–inducing drugs,[43] such as phenobarbital, phenytoin, or rifampin, and inhibition of disopyramide metabolism with erythromycin.[44]

Moricizine

Moricizine is well absorbed after oral administration but undergoes first-pass metabolism that reduces the bioavailability to 35% to 40%. It has a high hepatic clearance (20 ml/min/kg), no renal clearance, a large V_D (3 L/kg), and a short $t_{1/2}$ of 2 to 6 hr.[45,46] There may be active metabolites since there is no apparent correlation between blood levels and effects, and the onset of antiarrhythmic effect is substantially delayed from the time of the peak plasma concentration. Whether heart failure influences the pharmacokinetics of moricizine is unknown.

Few drug interactions have been reported with moricizine. Cimetidine inhibits the metabolism of moricizine.[47] Because active metabolites as well as the parent drug may be important to the effects of moricizine, it is impossible to predict the outcome of such an interaction, but it does not appear to have much clinical importance. Moricizine may enhance the metabolism and reduce the plasma concentration of theophylline.[47]

Lidocaine

Lidocaine has been used frequently as an example in the discussion above because it has been well studied in patients with heart failure. Its V_D (normally 1.5 L/kg) is reduced by as much as 50%, and its clearance (normally 11 ml/min/kg), which is entirely hepatic, is reduced by 50% or more, largely because of the decreased hepatic blood flow as a consequence of a low cardiac output.[17,48–50] The $t_{1/2}$ may be prolonged or it may be unchanged. As a consequence of these changes, lidocaine loading doses and maintenance infusion rates should be reduced by half in patients with heart failure, and signs of toxicity must not be overlooked. Blood concentrations of lidocaine may be helpful in determining the proper maintenance dose in individual patients.

Drug interactions with lidocaine are relatively rare. β-adrenergic receptor antagonists can reduce hepatic blood flow and some may also reduce the Cl_{int} of lidocaine, resulting in a reduction of lidocaine clearance of 15% to 45%.[51] Cimetidine also has been reported to reduce lidocaine clearance.[26] This is probably because of cimetidine's effect on hepatic drug metabolism (i.e., the Cl_{int} of lidocaine). Cimetidine also may reduce hepatic blood flow in some circumstances.

Mexiletine

Oral absorption of mexiletine is not affected by heart failure. Its V_D is large (normally 4.9 L/kg). The drug is metabolized almost entirely by the liver as a low to moderate clearance drug (normally 6.3 ml/min/kg). Heart failure does not affect mexiletine clearance unless it is severe, in which case $t_{1/2}$ (normally 9–12 hr) can be prolonged.[52]

Mexiletine's hepatic clearance can by enhanced by the enzyme inducers rifampin[53] or phenytoin.[54] Smokers have a higher clearance than nonsmokers.[55] Mexiletine can reduce the clearance of theophylline, occasionally resulting in theophylline toxicity.[56]

Tocainide

Tocainide pharmacokinetics is little changed by mild to moderate heart failure.[57] The drug is well absorbed and is eliminated by the liver (60%) and the kidneys (40%). Some studies suggest a reduction in clearance (normally 2.6 ml/min/kg) in severe heart failure associated with renal dysfunction and there also may be a reduction in the V_D (normally 3.0 L/kg) with no change in $t_{1/2}$ (normally 14 hr). However, the interpatient variability of $t_{1/2}$ in a group of patients with heart failure is large and some patients can have a markedly prolonged $t_{1/2}$.[58,59]

Tocainide does not interact with many other drugs. There is one study in healthy volunteers suggesting that cimetidine can inhibit the absorption of tocainide,[60] and another that rifampin may increase the hepatic metabolism of tocainide,[61] but the clinical significance of these studies is uncertain.

Encainide

Encainide displays complex pharmacokinetics.[62,63] The drug is well absorbed but in about 93% of the population, who are extensive metabolizers of encainide, first-pass metabolism reduces the bioavailability to 50% or less. The metabolites ODE and MODE formed in these patients are active and account for most of the overall antiarrhythmic activity attributed to encainide. The hepatic clearance of encainide is very high in these patients 25 ml/min/kg), and the $t_{1/2}$ is short (2 hr), whereas the active metabolites have lower clearances and longer half-lives. CHF may reduce the conversion rate of encainide to active metabolites, but whether an adjustment in dosing is necessary is unknown.[18] Because of the multiple active species in the blood after encainide administration, plasma concentrations have not been useful in adjusting dosage. Severe renal impairment results in excessive accumulation of active metabolites necessitating a reduction in dosage to avoid toxicity.[62] In the 7% of the population who are poor metabolizers encainide is a low clearance drug (2.6 ml/min/kg) with high bioavailability and a much longer $t_{1/2}$ (11.3 hr).

Active metabolites are not formed to any significant degree, and the antiarrhythmic activity is attributable to the parent drug. Whether adjustments in dose need to be made in poor metabolizers who have heart failure is unknown.

The interaction of encainide with quinidine has been mentioned above. Cimetidine can reduce encainide's metabolism but the clinical relevance is unknown.[26,63]

Flecainide

Because of its negative inotropic activity, flecainide usually is not given to patients with severe heart failure.[64] Flecainide is well absorbed and has a high bioavailability after oral administration. Its clearance is relatively low (5.6 ml/min/kg), its V_D is large (4.9 L/kg), it is metabolized to inactive metabolites, and renal elimination accounts for about 40% of the dose. The average $t_{1/2}$ in patients with heart failure (19 hr) is somewhat longer than in normals (14 hr), which may be due to a reduction in the renal elimination of the drug.[65,66] An occasional patient with heart failure can have a markedly reduced clearance and prolonged $t_{1/2}$.[67,68] Blood levels of flecainide correlate with effects and toxicity and can be used to guide dosage in patients with arrhythmias.

Cimetidine, quinidine, and amiodarone reduce the hepatic metabolism of flecainide, thus decreasing clearance and increasing plasma concentrations at steady state. Flecainide may slightly increase the serum levels of digoxin. The clinical significance of these interactions is not known.[66]

Propafenone

Although well absorbed, propafenone undergoes extensive first-pass metabolism in 93% of the population to active metabolites, which reduces the bioavailability of propafenone to 10% to 15%.[69] The drug is a weak β-adrenergic receptor antagonist.[69,70] This property, along with its negative inotropic effect, suggests that propafenone must be given with caution to patients with decompensated heart failure.[71,72] Propafenone has a high, but variable, hepatic clearance and a $t_{1/2}$ of 2 to 10 hr in the extensive metabolizers.[69] In the poor metabolizers, who make up 7% of the population, the hepatic clearance is low and the $t_{1/2}$ is much longer (12–32 hr). There are no data on the changes in pharmacokinetics produced by heart failure.

Rifampin has been reported to increase the clearance of propafenone and to reduce its antiarrhythmic effect.[73] Propafenone can increase digoxin concentration in normal volunteers and patients, perhaps increasing the effects of digoxin.[74,75] The metabolism of warfarin may be inhibited by propafenone thereby increasing the anticoagulant effect.[76] The metabolism of propranolol and metoprolol can be inhibited by propafenone, resulting in increased concentrations of these β-adrenergic antagonists.[77] Quinidine can reduce the metabolism of propafenone to one of its active metabolites, but the clinical significance of this observation is unknown.[69]

Amiodarone

Amiodarone has a low and variable oral bioavailability, which may be due in part to first pass metabolism by the gut mucosa. The V_D of amiodarone is extremely large (66 L/kg), which, combined with a low clearance (1.9 ml/min/kg, entirely hepatic), results in a very long $t_{1/2}$ of 1 to 2 months.[78] It is unlikely that heart failure will alter the pharmacokinetics of amiodarone, but this has not been specifically studied.

Amiodarone interacts with many other drugs to inhibit their metabolism or excretion.[78,79] This results in a reduced clearance and increased plasma concentration of the other drug. Drugs documented to be affected include digoxin, flecainide, phenytoin, warfarin, quinidine, encainide, procainamide, diltiazem, and benzodiazepines. Undoubtedly this list is not complete. A good rule is to assume that amiodarone will reduce the clearance of all other drugs coadministered and to monitor carefully blood levels and/or effects when amiodarone is added to any other drug regimen.

Inotropic Drugs

Digoxin

Digoxin in tablet form is absorbed slowly from the gut to the extent of about 65% to 70%. CHF does not consistently alter the rate or extent of absorption,[80,81] but absorption can be delayed in some patients with heart failure, particularly after a myocardial infarction.[82] This is probably related to a change in bowel motility. The V_D of 7 L/kg is similar in patients with or without heart failure. Since the drug is predominantly eliminated by the kidney, the clearance of the drug and the $t_{1/2}$ are not altered unless renal function is affected by heart failure. Thus, renal function can be used as a guide to selecting the maintenance dose of digoxin in heart failure.

A number of drugs reduce digoxin clearance and increase plasma digoxin concentration; these drugs include quinidine, amiodarone, verapamil, flecainide, and propafenone.[30,75,83,84] The best studied and probably most important and consistent of these interactions is that of quinidine and digoxin.[30] When a patient who is receiving digoxin is begun on quinidine, the maintenance dose of digoxin should be reduced by half. The plasma digoxin concentration should be monitored, but it is not worthwhile to obtain a level sooner than 5 days (about 3 half-lives of digoxin) after beginning the quinidine, unless clinical signs and symptoms warrant it. The next most significant of these interactions is that with amiodarone.[85,86] Amiodarone may increase digoxin absorption by an unknown mechanism as well as reduce digoxin clearance. This interaction may be gradual as the body load of amiodarone very gradually increases. The dose of digoxin need not be reduced initially, but the plasma digoxin concentration should be monitored weekly for 2 weeks to determine if there is an interaction occurring that requires a dosage adjustment. For the interaction of digoxin with the other drugs listed, a single blood level drawn 1 week after beginning the interacting drug should be adequate to determine whether the digoxin dosage needs to be adjusted.

Dobutamine

Used as an acute inotropic agent, dobutamine is given intravenously and titrated to produce a specific effect. In patients with CHF, dobutamine has a small V_D (0.2 L/kg) that may be somewhat larger in patients with edema, a large clearance (2350 ml/min/m^2) that is independent of cardiac output or liver blood flow, and a short $t_{1/2}$ (2.37 min).[87] With drugs like dobutamine, knowledge of pharmacokinetic changes in disease is not particularly helpful since the drug is given until it produces the hemodynamic end-point desired.[88]

Pharmacokinetic drug interactions are not important for the use of dobutamine.

Amrinone

The first of the phosphodiesterase inhibitors, amrinone is used intravenously for its acute inotropic and vasodilator affects. Although well absorbed orally, amrinone is not used for chronic therapy because of its toxicities. The drug has a V_D of 1.3 L/kg[89] that is not altered in heart failure.[88] It is cleared by renal and hepatic mechanisms. Part of hepatic metabolism is by N-acetylation at a genetically determined rate. About half the U.S. population are fast acetylators and have a substantially increased total clearance (9 ml/kg/min) and shorter $t_{1/2}$ (2 hr) compared to the slow acetylators (4 ml/kg/min and 4.4 hr).[90] Clearance is reduced by about half, and $t_{1/2}$ is doubled in patients with heart failure.[88,91,92] Whether this is due to reduced hepatic or renal function is not known.

Pharmacokinetic drug interactions are not important in the use of amrinone.

Milrinone

Another phosphodiesterase inhibitor, milrinone is still experimental in the U.S. It can be administered orally or intravenously. Oral bioavailability of amrinone in normal volunteers is >0.9. Patients with severe heart failure have delayed absorption and slightly reduced bioavailability (0.75). The V_D of milrinone is 0.25 to 0.45 L/kg and is little affected by heart failure.[88,92] The drug is eliminated mainly by the kidneys with a total clearance of 6 ml/min/kg that is reduced by half in patients with heart failure who have renal dysfunction.[92] The $t_{1/2}$ of milrinone is 0.9 hr in normals and twice as long in patients with severe heart failure.[93]

Drug interaction with milrinone is not known to be of importance.

Diuretics

Furosemide

Furosemide pharmacokinetics and pharmacodynamics have been particularly well studied in CHF. The oral absorption of furosemide is considerably delayed in patients with severe heart failure so that the peak concentration achieved is lower and occurs later. However, contrary to general belief, the extent of absorption (normal bioavailability of 0.5) is not consistently changed in patients with heart failure.[94,95] The V_D is small (0.15–0.2 L/kg) and is not changed in heart failure.[94] Sixty percent of the absorbed dose is eliminated by the kidneys. The renal clearance (normally 1 ml/min/kg) is reduced in patients with heart failure who have a reduced creatinine clearance, but the nonrenal clearance is unchanged.[94] The $t_{1/2}$ (normally 90 min) is increased up to twice normal in patients with heart failure because of the reduction in renal clearance.[94,96] Because the response to furosemide requires the drug to gain access to the tubular fluid, patients who have a diminished renal function due to heart failure will have a reduced response to the diuretic. However, other factors also are important, such as the time course of delivery of furosemide into the tubular fluid; therefore, the delay in oral absorption of furosemide also is a factor in the diminished response to the drug that is sometimes seen in patients with severe heart failure.[12,97,98] For a prompt diuretic response, intravenous drug is preferred.

Part of furosemide's diuretic effect and its ability to increase venous capacitance after intravenous administration are inhibited by nonsteroidal antiinflammatory drugs that inhibit prostaglandin synthesis.[99] Another important interaction is enhanced otic or renal toxicity with aminoglycosides.

Bumetanide

Although bumetanide is about 40 times more potent and is better absorbed (normal bioavailability is 0.8) than furosemide, there is no important reason to choose one of these diuretics over the other for use in patients with CHF.[98,100,101] Heart failure affects the absorption, clearance, and $t_{1/2}$ of bumetanide to the same extent as furosemide.[102] Thus, absorption is delayed but the extent of absorption is not affected.[103] Bumetanide's V_D

of 0.15 L/kg is unchanged in heart failure, but its renal clearance (normally 2.6 ml/min/kg) may be reduced and its $t_{1/2}$ (normally 0.8 hr) prolonged two- to threefold in patients with heart failure who have renal dysfunction similar to the effect of heart failure on the kinetics of furosemide.

Drug interactions with bumetanide are the same as with furosemide.

Hydrochlorothiazide

Hydrochlorothiazide absorption may be diminished in some patients with CHF, but this drug has not been studied extensively. Hydrochlorothiazide is cleared almost entirely by the kidney so that its clearance (normally 5 ml/min/kg) is reduced and its $t_{1/2}$ (normally 2.5 hr) is prolonged in patients who have CHF with renal dysfunction.[7,104]

In general, drug interactions are not important with thiazide diuretics. Lithium clearance may be reduced in patients with heart failure, particularly if they are on thiazide diuretics, which can result in lithium toxicity in patients receiving lithium carbonate therapy.[105]

Vasodilators

Captopril

The oral bioavailability of captopril is about 65% and this does not appear to be altered by heart failure. The V_D of 0.8 L/kg may be increased in heart failure.[106] The normal $t_{1/2}$ is 2 hr and the total clearance is 12 ml/min/kg, which is 40% renal. The renal clearance can be reduced and $t_{1/2}$ prolonged if renal insufficiency is present. The metabolites of captopril, which is a sulfhydryl-containing compound, include mixed disulfides that may act as a reservoir for the active drug.[107] Captopril metabolism is not influenced by heart failure. Heart failure may increase the response to captopril and other converting enzyme inhibitors, but this is not due to a pharmacokinetic change. Rather, it is related to the fact that plasma renin activity often is elevated in patients with heart failure.[108]

Enalapril

Unlike captopril, enalapril is a "pro-drug" that must be activated by hydrolysis to enalaprilic acid, a diacid that is the active compound.[109] The absorption of enalapril is about 70%, and about 55% of that is hydrolyzed to the diacid so that 35% to 40% of an oral dose is converted into active compound.[110,111] Most of the diacid is eliminated in the urine with a $t_{1/2}$ of 11 hr. CHF does not alter these pharmacokinetic parameters, although if renal dysfunction is present, the clearance will be reduced and the active metabolite will accumulate.[110]

Lisinopril

Lisinopril is a lysine analogue of enalaprilic acid, which, unlike enalapril, does not require activation before it can inhibit angiotensin-converting enzyme (ACE). After oral administration lisinopril is absorbed slowly (peak level at 6 hr) and incompletely (about 30%). The drug is cleared solely by the kidneys with a $t_{1/2}$ of about 12 hr. The clearance of lisinopril is correlated with creatinine clearance, both of which are reduced in the elderly.[112,113] Patients with CHF may have a reduced total absorption of lisinopril as well as a reduced renal clearance, and because of these two opposing effects, the plasma concentration achieved after oral dosing may not be altered much by heart failure.[114] However, some patients with heart failure and marked renal dysfunction may achieve higher than expected plasma concentrations with the usual doses.[112,113] The $t_{1/2}$ is similar in normal individuals and patients with heart failure despite the reduced drug clearance, suggesting that the V_D may be reduced in these patients.[114]

There are a few important drug interactions with the ACE inhibitors. Potassium supplements, potassium containing salt substitutes, and potassium-retaining diuretics (amiloride, spironolactone, or triamterene) must be used with great caution since aldosterone is reduced and hyperkalemia may occur readily. Nonsteroidal anti inflammatory drugs have been reported to reduce the antihypertensive efficacy of the ACE inhibitors, particularly captopril.[115]

Hydralazine

Hydralazine is acetylated to an inactive metabolite during its absorption after oral dosing. The acetylation rate is genetically determined with about 50% of the U.S. population being slow or fast acetylators. The bioavailability of hydralazine is 16% in the fast acetylators and 35% in the slow acetylators. The systemic clearance of hydralazine is very high (normally 56 ml/min/kg) and approaches cardiac output. The V_D is 1.5 L/kg and the $t_{1/2}$ is 1 hr. CHF does not consistently alter the kinetics of hydralazine,[116] but some patients with heart failure have been described who have a reduced clearance and an increased $t_{1/2}$.[117]

Hydralazine is not subject to known pharmacokinetic drug interactions.

Nitrates

There is a poor correlation between the plasma levels of the nitrates and the clinical effects because of the complex pharmacokinetics, the formation of active metabolites, and the rapid development of tolerance to these drugs when they are administered continuously.[118,119] After oral administration less than 1% of nitroglycerin reaches the circulation, and activity seen after oral dosing is likely due to dinitrate metabolites.[120–122] Sublingual bioavailability averages 31%,[123] and transdermal bioavailability from ointment is variable but substantial (70%), despite some presystemic metabolism by the skin.[124] Transdermal bioavailability particularly from patches seems to be reduced in some patients with heart failure, possibly related to tissue edema or poor subcutaneous blood flow.[125,126] Nitroglycerin has a very large metabolic clearance (200 ml/min/kg), which may be depressed in some patients with severe heart failure.[127] However, since there is a poor correlation between the therapeutic effects or toxicity and the plasma levels, these changes are of limited clinical relevance.

Isosorbide dinitrate is well absorbed orally but is only 25% bioavailable because of substantial first-pass elimination. Its clearance is high (normally 45 ml/min/kg), the V_D is 1.5 L/kg, and the $t_{1/2}$ is 0.8 hr. Isosorbide dinitrate is metabolized to active metabolites, isosorbide 2-mononitrate and isosorbide 5-mononitrate, which have longer half-lives than the parent compound. Neither the pharmacokinetics of isosorbide dinitrate nor its metabolites are altered by heart failure.[7,118]

Drug interactions with nitrates are not of clinical importance. There is some interest in the possibility that N-acetylcysteine can reduce the development of tolerance to nitrates, but this is not a clinically significant drug interaction.

Other Drugs

Theophylline

Theophylline is a drug with a narrow therapeutic window for which there is a good correlation between the plasma concentration and therapeutic and toxic effects. The drug is well absorbed orally with or without heart failure. Theophylline is a low clearance drug (normally 0.65 ml/min/kg) that is eliminated entirely by hepatic metabolism. The V_D is 0.5 L/kg, and the $t_{1/2}$ is 9 hr. Heart failure with hepatic congestion and pulmonary edema can reduce the clearance by half and prolong the $t_{1/2}$ by twofold or more.[128] Because of substantial interpatient variability, plasma levels must be used for safe and effective intravenous use of theophylline, not only in patients with heart failure, but with all patients receiving the drug.

Theophylline is subject to many important drug interactions affecting its metabolic clearance.[129,130] Theophylline clearance is inhibited by cimetidine, erythromycin, verapamil, ciprofloxacin and other fluoroquinolones, mexiletine, thiabendazole, and troleandomycin. Any of these drugs can increase theophylline plasma concentration and produce theophylline toxicity. Inducers of theophylline clearance, thereby reducing plasma concentrations, are barbiturates, carbamazepine, phenytoin, and rifampin. Smokers also have an increased theophylline clearance and require larger doses to achieve therapeutic concentrations and effects.

Warfarin

The effect of heart failure on the pharmacokinetics of warfarin has not been carefully examined. Warfarin is a mixture of two stereoisomers. S-warfarin is more potent than R-warfarin. There are no data regarding the influence of heart failure on the kinetics of the isomers of warfarin. Increased sensitivity to the anticoagulant effect of warfarin has been reported in CHF,[131] but this may not be due to an alteration in the pharmacokinetics of warfarin since no effect of heart failure on warfarin $t_{1/2}$ has been found.[132,133] Although the limitations of $t_{1/2}$ as an index of drug elimination must be kept in mind, warfarin has a small V_D (0.14 L/kg) that is unlikely to be affected by heart failure so that an unchanged $t_{1/2}$ (normally 37 hr) probably indicates that clearance (normally 0.045 ml/min/kg) is not changed by heart failure. Nonetheless, because of the increased sensitivity in some patients, the initial doses should be small and the dose titrated to the desired effect on prothrombin time.

Many, many drugs interact with warfarin to increase or decrease its metabolism and/or effect.[134,135] Some of these drugs have differential effects on the two isomers of warfarin. Drugs that affect the S isomer produce the greatest change in the effects of warfarin. The most important drugs that reduce the clearance of warfarin and thereby enhance its hypoprothrombinemic effect are amiodarone, cimetidine, some sulfonamides (e.g., sulfamethoxazole), ciprofloxacin and other fluoroquinolones, disulfiram, erythromycin, metronidazole, phenylbutazone, and sulfinpyrazone. Clofibrate and some anabolic steroids also increase warfarin's anticoagulant effect but by poorly understood mechanisms that do not involve warfarin's metabolism. Drugs that increase the clearance of warfarin and reduce its hypoprothrombinemic effect include barbiturates, phenytoin, rifampin, and carbamazepine. Many other drugs have been the subject of case reports that suggest an interaction with warfarin, but the clinical significance of these is uncertain.

General Pharmacokinetic Principles to Guide Therapy in Heart Failure

Based on the concepts outlined, a few generalizations can be made regarding the influence of CHF on pharmacokinetics.

1. Oral absorption of drugs that are normally rapidly absorbed in the upper small intestine may be delayed, but the extent of absorption is less likely to be affected. Drugs that are normally slowly absorbed will be influenced less by heart failure.
2. Transdermal drug absorption can be delayed and the extent of absorption may be reduced as a consequence of a reduction in blood flow and subcutaneous edema.
3. The V_D of drugs that are extensively distributed is likely to be reduced such that smaller loading doses will be required to produce therapeutic effects. For drugs with relatively small V_D, heart failure will not produce much change in the V_D, which may even increase slightly.
4. Hepatic clearance of high clearance drugs will be reduced as a consequence of the reduced hepatic blood flow. This is of particular importance for those drugs given intravenously, such as lidocaine. With very severe heart failure accompanied by hepatocellular damage, the intrinsic hepatic clearance of drugs will be reduced. This will result in higher blood levels at a given intravenous dose of low clearance drugs and higher blood levels after oral dosing for both low and high clearance drugs, so that smaller maintenance doses will be required for therapy.
5. Renal clearance of drugs and their metabolites will be influenced only if renal function is depressed by heart failure.
6. Drug $t_{1/2}$ may or may not be prolonged in patients with heart failure depending on the effects of the disease on the V_D and clearance. Half-life is a poor indicator of effects of heart failure on drug elimination.
7. For many drugs used in heart failure, the doses are titrated to effect. This is true for the inotropic agents, diuretics, vasodilators, and oral anticoagulants. For such drugs pharmacokinetic changes produced by heart failure are of less clinical relevance since the individual patient's response rather than the blood levels are the primary guide to therapy.
8. For some drugs, the real end-point of therapy may be difficult to determine and plasma levels become a useful surrogate end-point to guide dosage adjustment. Theophylline is the prime example where successful intravenous therapy requires the frequent monitoring of plasma levels to aid in adjustment of the infusion rate as heart failure or infection progresses or improves. Determination of plasma levels also is useful for many antiarrhythmic drugs (quinidine, procainamide, disopyramide, mexiletine, tocainide, lidocaine, and flecainide). However, some antiarrhythmic drugs are metabolized to several active metabolites so that plasma concentration measurements, at least as performed currently, are not helpful (encainide and propafenone). The utility of plasma level monitoring for digoxin therapy is less clear. In most patients, routine monitoring of digoxin plasma concentrations is not worthwhile. However, in patients where noncompliance, renal dysfunction, drug interaction, or drug overdose is suspected, the measurement of plasma digoxin concentration may be helpful for patient management.

The timing of blood sampling is important in interpretation of the results of a blood level measurement. In general, the most useful concentration is that determined at steady state (at least 3 half-lives after the last dosage adjustment) and obtained just prior to a dose (trough level) or during a continuous infusion (as with theophylline and lidocaine). In the interpretation of blood level data, it is important to remember that the plasma concentration is only one piece of information about the drug in an individual patient and, by itself, cannot be diagnostic of adequate therapy or toxicity of a drug.

9. Although some of the changes produced by heart failure may be anticipated, the interpatient variability may exceed the alteration produced by heart failure. The principles outlined are derived from populations with heart failure and can only give an approximation of initial dosing recommendations for a single patient. Thereafter, the drug's therapeutic effect or the blood concentrations produced by the dosing regimen must be evaluated and the dose adjusted based on the individual patient's response.

References

1. Rowland M, Benet LZ, Graham GG. Clearance concepts in pharmacokinetics. *J Pharmacokinet Biopharm.* 1973;1:123–136.
2. Wilkinson GR, Shand DG. A physiological approach to hepatic drug clearance. *Clin Pharmacol Ther.* 1975;18:377–390.
3. Nies AS, Shand DG, Wilkinson GR. Altered hepatic blood flow and drug disposition. *Clin Pharmacokinet.* 1976;1:135–55.
4. Wilkinson GR. Clearance approaches in pharmacology. *Pharmacol Rev.* 1987;39:1–47.
5. Benowitz NL, Meister W. Pharmacokinetics in patients with cardiac failure. *Clin Pharmacokinet.* 1976;1:389–405.
6. Williams RL, Benet LZ. Drug pharmacokinetics in cardiac and hepatic disease. *Annu Rev Pharmacol Toxicol.* 1980;20:389–413.
7. Shammas FV, Dickstein K. Clinical pharmacokinetics in heart failure. An updated review. *Clin Pharmacokinet.* 1988;15:94–113.
8. Nies AS. Principles of drug therapy. In: Wyngaarden JB, Smith LH, Jr, eds. *Cecil's Textbook of Medicine.*. 19th ed. Philadelphia: Saunders; 1991.
9. Winne D. The influence of villous counter current exchange on intestinal absorption. *J Theor Biol.* 1975;53:145–176.

10. Berkowitz D, Droll MN, Likoff W. Malabsorption as a complication of congestive heart failure. *Am J Cardiol.* 1963;11:43–47.

11. Benet LZ, Greither A, Meister W. Gastrointestinal absorption of drugs in patients with congestive heart failure. In: Benet LZ, ed. *The Effect of Disease States on Pharmacokinetics.* Washington, DC: American Pharmaceutical Association Academy of Pharmaceutical Sciences; 1976:33–50.

12. Kaojarern S, Day B, Brater DC. The time course of delivery of furosemide into urine: an independent determinant of overall response. *Kidney Int.* 1982;22:69–74.

13. Gibb I, Cowan JC, Parnham AJ, Thomas TH. Use and misuse of a digoxin assay service. *Br Med J.* 1986;293:678–680.

14. Benowitz N, Forsyth RP, Melmon KL, Rowland M. Lidocaine disposition kinetics in monkey and man. I. Prediction by a perfusion model. *Clin Pharmacol Ther.* 1974;16:87–98.

15. Benowitz N, Forsyth RP, Melmon KL, Rowland M. Lidocaine disposition kinetics in monkey and man. II. Effects of hemorrhage and sympathomimetic drug administration. *Clin Pharmacol Ther.* 1974;16:99–109.

16. Hepner GW, Vesell ES, Tantum KR. Reduced drug elimination in congestive heart failure. Studies using aminopyrine as a model drug. *Am J Med.* 1978;65:271–276.

17. Thomson PD, Rowland M, Melmon KL. The influence of heart failure, liver disease, and renal failure on the disposition of lidocaine in man. *Am Heart J.* 1971;82:417–421.

18. Woosley RL. Pharmacokinetics and pharmacodynamics of antiarrhythmic agents in patients with congestive heart failure. *Am Heart J.* 1987;114:1280–1290.

19. Bellet S, Roman LR, Boza A. Relation between serum quinidine levels and renal function. Studies in normal subjects and patients with congestive failure and renal insufficiency. *Am J Cardiol.* 1971;27:368–371.

20. Crouthamel WG. The effect of congestive heart failure on quinidine pharmacokinetics. *Am Heart J.* 1975;90:335–339.

21. Conrad KA, Molk BL, Chidsey CA. Pharmacokinetic studies of quinidine in patients with arrhythmias. *Circulation.* 1977;55:1–7.

22. Ochs HR, Greenblatt DJ, Woo E. Clinical pharmacokinetics of quinidine. *Clin Pharmacokinet.* 1980;5:150–168.

23. Kessler KM, Lowenthal DT, Warner H, Gibson T, Briggs W, Reidenberg M. Quinidine elimination in patients with congestive heart failure or poor renal function. *N Engl J Med.* 1974;290:706–709.

24. Data JL, Wilkinson GR, Nies AS. Interaction of quinidine with anticonvulsant drugs. *N Engl J Med.* 1976;294:699–702.

25. Twum-Barima Y, Carruthers SG. Quinidine-rifampin interaction. *N Engl J Med.* 1981;304:1466–1469.

26. Baciewicz AM, Baciewicz FA Jr. Effect of cimetidine and ranitidine on cardiovascular drugs. *Am Heart J.* 1989;118:144–154.

27. Edwards DJ, Lavoie R, Beckman H, Blevins R, Rubenfire M. The effect of coadministration of verapamil on the pharmacokinetics and metabolism of quinidine. *Clin Pharmacol Ther.* 1987;41:68–73.

28. Saal AK, Werner JA, Greene HL, Sears GK, Graham EL. Effect of amiodarone on serum quinidine and procainamide levels. *Am J Cardiol.* 1984;53:1264–1267.

29. Maisel AS, Motulsky HJ, Insel PA. Hypotension after quinidine plus verapamil. Possible additive competition at alpha-adrenergic receptors. *N Engl J Med.* 1985;312:167–170.

30. Bigger JT Jr, Leahey EB Jr. Quinidine and digoxin. An important interaction. *Drugs.* 1982;24:229–239.

31. Kuhlmann J, Dohrmann M, Marcin S. Effects of quinidine on pharmacokinetics and pharmacodynamics of digitoxin achieving steady-state conditions. *Clin Pharmacol Ther.* 1986;39:288–294.

32. Funck-Brentano C, Kroemer HK, Pavlou H, Woosley RL, Roden DM. Genetically-determined interaction between propafenone and low dose quinidine: role of active metabolites in modulating net drug effect. *Br J Clin Pharmacol.* 1989;27:435–444.

33. Turgeon J, Pavlou HN, Wong W, Funck-Brentano C, Roden DM. Genetically determined steady-state interaction between encainide and quinidine in patients with arrhythmias. *J Pharmacol Exp Ther.* 1990;255:642–649.

34. Koch-Weser J, Klein SW. Procainamide dosage schedules, plasma concentrations, and clinical effects. *JAMA.* 1971;215:1454–1460.

35. Kessler KM, Kayden DS, Estes DM, et al. Procainamide pharmacokinetics in patients with acute myocardial infarction or congestive heart failure. *J Am Coll Cardiol.* 1986;7:1131–1139.

36. Benet LZ, Williams RL. Appendix II. Design and optimization of dosage regimens: pharmacokinetic data. In: Gilman AG, Rall TW, Nies AS, Taylor P, eds. *Goodman and Gilman's The Pharmacological Basis of Therapeutics.* 8th ed. New York: Pergamon Press, 1990:1650–1735.

37. Drayer DE, Lowenthal DT, Woosley RL, Nies AS, Schwartz A, Reidenberg MM. Cumulation of N-acetylprocainamide, an active metabolite of procainamide, in patients with impaired renal function. *Clin Pharmacol Ther.* 1977;22:63–69.

38. Vlasses PH, Kosoglou T, Chase SL, et al. Trimethoprim inhibition of the renal clearance of procainamide and N-acetylprocainamide. *Arch Intern Med.* 1989;149:1350–1353.

39. Kowey PR, Friedman PL, Podrid PJ, et al. Use of radionuclide ventriculography for assessment of changes in myocardial performance induced by disopyramide phosphate. *Am Heart J.* 1982;104:769–774.

40. Di Bianco R, Gottdiener JS, Singh SN, Fletcher RD. A review of the effects of disopyramide phosphate on left ventricular function and the peripheral circulation. *Angiology.* 1987;38:174–183.

41. Podrid PJ, Schoeneberger A, Lown B. Congestive heart failure caused by oral disopyramide. *N Engl J Med.* 1980;302:614–617.

42. Landmark K, Bredesen JE, Thaulow E, Simonsen S, Amlie JP. Pharmacokinetics of disopyramide in patients with imminent to moderate cardiac failure. *Eur J Clin Pharmacol.* 1981;19:187–192.

43. Aitio ML, Mansury L, Tala E, Haataja M, Aitio A. The effect of enzyme induction on the metabolism of disopyramide in man. *Br J Clin Pharmacol.* 1981;11:279–285.

44. Ragosta M, Weihl AC, Rosenfeld LE. Potentially fatal interaction between erythromycin and disopyramide. *Am J Med.* 1989;86:465–466.

45. Woosley RL, Morganroth J, Fogoros RN, et al. Pharmacokinetics of moricizine HCl. *Am J Cardiol.* 1987; 60:35F–39F.

46. Fitton A, Buckley MM-T. Moricizine A review of its pharmacological properties, and therapeutic efficacy in cardiac arrhythmias. *Drugs.* 1990;40:138–167.

47. Siddoway LA, Schwartz SL, Barbey JT, Woosley RL. Clinical pharmacokinetics of moricizine. *Am J Cardiol.* 1990;65:21D–25D.

48. Stenson RE, Constantino RT, Harrison DC. Interrelationships of hepatic blood flow, cardiac output, and blood levels of lidocaine in man. *Circulation.* 1971;43:205–211.

49. Thomson PD, Melmon KL, Richardson JA, et al. Lidocaine pharmacokinetics in advanced heart failure, liver disease and renal failure in humans. *Ann Intern Med.* 1973;78:499–508.

50. Zito RA, Reid PR. Lidocaine kinetics predicted by indocyanine green clearance. *N Engl J Med.* 1978; 298:1160–1163.

51. Schneck DW, Luderer JR, Davis D, Vary J. Effects of nadolol and propranolol on plasma lidocaine clearance. *Clin Pharmacol Ther.* 1984;36:584–587.

52. Campbell RWF. Mexiletine. *N Engl J Med.* 1987; 316:29–34.

53. Pentikainen PJ, Koivula IH, Hiltunen HA. Effect of rifampicin treatment on the kinetics of mexiletine. *Eur J Clin Pharmacol.* 1982;23:261–266.

54. Begg EJ, Chinwah PM, Webb C, Day RO, Wade DN. Enhanced metabolism of mexiletine after phenytoin administration. *Br J Clin Pharmacol.* 1982;14:219–223.

55. Grech-Belanger O, Gilbert M, Turgeon J, LeBlanc PP. Effect of cigarette smoking on mexiletine kinetics. *Clin Pharmacol Ther.* 1985;37:638–643.

56. Stanley R, Comer T, Taylor JL, Saliba D. Mexiletine-theophylline interaction. *Am J Med.* 1989;86:733–734.

57. MacMahon B, Bakshi M, Branagan P, Kelly JG, Walsh MJ. Pharmacokinetics and haemodynamic effects of tocainide in patients with acute myocardial infarction complicated by left ventricular failure. *Br J Clin Pharmacol.* 1985;19:429–434.

58. Mohiuddin SM, Esterbrooks D, Hilleman DE, et al. Tocainide kinetics in congestive heart failure. *Clin Pharmacol Ther.* 1983;34:596–603.

59. Graffner C, Conradson TB, Hofvendahl S, Ryden L. Tocainide kinetics after intravenous and oral administration in healthy subjects and in patients with acute myocardial infarction. *Clin Pharmacol Ther.* 1980;27: 64–71.

60. North DS, Mattern AL, Kapil RP, Lalonde RL. The effect of histamine$_2$ receptor antagonists on tocainide pharmacokinetics. *J Clin Pharmacol.* 1988;28:640–643.

61. Rice TL, Patterson JH, Celestin C, Foster JR, Powell JR. Influence of rifampin on tocainide pharmacokinetics in humans. *Clin Pharm.* 1989;8:200–205.

62. Roden DM, Woosley RL. Clinical pharmacokinetics of encainide. *Clin Pharmacokinet.* 1988;14:141–147.

63. Woosley RL, Wood AJJ, Roden DM. Encainide. *N Engl J Med.* 1988;318:1107–1115.

64. de Paola AA, Horowitz LN, Morganroth J, et al. Influence of left ventricular dysfunction on flecainide therapy. *J Am Coll Cardiol.* 1987;9:163–168.

65. Conard GJ, Ober RE. Metabolism of flecainide. *Am J Cardiol.* 1984;53:41B–51B.

66. Roden DM, Woosley RL. Flecainide. *N Engl J Med.* 1986;315:36–41.

67. Nitsch J, Neyses L, Kohler U, Luderitz B. [Elevated plasma flecainide concentrations in heart failure]. *Dtsch Med Wochenschr.* 1987;112:1698–1700.

68. Cavilli A, Maggioni AP, Marchi S, Volpi A, Latini R. Flecainide half-life prolongation in 2 patients with congestive heart failure and complex ventricular arrhythmias. *Clin Pharmacokinet.* 1988;14:187–188.

69. Funck-Brentano C, Kroemer HK, Lee JT, Roden DM. Propafenone. *N Engl J Med.* 1990;322:518–525.

70. Burnett DM, Gal J, Zahniser NR, Nies AS. Propafenone interacts stereoselectively with β_1 and β_2-adrenergic receptors. *J Cardiovasc Pharmacol.* 1988; 12:615–619.

71. Harron DWG, Brogden RN. Propafenone. A review of its pharmacodynamic and pharmacokinetic properties and therapeutic use in the treatment of arrhythmias. *Drugs.* 1987;34:617–647.

72. Ravid S, Podrid PJ, Lampert S, Lown B. Congestive heart failure induced by six of the newer antiarrhythmic drugs. *J Am Coll Cardiol.* 1989;14:1326–1330.

73. Castel JM, Cappiello E, Leopaldi D, Latini R. Rifampicin lowers plasma concentrations of propafenone and its antiarrhythmic effect. *Br J Clin Pharmacol.* 1990;30: 155–156.

74. Nolan PE Jr, Marcus FI, Erstad BL, Hoyer GL, Furman C, Kirsten EB. Effects of coadministration of propafenone on the pharmacokinetics of digoxin in healthy volunteer subjects. *J Clin Pharmacol.* 1989;29: 46–52.

75. Calvo MV, Martin-Suarez A, Martin Luengo C, et al. Interaction between digoxin and propafenone. *Ther Drug Monit.* 1989;11:10–15.

76. Kates RE, Yee YG, Kirsten EB. Interaction between warfarin and propafenone in healthy volunteer subjects. *Clin Pharmacol Ther.* 1987;42:305–311.

77. Wagner F, Kalusche D, Trenk D, Jahnchen E, Roskamm H. Drug interaction between propafenone and metoprolol. *Br J Clin Pharmacol.* 1987;24:213–220.

78. Mason JW. Amiodarone. *N Engl J Med.* 1987;316: 455–466.

79. Wilson JS, Podrid PJ. Side effects from amiodarone. *Am Heart J.* 1991;121:158–171.

80. Applefeld MM, Adir J, Crouthamel WG, Roffman DS. Digoxin pharmacokinetics in congestive heart failure. *J Clin Pharmacol.* 1981;21:114–120.

81. Ohnhaus EE, Vozeh S, Nuesch E. Absorption of digoxin in severe right heart failure. *Eur J Clin Pharmacol.* 1979;15:115–120.

82. Korhonen UR, Jounela AJ, Pakarinen AJ, Pentikainen PJ, Takkunen JT. Pharmacokinetics of digoxin in pa-

tients with acute myocardial infarction. *Am J Cardiol* 1979;44:1190–1194.

83. Marcus FI. Pharmacokinetic interactions between digoxin and other drugs. *J Am Coll Cardiol.* 1985;5:82A–90A.

84. Brodie MJ, Feely J. Adverse drug interactions. *Br Med J.* 1988;296:845–849.

85. Nademanee K, Kannan R, Hendrickson J, Ookhtens M, Kay I, Singh BN. Amiodarone-digoxin interaction: clinical significance, time course of development, potential pharmacokinetic mechanisms and therapeutic implications. *J Am Coll Cardiol.* 1984;4:111–116.

86. Robinson K, Johnston A, Walker S, Mulrow JP, McKenna WJ, Holt DW. The digoxin-amiodarone interaction. *Cardiovasc Drugs Ther.* 1989;3:25–28.

87. Kates RE, Leier CV. Dobutamine pharmacokinetics in severe heart failure. *Clin Pharmacol Ther.* 1978;24:537–541.

88. Rocci ML Jr, Wilson H. The pharmacokinetics and pharmacodynamics of newer inotropic agents. *Clin Pharmacokinet.* 1987;13:91–109.

89. Park GB, Kershner RP, Angellotti J, Williams RL, Benet LZ, Edelson J. Oral bioavailability and intravenous pharmacokinetics of amrinone in humans. *J Pharm Sci.* 1983;72:817–819.

90. Hamilton RA, Kowalsky SF, Wright EM, et al. Effect of the acetylator phenotype on amrinone pharmacokinetics. *Clin Pharmacol Ther.* 1986;40:615–619.

91. Wilson H, Rocci ML Jr, Weber KT, Andrews V, Likoff MJ. Pharmacokinetics and hemodynamics of amrinone in patients with chronic cardiac failure of diverse etiology. *Res Commun Chem Pathol Pharmacol.* 1987;56:3–19.

92. Edelson J, Stroshane R, Benziger DP, et al. Pharmacokinetics of the bipyridines amrinone and milrinone. *Circulation.* 1986;73(suppl III):III145–III152.

93. Benotti JR, Lesko LJ, McCue JE, Alpert JS. Pharmacokinetics and pharmacodynamics of milrinone in chronic congestive heart failure. *Am J Cardiol.* 1985;56:685–689.

94. Brater DC, Seiwell R, Anderson S, Burdette A, Dehmer GJ, Chennavasin P. Absorption and disposition of furosemide in congestive heart failure. *Kidney Int.* 1982;22:171–176.

95. Vasco MR, Brown-Cartwright D, Knochel JP, Nixon JV, Brater DC. Furosemide absorption altered in decompensated congestive heart failure. *Ann Intern Med.* 1985;102:314–318.

96. Chaturvedi PR, O'Donnell JP, Nicholas JM, Shoenthal DR, Waters DH, Gwilt PR. Steady state absorption kinetics and pharmacodynamics of furosemide in congestive heart failure. *Int J Clin Pharmacol Ther Toxicol.* 1987;25:123–128.

97. Brater DC, Chennavasin P, Seiwell R. Furosemide in patients with heart failure: shift in dose-response curves. *Clin Pharmacol Ther.* 1980;28:182–186.

98. Brater DC. Resistance to loop diuretics. Why it happens and what to do about it. *Drugs.* 1985;30:427–443.

99. Favre L, Glasson P, Riondel A, Vallotton MB. Interaction of diuretics and non-steroidal anti-inflammatory drugs in man. *Clin Sci.* 1983;64:407–415.

100. Brater DC. Disposition and response to bumetanide and furosemide. *Am J Cardiol.* 1986;57:20A–25A.

101. Ward A, Heel RC. Bumetanide. A review of its pharmacodynamic and pharmacokinetic properties and therapeutic use. *Drugs.* 1984;28:426–464.

102. Cook JA, Smith DE, Cornish LA, Tankanow RM, Nicklas JM, Hyneck ML. Kinetics, dynamics, and bioavailability of bumetanide in healthy subjects and patients with congestive heart failure. *Clin Pharmacol Ther.* 1988;44:487–500.

103. Brater DC, Day B, Burdette A, Anderson S. Bumetanide and furosemide in heart failure. *Kidney Int.* 1984;26:183–189.

104. Beermann B, Groschinsky-Grind M. Pharmacokinetics of hydrochlorothiazide in patients with congestive heart failure. *Br J Clin Pharmacol.* 1979;7:579–583.

105. Kerry RJ, Ludlow JM, Owen G. Diuretics are dangerous with lithium. *Br Med J.* 1980;281:371.

106. Duchin KL, McKinstry DN, Cohen AI, Migdalof BH. Pharmacokinetics of captopril in healthy subjects and in patients with cardiovascular diseases. *Clin Pharmacokinet.* 1988;14:241–259.

107. Brogden RN, Todd PA, Sorkin EM. Captopril. An update of its pharmacodynamic and pharmacokinetic properties, and therapeutic use in hypertension and congestive heart failure. *Drugs.* 1988;36:540–600.

108. Belz GG, Kirch W, Kleinbloesem CH. Angiotensin-converting enzyme inhibitors. Relationship between pharmacodynamics and pharmacokinetics. *Clin Pharmacokinet.* 1988;15:295–318.

109. Todd PA, Heel RC. Enalapril. A review of its pharmacodynamic and pharmacokinetic properties, and therapeutic use in hypertension and congestive heart failure. *Drugs.* 1986;31:198–248.

110. Dickstein K, Till AE, Aarsland T, et al. The pharmacokinetics of enalapril in hospitalized patients with congestive heart failure. *Br J Clin Pharmacol.* 1987;23:403–410.

111. Dickstein K. Pharmacokinetics of enalapril in congestive heart failure. *Drugs.* 1986;32:40–44.

112. Gautam PC, Vargas E, Lye M. Pharmacokinetics of lisinopril (MK521) in healthy young and elderly subjects and in elderly patients with cardiac failure. *J Pharm Pharmacol.* 1987;39:929–931.

113. Thomson AH, Kelly JG, Whiting B. Lisinopril population pharmacokinetics in elderly and renal disease patients with hypertension. *Br J Clin Pharmacol.* 1989;27:57–65.

114. Till AE, Dickstein K, Aarsland T, Gomez HJ, Gregg H, Hichens M. The pharmacokinetics of lisinopril in hospitalized patients with congestive heart failure. *Br J Clin Pharmacol.* 1989;27:199–204.

115. Breckenridge AM. Drug interactions with ACE inhibitors. *J Hum Hypertens.* 1989;3:133–138.

116. Mulrow JP, Crawford MH. Clinical pharmacokinetics and therapeutic use of hydralazine in congestive heart failure. *Clin Pharmacokinet.* 1989;16:86–89.

117. Hanson A, Johansson BW, Wernersson B, Wahlander LA. Pharmacokinetics of oral hydralazine in chronic heart failure. *Eur J Clin Pharmacol.* 1983;25:467–473.

118. Thadani U, Whitsett T. Relationship of pharmacokinetic and pharmacodynamic properties of the organic nitrates. *Clin Pharmacokinet.* 1988;15:32–43.

119. Bogaert MG. Clinical pharmacokinetics of organic nitrates. *Clin Pharmacokinet.* 1983;8:410–421.

120. Lee FW, Salmonson T, Metzler CH, Benet LZ. Pharmacokinetics and pharmacodynamics of glyceryl trinitrate and its two dinitrate metabolites in conscious dogs. *J Pharmacol Exp Ther.* 1990;255:1222–1229.

121. Nakashima E, Rigod JF, Lin ET, Benet LZ. Pharmacokinetics of nitroglycerin and its dinitrate metabolites over a thirtyfold range of oral doses. *Clin Pharmacol Ther.* 1990;47:592–598.

122. Noonan PK, Benet LZ. The bioavailability of oral nitroglycerin. *J Pharm Sci.* 1986;75:241–243.

123. Noonan PK, Benet LZ. Incomplete and delayed bioavailability of sublingual nitroglycerin. *Am J Cardiol.* 1985;55:184–187.

124. Nakashima E, Noonan PK, Benet LZ. Transdermal bioavailability and first-pass skin metabolism: a preliminary evaluation with nitroglycerin. *J Pharmacokinet Biopharm.* 1987;15:423–437.

125. Armstrong PW. Pharmacokinetic-hemodynamic studies of transdermal nitroglycerin in congestive heart failure. *J Am Coll Cardiol.* 1987;9:420–425.

126. Armstrong PW, Armstrong JA, Marks GS. Pharmacokinetic-hemodynamic studies of nitroglycerin ointment in congestive heart failure. *Am J Cardiol.* 1980; 46:670–676.

127. Armstrong PW, Armstrong JA, Marks GS. Pharmacokinetic-hemodynamic studies of intravenous nitroglycerin in congestive cardiac failure. *Circulation.* 1980; 62:160–166.

128. Piafsky KM, Sitar DS, Rangno RE, Ogilvie RI. Theophylline kinetics in acute pulmonary edema. *Clin Pharmacol Ther.* 1977;21:310–316.

129. Upton RA. Pharmacokinetic interactions between theophylline and other medication. 1. *Clin Pharmacokinet.* 1991;20:66–80.

130. Upton RA. Pharmacokinetic interactions between theophylline and other medication. 2. *Clin Pharmacokinet.* 1991;20:135–150.

131. O'Reilly RA, Aggeler PM. Determinants of the response to oral anticoagulant drugs in man. *Pharmacol Rev.* 1970;22:35–96.

132. Ristola P, Pyorala K. Determinants of the response to coumarin anticoagulants in patients with acute myocardial infarction. *Acta Med Scand.* 1972;192:183–188.

133. Kelly JG, O'Malley K. Clinical pharmacokinetics of oral anticoagulants. *Clin Pharmacokinet.* 1979;4:1–15.

134. O'Reilly RA. Warfarin metabolism and drug-drug interactions. *Adv Exp Med Biol.* 1987;214:205–212.

135. Serlin MJ, Breckenridge AM. Drug interactions with warfarin. *Drugs.* 1983;25:610–620.

21
Diuretics

Stephen S. Gottlieb

Diuretic medications are deemed essential for the treatment of most patients with congestive heart failure (CHF). The underlying abnormality present in patients with heart failure leads to neurohormonal activation and salt and water retention. Medicines that cause increased sodium, and therefore water, excretion can be extremely effective. Indeed, symptoms of CHF may be completely relieved by this simple and inexpensive intervention. However, the adverse consequences associated with the use of diuretic medications are rarely considered. Knowledge of both potential problems and benefits can lead to safer and more effective use of these agents.

Effects of Diuretics on Cardiac Performance

Diuretics decrease many of the symptoms associated with heart failure. Decreased peripheral edema can be beneficial, as patients may present with painful extremities. Decreased pulmonary edema (if previously present) may improve oxygenation. Even more important, however, are the decreases in right and left ventricular filling, atrial, and pulmonary pressures. Lowering pulmonary pressure decreases the sensation of dyspnea, the major complaint of most patients with heart failure. Although this may occur without increasing cardiac index,[1] diuretic medications also have been reported to improve cardiac performance at rest and during exercise.[2] No direct inotropic effect has been ascribed to any diuretic, but there are multiple explanations as to why diuresis may increase cardiac performance.

It is possible that some of the benefits seen with diuretics are secondary to a reduction in systemic vascular resistance. Lower extravascular pressure may lead to vasodilation, and improved cardiac performance could lead to changes in neurohormonal activation with sub-sequent vasodilation. In addition, venous capacitance increases within 5 min of furosemide administration, suggesting an acute mechanism of vasodilation as well.[3] In contrast to the decreased peripheral resistance that is frequently observed after diuresis, some of the neurohormonal changes associated with diuretics may cause vasoconstriction. Thus, blood pressure may increase acutely with diuretics, with the beneficial hemodynamic effects of diuresis developing only later.[4] Nevertheless, in most patients chronic diuretic use causes decreased symptoms of heart failure, improved cardiac performance, and vasodilation.[5] The decreased afterload probably explains many of the reported improvements in cardiac index and other load-dependent indices of cardiac performance after diuresis.[6] The importance of afterload reduction as the cause of the improved cardiac performance is supported by the finding that the increased stroke volume often seen with diuretics is closely related to decreases in systemic vascular resistance, but not to decreases in preload.[7]

Despite the importance of afterload reduction, actions on preload could also improve cardiac performance. The abnormal valvular and papillary muscle geometry caused by ventricular enlargement can lead to abnormal mitral valve function and significant regurgitation.[8] Even abnormal atrial geometry may lead to mitral regurgitation.[9] Decreases in ventricular (and perhaps atrial) size therefore could increase forward flow by reducing backward flow. The importance of reversing mitral regurgitation has been clearly demonstrated with vasodilators.[10] Presumably, diuretic-induced volume reduction also decreases mitral regurgitation and thereby increases cardiac output. This concept could explain why diuretics improve cardiac output in patients with CHF, but not in individuals with normal cardiac size and function.[11]

While frequently hypothesized, it is unlikely that a decreased preload shifts the ventricle to a more optimal position on Starling's curve. A descending limb of the curve has been noted only at extremely high pressures (above 60 mm Hg)[12] and sarcomere length in a dilated canine heart is close to optimal.[13] However, it is likely that decreased systolic wall stress with reduced left ventricular size (the LaPlace effect) is beneficial. Not only would a decreased afterload improve cardiac performance, but the lower filling pressures associated with diuretics might limit ischemia.[14] Neurohormonal activation and a consequent positive inotropic effect could be another possible explanation of the improved cardiac performance frequently noted with the administration of diuretics to patients with heart failure.

Diuretics, of course, can lead to decreased cardiac output if the left ventricular filling pressure is decreased excessively. In contrast to the upper end of Starling's curve, the lower end of the curve is clinically important and has been demonstrated in man.[15] While neurohormonal activation may minimize the effects of the Starling phenomenon in normal individuals, in the severely compromised heart failure patient overdiuresis may cause devastating effects and should be avoided.

Neurohormonal Effects

Neurohormonal activation is important to the pathophysiology of CHF. It may reflect the severity of disease, as well as alter its natural history. These issues are discussed elsewhere in this book but are important to any discussion of diuretics, as neurohormones may be affected by their administration. Whether these neurohormonal changes directly cause benefit or harm, or whether they merely reflect changes in physiology, is often debated.

Renin-Angiotensin-Aldosterone System

Stimulation of the renin-angiotensin-aldosterone system is commonly found in patients with CHF, is associated with increased mortality, and may have both beneficial and detrimental effects. While stimulation of this system usually is assumed to be secondary to the severity of illness, increased angiotensin II (AII) concentrations and plasma renin activity actually often reflect the intensity of diuretic treatment. Renin release may be caused by volume contraction and stimulation of baroreceptors and the macula densa.[16] Thus, it is not surprising that many studies document increased plasma renin activity and plasma concentrations of AII in heart failure patients after diuretic therapy.[17,18] (Fig. 21.1) Indeed, concentrations may be normal in heart failure patients not treated with diuretics.[17,19]

Aldosterone concentrations are similarly affected by diuretics. Normal concentrations before treatment may

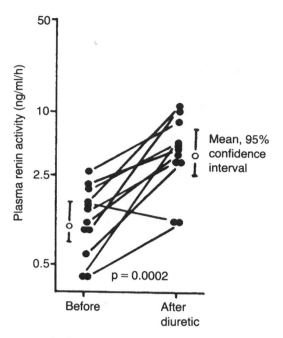

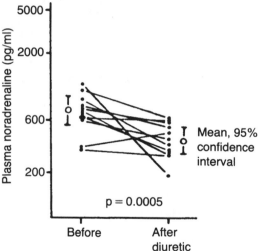

FIGURE 21.1. Neurohormonal concentrations before and after treatment with diuretics for 1 month. Plasma noradrenaline (norepinephrine) concentrations were elevated at baseline and decreased with diuretics. In contrast, plasma renin activity was normal or slightly elevated at baseline and increased with diuretics. Adapted, with permission, from Bayliss et al.[19]

be followed by increases with diuresis.[19,20] Interestingly, though, patients with elevated aldosterone concentrations before treatment with diuretics may exhibit decreases after their administration.[17] The varying response of aldosterone may reflect the conflicting consequences of the effects of diuretics on the severity of illness and their effects on delivery of sodium to the distal tubule. The importance of both of these factors is suggested by a report that patients with elevated baseline aldosterone concentrations demonstrate decreased concentrations with initial diuretic treatment (and improvement in symptoms), but increased concentrations as dry weight approaches and less sodium is delivered to the renal tubule.[21]

The ramifications of the stimulation of the renin-angiotensin-aldosterone axis with diuretics are not clearly understood. While increased plasma renin activity has important prognostic and clinical implications, the impact of diuretic-induced neurohormonal activation is not clear. For example, elevated concentrations of AII theoretically could increase mortality and symptoms by vasoconstrictive effects and direct actions (including arrhythmic) on myocardial tissue.[22] On the other hand, stimulation of the renin-angiotensin system may help to maintain renal function. There are other consequences of this neurohormonal stimulation that also could be important. Aldosterone stimulates collagen production,[23] and aldosterone antagonists could have an impact unrelated to actions on electrolytes or diuresis. The implications of the effects of diuretics on the renin-angiotensin-aldosterone axis mandate further investigation of the consequences of these actions.

Arginine Vasopressin

After diuretic administration, both stimulation and inhibition of the release of arginine vasopressin (ADH) have been reported. The complex regulation of ADH is probably responsible for these conflicting studies. Arginine vasopressin concentrations are affected by both osmotic and baroreceptor stimuli, and diuretics could increase the concentrations because of actions on these parameters. However, the physiologic effects of diuretics are not extensive enough to cause a consistent increase in ADH. While the decreased blood volume and increased plasma osmolality noted with furosemide[24] might be expected to result in increased ADH concentrations, a decrease in volume of 10% is needed to stimulate the baroreceptors, and the relative isoosmotic diuresis observed after the use of most diuretics should not alter ADH concentrations. It is therefore unclear whether diuretics directly cause the increased ADH concentrations often found in individuals with left ventricular dysfunction.

Indirect effects of diuretics, however, could impact on ADH regulation; changes in the activity of other neurohormonal systems may alter ADH concentrations. For example, AII may directly effect its release, and this mechanism may explain the increased ADH concentration noted with acute diuresis, even if the diuresis is isoosmotic and there is no change in oncotic pressure.[4] In contrast, normalization of the hemodynamic status with diuresis may return ADH concentrations to the normal range.[17] Most likely, alterations in ADH secretion are not important consequences of diuretic administration.

Atrial Natriuretic Peptide

An individual's volume status is related to secretion of atrial natriuretic peptide (ANP). Atrial stretch causes release of this peptide which, in turn, may cause natriuresis and vasodilation.[25,26] Diuretics would therefore be expected to lead to lower ANP concentrations and potential mitigation of the peptide's diuretic and vasodilatory effects. However, not only have decreased ANP concentrations not necessarily been noted after diuretic administration,[18] but the very high ANP concentrations seen in patients with severe heart failure appear to have little clinical effect; downregulation of receptor sites may prevent most of the response to ANP in these patients.[27] As with many neurohormones, ANP has prognostic importance in patients with heart failure,[28] but hemodynamic tolerance to chronic marked elevations in concentration have suggested that any impact of diuresis on ANP secretion may be clinically unimportant in these individuals.[29]

Prostaglandins

Prostaglandins affect the vasculature, and diuretic medications may alter prostaglandin concentrations by both direct and indirect means. Therefore, diuretics may exert beneficial or detrimental actions via this little appreciated mechanism. For example, furosemide, which increases venous capacitance, does not have the same effect in the presence of indomethacin concentrations known to inhibit prostaglandin production.[30] This suggests that its direct actions on prostaglandin production, such as stimulation of the renal production of prostaglandin E_2 (PGE_2) may have important therapeutic effects. Indeed, the clinical importance of the effects of furosemide on prostaglandin synthesis has been noted in disorders other than CHF. In premature infants, for example, furosemide increases the incidence of patent ductus arteriosus, presumably via prostaglandin stimulation.[31] Other diuretics also may cause alterations in prostaglandin production; various diuretics increase the production of PGI_2 from arachidonic acid in aortic smooth muscle cells.[32] Although the actions of diuretics on prostaglandins is rarely recognized, it is conceivable that some of the beneficial effects observed with diuretics may result from increased concentrations of prostaglandins.

The use of nonsteroidal antiinflammatory drugs therefore may affect the actions of diuretics, especially regarding renal function. Renal prostaglandins help to maintain renal blood flow in the presence of countervailing influences. Thus, if diuresis leads to neurohormonal activation limiting renal plasma flow, prostaglandins may be essential for the maintenance of renal function. The combination of diuretics and nonsteroidal antiinflammatory drugs would then decrease renal plasma flow and glomerular filtration. Indeed, in normal individuals in whom diuretics and aspirin individually had no effect on renal function, the combination caused marked decreases in the glomerular filtration rate.[33] In patients with CHF and compromised renal plasma flow, the effects might be even greater.

Catecholamines

In contrast to investigations of the renin-angiotensin system, studies of the sympathetic nervous system have consistently reported increased norepinephrine concentrations in patients with heart failure before treatment with diuretics.[18,19] Also in contrast to the renin-angiotensin system, catecholamine concentrations frequently decrease coincident with the symptomatic improvement caused by diuresis[19] (Fig. 21.1); norepinephrine concentrations are a sensitive reflector of poor cardiac performance.[34] This decrease in catecholamines could be an extremely important benefit of diuretic therapy. If catecholamines are responsible for arrhythmogenesis or cardiac deterioration, as is commonly believed,[35] diuretics (or any intervention that improves left ventricular performance) may lead to improved myocardial function and survival.

Diuretic-Induced Electrolyte Abnormalities

In addition to the neurohormonal effects, diuretics also have important metabolic actions. Volume contraction leads to avid sodium reabsorption and (when secondary to diuretics other than carbonic anhydrase inhibitors and potassium sparing agents) bicarbonate reabsorption and metabolic alkalosis. Uric acid excretion is inhibited by the commonly used diuretic medications, and this explains the high prevalence of gout in patients with CHF. The most problematic consequences of diuretic usage, however, are marked and potentially serious direct and indirect effects on electrolytes. Diuretic medications disturb electrolyte homeostasis, most notably altering potassium, magnesium, sodium, and calcium concentrations. The implications of most of these alterations remain controversial.

Potassium

Most diuretics (other than potassium-sparing agents) increase sodium delivery to the distal renal tubule, where potassium is excreted as sodium is reabsorbed; potassium depletion may therefore result. While even acute diuresis may cause hypokalemia, total body potassium depletion is associated with the duration of diuretic use.[36] Yet, the hypokalemia commonly observed in patients with heart failure cannot be attributed to diuretics alone, as hypokalemia is noted more frequently in patients receiving these medications for heart failure than in those receiving them for hypertension. Metabolic alkalosis resulting from intensive diuresis, decreased sodium intake, and neurohormonal activation may contribute to the hypokalemic effects of diuretics in patients with heart failure. Activation of the sympathetic nervous system and elevated aldosterone concentrations also are common in patients with severe heart failure and can lead to hypokalemia. Importantly, these factors may stimulate the kaliuretic actions of diuretics even when they do not directly increase potassium excretion. For example, diuretics may potentiate the hypokalemia caused by epinephrine or albuterol.[37,38] Thus, whereas diuretics themselves do not necessarily cause marked hypokalemia, in combination with the abnormal physiology of patients with CHF, most diuretics may induce potassium depletion.

Hypokalemia can cause symptoms, such as muscle aches, but of most concern are the potential arrhythmogenic effects of this state. In the hypertension literature the effect of hypokalemia on mortality has been controversial,[39,40] but it is generally accepted that hypokalemia increases the risk of arrhythmia in patients with heart failure. Most investigators assume that studies of hypertensive patients are not relevant to patients with CHF because of marked differences in anatomy and physiology. Although the concern about the dangers of hypokalemia in patients with heart failure is based on indirect evidence, it is convincing. For example, hypokalemia increases the frequency of early afterdepolarizations caused by quinidine[41] and the risk of arrhythmias associated with digoxin.[42] Low serum potassium concentrations also are associated with increased risk of arrhythmias after a myocardial infarction.[43] More important than the degree of hypokalemia, however, is probably the rate of change of the serum potassium[44]; hypokalemia associated with rapid diuresis may be more detrimental than that associated with chronic use of diuretics.

When discussing diuretics, the risks of *hyper*kalemia frequently are neglected. Not only may the use of potassiumsparing agents lead to hyperkalemia, but the routine prescription of potassium supplements with initiation of diuretics also can cause this fatal complication. Poor renal function, concomitant use of angiotensin-converting enzyme (ACE) inhibitors, and excessive potassium intake can produce hyperkalemia and consequent ventricular arrhythmias and sudden death.[45] Therefore, the serum potassium concentration should be followed carefully in all patients receiving diuretics.

Considering the problems associated with abnormal potassium concentrations, it is wise to keep the serum concentration above 4.0 mEq/l, but within the normal range. Although potassium-sparing diuretics or ACE inhibitors may be used to help achieve this goal, it should be realized that the combination of these two interventions increases the risk of hyperkalemia. Salt substitutes contain potassium and should also be considered as a cause of hyperkalemia in patients receiving potassium sparing agents. The use of any diuretic mandates close follow-up of the patient to maintain the potassium concentration within the normal range.

Magnesium

While reports of the prevalence of magnesium deficiency in patients with CHF range from 7% to more than 37%, the true prevalence is disputed for many reasons.[46] First, there is no "gold standard" measurement of magnesium deficiency. Determination of the serum magnesium concentration is easy, but it may not reflect total body stores of the electrolyte. Serum, myocardial, lymphocyte, and muscle magnesium concentrations do not correlate,[47] and the concentration (if any) that is most clinically relevant is unknown. There are other factors that also prevent determination of the true prevalence of magnesium deficiency. Diverse definitions of normal magnesium concentrations, differing nutritional intake, and analyses of patients with varying severity of disease have led to wide-ranging estimates of the prevalence of magnesium depletion. Nevertheless, investigations consistently demonstrate that a large percentage of patients with heart failure are magnesium deficient.

It is often assumed that diuretics are the cause of magnesium depletion in patients with heart failure, and chronic diuretic use probably does lead to magnesium depletion,[48] with the duration of therapy an important determinant of the extent of depletion.[36] However, other factors also affect magnesium excretion. Some studies suggest that low magnesium concentrations are common in heart failure patients even before treatment with diuretics,[49] possibly caused by aldosterone-induced magnesium excretion.[50] In contrast, other neurohormonal mechanisms may limit the excretion of magnesium caused by diuretics; renal denervation leads to increased magnesium excretion after the administration of diuretics.[51] Despite these confounding factors, it is likely that diuretics are the predominant cause of hypomagnesemia in CHF patients.

The clinical implications of magnesium depletion in patients with CHF are controversial. There are reports of various symptoms related to hypomagnesemia, ranging from muscle weakness to depression.[52] It is also possible that magnesium depletion impairs cardiac performance, either by directly reducing cardiac contractility[53] or by causing peripheral vasoconstriction.[54] However, the consequence of most concern is the possibility that magnesium depletion causes ventricular arrhythmias and sudden death.

There are reasons to suspect that magnesium depletion increases the frequency of ventricular arrhythmias. A low magnesium concentration decreases the threshold needed to induce ventricular tachycardia and ventricular fibrillation in normal and digitalis-treated dogs,[55] and hypomagnesemia potentiates the development of digitalis-induced arrhythmias.[56] Furthermore, administration of intravenous magnesium suppresses early afterdepolarizations and ventricular tachycardia induced by cesium in dogs[57] and may prevent the clinical occurrence of ventricular tachycardia in patients.[58,59] These actions of magnesium may be related to its function as a critical cofactor in the cellular functions that regulate intracellular electrolyte concentrations.[60] Hypomagnesemia also may exacerbate the development of hypokalemia and cause arrhythmias indirectly.[61]

Despite the multiple reasons to suspect that hypomagnesemia may be clinically important, this hypothesis has not been proven. Some studies suggest an association of hypomagnesemia and arrhythmias,[62] whereas others do not.[63] There are no large prospective well controlled studies evaluating the significance of magnesium, and there is no proof that magnesium supplementation is beneficial. It is thus currently unknown whether the actions of diuretics on magnesium excretion need to be countered. However, magnesium administration should be considered in the settings of intractable ventricular arrhythmias or refractory hypokalemia coincident with hypomagnesemia.

Sodium

Hyponatremia may be observed in patients with heart failure, and often is ascribed to diuretic therapy. While heart failure patients not on diuretics can experience hyponatremia secondary to total body fluid overload (not sodium depletion),[64] diuretics clearly can exacerbate hyponatremia. Direct renal actions lead to sodium excretion which, in the presence of inappropriately elevated arginine vasopressin concentrations (perhaps partially caused by the diuretic itself), may lead to hyponatremia.[65-67] Usually, however, the diuresis associated with potent diuretics is relatively isoosmotic and does not cause hyponatremia. Indeed, only patients receiving diuretics will experience reversal of hyponatremia with ACE inhibition.[68] Similarly, loop diuretics inhibit the ability of the medullary interstitium to concentrate and therefore may correct the hyponatremia associated with SIADH. Therefore, diuretics, which may cause hyponatremia, also may correct hyponatremia induced by severe heart failure.

Hyponatremia itself generally does not cause symptoms in patients with CHF. It is gradual in onset, and thus nervous system complications do not occur. There is no evidence that chronic hyponatremia is dangerous and needs to be treated. Even though hyponatremia is rarely directly deleterious, it does reflect stimulation of the renin-angiotensin system and has prognostic implications.[69] It also may reflect overdiuresis, a situation in which it should be accompanied by evidence of renal dysfunction, hypotension, or other clinical problems and that can be treated, if necessary, by adjustment of diuretics. In contrast to the chronic development of hyponatremia, acute hyponatremia (while rare) could be dangerous. When secondary to overdiuresis, it is corrected easily with modification of the treatment regimen and without administration of sodium. When severe hyponatremia progresses despite diuretic modification, a syndrome of inappropriate ADH secretion should be considered.

Calcium

Diuretic medications alter urinary calcium excretion in various ways. Some diuretics, such as furosemide, increase calcium excretion,[70] whereas others, such as thiazides, depress it.[71] The combination of these medications may minimize changes (e.g., metolazone decreases furosemide-induced calciuria).[72] Whether these urinary changes reflect important physiologic perturbations is unknown, as compensatory actions, such as alteration of parathyroid hormone secretion, may occur and prevent clinical harm. Since the measurement of low serum concentrations of calcium may not adequately reflect ionized calcium or intracellular concentrations, it is difficult to determine the significance of altered calcium excretion.

Nevertheless, there are reasons to be concerned that diuretic-induced alterations of calcium concentrations could have important physiologic effects. Myocardial function is dependent on calcium, and, although total serum calcium concentration does not correlate with cardiac performance, the influence of ionized calcium concentrations on myocardial function has been suggested.[73] There is even a case report of myocardial function varying with the serum-ionized calcium concentration. It was hypothesized that myocardial function in severely ill patients is particularly dependent on calcium concentration because of beta-receptor downregulation.[74] However, at present it is unclear if the actions of diuretics on calcium excretion alter myocardial function.

Renal Effects

Alterations in glomerular filtration are commonly noted after the administration of diuretic medications, and frequently they mandate modification of the treatment regimen. Most often, the indirect actions consequent to intravascular sodium and volume depletion explain these renal effects of diuretics, but direct renal actions also may have important ramifications. If the volume contraction is severe or chronic enough, the physiologic alterations that maintain blood pressure can cause decreased glomerular filtration and, ultimately, renal failure. Neurohormonal activation is the most likely cause of the resultant renal dysfunction. The importance of neurohormonal factors is suggested by the commonly noted diuresis that occurs with reclining. The increased glomerular filtration rate and sodium, potassium, and volume excretion in patients who are reclining (as compared to standing) is associated with less stimulation of the sympathetic and renin-angiotensin-aldosterone systems.[75]

Diuresis need not lead to intravascular depletion.[76] Plasma volume actually may increase, perhaps secondary to increased venous capacitance, decreased capillary hydrostatic pressure, and increased colloid pressure. In such patients, effects of diuretics on glomerular filtration may be secondary to direct actions on renal vascular resistance and renal plasma flow. For example, renal vascular resistance has been reported to increase after the administration of hydrochlorothiazide.[77] However, renal vascular resistance also may decrease after the administration of diuretics. Renal artery vasodilation with furosemide and ethacrynic acid probably explains the acute increases in both renal plasma flow and glomerular filtration caused by these agents.[78,79] Increased prostaglandin production, reflected by increased urinary excretion of PGE_2 and $PGF_{2\alpha}$, may be the cause of these acute renal effects.[77]

Practical Implications of the Multiple Effects of Diuretics

There is no doubt that diuretic medications are and will continue to be a primary tool in the treatment of CHF. The rapid and dramatic clinical effects caused by these agents will continue to mandate their prescription. However, the obvious symptomatic benefits derived from the correct use of diuretics have blinded us to a careful evaluation of their risks and benefits. An analysis of the multiple neurohormonal, electrolyte, renal, and cardiac performance effects of diuretics should alter the way we prescribe these and concomitant medications. Although not all of the answers are in, the data increasingly suggest that we can achieve an optimal level of diuresis while minimizing adverse effects.

The neurohormonal effects of diuretics probably are very important. For example, the activation of the renin-angiotensin system by diuretics may be detrimental; blockade of the renin-angiotensin system improves symptoms and survival. This suggests that ACE inhibitors should be started in the early stages of heart failure, when initiation of diuretics increases plasma renin activity. Studies to test the hypothesis that ACE inhibitors improve survival in the early stages of heart failure are underway, and should be analyzed to test the effect of ACE inhibition on patients receiving diuretics as compared to those not receiving diuretics. In contrast to the actions on the renin-angiotensin system, however, diuretics act to inhibit the sympathetic nervous system in patients with mild heart failure. Early use of diuretics therefore may preclude benefits of beta-blockade in the early stages of CHF.

Extent of Diuresis

Measurement of activation of neurohormonal systems may be the indicator of the optimal level of diuresis for which we have searched. Currently the absence of peripheral edema is the most widely used gauge of adequate diuresis; however, it may make more sense to analyze the physiologic parameters reflected by neurohormones. With initiation of diuresis, catecholamine and aldosterone concentrations decrease coincident with the observed improvement of symptoms. However, the concentrations of these neurohormones increase as dry weight is approached. Perhaps the lowest level of neurohormonal activation is the best indicator of optimal volume status.

Even if the optimal extent of diuresis is not certain, clinical experience provides us with tools to assess fluid status. Lung sounds are poor indicators of optimal fluid status; clear lungs do not necessarily indicate adequate diuresis and rales may not be able to be resolved with diuresis. Rather, assessment of total body fluid (using peripheral edema, ascites, and sacral edema as guides) is easy and should indicate the necessity for diuresis. Nevertheless, inadequate diuresis probably is the most common mistake made in the treatment of CHF. Many physicians are reluctant to treat patients aggressively with diuretics. Hospitalized patients often are diuresed enough to eliminate pulmonary edema, but are then sent home despite obvious total body fluid overload. With inadequate diuretic doses at home, increased edema and severe symptoms soon return.

A patient should be diuresed until no edema is present or other complications occur. Decreased renal function or increased blood urea nitrogen (BUN)/serum creatinine ratio after diuresis usually is a reflection of the rate of diuresis, and not the extent. Hospitalized, massively overloaded patients usually can be diuresed safely, losing approximately 1 kg/day, with slight, but clinically insignificant, deterioration in renal function. An elevated BUN concentration usually can be ignored in such circumstances; the patient is intentionally being made intravascularly deplete while being diuresed and the elevated BUN will not have clinical consequences. Even a slightly elevated serum creatinine

concentration can be tolerated with no important loss of renal function. When the patient's weight stabilizes with the resolution of intravascular depletion, the indices of renal function generally will improve. Even in stable patients, however, BUN and creatinine concentrations that are elevated from baseline, but stable, may be tolerated if the resultant fluid status results in improved symptomatology.

Prevention of Complications

Although renal dysfunction usually does not occur with diuretic use, marked increases in serum creatinine concentrations and decreases in glomerular filtration rate can be worrisome. When this occurs, simple measures usually resolve the problem. A slower rate of diuresis often is sufficient. It also may be advisable to limit the use of ACE inhibitors while aggressively diuresing a patient. The patients who develop renal failure with ACE inhibition usually are sodium and volume intravascularly deplete,[80] and initiation of ACE inhibitors after the patient is euvolemic may prevent the renal failure, which occurs occasionally with the combination of these drugs and diuretics.

The various electrolyte abnormalities that can occur with diuretic use have been discussed, but it is only the potassium concentration that, according to general wisdom, must be kept within the normal range (usually above 4.0 mEq/l). Even with aggressive diuresis this can be accomplished with frequent measurement of serum concentrations and appropriate potassium replacement. However, methods that counteract the underlying causes of potassium loss may prevent hypokalemia more efficiently and safely as well as other potentially important electrolyte abnormalities. The potassium-sparing diuretics are not potent, but may be helpful for electrolyte conservation. ACE inhibition similarly may prevent the electrolyte depletion associated with most diuretics. However, the effects of the combined use of these two modalities may be unpredictable, and patients need to be followed carefully in such a situation. Although such a combination may be helpful for maintaining a normal potassium concentration in some patients with refractory hypokalemia, it may lead to hyperkalemia in other patients.

The best means of keeping patients euvolemic would be the avoidance of the causes of fluid and sodium retention. Decreased sodium intake can decrease the need for high doses of diuretics, and should be encouraged in all patients, but fluid restriction is rarely beneficial. While the hyponatremia and fluid overload associated with CHF makes fluid restriction appealing, such an approach rarely is successful. First, the drive to drink water is strong, and it is virtually impossible to fluid restrict a patient successfully. Second, diuresis can be successful without fluid restriction. Third, hyponat-

TABLE 21.1. Comparison of diuretic medications, listed according to site of action.

Diuretic	FENa+ (max) (%)	Dosage (mg/day)	Onset of action Oral (hr)	Onset of action IV (min)	Action duration Oral (hr)	Action duration IV (hr)	Peak oral effect (hr)	Comments
Ascending loop of Henle								
Furosemide	20–25	40–400	1	5	6	2–3	1–3	
Bumetanide	20–25	1–5	0.5	5	6	2–3	1–3	
Ethacrynic acid	20–25	50–100	0.5	5	6–8	3	2	High ototoxicity risk, but (unlike other loop diuretics) can use in sulfa-allergic patients
Early distal tubule								
Metolazone	5–8	2.5–20	1	—	12–24	—	2–4	Greatest potential for potassium loss; also slight actions in proximal tubule
Chlorthalidone	5–10	25–200	2	—	24–48	—	6	Ineffective when GFR < 30
Hydrochlorothiazide	5–8	25–100	2	—	12	—	4	Ineffective when GFR < 30
Chlorothiazide	5–8	500–1000	1	15–30	8	—	4	Ineffective when GFR < 30
Late distal tubule								
Spironolactone	2	50–400	48–72	—	48–72	—	1–2 days	Efficacy dependent on aldosterone presence

GFR = Glomerular Filtration Rate (ml/min/1.73 M²).

remia rarely causes problems, and excessive hyponatremia can be treated successfully by modifying the diuretic regimen.

Comparisons of Diuretics

There are many excellent reviews of the pharmacokinetics and pharmacodynamics of the various diuretic medications.[81-84] These are summarized in Table 21.1. Figure 21.2 demonstrates the four areas where these agents work; the efficacy and side effects of most agents in large part can be ascribed to the sites of action of the drugs. However, the efficacy of any particular agent also depends on the particular pharmacokinetics of that agent, and, as discussed elsewhere in this book, CHF significantly alters the pharmacokinetics of most medications. Gastrointestinal absorption, volume of distribution, and delivery of the drug to its active site may alter with CHF.[85] In addition, the efficacy of any agent is limited by the severity of heart failure. Diuresis cannot exceed the filtered sodium, and the renal function often is limited by the multiple physiologic alterations that occur in heart failure. Effective use of diuretics in patients with CHF mandates knowledge of the actions of the drugs in these particular patients.

The loop diuretics are the agents most frequently used in patients with heart failure because of efficacy and potency, and there appear to be minimal clinically significant differences between furosemide and bumetanide.[86] However, inadequate doses of these agents often are prescribed in heart failure patients. Since loop diuretics are secreted in the proximal tubule and act from the luminal side of the loop of Henle, increasing doses of these drugs are needed as glomerular filtration rate decreases. The effective doses of these agents in normal individuals, therefore, often are inadequate in patients with heart failure who frequently exhibit decreased renal function. Physicians should not hesitate to use doses at the upper end of the therapeutic range in patients refractory to lower doses.

There are other reasons why high doses of loop diuretics may be needed in patients with heart failure. Contrary to popular belief, it appears as if the total bioavailability of the drugs is the same in these individuals as in normal controls, but the time course of oral absorption varies.[86] Poor absorption is not the mechanism of decreased activity of diuretic medications in heart failure. Rather, the increased absorption time results in lower peak plasma concentrations of loop diuretics, and high oral doses of the agents may be needed to achieve a therapeutic effect. The lower peak serum concentration, however, indicates that the risk of ototoxicity from a large oral dose of loop diuretics given to a patient with heart failure is no higher than a lower dose given to a normal individual. In contrast, a big dose, when given intravenously, will result in higher peak concentrations, and both increased efficacy and increased risk of toxicity. Continuous infusions of loop diuretics have been advocated,[87] but, considering the prolonged half-life of these agents in heart failure, probably are not needed. In fact, the elimination half-life of loop diuretics is increased two to three times in patients with heart failure as compared to normal individuals. The mechanism of action of loop diuretics means that treatment of heart failure, which often in-

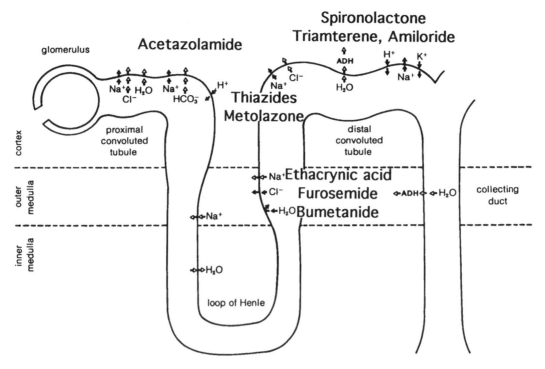

FIGURE 21.2. Fluid and electrolyte transport within the nephron, with sites of action of most commonly used diuretics. Solid arrow indicates active transport and open arrow indicates passive reabsorption. Adapted, with permission, from Puschett.[98]

creases renal flow and the clearance of the drug, may increase the efficacy of diuretic medications; the ability of hydralazine to increase furosemide clearance and diuresis has indeed been demonstrated.[88] Diuretic doses should be evaluated and adjusted frequently when the patient's overall status and fluid state are changing.

The thiazides are used rarely in patients with heart failure for a number of reasons. First and foremost, they are not as potent as the loop diuretics, and therefore not desirable when extensive diuresis is necessary. Second, renal clearance decreases in patients with CHF,[89] and thiazides are ineffective when the glomerular filtration rate is below approximately 30 ml/min. Third, thiazide diuretics cause a greater decrease in potassium than loop diuretics for the same quantity of diuresis.[39]

Spironolactone is not a potent diuretic, partially because its actions are countered by a compensatory increase in aldosterone concentration.[90] Other potassium-sparing agents, therefore are used often when a potent agent is desired. However, the consequences of spironolactone's antagonism of aldosterone may be important in many ways. Spironolactone conserves potassium and is the chief reason for much of its present use; it can help maintain serum potassium concentration in a patient who excretes a large quantity of the electrolyte. Like other potassium-sparing agents, it also is used often for its synergistic effects when combined with other diuretic medications. However, there are sugges-

tions of other effects of spironolactone that may be even more important and that need further investigation. For example, not only does spironolactone limit potassium excretion, but it reportedly prevents the exacerbation of hypokalemia, which is normally associated with epinephrine infusion.[37] Spironolactone also may be able to prevent digoxin toxicity, not only by conserving potassium, but perhaps by directly countering the actions of digoxin.[91] A metabolite of spironolactone, canrenone, may even have direct effects on the sodium-potassium pump.[92] Spironolactone also has been reported to decrease digoxin clearance, but many of these reports may be secondary to interference in the assay and increased digoxin levels have not always been found after spironolactone administration.[93]

The toxicities of the commonly used diuretic agents are listed in Table 21.2. Some, such as the effects on acid-base status and potassium, are avoidable if the patient is observed carefully and diuretic dosage adjusted as necessary. Others are rarer, but the potential of diuretics to cause these problems needs to be remembered.

Combination of Diuretics

It often is difficult to get effective diuresis in patients with heart failure. The physiologic stimulus to retain fluid may be strong enough to overwhelm the diuretic

TABLE 21.2. Common toxicities associated with diuretic use.

Hypersensitivity reactions
    Various skin rashes—most agents
    Interstitial nephritis—furosemide, thiazides
    Pancreatitis—thiazides
Deafness
    Loop diuretics
Renal calculi
    Acetazolamide
    Triamterene
Hyperuricemia, gout
    Thiazides
    Loop diuretics
Gynecomastia
    Spironolactone
Carbohydrate intolerance
    Thiazides
    Furosemide, bumetanide
Potassium abnormalities
    Hypokalemia—loop diuretics, thiazides
    Hyperkalemia—spironolactone, triamterene, amiloride
Acid-base abnormalities
    Acidosis—acetazolamide, spironolactone, triamterene, amiloride
    Alkalosis—loop diuretics, thiazides

Adapted with permission from Dirks JH, Sutton RAL.[99]

actions of any single agent. Thus, potent diuretics (such as the loop diuretics) may be rendered ineffective by distal reabsorption. In contrast, the agents that act distally, such as the potassium sparing agents, may not be potent enough to yield the desired results. In such patients, the synergistic effects of combining diuretics can have many beneficial consequences.

The combination of loop diuretics and metolazone has proved to be particularly potent.[94,95] With the combined use of these agents, effective diuresis may be produced in patients who have been resistant to other interventions. However, it may take days to see the results of the addition of metolazone because of the pharmacokinetics of the drug. It also is important to realize that the hypokalemia that results from the combined use of loop diuretics and metolazone may be severe; serum potassium concentrations need to be watched especially carefully in these patients. The other useful method of combining diuretics is to add a potassium-sparing agent to the diuretic regimen. Not only does this potentiate the diuretic actions of the original regimen, but it also prevents extreme potassium loss and simplifies electrolyte management.

Other Methods

Since fluid retention develops because of the abnormal hemodynamic status of patients with heart failure, enhancement of that status is an obvious means of improving diuresis. Interestingly, dobutamine alone, while improving the cardiac output and left ventricular filling pressure, at times does not improve renal function. The addition of low dose dopamine (approximately 2 μg/min/M^2), however, can increase the glomerular filtration rate, urine flow rate, and the fractional excretion of sodium by direct vasodilatory actions on the renal vasculature.[96] Administration of low dose dopamine is very effective for increasing diuresis in patients whose renal function is limited by severe heart failure.

When all else fails, ultrafiltration may improve the fluid status of a patient. Perhaps the many actions of diuresis on cardiac performance and neurohormones explain the reports of the chronic benefit of this intervention.[97] Ultrafiltration is discussed further elsewhere in this book.

Conclusions

Diuretic medications are valuable tools in our armamentarium for the treatment of CHF. They acutely improve symptoms and cardiac performance by multiple mechanisms. However, their chronic ramifications have not been adequately evaluated. Neurohormonal, electrolytic, and renal effects may have unintended consequences. Increased study and application of the results of these studies to the clinical arena should provide a more rational approach to the magnitude of diuresis and choice of diuretics prescribed for patients with CHF.

References

1. Achhammer I, Podszuz T. Effect of furosemide on pulmonary and cardiac haemodynamics after treatment of chronic heart failure. In: Puschett JB, Greenberg A, eds. *Diuretics III: Chemistry, Pharmacology, and Clinical Applications.* New York: Elsevier Science Publishing Co; 1990:331–333.
2. Stampfer M, Epstein SE, Beiser GD, Braunwald E. Hemodynamic effects of diuresis at rest and during intense upright exercise in patients with impaired cardiac function. *Circulation.* 1968;37:900–911.
3. Dikshit K, Vyden JK, Forrester JS, Chatterjee K, Prakash R, Swan HJC. Renal and extrarenal hemodynamic effects of furosemide in congestive heart failure after acute myocardial infarction. *N Engl J Med.* 1973;288:1087–1090.
4. Francis GS, Siegel RM, Goldsmith SR, Olivari MT, Levine TB, Cohn JN. Acute vasoconstrictor response to intravenous furosemide in patients with chronic congestive heart failure. *Ann Intern Med.* 1985;103:1–6.
5. Biddle TL, Yu PN. Effect of furosemide on hemodynamics and lung water in acute pulmonary edema secondary to myocardial infarction. *Am J Cardiol.* 1979;43:86–90.
6. Hutcheon D, Nemeth E, Quinlan D. The role of furosemide alone or in combination with digoxin in the

relief of symptoms of congestive heart failure. *J Clin Pharmacol*. 1980;20:59–68.

7. Wilson JR, Reichek N, Dunkman WB, Goldberg S. Effect of diuresis on the performance of the failing left ventricle in man. *Am J Med*. 1981;70:234–239.

8. Perloff JK, Roberts WC. The mitral apparatus: functional anatomy and mitral regurgitation. *Circulation*. 1972; 46:227–239.

9. Stevenson LW, Dadourian BJ, Child JS, Clark SH, Laks H. Mitral regurgitation after cardiac transplantation. *Am J Cardiol*. 1987;60:119–122.

10. Stevenson LW, Brunken RC, Belil D, et al. Afterload reduction with vasodilators and diuretics decreases mitral regurgitation during upright exercise in advanced heart failure. *J Am Coll Cardiol*. 1990;15:174–180.

11. Ramirez A, Abelmann WH. Hemodynamic effects of diuresis by ethacrynic acid. *Arch Intern Med*. 1968; 121:320–326.

12. MacGregor CD, Covell JW, Mahler F, Dilley RB, Rose J Jr. Relations between afterload, stroke volume, and the descending limb of Starling's curve. *Am J Physiol*. 1975;227:884–890.

13. Ross J Jr, Sonnenblick EH, Taylor RR, Spotnitz HM, Covell JW. Diastolic geometry and sarcomere length in the chronically dilated canine left ventricle. *Circ Res*. 1971;28:49–61.

14. Nechwatal W, Stange A, Sigel H, et al. Der Einfluss von Piretanid auf die zentrale Hamodynamik und Belastung-stoleranz von Patienten mit angina pectoris. *Herz Kreis-lauf*. 1982;14:91–96.

15. Ross J Jr. The assessment of myocardial performance in man by hemodynamic and cineangiographic technics. *Am J Cardiol*. 1969;23:511–515.

16. Keeton TK, Campbell WB. The pharmacologic alteration of renin release. *Pharmacol Rev*. 1980;32:81–227.

17. Broqvist M, Dahlstrom U, Karlberg BE, Karlsson E, Marklund T. Neuroendocrine response in acute heart failure and the influence of treatment. *Eur Heart J*. 1989;10:1075–1083.

18. Francis GS, Benedict C, Johnstone DE, et al. Comparison of neuroendocrine activation in patients with left ventricular dysfunction with and without congestive heart failure: a substudy of the Studies of Left Ventricular Dysfunction (SOLVD). *Circulation*. 1990;82:1724–1729.

19. Bayliss J, Norell M, Canepa-Anson R, Sutton G, Poole-Wilson P. Untreated heart failure: clinical and neuroendocrine effects of increasing diuretics. *Br Heart J*. 1987;57:17–22.

20. Verho M, Heintz B, Nelson K, Kirsten R. The effects of piretanide on catecholamine metabolism, plasma renin activity and plasma aldosterone: a double-blind study versus furosemide in healthy volunteers. *Curr Med Res Opin*. 1985;7:461–467.

21. Knight RK, Miall PA, Hawkins LA, Dacombe J, Edwrads CRW, Hamer J. Relation of plasma aldosterone concentration to diuretic treatment in patients with severe heart disease. *Br Heart J*. 1979;42:316–325.

22. de Langen CDJ, van Gilst WH, de Graeff PA, Kingma JH, Wesseling H. Effects of the renin-angiotensin system on sustained ventrlcular tachycardia after myocardial infarction. *Circulation*. 1986;74:II-351.

23. Brilla CG, Janicki JS, Weber KT. Myocardial fibrosis in systemic hypertension: role of mineralocorticoids, dietary sodium and hypertension. *Clin Res*. 1990;38:868A.

24. Bayliss PH, DeBeer FC. Human plasma vasopressin response to potent loop-diuretic drugs. *Eur J Clin Pharmacol*. 1981;20:343–346.

25. Genest J. The atrial natriuretic factor. *Br Heart J*. 1986;56:302–316.

26. Edwards BS, Zimmerman RS, Burnett JC Jr. Atrial natriuretic factor: physiologic actions and implications in congestive heart failure. *Cardiovasc Drugs Ther*. 1987; 1:89–100.

27. Schiffrin EL. Decreased density for binding sites of atrial natriuretic peptide on platelets of patients with severe congestive heart failure. *Clin Sci*. 1988;74:213–218.

28. Gottlieb 55, Kukin ML, Ahern D, Packer M. Prognostic importance of atrial natriuretic peptide in patients with chronic heart failure. *J Am Coll Cardiol*. 1989;13:1534–1539.

29. Riegger GAJ, Elsner D, Kromer EP, et al. Atrial natriuretic peptide in congestive heart failure in the dog: plasma levels, cyclic guanosine monophosphate, ultrastructure of atrial myoendocrine cells, and hemodynamic, hormonal, and renal effects. *Circulation*. 1988;77:398–406.

30. Johnston GD, Hiatt WR, Nies AS, Payne A, Murphy RC, Gerber JG. Factors modifying the early non-diuretic vascular effects of furosemide in man. *Circ Res*. 1983;53:630–635.

31. Green TP, Thompson TR, Johnson DE, Lock JE. Furosemide promotes patent ductus arteriosus in premature infants with the respiratory distress syndrome. *N Engl J Med*. 1983;308:743–748.

32. Dorian B, Larrue J, Defeudis FV Salari H, Borgeat P, Braquet P. Activation of prostacyclin synthesis in cultured aortic smooth muscle cells by diuretic-antihypertensive drugs. *Biochem Pharmacol*. 1984;33:2265–2269.

33. Multher RS, Potter DM, Bennett WM. Aspirin-induced depression of glomerular filtration rate in normal humans: role of sodium balance. *Ann Intern Med*. 1981;94:317–321.

34. Kao W, Gheorghiade M, Hall V, Goldstein S. Relation between plasma norepinephrine and response to medical therapy in congestive heart failure secondary to coronary artery disease or idiopathic dilated cardiomyopathy. *Am J Cardiol*. 1989;64:609–613.

35. Packer M, Lee WH, Kessler PD, Gottlieb SS, Bernstein JL, Kukin ML. Role of neurohormonal mechanisms in determining surnval in patients with severe chronic heart failure. *Circulation*. 1987;75:IV-80–IV-92.

36. Abraham AS, Meshulam Z, Rosenmann D, Eylath U. Influence of chronic diuretic therapy on serum, lymphocyte and erythrocyte potassium, magnesium and calcium concentrations. *Cardiology*. 1988;75:17–23.

37. Whyte KF, Whitesmith R, Reid JL. The effect of diuretic therapy on adrenaline-induced hypokalemia and hypomagnesemia. *Eur J Clin Pharmacol*. 1988;34:333–337.

38. Lipworth BJ, McDevitt DG, Struthers AD. Prior treatment with diuretic augments the hypokalemic and electrocardiographic effects of inhaled albuterol. *Am J Med*. 1989;86:653–657.

39. Morgan DB, Davidson C. Hypokalemia and diuretics: an analysis of publications. *Br Med J.* 1980;280:905–908.

40. Papademetriou V, Burris JF, Notargiacomo A, Fletcher RD, Freis ED. Thiazide therapy is not a cause of arrhythmia in patients with systemic hypertension. *Arch Intern Med.* 1988;148:1272–1276.

41. Roden DM, Hoffman BF. Action potential prolongation and induction of abnormal automaticity by low quinidine concentrations in canine purkinje fibers: relationship of potassium and cycle length. *Circ Res.* 1985;56:857–867.

42. Steiness E, Olesen KH. Cardiac arrhythmias induced by hypokalemia and potassium loss during maintenance digoxin therapy. *Br Heart J.* 1976;38:167–172.

43. Dyckner T, Helmers C, Lundman T, Wester PO. Initial serum potassium level in relation to early complications and prognosis in patients with acute myocardial infarction. *Acta Med Scand.* 1975;197:207–210.

44. Pelleg A, Mitamura H, Price R, et al. Extracellular potassium ion dynamics and ventricular arrhythmias in the canine heart. *J Am Coll Cardiol.* 1989;13:941–950.

45. Packer M, Lee WH. Provocation of hyper- and hypokalemic sudden death during treatment with and withdrawal of converting enzyme inhibition in severe chronic congestive heart failure. *Am J Cardiol.* 1986;57:347–348.

46. Gottlieb SS. Importance of magnesium in congestive heart failure. *Am J Cardiol.* 1989;63:39G–42G.

47. Ralston MA, Murnane MR, Kelley RE, Altschuld RA, Unverferth DV, Leier CV. Magnesium content of serum, circulating mononuclear cells, skeletal muscle, and myocardium in congestive heart failure. *Circulation.* 1989;80:573–580.

48. Dorup I, Skajaa K, Clausen T, Kjeldsen K. Reduced concentrations of potassium, magnesium, and sodium-potassium pumps in human skeletal muscle during treatment with diuretics. *Br Med J.* 1988;296:455–458.

49. Lim P, Jacob E. Magnesium deficiency In patients on long-term diuretic therapy for heart failure. *Br Med J.* 1972;3:60–62.

50. Mulder H, Schopman W, van der Lely AJ, Schopman W Sr. Acute change in plasma renin activity, plasma aldosterone concentration and plasma electrolyte concentrations following furosemide administration in patients with congestive heart failure—interrelationships and diuretic response. *Horm Metab Res.* 1987;19:80–83.

51. Girchev RA, Natcheff ND. Excretory function after renal denervation and administration of diuretic to unanesthetized dogs. *Biomed Biochim Acta.* 1988;6:507–514.

52. Sheehan J, White A. Diuretic-associated hypomagnesemia. *Br Med J.* 1982;285:1157–1159.

53. Polimeni PI, Page E. Magnesium in heart muscle. *Circ Res.* 1973;33:367–374.

54. Dagirmanjian R, Goldman H. Magnesium deficiency and distribution of blood in the rat. *Am J Physiol.* 1970;218:1464–1467.

55. Ghani MF, Rabah M. Effect of magnesium chloride on electrical stability of the heart. *Am Heart J.* 1977;94:600–602.

56. Flink EB. Hypomagnesemia in patients receiving digitalis. *Arch Intern Med.* 1985;145:625–626.

57. Bailie DS, Inoue H, Kaseda 5, Ben-David J, Zipes DP. Magnesium suppression of early afterdepolarizations and ventricular tachyarrhythmias induced by cesium in dogs. *Circulation.* 1988;6:1395–1402.

58. Iseri LT, Freed J, Bures AR. Magnesium deficiency and cardiac disorders. *Am J Med.* 1975;58:837–846.

59. Ramee SR, White CJ, Svinarich JT, Watson TD, Fox RF. Torsades des pointe and magnesium deficiency. *Am Heart J.* 1985;109:823–828.

60. White RE, Hartzell HC. Magnesium ions in cardiac function regulator of ion channels and second messengers. *Biochem Pharmacol.* 1989;38:859–867.

61. Shils ME. Experimental human magnesium deficiency. *Medicine.* 1969;48:61–85.

62. Gottlieb SS, Baruch L, Kukin ML, Bernstein JL, Fisher ML, Packer M. Prognostic importance of the serum magnesium concentration in patients with congestive heart failure. *J Am Coll Cardiol.* 1990;16:827–831.

63. Ralston MA, Murnane MR, Unverferth DV, Leier CV. Serum and tissue magnesium concentrations in patients with heart failure and serious ventricular arrhythmias. *Ann Intern Med.* 1990;113:841–846.

64. Anand IS, Ferrari R, Kalra GS, Wahi PL, Poole-Wilson PA, Haris PC. Edema of cardiac origin. Studies of body water and sodium, renal function, hemodynamic indexes, and plasma hormones in untreated congestive cardiac failure. *Circulation.* 1989;80:299–305.

65. Gross P, Ketteler M, Hausmann C, et al. Role of diuretics, hormonal derangements, and clinical setting of hyponatremia in medical patients. *Klin Wochenschrift.* 1988;66:662–669.

66. Kennedy RM, Earley LE. Profound hyponatremia resulting from a thiazide-induced decrease in urinary diluting capacity in a patient with primary polydypsia. *N Engl J Med.* 1970;282:1185–1186.

67. Schrier RW, Berl T, Anderson RJ. Osmotic and nonosmotic control of vasopressin release. *Am J Physiol.* 1979;236:F321–F332.

68. Dzau VJ, Hollenberg NK. Renal response to captopril in severe heart failure: role of furosemide in natriuresis and reversal of hyponatremia. *Ann Intern Med.* 1984;100:777–782.

69. Lee WH, Packer M. Prognostic importance of serum sodium concentration and its modification by converting-enzyme inhibition in patients with severe chronic heart failure. *Circulation.* 1986;73:257–267.

70. White MG, van Gelder J, Estes G. The effect of loop diuretics on the excretion of Na^+, Ca^{2+}, Mg^{2+}, and Cl^-. *J Clin Pharmacol.* 1981;21:610–614.

71. Breslau N, Moses AM, Weiner IM. The role of volume contraction in the hypocalciuric action of chlorothiazide. *Kidney Int.* 1976;10:164–170.

72. Marone C, Muggli F, Lahn W, Frey FJ. Pharmacokinetic and pharmacodynamic interaction between furosemide and metolazone in man. *Eur J Clin Invest.* 1985;15:253–257.

73. Bristow MR, Schwartz HD, Binetti G, Harrison DC, Daniels JR. Ionized calcium and the heart: elucidation of in vivo concentration-response relationships in the open-chest dog. *Circ Res.* 1977;41:565–574.

74. Ginsburg R, Esserman LJ, Bristow MR. Myocardial performance and extracellular ionized calcium in a severely

failing human heart. *Ann Intern Med*. 1983;98:603–606.

75. Ring-Larsen H, Henriksen JH, Wilken C, Clausen J, Pals H, Christensen NJ. Diuretic treatment in decompensated cirrhosis and congestive heart failure: effect of posture. *Br Med J*. 1986;292:1351–1353.

76. Schuster CJ, Weil MH, Besso J, Carpio M, Henning RJ. Blood volume following diuresis induced by furosemide. *Am J Med*. 1984;76:585–592.

77. Hook JB, Blatt AH, Brody MJ, Williamson HE. Effects of several saluretic-diuretic agents on renal hemodynamics. *J Pharmacol Exp Ther*. 1966;154:667–673.

78. Scherer B, Weber PC. Time-dependent changes in prostaglandin excretion in response to frusemide in man. *Clin Sci*. 1979;56:77–81.

79. Kim KE, Onesti G, Moyer J, Swartz C. Ethacrynic acid and furosemide: diuretic and hemodynamic effects and clinical uses. *Am J Cardiol*. 1971;27:407–415.

80. Hricik DE. Captopril-induced renal insufficiency and the role of sodium balance. *Ann Intern Med*. 1985;103:222–223.

81. Sica DA, Gehr T. Diuretics in congestive heart failure. *Cardiol Clin*. 1989;7:87–96.

82. Puschett JB, Greenberg A, eds. *The Diuretic Manual*. New York: Elsevier; 1984.

83. Dirks JH, Sutton RAL, eds. *Diuretics: Physiology, Pharmacology, and Clinical Use*. Philadelphia: Saunders; 1986.

84. Puschett JB. Clinical pharmacologic implications in diuretic selection. *Am J Cardiol*. 1986;57:6A–13A.

85. Tilstone WJ, Dargie H, Dargie EN, Morgan HG, Kennedy AC. Pharmacokinetics of metolazone in normal subjects and in patients with cardiac or renal failure. *Clin Pharmacol Ther*. 1976;16:322–329.

86. Brater DC, Day B, Burdette A, Anderson S. Bumetanide and furosemide in heart failure. *Kidney Int*. 1984;26:183–189.

87. Lawson DH, Gray JMB, Henry DA, Tilstone WJ. Continuous infusion of frusemide in refractory oedema. *Br Med J*. 1978;2:476.

88. Nomura A, Yasuda H, Minami M, Akimoto T, Miyazaki K, Arita T. Effect of furosemide in congestive heart failure. *Clin Pharmacol Ther*. 1981;30:177–182.

89. Beermann B, Groschinsky-Grind M. Pharmacokinetics of hydrochlorothlazide in patients with congestive heart failure. *Br J Clin Pharmacol*. 1979;7:579–583.

90. Nicholls MG, Espiner EA, Hughes H, Rohers T. Effect of potassium-sparing diuretics on the renin-angiotensin-aldosterone system and potassium retention in heart failure. *Br Heart J*. 1976;38:1025–1039.

91. Waldorff S, Hansen PB, Egeblad H, et al. Interactions between digoxin and potassium-sparing diuretics. *Clin Pharmacol Ther*. 1983;33:418–423.

92. Garay RP, Diez J, Nazaret C, Dagher G, Abitol JP. The interaction of canrenone with the Na$^+$, K$^+$ pump in human red blood cells. *Arch Pharmacol*. 1985;329:311–315.

93. Finnegan TP, Spence JD, Cape RD. Potassium sparing diuretics: interaction with digoxin in elderly men. *J Am Geriatr Soc*. 1984;32:129–131.

94. Kiyingi A, Field MJ, Pawsel CC, Yiannikas J, Lawrence JR, Arter WJ. Metolazone in treatment of severe refractory congestive heart failure. *Lancet*. 1990;335:29–31.

95. Ghose RR, Gupta SK. Synergistic actions of metolazone with "loop" diuretics. *Br Med J*. 1981;812:1432–1433.

96. Pabico RC, Rogal GJ, McKenna BA, Richeson JF, Hood WB. Renal effects of dobutamine and dopamine in congestive heart failure. In Puschett JB, Greenberg A, eds. *Diuretics III: Chemistry, Pharmacology, and Clinical Applications*. New York: Elsevier Science Publishing Co; 1990:302–312.

97. L'Abbate A, Emdin M, Piacenti M, et al. Ultrafiltration: a rational treatment for heart failure. *Cardiology*. 1989;76:384–390.

98. Puschett JB. Physiologic basis for the use of new and older diuretics in congestive heart failure. *Cardiovasc Med*. 1977;2:119–134.

99. Dirks JH, Sutton RAL, eds. *Diuretics: Physiology, Pharmacology, and Clinical Use*. Philadelphia: Saunders; 1986.

22
Digitalis Glycosides

Ralph A. Kelly and Thomas W. Smith

Historical Perspectives

Cardiac glycosides have played a prominent role in the therapy of congestive heart failure since William Withering codified its use in his classic monograph on the efficacy of the leaves of the common foxglove plant (*Digitalis purpurea*) in 1785. However, a controversy has arisen in the past two decades about whether the risks of digitalis preparations outweigh their benefits, particularly in patients with heart failure in sinus rhythm.[1] The standard for clinical use of the cardiac glycosides in modern medicine was reflected in a debate between two eminent clinicians, who were also the coeditors of the *Oxford Medicine*, Henry Christian and Sir James Mackenzie. Sir James Mackenzie advocated the use of digitalis preparations only in those patients with heart failure who also had atrial arrhythmias, prompting the following response from Christian: "My views evidently differ from those of my fellow editor of the *Oxford Medicine*. The views of Sir James MacKenzie have been concurred in by numerous observers, with the result that there is a growing feeling that, unless the pulse is absolutely irregular and rapid, little is to be gained from digitalis therapy. My own experience is so directly contrary to this that is seems worthwhile to restate the views already expressed by me . . . My own view with regard to digitalis, as a rule, is that it has a striking effect on those changes in the patient which are brought on by cardiac insufficiency, and this effect appears irrespective of whether or not the pulse is irregular."[2]

Within the United States at least, Dr. Christian's views prevailed until several retrospective and uncontrolled trials in the 1970s pointed to a lack of efficacy of digitalis preparations in many patients for whom they were prescribed. This debate has become more relevant with the availability of other, potentially less toxic remedies for heart failure, most notably the introduction of loop diuretics in the 1960s, followed by the devel-

opment of new classes of vasodilators, which enabled the clinician to optimize ventricular loading while alleviating congestive symptoms. Over the past 10 years, however, a number of prospective controlled trials have appeared, discussed in more detail below, that document the safety and efficacy of digitalis in patients with moderate and severe congestive heart failure (CHF), whether prescribed alone or in combination with newer therapeutic modalities.

In this chapter, we begin with a brief overview of the basic pharmacology and cardiac cell biology of the actions of cardiac glycosides, including research in the past decade that has documented the mechanism of the positive inotropic effect of these drugs. This is followed by a review of the pharmacokinetics of several cardiac glycosides with important drug interactions. The data justifying the use of digoxin in patients with moderate to severe CHF are reviewed in some detail, followed by a description of the mechanisms underlying the toxic manifestations of this class of drugs and their treatment. The chapter ends with a discussion of the role of Fab fragments of antidigoxin antibodies in the treatment of digoxin toxicity, and the relevance of serum levels of digoxin to clinical practice.

Cardiac Glycosides: Natural Sources and Chemical Structure

The terms "digitalis" or "cardiac glycosides" are used in this chapter to refer to any of the steroid or steroid glycoside compounds that exert characteristic positive inotropic and electrophysiological effects on the heart. Although there are important differences in pharmacokinetics among the more than 300 known compounds with these properties, their pharmacological actions are fundamentally similar, and detailed consideration therefore will be limited to those agents that are in current clinical use. Optimal use of digitalis requires considerable knowledge and skill on the part of the physician because of the unusually narrow therapeutic/toxic dose ratio of this group of drugs. A sound understanding of the actions and pharmacokinetics of digitalis preparations is essential to minimize the ever-present risk of toxicity and to provide maximum benefit to the patient.

The cardiac glycosides comprise a group of compounds found in plants and in the venom and skin of certain toads. Clinically useful preparations are derived from the leaves and seeds of plants in the genera *Digitalis* and *Strophanthus*. From the leaves of *Digitalis purpurea* is derived digitoxin, and from those of *Digitalis lanata*, digoxin is derived after a mild alkaline hydrolysis step, as well as lanatoside C and deslanoside. From the seeds of *Strophanthus gratus* comes ouabain, a hydrophilic, relatively rapidly acting cardiac glycoside. In the 1990s, digoxin is by far the most commonly prescribed of these drugs because of the ready availability of techniques for measuring serum levels, flexibility in its routes of administration, and its intermediate duration of action.

A detailed description of sources of cardiac glycosides, their chemistry, and structure-activity relationships are extensively considered in standard texts.[3-5] The steroid nucleus common to all cardiac glycosides contains an α, β-unsaturated lactone ring attached at the C-17 position. Without the sugar moieties, the steroid and unsaturated lactone part of the molecule is called a "genin" or an "aglycone." The genins usually are less potent and have more transient actions due to altered pharmacokinetics than do the parent glycosides. It is apparent from structure-activity comparisons that the cardioactive glycosides demonstrate considerable variation in the structure of the steroid nucleus, as well as the sugar substitutes attached at the C-3 position. The structure of digoxin is illustrated in Figure 22.1. Digitoxin differs from digoxin only by the absence of a hydroxyl groups at C-12. This absent hydroxyl group reduces the hydrophilicity of the compound and results in markedly different metabolism and protein binding compared to digoxin. Potent cardioactivity traditionally has been thought to require the unsaturated lactone ring, the C-14 β-hydroxyl group, and *cis* fusion of the A-B and C-D rings. However, the recent review of Thomas et al.[6] prompts reconsideration of these and other unduly restrictive views regarding requirements for cardioactivity. For example, although an important determinant, the *cis* β configuration of the C and D rings appears to be less than absolutely necessary, because synthetic derivatives of prednisone and prednisolone have biological activity despite their typical mammalian steroid 14α-H structures. 14β-Hydroxyprogesterone binds to and inhibits the sodium pump with about one tenth the potency of ouabagenin, and increases contractile force of isolated cardiac muscle. Ultimately, continued research into

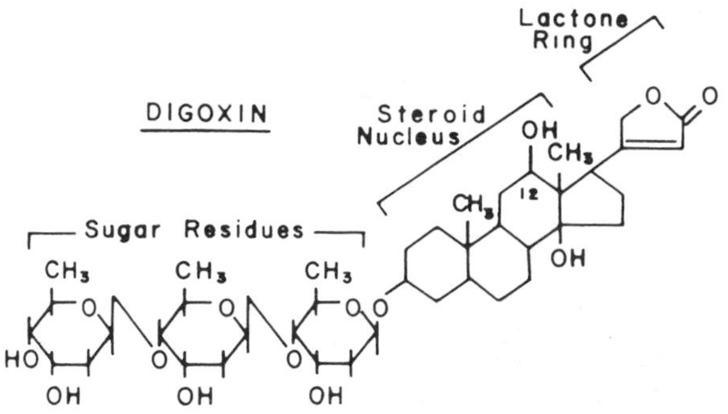

FIGURE 22.1. Molecular structure of digoxin.

digitalis structure-activity relationships is designed to lead to improved cardiac glycoside molecules with reduced adverse side effects and enhanced selectivity of action.[6]

Mechanism of Action

Positive Inotropic Effect

By the late 1920s, it became clear that digitalis preparations caused a positive inotropic effect on the intact ventricle, resulting in an increase in the rate of rise of intracavitary pressure during isovolumic systole at constant heart rate and aortic pressure.[7] This effect could be demonstrated in normal as well as failing cardiac muscle. Cardiac glycoside administration caused the ventricular function (Frank-Starling) curve of the intact heart to shift upward and to the left, so that more stroke work is generated at a given filling pressure (Fig. 22.2). This was found to be true of both right and left ventricles, and of atrial as well as ventricular myocardium. Force-velocity curves for isolated cardiac muscle are shifted in parallel upward and to the right by cardioactive steroids.[8] These effects appear to be sustained during in vivo administration of digitalis, for periods of weeks to months, without any evidence of desensitization or tachyphylaxis.[9,10] The time to peak force generation and the relaxation rates are altered little by subtoxic doses or concentrations of cardioactive steroids,[11] but the positive inotropic effect observed is highly dependent on contraction frequency,[12] declining on either side of an intermediate frequency that yields the maximal inotropic response.

It is now generally believed that digitalis compounds bring about an increase in the availability of activator Ca^{2+} in heart cells,[5,13-15] and that this increase in intracellular Ca^{2+} activity is sufficient to explain both the inotropic and arrhythmogenic effects of these drugs (Fig. 22.3). Importantly, it also is now accepted that the rise in intracellular Ca^{2+} is a consequence of the "direct" effect of cardiac glycosides on transmembrane Na^+ transport.[5,16-20]

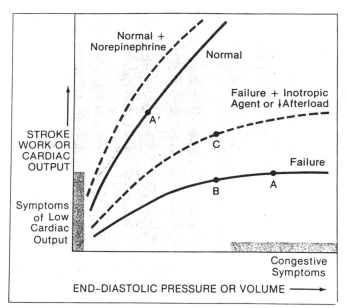

FIGURE 22.2. Relationship between ventricular filling pressure or volume and stroke work (or cardiac output). The points labeled A and A' are the operating points for a patient with congestive symptoms and a decreased cardiac output and a normal patient, respectively. The dashed lines indicate the effects of an agent that increases inotropic state, such as norepinephrine in the normal person during exercise, or in a patient with CHF given a digitalis glycoside. Administration of a diuretic often results in a decline in end-diastolic pressure or preload, as shown in the figure by moving from point A to point B. Either a balanced vasodilator or an inotropic agent will result in improved forward output and reduced filling pressures, as illustrated by moving from point A to point C on the dashed line. Reprinted from Smith TW, In *Cecil's Textbook of Medicine*. 18th ed. Saunders, 1988; with permission.

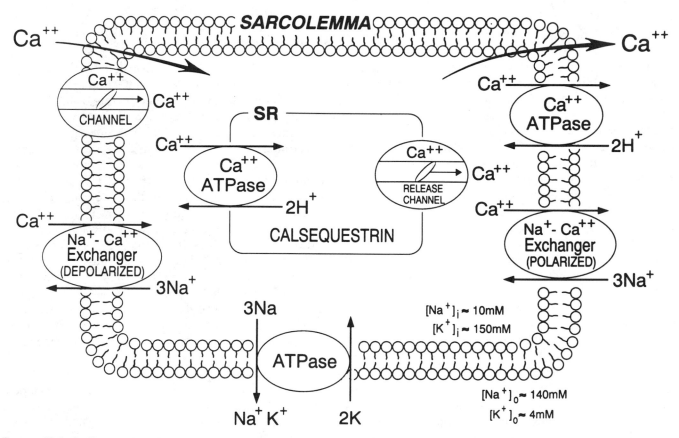

FIGURE 22.3. Sodium and calcium pathways relevant to the inotropic effect of the cardiac glycosides. The diagram represents an isolated cardiac muscle cell in which the various transmembrane ion pumps, channels, and exchangers that are discussed in the text as important in regulating intracellular Na^+ and Ca^{2+} activities and in mediating the positive inotropic effect of cardiac glycosides. The digitalis binding site is on the extracellular aspect of the Na and K transporting ATPase sites. The movement of Ca^{2+} via the Na^+-Ca^{2+} exchange protein is illustrated in two formulations, depending on membrane potential. SR = sarcoplasmic reticulum; calsequestrin = SR calcium binding protein. Reprinted from Smith TW, et al, In Braunwald EB, ed. *Heart Disease*. 4th ed. 1991; with permission.

Inhibition of NaK-ATPase

The lack of any well defined effects of digitalis on other basic cellular functions led to intense investigative interest in the specific ability of cardioactive steroids to inhibit the active transmembrane transport of the monovalent cations Na^+ and K^+. All cardioactive steroids share the property of being potent and highly specific inhibitors of the intrinsic membrane protein NaK-ATPase. The plasma membrane NaK-ATPase, the molecular machinery that comprises the cellular sodium pump, is representative of a family of evolutionarily ancient enzymes in which membrane ion translocation is coupled to the hydrolysis of a high-energy ATP phosphate.[21] With the advent of new molecular biological methods that allow the primary structure of proteins to be deduced from cDNA sequences, a remarkably high degree of homology has been found among those ion-translocating ATPases that form a covalent phosphorylated intermediate ("P-type" ATPases).[22-24] The α or catalytic subunit component of the sodium pump, the roughly 100-kDa integral membrane protein that almost certainly contains the Na^+, K^+, and ATP binding sites of the intact enzyme, has been highly conserved in eukaryotes for the establishment and maintenance of transmembrane Na^+ and K^+ gradients, and shows considerable sequence homology with the sarcoplasmic reticular and plasmalemmal Ca^{2+}-ATPases and the H^+-K^+-ATPase of gastric mucosa, particularly at the phosphorylation site.[25-29] There is even sequence homology at this site with K^+-ATPases from prokaryotes, reflecting the long history of success of this molecular design.[26] Unique to the NaK-ATPase is the presence of an approximate 40,000-kDa glycosylated subunit termed the β subunit, the function of which is as yet unknown. This subunit too has been highly conserved as indicated by nucleotide sequence analysis from phylogenetically diverse species ranging from the electric fish *Torpedo californica* to humans.[30,31] Evidence supporting the existence of a much smaller, third subunit termed the γ subunit, originally described by Forbush et al.,[32] remains controversial. This amphiphilic protein appears to contain two distinct structural domains with a total of 68 amino acids.[33] It is unclear whether this protein, if it is part of the quaternary structure of the mature enzyme, is necessary for ion-translocating activity.

Aside from its α, β heterodimer structure, another characteristic of the NaK-ATPase that is unique among the P-type ATPases is the presence of a binding site on the extracytoplasmic face of the α subunit for the cardiac glycosides.[34,35] Although the binding affinity varies among isoforms of the enzyme and from species to species, the ability of the enzyme to bind and to be inhibited by cardiac glycosides has been very highly conserved; it is so highly conserved, in fact, that cardiac glycoside binding is a sine qua non for identifying functional NaK-ATPase and is used to define the contribution of the sodium pump to plasmalemmal monovalent cation fluxes. One cardiac glycoside binding site facing the extracellular surface is present per α chain. Optimal binding requires Na^+, $Mg,^{2+}$ and ATP, and is inhibited by extracellular K^+. Cardiac glycoside binding results in complete inhibition of enzymatic and transport functions of each NaK-ATPase site occupied. In addition to a wealth of evidence from animal, whole heart, isolated muscle, single cell, and molecular studies, inhibition of the sodium pump in atrial tissue of patients treated with conventional doses of digoxin also has been demonstrated. Indeed, the highly selective action of the cardiac glycosides to bind to the "digitalis binding site" on the extracellular face of the α subunit of NaK-ATPase has engendered much speculation about the possible existence of endogenous ligands, simply because the amino acid sequence and conformation that forms their binding site has been so highly conserved over many phyla and millennia. There is no proof yet that any "endogenous digitalis" exists that has a well defined biologic role in regulating NaK-ATPase function (vide infra).

Na^+-Ca^{2+} Exchange and Increased Intracellular Calcium

Compelling direct evidence supporting cardiac glycoside-induced increases in intracellular Na^+ concentration or activity ($[Na^+]_i$) is now available from studies of cardiac cells impaled with Na^+-sensitive microelectrodes.[19,20] The relation of $[Na^+]_i$ to tension development is direct and remarkably steep,[19] which may explain why an increase in $[Na^+]_i$ was difficult to demonstrate at subtoxic cardiac doses using older and less sensitive methods. Data from these and other experiments support the view that inhibition of active cellular Na^+ transport results in augmentation of myocyte Ca^{2+} content which, in turn, produces a positive inotropic response (see Fig. 22.3). This is analogous to the increase in contractility that follows an increase in $[Na^+]_i$ due to increased contraction frequency, a phenomenon termed "treppe" or "Bowditch staircase."[36] The mechanism of both digitalis-induced positive inotropy and the staircase phenomenon appears to involve an altered balance between intracellular Na^+ and Ca^{2+}, as shown in schematic form in Figure 22.3. The transmembrane Na^+ influx occurring with each action potential, in the presence of diminished outward Na^+ pumping due to digitalis, leads to the increased intracellular Na^+ concentration proposed to promote increased intracellular Ca^{2+} stores, either through enhanced Ca^{2+} entry, reduced Ca^{2+} efflux, or both. These effects are thought to be mediated via Na^+-Ca^{2+} exchange. At rapid heart rates, Na^+ influx in the presence or absence of digitalis may be sufficiently great to approach the maximum inotropically effective intracellular Na^+. This is consistent with the diminished effects of cardiac glycosides at high contraction frequencies.

Studies with spontaneously contracting, isolated, and cultured ventricular cells have demonstrated direct correlations between ouabain-induced enhancement of the contractile state, inhibition of Na^+ and K^+ transport, and increased cellular content of both Na^+ and Ca^{2+}.[17] These data support the hypothesis that inhibition of the Na^+ pump by digitalis leads to a positive inotropic response, and are consistent with modulation of Ca^{2+} content by Na^+ via the Na^+-Ca^{2+} exchange carrier mechanism. A similar effect can be achieved by decreasing extracellular $[K^+]$, which can produces equivalent positive inotropic effects accompanied by inhibition of Na^+ and K^+ transport and an increase in intracellular $[Na^+]$ and intracellular calcium activity, $[Ca^{2+}]_i$, via Na^+-Ca^{2+} exchange.[37] Direct evidence for a rise in $[Ca^{2+}]_i$ after digitalis comes from studies using the Ca-activated photoprotein aequorin,[15] as well as more recently developed Ca^{2+}-specific fluorescent probes. During the inotropic effect of digitalis, there is a close association between the increase in peak systolic aequorin luminescence, which is directly related to intracellular $[Ca^{2+}]$ over the relevant range, and the increase in twitch force.[14,15]

In addition to increased $[Ca^{2+}]_i$ accumulation via Na^+-Ca^{2+} exchange, digitalis under some circumstances also may increase Ca^{2+} influx through sarcolemmal voltage-sensitive Ca channels. An increase in Ca^{2+}, current accompanies digitalis inotropy in both isolated Purkinje fibers and in isolated cells from mammalian ventricle. Marban and Tsien proposed a mechanism for this increase in Ca^{2+} current (I_{Ca}): a small increase in intracellular free $[Ca^{2+}]$ (by Na pump inhibition or any other means) could act as a positive feedback signal to increase I_{Ca}.[13] A similar mechanism was proposed by Lederer and Eisner to explain changes in the membrane current that they observed during NaK-ATPase inhibition by extracellular K^+ withdrawal.[38]

The relative contribution of increased I_{Ca} to the inotropic effect of digitalis is still undetermined, but is not thought to be a primary mechanism. $[Ca^{2+}]_i$ also has negative feedback effects on I_{Ca}. Ca channel inactivation is partly Ca-dependent,[39] so that increased $[Ca^{2+}]_i$ actually may lead to a net decrease in I_{Ca} at higher $[Ca^{2+}]_i$ levels.

The issue of whether or not diastolic $[Ca^{2+}]_i$ rises with digitalis has important mechanistic implications, in that most theories predict increases in both diastolic and systolic $[Ca^{2+}]_i$. There is no compelling evidence that a rise in diastolic $[Ca^{2+}]_i$ is invariably associated with the positive inotropic effect, and indeed careful mechanical measurements at positively inotropic but subtoxic cardiac glycoside levels show no diastolic con-

tracture. Experiments using techniques in beating heart tissue (e.g., Ca-sensitive microelectrodes[40] or $^{45}Ca^{2+}$ accumulation[17,18]) confirm that there is a rise in overall $[Ca^{2+}]_i$ during the positive inotropic effect, but the limited time resolution of the measurements has thus far precluded further analysis. These and related mechanistic issues are discussed in greater detail elsewhere.[5]

Electrophysiologic Effects

A thorough discussion of the major electrophysiologic effects of digitalis is beyond the scope of this chapter, and the interested reader is referred to several comprehensive reviews.[5,41,42] As with the positive inotropic effect of these drugs, the major effect on cardiac rhythm of digitalis preparations is believed to be due to inhibition of the sodium pump. The 80- to 90-mV transmembrane resting potential of cardiac cells is maintained by Na^+ and K^+ gradients (particularly the latter) which, in turn, are dependent on the integrity of the active Na-K pump mechanism. There is general agreement that inhibition of NaK-ATPase underlies the direct toxic effects of digitalis preparations on cardiac rhythm, and thus represents an extension of the drugs' therapeutic effects. Cells in various parts of the heart show differing sensitivities to digitalis, and both direct and neurally mediated effects must be dissected before conclusions can be drawn about the mechanisms involved.[43,44] For example, digoxin does not produce significant changes in atrial effective or functional refractory periods in denervated hearts, nor does it change sinus node cycle length.[45,46] These findings point to the importance of the autonomic nervous system in the modulation of automaticity and conduction by digitalis. Indeed, at the lower concentrations associated with the therapeutic levels of digoxin, the drugs decrease automaticity and increase maximum diastolic potential, effects that can be blocked by atropine, whereas higher concentrations decrease diastolic potentials and increase automaticity.

Similarly, the toxic arrhythmogenic effect of the cardiac glycosides are due to a combination of direct effects on the myocardium and neurally mediated increases in autonomic activity. During exposure to high concentrations of digitalis, isolated myocardial preparations demonstrate small unstimulated depolarizations and contractions after action potentials. These oscillatory events coincide with the development of digitalis-toxic arrhythmias in intact animals exposed to similar levels of digitalis. Both systolic and diastolic $[Ca^{2+}]_i$ increase during digitalis-induced arrhythmias, increases that were first inferred from changes in tension, leading to the idea that intracellular "Ca overload" contributes to the observed arrhythmogenic effects. These occur presumably because $[Ca^{2+}]_i$ increases progressively until the sarcoplasmic reticulum, the major intracellular organelle responsible for Ca^{2+} sequestration, is no longer capable of retaining all the Ca^{2+} taken up with each depolarization. Spontaneous cycles of Ca release and reuptake then ensue, resulting in afterdepolarizations and aftercontractions. The afterdepolarization is the result of a Ca^{2+}-activated transient inward current, and is thought to be the macroscopic manifestation of Ca-activated nonspecific cation channels, plus Na-Ca exchange current[5] (Fig. 22.3). In this formulation, the inotropic and arrhythmic effects of digitalis constitute a spectrum dependent on the overall level of intracellular Ca loading.

The effects of antiarrhythmic drugs that decrease transient inward current often appear to be attributable to a decrease in cellular Ca loading. For example, the reduction in transient inward current produced by lidocaine is thought to occur because it blocks Na influx, thus reducing Na^+ loading which, in turn, prevents Ca^{2+} loading, thereby decreasing the likelihood for oscillatory Ca release. Ca channel blockers, which reduce digitalis-induced afterdepolarizations, probably do so directly by inhibiting Ca^{2+} influx, thereby decreasing intracellular $[Ca^{2+}]$.

Neurally Mediated Actions of Cardiac Glycosides

The toxic electrophysiologic effects of digitalis also involve neural mechanisms. β-Blockers will inhibit neural hyperactivity and may prevent some digitalis-induced ventricular arrhythmias. Sympathetic nerve activity is substantially augmented by toxic doses of cardiac glycosides, and animal experimental studies document that spinal cord section at the C_1 level can prevent or delay some digitalis-induced arrhythmias.[47,48] The reader is referred to several comprehensive reviews of interactions between the autonomic nervous system and digitalis.[42,49,50]

It is important to understand the pathophysiology of heart failure and the role of digitalis glycosides in modifying the abnormal autonomic nervous system activity characteristic of advanced heart failure, including altered baroreflex activity. The responsiveness of the baroreflex system is diminished in CHF. As stimulation of this reflex normally inhibits sympathetic outflow, the result of diminished baroreflex activity in these patients is increased sympathetic nerve activity, as well as increased vasopressin and renin release. Several reports have demonstrated recently that digitalis, at therapeutic concentrations, reduces sympathetic nerve activity (in contrast to toxic levels, noted above). This may be due to activation of either low- or high-pressure baroreceptors[51] and not be simply due to a drug-mediated increase in stroke volume.

Pharmacology

Although a number of cardiac glycoside preparations remain available, digoxin is the most commonly prescribed and its pharmacology will be described in detail, although other preparations will be mentioned briefly. Note that the values for pharmacokinetic data given below represent averages and the clinician should be aware of the possibility of substantial interindividual variation.

Digoxin

Because of flexibility in routes of administration and its intermediate duration of action, digoxin has become the preferred digitalis preparation. Digoxin is excreted exponentially, with an elimination half-life of 36 to 48 hr in patients with normal renal function, resulting in the daily loss of about one third of body stores. The drug is excreted for the most part unchanged, although some patients excrete detectable quantities of the inactive metabolite dihydrodigoxin, which arises through bacterial biotransformation in the gut lumen.[52] Renal excretion of digoxin is proportional to the glomerular filtration rate (and hence to creatinine clearance) and is largely independent of the urine flow rate in patients with reasonably intact renal function. In patients with prerenal azotemia, digoxin clearance may correlate more closely with urea clearance, suggesting that the drug may undergo some degree of tubular reabsorption.[53]

With daily maintenance therapy, a steady state is reached when daily losses are matched by daily intake. For patients not previously given digitalis, institution of daily maintenance therapy without a loading dose results in development of steady-state plateau concentrations after four to five half-lives, or about 7 days, in persons with normal renal function. If the half-life of the drug is prolonged, the length of time before a steady state is reached on a daily maintenance dose also would be prolonged proportionately. Because of the high degree of tissue binding of digoxin (i.e., a large volume of distribution, averaging 4–7 L/kg), the drug is not removed effectively from the body by dialysis. Serum digoxin levels and pharmacokinetics are essentially the same before and after the loss of large amounts of adipose tissue in massively obese persons, suggesting that a patient's estimated lean body mass should be used in the calculation for maintenance dosing (vide infra). Acute vasodilator therapy with nitroprusside or hydralazine tends to increase renal digoxin clearance and may necessitate adjustment of the maintenance digoxin dosage.[54] Infants and children absorb and excrete digoxin in much the same way as adults do, although recent evidence suggests that secretion at the renal tubular level may be quantitatively more important in children before puberty. Digoxin doses in neonates and infants are substantially larger than those in adults when calculated on the basis of milligrams per kilogram of body weight or per square meter of body surface area.[55] These higher doses result in relatively higher serum digoxin concentrations, which are generally well tolerated. Digoxin does cross the placenta and fetal umbilical cord venous blood levels of the drug are similar to maternal blood levels.

Numerous studies over several decades have documented incomplete absorption of digoxin after oral administration with the bioavailability of currently marketed tablet preparations averaging about 65% to 75%. Individual patient variation, interactions with other concurrently administered drugs, and the characteristics of the digoxin preparation ingested are all known to affect the drug's bioavailability. Patients with malabsorption syndromes often absorb digoxin poorly and erratically. However, patients with pancreatic insufficiency, despite steatorrhea, appear to absorb the drug normally. Administration of digoxin after meals is likely to delay absorption, thus diminishing peak serum levels, but absolute bioavailability is not affected to any noteworthy degree. Absorption of digoxin tends to be reduced by drugs that increase motility, particularly if a particular formulation releases the active drug slowly. In addition, nonabsorbed substances, such as cholestyramine, colestipol, neomycin, kaolin, and pectin (Kaopectate), and nonabsorbable antacids, when taken concurrently with digoxin, can interfere with gastrointestinal absorption of digoxin. Because of documented large variations in the bioavailability of commercially available digoxin preparations in the past,[56] bioavailability specifications are now mandated by both the FDA and USP.

The highest bioavailability is currently available in an encapsulated gel preparation that is reported to have 90% to 100% absorption with reduced variation among subjects.[57] Clinicians who use this formulation should reduce the dose prescribed accordingly. Intramuscular digoxin (not recommended) typically causes severe pain at the injection site and bioavailability is not highly predictable. Digoxin elixir is somewhat better absorbed than most tablet formulations.

An important interaction between digoxin and quinidine leads to an approximately twofold increase in serum digoxin concentrations with addition of quinidine at conventional doses.[58] Quinidine alters both renal clearance and tissue binding of digoxin by unknown mechanisms. The increase in serum digoxin concentration can be associated with the development of digoxin-toxic rhythm disturbances. A decrease in the maintenance digoxin dose of about 50%, in addition to frequent assessment of serum digoxin concentration and clinical status, is advisable when quinidine is given con-

currently. Interactions of digoxin with verapamil and amiodarone (among other drugs) tend to raise serum digoxin levels and necessitate drug monitoring when these agents are prescribed concurrently. Neomycin, cholestyramine, Kaopectate, and nonabsorbable antacids can interfere with digoxin absorption, lowering steady-state digoxin levels.

Digitoxin

Digitoxin, a cardiac glycoside that is the principal active agent in digitalis leaf preparations, is the least polar and most slowly excreted of the available cardiac glycosides. Gastrointestinal absorption of digitoxin is essentially complete. About 9% of the serum or plasma content of the drug is bound to albumin at clinically relevant concentrations, in contrast to digoxin, which is only about 25% bound to plasma proteins. Extensive metabolism of digitoxin occurs, presumably in the liver, with minimal renal clearance of unchanged drug. An enterohepatic cycle exists for digitoxin that can be interrupted by resins, such as cholestyramine, that bind digitoxin in the gut lumen. Although displacement of digitoxin from serum proteins does occur with high concentrations of other drugs that are also highly protein bound, including warfarin, tolbutamide, and clofibrate, these effects probably are not clinically important at the plasma concentrations of digitoxin encountered in clinical use. Oral absorption of digitoxin is virtually 100%, although cholestyramine and ion-exchange resins can diminish uptake.

Half-lives of digitoxin in plasma are in the range of 4 to 6 days irrespective of renal function, with estimates as long as 8 days in selected patients. Therefore, without a loading dose, continuous administration of a daily maintenance dose will result in stable plasma levels after 3 to 4 weeks.

Ouabain

Ouabain is the most polar and rapidly acting of the cardiac glycosides commonly available. The plasma half-life of ouabain in normal persons is about 21 hr, although impairment of renal function will diminish clearance of the drug. Although ouabain is predominantly excreted unchanged via the renal route, its gastrointestinal excretion is substantial even after intravenous administration.[59] It is poorly absorbed from the gastrointestinal tract, and therefore is not available for oral use. Detailed reviews of the pharmacokinetics and metabolism of these and other cardiac glycosides are available.[42,60]

Cardiac glycosides may transiently raise systemic vascular resistance and decrease venous capacitance due to direct vasoconstrictor effects in vascular smooth muscle, presumably due in part to inhibition of NaK-

ATPase, resulting in greater intracellular Ca^{2+} via Na^{+}-Ca^{2+} exchange, and to increased sympathetic nerve-mediated vasoconstriction, including vasoconstriction of the coronary arteries.[61,62] These vasoconstrictor effects may be seen after bolus injections of any cardiac glycoside, but may be more likely to be seen after acute bolus injections of ouabain (not recommended). The vasoconstrictor effects are rapid in onset, precede any discernable inotropic effect of cardiac glycosides, and can be diminished partially, but not completely, by α_1-adrenergic antagonists.

Digoxin Dosing Schedules

There usually is no need to treat patients with a loading dose of digoxin except in the setting of certain supraventricular arrhythmias when other drugs useful in treating these arrhythmias are contraindicated or have not been effective. This is due to the narrow therapeutic "window" of cardiac glycosides, which often makes it difficult to judge accurately an effective loading dose of digoxin that will also minimize the risk of toxicity. Often, the patients who would benefit most from the addition of a cardiac glycoside also are those at greatest risk of exhibiting toxic effects of these drugs (see below). Nevertheless, if a loading dose is to be given, assuming a bioavailability of 75% to 80% for most digoxin tablet formulations, 0.9 and 1.8 mg given in divided doses over 24 hr will result in plasma levels that approximate those achieved by either 0.25 or 0.50 mg of digoxin respectively, given daily for about a week in patients with normal renal function. Lean body mass should be used in the calculation of both loading and maintenance digoxin doses. In adults, intravenous loading doses of 0.50 to 0.75 mg/45 kg (i.e., 100 lbs.) of body weight, in divided doses over 24 hr, are unlikely to cause toxicity and can be supplemented as required by the patient's clinical condition. The loading dose of digoxin should be reduced in patients with renal insufficiency due to a reduction in the drug's volume of distribution in this condition.

The calculation of the regular maintenance dose is determined by the drug's clearance rate from the body which, in the case of digoxin, is closely related to the rate of clearance of creatinine. A reasonable approximation of the daily percentage loss of digoxin is given by:

$$\% \text{ Daily loss} = 14 + \frac{C_{Cr} \text{ in ml/min}}{5}$$

The daily maintenance dose, therefore, is calculated by multiplying the percent daily loss and the loading dose given that yielded effective therapeutic drug levels (adjusting for reduced bioavailability if the maintenance dose is to be given orally, but the loading dose was given intravenously). Useful nomograms have been published that provide loading and maintenance doses of digoxin based on estimates of lean body weight and renal function.[63,64] Daily maintenance doses for children with normal renal function are estimated at 20% to 30% of the oral loading dose for premature infants and 25% to 30% of the oral loading dose for full-term infants through children of 10 years of age and older. As in adults, parenteral (intravenous) loading and maintenance dose recommendations are approximately 75% of the oral dosages. These estimates of loading and maintenance doses are average values intended only for use as initial approximations, and in no way diminish the need for further adjustments based on frequent and careful observation of the patient.

Optimal Dosing Strategies: Therapeutic End-Points

The optimal dose of digitalis is not necessarily the largest dose that can be tolerated without the emergence of overt toxicity. The availability of other effective pharmacologic therapies for treating heart failure usually obviates balancing therapy at the edge of toxicity. Electrocardiographic ST-segment and T-wave changes of the "digitalis effect" are, unfortunately, limited indicators of the state of digitalization. It is also inappropriate to depend on the slowing of a sinus tachycardia to gauge the adequacy of digitalis dosage in patients with sinus rhythm with CHF.

In patients with atrial flutter or fibrillation, control of the ventricular response provides a relatively straightforward end-point. Although the failure of atropine or exercise to increase the ventricular response has been used as an additional indicator of "full digitalization" in such patients, achieving this goal may result in unduly slow resting heart rates or evidence of overt toxicity.

In the treatment of CHF, it is helpful to remember that the positive inotropic effect of digitalis is a graded response that results in clinical improvement at doses well below the "maximally tolerated doses." Available data suggest that further inotropic benefit may not occur clinically beyond serum digoxin levels in the 1.0 to 2.0 ng/ml range. Carotid sinus massage can provide useful bedside clues to impending digitalis excess. Rhythm disorders such as increased atrioventricular (AV) block or evidence of increased automaticity may emerge in response to carotid sinus stimulation before they occur spontaneously.

Drug Interactions

Concomitant drug administration may directly alter the pharmacokinetics of digitalis preparations, or indirectly alter their action on the heart by pharmacodynamic interactions (Table 22.1). As noted above, certain drugs such as cholestyramine, neomycin, nonabsorbable anta-

TABLE 22.1. Interactions with digoxin.

Drug	Magnitude of interaction	Proposed mechanism
Antacids Kaolin-pectin Cholestyramine	Minimal decrease in blood levels	Decreased absorption
Amiodarone Quinidine Verapamil Tiapamil Propofenone Indomethacin	50–100% increase in blood levels	Multifactorial, including decreased renal and nonrenal clearance and diminished volume of distribution
Bran Sulfasalazine Bepridil Phenytoin	Moderate decrease in blood levels (20–40%)	Unknown
Erythromycin Tetracyclines	40–100% increase in blood levels in small (<10%) subset of patients	Decreased metabolism of oral digoxin by intestinal bacteria, resulting in effectively higher bioavailability

cids, and Kaopectate may decrease the oral absorption of digoxin.

Quinidine reduces both the renal and nonrenal elimination of digoxin and also decreases its volume of distribution.[65,66] The net result is an increase in serum digoxin concentration that averages twofold in patients given conventional doses of quinidine. Unfortunately, individual responses to quinidine may vary and close surveillance of clinical status and the serum digoxin concentration is warranted. Procainamide and disopyramide do not appear to alter serum digoxin levels, but verapamil does increase the serum digoxin concentration by an average of 35%,[67] again by decreasing digoxin's volume of distribution and clearance rate. Nifedipine and diltiazem have no reproducible effect on digoxin clearance.[68,69] Both short-term and long-term amiodarone administration has been found to increase the steady-state digoxin concentration.[70,71] Other newly introduced drugs will require close surveillance for interactions with cardiac glycosides.

Examples of pharmacodynamic interactions include concomitantly administered diuretic agents that may increase the incidence of digitalis toxicity both by decreasing the glomerular filtration rate due to volume depletion and by inducing a variety of electrolyte disturbances, including hypokalemia, hypomagnesemia, and (for thiazide diuretics) hypercalcemia. Also, concurrent administration of some antiarrhythmic agents may increase the possibility of proarrhythmic events, an outcome that often is unpredictable in an individual patient.

Several anesthetic agents may demonstrate additive or synergistic proarrhythmic effects when coadministered with digitalis, such as cyclopropane and succinylcholine. Experimental studies demonstrate that catecholamine-induced increases in ventricular automaticity add to the arrhythmogenic effects of digitalis. Therefore, it is reasonable to assume that sympathomimetic agents increase the likelihood of enhanced automaticity of atrial and ventricular tissue in patients receiving digitalis.

Therapeutic Indications for Digitalis Glycosides

Congestive Heart Failure

Hemodynamics

Despite the fact that digitalis has been used for the treatment of symptoms of CHF for at least 200 years, it was not until early in this century that a series of clinical observations led to the recognition that these drugs could be useful in patients with a normal sinus rhythm. The underlying mechanism of action, the drug's inotropic effect on cardiac muscle, was not appreciated until improved techniques for quantitating physiologic parameters became available in the 1930s. Wiggers and Stimson showed that digitalis increased the rate of rise in intraventricular pressure during isovolumetric systole when heart rate and aortic pressure were kept constant.[7] The inotropic action of digitalis is manifest in normal, as well as in failing, heart muscle.

The effect of digitalis on the intact heart is demonstrated in the ventricular function curve (illustrated by Fig. 22.2). Cardiac glycosides cause the curve to shift upward and to the left so that, at any given ventricular filling pressure, more stroke work is generated. Experimental studies demonstrate a shift in the force-velocity relation such that the velocity of muscle shortening is greater at any given load imposed.

Administration of cardiac glycosides results in either no change or a slight decline in cardiac output in normal persons. This is not surprising since cardiac output is determined not only by contractile state, but also by preload, afterload, and heart rate. Although digitalis augments the contractile state of the nonfailing myocardium in the intact human heart, adjustments in other determinants of cardiac output usually prevent a detectable increase in cardiac output.[72a]

Aside from reducing the ventricular response rate in patients with supraventricular tachyarrhythmias, discussed in more detail below, other mechanisms may contribute to digitalis' effect in patients with CHF in addition to the drug's inotropic effect. Digitalis glycosides have been shown to induce a natriuresis in some experimental models, presumably by directly inhibiting NaK-ATPase in renal tubular epithelial cells, thus reducing Na^+ reabsorption. Although this effect can be demonstrated easily perfused mammalian kidneys or isolated tubule preparations, it is very difficult to demonstrate any direct natriuretic effect of these drugs in the intact animal at doses relevant to clinical therapeutics, presumably because of the many compensatory mechanisms within the kidney that can be recruited to maintain sodium homeostasis. Digitalis does have important effects on baroreflex sensitivity, as noted above, and thus may indirectly affect central nervous system control of both sympathetic outflow and the release and appearance of vasoactive and antidiuretic hormones such as vasopressin[72b] as well as locally acting autacoids and cytokines such as bioactive eicosanoids and angiotensins.

As various pathological processes (such as ischemia, volume or pressure loading, or intrinsic cardiac muscle defects) decrease contractility, compensatory mechanisms are brought into play. Elevations in end-diastolic pressure and volume result in increased contractile force through the Frank-Starling mechanism. Hypertrophy of contractile elements occurs, and increased sympathetic tone tends to increase contractile state. A number of neurohumoral systems respond to the decrease in cardiac output by reducing salt and water excretion by the kidney and increasing systemic vascular resistance. However, each of these compensatory mechanisms exacts a price: pulmonary or peripheral edema occurs when end-diastolic ventricular pressures rise excessively, and tachycardia may be an undesirable effect of excessive sympathetic tone. An increase in myocardial oxygen consumption tends to occur with all of these compensatory mechanisms. If cardiac disease progresses and contractility continues to diminish, the consequences of one of these compensatory responses will become dominant (e.g., pulmonary edema) and eventually, the compensatory mechanisms will become insufficient to maintain cardiac output.

Under these circumstances, administration of cardiac glycosides will improve the depressed contractile state, decreasing encroachment on compensatory mechanisms and improving cardiac reserve (see Table 22.2). The ventricular function curve is shifted upward, so that for any given ventricular end-diastolic pressure, cardiac output is greater. The clinical consequence is a reduction in end-diastolic pressure (and hence, diminished pulmonary and systemic venous pressure) and increased cardiac output.[9] As would be expected, the favorable hemodynamic effects of digoxin are additive to those of vasodilators, including angiotensin-converting enzyme inhibitors[73] (vide infra) and also to those of β-adrenoceptor agonists.[74]

TABLE 22.2. Action of cardiac glycosides in CHF (for patients in sinus rhythm).

Primary actions of digitalis compounds are to:
— increase myocardial contractility
— increase baroreflex sensitivity

These primary actions lead to:
— increased stroke volume, leading in turn to:
— a decrease in end-systolic ventricular volume
— this may cause a decrease in ventricular filling pressures
— reduced chamber size and improved systolic function favor a decrease in ventricular wall tension, which tends to
— reduce myocardial oxygen consumption and may lower heart rate (both by reflex mechanisms and directly)

Digitalis in Patients with Congestive Heart Failure in Sinus Rhythm: Clinical Trials

Clinical studies appeared in the 1960s and 1970s that questioned Henry Christian's assertion that patients in sinus rhythm with heart failure clearly benefited from digitalis. These studies suggested that many patients receiving chronic maintenance doses of digoxin did not benefit from the drug. In 1969, Starr and Luchi[75] questioned the efficacy of chronic digoxin therapy on the basis of a placebo-controlled, double-blind study of 11 elderly patients in normal sinus rhythm. During the following decade, studies from both Europe and the United States recorded similar conclusions. Nevertheless, these data were not convincing. In several studies, the diagnosis of CHF was not documented. In addition, in a study by Dobbs et al.,[76] a well designed, double-blind, placebo-controlled, single crossover study, nearly one third of the 46 patients studied had atrial fibrillation, and their outcome was not differentiated from those who were in sinus rhythm.

The data from randomized controlled trials of digoxin in patients with heart failure and normal sinus rhythm are still somewhat limited, but a number of studies meeting current criteria for such investigations have been published in the period from 1980 to 1992. Several smaller trials used a crossover design and involved 22 to 44 patients, with observations that included clinical end-points and follow-up for 7 to 12 weeks. Three studies were attempted in the early 1980s. All were well designed and well executed, but yielded conflicting results. The first, a double-blind, placebo-controlled, crossover trial in 30 patients by Fleg et al.,[77] found that over 3 months there was no difference in a variety of clinical end-points, including no change in the incidence of orthopnea, paroxysmal nocturnal dyspnea, or exercise capacity between digoxin and placebo phases, although small differences favoring digoxin were noted in echocardiographic indexes of left ventricular function. All patients were in New York Heart Association (NYHA) class II or III at the start of the study. Similarly, in 22 ambulatory patients studied by Taggart et al.[78] in a randomized, placebo-controlled, crossover trial, although systolic time intervals shortened during the active drug phase, this was not accompanied by any significant symptomatic improvement.

The results of these two controlled trials are in contrast with those reported by Lee et al.,[10] in a double-blind, placebo-controlled crossover trial of 25 outpatients with heart failure in sinus rhythm. Although these investigators evaluated both echocardiographic and inotropic measures of left ventricular dysfunction, the most dramatic differences between active drug and placebo were recorded in a heart failure score that combined a physician's assessment of dyspnea, as well as the presence of rales, the heart rate, signs of right-sided cardiac failure, and the presence of abnormalities on the chest roentgenogram. Fourteen of the 25 patients' conditions improved with digoxin. The clinical finding that best separated responders from nonresponders was the presence of a third heart sound on auscultation of the chest. Indeed, if one excludes from the analysis those patients whose ejection fraction was normal at the beginning of the study, as well as those patients who had subtherapeutic digoxin levels continuously throughout the duration of the protocol (i.e., always <0.5 ng/ml), then 14 of 16 patients were digoxin responders. These investigators concluded that patients with advanced CHF were most likely to benefit from digoxin, although none of the patients recruited for this trial was in NYHA functional class IV at the beginning of the study.

Guyatt[79] reviewed the data from these three reports that had investigated the efficacy of digoxin in patients in sinus rhythm with CHF. Although there was no one factor that, in retrospect, could explain the different outcomes reported, it is possible that the patients in the study that supported digoxin use[10] had somewhat more severe CHF (e.g., the mean ejection fraction was lower in the study by Lee et al.,[10] and only one patient in the study of Fleg et al.[77] had a third heart sound). Also, there was another important distinguishing characteristic of the one positive study: the daily dose of digoxin was about twice as high in the report by Lee et al.[10] (averaging 0.435 mg/day) than in the study by Fleg et al.[77] (averaging 0.240 mg/day), even though the stated target for serum digoxin concentrations was similar in both trials.

The consensus that has emerged from these reports is that a number of patients in sinus rhythm with mild to moderate CHF do not derive evident symptomatic benefit from the addition of a cardiac glycoside. On the other hand, there appears to be a subset of patients who clearly respond to digoxin therapy. The efficacy of digoxin in patients with more disabling heart failure had been described in 1980 by Arnold et al.[9] in a small number of patients who had moderate to severe left ventricular dysfunction, as evidenced by an ejection fraction (while taking no cardiac glycosides) of $30 \pm 14\%$. On withdrawal of digoxin, left ventricular filling pressures increased from 21 to 29 mm Hg, and the mean cardiac index declined from 2.4 to 2.1 L/min. All four of the patients who were in NYHA class IV while in the placebo phase of the trial improved to stage III when given active drug, but no patient in stage II on placebo improved symptomatically when given digoxin.

Changes in quantitative measures of contractile function in these studies were variably correlated with symptoms or exercise performance where such correlations were sought; in general, patients with more severe contractile dysfunction demonstrated the most pronounced beneficial response to digoxin. This was particularly evident in the study of Gheorghiade et al.,[80] in which marked improvements in mean cardiac output ($+48\%$), left ventricular filling pressure (-36%), and ejection fraction ($+8\%$) were observed in the subset of patients who remained in overt failure after diuretic and vasodilator treatment, whereas no significant further improvement was observed in the subset who were relatively well compensated at the completion of the diuretic-vasodilator treatment period.

Three prospective trials have compared digoxin with either placebo or a converting enzyme inhibitor in the therapy of mild to moderate CHF. The study of Alicandri et al.,[81] a double-blind, randomized, crossover trial, compared digoxin with captopril. Importantly, each active drug phase was preceded by a placebo phase. The patients had mild heart failure (13 of 16 were in NYHA class II). The captopril dose was 25 mg, administered 3 times daily, and the average digoxin dose was 0.25 mg/day; all patients continued taking their pretrial doses of diuretics. Both exercise duration and total work performed during a standard exercise protocol were significantly higher in patients taking either active drug than in the placebo phase. The blood pressure was significantly lower in patients receiving captopril, but this did not result in any symptomatic hypotension. The investigators concluded that both captopril and digoxin were effective in mild to moderate CHF in patients in normal sinus rhythm.

A second small but carefully controlled study completed in 20 patients with CHF was carried out by Guyatt et al.[82] This was a randomized, placebo-controlled and double-blinded crossover trial that, among other measures of outcome, included a multifactorial heart failure score similar to that used by Lee et al.[10] These investigators also chose to titrate their patients' digoxin serum levels to between 1.2 and 2.1 ng/ml, yielding an average daily dose—0.39 mg/day—very close to that reported by Lee et al. in the earlier study.[10] Seven of the 20 participants required treatment during the placebo period because of worsening CHF, whereas no patient during the active drug (digoxin) phase had worsening symptoms; these patients were termed "digoxin responders." Interestingly, there was no significant change in echocardiographic measures of left ventricular function, although exercise tolerance, as judged by a 6-min walk test, was marginally better during the digoxin phase. Of the variables that were predictive of a response to digoxin, a third heart sound was heard in six of the seven responders, but in half of the nonresponders. Similarly, six of seven patients in NYHA class III or IV were responders, but several nonresponders fell into this category as well. The most specific criterion was a heart failure score of 2 or greater (no nonresponders fell into this category), although it missed two of seven responders. This study, although well designed and executed, used a dose of digoxin somewhat higher than that typically used in clinical practice. Although none of these patients was deemed to be digoxin toxic, this higher dose would obviously increase the risk of toxicity when prescribed to the large population of patients with advanced CHF. These data highlight the importance of being able to select those patients who are more likely to respond clinically to a cardiac glycoside, since more than half the patients in this study had no evident clinical response despite receiving a relatively high dose of drug.

Three larger multicenter trials have appeared since 1988. Of these, the digoxin-xamoterol study by a German and Austrian study group[83] is the most difficult to assess because the 433 patients enrolled in the trial were not well characterized at entry; indeed, 106 were stated to be NYHA class I and 87% were NYHA class I or II. Xamoterol is a partial, β_1-selective agonist with some β-antagonist activity. Patients were randomized to placebo, xamoterol, or digoxin in a 1:2:1 ratio; diuretics were continued but were limited to no more than 80 mg/day of furosemide or equivalent. Three hundred patients completed the double-blind phase with valid exercise tests at entry and at 3 months, and among these, only xamoterol (and not digoxin) improved exercise duration and work done on a bicycle ergometer. The extent to which this may have reflected the beneficial effects of partial β-adrenergic blockade in patients with underlying ischemic heart disease is unclear, since the etiology of heart failure was unspecified in more than half of the patients in the study. However, both digoxin and xamoterol demonstrated significant improvement in symptoms compared to placebo. Xamoterol subsequently has been reported to cause excess mortality in patients with heart failure.[84,85]

The captopril-digoxin trial[86] compared captopril, digoxin, and placebo during maintenance diuretic therapy in 196 patients, 85% of whom were judged to be in NYHA class I or II. An important feature of the study design tended to favor captopril in this comparison, since patients who did not tolerate withdrawal from digoxin were not randomized, thus excluding the sub-

set of patients who were presumably the most likely to demonstrate benefit from digoxin. Three major conclusions emerged from this trial: First, digoxin but not captopril significantly improved the left ventricular ejection fraction. Second, captopril significantly prolonged exercise time by 14% compared to 6% for placebo; digoxin was intermediate with a 10% improvement, not significantly different at the 0.05 level from either captopril or placebo. Third, digoxin and captopril were both similarly effective in reducing morbidity (by about half) compared to placebo in terms of increased diuretic requirements and hospitalization and emergency room visits.

The milrinone-digoxin trial[87] randomly assigned 230 patients in sinus rhythm with moderately severe heart failure to treatment with digoxin, milrinone, both drugs, or placebo added to baseline diuretic therapy. Milrinone is both a vasodilator and a positively inotropic agent with a mechanism of action quite distinct from that of the cardiac glycosides [i.e., it decreases the rate of intracellular metabolism of cyclic adenosine monophosphate (cAMP) by inhibiting a phosphodiesterase]. After 3 months, digoxin improved the average ejection fraction by +1.7%, compared to −2% in the placebo group ($p < .01$), while exercise tolerance improved by 14% ($p < .05$) compared to placebo. There was a marked benefit of digoxin over placebo or milrinone as judged by the frequency of decompensation within the initial 2 weeks and also at 3 months. Importantly, there was a significantly lower incidence of ventricular ectopy in the digoxin-treated group, compared to those patients randomized to receive milrinone.

Several other prospective trials have examined the effects of adding digoxin to vasodilators in patients with chronic heart failure. A recent study by Gheorghiade and coworkers[88] demonstrated that digoxin administered with captopril produced favorable additive effects in patients with severe CHF in sinus rhythm. A significant increase in mean exercise time was apparent only when captopril was combined with digoxin, but not when either drug was given alone. The improvement in clinical status was reflected by a reduction in plasma norepinephrine levels, which had not declined in response to captopril alone, and by a decrease in plasma aldosterone levels. Studies by Ribner et al.,[89] Cantelli et al.,[90] Sullivan et al.,[91] Pugh et al.,[92] and Fleg et al.,[93] also demonstrated that the addition of digoxin to a regimen of diuretics and vasodilators increased cardiac output and exercise capacity and reduced ventricular filling pressures, while minimizing the symptomatic hypotension often observed with higher doses of vasodilators. In a prospective trial that examined clinical outcomes such as length of hospitalization in patients with congestive heart failure, those patients receiving digoxin with or without an ACE-inhibitor at the time of admission tended to require fewer drugs in the hospital.[94]

Finally, data from two trials, which will be published in early 1993, have been presented in preliminary form and support the conclusion that digoxin improves symptoms in patients with congestive failure. The PROVED (Prospective Randomized Study of Ventricular Failure and Efficacy of Digoxin)[95] and the RADIANCE (Randomized Assessment of Digoxin on Inhibitors of Angiotensin Converting Enzyme)[96] were both multicenter, placebo-controlled trials that examined the effect of withdrawing digoxin therapy in patients with clinically stable congestive heart failure. All patients were in New York Heart Association (NYHA) classes II and III. Patients with severe or poorly controlled symptoms of CHF (i.e., NYHA class IV) were excluded. No patient in the PROVED study received concurrent ACE-inhibitor therapy, while all patients in the RADIANCE trial received a stable dose of an ACE-inhibitor. Although the number of patients studied in either trial was not large, there was a significant increase in worsening heart failure symptoms during the digoxin withdrawal, placebo phase of both studies.

None of these trials had sufficient power to allow any assessment of the effects of digoxin on mortality, a goal that would likely require the randomization of 5000 to 10,000 patients with left ventricular dysfunction and symptoms of heart failure if, for example, a 10% to 15% alteration in mortality were to be discerned.[97] The Digoxin Investigators Group (DIG) trial, organized by the National Heart, Lung and Blood Institute of the NIH, has been designed to answer the question of whether digoxin improves mortality in patients with heart failure, and enrollment of patients is well underway.

Digitalis in Congestive Heart Failure: Therapeutic End-Points

Of major clinical importance is the selection of appropriate end-points or therapeutic goals in the use of digitalis. Although experimental studies have indicated that the positive inotropic action of cardiac glycosides increases progressively until toxic arrhythmias appear, the limited evidence from clinical trials suggests that little, if any, further benefit is to be expected by increasing digoxin doses to levels that result in serum concentrations greater than about 1.5 to 2.0 ng/ml in patients with CHF and normal sinus rhythm. As indicated by several of the studies noted above, particularly those of Lee et al.[10] and Guyatt et al.,[82] patients receiving somewhat higher doses of digoxin (averaging about 0.400 mg/day) appeared to sustain the greatest benefit, although the target serum concentration remained in the range of from 1.5 to 2.0 ng/ml.

In mitral stenosis, cardiac glycosides are clearly beneficial in slowing the ventricular response to atrial fibrillation, thereby allowing more effective diastolic filling of the left ventricle. In the presence of right ventricular failure, benefit also results from increased contractility and reduced end-diastolic pressure. However, in a study of patients with mitral stenosis and normal sinus rhythm, ouabain given acutely produced no significant change in heart rate and had no beneficial effect on cardiac output, oxygen consumption, or severity of pulmonary hypertension at peak exercise.[98]

The therapeutic value of digitalis in the hypertrophied or dilated nonfailing heart remains unclear. With the development of hypertrophy, and before the onset of overt failure, the work capacity of the myocardium at any given left ventricular end-diastolic pressure tends to be decreased. By exerting a positive inotropic action, digitalis augments the capacity for cardiac work and reduces end-diastolic volume and end-diastolic pressure[72,72a] (Table 22.2). If cardiac output is not significantly reduced because of the underlying disease process, then cardiac glycosides will not increase it further, but the same stroke work and cardiac output can be delivered from a lower ventricular filling pressure. Thus, digitalis should provide for a greater inotropic reserve in these patients.

There is no evidence that digitalis provides any benefit in patients whose hearts have well maintained systolic function but, nevertheless, exhibit congestive symptoms due to "diastolic dysfunction" or restrictive or constrictive physiology. Indeed, the rise in intracellular Ca^{2+} that is central to digitalis' inotropic effect could conceivably worsen abnormal myocardial relaxation during diastole. Also, patients with hypertrophic cardiomyopathy, and in particular those with asymmetric septal hypertrophy with subaortic outflow obstruction, may increase their subaortic gradient in response to the addition of a cardiac glycoside. Although slowing of the ventricular rate is an important component of the therapeutic strategy in treating diastolic dysfunction in patients with atrial arrhythmias, drugs other than cardiac glycosides usually are preferable for this purpose.

Digitalis glycosides may improve symptoms of angina pectoris when it coexists with cardiomegaly and CHF. However, an increase in angina frequency may occur unless oxygen consumption is reduced by decreased ventricular size and wall tension as a result of the direct and indirect actions of the cardiac glycosides.

Prophylactic digitalization of patients with diminished cardiac reserve about to undergo a major stress such as surgery remains controversial.[99] In the absence of obvious cardiomegaly or other evidence of overt CHF, most clinicians prefer to withhold digitalis until a specific indication arises. Prophylactic digitalization has been recommended for patients undergoing aortocoronary bypass surgery on the basis of a significant reduction in supraventricular arrhythmias.[100] Evidence of a difference in ultimate outcome between digitalized and nondigitalized patients has not been documented, however, and another study of 140 consecutive patients undergoing myocardial revascularization showed a higher incidence of supraventricular tachyarrhythmias in patients receiving prophylactic digitalis.[101]

Cardiac Glycosides and Arrhythmia Management

A detailed description of the use of digitalis in arrhythmic management is beyond the scope of this chapter. The reader is referred to refs. 41, 102, 103, and 104 for a comprehensive treatment of this topic. Briefly, digitalis is useful in treating four types of supraventricular tachyarrhythmias.

Paroxysmal supraventricular tachycardia usually will respond to digitalis, although most clinicians now would prefer to use adenosine, verapamil, or possibly a β-blocker for this indication. The combination of carotid sinus massage and digitalis often will succeed if administration of the drug alone is insufficient. Of course, in patients already receiving a cardiac glycoside, digitalis toxicity must be excluded as a cause of the arrhythmia.

Atrial fibrillation complicated by a rapid ventricular response probably is the most common indication for digoxin's prescription as an antiarrhythmic. Although conversion to normal sinus rhythm may occur after digitalis, at least one controlled trial failed to document any increased likelihood of conversion in patients with recent onset atrial fibrillation given this class of drugs.[105] Digoxin, given in doses sufficient to maintain the serum level within the therapeutic range of 1.0 to 2.0 ng/ml, usually is insufficient to control the ventricular rate alone, especially during exercise.[106,107] Therefore, addition of a β-blocker,[108] or verapamil[109] may allow better rate control in patients without severely compromised left ventricular function.[110]

Atrial flutter, usually accompanied by some degree of AV block, often can be managed by a digitalis-induced increase in the degree of AV block from 2:1 to 4:1 or greater, with a resulting ventricular response between 60 and 100 beats/min. Digitalis may be of particular benefit in patients with CHF who experience paroxysmal atrial fibrillation or atrial flutter.

Wolff-Parkinson-White tachyarrhythmias may be terminated or prevented by digitalis administration in selected patients with this syndrome. However, digitalis usually is contraindicated in Wolff-Parkinson-White patients with a history of atrial fibrillation or atrial flutter. In a detailed electrophysiologic assessment of cardiac glycosides in Wolff-Parkinson-White syndrome, Sellers et al. concluded that it was difficult to predict a priori which patients would benefit from digitalis, and suggested that formal electrophysiologic testing be done before prescribing a cardiac glycoside to patients with this syndrome.[111]

Digitalis Toxicity

Although the appropriateness of digoxin administration as a first-line agent to patients with mild CHF remains controversial, there is little doubt that cardiac glycosides are efficacious in some patients with moderate to severe left ventricular dysfunction.[112] However, it is this particular group of patients, many of whom are elderly with underlying ischemic heart disease and often diseases of other organ systems as well, who are at greatest risk for digoxin toxicity. The most prevalent and dangerous manifestations of digoxin toxicity are the toxic electrophysiologic effects of the drug.[113,114]

Cardiac Toxicity

Atrium and Atrioventricular Node

The effect of therapeutic serum levels of the cardiac glycosides in patients in sinus rhythm often is a minor slowing of the atrial rate, in part due to a diminution of adrenergic tone as a result of enhanced cardiac performance and to a direct effect of the drug on baroreceptor activity. Toxic levels of cardiac glycosides occasionally lead to sinus arrest or sinus exit block, probably due to a direct effect of the drug on sinoatrial nodal conduction tissue.[45] The atrium is little affected by therapeutic doses of digoxin, but toxic levels can produce profound electrophysiologic effects on atrial tissue, especially an increased automaticity and a decline in conduction velocity. The effects of the cardiac glycosides on the AV node (slowing conduction and prolonging AV nodal refractoriness) constitute a major antiarrhythmic action of these drugs and are largely mediated by enhanced parasympathetic and decreased adrenergic tone. At toxic levels, however, the direct actions of these drugs on AV nodal tissue prolong the AV nodal refractory period, and this effect (along with the heightened parasympathetic tone) may lead to advanced AV junctional conduction block.

The electrocardiographic manifestations of digoxin toxicity are numerous but, unfortunately, too nonspecific in most instances to be diagnostic. Whereas sinoatrial exit block may occur in digitalized patients, its frequency is low and even patients with sick sinus syndrome usually tolerate the drug well. In atrial fibrillation, patients receiving digitalis typically show a gradual slowing of the ventricular response. At higher doses, junctional pacemakers may begin to discharge at increasing frequency, resulting in a nonparoxysmal AV junctional tachycardia. This is recognized clinically as a paradoxical regularization of the ventricular rate despite persistent atrial fibrillation. Common supraventricular arrhythmias associated with digitalis toxicity include AV nodal reentrant tachycardias and tachycardias that originate because of enhanced atrial automaticity. Although paroxysmal atrial tachycardia with block ("PAT with block") often is recognized as being a classic digitalis-toxic arrhythmia, there are no electrocardiographic features that clearly distinguish whether this supraventricular arrhythmia is or is not due to digitalis.[115]

After ventricular arrhythmias, AV junctional block of varying degrees is probably the most common manifestation of digoxin toxicity, occurring in 30% to 40% of patients with recognized digoxin toxicity. First-degree AV block often may be a simple manifestation of digitalis effect, but higher degrees of AV block should suggest the possibility of digoxin toxicity. Second-degree AV block with Wenckenbach periodicity (Mobitz type I) may be present in sinus rhythm or in an automatic atrial tachycardia and should strongly suggest the possibility of digitalis excess. Mobitz type II second-degree AV block due to digitalis intoxication alone is rare. Third-degree AV block is consistent with advanced digitalis toxicity, but should be distinguished electrocardiographically from apparent AV dissociation due to an accelerated idioventricular or AV junctional pacemaker.

Purkinje Fibers and Ventricular Muscle

The nonspecific ST- and T-wave changes in the electrocardiograms of patients treated with cardiac glycosides probably reflect alterations in the time course of ventricular repolarizations that occur with therapeutic doses of these drugs. The toxic manifestations of the cardiac glycosides are primarily due to enhanced automaticity and triggered activity. However, ventricular arrhythmias are uncommon in young patients with healthy hearts even after the suicidal injection of a large quantity of digoxin, suggesting that enhanced Purkinje fiber automaticity (or reentry) in older patients with underlying heart disease may account for digitalis toxicity that in addition may be exacerbated by ischemia, fiber stretch, or other injury.

The degree of diastolic depolarization observed experimentally with digitalis toxicity also increases with the ventricular rate and the drug level, and probably contributes to the development of atrial and ventricular tachyarrhythmias. A second contributing mechanism, described in more detail earlier in this chapter, includes spontaneous depolarizations triggered by previous action potentials, or "delayed afterdepolarizations." These may be related to a transient reduction in membrane potential late in phase 3 or early in phase 4 that reaches threshold and depolarizes the ventricle. The magnitude of afterdepolarizations and the likelihood that they will reach threshold are enhanced by hypokalemia or hypercalcemia, and may be induced experimentally by catecholamines and by digitalis glycosides in isolated Purkinje fibers. Although the presence of triggered activity may conveniently explain the de-

velopment of many digitalis-induced ventricular (and perhaps atrial) arrhythmias, this mechanism has not been proved in humans.[116]

Almost every variety of ventricular arrhythmia has been associated with digitalis toxicity. The most common manifestation is an increase in the frequency of ventricular premature beats of any morphology, with either fixed or varying coupling intervals to preceding supraventricular beats. One uncommon ventricular arrhythmia that is associated with digoxin toxicity is ventricular bigeminy with alternating left- and right-axis deviation. Rarely, bidirectional or "fascicular" ventricular tachycardia may occur, an arrhythmia that is very suggestive of digitalis toxicity. Another characteristic, but less specific, pattern is multiform and repetitive ventricular premature beats occurring during atrial fibrillation. Ventricular fibrillation is rarely the first electrophysiologic manifestation of digitalis toxicity. Although there is no one electrocardiographic abnormality that is pathognomonic of digitalis excess, the combination of enhanced automaticity and impaired conduction (e.g., AV block accompanied by an accelerated junctional pacemaker) is highly suggestive of toxicity even in patients whose serum levels are within the accepted therapeutic range.

Extracardiac Manifestations

Gastrointestinal Symptoms

Anorexia often is an early manifestation of digitalis intoxication; nausea and vomiting result from central nervous system mechanisms and follow as clear consequences of digitalis overdose. Unfortunately, often it is difficult to attribute these symptoms unequivocally to digitalis excess, since they also may be exacerbated by cardiac failure, associated illnesses, or concomitant drug administration.

Neurological Symptoms

Neurological symptoms include headache, fatigue, malaise, neuralgic pain, disorientation, confusion, delirium,[117] and seizures. Visual symptoms are not infrequent and include scotomas, flickering, halos, and changes in color perception.[118] As with gastrointestinal symptoms, it often is difficult to determine whether these neurological symptoms are a direct consequence of digitalis excess, or are due to associated fluid and electrolyte disturbances, other drugs, or associated illness.

Increased Sensitivity to Toxic Manifestations of Digitalis: Risk Factors

Electrolyte and Acid-Base Disturbances

Disturbances of potassium homeostasis clearly influence the action of digitalis (Table 22.3). The ability of potas-

TABLE 22.3. Electrolyte abnormalities and digitalis toxicity.

Increased sensitivity	Decreased sensitivity
Hypokalemia	Hyperkalemia
Hypercalcemia	
Hypomagnesemia	

TABLE 22.4. Acute potassium administration in suspected digitalis toxicity.

Indications
 Serum potassium <4.0 mEq/L:
  VPCs; ventricular tachycardia
  SVT with AV block
 Serum potassium <3.0 mEq/L:
  First-degree AV block
Relative contraindication
 Serum potassium >5.0 mEq/L (particularly if AV block is present)

AV = atrioventricular; SVT = supraventricular tachycardia; VPCs = ventricular premature complexes.

TABLE 22.5. Guidelines for potassium administration concurrent with chronic cardiac glycoside therapy.

Indications
 Serum potassium <3.5 mEq/L
 Combined diuretic/cardiac glycoside therapy
Use particular caution with the following:
 Concurrent administration of:
  Potassium-sparing diuretics
  β-Blockers
  ACE inhibitors
  Nonsteroidal antiinflammatory drugs
 Chronic renal insufficiency (GFR < 20 ml/min)
 Hyporeninism (type IV RTA; diabetes mellitus)

GFR = glomerular filtration rate; RTA = renal tubular acidosis; ACE = angiotensin-converting enzyme.

sium depletion to increase the risk of digoxin toxicity is due to several factors. Cardiac glycoside binding to sarcolemmal NaK-ATPase is favored by phosphorylation of the enzyme in the presence of sodium. The association of potassium with this conformation of the enzyme results in dephosphorylation and a reduction in the likelihood that a cardiac glycoside will bind to and inhibit this enzyme. In addition to this effect of potassium on digitalis binding to NaK-ATPase, potassium also is a necessary cofactor for the normal operation cycle of NaK-ATPase; thus, severe hypokalemia (<2.5 mEq/liter) itself will reduce the turnover rate of the enzyme, exacerbating sodium pump inhibition due to cardiac glycosides. Also, chronic hypokalemia has been shown to reduce the number of NaK-ATPase units in skeletal muscle,[119] but not in myocardium, thus reducing the binding of the drug to peripheral tissues, and thereby decreasing the volume of distribution of the drug. Finally, hypokalemia has primary arrhythmogenic effects separate from a toxic effect of digitalis. The enhanced automaticity of cardiac tissue in response to toxic levels of cardiac glycosides is increased by hypokalemia in experimental animals, whereas the appearance of delayed afterdepolarizations that could reach threshold is antagonized by hyperkalemia.[120] Although most of these electrophysiologic effects of hypokalemia have been observed in vitro or in experimental animal preparations, clinical experience suggests that such electrophysiologic effects also may occur in humans.

In contrast to hypokalemia, when the serum potassium concentration is normal or elevated (>5.5 mEq/liter), any further increase in extracellular potassium necessarily will result in a further depolarization of myocardial conduction tissue. This effect may be most pronounced in AV nodal tissue, where conduction is relatively slow, leading to an exacerbation of digitalis-induced conduction delays. Thus, extracellular potassium exhibits a "bimodal" effect on AV conduction depending on the extracellular concentration; hypokalemia may exacerbate digitalis-induced AV block, whereas hyperkalemia may worsen nodal conduction delays of any etiology (Table 22.4). For this reason, potassium should be administered cautiously to any patient with first- or second-degree AV block, as well as third-degree block, and facilities for external or transvenous cardiac pacing should be readily available. Similarly, sinoatrial conduction defects due to digitalis may be exacerbated by potassium. Potassium is particularly efficacious for treatment of cardiac glycoside–induced ventricular arrhythmias and may be effective even when the serum potassium concentration is in the normal range (Table 22.4).

The routine administration of potassium supplements to digitalized patients with moderate to severe CHF who are also receiving loop diuretics probably is justified. However, several classes of drugs often prescribed in these patients also may raise the serum potassium concentration, including potassium-sparing diuretics, ACE inhibitors, and nonselective β-blockers. Guidelines for administration of potassium salts in proven or suspected digitalis toxicity are given in Tables 22.4 and 22.5.

Disturbances in serum levels of other electrolytes also can influence myocardial sensitivity to digitalis, although less profoundly than K^+ concentration (Table 22.2). Administration of Mg^{2+} salts suppresses digitalis-induced arrhythmias and hypomagnesemia appears to predispose to digitalis toxicity.[41] Magnesium depletion may become clinically important in patients chronically treated with diuretic agents,[41] and in those with gastrointestinal disease, diabetes mellitus, or poor nutritional status. The clinical importance of Mg^{2+} depletion in digitalis therapy remains controversial. Nevertheless, hypomagnesemia appears to be a frequent occurrence in CHF patients, with a reported incidence of 19% in one series.[121] However, there is little correlation between serum Mg^{2+} and tissue Mg^{2+} concentration as measured in peripheral blood mononuclear cells, skeletal muscle, or, presumably, myocardium, leaving unresolved the question of the relevance of blood Mg^{2+} levels to digitalis toxicity.

Elevated serum Ca^{2+} levels increase ventricular automaticity, and this effect is at least additive to, and perhaps synergistic with, the effects of digitalis. Administering intravenous calcium parenterally to digitalized patients may provoke lethal ventricular arrhythmias.

The interactions of cardiac glycosides with acid-base disturbances are complex. Perturbations in potassium homeostasis that follow a shift in blood pH will affect myocardial binding of cardiac glycosides. Similarly, acid-base status will influence the serum levels of ionized Ca^{2+}, with subsequent effects on automaticity. Whether acid-base balance, independent of these changes, alters myocardial sensitivity to digitalis is unclear.

Type and Severity of Underlying Heart Disease

The effects of digitalis on the heart are modified by the type and severity of the underlying heart disease. As mentioned above, this is demonstrated perhaps most dramatically in otherwise healthy persons who ingest massive doses of digitalis. Toxicity in these persons usually is characterized by diminished AV conduction or by sinoatrial exit block, rather than by enhanced automaticity and ventricular ectopic activity, as seen in patients with underlying heart disease.[124] In patients with ischemic heart disease, valvular heart disease, or cardiomyopathies, the effects of digitalis often are superimposed on an electrophysiologically unstable condition with preexisting abnormalities of impulse formation and conduction. The clinical impression that digitalis toxicity is particularly common in patients with cardiac involvement by amyloidosis may be accounted for, at least in part, by digoxin binding by amyloid fibrils.[125]

Changes in myocardial oxygen consumption with cardiac glycosides in patients with underlying ischemic heart disease, and thus the issue of whether these drugs will improve or exacerbate the underlying disease process, always is the net result of two opposing effects of digitalis: a potential reduction in wall tension and an increase in contractility (see Table 22.1). In the failing heart, a decrease in myocardial oxygen consumption usually occurs when some therapeutic intervention leads to a decrease in left ventricular end-diastolic pressure and volume and, consequently, a decline in intramyocardial tension. Thus, angina pectoris may improve after digitalization in patients with heart failure, especially with ventricular dilation, but the frequency of anginal symptoms in other instances may increase, par-

ticularly in those patients who initially were relatively well compensated, and thus did not have very elevated end-diastolic ventricular pressures and dimensions. These considerations are of clinical importance when a decision must be made about whether to use digitalis in patients with ischemic heart disease. Improved myocardial perfusion judged by means of thallium-210 scans was found in one study in response to digoxin in patients with coronary artery disease and left ventricular dysfunction.[124] The combination of propranolol and digoxin also was found to be advantageous in a subgroup of patients with angina pectoris and abnormal ventricular function.[125]

Digitalis in Acute Myocardial Infarction

There is no indication for administration of the drug to patients who have uncomplicated infarction without signs or symptoms of heart failure. There is limited clinical documentation of its value in cardiogenic shock, except in the management of supraventricular arrhythmias. Indeed, rapid digitalization occasionally may be harmful, owing to the transient initial vasoconstrictor properties of the drug. However, in a study of patients with acute myocardial infarction, 89% tolerated a full dose of acetylstrophanthidin, suggesting no significant enhancement of sensitivity to the drug.[126] In patients with acute myocardial infarction treated with intravenous digoxin using a double-blind randomized protocol, no difference in the incidence of rhythm disturbances was found between digoxin-treated and control patients.[127] Thus, there appears to be no convincing evidence for an increased incidence of arrhythmias complicating digitalization in patients with acute infarction when serum levels do not exceed the conventional therapeutic range. Evidence based on retrospective analyses by Moss et al.[128] and Bigger and colleagues[129] suggested that mortality within the first several months after myocardial infarction may be increased in a high-risk subset of patients with CHF and ventricular arrhythmias. However, in other large retrospective data analyses that have demonstrated the increased mortality after myocardial infarction among patients with chronic heart failure or cardiac arrhythmias that one would expect, there was no statistically significant increment in mortality independently attributable to digoxin.[130–133]

Thus, the available data do not indicate that digoxin therapy is unusually hazardous after myocardial infarction, but the existence of an undetected harmful effect can be excluded only with a large randomized study. Given the evidence available in 1993, we would recommend the following: (a) careful consideration of whether any treatment of ventricular systolic dysfunction is needed, (b) consideration of alternatives to digoxin therapy, and (c) restriction of digoxin use to the subgroup of patients with chronic CHF and a dilated left ventricle, or to those for whom digoxin is indicated because of a supraventricular tachyarrhythmia and CHF.

Advanced Age

Advanced age, per se, has been considered by some to be a risk factor in the development of digitalis toxicity. However, advanced age is associated with many factors that increase the likelihood of digitalis intoxication, including more severe heart disease, impairment of pulmonary and neurologic function, an increase in the number of concurrent medications, and a diminished glomerular filtration rate that would predispose to the accumulation of digoxin.

End-Stage Renal Insufficiency

In patients requiring hemodialysis, a transient decrease in serum potassium during the dialysis procedure will increase the likelihood of digitalis-induced arrhythmias. Depending on the magnesium content of the dialysate and the use of magnesium-containing antacids by the patients, there may be significant aberrations of serum magnesium levels in dialyzed patients as well. Clinicians are advised to use the minimum drug dosage that produces the desired clinical effects in this condition because of marked fluctuations in fluid and electrolyte balance. As mentioned previously, the volume of distribution for digoxin in serum is decreased in renal failure,[134] and thus the loading dose, as well as maintenance dose, will need to be adjusted downward accordingly.

Thyroid Disease

In hypothyroid patients, the elimination half-life of digoxin is consistently prolonged while in those with hyperthyroidism, serum digoxin levels tend to be decreased, due at least in part to an increased volume of distribution. This apparent increase in either resistance or sensitivity to digitalis in thyroid disease thus appears to depend on changes in both target organ responsiveness and the pharmacokinetics of digoxin. Changes in autonomic tone also may contribute to the apparent resistance to digitalis effects seen in thyrotoxicosis.

Pulmonary Disease

Ventricular ectopic activity consistent with digitalis toxicity often occurs in patients with respiratory disease. However, respiratory failure and hypoxemia frequently provoke arrhythmias indistinguishable from those associated with digitalis excess. Excessive sensitivity to digitalis in patients with pulmonary disease generally correlates with overt right heart failure, hypercapnia, and hypoxemia. As a result of diuretic therapy, these patients also are subject to derangements in potassium homeostasis and the development of metabolic alkalosis—both of which predispose to digitalis toxicity.

Exogenous catecholamine and sympathomimetic agents commonly used in the therapy of chronic airways disease also may increase the incidence of digitalis-related arrhythmias.

Individual Sensitivity to Digitalis

It is considerably easier to calculate body pools of cardiac glycosides than to judge clinically whether optimal digitalization has been achieved in a specific patient. Changes in absorption or bioavailability may increase the probability of suboptimal digitalization even in patients on a fixed dosage regimen. Such changes should be reflected in the serum glycoside concentration, however, and do not represent a change in sensitivity to the drug's effects. Distinct from the problem of variable bioavailability is an increased sensitivity to lower serum concentrations of cardiac glycosides noted in a small minority of patients who have serum digoxin concentrations within the "therapeutic range."

Treatment of Digitalis Toxicity

The key to successful treatment of digitalis toxicity is early recognition that an arrhythmia is related to digitalis intoxication. The more common manifestations—including occasional ectopic beats, marked first-degree AV block, or atrial fibrillation with a slow ventricular response—require only temporary withdrawal of the drug, electrocardiographic monitoring (if indicated), and subsequent adjustment of the dosage schedule to prevent recurrence. Rhythm disturbances that impair cardiac output require more active intervention. Ventricular tachycardia due to digitalis intoxication demands immediate vigorous treatment. Sinus bradycardia, sinoatrial arrest, and AV block of second or third degree sometimes are treated effectively with atropine. On occasion, electrical pacing will be required. Nonparoxysmal accelerated AV junctional rhythms with rates greater than 90, or those associated with exit block, ought to be followed closely and treated actively if hemodynamic impairment is evident. AV junctional escape rhythms may simply be monitored if the rate is satisfactory.

Potassium

Both hypokalemia and hyperkalemia may exacerbate digitalis-induced arrhythmias. Hyperkalemia can occur as a consequence of massive digitalis overdose, usually after attempted suicide, but rarely complicates the more common forms of digitalis toxicity in patients with underlying heart disease. Administration of potassium salts, as indicated in Table 22.3, is recommended for ectopic ventricular arrhythmias, even when the serum potassium is within the "normal" range. Potassium also may improve digitalis-induced AV block in the presence of hypokalemia, although it should be given cautiously, with continuous electrocardiographic monitoring, and with either an external pacemaker or facilities for transvenous pacing close at hand.

Antiarrhythmics

The drugs most useful for treatment of digitalis-induced ventricular arrhythmias are phenytoin and lidocaine, each of which has relatively little effect on the sinus node or on sinoatrial, AV, or His-Purkinje conduction. Phenytoin may improve sinoatrial or AV conduction under some circumstances. Both quinidine and procainamide can depress AV and sinoatrial conduction, as well as occasionally exhibiting proarrhythmic effects in the presence of digitalis-toxic arrhythmias. Quinidine, as mentioned above, can reduce tissue binding and renal clearance of digoxin. β-Blockers also may exacerbate AV conduction disturbances due to digitalis, although they are likely to be effective in decreasing catecholamine-induced automaticity. β-Blockers also shorten the refractory period of atrial and ventricular muscle and slow conduction velocity, effects that would tend to improve some digitalis-induced arrhythmias. They may, of course, exert a negative inotropic effect that would be undesirable in patients with marginal ventricular function. Due to these considerations, use of an ultra–short-acting β-blocker, such as esmolol, may be appropriate initially if indicated in severely ill patients monitored in an intensive care unit.

Electrical Cardioversion

In the absence of digitalis-induced arrhythmias, DC cardioversion is safe, particularly if lower energy levels are employed.[135,136] Electrical cardioversion is potentially hazardous in severe arrhythmias caused by digitalis toxicity, and should be avoided if other measures are available and effective.

Binding Resins and Hemodialysis

Selected cardiac glycosides such as digitoxin, which undergo some enterohepatic circulation, may be trapped by binding resins during transit through the gut lumen. Both cholestyramine and colestipol can reduce serum digitoxin levels by this means, but the decrease is not of sufficient magnitude or rapidity to affect life-threatening toxicity. Hemodialysis is ineffective both in the case of digitoxin toxicity, because of its extensive binding by serum proteins, and in the treatment of digoxin toxicity, because of the drug's large volume of distribution.

Digoxin-Specific Fab Fragments

The widespread availability of Fab fragments of high-affinity polyclonal digoxin-specific antibodies ("Digi-

TABLE 22.6. Calculation of dose of antidigoxin Fab fragments.

Step 1. Estimate total body digitalis content (in mg)
    A. Acute digitalis poisoning:
        Estimating amount ingested acutely (mg) × 0.80

    B. Known or suspected toxicity during chronic digoxin therapy:

$$\frac{\text{Serum digoxin concentration} \times (5.6) \times (\text{weight in kg})}{1000}$$

Step 2. Calculate dose of Fab fragments, by either:
    A. Mol. mass Fab frag. = 50,000 × 64 × total body dig content

$$\frac{\text{Mol. mass digoxin} = 781}{} = \text{dose of Fab fragments (mg)}$$

OR, if using a standard formulation (e.g., "Digibind")

    B. $\dfrac{\text{Estimated total body load of digoxin (mg)}}{0.6 \text{ (mg/vial)}}$
        = "Digibind" dose numbers of vials

bind," Burroughs Wellcome, Inc.) provides the clinician with a means of rapidly and selectively reversing digoxin toxicity with little risk of adverse effects (Table 22.6). Fab fragments of antidigoxin antibodies also have been used to reverse life-threatening digitoxin toxicity. The use of Fab fragments, as opposed to intact IgG molecules, results in rapid clearance of the antibody fragment-digitalis complex, a property that reduces the immunogenicity of this foreign (i.e., sheep) protein (see Fig. 22.4). Digoxin-specific Fab fragments also have a large volume of distribution and result in rapid binding of digoxin from myocardial and other tissue-binding sites. Several thousand patients including infants and children have now been treated who had life-threatening digoxin or digitoxin toxicity, most successfully with few adverse effects.[137,138,139] A few patients have now been treated on more than one occasion for suicidal digitalis overdose with no evidence of a hypersensitivity reaction to the injection of foreign protein. Of course, administration of antidigoxin Fab also will reverse the inotropic and antiarrhythmic effects of cardiac glycosides, although this usually can be managed in the short run with other medications. Digitalis therapy usually can be reinitiated safely several days after infusion of Fab fragments if indicated.

Neither a prospective trial of the use of Fab fragments of digoxin-specific antibodies nor a recently published observational surveillance study of the postmarketing use of the antibody preparation addressed the issue of whether this drug ought to be given to patients with moderate digoxin toxicity. Also, the efficacy of antidigoxin Fab fragments as a diagnostic agent in patients with suspected digitalis toxicity has not been studied, nor is it likely that a prospective clinical trial of sufficient magnitude to examine this issue will be carried out. This is due, in large part, to the declining incidence

FIGURE 22.4. Antidigoxin antibodies. A schematic illustration of intact antidigoxin IgG, as well as the Fab fragments derived from IgG.

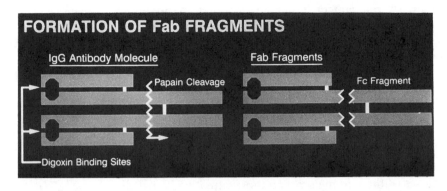

FORMATION OF Fab FRAGMENTS

IgG Antibody Molecule — Papain Cleavage — Fab Fragments — Fc Fragment — Digoxin Binding Sites

of digoxin toxicity over the past 20 years[140] since the introduction of the radioimmunoassay for digoxin, improved understanding of digoxin pharmacokinetics by clinicians, and the development of other classes of drugs effective in the treatment of heart failure.[141] Nevertheless, the good safety record of the antidigoxin Fab preparation, and its specificity and clear efficacy, argue for the use of this agent in the treatment of known cases of advanced and potentially life-threatening digitalis toxicity. The preparation is expensive, however. The average patient in the postmarketing surveillance study received 80 mg of the antibody preparation,[138] which in 1993 would result in a charge to the patient of more than $2000 at many hospitals. On the other hand, if administration of the antibody preparation could safely avoid admission to an intensive care unit, the cost/benefit ratio would appear to favor the use of the antibody preparation. In any case, the widespread availability of a highly selective and safe antidote to cardiac glycoside toxicity provides the clinician with a useful and reassuring safety net, especially in those patients at somewhat higher risk for digitalis toxicity, but for whom the drug is clearly indicated.

Therapeutic Drug Monitoring

The relatively narrow margin between therapeutic and toxic doses of digitalis obviously defines the risk of clinical toxicity. This problem has stimulated the development of methods for determining circulating cardiac glycoside concentrations. Measurements of serum or plasma concentration have clinical utility, but the inappropriate interpretation of these laboratory values can limit their usefulness. A useful relationship exists between serum levels of cardiac glycosides and their pharmacologic effect, and in the case of digoxin, experimental and clinical studies have shown a relatively constant ratio of serum digoxin levels to myocardial or other tissue concentrations, provided adequate equilibration between the vascular and peripheral compartments has taken place after acute dosing. However, as discussed above, the type and severity of existing heart disease and many other variables interact to de-

termine an individual patient's response to a given serum cardiac glycoside concentration. From analysis of a number of studies (reviewed in ref. 142), the mean serum digoxin level in patients judged clinically to be receiving an appropriate dose was determined to be about 1.4 ng/ml (or 1.8 nmol/L), whereas patients with overt signs of toxicity had serum levels usually two- to threefold higher. Despite this difference, which is still a rather narrow toxic/therapeutic ratio, considerable overlap exists in serum levels of digoxin between patients with and without toxicity.

Data from a similar series of studies involving patients receiving digitoxin (also reviewed in ref. 142) found that serum digitoxin levels were about 10-fold higher than analogous serum digoxin concentrations because of the extensive serum protein binding of this hydrophobic cardiac glycoside. As in the case of digoxin, mean values for groups of patients considered to be receiving optimal therapeutic doses are significantly less than mean values for patients with symptoms and signs of toxicity, but there was still considerable overlap between the two groups.

Establishment of an accurate diagnosis of digitalis toxicity often is difficult, since virtually any abnormality of cardiac impulse formation or conduction that might result from digitalis excess can be caused by intrinsic heart disease as well. For these reasons, serum glycoside concentration values should be used along with all other relevant clinical data before one can arrive at appropriate management decisions. Even so, therapeutic cardiac glycoside effects may be difficult to correlate with serum levels in humans. The correlation between serum digoxin concentration and slowing of previously rapid ventricular rates in patients with atrial fibrillation is rough at best. Nevertheless, the ventricular response rate and the absence of other signs or symptoms of digitalis toxicity usually can serve as an appropriate guide to dosage under these circumstances.

Patients with CHF and normal sinus rhythm present a more difficult problem. Although evidence in experimental animal models indicates that the inotropic effect of acutely administered cardiac glycosides will increase with dose, ultimately limited by the emergence of overt rhythm disturbances, this conclusion is not particularly relevant in the clinical context. Available studies suggest that, with regard to digoxin's inotropic response, a point of diminishing returns may be reached at serum digoxin levels approaching 2 ng/ml. Since the risk of digitalis-toxic arrhythmias clearly increases at serum concentrations beyond this range, the risk/benefit ratio appears to be optimal in the range of 1 to 2 ng/ml. Unfortunately, the available data on this important issue are quite limited, particularly regarding patients with advanced heart failure. As noted above, several small but well designed studies have indicated that doses of digoxin higher than those often employed clinically at the present time (i.e., about 0.400 mg/day on average) did result in improved symptoms in patients with sinus rhythm with CHF, whereas serum digoxin levels remained at or below 2 ng/ml.[10,82]

Relatively limited data are available correlating noncardiac symptoms of toxicity with serum digitalis levels. In an extensive study of 1148 patients, there was considerable overlap among serum digoxin levels in patients with and without extracardiac symptoms of toxicity, although the mean digoxin levels of the groups with and without toxicity were significantly different.[143]

Eraker and Sasse[144] developed a Bayesian approach to using serum digoxin levels in clinical decision making. The relation between the estimated risk of toxicity in a patient population at risk of digitalis toxicity and the predictive value of the serum digoxin concentration was established and used to analyze the importance of the degree of elevation of the serum digoxin level in a given patient. This study formalized the approach we have long advocated in the use of serum digoxin concentration data; that is, that the values be used in an overall clinical context in formulating clinical decisions.

Digitalis-Like Factors: Relevance to Therapeutic Drug Monitoring

The universal presence of a binding site for cardiac glycosides on NaK-ATPase has resulted in much speculation as to whether it also serves as a receptor for an endogenous digitalis-like hormone or autacoid.[145,146] Indeed, ouabain itself has been identified by one laboratory as an endogenously synthesized ligand for this binding site,[147] and that elevated serum levels of endogenous ouabain are elevated in patients with congestive heart failure.[148,149] While the evidence for such "endogenous digitalis-like hormones" remains inconclusive and controversial, the presence of compounds in plasma with "digoxin-like immunoreactivity" may complicate determination of digoxin levels in some patients, particularly when radioimmunoassay kits of limited specificity are used. The patient population at greatest risk for exhibiting this artifact are uremic patients, newborn and premature infants, and some pregnant women.[150–162] Techniques for avoiding this problem and guidelines for screening patients who might have falsely positive plasma levels of digoxin due to interfering chemical constituents in plasma have been discussed at length in the clinical chemistry literature.[146,163–172]

References

1. Withering W. An account of the foxglove and some of its medical uses, with practical remarks on dropsy, and other disease. In: Willius FA, Keys TE, eds. *Classics of Cardiology*. New York: Henry Schuman, Dover Publications; 1941;I:231–252.
2. Christian HA. Digitalis effects in chronic cardiac cases with regular rhythm in contrast to auricular fibrillation. *Med Clin North Am*. 1922;5:117–119.
3. Guntert TW, Linde HHA. Chemistry and structure-activity relationships of cardioactive steroids. In: Greeff K, ed. *Handbook of Experimental Pharmacology, Vol. 56/I, Cardiac Glycosides*. Berlin: Springer-Verlag; 1981: 13–24.
4. Marshall PG. Steroids: cardiotonic glycosides and aglycones; toad poisons. In: Coffy S, ed. *Rodd's Chemistry of Carbon Compounds, Vol. 2D, Steroids*. Amsterdam: Elsevier; 1970.
5. Eisner DA, Smith TW. The Na-K pump and its effectors in cardiac muscle. In: Fozzard HA, Haber E, Katz AM, Morgan HE, eds. *The Heart and Cardiovascular System*. New York: Raven Press; 1992.
6. Thomas R, Gray P, Andrews J. Digitalis: its mode of action, receptor, and structure-activity relationships. In: Testa B, ed. *Advances in Drug Research*. New York: Academic Press; 1989:19.
7. Wiggers CJ, Stimson B. Studies on cardiodynamic action of drugs. III. The mechanism of cardiac stimulation by digitalis and g-strophanthin. *J Pharmacol Exp Ther*. 1927;30:251–269.
8. Sonnenblick EH, Williams JF Jr, Glick G, et al. Studies on digitalis. XV. Effects of cardiac glycosides on myocardial force-velocity relations in the nonfailing human heart. *Circulation*. 1966;34:532–539.
9. Arnold SB, Byrd RC, Meister W, et al. Long-term digitalis therapy improves left ventricular function in heart failure. *N Engl J Med*. 1980;303:1443–1448.
10. Lee DC-S, Johnson RA, Bingham JB, et al. Heart failure in outpatients. A randomized trial of digoxin versus placebo. *N Engl J Med*. 1982;306:699–705.
11. Reiter M. The positive inotropic action of cardiac glycosides on cardiac ventricular muscle. In: Greeff K, ed. *Handbook of Experimental Pharmacology, Vol. 56/I, Cardiac Glycosides*. Berlin: Springer-Verlag; 1981:187–210.
12. Koch-Weser J, Blinks JR. Analysis of the relation of the positive inotropic action of cardiac glycosides to the frequency of contraction of heart muscle. *J Pharmacol Exp Ther*. 1962;136:305–317.
13. Marban E, Tsien RW. Enhancement of cardiac calcium current during digitalis inotropy: positive feedback regulation by intracellular calcium? *J Physiol (Lond)*. 1982;329:589–614.

14. Wier WG, Hess P. Excitation-contraction coupling in cardiac Purkinje fibers. Effects of cardiotonic steroids on the intracellular [Ca^{2+}] transient, membrane potential, and contraction. *J Gen Physiol*. 1984;83:395–415.

15. Morgan JP, Blinks JR. Intracellular Ca^{2+} transients in the cat papillary muscle. *Can J Physiol Pharmacol*. 1982;60:524–528.

16. Kim D, Barry WH, Smith TW. Kinetics of ouabain binding and changes in cellular sodium content, ^{42}K$^+$ transport, and contractile state during ouabain exposure in cultured chick heart cells. *J Pharmacol Exp Ther*. 1984;231:326–333.

17. Biedert S, Barry WH, Smith TW. Inotropic effects and changes in sodium and calcium contents associated with inhibition of monovalent cation active transport by ouabain in cultured myocardial cells. *J Gen Physiol*. 1979;74:479–494.

18. Barry WH, Hasin Y, Smith TW. Sodium pump inhibition, enhanced Ca-influx via Na-Ca exchange, and positive inotropic response in cultured heart cells. *Circ Res*. 1985;56:231–241.

19. Eisner DA, Lederer WJ, Vaughan-Jones RD. The quantitative relationship between twitch tension and intracellular sodium activity in sheep cardiac Purkinje fibers. *J Physiol*. 1984;355:251–266.

20. Grupp I, Im WB, Lee CO, et al. Relation of sodium pump inhibition to positive inotropy at low concentrations of ouabain in rat heart muscle. *J Physiol*. 1985;360:149–160.

21. Skou JC. The Na,K-pump. In: Fleischer S, Fleischer B, eds. *Methods in Enzymology*. San Diego, CA: Academic Press; 1988;156:1–28.

22. Pedersen PL, Carafoli E. Ion motive ATPases. *Trends Biol Sci*. 1987;12:146–150, 186–189.

23. Shull GE, Lingrel JB. Molecular cloning of the rat stomach (H$^+$-K$^+$)-ATPase. *J Biol Chem*. 1986;261:16788–16791.

24. Shull GE, Young RM, Greeb G, et al. Amino acid sequences of the alpha and beta subunits of the Na,K-ATPase. In: Skou JC, Norby JG, Maunsbach AB, Esmann M, eds. *The Na$^+$,K$^+$-Pump, Molecular Aspects*. New York: Alan R Liss; 1988;1(Pt. A):3–18.

25. Gunteski-Hamblin AM, Greeb J, Shull GE. A novel Ca^{2+} pump expressed in brain, kidney and stomach is encoded by an alternative transcript of the slow-twitch muscle sarcoplasmic reticulum Ca-ATPase gene. *J Biol Chem*. 1988;263:15032–15040.

26. Jorgensen PL, Collins JH. Localization of tryptic and chymotryptic cleavage sites in alpha-subunit of Na,K-ATPase. In: Skou JC, Norby JG, Maunsbach AB, Esmann M, eds. *The Na$^+$,K$^+$-Pump, Molecular Aspects*. New York: Alan R Liss; 1988; 1(Pt. A):85–92.

27. Lytton J, MacLennan DH. Molecular cloning of cDNAs from human kidney coding for two alternatively spliced products of the cardiac Ca^{2+}-ATPase gene. *J Biol Chem*. 1988;263:15024–15031.

28. MacLennan DH, Brandl CJ, Korczak B, et al. Amino-acid sequence of a Ca^{2+} + Mg^{2+}-dependent ATPase from rabbit muscle sarcoplasmic reticulum, deduced from its complementary DNA sequence. *Nature*. 1985; 316:696–700.

29. Shull GE, Schwartz A, Lingrel JB. Amino-acid sequence of the catalytic subunit of the (Na$^+$ + K$^+$)ATPase deduced from a complementary DNA. *Nature*. 1985; 316:691–695.

30. Shull GE, Lane LK, Lingrel JB. Amino-acid sequence of the beta-subunit of the (Na$^+$ + K$^+$)ATPase deduced from a cDNA. *Nature*. 1986;321:429–431.

31. Young RM, Shull GE, Lingrel JB. Multiple mRNAs from rat kidney and brain encode a single Na$^+$,K$^+$-ATPase beta subunit protein. *J Biol Chem*. 1987;262: 4905–4910.

32. Forbush B, Kaplan J, Hoffman JF. Characterization of a new photoaffinity derivative of ouabain labeling of the large polypeptides and of a proteolipid compound of the NaK-ATPase. *Biochemistry*. 1978;17:3667–3675.

33. Collins JH, Leszyk J. The "gamma subunit" of Na,K-ATPase: a small amphiphilic protein with a unique amino acid sequence. *Biochemistry*. 1987;26:8665–8668.

34. Forbush B. Cardiotonic steroid binding to NaK-ATPase. In: Hoffman JF, Forbush B, eds. *Current Topics in Membrane Transport*. New York: Academic Press; 1983:167–201.

35. Wallick ET, Schwartz A. Interaction of cardiac glycosides with Na$^+$,K$^+$-ATPase. In: Fleischer S, Fleischer B, eds. *Methods in Enzymology*. San Diego, CA: Academic Press; 1988;156:201–213.

36. Langer GA. Relationship between myocardial contractility and the effects of digitalis on ionic exchange. *Fed Proc*. 1977;36:2231–2234.

37. Eisner DA, Lederer WJ. The role of the sodium pump in the effects of potassium-depleted solutions on mammalian cardiac muscle. *J Physiol*. 1979;294:279–301.

38. Lederer WJ, Eisner DA. The effects of sodium pump activity on the slow inward current in sheep cardiac Purkinje fibers. *Proc R Soc Lond*. 1982;B214:249–262.

39. Lee KS, Marban E, Tsien RW. Inactivation of calcium channels in mammalian heart cells. Joint dependence on membrane potential and intracellular calcium. *J Physiol*. 1985;364:395–411.

40. Dagostino M, Lee CO. Neutral carrier Na$^+$- and Ca^{2+}-selective microelectrodes for intracellular application. *Biophys J*. 1982;40:199–207.

41. Smith TW, Braunwald E, Kelly RA. Management of congestive heart failure. In: Braunwald E, ed. *Heart Disease*. 4th ed. Philadelphia: Saunders; 1992.

42. Smith TW, ed. *Digitalis Glycosides*. Orlando: Grune & Stratton; 1986.

43. Watanabe AM. Digitalis and the autonomic nervous system. *J Am Coll Cardiol*. 1985;5(Suppl A):35A–42A.

44. Rosen MR. Cellular electrophysiology of digitalis toxicity. *J Am Coll Cardiol*. 1985;5(Suppl A):22A–34A.

45. Dhingra RC, Amat-Y-Leon F, Wyndham C, et al. The electrophysiological effects of ouabain on sinus node and atrium in man. *J Clin Invest*. 1975;56:555–562.

46. Goodman DJ, Rossen RM, Ingham R, et al. Sinus node function in the denervated human heart: effects of digitalis. *Br Heart J*. 1975;37:612–618.

47. Somberg JC, Smith TW. Localization of the neurally-mediated arrhythmogenic properties of digitalis. *Science*. 1979;204:321–323.

48. Somberg JC, Risler TG, Smith TW. Neural factors in

digitalis toxicity: protective effect of C-1 spinal cord transection. *Am J Physiol*. 1978;235:H531–H536.

49. Rosen MR. Interactions of digitalis with the autonomic nervous system and their relationship to cardiac arrhythmias. In: *Disturbances in Neurogenic Control of the Circulation*. Bethesda, MD: American Physiological Society; 1981:251–263.

50. Packer M, ed. Role of the sympathetic nervous system in heart failure: basic mechanisms and clinical directions. *Circulation*. 1990;82(Suppl I):I-1–I-13.

51. Ferguson DW, Berg WJ, Sanders JS, et al. Sympathoinhibitory responses to digitalis glycosides in heart failure patients: direct evidence from sympathetic neural recordings. *Circulation*. 1989;80:65–77.

52. Lindenbaum J, Rund DG, Butler VP Jr. Inactivation of digoxin by the gut flora: reversal by antibiotic therapy. *N Engl J Med*. 1981;305:789–794.

53. Halkin H, Sheiner LB, Peck CC, et al. Determinants of the renal clearance of digoxin. *Clin Pharmacol Ther*. 1975;17:385–394.

54. Cogan JJ, Humphreys MH, Carlson CJ, et al. Acute vasodilator therapy increases renal clearance of digoxin in pateints with congestive heart failure. *Circulation*. 1981;64:973–976.

55. Linday LA, Drayer DE, Khan MAA, et al. Pubertal changes in net renal tubular secretion of digoxin. *Clin Pharmacol Ther*. 1984;35:438–446.

56. Lindenbaum J, Mellow MH, Blackstone MO, et al. Variation in biologic availability of digoxin from four preparations. *N Engl J Med*. 1971;285:1344–1347.

57. Johnson BF, Lindenbaum J, Budnitz E, et al. Variability of steady-state digoxin kinetics during administration of tablets or capsules. *Clin Pharmacol Ther*. 1986;39:306–312.

58. Leahey EB Jr, Reiffel JA, Drusin RE, et al. Interaction between quinidine and digoxin. *JAMA*. 1978;240:533–534.

59. Selden R, Margolies MN, Smith TW. Renal and gastrointestinal excretion of ouabain in dog and man. *J Pharmacol Exp Ther*. 1974;188:615–623.

60. Cardiac Glycosides. Part II: pharmacokinetics and clinical pharmacology. In: Greeff K, ed. *Handbook of Experimental Pharmacology*. Berlin: Springer-Verlag; 1981; 56.

61. Blatt CM, Marsh JD, Smith TW. Extracardiac effects of digitalis. In: Smith TW, ed. *Digitalis Glycosides*. Orlando: Grune & Stratton; 1985:209–215.

62. Sagar KB, Hanson EC, Powell WJ. Neurogenic coronary vasoconstrictor effects of digitalis during acute global ischemia in dogs. *J Clin Invest*. 1977;60:1248–1257.

63. Jelliffe RW, Brooker G. A nomogram for digoxin therapy. *Am J Med*. 1974;57:63–68.

64. Hougen TJ. Use of digoxin in the young. In: Smith TW, ed. *Digitalis Glycosides*. Orlando: Grune & Stratton; 1985:169–208.

65. Antman EM, Smith TW. Drug interactions with digitalis glycosides. In: Smith TW, ed. *Digitalis Glycosides*. Orlando: Grune & Stratton; 1985:65–82.

66. Marcus FI. Pharmacokinetic interactions between digoxin and other drugs. *J Am Coll Cardiol*. 1985;5:82A–90A.

67. Kuhlmann J, Marcin S. Effects of verapamil on pharmacokinetics and pharmacodynamics of digitoxin in patients. *Am Heart J*. 1985;110:1245–1250.

68. Elkayam U, Parikh K, Torkan B, et al. Effect of diltiazem on renal clearance and serum concentration of digoxin in patients with cardiac disease. *Am J Cardiol*. 1985;55:1393–1395.

69. Lessem J, Bellinetto A. Interaction between digoxin and calcium antagonists. *Am J Cardiol*. 1982;49:1025.

70. Moysey JO, Jaggarao NSV, Grundy EN, et al. Amiodarone increases plasma digoxin concentrations. *Br Med J*. 1981;282:272.

71. Nademanee K, Kannan R, Hendrickson J, et al. Amiodarone-digoxin interaction during treatment of resistant cardiac arrhythmias. *Am J Cardiol*. 1982;49:1026.

72a. Braunwald E. Effects of digitalis on the normal and the failing heart. *J Am Coll Cardiol*. 1985;5:51A–59A.

72b. Gheorghiade M, Ferguson D. Digoxin. A neurohormonal modulation in heart failure. *Circulation*. 1991; 84:2181–2186.

73. Cantelli I, Vitolo A, Lombardi G, et al. Combined hemodynamic effects of digoxin and captopril in patients with congestive heart failure. *Curr Ther Res*. 1984;36: 323–331.

74. Bostrom PA, Andersson J, Johansson BW, et al. Hemodynamic effects of prenalterol and cardiac glycosides in patients with recent myocardial infarction. *Eur J Clin Invest*. 1984;14:175–180.

75. Starr I, Luchi RJ. Blind study on the action of digitoxin on elderly women. *Am Heart J*. 1969;78:740–751.

76. Dobbs SN, Kenyon WI, Dobbs RJ. Maintenance digoxin after an episode of heart failure. Placebo controlled trial in outpatients. *Br Med J*. 1977;1:749–752.

77. Fleg L, Gottlieb SH, Lakatta EG. Is digoxin really important in compensated heart failure? *Am J Med*. 1982;73:244–250.

78. Taggart AJ, Johnston GD, McDevitt DG. Digoxin withdrawal after cardiac failure in patients with sinus rhythm. *J Cardiovasc Pharmacol*. 1983;5:229–234.

79. Guyatt GH. The treatment of heart failure. A methodological review of the literature. *Drugs*. 1986;32:538–568.

80. Gheorghiade M, St. Clair J, St. Clair C, et al. Hemodynamic effects of intravenous digoxin in patients with severe heart failure initially treated with diuretics and vasodilators. *J Am Coll Cardiol*. 1987;9:849–857.

81. Alicandri C, Fariello R, Boni E, et al. Captopril versus digoxin in mild-moderate chronic heart failure: a crossover study. *J Cardiovasc Pharmacol*. 1987;9:S61–S67.

82. Guyatt GH, Sullivan MJJ, Fallen EL, et al. A controlled trial of digoxin in congestive heart failure. *Am J Cardiol*. 1988;61:371–375.

83. German and Austrian Xamoterol Study Group. Double-blind placebo-controlled comparison of digoxin and xamoterol in chronic heart failure. *Lancet*. 1988;1:489–493.

84. Xamoterol in Severe Heart Failure Study Group. Xamoterol in severe heart failure. *Lancet*. 1990;336:1–6.

85. Anon. Editorial. New evidence on xamoterol. *Lancet*. 1990;336:24.

86. Captopril-Digoxin Multicenter Research Group. Comparative effects of therapy with captopril and digoxin in

patients with mild to moderate heart failure. *JAMA.* 1988;259:539–544.

87. DiBianco R, Shabetai R, Kostuk W, et al. A comparison of oral milrinone, digoxin, and their combination in the treatment of patients with chronic heart failure. *N Engl J Med.* 1989;320:677–683.

88. Gheorghiade M, Hall V, Lakier JB, et al. Comparative hemodynamic and neurohormonal effects of intravenous captopril and digoxin and their combinations in patients with severe heart failure. *J Am Coll Cardiol.* 1989; 13:134–142.

89. Ribner HS, Zucker MJ, Stasior C, et al. Vasodilators as first-line therapy for congestive heart failure: a comparative hemodynamic study of hydralazine, digoxin and their combination. *Am Heart J.* 1987;114:91–96.

90. Cantelli I, Vitolo A, Lombardi G, et al. Combined hemodynamic effects of digoxin and captopril in patients with congestive heart failure. *Curr Ther Res.* 1984; 36:323–331.

91. Sullivan M, Atwood JE, Myers J, et al. Increased exercise capacity after digoxin administration in patients with heart failure. *J Am Coll Cardiol.* 1989;13:1138–1142.

92. Pugh SE, White NJ, Aronson JK, et al. Clinical, hemodynamic, and pharmacological effects of withdrawal and reintroduction of digoxin in patients with heart failure in sinus rhythm after long-term treatment. *Br Heart J.* 1989;61:529–539.

93. Fleg JL, Rothfeld B, Gottlieb SH. Effect of maintenance digoxin Therapy on aerobic performance and exercise left ventricular function in mild to moderate heart failure due to coronary artery disease: a randomized, placebo-controlled crossover trial. *J Am Coll Cardiol.* 1991;17: 743–751.

94. Mohan P, Hii JTY, Wuttke RD, et al. Acute heart failure: determinants of outcome. *Int J Cardiol.* 1991; 32:365–376.

95. Young JB, Uretsky BF, Shahidi E, et al. Multicenter, double-blind, placebo-controlled randomized withdrawal trial of the efficacy and safety of digoxin in patients with mild to moderate chronic heart failure not treated with converting enzyme inhibitors. *J Am Coll Cardiol.* 1992; 19:259A.

96. Packer M, Gheorghiade M, Young JB, et al. Randomized, double-blind, placebo-controlled, withdrawal study of digoxin in patients with chronic heart failure treated with converting-enzyme inhibitors. *J Am Coll Cardiol.* 1992;19:260A.

97. Kelly RA, Smith TW. Digoxin in heart failure: Implications of recent trials. *J Am Coll Cardiol.* 1993; (in Press).

98. Beiser GD, Epstein SE, Stampfer M, et al. Studies on digitalis. XVII. Effects of ouabain on the hemodynamic response to exercise in patients with mitral stenosis in normal sinus rhythm. *N Engl J Med.* 1968;278:131–137.

99. Antman E. Medical management of the patient undergoing cardiac surgery. In: Braunwald E, ed. *Heart Disease.* 4th ed. Philadelphia: Saunders; 1992.

100. Johnson LW, Dickstein RA, Freuhan CT, et al. Prophylactic digitalization for coronary artery bypass surgery. *Circulation.* 1976;53:819–822.

101. Tyras DH, Stothert JC Jr, Kaiser GC, et al. Supraventricular tachyarrhythmias after myocardial revascu-

larization: a randomized trial of prophylactic digitalization. *J Thorac Cardiovasc Surg.* 1979;77:310–314.

102. Antman EM, Friedman PL. Use of digitalis glycosides in the management of cardiac arrhythmias. In: Smith TW, ed. *Digitalis Glycosides.* Orlando: Grune & Stratton; 1985:127–151.

103. Surawicz B. Supraventricular arrhythmias. In: Messerli FH, ed. *Cardiovascular Drug Therapy.* Philadelphia: Saunders; 1990:1150–1166.

104. Bigger JT Jr, Hoffman BF. Antiarrhythmic drugs. In: Gilman AG, Rall TW, Nies AS, Taylor P, eds. *The Pharmacological Basis of Therapeutics.* 8th ed. New York: Pergamon Press; 1990:840–873.

105. Falk RH, Knowlton AA, Bernard SA, et al. Digoxin for converting recent-onset atrial fibrillation to sinus rhythm: a randomized, double-blinded trial. *Ann Intern Med.* 1987;106:503–506.

106. Simpson RJ, Foster JR, Woelfel AK, et al. Management of atrial fibrillation and flutter—a reappraisal of digitalis therapy. *Postgrad Med.* 1986;79:241–253.

107. Beasley R, Smith DA, McHaffie DJ. Exercise heart rates at different serum digoxin concentrations in patients with atrial fibrillation. *Br Med J.* 1985;290:9–11.

108. Zoble RG, Brewington J, Olukotun AY, et al. Use of beta-blockers as antiarrhythmic agents. Comparative effects of nadolol-digoxin combination therapy and digoxin monotherapy for chronic atrial fibrillation. *Am J Cardiol.* 1987;60:39D–45D.

109. Ahuja RC, Sinha N, Saran RK, et al. Digoxin or verapamil or metoprolol for heart rate control in patients with mitral stenosis—a randomized crossover study. *Int J Cardiol.* 1989;25:325–331.

110. Rawles JM, Metcalfe MJ, Jennings K. Time of occurrence, duration, and ventricular rate of paroxysmal atrial fibrillation: the effect of digoxin. *Br Heart J.* 1990;63:225–227.

111. Sellers TD, Bashore TM, Gallagher JJ. Digitalis in pre-excitation syndrome—analysis during atrial fibrillation. *Circulation.* 1977;56:260–267.

112. Kelly RA. Cardiac glycosides and congestive heart failure. *Am J Cardiol.* 1990;65:10E–16E.

113. Smith TW, Antman EM, Friedman PL, et al. Digitalis glycosides: mechanisms and manifestations of toxicity. Part I. *Prog Cardiovasc Dis.* 1984;26:414–458.

114. Hoffman BF, Bigger JT Jr. Digitalis and allied cardiac glycosides. In: Gilman AG, Rall TW, Nies AS, Taylor P, eds. *The Pharmacological Basis of Therapeutics.* 8th ed. New York: Pergamon Press; 1990:814–839.

115. Lown B, Wyatt NF, Levine HD. Paroxysmal atrial tachycardia with block. *Circulation.* 1960;21:129–143.

116. Fisch C, Knoebel SB. Accelerated junctional escape: a clinical manifestation of "triggered" automaticity. In: Zipes DP, Jalife J, eds. *Cardiac Electrophysiology and Arrhythmias.* New York: Grune & Stratton; 1985:467.

117. Eisendrath SJ, Sweeney MA. Toxic neuropsychiatric effects of digoxin at therapeutic serum concentrations. *Am J Psychiatry.* 1987;144:506–507.

118. Blatt CM, Marsh JD, Smith TW. The role of neural factors in digitalis intoxication. In: Smith TW, ed. *Digitalis Glycosides.* Orlando: Grune & Stratton; 1985:277–294.

119. Klausen T, Kjeldsen K, Norgaard A. Effects of denervation on sodium, potassium and [H³]ouabain binding in

muscles of normal and potassium depleted rats. *J Physiol.* 1983;345:123–134.

120. Ferrier GR, Saunders JH, Mendez C. A cellular mechanism for the generation of ventricular arrhythmias by acetylstrophanthidin. *Circ Res.* 1973;32:600–609.

121. Whang R, Qei TO, Watanabe A. Frequency of hypomagnesemia in hospitalized patients receiving digitalis. *Arch Intern Med.* 1985;145:655–656.

122. Smith TW, Butler VP Jr, Haber E, et al. Treatment of life-threatening digitalis intoxication with digoxin-specific Fab fragments: experience in 26 cases. *N Engl J Med.* 1982;307:1357–1362.

123. Rubinow A, Skinner M, Cohen AS. Digoxin sensitivity in amyloid cardiomyopathy. *Circulation.* 1981;63:1285–1288.

124. Vogel R, Kirch D, LeFree M, et al. Effects of digitalis on resting and isometric exercise myocardial perfusion in patients with coronary artery disease and left ventricular dysfunction. *Circulation.* 1977;56:355–359.

125. Crawford MH, LeWinter MM, O'Rourke RA, et al. Combined propranolol and digoxin therapy in angina pectoris. *Ann Intern Med.* 1975;83:449–455.

126. Lown B, Klein MD, Barr I, et al. Sensitivity to digitalis drugs in acute myocardial infarction. *Am J Cardiol.* 1972;30:388–395.

127. Reicansky I, Conradson TB, Holmberg S, et al. The effect of intravenous digoxin on the occurrence of ventricular tachyarrhythmias in acute myocardial infarction in man. *Am Heart J.* 1976;91:705–711.

128. Moss AJ, Davis HT, Conard DL, et al. Digitalis-associated cardiac mortality after myocardial infarction. *Circulation.* 1981;64:1150–1156.

129. Bigger JT, Fleiss JL, Rolnitzky LM, et al. Effect of digitalis treatment on survival after acute myocardial infarction. *Am J Cardiol.* 1985;55:623–630.

130. Ryan TJ, Bailey KR, McCabe CH, et al. The effects of digitalis on survival in high-risk patients with coronary artery disease. *Circulation.* 1983;67:735–742.

131. Madsen EB, Gilpin E, Henning H, et al. Prognostic importance of digitalis after acute myocardial infarction. *J Am Coll Cardiol.* 1984;3:681–689.

132. Byington R, Goldstein S, and the BHAT Research Group. Association of digitalis therapy with mortality in survivors of acute myocardial infarction: observations in the beta-blocker heart attack trial. *J Am Coll Cardiol.* 1985;6:976–982.

133. Muller JE, Turi ZG, Stone PH, et al. Digoxin therapy and mortality after myocardial infarction: experience in the MILIS study. *N Engl J Med.* 1986;314:265–271.

134. Szefler SJ, Jusko WJ. Decreased volume of distribution of digoxin in a patient with renal failure. *Res Commun Chem Pathol Pharmacol.* 1973;6:1095–1098.

135. Friedman PL, Antman EM, Smith TW. Clinical management of digitalis toxicity. In: Smith TW, ed. *Digitalis Glycosides.* Orlando: Grune & Stratton; 1985:295–309.

136. Ditchey RV, Karliner JS. Safety of electrical cardioversion in patients without digitalis toxicity. *Ann Intern Med.* 1981;95:676–679.

137. Antman EM, Wenger TL, Butler VP Jr, et al. Treatment of 150 cases of life-threatening digitalis intoxication with digoxin-specific Fab antibody fragments: final re-

port of a multicenter study. *Circulation.* 1990;81:1744–1752.

138. Hickey AR, Wenger TL, Carpenter VP, et al. Digoxin immune Fab therapy in the management of digitalis intoxication: safety and efficacy results of an observational surveillance study. *J Am Coll Cardiol.* 1991;17:590–598.

139. Woolf AD, Wenger T, Smith TW, Lovejoy FH. The use of digoxin-specific Fab fragments for severe digitalis intoxication in children. *N Engl J Med.* 1992;326:1739–1744.

140. Mahdyoon H, Battilana G, Rosman H, et al. The evolving pattern of digoxin intoxication: observations at a large urban hospital from 1980 to 1988. *Am Heart J.* 1990;120:1189–1194.

141. Kelly RA, Smith TW. Recognition and management of digitalis toxicity. *Am J Cardiol.* 1992;69:1086–1196.

142. Smith TW. Serum and plasma cardiac glycoside concentrations: clinical use and misuse. In: Smith TW, ed. *Digitalis Glycosides.* Orlando: Grune & Stratton; 1985:153–167.

143. Doering W, Konig E, Sturm W. Digitalis intoxication: specificity and significance of cardiac and extracardiac symptoms. I. Patients with digitalis-induced arrhythmias. *Z Kardiol.* 1977;66:121–128.

144. Eraker SA, Sasse L. The serum digoxin test and digoxin toxicity: a Bayesian approach to decision making. *Circulation.* 1981;64:409–420.

145. Kelly RA, Smith TW. The search for the endogenous digitalis: an alternative hypothesis. *Am J Physiol.* 1989; 25:C737–C950.

146. Goto A, Yamada K, Yagi N, et al. Physiology and pharmacology of endogenous digitalis-like factors. *Pharmacol Rev.* 1992;44:377–399.

147. Hamlyn JM, Blaustein MP, Bova S, et al. Identification and characterization of a ouabain-like compound from human plasma. *Proc Natl Acad Sci USA.* 1991;88:6259–6263.

148. Gottlieb SS, Rogowski AC, Weinberg M, et al. Elevated concentrations of endogenous ouabain in patients with congestive heart failure. *Circulation.* 1992;86:420–425.

149. Kelly RA, Smith TW. Is ouabain the endogenous digitalis? *Circulation.* 1992;86:694–697.

150. Graves SW, Brown B, Valdes R. An endogenous digoxin-like substance in patients with renal impairment. *Ann Intern Med.* 1983;99:604–608.

151. Kramer HJ, Heppe M, Weiler E, et al. Further characterization of the endogenous natriuretic and digoxin-like immunoreacting activities in human urine: effects of changes in sodium intake. *Renal Physiol.* 1985;8:80–89.

152. Graves SW, Williams GH. An endogenous ouabain-like factor associated with hypertensive pregnant women. *J Clin Endocrinol Metab.* 1984;59:1070–1074.

153. Seccombe DW, Pudek MR, Whitfield et al. Perinatal changes in a digoxin-like immunoreactive substance. *Pediatr Res.* 1984;18:1097–1099.

154. Graves SW, Valdes R, Brown BA, et al. Endogenous digoxin-immunoreactive substance in human pregnancies. *J Clin Endocrinol Metab.* 1984;58:748–751.

155. Vinge E, Helgessen-Rosendal S, Backstrom T. Progesterone, some progesterone derivatives and urinary digoxin-like substances from pregnant women in radio-

immuno- and ^{85}Rb uptake assays of digoxin. *Pharmacol Toxicol*. 1988;63:277–280.

156. Koren G, Farine D, Grundmann H, et al. Endogenous digoxin-like substance(s) associated with uneventful and high-risk pregnancies. *Dev Pharmacol Ther*. 1988;11:82–87.

157. Shrivastav P, Gill DS, D'Souza V, et al. Secretion of atrial natriuretic peptide and digoxin-like immunoreactive substance during pregnancy. *Clin Chem*. 1988;34:977–980.

158. Longerich L, Brent DA, Johnson RL, et al. Identification of progesterone and cortisol as immunoreactive plasma digitalis-like factors in pregnancy. *Res Commun Chem Pathol Pharmacol*. 1988;59:383–393.

159. Goodlin RC. Fetal endoxin and pregnancy complication. *Am J Obstet Gynecol*. 1988;158(Pt 1):529–530.

160. Phelps SJ, Cochran EB, Gonzalez-Ruiz A, et al. The influence of gestational age and preeclampsia on the presence and magnitude of serum endogenous digoxin-like immunoreactive substance(s). *Am J Obstet Gynecol*. 1988;158:34–39.

161. Weiner CP, Robillard JE. Atrial natriuretic factor, digoxin-like immunoreactive substance, norepinephrine, epinephrine, and plasma renin activity in human fetuses and their alteration by fetal disease. *Am J Obstet Gynecol*. 1988;159:1353–1360.

162. Gonzalez AR, Phelps SJ, Cochran EB, et al. Digoxin-like immunoreactive substance in pregnancy. *Am J Obstet Gynecol*. 1987;157:660–664.

163. Rauch AL, Buckalew VM Jr. Characterization of a competitive and reversible ligand to E_2 conformation of Na,K-ATPase molecule. *Biochem Biophys Res Commun*. 1988;150:648–654.

164. Kelly RA. Excretion of artifactual endogenous digitalis-like factors. *Am J Physiol*. 1986;251:H205–H209.

165. Diamandis EP, Papanastasiou-Diamandis A, Soldin SJ. Digoxin immunoreactivity in cord and maternal serum and placental extracts: partial characterization of immunoreactive substances by high-performance liquid chromatography and inhibition of Na$^+$,K$^+$-ATPase. *Clin Biochem*. 1985;18:48–55.

166. Soldin SJ. Digoxin—issues and controversies. *Clin Chem*. 1986;32:5–12.

167. Stone JA, Soldin SJ. Improved liquid chromatographic/immunoassay of digoxin in serum. *Clin Chem*. 1988;34:2547–2551.

168. Longerich L, Vasdev S, Johnson E, et al. Disposable-column radioimmunoassay for serum digoxin with less interference from metabolites and endogenous digitalis-like factors. *Clin Chem*. 1988;34:2211–2216.

169. Vinge E, Ekman R. Evaluation of crossreactivity of urinary digoxin-like substance in different radioimmunoassay. *Ther Drug Monit*. 1988;10:316–320.

170. Lau BW, Valdes R Jr. Criteria for identifying endogenous compounds as digoxin-like immunoreactive factors in humans. *Clin Chim Acta*. 1988;175:67–77.

171. Dasgupta A, Malik S, Ahmad S, et al. Mass spectrometry studies of a novel digoxin-like substance (DLIS-2) isolated from human plasma ultrafiltrate. *Biochem Biophys Res Commun*. 1988;152:1435–1440.

172. Yannakou L, Diamandis EP, Souvatzoglou A. Effect of incubation time and temperature on the interference of digoxin-like immunoreactive substances in digoxin immunoassays. *Ther Drug Monit*. 1987;9:461–463.

23
Angiotensin-Converting Enzyme Inhibitor Therapy for Congestive Heart Failure: Rationale, Results, and Current Recommendations

Barry M. Massie and Thomas Amidon

The treatment of congestive heart failure (CHF) has undergone significant changes in recent years.[1] This has occurred as a result of both our improved understanding of the hemodynamic and neurohormonal alterations that underlie the pathophysiology of CHF and the availability of new therapeutic agents. In particular, heart failure is now recognized as a complex syndrome, involving the central and peripheral circulations, neurohormonal responses, and alterations of renal and skeletal muscle function, rather than a simple hemodynamic derangement.[2] In this chapter we review the neuroendocrine changes that characterize CHF and focus on the use of angiotensin-converting enzyme (ACE) inhibition in its treatment. This discussion is limited to CHF resulting from left ventricular systolic dysfunction, characterized by reduced indices of contractility and left ventricular dilatation. CHF resulting from left ventricular diastolic dysfunction, although now more commonly recognized than previously, is beyond the scope of this chapter.

Background and Rationale for the Use of ACE Inhibitors in CHF

Hemodynamic Alterations in Congestive Heart Failure

The primary abnormality in most patients with CHF is impaired left ventricular systolic function.[3] This usually is caused by processes that cause global or regional left ventricular damage, or less frequently, depressed function of viable myocardium. In response, a number of compensatory mechanisms are called into play, which serve primarily to maintain arterial pressure and cardiac output.[2] These include an increase in heart rate, left ventricular preload, and left ventricular afterload. Heart rate rises both in response to increased sympathetic nervous system activity and diminished parasym-

pathetic tone. The rise in heart rate serves to maintain cardiac output when stroke volume is diminished. Left ventricular preload rises as a result of the increased residual left ventricular volume at end-systole, an increase in intravascular volume, and a further increase in central blood volume due to neurohormonally mediated venoconstriction. The increase in preload, or left ventricular volume, allows the Frank-Starling mechanism to operate, providing enhanced contractility. Impedance to left ventricular ejection also rises because of systemic vasoconstriction and diminished vascular compliance. These latter changes are mediated by increased sympathetic and renin-angiotensin system activity, as well as other circulating vasoconstricting substances and intrinsic changes in the blood vessels.

Although these changes preserve arterial blood pressure and cardiac output, they do so at the cost of elevated ventricular filling pressures, increased systolic wall stress, and excessive energy requirements. As illustrated in Figure 23.1, these compensatory mechanisms themselves may become deleterious, causing further depression in myocardial function and progression of the heart failure syndrome. In addition, the elevated left atrial and systemic venous pressures are responsible for many of the congestive symptoms in patients with heart failure, and the changes in the peripheral circulation may play a role in the accompanying renal dysfunction and impaired exercise tolerance.

Neurohormonal Alterations in Congestive Heart Failure

As indicated in the previous section, the hemodynamic alterations in CHF both activate and reflect alterations in neurohormonal activity. The hormonal changes play both a compensatory and deleterious role in the syndrome of CHF.[4–7] Recent studies indicate that the first response in many patients with CHF is increased

FIGURE 23.1. This figure illustrates how many of the compensatory mechanisms that come into play after the onset of left ventricular dysfunction can themselves lead to further left ventricular dysfunction.

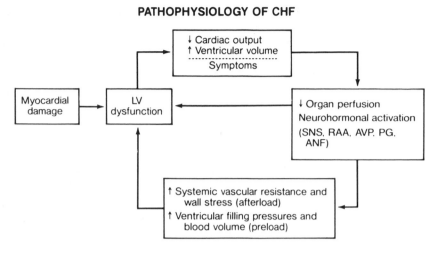

PATHOPHYSIOLOGY OF CHF

systemic concentrations of atrial natriuretic peptides (ANPs), which can both facilitate natriuresis and diuresis and produce systemic vasodilation.[8,9] Elevated levels of this hormone are detectable in people with left ventricular dysfunction before the onset of symptoms. Plasma norepinephrine levels rise later and primarily in patients with symptomatic CHF[8,9]; high levels are associated with a poor prognosis.[10] Increased activity of the circulating renin-angiotensin-aldosterone system appears to be a relatively late phenomenon, as is increased activity of the arginine vasopressin system.[8,9] The presence of a functional renin-angiotensin system in many tissues is now well documented.[11–13] It is uncertain what role these tissue systems play and when they become activated, but favorable responses to ACE inhibitors in patients with normal plasma renin activity suggest that local renin-angiotensin systems, particularly those in the vasculature, myocardium, and kidneys, may play an important role in the pathophysiology of CHF. In addition to ANP, other vasodilating hormones, such as the prostaglandins, are also often increased.[14]

The occurrence of these neurohormonal alterations has been well characterized, but their role in the pathophysiology of CHF is more difficult to pinpoint. Clearly, there is a balance between vasodilating and natriuretic hormones on the one hand, and those that cause vasoconstriction and salt and fluid retention on the other. Many of these systems also are interrelated, often in very complex ways. Thus, the sympathetic nervous system modulates renin release, and conversely, angiotensin can enhance the release of norepinephrine from sympathetic nerves and, possibly, increase central nervous system sympathetic outflow. Angiotensin II stimulates the vasopressin secretion, while ANPs can counteract both the vasoconstricting and some sodium-retaining actions of other neurohormones. Thus, the neurohormonal milieu in patients with CHF can be seen as a dynamic interplay between vasoactive and renoactive substances with opposing effects, which is both

responsive to—and an important determinant of—the hemodynamic status of the patient.

There are a number of important ramifications of these neurohormonal alterations in CHF. First, although they may be important in the initial compensation to cardiac dysfunction, excessive responses clearly have negative prognostic significance. Elevated levels of plasma norepinephrine, plasma renin, and ANP are all associated with poorer outcome.[7,10,15] What is uncertain is whether these substances are involved in the progression of CHF and are responsible for increased mortality, or whether they are primarily markers of patients at risk for these complications. This key question has important therapeutic consequences, since agents are available that can interdict or enhance the activity of many of these systems.

Rationale for Vasodilator Therapy in Congestive Heart Failure

From the foregoing discussion, the rationale for using vasodilators in patients with heart failure becomes clear. The initially compensatory vasoconstriction may exacerbate many of the symptoms of CHF and accelerate its progression. Arteriolar constriction increases impedance to left ventricular ejection, reducing stroke volume and enhancing left ventricular wall stress. Venous constriction shifts blood centrally from the peripheral and splanchnic beds, contributing to congestive symptoms. Vasodilation improves systemic hemodynamics and cardiac performance, as judged by the relationship between stroke volume or stroke work and left ventricular filling volume and pressure. These hemodynamic responses may be similar to those obtained with inotropic stimulation or, even substantially greater in patients with diminished contractile reserve. In addition, unloading the heart may decrease myocardial oxygen demand and improve diastolic compliance.

Numerous vasodilators have been investigated in the treatment of CHF.[1] Although virtually all are associated with improved hemodynamic measurements, clinical benefit has been more difficult to demonstrate. In part, this discordance probably is explained by the loss of efficacy during continued therapy because of pharmacologic or hemodynamic tolerance. Tolerance occurs so rapidly with α-adrenergic blocking agents, such as prazosin, that initial hemodynamic responses are no longer demonstrable after several days of treatment.[16] Nitrate tolerance is a frequent occurrence, but although the response is blunted, it is not obliterated in most patients.[17] While one mechanism of tolerance to vasodilators relates to changes in vascular receptors, it is also clear that these agents may evoke neurohormonal responses, which lead to vasoconstriction and fluid retention. Increased plasma norepinephrine concentrations and renin-angiotensin activity have been demonstrated during treatment with several vasodilators, and the tachycardia associated with hydralazine therapies suggests increased sympathetic nervous system stimulation of the heart. Thus, although the combination of hydralazine and isosorbide dinitrate have been shown to reduce mortality in patients with CHF, these agents may not represent the optimal therapeutic approach.

Rationale for ACE Inhibition in Congestive Heart Failure

Based on theoretical considerations, the ACE inhibitors would appear to be ideal agents for the treatment of heart failure. In addition to being potent vasodilators, they are less likely than the direct acting agents of this class to provoke vasoconstrictor and antinatriuretic responses. There is no evidence that the renin-angiotensin-aldosterone system escapes from the effects of ACE inhibitors. Because of the interaction between the renin-angiotensin and sympathetic nervous systems, reflex sympathetic activation also is less likely. Furthermore, because of the potentially deleterious consequences of neurohormonal activation on the heart and on the progression of CHF, interdiction of this process itself is a worthwhile goal.

Hemodynamic and Neurohormonal Responses to ACE Inhibition

Hemodynamic Response

Numerous studies have evaluated the acute hemodynamic effects of ACE inhibition in heart failure patients,[18-23] and these have shown remarkably consistent results despite differences in the patient population studied and the agent employed. Acutely, ACE inhib-

itors produce relatively modest increases in cardiac, stroke, and stroke work indices, ranging from 15% to 35% in most studies (Fig. 23.2). In contrast, direct-acting arteriolar dilators, such as hydralazine, increase cardiac index by 30% to 50% or even more in most patients. The decreases in left ventricular filling pressures and right atrial pressure observed with ACE inhibitors, in contrast, are as prominent as those obtained with any other nonparenteral agents. In most studies, these fall by 25% to 45%. Some decrease in arterial pressure is observed in almost all patients treated with ACE inhibitors, and in some this may be marked. Of note is that rather than provoking reflex tachycardia, modest decreases in heart rate averaging approximately 5 beats/min usually occur. Presumably this indicates a lack of reflex sympathetic activation, and in fact suggests a withdrawal of sympathetic tone, perhaps due to interactions between angiotensin II and the sympathetic nervous system. This may explain why the hypotension associated with the initiation of ACE inhibitors is relatively well tolerated, and why myocardial ischemia usually is not precipitated.

In addition to the acute hemodynamic changes at rest, similar improvements are observed during exercise.[21,23,24] At matched workloads, on ACE inhibitors there are smaller rises in arterial pressure, pulmonary artery pressure, and ventricular filling pressures, as well as greater increases in cardiac and stroke output. These hemodynamic responses are accompanied by modest decreases in left and right ventricular end diastolic and systolic volumes, both at rest and during exercise (Fig. 23.3).[21] However, the change in ejection fraction is relatively small. These changes could all be expected to decrease myocardial energy requirements, and indeed a decrease in myocardial oxygen consumption has been demonstrated after the acute administration of captopril.[25]

Although it appears that all of the ACE inhibitors that have been studied produce similar hemodynamic responses, there are important differences in the time course of these effects. A hemodynamic response to captopril is apparent within 30 min after oral administration, peaks at approximately 60 min postdosing, and persists from 4 to 8 hr.[19-22] Lisinopril, which like captopril is pharmacologically active without deesterification, has a peak effect after 2 to 4 hr, and the duration of effect is considerably longer. The onset of enalapril action is much more variable for patients with heart failure, presumably because of the variable rate of hepatic metabolism to the active moiety, enalaprilat. During acute studies of most ACE inhibitors, after achieving a relatively low threshold dose, there is not a clear-cut dose response relationship, but the duration of action lengthens as the dosages are increased.[19,20] This lack of a dose response relationship during acute studies, however, may not be applicable to long-term

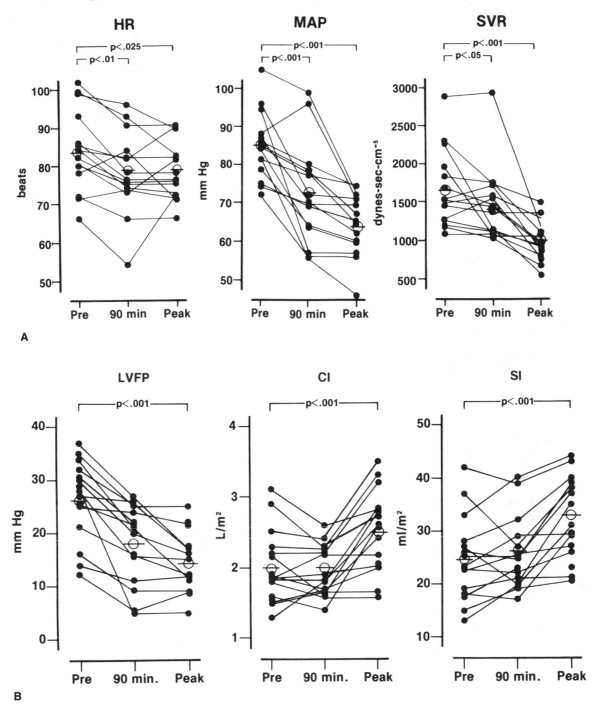

FIGURE 23.2. Acute hemodynamic effect of captopril at rest. **A:** Illustrates the changes in heart rate (*HR*), mean arterial pressure (*MAP*), and systemic vascular resistance (*SVR*) after the administration of a 25-mg oral dose of captopril. By 90 min, there are significant decreases in heart rate, *MAP*, and *SVR*. These changes reach their peak 2–3 hr postdosing. **B:** Shows the changes in left ventricular filling pressure (*LVFP*) and cardiac index (*CI*), and stroke volume index (*SI*). Again, significant changes in *LVFP* are seen early and persist. *CI* and *SI* increase somewhat later, and are significantly elevated by 2–3 hr. The most marked changes are the decrease in *LVFP* and *MAP*; most notably, there is no reflex rise in heart rate, but rather, a modest decline. Reprinted, with permission, from Topic et al. *Am Heart J.* 1982;104:1172.

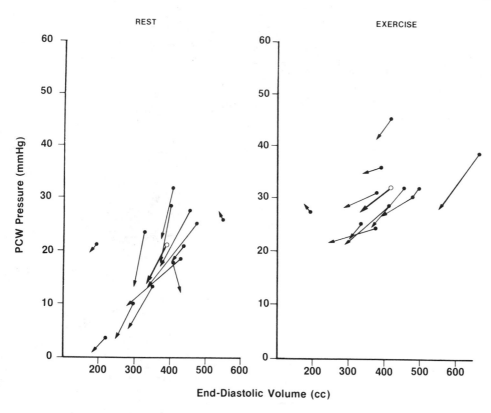

REST   EXERCISE

FIGURE 23.3. The acute changes in pulmonary capillary wedge pressure (*PCW*) and left ventricular and diastolic volume after captopril administration are shown. Both at rest and during exercise, there are significant decreases in both filling pressure and volume. Reprinted, with permission, from Massie et al. *Circulation.* 1982;65:1374. Copyright by the American Heart Association.

treatment, since some data indicate greater hemodynamic and clinical responses with higher dosages.[26]

There is less information about the long-term hemodynamic effect of ACE inhibitors in patients with heart failure, but the available data indicate that the acute hemodynamic responses were maintained for weeks to months (Fig. 23.4).[19,20,22,23,27] Indeed, the declines in left and right ventricular filling pressures may be greater during maintenance therapy than after acute dosing. In any case, unlike other vasodilators, hemodynamic tolerance to ACE inhibitors appears to be unusual.

Several studies have sought to determine whether there are measurable predictors of the acute and chronic hemodynamic response to ACE inhibition. Most data indicate that acutely, there are significant, but by no means very strong, relationships between pretreatment plasma renin activity and the magnitude of the declines in systemic vascular resistance and arterial pressure, and rise in cardiac output.[20,28,29] The same could be said for the relationship between the magnitude of response and the severity of pretreatment hyponatremia, which is a useful marker for activation of the renin-angiotensin system.[30] However, relationships between long-term hemodynamic changes and plasma renin activity at the onset of therapy are weak at best. Thus, hyponatremia, prerenal azotemia secondary to acute diuresis, and clinical evidence of intravascular hypokalemia are all markers for a greater hemodynamic response acutely, and therefore delineate groups of pa-

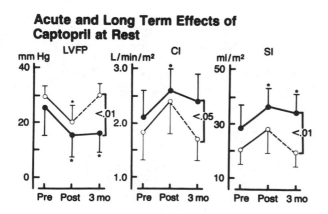

Acute and Long Term Effects of Captopril at Rest

FIGURE 23.4. This figure indicates the hemodynamic changes after 48 hr of captopril therapy (*post*) and after 3 months (*3 mo*). All patients received captopril initially, but after the first 48 hr only those indicated by the darker line continued on active drug. The group of patient illustrated by the lighter line and open circles was subsequently converted to placebo in a double-blind protocol. Their initial hemodynamic improvement disappeared. In contrast, the captopril group, shown by the solid circles and darker line, exhibited long-term benefit. It can be appreciated that the acute improvements in left ventricular filling pressure (*LVFP*), cardiac index (*CI*), and stroke volume index (*SI*) persist. Reprinted, with permission, from Kramer et al. *Circulation.* 1983;67:807. Copyright by the American Heart Association.

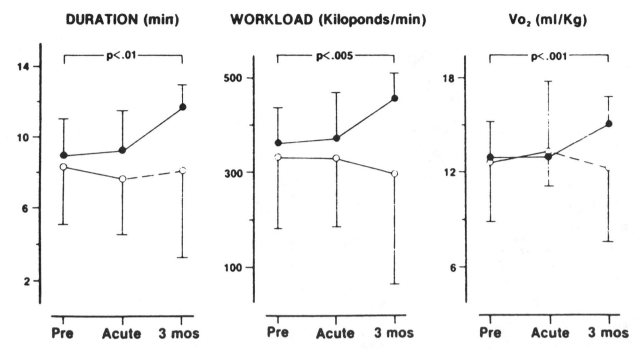

FIGURE 23.5. Utilizing the same format as Fig. 23.3, the initial and long-term (*3 mos*) changes in measurements of exercise capacity are shown. While there is no significant acute change, during follow-up exercise duration, maximum workload, and peak VO$_2$ all rise significantly. Reprinted, with permission, from Kramer et al. *Circulation*. 1983;67:807. Copyright by the American Heart Association.

tients who may be at greatest risk for acute hypotension, but none of these are accurate indicators of the efficacy of long-term treatment.

Effects on Exercise Tolerance

Since exercise intolerance is a primary symptom in patients with mild and moderate CHF, many studies have examined the effect of ACE inhibitor therapy on exercise capacity.[23,27,31–33] Despite immediate hemodynamic improvement, exercise tolerance does not change acutely[27] (Fig. 23.5). Rather, it increases slowly, with the maximum benefit appearing after 3 to 6 months. ACE inhibitors both increase maximal exercise capacity (as assessed by peak VO$_2$) and reduce symptoms during submaximal exercise. Of note is that there is no correlation between the acute hemodynamic response and subsequent improvement in exercise tolerance or symptoms (Fig. 23.6).

The gradual time course of improvement suggests that peripheral adaptations are required before the improved hemodynamics can be translated into enhanced work capacity of the exercising muscles.[34] Individuals exhibiting an increase in their exercise tolerance have been shown to have increased muscle blood flow, improved muscle metabolism, and normalization of their mitochondrial structure (Fig. 23.7).[30,35,36] These changes permit the exercising muscle not only to receive a higher blood flow, but also to increase O$_2$ extraction.

The mechanism of these peripheral adaptations is unclear. It seems unlikely that they are simply a "training" effect due to increased activity, since few patients markedly increase their activity level. It is possible that a reduction in neurohormonal activation could cause significant changes in muscle, or that the initiating change is an increase in muscle blood flow.

Neurohormonal Responses

Clearly, one of the unique features of ACE inhibition is its ability to alter the neurohormonal milieu in patients with heart failure. ACE inhibitors all produce significant reductions in plasma angiotensin II concentrations and aldosterone secretion, with an accompanying rise in plasma renin activity. However, as noted above, neither the chronic hemodynamic nor clinical effects of these agents are dependent on pretreatment activation of the renin-angiotensin system. This discordance supports the involvement of either tissue-based renin-angiotensin systems or the involvement of other neurohormonal mechanisms. Evidence for the presence and importance of converting enzyme in numerous tissues, including blood vessels, kidneys, and the heart, is growing.[11–13] It seems likely that ACE inhibitors may achieve some of their response by blocking the generation of angiotensin II in these tissues, and this may not be reflected by assays of the circulating components of the renin-angiotensin system. Converting enzyme also

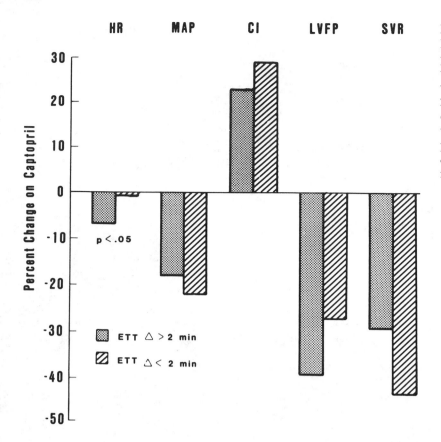

FIGURE 23.6. The relationship between the acute hemodynamic changes and the subsequent improvement or lack of improvement in exercise tolerance is shown. Of note is that patients whose exercise duration increased by more than 2 min did not show significantly greater hemodynamic responses than those whose exercise tolerance did not improve by that degree. Reprinted, with permission, from Massie et al. *Circulation*. 1984;69:1135. Copyright by the American Heart Association.

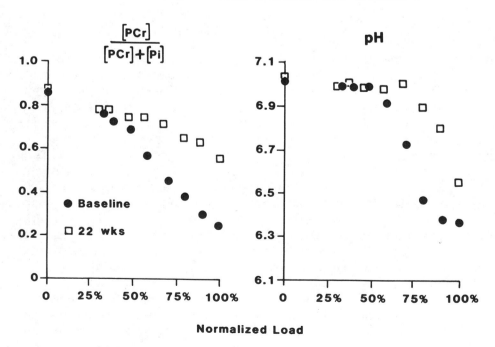

FIGURE 23.7. This figure illustrates measurements of phosphocreatinine (*PCr*), which is normalized to the sum of PCr + inorganic phosphate (*PI*), and pH performed during an incremental exercise protocol in a CHF patient before and 5 months after the institution of ACE inhibitor therapy. The metabolic measurements are shown in relationship to the percent of maximal exercise. Of note is that during the repeat study at the end of the 5-month treatment period, which is shown by the open squares, the patients was able to exercise to a 30% higher load. Despite the greater work at each stage, the metabolic changes were much less for PCr, and the decline in pH occurred at a higher levei of exercise. This type of change indicates metabolic adaptation in muscle, which is most likely an indirect effect of chronic ACE inhibitor therapy. Reprinted, with permission, from Massie BM. *Am J Med*. 1988;84(Suppl 3A):75.

is an important mechanism of degradation of tissue kinins. Inhibition of kinin degradation can not only produce a vasodilator response, but also will stimulate production of vasodilating prostaglandins. Increased levels of prostaglandins have been demonstrated after the administration of ACE inhibitors, and several studies have shown that concomitant administration of inhibitors of prostaglandin synthesis can substantially mitigate the acute hemodynamic response to ACE inhibitors.[14,37,38] The importance of these non-renin actions of ACE inhibitors is unclear at this time, but warrants study in light of the observation that concurrent aspirin therapy may have limited the benefit of enalapril in the SOLVD Trial.[39]

Interactions between the renin-angiotensin system and the sympathetic nervous system have been demonstrated,[40,41] but again the importance of these in the response to ACE inhibition in heart failure is unclear. Several studies have demonstrated that ACE inhibitors can reduce plasma norepinephrine activity and reestablish baroreceptor responsiveness.[42–45] These could be explained by the modulating effect of angiotensin II on norepinephrine release from presynaptic nerves or by a regulatory role of angiotensin II on central nervous system sympathetic output. In addition, chronic ACE inhibition may affect adrenergic receptor–adenylate cyclase coupling.[46] Alternatively, changes in sympathetic activity may reflect improvement in CHF due to ACE inhibitor therapy.

Clinical Trials of ACE Inhibitors in CHF

The favorable hemodynamic responses to ACE inhibitors, together with the conceptual advantages of this approach to treatment, have led to a large number of clinical studies. Several small, well designed clinical trials quickly established the benefit of this approach to therapy by demonstrating sustained hemodynamic improvements and beneficial effects on symptomatology and exercise capacity.[23,27,32,33] However, more than any other group of therapeutic agents for heart failure, the ACE inhibitors have been assessed in major multicenter trials, which have established their role in a wide variety of patients. These will be summarized, since they provide the best available information on how and when to use these agents.

Captopril Multicenter Trial (1983)[31]

This was the first major clinical trial of an ACE inhibitor in CHF, and its results led not only to the approval of this agent for the treatment of CHF, but also established a study methodology that has been employed in many subsequent studies. Ninety-two patients who remained moderately to severely symptomatic (NYHA Class III or II) despite chronic treatment with digitalis and diuretics were studied in a randomized, double-

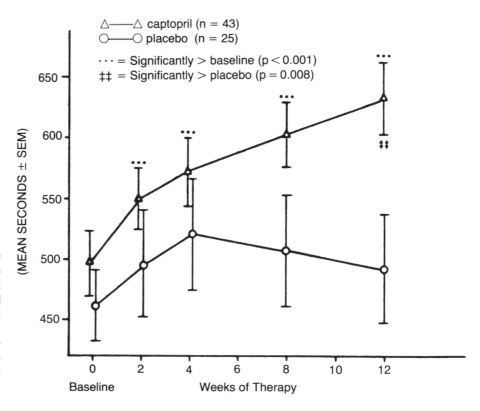

FIGURE 23.8. The changes in exercise time during serial treadmill exercise tests after the initiation of captopril in a placebo-controlled, double-blind study of patients with NYHA Class II and III CHF on diuretics and digoxin. Exercise capacity increased progressively over the 3-month study. Reprinted, with permission, from *J Am Coll Cardiol.* 1983;2:755.

blind trial of 3 months' duration. Patients were commenced on 25 mg/tid, but increased to 50 mg three times daily if tolerated on the next day. The dosage was then increased to 100 mg three times daily after 2 weeks if tolerated. Captopril was remarkably effective in this trial. The duration of treadmill exercise, the primary study end-point, increased by nearly 25% on captopril and was unchanged in the placebo group (Fig. 23.8). Assessment of symptoms by both patients and physicians also significantly improved in the captopril group, but not in the placebo patients. Of note is that 12 of 42 patients in the placebo group withdrew due to worsening heart failure (8) or died (4), as compared to only 2 of 50 patients in the captopril group. Despite the high doses employed, captopril was generally well tolerated. Three patients were unable to tolerate the initial 25-mg dosage due to hypotension, and an additional 36% of patients randomized to captopril experienced symptoms consistent with hypotension during double-blind therapy, but were able to continue the drug. Indeed, 25% of the placebo-treated patients also had similar symptoms. Otherwise, the drug was generally well tolerated, with only one patient experiencing significant renal dysfunction and several others developing skin rashes or taste alterations. This landmark study established the efficacy of captopril in moderate to severe heart failure, and also suggested that ACE inhibition might have a beneficial effect on survival and on the natural history of heart failure.[47]

The CONSENSUS I Trial (1987)[48]

The second major trial that confirmed the efficacy of ACE inhibitors in heart failure was the Scandinavian CONSENSUS study. In this trial, 253 patients with very severe heart failure (NYHA Class IV), despite hospitalization and an intensive therapy, were randomized to treatment with enalapril or placebo with the primary end-point of survival. Most patients were receiving diuretics and digoxin, and many were receiving other vasodilators as well. Blinded therapy was commenced with enalapril 5 mg twice daily, or matching placebo, and the dosage was increased to 10 mg twice daily if tolerated. Additionally, increases up to 20 mg twice daily were permitted if clinically indicated. Mortality rates were very high in the severely ill group, but enalapril decreased 6- and 12-month mortality rates from 44% and 52% in the placebo group, to 26% and 36% (Fig. 23.9). This beneficial effect was entirely due to a reduction in deaths classified as being due to progression of CHF; no reduction in sudden cardiac death was noted. In addition, patients randomized to enalapril therapy exhibited significantly greater improvement in their symptoms. The final mean dosage of enalapril was 18.4 mg, and in general it was less tolerated, with only seven patients experiencing symptoms of hypotension. This study demonstrated conclusively that ACE inhibition could reduce mortality in patients with severe heart failure.

Captopril-Digoxin Multicenter Study (1988)[49]

This multicenter trial was designed to compare the effects of treatment with captopril or digoxin with those of placebo in patients with mild to moderate heart failure and left ventricular ejection fractions below 40% who were in normal sinus rhythm. It was a randomized, double-blind study conducted in 300 patients with pre-

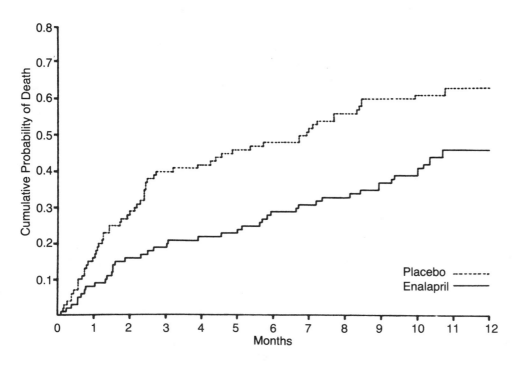

FIGURE 23.9. The mortality curve during the CONSENSUS Study is shown. There is a significant decrease in mortality in the group treated with enalapril; nonetheless, beyond 1 yr, mortality is high in both groups. Reprinted, with permission, from *N Engl J Med.* 1987;316:1429.

FIGURE 23.10. **A:** Shows the changes in treadmill exercise time over the 6 months of double-blind, randomized therapy in the Captopril-Digoxin Multicenter Study. The captopril group (*solid bars*) exhibited a significant increase in exercise time, both compared to baseline and to the placebo group (*open bars*). The digoxin group (*hatched bars*) showed intermediate results. **B:** Utilizes the same format and shows the proportion of patients showing improvement in NYHA classification. Captopril caused a significantly greater number of patients to exhibit improvement in their NYHA functional class, compared to the placebo group. Again, the digoxin patients were intermediate. Reprinted, with permission, from *JAMA*. 1988;259:539. Copyright by the American Medical Association.

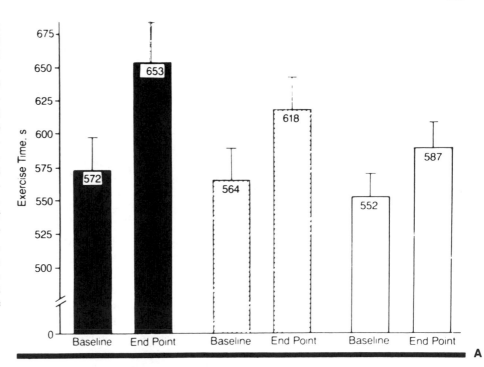

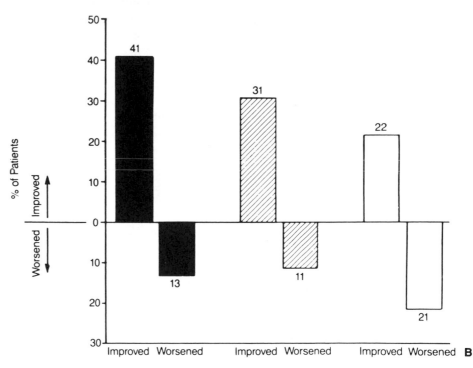

dominantly NYHA Class II CHF who could be stabilized either on diuretics alone or no treatment. Of note is that most of these patients had been withdrawn from previous digoxin therapy before entry in the study, which may have biased the study against digoxin if patients who deteriorated after withdrawal were not entered. Captopril was initiated at 25 mg three times a day and increased after 1 week to 50 mg three times a day if tolerated. Patients were followed for 6 months, with the primary end-points being exercise tolerance, symptoms, diuretic requirements, and deterioration of heart failure. Compared to placebo, the captopril group showed a significantly greater increase in exercise tolerance and more frequent improvement in clinical class (Fig. 23.10). The digoxin group showed intermediate results, and was not significantly different from either placebo or captopril. Both captopril and digoxin were associated with a less frequent need for increased diuretic treatment and markedly fewer hospitalizations and emergency room visits for worsening heart failure.

The SOLVD Treatment Trial (1991)[50]

The SOLVD Study (Studies on Left Ventricular Dysfunction) consisted of two parallel studies conducted simultaneously in the U.S., Canada, and Europe. These included patients with left ventricular dysfunction, as defined by an ejection $\leq 35\%$, due to ischemic heart disease in most patients, or nonischemic cardiomyopathy. One study, designated as the Treatment Trial, randomized 2569 patients with primarily NYHA Class II and III CHF, to treatment with enalapril or placebo for a mean follow-up of 41 months. The primary end-points were total mortality and the combination of death or hospitalization for heart failure. Enalapril or matching placebo was commenced at 2.5 or 5 mg twice daily, and the medication was titrated to a maximum 10 mg twice daily if tolerated. The average prescribed dose of the active drug was 16.6 mg daily. Approximately 85% of these patients were receiving diuretics, and 67% digoxin. In addition, approximately 40% were receiving nitrates and another 30%, calcium channel blockers. Overall, enalapril treatment was associated with a 16% reduction in mortality and 26% reduction in combined deaths and hospitalizations for heart failure (Fig. 23.11). This benefit was seen across most subgroups, including those taking vasodilators, those with and without ischemic heart disease, and patients with both NYHA Class II and III CHF. Of note is that, like the CONSENSUS Trial, the primary reduction was in death due to progressive heart failure, and a reduction in sudden death mortality was not demonstrated. Interestingly, there was a strong trend toward a decrease in myocardial infarctions and episodes of unstable angina.

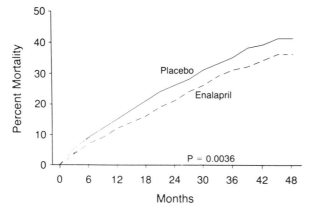

FIGURE 23.11. This figure illustrates the mortality curves from the SOLVD Treatment Trial. Although this group was less ill and more diverse than the patients in the CONSENSUS Study, enalapril significantly reduced mortality over a much longer period of follow-up. Reprinted, with permission, from *N Engl J Med.* 1991;325:293.

The SOLVD Prevention Trial (1992)[51]

The second component of the SOLVD Trial was called the Prevention Trial. This component included 4226 patients with left ventricular dysfunction (mean ejection fraction 28%), but no symptoms of heart failure. These patients did not require treatment with digitalis, diuretic, or vasodilators for heart failure, although they may have been taking these drugs for other indications. Approximately 80% of these patients had prior myocardial infarction; many were identified during routine postinfarction assessment of left ventricular function. Enalapril or placebo were administered in the same manner as in the Treatment Trial, but the primary study end-point for the Prevention patients was a combination of mortality and the onset of clinical heart failure. Thirty-seven percent fewer patients in the enalapril group developed clinical heart failure, and 20% fewer experienced the combined end-point of mortality or hospitalization for heart failure. Once heart failure occurred, the mortality curves in the affected patients showed a similar benefit from ACE inhibitor treatment as observed in the Treatment arm, with the overall 15% reduction approaching statistical significance. Again, there was a trend toward a reduction in myocardial infarctions (29% fewer) and angina (21% fewer).

Taken together, the combined results of the SOLVD Trial indicate a beneficial effect of ACE inhibitor therapy on survival and on the natural history of CHF in virtually all patients with significant left ventricular dysfunction.

SAVE (1992)[52]

The SAVE investigators similarly evaluated the effect of ACE inhibitor treatment in patients with left ventricular dysfunction but no overt heart failure. A total of 2,231 patients with ejection fractions below 40%, but free of clinical CHF, were randomized to captopril 50 mg tid or placebo. Treatment commenced 3 to 16 days postinfarct and patients were followed up to 42 months. The results were strikingly positive: all-cause mortality was reduced by 19%, cardiovascular mortality by 21%, and progression to CHF by 37%.

CONSENSUS II (1992)[53]

The CONSENSUS Study Group has recently terminated a trial in which patients with acute myocardial infarction were randomized at the time of admission to treatment with enalapril (initially administered intravenously and then orally) or placebo. As with SOLVD, the end-points were mortality and progression to heart failure. The study was terminated prematurely because there was no trend toward a beneficial effect, and given the results to that point, it was not considered possible to obtain a positive outcome. Obviously, the results of the study will require further scrutiny, but they raised the possibility that ACE inhibitor therapy commencing immediately postinfarction may not be beneficial.

V-HeFT II (1991)[54]

V-HeFT II represented the logical extension of the VA Cooperative Heart Failure study group, following the results of V-HeFT I, where the combination of hydralazine and isosorbide dinitrate produced a significant reduction in mortality in patients with NYHA Class II and III heart failure.[55] In V-HeFT II, this combination vasodilator regimen was compared to enalapril in a double-blind, randomized study involving 804 patients with NYHA Class II and III symptoms of CHF and either an ejection fraction less than 45% or evidence of cardiac dilatation. Treatment with enalapril was commenced with 5 mg twice daily and was titrated to 10 mg twice daily if tolerated, with the average daily dosage being 15 mg. The enalapril group exhibited a significantly lower mortality rate, the primary study endpoint, over the follow-up period, which ranged from 6 months to 5.7 yr. The mortality reduction in the enalapril group was 34% after 1 year, 28% after 2 years, and fell to 10% to 15% thereafter (Fig. 23.12). In this study, the greatest relative benefit was seen in patients with primary cardiomyopathy and in those with milder (NYHA Class II) CHF. These trends differ from the placebo-controlled SOLVD Study, in which substantial benefit was seen in patients with ischemic heart disease

and NYHA Class III symptoms. Of note is that the primary difference between the two groups was in the number of sudden deaths, with essentially equal numbers of patients dying from progressive heart failure. This latter result differs from those reported by the SOLVD and CONSENSUS studies, and raises the possibility that treatment with hydralazine and isosorbide dinitrate, while reducing overall mortality and, particularly, mortality related to progressive heart failure, may be increasing the numbers of sudden deaths. ACE inhibitors, by interfering with the neurohormonal activation which, if anything, may be exacerbated by direct-acting vasodilators, may prevent these sudden deaths. In any case, since enalapril was at least as well tolerated as hydralazine and isosorbide dinitrate, this study indicates that ACE inhibition should be the vasodilator regimen of choice for most patients with CHF.

Comparison of ACE Inhibitors with Other Therapeutic Modalities in Heart Failure

Diuretics

Diuretics often are considered the first line of therapy in patients with symptomatic CHF, particularly in the presence of manifest fluid retention[1]; however, diuretic therapy carries the risk of excessive electrolyte depletion and has the potential to activate potentially deleterious neurohormonal systems.[56,57] Data comparing ACE inhibitors and diuretics as initial therapy in heart failure are relatively limited. In one small double-blind study, diuretic proved superior to captopril in patients with mild heart failure.[58] Indeed, the addition of an ACE inhibitor to a low dose of diuretic was not as effective as raising the diuretic dose in a group of patients with edematous heart failure.[59] In patients with more severe heart failure and hyponatremia, an adequate diuresis could not be obtained and hyponatremia could not be corrected without adding a diuretic to ACE inhibitor therapy.[60] Finally, in a small study in which patients with previously untreated heart failure, some of whom had clinical evidence of fluid retention, were treated with enalapril alone, neither adequate clinical nor hemodynamic responses were observed, even though some diuresis occurred.[61] All five patients ultimately required the addition of diuretics.

Although not definitive, the results of these small studies indicate that diuretics remain an essential part of the treatment of patients with symptomatic heart failure. ACE inhibitors as sole therapy are not adequate but, based on other results of the previously cited multicenter studies, they clearly have a complementary role.

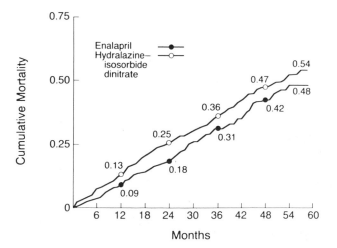

FIGURE 23.12. These mortality curves are derived from V-HeFT II, the randomized comparison of enalapril vs. the combination of hydralazine and isosorbide dinitrate. Again, the ACE inhibitors significantly reduced mortality over a very long period of follow-up in these predominantly NYHA Class II and III heart failure patients. Reprinted, with permission, from Cohn et al. *N Engl J Med.* 1991;325:303.

Digoxin

Until the advent of ACE inhibitors, digoxin was considered by many to be an essential part of the management of patients with symptomatic CHF, although questions remained concerning its role in patients in sinus rhythm. Although recent data have confirmed the efficacy of digoxin in such patients, the advent of ACE inhibitors has reopened the question of the appropriate role of digitalis glycosides. The Captopril-Digoxin Multicenter Study discussed previously demonstrated that both agents were effective by clinical criteria, and failed to demonstrate significant advantages of one agent over the other.[49] Similar results were obtained in a Canadian multicenter trial comparing digoxin and enalapril.[62] One hundred forty-five patients with NYHA Class II and II CHF were randomized to enalapril (5–20 mg twice daily) or digoxin for 14 weeks. Although exercise tolerance improved comparably with both agents, those taking enalapril experienced a lessening of dyspnea at submaximal exercise, which was not seen with digoxin. A greater number of patients experienced worsening of heart failure in the digoxin group, as well. These data, together with the well documented improvement of prognosis during ACE inhibitor therapy in the absence of similar data with digoxin, suggest that ACE inhibitors should be the second line of therapy in most heart failure patients who remain in sinus rhythm.

Both digoxin and the ACE inhibitors produce significant hemodynamic and clinical benefit in patients with CHF. Several trials have shown that ACE inhibitors produce further clinical improvement when added to digoxin. Although in one acute hemodynamic study, captopril and digoxin produced independent and additive hemodynamic benefits, both at rest and during exercise,[63] there are fewer data concerning clinical responses when digoxin is added in patients maintained on ACE inhibitors. A recent preliminary report of a multicenter placebo-controlled trial has now demonstrated that digoxin withdrawal in patients maintained on diuretics and ACE inhibitors is associated with frequent clinical deterioration and a decline in exercise capacity.[64] Thus, diuretics, ACE inhibitors, and digoxin appear to be complementary in their activity, and most symptomatic patients should be treated with all three in combination. The primary remaining question is whether digoxin has a positive or negative effect on survival.

ACE Inhibitors Versus Other Vasodilators

The most important trial comparing different approaches to vasodilator therapy, V-HeFT II, has been discussed previously.[53] In this study, the ACE inhibitor showed a significant advantage in terms of reducing mortality. A recent preliminary report in patients with more severe heart failure also demonstrated a reduction in sudden death mortality with ACE inhibitors compared to regimens utilizing hydralazine and nitrates.[65] However, it should be noted that in V-HeFT II, there is a trend toward greater symptomatic and exercise tolerance improvement as the hydralazine-isosorbide dinitrate regimen.[54]

A number of small studies also have compared the efficacy of ACE inhibitors and other vasodilators. In a double-blind, crossover study of 16 patients comparing captopril with the α-adrenergic blocking agent, prazosin, clinical improvement was seen only with the ACE inhibitor.[66] On prazosin, increased activity of the renin-angiotensin system and higher levels of plasma catecholamines were observed. These findings were confirmed by another group, which concluded that although both agents block vasoconstrictive neurohormonal systems, further activation of these systems after α-adrenergic blockade overcomes the potential benefit of this approach.[67]

Studies also have been conducted comparing captopril with hydralazine and with isosorbide dinitrate. In a study in which 50 patients are randomized to hydralazine or captopril, the ACE inhibitor produced greater improvements in exercise tolerance and symptoms.[68] Similarly, in a study of 21 patients randomized to captopril or isosorbide dinitrate, the ACE inhibitor improved symptoms and significantly lessened the requirements for additional diuretic compared to isosorbide dinitrate.[69] The calcium channel blockers generally are not recommended for the treatment of heart failure, since they increase the incidence of CHF and may increase mortality in patients with left ventricular dysfunction.[70–72] However, they are potent peripheral vasodilators and continue to be studied for this indication. As with the other direct-acting vasodilators, a comparative study of captopril with nifedipine showed significant beneficial responses to the former agent and no effect to the latter.[73] Again, this difference appeared to be due at least in part to activation of neurohormonal mechanisms with nifedipine.

The results of these studies clearly support the use of ACE inhibitors before other vasodilators in most patients with CHF. However, they also raise the provocative question as to whether the combination of ACE inhibitors and direct-acting vasodilators may provide additional benefit. This can be justified on hemodynamic grounds, since the ACE inhibitors are relatively less potent vasodilators,[74a] but they could prevent the neurohormonal activation associated with other agents. A recently reported study, FACET, has now shown that exercise tolerance and indices of quality of life are improved when the newly approved direct acting vasodilator flosequinan is added to a regimen of an ACE inhibitor, diuretic, and digoxin.[74b] This hypothesis also will be tested in the V-HeFT III study.

Indications for ACE Inhibitors in CHF

Based on the studies described in the previous sections, it is possible to develop guidelines for the use of ACE inhibitors in most patients with CHF and left ventricular dysfunction. Patients with severe heart failure, as defined by the need for frequent hospitalizations, NYHA Class III to IV symptoms, and marked neurohormonal activation, should be treated with ACE inhibitors if at all possible. ACE inhibitors reduce mortality, prevent hospitalizations, and improve symptoms in this group. Patients with CHF of moderate severity, as defined by significant activity limitation despite the treatment with diuretics or diuretics plus digoxin, also benefit from ACE inhibitor therapy. In these patients, mortality and hospitalizations are reduced and symptoms improved. These patients also benefit from digoxin, so most should be treated with a combination of diuretics, ACE inhibitors, and glycosides.

ACE inhibitors have now been proven effective in patients with mild symptoms from heart failure. In these, ACE inhibitors improve prognosis, preventing both death and progression of heart failure. Based on the results of many studies, it may be harder to demonstrate symptomatic improvement in these less ill patients. Nonetheless, since this represents most patients with heart failure and since they may still benefit from an improved prognosis, this is an important group to treat with ACE inhibitors. Thus, although diuretics remain an important therapeutic modality in mild heart failure, ACE inhibitors should be used concomitantly in most patients. By and large, until the effect of digoxin on prognosis is established, this agent should be held in reserve for patients who remain symptomatic on diuretics and ACE inhibitors, or who have associated supraventricular arrhythmias.

The most exciting new indication for ACE inhibitors is in patients with asymptomatic left ventricular dysfunction,[75] but this approach should be undertaken with some caution. The SOLVD Prevention Trial shows that ACE inhibitors can prevent or delay the onset of clinical heart failure in patients with left ventricular ejection fractions < 35%. ACE inhibitors also appear to prolong survival in this group, but primarily in those individuals who first manifest heart failure. Thus, it is unclear whether initiation of ACE inhibitors after the onset of heart failure would not be an adequate approach, although clearly it would be optimal to prevent the initial episodes. Furthermore, it will need to be determined whether all patients with left ventricular ejection fractions < 35% benefit, or whether most of the effect is found in those with lower ejection fractions or greater left ventricular dilatation.

The hypothesis that early treatment in individuals with recent myocardial damage and new left ventricular destruction can prevent a further decline in ejection fraction, presumably by affecting the process of left ventricular remodelling and dilatation, and improve prognosis has now been evaluated.[76] Several small, controlled studies have proved that the administration of captopril commencing within several weeks of a large myocardial infarction can prevent left ventricular dilatation.[77-80] The SAVE study was designed to determine whether captopril commenced early but not immediately postinfarction prevents progression to CHF and prolongs survival.[52] Administration of captopril was associated with improvement in overall survival and decreased morbidity and mortality due to cardiovascular events. This occurred independent of concomitant treatment with thrombolysis and β-blockers, but may have been mitigated by concommitant aspirin. These findings, taken together with the SOLVD Prevention Trial, support a strategy of commencing ACE inhibitor therapy in patients with asymptomatic left ventricular dysfunction (ejection fraction of $\leq 35-40\%$).

Differential Pharmacology of ACE Inhibitors

Since a peptide component of the venom of the Brazilian snake, *Barthrops jararaca*, was found to inhibit the conversion of angiotensin I and angiotensin II in the 1960s, and orally active ACE inhibitors were subsequently synthesized, the number of agents in this class has grown continuously.[81,82] The active site of ACE was found to contain a zinc ion and all current ACE inhibitors are known to bind with the zinc moiety. The potency of the various ACE inhibitors is determined by the strength of their binding to the zinc ligand and the number of additional binding sites.[83] Other properties of these compounds, such as their size, conformation, and lipophilicity, determine their metabolism, routes of elimination, and tissue penetration properties. There currently are three classes of ACE inhibitors as defined by their active site: (a) captopril, the first orally active agent of this class, contains a sulfhydryl group that binds to the zinc atom of ACE. Other sulfhydryl-containing ACE inhibitors that currently are in use abroad or under investigation are converted to captopril, which is the active compound; (b) the second class of ACE inhibitors contains carboxyl groups, which bind to the zinc atom in ACE. Enalapril and lisinopril are representatives of this group, as are a number of recently released or soon to become available agents, such as benazepril, spirapril, quinapril, ramipril, cilazapril, perindopril, and delapril; (c) the third class of ACE inhibitors contains a phosphoryl group; fosinopril is the only available member of this group.

There are a number of important pharmacological differences among the ACE inhibitors.[82,84,85] With regard to heart failure patients, probably the most important of these is whether the drug is active in its native form or functions as a prodrug, requiring biotransformation primarily in the liver. Only captopril and lisinopril fall into the former category, and therefore these have more predictable pharmokinetics in patients with heart failure. Captopril has a rapid onset of effect and reaches peak serum activity within 1 hr. Lisinopril absorption is somewhat slower, but peak activity occurs within 2 to 6 hr. All of the other agents are prodrugs, and their peak effect may be considerably more variable.[86,87]

The ACE inhibitors also differ in their route of elimination.[82,85] Most are excreted primarily by the kidneys, but fosinopril and benazapril have significant hepatic excretion. Therefore, these agents may be preferable in patients with significant renal dysfunction. Aside from captopril, most of the ACE inhibitors have a relatively long duration of action. All can be given once, or at most twice, daily.

Another important potential difference between the different ACE inhibitors is their ability to inhibit tissue ACE.[11–13] As discussed above, the role of tissue renin-angiotensin systems is not yet known, but differences between the various agents and their ability to penetrate tissues and inhibit ACE activity in various organs are beginning to be recognized.[88] It has been speculated that these differences may explain a higher incidence of renal dysfunction with some agents or even differential effects on mortality,[89,90] but supportive evidence for these assertions is lacking. Nonetheless, the role of tissue ACE and the tissue specificity of various compounds remain important areas of investigation.

Clinical Studies with the Newer ACE Inhibitors

All of the clinical studies discussed thus far have involved captopril or enalapril, the first two ACE inhibitors to be investigated. Recently, two additional ACE inhibitors, lisinopril and quinopril, have been approved for the treatment of CHF in the U.S. Several others have also undergone clinical evaluation. Although a number of studies with both older and newer agents have failed to yield positive results, these negative outcomes may be explained by inadequate sample size, inappropriate patient selection, or protocol deficiencies. With the growing use of ACE inhibitors, it has become increasingly difficult to conduct well designed trials.[91,92] Nonetheless, most of the negative studies have shown favorable trends in at least some of the efficacy measurements, and there are no data to indicate that the efficacy of ACE inhibitors in patients with heart failure is not a class effect shared by all of these drugs.

Lisinopril has undergone several clinical trials. In one study of 189 patients with NYHA Class II to IV CHF and ejection fractions <45%, who were receiving diuretics and digoxin, lisinopril was compared to captopril. Lisinopril was commenced at 5 mg od and captopril at 12.5 mg tid; the dosages were titrated to a maximum of 20 mg od and 50 mg tid, respectively, as tolerated if the patients remained symptomatic. In this trial, lisinopril produced a significantly greater increase in exercise tolerance and improvement in functional capacity and symptoms over the 12-week double-blind treatment period. In a trial with similar entry criteria, lisinopril was compared to placebo in 193 patients. There was a trend toward greater improvement in exercise tolerance, which was significant in the subgroup of patients with ejection fractions <35%, and the active treatment group showed significant improvement in symptoms.

Studies also continue to appear with the newer ACE inhibitors.[26,93] Of note is a double-blind, placebo-controlled trial of quinopril, because this study included parallel treatment of groups randomly assigned to three different dosages of the drug or placebo.[26] This is the only study thus far in which the dose-response relationship can be assessed during chronic therapy. By serial measurements of exercise tolerance, greater responses were observed with the higher dosages. Since most ACE inhibitor trials have used relatively high dosages compared to those employed in clinical practice, these findings raise the possibility that physicians may not be utilizing optimal regimens of many ACE inhibitors.

Possible Differences Between ACE Inhibitors in CHF

Although there are significant pharmacological differences among the available ACE inhibitors, it is not clear that these lead to clinically important distinctions among drugs. Certainly captopril, because of its rapid onset of effect, lends itself well to test-dosing in outpatients.[87] Its relatively short duration of effect may also lead to incomplete ACE inhibition during some intervals over the 24-hr day, especially when bid dosing is employed.[84,85] This also may result in less sustained reductions in blood pressure in susceptible individuals. In a study in which 42 patients were randomly assigned to either captopril 50 mg tid or enalapril 20 mg bid, a greater rise in serum creatinine and potassium levels was noted with the longer acting agent, enalapril.[89] However, diuretic and ACE inhibitor dose adjustments were not permitted in this trial, so its clinical relevance is unclear. Nonetheless, the differential pharmacology of captopril and the more long-acting ACE inhibitors suggest that the former agent may be more appropriate for the initial treatment of patients with borderline blood pressures or abnormal renal function.

In a recent post hoc analysis of a trial of investigational β-adrenergic agonist, xamoterol, in patients with Class III or IV heart failure, it was found that patients being treated with captopril exhibited a higher mortality rate than those receiving enalapril.[90] Since the choice of ACE inhibitors was not randomized and the analysis was retrospective, it is impossible to be sure whether this mortality difference reflected a true difference between the drugs or differences in the patient populations receiving them. Nonetheless, this study raises the possibility that sustained inhibition of ACE may be advantageous.

As mentioned earlier, there may be differences among ACE inhibitors in their activity against tissue ACE. Such differences could reflect variable tissue penetration or different affinities to the tissue enzyme. One might postulate that differences between the drugs, such as those seen in renal function or even in mortality, could reflect differences in tissue effects, as well as in pharmacodynamics.

Side Effects and Toxicity

Hypotension and Renal Dysfunction

In clinical practice, the major limiting effect of ACE inhibitor therapy in patients with heart failure is hypotension. As noted earlier, ACE inhibitors produce a consistent decline in arterial pressure. This occurs acutely, but persists to a lesser extent during chronic therapy. In general, the hypotension is associated with few or no symptoms, although dizziness and light headedness occur in 5% to 20% of patients and require downward dose adjustment or discontinuation in up to 10%.[50,94] However, in some cases hypotension can be severe and life-threatening.[95]

Of more concern are the changes in renal function, which may occur in patients treated with ACE inhibitors, especially in those who have relatively low pretreatment blood pressures and experience further declines. ACE inhibitor–induced renal dysfunction occurs on a functional hemodynamic basis, and is reversible if the drugs are discontinued in a timely manner.[96] The renin-angiotensin system plays an important role in renal blood flow autoregulation. When renal perfusion pressure decreases, glomerular filtration is maintained in part by postglomerular arteriolar constriction mediated by angiotensin II.[96–98] The combination of systemic hypotension and ACE inhibition may cause significant elevations of BUN and creatinine, together with hyperkalemia.[89,99] Such changes may be more frequent in patients with renal vascular disease,[100] diabetes, or intrinsic renal disease,[100] but they may occur in patients with apparently normal renal function as well. The combination of ACE inhibitors and prostaglandin inhibitors, such as the nonsteroidal antiinflammatory agents, may be particularly dangerous. Since these

latter agents interfere with prostaglandin-mediated efferent arteriolar dilatation, the combination can completely interfere with all renal autoregulatory mechanisms.[96] Thus, nonsteroidal agents should be avoided completely in patients with borderline arterial pressure on ACE inhibitors, or if they must be given, careful monitoring of renal function is essential. Overall, approximately 10% of patients with CHF treated with ACE inhibitors may exhibit increases in serum BUN and creatinine, but a smaller number will require significant dose reductions or drug discontinuation.

ACE Inhibitor Side Effects

Aside from symptoms of cerebral hypoperfusion, the most common side effects of ACE inhibitors in heart failure are those seen in the hypertensive population. Cough is the most problematic of these and appears to occur in equal numbers of patients with all available ACE inhibitors.[101] Cough may be more common, but also more difficult to recognize, in heart failure patients. Estimates of the incidence of cough range from 5% to 20% of patients, but a smaller number require drug discontinuation. Other side effects include skin rashes, taste alteration, and gastrointestinal side effects. The former two problems may be more common with captopril, because of its sulfhydryl group. Angioneurotic edema occurs as a result of the increase in tissue kinin levels and their interaction with the complement system in predisposed individuals, rather than as an allergic reaction.[102,103] Angioneurotic edema is seen with all ACE inhibitors, but may not appear until after many months of therapy. Because it may result in airway compromise, further ACE inhibitor therapy is contraindicated.

Guidelines for the Initiation and Monitoring of ACE Inhibitor Therapy

ACE inhibitors can be initiated safely and successfully in the vast majority of heart failure patients. Individuals at high risk for hypotension or renal dysfunction should be identified before therapy. These include patients with borderline blood pressure (systolic pressure < 100 mm Hg), those with preexisting renal dysfunction, those with prerenal azotemia, and those with evidence of excessive neurohormonal activation, as indicated by hyponatremia. In general, ACE inhibitors should not be commenced after a rapid diuresis; in patients with clinical evidence of intravascular volume depletion, diuretics should be withheld or decreased in dosage for one or more days beforehand. Patients in these high-risk categories should be commenced with particularly low doses, such as 6.25 mg captopril tid, 2.5 mg enalapril od or bid, or 2.5 to 5 mg of lisinopril od. Captopril has the advantage of causing the peak hemodynamic response within 1 hr, so the patient can be conveniently monitored. Patients in lower risk groups can be commenced at approximately twice these initial dosages. Renal function and serum potassium levels should be monitored early, after the initiation of ACE inhibitors; this should occur within 48 hr in high-risk patients and within 1 week in virtually all patients. Early communication with patients to determine whether they have symptoms of hypotension can be helpful in detecting those who need medication adjustment or early renal function monitoring. In addition to diuretic adjustment, it may be helpful to reduce or discontinue other hypotensive medications at the time of ACE inhibitor initiation. Potassium-sparing agents should be withdrawn, and potassium supplements should be reduced in dosage until need for further potassium supplementation can be confirmed.

The optimal dose of ACE inhibitors for maintenance therapy is unknown. However, there is marked discordance between the relatively high dosages employed in all the major clinical trials (150–300 mg captopril, 20 mg enalapril, 20 mg lisinopril) and those often used in clinical practice. Until further data are available about the efficacy of lower doses of ACE inhibitors, patients generally should be titrated to these levels if tolerated.

Remaining Questions Concerning ACE Inhibitors in CHF

From the foregoing, it is clear that ACE inhibitors have undergone extensive evaluation in patients with CHF. Indeed, more is known about their efficacy and their appropriate clinical use than about any other treatment for CHF. Nonetheless, important questions remain. The most vital of these concerns the mechanism about which ACE inhibitors produce clinical benefit and improve prognosis. Do they work through the circulating renin-angiotensin system, tissue-based systems, or indirectly through non–renin-related pathways? Do they exert their benefit through their hemodynamic actions or their endocrine effects? What is the mechanism of their apparent beneficial effect in preventing ischemic events due to coronary disease?

Although ACE inhibitors appear to have a benefit in virtually all patients with symptomatic CHF, and in most with asymptomatic left ventricular systolic dysfunction, can we identity subsets who are less likely to benefit? These appear to include patients with relatively preserved left ventricular function, such as those with ejection fractions >30% to 40%. The importance and mechanism of the interaction between aspirin and ACE inhibitors that may mitigate their benefited effects on prognosive need to be defined. In asymptomatic individuals, how much is lost by delaying therapy until symptoms occur? Does digoxin prolong survival in

stable patients on ACE inhibitors? What about β-blockers? And, importantly, what is the minimum effective dose and the optimal dose of these agents? It would be tragic if the impact of the dramatic trials with ACE inhibitors is minimized or lost in clinical practice because subtherapeutic dosages are utilized.

References

1. Christoph I, Minotti J, Massie BM. Current status of treatment for congestive heart failure. *Prog Cardiol.* 1991;4/2:3–42.
2. Cohn JN. Overview of pathophysiology of congestive heart failure. In: Hosenpud JD, Greenberg BH, eds. *Congestive Heart Failure: Pathophysiology, Differential Diagnosis, and Comprehensive Approach to Therapy.* New York: Springer-Verlag; 1993.
3. Casabello BA. Abnormalities in cardiac contraction: systolic dysfunction. In: Hosenpud JD, Greenberg BH, eds. *Congestive Heart Failure: Pathophysiology, Differential Diagnosis, and Comprehensive Approach to Therapy.* New York: Springer-Verlag; 1993.
4. Colucci WS. The sympathetic nervous system in congestive heart failure. In: Hosenpud JD, Greenberg BH, eds. *Congestive Heart Failure: Pathophysiology, Differential Diagnosis, and Comprehensive Approach to Therapy.* New York: Springer-Verlag; 1993.
5. Packer M. Nonadrenergic hormonal alterations in congestive heart failure. In: Hosenpud JD, Greenberg BH, eds. *Congestive Heart Failure: Pathophysiology, Differential Diagnosis, and Comprehensive Approach to Therapy.* New York: Springer-Verlag; 1993.
6. Francis GS, Goldsmith SR, Levine TB, et al. The neurohormonal axis in congestive heart failure. *Ann Intern Med.* 1984;101:370–377.
7. Packer M, Lee WH, Kessler PD, et al. Role of neurohormonal mechanisms in determining survival in patients with severe chronic heart failure. *Circulation.* 1987;75(Suppl II):IV80–IV92.
8. Francis GS, Benedict C, Johnson DE, et al. Comparison of neurohormonal activation in patients with left ventricular dysfunction with and without congestive heart ailure. *Circulation.* 1990;82:1724–1729.
9. Remes J, Tikkanen I, Fyhrquist F, et al. Neuroendocrine activity in untreated heart failure. *Br Heart J.* 1991;65:249–255.
10. Cohn JN, Levine TB, Oliveri MT, et al. Plasma norepinephrine as a guide to prognosis in patients with chronic congestive heart failure. *N Engl J Med.* 1984;311:819–823.
11. Dzau VJ. Circulating versus local renin-angiotensin system in cardiovascular homeostasis. *Circulation.* 1988;77(Suppl I):I4–I113.
12. Hirsch AT, Pinto YM, Schunkeat H, et al. Potential role of the tissue renin-angiotensin system in the pathophysiology of congestive heart failure. *Am J Cardiol.* 1990;66:220–300.
13. Lindpaintner K, Ganten D. The cardiac renin-angiotensin system: an appraisal of present experimental and direct evidence. *Circ Res.* 1991;68:905–921.

14. Dzau VJ, Packer M, Lilly LS, et al. Prostaglandins in severe congestive heart failure. Relation to activation of the renin-angiotensin system and hyponatremia. *N Engl J Med.* 1984;310:347–352.

15. Swedberg K, Eneroth P, Kjekshus J, et al. Hormone regulation of cardiovascular function in patients with severe congestive heart failure and their relation to mortality. *Circulation.* 1990;82:1730–1736.

16. Arnold SB, Williams RL, Ports TH, et al. Attenuation of prazosin effect on cardiac output in chronic heart failure. *Ann Intern Med.* 1979;91:345–349.

17. Flaherty JT. Nitrate tolerance—a review of the evidence. *Drugs.* 1989;37:523–550.

18. David R, Ribner HS, Keung E, et al. Treatment of chronic congestive heart failure with captopril, an oral inhibitor of angiotensin converting enzyme. *N Engl J Med.* 1979;301:117–121.

19. Ader R, Chatterjee K, Ports T, et al. Immediate and sustained hemodynamic and clinical improvement in chronic heart failure by angiotensin-converting enzyme inhibitors. *Circulation.* 1980;61:931–937.

20. Levine TB, Franciosa JA, Cohn JN. Acute and long-term response to an oral converting enzyme inhibitor, captopril, in congestive heart failure. *Circulation.* 1980;62:35–41.

21. Massie B, Kramer BL, Topic N, et al. Hemodynamic and radionuclide effects of acute captopril therapy for heart failure: changes in left and right ventricular volumes and function at rest and during exercise. *Circulation.* 1982;65:1374–1381.

22. Captopril Multicenter Research Group. A cooperative multicenter study of captopril in congestive heart failure: hemodynamic effects and long-term response. *Am Heart J.* 1985;110:439–447.

23. Creager MA, Massie BM, Faxon DP, et al. Acute and long term effects of enalapril on the cardiovascular response to exercise and exercise tolerance in patients with congestive heart failure. *J Am Coll Cardiol.* 1985;6:163–170.

24. Topic N, Kramer B, Massie B. Acute and long-term effects of captopril on exercise cardiac performance and exercise capacity in congestive heart failure. *Am Heart J.* 1982;104:1172–1179.

25. Chatterjee K, Rouleau JL, Parmley WW. Haemodynamic and myocardial metabolic effects of captopril in chronic heart failure. *Br Heart J.* 1982;47:233–388.

26. Rieger GA. The effects of ACE inhibitor on exercise capacity in the treatment of congestive heart failure. *J Cardiovasc Pharmacol.* 1990;15(Suppl 2):541–546.

27. Kramer BL, Massie BM, Topic N. Controlled trial of captopril in chronic heart failure: a rest and exercise hemodynamic study. *Circulation.* 1983;67:807–816.

28. Cody RJ, Laragh JH. Use of captopril to estimate renin-angiotensin-aldosterone activity in the pathophysiology of chronic heart failure. *Am Heart J.* 1982;104:1184–1189.

29. Packer M, Medina N, Yushak M, et al. Hemodynamic patterns of response during long-term captopril therapy for severe chronic heart failure. *Circulation.* 1983;68:803–812.

30. Packer M, Medina N, Yushak M. Relationship between serum sodium concentrations and the hemodynamic and clinical response to converting enzyme inhibition with captopril in severe heart failure. *J Am Coll Cardiol.* 1984;3:1035–1043.

31. Captopril Multicenter Research Group. A placebo-controlled trial of captopril in refractory chronic congestive heart failure. *J Am Coll Cardiol.* 1983;2:755–763.

32. Sharpe DN, Murphy J. Enalapril in patients with chronic heart failure: a placebo-controlled, randomized, double-blind study. *Circulation.* 1984;70:271–278.

33. Cleland JGF, Dargie HJ, Hodsman GP, et al. Captopril in heart failure. A double blind controlled trial. *Br Heart J.* 1984;52:530–535.

34. Massie BM. Exercise tolerance in congestive heart failure: role of cardiac function, peripheral blood flow and muscle metabolism, and effect of treatment. *Am J Med.* 1988;84(Suppl 3A);75–82.

35. Mancini DM, Davis L, Wexler JP, et al. Dependence of enhanced maximal exercise performance on increased peak skeletal muscle perfusion during long-term captopril therapy in heart failure. *J Am Coll Cardiol.* 1987;845–850.

36. Drexler H, Banhardt U, Meinhertz T, et al. Contrasting peripheral short-term and long-term effects of converting enzyme inhibition in patients with congestive heart failure. A double-blind, placebo-controlled trial. *Circulation.* 1989;79:491–502.

37. Swartz SL, Williams GH. Angiotensin converting enzyme inhibition and prostaglandins. *Am J Cardiol.* 1982;49:1405–1409.

38. Silberhauer K, Punzengruber C, Sinzinger H. Endogenous prostaglandin E_2 metabolite levels, renin-angiotensin system and catecholamines versus acute hemodynamic response to captopril in chronic congestive heart failure. *Cardiology.* 1983;70:297–307.

39. Pitt B. Personal communication.

40. Zimmerman BG, Sybertz EJ, Wong PC. Interrelationship between sympathetic and renin-angiotensin systems. *J Hypertens.* 1984;2:581.

41. Crozier IG, Teoh R, Kay R, et al. Sympathetic nervous system during converting enzyme inhibition. *Am J Med.* 1989;87(Suppl 6B):295–325.

42. Cody RJ, Franklin RW, Kluger J, et al. Mechanisms governing the postural response and baroreceptor abnormalities in chronic congestive heart failure. Effects of acute and long-term converting-enzyme inhibition. *Circulation.* 1982;66:135–142.

43. Riegger GAJ, Kochsiek K. Vasopressin, renin and norepinephrine levels before and after captopril administration in patients with congestive heart failure due to idiopathic dilated cardiomyopathy. *Am J Cardiol.* 1986;58:300–303.

44. Osterziel KJ, Rohrig N, Dietz R, et al. Influence of captopril on the arterial baroreceptor reflex in patients with heart failure. *Eur Heart J.* 1988;9:1137–1145.

45. Osterziel KJ, Dietz R, Schmid W, et al. ACE inhibition improves vagal reactivity in patients with heart failure. *Am Heart J.* 1990;1120–1129.

46. Horn EM, Corwin SJ, Steinberg SF, et al. Reduced lymphocyte stimulating guanine nucleotide regulatory protein and beta-adrenergic receptors in congestive heart

failure and reversal with angiotensin converting enzyme inhibitor therapy. *Circulation.* 1988;78:1373–1379.

47. Newman TJ, Maskin CJ, Dennick LG, et al. Effects of captopril on survival in patients with heart failure. *Am J Med.* 1988;84(Suppl 3H):140–144.

48. The CONSENSUS Trial Study Group. Effects of enalapril on mortality in severe congestive heart failure: results of the Cooperative North Scandinavian Enalapril Survival Study (CONSENSUS). *N Engl J Med.* 1987;316:1429–1435.

49. The Captopril-Digoxin Multicenter Research Group. Comparative effects of therapy with captopril and digoxin in patients with mild to moderate heart failure. *JAMA.* 1988;259:539–544.

50. The SOLVD Investigators. Effect of enalapril on survival in patients with reduced left ventricular ejection fractions and congestive heart failure. *N Engl J Med.* 1991;325:293–302.

51. The SOLVD Investigators. Effect of enalapril on mortality and the development of heart failure in asymptomatic patients with reduced left ventricular ejection fractions. *N Engl J Med.* 1992;327:685–691.

52. Pfeffer MA, Braunwald E, Moye LA, et al. Effect of captopril on mortality and morbidity in patients with left ventricular dysfunction after myocardial infarction— results of the survival and ventricular enlargement trial. *N Engl J Med.* 1992;327:669–677.

53. Swedberg K, Held P, Kjekshus J, et al. Effects of the early administration of enalapril on mortality in patients with acute myocardial infarction. Results of the Cooperative New Scandinavian Enalapril Survival Study II (CONSENSUS II). *N Engl J Med.* 1992;327:678–684.

54. Cohn JN, Johnson G, Ziesche S, et al. A comparison of enalapril with hydralazine-isosorbide dinitrate in the treatment of chronic congestive heart failure. *N Engl J Med.* 1991;325:303–310.

55. Cohn JN, Archibald DG, Zresche S, et al. Effect of vasodilator therapy mortality in chronic congestive heart failure: results of a VA Cooperative study. *N Engl J Med.* 1986;314:1547–1552.

56. Bayliss J, Norell M, Canepa-Anson R, et al. Untreated heart failure: Clinical and neuroendocrine effects of introducing diuretics. *Br Heart J.* 1987;57:17–22.

57. Ikram H. Haemodynamic and humoral response to acute and chronic furosemide therapy in congestive heart failure. *Clin Sci.* 1980;59:443–449.

58. Richardson A, Bayliss J, Scriven AJ, et al. Double-blind comparison of captopril alone against furosemide plus amiloride in mild heart failure. *Lancet.* 1987;2:709–711.

59. Cowley AJ, Stainer K, Wynne, et al. Symptomatic assessment of patients with heart failure: double blind comparison of increasing doses of diuretics and captopril in moderate heart failure. *Lancet.* 1986;2:770–772.

60. Dzau VJ, Hollenberg NK. Renal response to captopril in severe heart failure: role of furosemide in natriuresis and reversal of hyponatremia. *Ann Intern Med.* 1984;100:777–782.

61. Anand IS, Kalka KS, Ferrari R, et al. Enalapril as sole treatment in severe chronic heart failure with sodium retention. *Int J Cardiol.* 1990;28:341–346.

62. Davies RF, Beanlands DS, Nadeu C, et al. Enalapril versus digoxin in patients with congestive heart failure: a multicenter study. *J Am Coll Cardiol.* 1991;18:1602–1609.

63. Gheorghiade M, Hall V, Lakier JB, et al. Comparative hemodynamic and neurohormonal effects of intravenous captopril and digoxin and their combination in patients with severe heart failure. *J Am Coll Cardiol.* 1989;13:134–142.

64. Packer M, Gheorghiade M, Young JB, et al. Randomized, double-blind, placebo-controlled, withdrawal study of digoxin in patients with chronic heart failure treated with converting-enzyme inhibitors. *J Am Coll Cardiol.* 1992;260A. Abstract.

65. Fonarow G, Chelinsky-Fallick C, Stevenson LW, et al. Reduction of sudden death by therapy with angiotensin-converting enzyme inhibition compared to direct vasodilation: a randomized trial. *Clin Res.* 1991;39:48A. Abstract.

66. Bayliss J, Norell MS, Canepa-Anson R, et al. Clinical importance of the renin-angiotensin system in chronic heart failure: double-blind comparison of captopril and prazosin. *Br Med J.* 1985;290:1861–1865.

67. Mettauer B, Rouleau J-L, Bichet D, et al. Differential long-term intrarenal and neurohormonal effects of captopril and prazosin in patients with chronic congestive heart failure: importance of initial plasma renin activity. *Circulation.* 1986;73:492–502.

68. Schofield PM, Brooke NH, Lawrence GP, et al. Which vasodilator drug in patients with chronic heart failure? A randomized comparison of captopril and hydralazine. *Br J Clin Pharmacol.* 1991;31:25–32.

69. Wilkes NPF, Barin E, Hoschl R, et al. Comparison of the immediate and long-term effects of captopril and isosorbide dinitrate as adjunctive treatment in mild heart failure. *Br J Clin Pharmacol.* 1989;28:427–434.

70. Goldstein RE, Boccuzzi SJ, Cruess D, et al. Diltiazem increases late-onset congestive heart failure in postinfarction patients with early reduction in ejection fraction. *Circulation.* 1991;83:52–60.

71. Elkayam U, Amin J, Mehra A, et al. A prospective, randomized double-blind crossover study to compare the efficacy and safety of chronic nifedipine therapy with that of isosorbide dinitrate and their combinations in the treatment of chronic congestive heart failure. *Circulation.* 1990;82:1954–1961.

72. The Multicenter Postinfarction Trial Research Group. The effect of diltiazem on mortality and reinfarction after myocardial infarction. *N Engl J Med.* 1988;319:385–392.

73. Agostoni PG, deCesare N, Doria E, et al. Afterload reduction: a comparison of captopril and nifedipine in dilated cardiomyopathy. *Br Heart J.* 1986;55:391–399.

74a. Massie BM, Packer M, Hanlon JT, et al. Combined captopril and hydralazine therapy for refractory heart failure. *J Am Coll Cardiol.* 1983;2:338–345.

74b. Massie BM, Berk MR, Brozena SC, et al. Can further benefit be achieved by adding flosequinan to patients with congestive heart failure who remain symptomatic on diuretics, digoxin, and an angiotensin converting enzyme inhibitor? Results of the Flosequinan plus ACE Inhibitor Trial. *Circulation.* 1993 (in press for September).

75. Massie BM. All patients with left ventricular systolic dysfunction should be treated with an angiotensin-converting enzyme inhibitor: a protagonist's viewpoint. *Am J Cardiol.* 1990;66:439–443.

76. Pfeffer MA, Braunwald E. Ventricular remodelling after myocardial infarction: experimental observations and clinical implications. *Circulation.* 1990;81:1161–1172.

77. Pfeffer MA, Lamas GA, Vaughen DE, et al. Effect of captopril and progressive ventricular dilatation after anterior myocardial infarction. *N Engl J Med.* 1988; 319:80–86.

78. Sharpe N, Murphy J, Smith H, et al. Treatment of patients with symptomless left ventricular dysfunction after myocardial infarction. *Lancet.* 1988;1:255–259.

79. Sharpe N, Smith H, Murphy J, et al. Early prevention of left ventricular dysfunction after myocardial infarction with angiotensin-converting-enzyme inhibition. *Lancet.* 1991;337:872–876.

80. Oldroyd KG, Rye MP, Ray SG, et al. Effects of early captopril administration on infarct expansion, left ventricular remodelling and exercise capacity after acute myocardial infarction. *Am J Cardiol.* 1991;68:713–718.

81. Ferreira SH. History of the development of inhibitors of angiotensin I conversion. *Drugs.* 1985;30(Suppl 1):1–5.

82. Salvetti A. Newer ACE inhibitors. A look to the future. *Drugs.* 1990;40:800–822.

83. Cushman DW, Cheung HS, Sabo EF. Design of new antihypertensive drugs: potent and specific inhibitors of angiotensin-converting enzyme. *Prog Cardiovasc Dis.* 1978;21:176–182.

84. Kubo SH, Cody RJ. Clinical pharmacokinetics of angiotensin converting enzyme inhibitors. *Clin Pharmacokin et.* 1985;10:377–391.

85. Cody RJ. Pharmacology of angiotensin-converting enzyme inhibitors as a guide to their use in congestive heart failure. *Am J Cardiol.* 1990;60(Suppl D):7D–11D.

86. Schwartz JB, Taylor A, Abernathy D. Pharmacokinetics and pharmacodynamics of enalapril in patients with congestive heart failure and patients with hypertension. *J Cardiovasc Pharmacol.* 1985;7:767–776.

87. MacFadyen RJ, Lees KR, Reid JL. Differences in first dose response to angiotensin converting enzyme inhibition in congestive heart failure in a placebo controlled study. *Br Heart J.* 1991;66:206–211.

88. Hirsch AT, Talsness CE, Smith AD, et al. Captopril vs enalapril: Differential effects on tissue converting enzyme in experimental heart failure. *Circulation.* 1990;82–274. Abstract.

89. Packer M, Lee WH, Yushak M, et al. Comparison of captopril and enalapril in patients with severe chronic heart failure. *N Engl J Med.* 1986;315:847–853.

90. Pouleur H, Rousseau MF, Oakley C, et al. Differences in mortality between patients treated with captopril or enalapril in the Xamaterol in Severe Heart Failure Study. *Am J Cardiol.* 1991;68:71–74.

91. Chalmers JP, West MJ, Cyran J, et al. Placebo-controlled study of lisinopril in congestive heart failure: a multicenter study. *J Cardiovasc Pharmacol.* 1987; 9(Suppl 3):S89–S97.

92. Giles TD, Katz R, Sullivan JM, et al. Short- and long-acting angiotensin-converting enzyme inhibition: a randomized trial of lisinopril vs captopril in the treatment of congestive heart failure. *J Am Coll Cardiol.* 1989;13:1240–1247.

93. Bounhoure JP, Bettineau G, Lechat P, et al. Value of perindopril in the treatment of chronic congestive heart failure. Multicenter double-blind placebo-controlled study. *Clin Exp Hypertens.* 1989;11(Suppl 2):575–586.

94. Kjekshus J, Swedberg K. Tolerability of enalapril in congestive heart failure. *Am J Cardiol.* 1988;62(Suppl A):67A–72A.

95. Cleland JGF, Dargie HJ, McAlpine H, et al. Severe hypotension after first dose of enalapril in heart failure. *Br Med J.* 1985;291:1309–1312.

96. Gottlieb SS, Weir MR. Renal effects of angiotensin-converting enzyme inhibition in congestive heart failure. *Am J Cardiol.* 1990;66(Suppl D):14D–20D.

97. Pierpont GL, Francis GS, Cohn JN. Effect of captopril on renal function in patients with congestive heart failure. *Br Heart J.* 1981;46:522–527.

98. Cleland JG, Dargie HJ, Gillen G. Captopril in heart failure: a double-blind study of the effects on renal function. *J Cardiovasc Pharmacol.* 1986;8:700–706.

99. Brown C, Rush J. Risk factors for the development of hyperkalemla in patients treated with enalapril for heart failure. *Clin Pharmacol Ther.* 1989;45:167. Abstract.

100. Packer M, Lee WH, Medina N, et al. Influence of diabetes mellitus on changes in left ventricular performance and renal function produced by converting enzyme inhibition in patients with severe chronic heart failure. *Am J Med.* 1987;82:1119–1126.

101. Sebastian JL, McKinney WP, Kaufman J, et al. Angiotensin-converting enzyme inhibitors and cough. Prevalence in an outpatient medical clinic population. *Chest.* 1991;99:36–39.

102. Chin HL, Buchan DA. Severe angioedema after long-term use of an angiotensin converting enzyme inhibitor. *Ann Intern Med.* 1990;112:312–313.

103. Orfan N, Patterson K, Dykewicz MS. Severe angioedema related to ACE inhibitors in patients with a history of idiopathy angioedema. *JAMA.* 1990;264: 1287–1289.

24
Vasodilators

Garrie J. Haas and Carl V. Leier

The primary objective of vasodilator therapy is to "un-load" the volume- or pressure-overloaded heart. The unloading can be aimed at diastole with interventions directed at reducing elevated ventricular diastolic pressure or volume (commonly referred to as "preload reduction") or at systole with interventions directed at reducing elevated aortic-pulmonic impedance and vascular resistance (referred to as "afterload reduction").

Burch[1] published the observation in 1956 that markedly increased venous tone and symptoms of congestive heart failure (CHF) can be reduced with sympatholytic (hexamethonium) vasodilatation; however, the introduction of vasodilator therapy as a major intervention for heart failure occurred in the late 1960s and early 1970s. Gould and colleagues[2] reported in 1969 that the α-adrenergic blocker, phentolamine, improved hemodynamics and the clinical status of patients with heart failure; these observations were confirmed in 1971 by Majid et al.[3] Nitroprusside was noted to augment hemodynamics and improve the clinical condition of postinfarction patients with heart failure, as reported in 1972 by Franciosa and colleagues.[4]

The recognition and acceptance by the medical community of vasodilator therapy as a major intervention for CHF can be attributed perhaps to four pivotal events. The introduction of the flow-directed pulmonary artery catheter, directed initially at the management of circulatory block, greatly facilitated the investigation of CHF and the role of vasodilators in therapeutics of this condition. Second, utilizing the vast distribution and readership of the *New England Journal of Medicine*, the article "Vasodilator Therapy of Cardiac Failure" by Cohn and Franciosa[5] in 1977 greatly disseminated this concept, particularly at academic medical centers. Third, the introduction and effectiveness of converting enzyme inhibitors in the management of heart failure expanded for many physicians the classic and almost sacred combination, digitalis-diuretics, into triple therapy, digitalis-diuretics-vasodilators. Last, the

reports of the V-HeFT[6] (1986) and CONSENSUS[7] (1987) trials, demonstrating in large heart failure populations that vasodilator therapy in the form of hydralazine-nitrates and converting enzyme inhibitors, respectively, also improves survival, have forced all physicians managing heart failure to consider whether it is ethical to withhold vasodilator therapy from any patient burdened with this high-mortality condition.

Unloading the failing heart, particularly in the form of preload reduction, was likely practiced on a regular basis by the very first person ever afflicted with CHF when he noted that most upright positions were associated with less dyspnea and greater overall comfort than any horizontal position. More "sophisticated" forms of preload reduction were developed over the ensuing millennia and included blood-letting, drainage procedures for ascites and tissue edema, hydragogue cathartics, and sudorific agents. Diuretics, introduced well over a century ago in the form of mercury-containing compounds (e.g., calomel), proved to be a very effective and a surviving form of preload reduction (and to some extent, afterload reduction as well). Digitalis, a complex agent used for more than 200 years in the management of heart failure, delivers much of its favorable pharmacologic effects via preload and afterload reduction.[8]

This chapter discusses the vasodilator drugs most commonly studied and employed in the management of heart failure. The converting enzyme inhibitor form of vasodilatation is presented elsewhere in this book.

Vasodilators: Rationale for Use in Congestive Heart Failure

The primary objective of vasodilator therapy in CHF is afterload and/or preload reduction of the failing ventricle. However, as depicted in Table 24.1 and discussed below, vasodilators can elicit a number of other favorable effects in this clinical setting.

TABLE 24.1. Objectives and potential benefits of vasodilator therapy in CHF.

*Primary objectives**
Afterload reduction (right and left heart)
Preload reduction (right and left heart)

   *General aim: improve clinical status, sense of well-being, activity/ exercise capacity, and survival.

Secondary objectives and other potential benefits
Improvement of ventricular diastolic function
Favorable effect on myocardial energetics
Reduction of valvular regurgitation
Reduction of ventricular remodeling
Regression of myocardial hypertrophy
Favorable effect on atrial size, function, and rhythms
Augmentation of regional blood flow
Less hospitalization
Favorable effect on survival

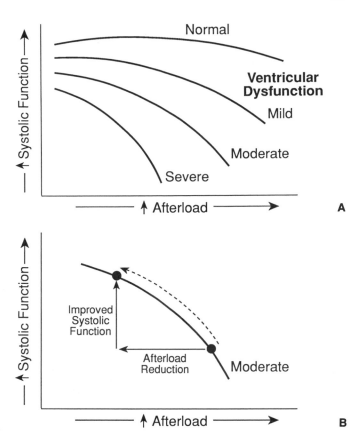

FIGURE 24.1. **A:** The relationship between ventricular afterload and systolic function for normal and failing ventricles. Adapted, with permission, from ref. 5. Copyright by the New England Journal of Medicine. **B:** Schematic representation of how vasodilator therapy augments ventricular systolic function by reducing ventricular afterload.

Primary Objectives of Vasodilator Therapy

Afterload Reduction

Ventricular afterload (ventricular wall stress during systole) has a major influence on ventricular systolic performance.[5,9–14] As discussed in several other sections of this book, ventricular afterload rises in most patients with heart failure because of an increase in one or more of the following determinants of afterload: ventricular systolic volume, characteristic aortic impedance, systemic vascular resistance, reflected arterial waves (earlier occurrence and accentuation), and for some, ventricular systolic pressure. Insufficient myocardial hypertrophy (inadequate relative to required ventricular work) may contribute as well.

Excessive afterload has a devastating effect on ventricular function in heart failure (Fig. 24.1A). The magnitude of the detrimental effect is proportional to the degree of ventricular failure. In addition, the ventricles with more severe dysfunction usually are afflicted with the greatest afterload and are those whose systolic function can least sustain any increase in afterload.

Afterload reduction via vasodilator therapy therefore is directed at reducing the excessive ventricular afterload or wall stress of CHF with resultant augmentation of ventricular systolic function, stroke volume, cardiac output, and overall cardiovascular performance (Fig. 24.1B). This therapeutic principle has now been well established in more than 500 publications addressing the hemodynamic responses of human heart failure to a wide variety of cardiovascular-active compounds. In addition to the general group of vasodilator drugs, afterload reduction is an important component of the cardiovascular pharmacology of the converting enzyme inhibitors, digitalis, some of the intravenously adminis-

tered positive inotropic drugs (e.g., dobutamine), diuretics, phosphodiesterase inhibitors, and others.

Preload Reduction

As presented elsewhere in this book ventricular preload (cardiomyocyte stretch at end-diastole) increases in most forms of CHF secondary to an expansion of intravascular (hence, intracardiac) volume via fluid retention by the kidney, neurogenic and hormonal venoconstriction, and elevated afterload. An increase in preload or end-diastolic actin-myosin stretch is generally accompanied by augmentation of ventricular systolic function (Fig. 24.2A), a concept commonly referred to as the Frank-Starling relationship.[15] For many patients with heart failure, this rise in ventricular preload evokes the essential improvement in ventricular systolic function to keep the patient in an adequately compensated state of cardiovascular performance despite an underlying cardiac disorder (Fig. 24.2B); in this setting, the rise in ventricular preload often is referred to as one of the "compensatory responses" to cardiac ventricular dysfunction.

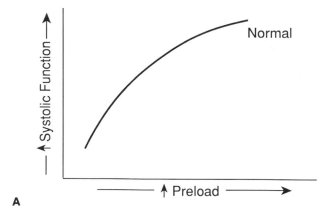

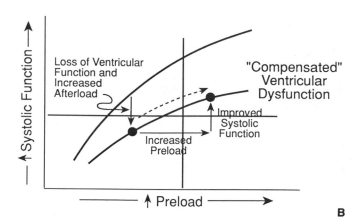

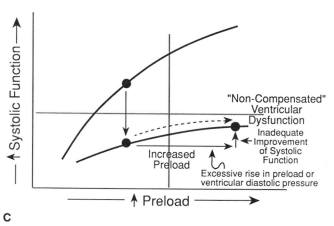

FIGURE 24.2. **A:** The Frank-Starling mechanism relating ventricular preload (as determined by ventricular diastolic volume and pressure) to ventricular systolic function. **B:** Schematic representation of how a rise in preload can improve systolic function and bring a patient into the range of "compensated" ventricular dysfunction after a myocardial insult and resultant rise in afterload. **C:** With severe loss of ventricular function, the marked rise in preload (to the point of large elevations in ventricular end-diastolic pressure and volume) is not capable of evoking an adequate increase in ventricular systolic function. The patient remains in a decompensated state of cardiac dysfunction, characterized by the clinical and hemodynamic manifestations of low cardiac output and markedly elevated ventricular filling pressures.

In patients with severe "decompensated" ventricular dysfunction, the rise in preload does not elicit a sufficient augmentation of ventricular systolic function, even with a marked increase in preload (Fig. 24.2C). In fact, for most of these patients, the systolic function/preload curve is relatively flat, such that any increase in ventricular end-diastolic pressure or volume (i.e., preload) is accompanied by only modest augmentation of systolic function. The persistent depression of stroke work and volume and cardiac output perpetuates the mechanisms responsible for fluid retention, venoconstriction, and excessive afterload such that preload increases further and enters the "excessive preload" stage (Figs. 24.2C, 24.3); this represents a stage in which any additional increase in preload evokes little to no improvement in systolic function (Fig. 24.2C) and represents the region of the ventricular diastolic pressure-volume curve in which any additional increase in intravascular volume or pressure is accompanied by a steep rise in intraventricular pressure with little to no additional increase in ventricular volume (Fig. 24.3). Basically, ventricular end-diastolic pressures rise to high levels (>20 mm Hg) with accompanying signs and symptoms of such ("congestion") without an adequate stroke volume and cardiac output.

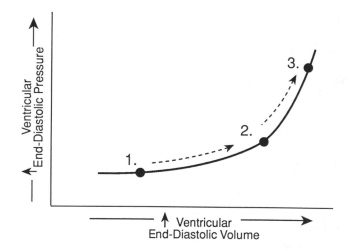

FIGURE 24.3. Graph relating left ventricular end-diastolic pressure to volume. At low to moderate levels of ventricular end-diastolic pressure or volume (*1* to *2*), mild changes in ventricular pressure effect a substantial increase in ventricular volume or preload. At high levels of ventricular end-diastolic pressure and volume (*2* to *3*), any additional increase in pressure is accompanied by only a modest increase in preload or volume [or any additional increase in preload or ventricular volume at this point (*3*) requires a marked increase in end-diastolic pressure].

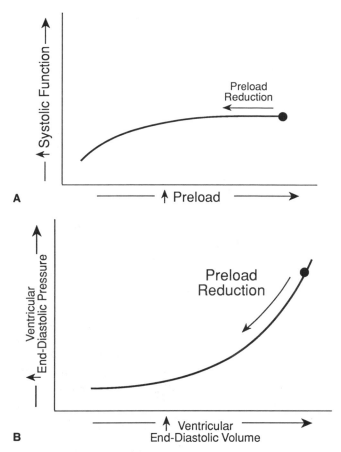

A

B

FIGURE 24.4. Preload reduction therapy is directed at decreasing excessive preload by reducing ventricular end-diastolic pressure and volume; schematically depicted on the Frank-Starling curve (**A**) and the ventricular diastolic pressure-volume curve (**B**). The fundamental therapeutic objective of preload reduction therapy is to lower excessively elevated ventricular end-diastolic (filling) pressures and control the accompanying "congestive" symptoms.

Preload reduction therapy therefore is directed at decreasing excessive preload (Fig. 24.4) and its accompanying signs and symptoms by intercepting the factors responsible for elevated ventricular end-diastolic pressure and volume; specifically, dietary measures (salt restriction) and diuretics are aimed at countering the fluid retention of CHF, venodilator drugs (e.g., nitrates) the venoconstriction, and afterload-reducing drugs the heightened ventricular afterload.

Combined Afterload-Preload Reduction

It is naive to think that vasodilator drugs can be distinctly separated into those that achieve only afterload reduction, and those directed at preload reduction alone. All agents with predominant afterload-reducing properties also drop preload via a number of mechanisms, including enhanced systolic emptying of the ven-

tricle and for many patients, less valvular regurgitation. Conversely, the predominantly preload-reducing drugs can favorably affect afterload by reducing ventricular volume, general sympathetic nervous system tone (by improving symptoms), and others. The separation of vasodilators into these two drug groups is made merely to facilitate a methodical presentation and a better understanding of the pharmacophysiology of these agents.

The conceptional separation of vasodilator therapy into drugs that predominantly alter afterload and those predominantly affecting preload also assists in the clinical application of these agents. Certain heart failure conditions (e.g., valvular regurgitation) are treated with drugs that have a major effect on ventricular afterload and other conditions (e.g., diastolic dysfunction) with agents having their primary effect on ventricular preload or filling pressures. In general, most patients with CHF are approached with vasodilator therapy directed at reducing both afterload and preload in varying degrees.

Secondary Objectives and Other Potential Benefits of Vasodilator Therapy in CHF

Improvement of Ventricular Diastolic Function

Diastolic dysfunction of the ventricle is secondary to impaired ventricular relaxation and/or reduced ventricular compliance.[16–19] Most heart failure patients with diastolic dysfunction have reduced ventricular compliance, graphically represented by a steep ventricular diastolic pressure-volume curve (Fig. 24.5A). With expansion of intravascular volume and/or venoconstriction, the shift in blood volume centrally is accompanied by a dramatic rise in ventricular diastolic pressure with little change in ventricular diastolic volume, cardiomyocyte lengthening, and actin-myosin stretch. Thus, actual cellular preload (actin-myosin stretch) in these patients is not substantially increased despite high ventricular end-diastolic pressures. The rather dramatic and large rise in ventricular filling pressures in these patients accounts for their symptoms and physical signs of "congestion" without cardiomegaly or even resting systolic dysfunction; this clinical condition is referred to as diastolic heart failure, CHF with normal systolic function, and a number of other similar terms. Most patients with CHF have some degree of ventricular diastolic dysfunction ranging from mild, even in the presence of severe systolic dysfunction, to marked, often noted in patients with little to no impairment of resting ventricular systolic function.

Preload-reducing agents in this condition are clinically directed at lowering excessively elevated ventricular diastolic pressures and diminishing the signs and symp-

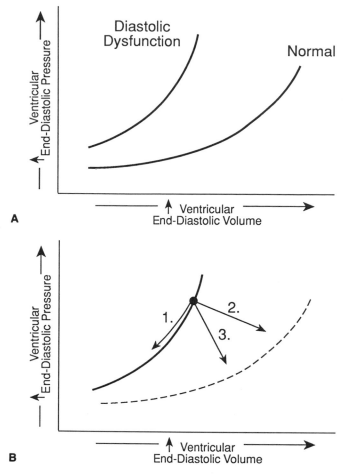

A

B

FIGURE 24.5. **A**: Diastolic pressure-volume curves of a normal ventricle and a ventricle with diminished compliance (diastolic dysfunction). **B**: Excessively elevated ventricular filling pressure (and associated symptoms) in patients with congestion secondary to diastolic dysfunction can be reduced by decreasing intraventricular volume via diuretics or venodilators (*1*), by improving ventricular diastolic function (*2*), or both (*3*).

toms of congestion. This is accomplished by two means (Fig. 24.5B).

First, one can move down the steep diastolic pressure-volume curve and thus drop the excessively elevated intraventricular diastolic pressure by reducing ventricular diastolic volume; this can be achieved by decreasing intravascular volume (e.g., diuretics) or by effecting a central-to-peripheral shift in blood volume via systemic venodilatation (e.g., nitrates). These two interventions represent the primary means of reducing high end-diastolic pressure and symptoms in the patient whose diastolic dysfunction is secondary to fixed structural myocardial disease (e.g., myocardial fibrosis, amyloidosis). It is important to note that these patients experience a rapid and marked rise in ventricular diastolic pressure with even mild increases in ventricular diastolic filling. Conversely, from a therapeutic standpoint, it is important to recognize that frequently it

takes little diuresis and/or venodilator therapy to effect a dramatic and potentially symptomatic (hypotension, weakness, malaise) fall in ventricular diastolic pressure in these patients. The "art" of therapeutics in this situation is to judiciously employ the aforementioned agents that drop the markedly elevated ventricular diastolic pressures for the purpose of ameliorating the symptoms of congestion, but avoid an excessive reduction in ventricular diastolic pressure, which leads to systolic dysfunction and accompaning low-output symptoms. The optimal ventricular filling pressures in patients with predominantly diastolic CHF usually fall into a very narrow range.

Second, therapy can be directed at reducing elevated ventricular diastolic pressures by improving ventricular compliance (Fig. 24.5B); this generally is accomplished only in patients with reversible "metabolic" ventricular stiffness. Myocardial ischemia is perhaps the most common cause of reversible, metabolic diastolic dysfunction.[16,20–22] Augmentation of myocardial perfusion is the likely mechanism explaining the favorable clinical response of patients with ischemic-diastolic dysfunction to chronic therapy with nitrates, calcium channel blocking drugs, and perhaps β-adrenergic blocking drugs. Improvement of calcium transport and exchange within the cardiomyocyte theoretically can serve as a contributory mechanism explaining the effectiveness of the aforementioned drug groups, particularly in patients not afflicted with myocardial ischemia.

Myocardial hypertrophy is another common cause of reduced ventricular compliance.[23–25] For most patients, myocardial hypertrophy is secondary to chronic pressure and/or volume overload and is, at least, partially reversible with proper management of the underlying causative condition (e.g., antihypertensive therapy for systemic hypertension, valve replacement for aortic stenosis).[26,27] Myocardial cellular hypertrophy and fibrosis may explain the development of varying degrees of diastolic dysfunction with age.[28]

Left ventricular compliance and filling can be affected adversely by a number of other conditions. The pericardium itself can restrict ventricular diastolic filling in cardiomegalic conditions. Right ventricular enlargement and filling within the confines of a fixed pericardial space can encroach on left ventricular diastolic volume via a leftward shift of the interventricular septum.[29,30] Elevated right heart pressures also increase coronary sinus pressure leading to a rise in intramyocardial venous and interstitial pressure with resultant reduced ventricular compliance.[31] Thus, preload reduction therapy with venodilators or diuretics also can favorably affect left ventricular compliance and filling by reducing right heart volume and pressure.

It is interesting to note that preload reduction therapy, which improves ventricular compliance (e.g., nitrates) in patients with reversible diastolic dysfunction, actually may increase preload. As ventricular compliance improves, the same or any rise in central blood volume effects a greater increase in ventricular diastolic volume, cardiomyocyte lengthening, and actin-myosin stretch. Cellular preload thus can be favorably increased at a lower ventricular filling pressure to maintain or improve ventricular systolic function.

Favorable Effect on Myocardial Energetics

By reducing ventricular systolic wall stress through afterload reduction and diastolic wall stress through preload reduction, vasodilator therapy invariably reduces myocardial oxygen consumption of the failing heart. This effect is obviously beneficial to patients with occlusive coronary artery disease and myocardial ischemia. Some of the vasodilators also may augment coronary blood flow and myocardial perfusion.

It is likely that myocardial energetics are disturbed in most advanced stages of dilated cardiomyopathy (DCM), even in the absence of occlusive coronary artery disease.[32,33] In this clinical setting, myocardial oxygen consumption is elevated relative to any ventricular work or power output because of elevated ventricular wall stress and heart rate. Coronary blood flow, myocardial perfusion, and oxygen delivery are reduced because of a decrease in coronary perfusion pressure (ventricular end-diastolic pressure rises while aortic diastolic pressure remains unchanged or falls) and coronary perfusion time (diastolic perfusion time falls as heart rate rises). Several lines of evidence support the hypothesis that patients in the very advanced stages of DCM are afflicted with subendocardial ischemia, which perpetuates the heart failure process.[32]

By reducing myocardial oxygen consumption and enhancing myocardial perfusion, vasodilatory therapy has a favorable effect on myocardial energetics in heart failure with resultant augmentation of systolic and diastolic performance.[32,33] It is likely that much of the sustained hemodynamic and clinical improvement noted after 72-hr infusions of nitrates or dobutamine in patients with end-stage DCM and severe CHF are secondary to the vasodilating properties of these drugs with consequent reduction of subendocardial ischemia and improvement of disturbed myocardial energetics.[32,34,35]

Reduction of Valvular Regurgitation

All forms of valvular regurgitation are burdensome to the failing heart.[36–45] These lesions not only reduce forward or "effective" cardiac output, but they also accentuate the problem of ventricular volume overload. Ventricular diastolic volume and wall stress rise further to accommodate the additional regurgitant volume.

Afterload reduction decreases the degree and clinical consequences of aortic and mitral valvular regurgitation.[36–45] This form of therapy is quite effective in ameliorating symptoms and controlling the hemodynamic deterioration of acute aortic or mitral regurgitation until the necessary diagnostic studies are completed and a definitive surgical procedure is performed; nitroprusside is employed most commonly for afterload reduction in these acute conditions.[39,41,44] Hydralazine and converting enzyme inhibitors currently are used to reduce afterload in patients with nonsurgical chronic valvular regurgitation.[42,45]

A relatively high percentage of patients with chronic CHF have some degree of mitral regurgitation. Strauss and colleagues[36] found at least moderate degrees of mitral regurgitation in each of 50 patients referred for heart failure management or cardiac transplantation. Patients with ischemic cardiac disease or DCM are particularly susceptible to the development of chronic mitral regurgitation. Papillary muscle dysfunction and regional wall motion abnormalities are the common mechanisms for mitral regurgitation in ischemic cardiac disease and distortion of the mitral valve complex from dilatation of the left ventricle, left atrium, and mitral annulus accounts for the regurgitation in DCM. Evidence is accruing to suggest that mitral regurgitation often is a hemodynamically and clinically significant lesion in chronic heart failure, that it can play a major role in the decompensation of these patients, and that much of the hemodynamic and clinical benefit derived from chronic vasodilator therapy probably is mediated through a reduction in the severity of mitral regurgitation.

Reduction of Ventricular Remodeling

Ventricular remodeling is a complication of a significant insult to the myocardium (e.g., myocardial infarction, myocarditis). After a sizable myocardial infarction, the ventricular cavity enlarges and assumes a spherical shape as it evolves into a state of dysfunction and failure.[46–48] Converting enzyme inhibition (specifically captopril) has been shown to be effective in preventing much of the cardiomegaly, remodeling, and heart failure after myocardial infarction.[49,49a] It is likely that this favorable effect is mediated through afterload and/or preload reduction. Long-term nitrate therapy averts ventricular remodeling in a canine model of discrete myocardial damage.[49b]

Although ventricular remodeling has been systematically studied primarily in the postinfarction setting,[46–49a] it is obviously the process whereby a normal ventricle evolves into a large spherical hypokinetic chamber when its myocardium becomes afflicted with the diseases causing DCM. It is likely that vasodilator therapy can avert this detrimental process when administered at the very earliest stages of this condition, but this hypothesis remains to be tested. From a practical standpoint, finding patients in the very early presymptomatic stage of DCM is a most difficult challenge and finding them in the predilated stage, when remodeling prevention therapy should be most effective, is yet more difficult. Long-term therapy with converting enzyme inhibitors appears to retard the progression of left ventricular enlargment and dysfunction in patients already afflicted with cardiomegaly and chronic heart failure.[49c]

Regression of Myocardial Hypertrophy

Interventions that successfully unload pressure- and volume-overloaded ventricles generally effect a regression of myocardial hypertrophy.[26,27,50–54] Ventricular hypertrophy can adversely affect overall cardiac performance and a patient's clinical status through a greater predisposition for myocardial ischemia, enhanced myocardial fibrosis, diastolic dysfunction, conversion of myosin type, eventual systolic dysfunction, myocardial inefficiency (less work output per myocardial mass or oxygen consumption), and enhanced cardiovascular morbidity and mortality.[23–27,53–57] Antihypertensive therapy evokes a regression of ventricular muscle mass in chronic systemic hypertension.[50–53] Chronic vasodilator therapy in CHF with hydralazine or the hydralazine-nitrate combination has been shown to reduce ventricular myocardial cell size and normalize the high energy phosphate content of the subendocardium.[54,58]

Favorable Effects on Atrial Size, Function, and Rhythm

Atrial enlargement is associated with atrial arrhythmias, atrial thrombi and embolization, and impaired contractility (atrial systolic dysfunction). Atrial enlargement occurs as a result of chronic volume or pressure overload and/or atrial myopathy.

Hamilton and colleagues[59] have shown that in patients with CHF, acute vasodilator and diuretic therapy can reduce atrial size by 18% to 24% secondary to a substantial therapy-induced fall in ventricular filling pressures and in the degree of tricuspid and mitral valvular regurgitation. Long-term vasodilator therapy is likely to have a favorable effect on atrial remodeling, volume, function, and rhythms via chronic preload and afterload reduction of the atria.

Augmentation of Regional Blood Flow

In the setting of CHF, certain vasodilators can selectively enhance regional or organ blood flow.[60] Nitroprusside evokes a favorable renal hemodynamic response with some accompanying improvement in overall renal function.[60–62] Hydralazine usually increases limb and renal blood flow,[63] and the calcium channel blocking agent, nifedipine, tends preferentially to increase limb

blood flow.[64] Vasodilation with α_1-adrenergic blocking drugs (e.g., prazosin) generally augments visceral (hepatic-splanchnic) blood flow.[60,63]

It is important to note that vasodilators also may have an adverse effect on regional blood flow and the distribution of cardiac output. Intravenously administered nitrates and oral isosorbide dinitrate in heart failure evoke a smaller reduction in renal vascular resistance than that of other regions, and thus may redistribute blood away from the kidneys.[61,65] This observation may account for some of the fluid retention, expanded intravascular volume, and pharmacodynamic tolerance to nitrates during continuous or long-term nitrate therapy.

Less Hospitalization

Proper vasodilator therapy reduces the frequency and duration of hospitalization for decompensated heart failure. Stevenson and colleagues[66] have convincingly shown that many patients referred for cardiac transplantation can forego this procedure, experience considerable improvement of heart failure symptoms, achieve an earlier hospital discharge, and attain a reasonable survival after a systematic analysis and selection of vasodilator therapy; this represents an important study and advance in an era of an insufficient number of heart donors, a larger population of heart failure victims, and accelerated cost of health care.[66–68]

Favorable Effect on Survival

The V-HeFT trial in a sizable heart failure population demonstrated that the vasodilator combination, hydralazine-isosorbide dinitrate, improved survival.[6] The mechanisms linking vasodilator therapy to improved survival are not known, but are likely related to the effects of "unloading". An increase in ejection fraction was observed in the hydralazine-nitrate–treated group compared to an unchanged ejection fraction for the placebo or prazosin-treated groups. Converting enzyme inhibition also improves survival in human heart failure[7] and may have a more favorable effect on this treatment endpoint than the hydralazine-nitrate combination.[68a]

The drug-induced improvement in survival[6,7] poses the question of whether it is ethical to treat anyone with symptomatic heart failure with a regimen that does not include a converting enzyme inhibitor or the hydralazine-nitrate combination. Ideally, improvement of survival should be a primary objective of heart failure treatment; but from a pragmatic (i.e., realistic) viewpoint, most physicians prescribe vasodilator therapy to reduce symptoms and improve the overall clinical status of their heart failure patients and simply hope also to improve survival as a secondary gain of the therapy.

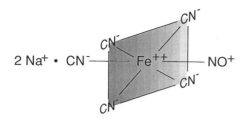

FIGURE 24.6. The sodium nitroprusside molecule.

Nitroprusside

Nitroprusside was one of the vasodilators used in many of the early reports presenting the beneficial clinical and hemodynamic effects of vasodilator therapy in heart failure.[4,5] Nitroprusside and intravenously administered nitroglycerin currently are the primary choices for acute afterload and/or preload reduction and of the two, nitroprusside delivers the most powerful vasodilation.

Basic Pharmacology, Metabolism, and Pharmacokinetics

Nitroprusside is a sodium (or potassium) salt of a complex molecule made up of ferricyanide (Fe^{2+} and five cyanide groups) and nitric acid (Fig. 24.6).[69-71] Although nitroprusside at high doses may evoke a relaxation effect on smooth muscle of other organ systems (e.g., esophagus), this agent displays an overwhelming preference for vascular (arterial and venous) smooth muscle.[69-73] This effect appears to be largely mediated via production of nitrosothiol in vasculature with subsequent generation of cyclic guanosine monophosphate (cGMP) in vascular smooth muscle to evoke relaxation.[72]

Nitroprusside has a rapid onset of action with vasodilating effects detectable within 60 to 90 s of initiating the infusion. Some of the administered nitroprusside decomposes after entering the blood stream with the release of cyanide into the circulation.[73] Additional cyanide is produced when nitroprusside is metabolized by vascular tissue and the liver. Circulating cyanide is metabolized by the liver to thiocyanate, which is then slowly cleared by the kidney (half-life about 3–4 days). Cyanide also is metabolized to prussic acid, which is bound to methemoglobin after it enters the circulation.

Cyanide therefore is a metabolite of nitroprusside that can become elevated to measurable serum concentrations during nitroprusside infusions. However, cyanide toxicity per se is not commonly noted. Prussic acid–methemoglobin and thiocyanate are the usual final metabolic products of nitroprusside. Because of its long half-life, thiocyanate can accumulate during prolonged or high-dose nitroprusside infusions or in the setting of renal dysfunction to evoke signs and symptoms of thiocyanate toxicity.

Cardiovascular Pharmacology in Heart Failure

In normotensive and hypertensive patients, nitroprusside lowers systemic blood pressure and systemic vascular resistance with a variable effect on cardiac output.[74,75] In CHF, a condition of multiple hemodynamic derangements (e.g., elevated systemic and pulmonic vascular resistances, increased ventricular filling pressures, depressed cardiac output), nitroprusside generally elicits a much more favorable overall hemodynamic response (Fig. 24.7).[4,5,14,61,70,76-93]

Preload Reduction

Nitroprusside invariably reduces the excessively elevated ventricular filling pressures and preload in patients with CHF; the mechanisms involved in this hemodynamic response are multiple. Nitroprusside diminishes heightened venous tone,[79] thereby increasing venous capacitance with a resultant peripheral shift of central blood volume. By reducing ventricular afterload, nitroprusside decreases ventricular systolic and diastolic volume and preload via greater ventricular systolic emptying and less valvular regurgitation.[5,39-42,79,83-87] Nitroprusside also may lower ventricular filling pressures by improving ventricular diastolic properties or negating the restraining effect of the pericardium (by lowering intracardiac pressures and volume).[88-91] Augmentation of renal function by nitroprusside may contribute, if accompanied by a diuretic-natriuretic effect, to preload reduction in certain patients[62]; suppressing the heightened neurohormonal responses in acute, severe heart failure by improving hemodynamics may favorably affect preload.[92]

Afterload Reduction

Since nitroprusside has no direct effect on ventricular contractility, the augmentation of stroke volume and cardiac output invariably elicited during its administration in heart failure is secondary to afterload reduction.[5,14,61,79,83-87] Nitroprusside is clinically regarded as one of the most effective and powerful afterload-reducing agents. Afterload reduction with this agent is accomplished by a drug-induced fall in aortic input impedance, systemic and pulmonic vascular resistance, and ventricular systolic volume.

Nitroprusside reduces the major components of aortic impedance, namely, mean vascular load (determined by systemic vascular resistance) and hydraulic vascular load (determined by aortic stiffness and arterial wave reflectance).[83,84] The improvement in ventricular performance, stroke volume, and cardiac output during nitroprusside administration is independent of any change in aortic pressure.[83] In fact, proper patient and dose selection achieves a fall in aortic impedance (↑ aortic compliance, ↓ wave reflectance, ↓ vascular re-

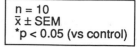

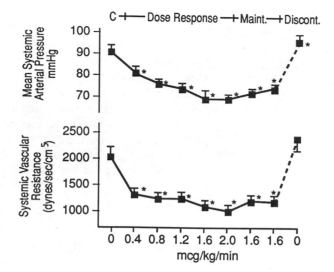

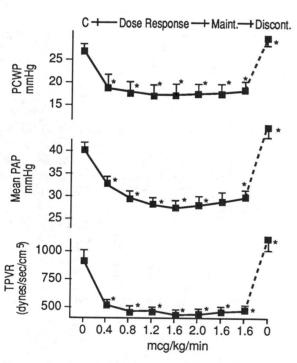

FIGURE 24.7. Central hemodynamic responses to nitroprusside in 10 patients with CHF. Abbreviations: C = baseline control; discont. = discontinuation of the infusion; maint. = maintenance infusion period; mean PAP = mean pulmonary artery pressure; PCWP = pulmonary capillary wedge (arterial occlusive) pressure; TPVR = total pulmonic vascular resistance. Adapted with permission, from ref. 61.

sistance), augmentation of cardiac function (↑ stroke volume, ↑ cardiac output, ↓ ventricular volume and filling pressures), and a drop in excessive preload without a significant reduction in systemic blood pressure or rise in heart rate.

Although often overlooked, afterload reduction of the right heart is likely to be just as important as that of the left heart.[85-87] If both right and left ventricles are burdened with a high afterload, it is unlikely that afterload reduction of the left ventricle alone (if this could be achieved) would evoke a substantial improvement in overall cardiovascular function. Fortunately, measures to "unload" the left heart (e.g., vasodilators, intraaortic balloon counterpulsation) invariably unload the right heart as well (e.g., dropping filling pressures of the left heart drops afterload of the right heart). Within a confined pericardial space, interventions that reduce excessive afterload and volume of the right heart have a favorable effect on the position of the interventricular septum, left heart filling, and thus, left heart diastolic and systolic function. Nitroprusside likely achieves some of its favorable hemodynamic effects through a combination and interaction of these mechanisms.

Effects on Diastolic Function

Although there are multiple methods available to assess ventricular diastolic function, the cumulative data support the general impression that nitroprusside has a favorable effect on overall diastolic function.[88–91] Relaxation time does not change or actually may increase secondary to a greater fall in the left atrial–ventricular diastolic pressure crossover point than in end-systolic pressure.[90] Nitroprusside generally increases early and late diastolic filling and evokes a downward shift in the ventricular diastolic pressure-volume curve (see Fig. 24.5B). Whether the downward shift in the diastolic pressure-volume curve is related to improvement in ventricular compliance, reduced ventricular diastolic volume within the pericardial constraint, or both has not been definitely resolved for human heart failure.

Myocardial Energetics and Coronary Blood Flow

In the setting of CHF, nitroprusside generally lowers myocardial oxygen consumption as measured directly or as estimated by the determination of double or triple product, systolic pressure–time index, systolic stress–time integral, pressure-volume work, and other indirect parameters.[61,93–95] Nitroprusside administration in heart failure has a very favorable effect on the major determinants of myocardial oxygen consumption, specifically systolic and diastolic wall stress, particularly if infused at doses that do not evoke a reflex increase in

neurohormones, renin-angiotensin, heart rate, and ventricular inotropy.

The effect of nitroprusside on coronary hemodynamics has not been extensively studied in human heart failure. In a preliminary report by Powers et al.,[95] nitroprusside (95 $\pm$ 19 μg/min) increased coronary sinus oxygen saturation in 33% of patients with severe CHF and mean coronary blood flow rose 6% despite an average fall in mean systemic arterial pressure of 18 mm Hg. These findings are best explained by a nitroprusside-induced reduction in myocardial oxygen requirements (double product fell 24%) and coronary vascular resistance (calculated coronary vascular resistance fell 22%).

Mechanistically, nitroprusside may favorably affect coronary hemodynamics in heart failure by lowering coronary vascular resistance (direct vasodilating effect plus a lower coronary venous pressure) or by increasing coronary perfusion pressure (at doses that elicit a greater fall in ventricular diastolic pressure than aortic-coronary diastolic pressure). Diastolic perfusion time itself is not significantly altered in heart failure by nitroprusside.[80] Data are available to suggest that the response of coronary blood flow to nitroprusside in heart failure also follows any evoked change in myocardial oxygen consumption.[95,96] In other words, a drop in myocardial oxygen consumption or in the indirect determinants of such can be accompanied by a fall in coronary blood flow (Fig. 24.8).[61,96]

The question of nitroprusside's effect on coronary blood flow and myocardial perfusion is particularly pertinent to heart failure patients with occlusive coronary artery disease. Nitroprusside administration asso-

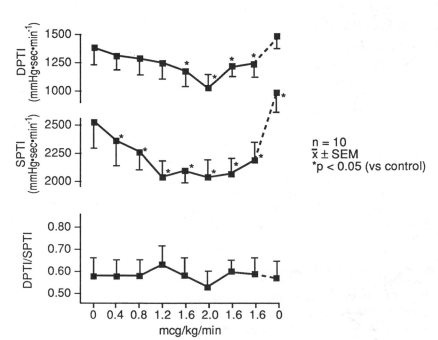

FIGURE 24.8. Changes in diastolic pressure-time index (*DPTI*) and systolic pressure-time index (*SPTI*) during nitroprusside administration in CHF. DPTI and SPTI represent formulations of major determinants of myocardial oxygen supply and demand respectively. Adapted, with permission, from ref. 61.

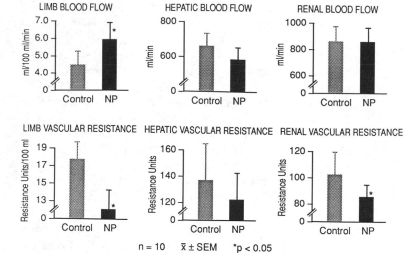

Figure 24.9. Regional hemodynamic responses to a standard maintenance infusion of nitroprusside (*NP*) in CHF. See Fig. 24.7 (*maint.*) for concomitant central hemodynamic responses. Adapted, with permission, from ref. 61.

ciated with a greater reduction in the determinants of myocardial oxygen consumption (excessive afterload and preload) than in the determinants of coronary blood flow and perfusion generally will have a favorable effect on myocardial viability and function and on overall cardiovascular performance.[4,77,78,93,95–98] An infusion-evoking fall in coronary perfusion pressure (by an excessive drop in aortic-coronary diastolic pressure) or diastolic perfusion time (by increasing heart rate), development of coronary "steal", or increase in myocardial oxygen consumption (by increasing heart rate, reflex neurohormonal activation) will adversely affect coronary blood flow and myocardial perfusion.[99,100] A reduction in oxygen-carrying capacity because of elevated methemoglobin levels can adversely affect myocardial oxygenation during prolonged or high-dose nitroprusside infusions.[73]

Regional Blood Flow

In the setting of human CHF, nitroprusside preferentially reduces limb vascular resistance with augmentation of limb blood flow comparable in degree to the rise in cardiac output (see Fig. 24.9).[61] Renal vascular resistance also is reduced in the therapeutic range of nitroprusside[61,101]; however, the resultant renal blood flow is heavily dependent on changes in systemic blood pressure and renal perfusion pressure.[61] Some patients can experience an improvement in overall renal function during a nitroprusside infusion.[62,101] Hepatic-splanchnic vascular resistance and blood flow are not altered significantly during therapeutic infusion rates of nitroprusside.[61]

Neurohormonal Responses

The neurohormonal responses to a nitroprusside infusion in heart failure varies considerably.[92,102] Olivari and colleagues[92] found disparate norepinephrine re-

sponses in a population of heart failure patients. Despite statistically similar resting hemodynamics and comparable hemodynamic responses to nitroprusside, one group (I) experienced an increase in plasma norepinephrine and the other group (II) a decrease during the infusion. The group II patients appeared to be in a more advanced and severe stage of heart failure with a higher mortality than that of group I. Differences in baroreceptor and mechanoreceptor sensitivity and responsivity likely account for the disparate norepinephrine responses of the two groups.

Although not statistically significant, nitroprusside numerically increased mean plasma renin activity 20% above baseline in 36 patients with heart failure.[102]

Clinical Application and Administration

Indications

Nitroprusside is employed most commonly in clinical situations requiring acute, rather aggressive, short-term preload and/or afterload reduction.[4,39,44,70,76–90,93,96–98,101,103–114] The typical patient has a relatively urgent, symptomatic presentation of elevated left ventricular filling and pulmonary capillary wedge pressures (≥ 20 mm Hg), inadequate or ineffective cardiac output with compromised peripheral perfusion, and an "adequate" systemic arterial pressure (≥ 90 mm Hg systolic), but with elevated systemic vascular resistance ($\uparrow\uparrow$ resistance = $\rightarrow$ or $\downarrow$ mean arterial pressure/ $\downarrow\downarrow\downarrow$ cardiac output). The underlying clinical conditions encountered most commonly in this clinical-hemodynamic presentation are a large or complicated acute myocardial infarction, acute valvular insufficiency, acute fulminating myocarditis, and postcardiac surgery/cardiopulmonary bypass.

Nitroprusside should be considered "short-term" intervention (hours to days), because of the potential toxicity of prolonged administration and the relatively poor prognosis of patients who are not advanced to more definitive interventions (e.g., cardiac surgical procedure) when feasible. Nitroprusside, like dopamine and dobutamine, therefore should be viewed generally as a "pharmacologic bridge" to a form of cardiovascular mechanical assist (e.g., intraaortic balloon counterpulsation, ventricular assist devices) and/or surgical repair (e.g., coronary bypass revascularization, valvular replacement). However, nitroprusside is used on occasion to support a patient's cardiovascular condition during an anticipated relatively short decompensated course (e.g., acute decompensation of chronic heart failure).

Acute Myocardial Infarction

Many of the early studies examining the application of afterload reduction in heart failure were performed in the setting of acute myocardial infarction.[4,77,78] Nitroprusside infusions were found to lower ventricular filling pressures into an acceptable range and increase stroke volume, cardiac output, and peripheral perfusion by lowering systemic vascular resistance. Proper dosing averted significant hypotension and reflex tachycardia.

Sublingual or intravenously administered nitroglycerin is generally considered preferable to nitroprusside for most ischemic syndromes because of a theoretically more favorable effect on coronary vasculature, less drug-induced hypotension and postinfusion "rebound," and less methemoglobinemia.[61,99,100,115] However, nitroprusside is indicated as short-term preload/afterload reduction therapy in myocardial infarction complicated by symptomatic, decompensated hemodynamics secondary to marked elevation of systemic blood pressure inadequately controlled with nitroglycerin and intravenously administered β-adrenergic blockade, marked mitral valvular regurgitation (e.g., ruptured papillary muscle), ruptured interventricular septum, and a large infarction symptomatically and hemodynamically refractory to nitroglycerin. Again, it is important to emphasize that for most of these patients, nitroprusside represents a stabilizing pharmacologic bridge to more effective and definitive interventions. Data on clinical status and postinfarction mortality do not convincingly support the routine use of nitroprusside for uncomplicated myocardial infarction, even when accompanied by simple elevation of left ventricular filling pressures.[116,117]

Valvular Regurgitation

Nitroprusside is the most effective pharmacologic intervention for symptomatic, acute valvular insufficiency and severely decompensated chronic valvular insufficiency.[39–42,44,59,103] For the aortic valve, the most common underlying diseases include infectious endocarditis, prolapsed cusp(s), aortic–right heart fistula, and aortic dissection. Acute severe mitral regurgitation can be secondary to ruptured chordae tendinae (e.g., connective tissue disorder, myxomatous disease, bacterial endocarditis, trauma) and papillary muscle dysfunction or rupture (generally ischemia-infarction). Again, nitroprusside often is required to improve and stabilize these patients en route to more definitive interventions.

In acute severe aortic regurgitation, afterload reduction with nitroprusside improves hemodynamics by decreasing the regurgitant volume and ventricular diastolic volume and pressure, and by augmenting cardiac systolic performance. For patients with acute severe insufficiency of a disrupted mitral valve, afterload reduction with nitroprusside reduces mitral regurgitant volume, left atrial pressure and volume, pulmonary venous and capillary wedge pressure and lung congestion, and diastolic ventricular pressure and volume. For patients whose severe mitral insufficiency is secondary to ventricular remodeling or enlargement, afterload reduction with nitroprusside reduces the mitral regurgitant volume by decreasing ventricular volume and perhaps, mitral annular dilatation, and by reducing aortic outflow impedance.

Chronic CHF

Nitroprusside offers rapid symptomatic relief for patients with chronic CHF who enter the hospital severely decompensated (resting dyspnea, pulmonary edema) or who decompensate while undergoing diagnostic or therapeutic procedures (e.g., noncardiac surgery).

Stevenson and colleagues[66] have successfully employed nitroprusside to improve, stabilize, and optimize the hemodynamic and clinical status of patients with severe chronic CHF in preparation for selecting the most effective orally administrable agents; the optimal hemodynamic response to nitroprusside serves as a guide or end-point for testing oral agents. This approach has been very effective in improving the clinical status of severely decompensated patients, facilitating their hospital discharge, and decompressing the rather voluminous cardiac transplantation "waiting lists."[66]

Nitroprusside also is employed in the evaluation of potential recipients of heart transplantation to determine the reversibility of elevated pulmonary vascular resistance.[113] Afterload reduction with nitroprusside is useful in characterizing ventricular performance through the generation of ventricular pressure-volume loops and end-systolic pressure-volume (dimension) relations.[114]

Administration

Nitroprusside is administered intravenously with an infusion pump or microdrip regulator system to ensure controlled, precise dosing. Nitroprusside is light sensitive; the infusion set therefore should be shielded.

In CHF, the initial dose is 0.10 to 0.20 μg/kg/min and is gradually advanced as needed to attain the clinical and hemodynamic objectives. The incidence of side effects and toxicity is directly related to the dose and duration of administration.

The optimally effective and safe administration of nitroprusside generally requires direct hemodynamic monitoring. To improve a patient's clinical status promptly in certain hemodynamically catastrophic conditions (e.g., rupture of papillary muscle), nitroprusside occasionally must be initiated before the placement of hemodynamic-monitoring catheters. The objectives of nitroprusside administration in heart failure are directed at improving a patient's clinical status (e.g., ↓ dyspnea) by bringing excessively elevated ventricular filling pressures into an acceptable range (≤18 mm Hg), dropping excessively elevated vascular resistances, decreasing valvular regurgitation, and bringing stroke volume, cardiac output, and oxygen delivery into an acceptable range without eliciting significant hypotension or reflex tachycardia. Repeated clinical assessment and hemodynamic monitoring (via triple-lumen, thermodilution pulmonary artery catheter and systemic intraarterial catheter) provide the database needed to proficiently deliver the optimal nitroprusside dose. It is important to note that drug-induced changes in systemic blood pressure recorded from a radial artery catheter do not always correspond to pressure changes within the aorta; for instance, nitroprusside can evoke a significant fall in central aortic pressure by reducing the amplitude of reflected waves and moving them farther from systole, with little to no change in the more peripherally recorded, radial artery pressure.[118]

Nitroprusside can effectively augment the hemodynamic effects of dopamine, dobutamine, and similar agents.[105–108,119] Combination pharmacologic support (e.g., dobutamine plus nitroprusside) is commonly employed in the intensive care setting to optimize clinical and hemodynamic responses in patients with severe low-output, high-ventricular filling pressures.[119]

Potential Adverse Effects and Toxicity

The most commonly encountered adverse effect of nitroprusside administration is systemic hypotension.[69,70,73,92,99,100,120–137] When accompanied by a fall in coronary perfusion pressure and a rise in heart rate, nitroprusside-induced hypotension can be particularly detrimental in patients with myocardial ischemia/infarction. Dysfunction of noncardiac organ systems (e.g., azotemia) has been noted in association with nitroprusside infusions, typically during periods of systemic hypotension or hypoperfusion. Hypotension usually can be averted with proper hemodynamic monitoring and dose selection.

Some patients may experience symptomatic, rebound hemodynamic deterioration after the withdrawal of nitroprusside.[61,134–136] Gradual discontinuation, switch to nitroglycerin, or the addition of a converting enzyme inhibitor or sympatholytic drug are considerations for achieving a smoother withdrawal.

Nausea, disorientation, confusion, psychosis, weakness, muscle spasm, hyperreflexia, and convulsions are side effects of thiocyanate toxicity, which may occur as plasma thiocyanate concentrations rise above 6 mg%.[120–123] Thiocyanate can be removed with hemodialysis.

Deaths from nitroprusside toxicity usually are associated with prolonged, high-dose administration, and most often are secondary to cyanide toxicity.[120–127] The early sign of cyanide toxicity is metabolic (lactic) acidosis secondary to cyanide binding of cytochrome C; if uncorrected, tissue hypoxia and death can eventuate. Cyanide toxicity has been managed successfully with infusions of thiosulfate, sodium nitrate, and hydroxocobalamin. Conversion of cyanide to prussic acid raises methemoglobin levels and, thus, lowers the oxygen-carrying capacity of blood.

Thiocyanate and cyanide toxicity is rare during the usual administration of nitroprusside in heart failure (≤3 μg/kg/min for ≤72 hr).

Nitroprusside can lower systemic arterial oxygen content by causing or exacerbating a pulmonary ventilation/perfusion mismatch, probably via dilatation of pulmonary arterioles in nonventilated areas.[130–132] However, for most patients receiving nitroprusside, oxygen delivery is still augmented during the infusion because the rise in cardiac output greatly exceeds the fall in arterial oxygen content.

Laboratory data suggest that nitroprusside is capable of diverting blood flow from ischemic or threatened myocardium to normal myocardium by dilating the arterioles in the normal region.[99,100] This potential for "coronary steal" has been an issue in the shift of acute vasodilator therapy from nitroprusside to nitroglycerin for many patients with occlusive coronary artery disease.

Other far less commonly encountered side effects of nitroprusside include reduced platelet number and function, hypothyroidism (thiocyanate impairs iodine transport), and vitamin B_{12} deficiency.[128,129,137]

Nitrates

Nitrates have been used for more than 100 years, predominantly in the treatment of angina pectoris. Although not officially approved for use in CHF by the

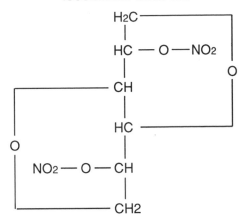

FIGURE 24.10. Molecular structure of the nitrates used most commonly in the management of CHF.

Food and Drug Administration, nitrates have earned a role in the therapeutics of this condition over the past two decades.[138-140] This section will focus on the clinical pharmacology and therapeutics of nitrates in the clinical setting of CHF.

Basic Pharmacology, Metabolism, and Pharmacokinetics

The molecular structures of the major nitrate preparations are presented in Figure 24.10.

The cardiovascular effects of nitrates are mediated through relaxation of vascular smooth muscle with consequent vasodilatation of venous and arterial structures. The precise cellular mechanisms, and relative contribution of each, of nitrate-induced vasodilatation have not been definitively established. The predominant mechanism is probably related to the formation of S-nitrosothiols, which are potent activators of guanylate cyclase. The resultant elevation of cGMP elicits relaxation of vascular smooth muscle.[72,141,142] Endothelial production and release of prostacyclin or prostaglandin E may contribute as well.[143-145]

Nitrates are cleared via extraction by vasculature, hydrolysis in blood, and hepatic metabolism by glutathione-nitrate reductase.[146,147]

Nitroglycerin (glyceryl trinitrate) has a half-life of 1 to 3 min; dinitrates, 40 to 45 min; and mononitrates, 2 to 5 hr. Since nitrates are cleared rather rapidly, blood levels are related predominantly to the rate and route of administration.[146-154] For intravenous administration, a good correlation exists between infusion rate and blood level.[148] Food may reduce the absorption of orally administered nitrates.[153] Site of topical application may have only a modest effect on blood levels in CHF.[151]

Because of the development of pharmacodynamic tolerance, the correlation between nitrate blood levels and pharmacodynamic effect is poor during continuous or repeated administration (discussed below).

Cardiovascular Pharmacology in Heart Failure

Nitrates evoke a number of circulatory responses; preload reduction is its major hemodynamic effect.[43,61,65,79,80,115,138-140,148-165]

Preload Reduction

In the clinical setting of CHF, nitrates drop ventricular filling pressures. A reduction in ventricular volume also has been detected during nitrate therapy.[161,166] The principle mechanism for this hemodynamic response is a nitrate-induced increase in venous capacitance, presumably via venodilatation, with a resultant shift of intracardiac blood volume into peripheral capacitance vessels. Improvement in ventricular relaxation and compliance likely contributes to the drop in ventricular filling pressures for some heart failure patients.

Since nitrates are less effective than nitroprusside in decreasing systemic vascular resistance,[61] nitrates are less effective in reducing the degree of valvular (aortic or mitral) regurgitation. Although nitrate-induced reduction in ventricular volume and augmentation of myocardial perfusion (with reversal of ischemic papillary muscle dysfunction in some patients) should favorably affect the degree of regurgitation across the mitral valve, the decrease in regurgitation noted during nitrate therapy in heart failure is related primarily to its peripheral vascular effects (↓ vascular resistance). At intravenous doses of nitroglycerin that dropped systemic vascular resistance, Keren and colleagues[38] noted a significant reduction in mitral regurgitation at rest and during isometric exercise in heart failure subjects. Elkayam et al.[167] found that nitrates, at doses that lowered pulmonary artery wedge pressures by 20% but did not affect systemic vascular resistance, had little to no effect on the mitral regurgitant volume.

Afterload Reduction

Although generally regarded as predominantly preload-reducing agents, sublingual, intravenous, and high-dose oral nitrates have been shown to reduce systemic and pulmonary vascular resistances.[61,65,148–150,153–165]

The ability of nitrates to reduce vascular resistance is related to the amount and rate of nitrate delivered to the blood, but with repeated or continuous dosing, this response becomes blunted by the development of pharmacodynamic tolerance. While considerable individual variation can be expected, intravenously administered nitroglycerin and isosorbide dinitrate drop systemic and pulmonic vascular resistances at ≥ 0.3 to 0.4 μg/kg/min.[61] The 20-mg dose of oral isosorbide dinitrate can reduce pulmonary vascular resistance,[65] but 30 mg generally is required to decrease systemic vascular resistance.[65,163,165,168,169] Nitrate-induced reduction of vascular resistance and afterload is generally accompanied by an augmentation of ventricular performance, stroke volume, and cardiac output.

Figure 24.11 illustrates the comparison of intra-venously administered nitroglycerin and nitroprusside relative to their ability to drop ventricular filling pressures and vascular resistances; for a given fall in ventricular filling pressure, nitroprusside evokes a greater reduction in pulmonic and systemic vascular resistances; stated another way, for any drug-induced fall in vascular resistance, intravenous nitroglycerin evokes a greater reduction in ventricular filling pressures.

Effects on Diastolic Function

Although not convincingly proven in the clinical setting of human CHF, a portion of the nitrates' capacity to drop ventricular filling pressures possibly is related to a favorable effect on diastolic function.[170–172] For patients whose diastolic dysfunction is secondary to subendocardial ischemia, nitrates may improve diastolic function by augmenting myocardial perfusion.[20–22,34] In patients

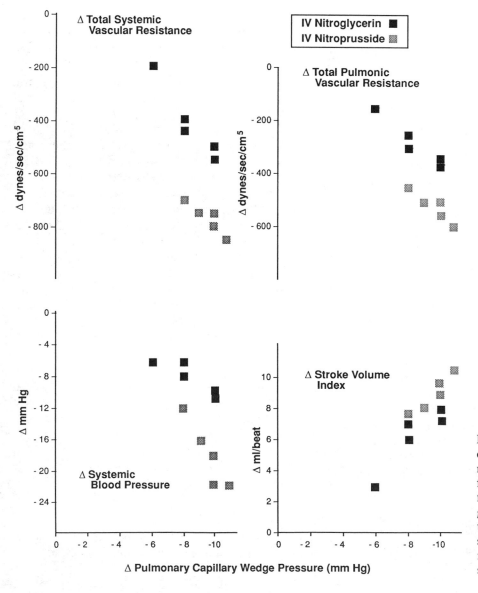

FIGURE 24.11. Relative hemodynamic effects of intravenous nitroglycerin and nitroprusside in patients with heart failure. For a given fall in ventricular filling pressure, nitroprusside evokes a greater reduction in vascular resistance; or for a given fall in vascular resistance, nitroglycerin elicits a greater reduction in ventricular filling pressures.

with high right atrial pressures, nitrates may improve left ventricular diastolic function by dropping right atrial pressure and, hence, coronary sinus pressure, myocardial venous pressure, and intramyocardial-interstitial pressure. Kingma and colleagues[166] have suggested that the improvement of diastolic function during nitrate therapy in heart failure is secondary to loss of the pericardial restraint as cardiac volume decreases.

Myocardial Energetics and Coronary Blood Flow

The effects of nitrates on myocardial energetics and coronary blood flow have not been studied extensively in human heart failure. The fall in myocardial oxygen consumption with nitrate therapy probably is secondary to nitrate-induced reduction in ventricular diastolic volume and pressure ($\downarrow$ diastolic wall stress) and the tendency of nitrates to decrease heart rate in the setting of CHF. Doses that drop ventricular afterload also contribute this factor to the fall in myocardial oxygen consumption. While nitrates should increase overall coronary blood flow by increasing coronary perfusion pressure, via a greater fall in ventricular than aortic diastolic pressure, and by tending to lengthen diastolic perfusion time,[61] coronary blood flow directionally follows myocardial oxygen consumption[162]; that is, as myocardial oxygen consumption falls with nitrates, so does overall coronary blood flow, but without an increase in oxygen extraction or lactate production. It is likely that nitrates favorably affect subendocardial perfusion and oxygenation in human heart failure.[32,34]

Regional Blood Flow

In the setting of CHF, nitrates reduce upper limb (musculocutaneous) vascular resistance with augmentation of limb blood flow.[61,65,156] Renal vascular resistance remains unchanged or may increase, resulting in little change or an actual fall in renal blood flow.[61,65] Hepatic-splanchnic vascular beds are not significantly affected by nitrate therapy.[61,65]

Neurohormonal Responses

Olivari et al.[173] reported that transdermal nitroglycerin doses that dropped ventricular filling pressures and pulmonic and systemic vascular resistances, but without a fall in systemic arterial pressure, did not change plasma norepinephrine concentrations or renin activity.

Exercise Hemodynamics and Performance

Acute and chronic nitrate administration has been associated with improved exercise performance and activity tolerance in heart failure.[163,174–177] The mechanism likely resides in the nitrate-induced improvement in central hemodynamics, particularly the reduc-

TABLE 24.2. Clinical uses of nitrates in CHF.

Acute intervention (intravenous, sublingual tablet, and lingual spray preparations)
Acute heart failure
Cardiogenic pulmonary edema
Acutely/severely decompensated chronic heart failure
Ischemic-myocardium syndromes
Addition of preload/afterload reduction to other agents (e.g., dobutamine, dopamine)

Chronic therapy (oral and transcutaneous preparations)
Combined with afterload-reducing agents (e.g., hydralazine)
Heart failure secondary to occlusive coronary artery disease
Heart failure accompanied by angina or angina-equivalent symptoms
Heart failure caused by metabolic or ischemic diastolic dysfunction of the ventricle.
Specifically timed preload reduction (e.g., paroxysmal nocturnal dyspnea, daytime dyspnea)

tion of ventricular filling pressures.[163,174–179] Studies by Wilson and colleagues[178,179] suggest that nitrates do not increase nutritional blood flow or oxygen delivery to working skeletal muscle during exercise.

Antiarrhythmic Properties

Nitroglycerin may have antiarrhythmic properties.[180] It is noteworthy that the improvement in survival for hydralazine-nitrate combination in the V-HeFT trial was better in the patients with ventricular arrhythmias at baseline than in those without arrhythmias, and better than the survival achieved by placebo or prazosin therapy (see section on hydralazine).

Clinical Application

A list of the clinical uses of nitrates in heart failure is presented in Table 24.2.

Acute Intervention

Acute nitrate administration is an effective form of therapy in the management of acute heart failure, cardiogenic pulmonary edema, and severely decompensated chronic CHF.[61,148,158,160,181–187] Intravenously administered nitroglycerin is the preparation used most commonly in these conditions, although sublingual tablets and lingual spray occasionally are employed until the intravenous preparation is infused and, less commonly, are used in place of the intravenous preparation. In the aforementioned conditions, these "acute preparations" reduce symptoms and improve hemodynamics by decreasing pulmonic and systemic venous pressures, ventricular filling pressures, pulmonic and systemic vascular resistances, right heart systolic/diastolic pressures and afterload, and in a mild to moderate degree, left heart afterload (Fig. 24.12).

Nitrates are particularly effective in controlling the

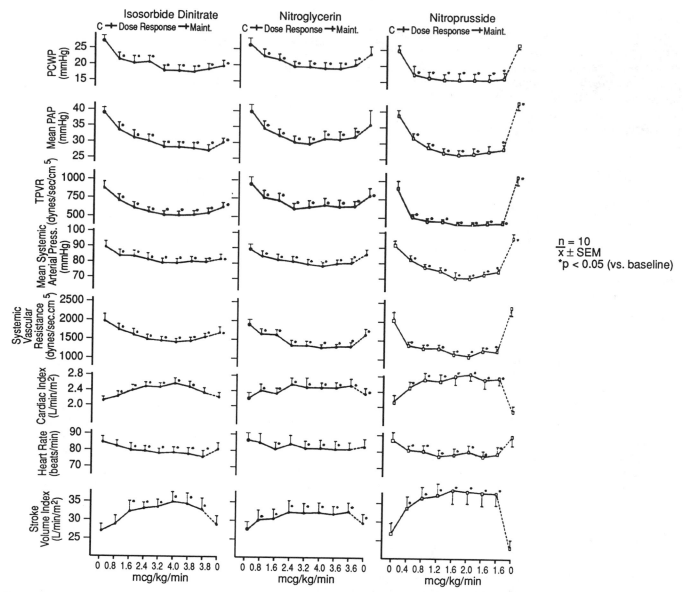

FIGURE 24.12. Hemodynamic responses to the intravenous administration of nitrates (nitroglycerin and isosorbide dinitrate) and nitroprusside (parallel control) in 10 patients with moderately severe CHF. The baseline control period (C) is followed in sequence by a dose response period, a 90-min constant maintenance dose period (*maint.*), and a discontinuation point. Pharmacodynamic tolerance developed for some hemodynamic parameters (e.g., cardiac index) by the second maintenance point for isosorbide dinitrate. Rebound at 30 min after drug withdrawal occurred only with nitroprusside. Abbreviations: mean PAP = mean pulmonary artery pressure; PCWP = pulmonary capillary wedge pressure; TPVR = total pulmonic vascular resistance. Adapted, with permission, from ref. 61.

symptoms and hemodynamic derangements of acute myocardial ischemia/infarction, particularly when accompanied by angina, elevated ventricular filling pressures, systolic or diastolic dysfunction, and heart failure.[158,160,181–187]

Severe CHF refractory to acute nitrate therapy or that caused by catastrophic events (e.g., ruptured papillary muscle, ruptured ventricular septum) usually will require nitroprusside.[61,182] Compared to acute nitrate therapy, nitroprusside is a more powerful afterload-reducing agent for the same degree of preload reduction (Figs. 24.11, 24.12), and is less likely to be accompanied by pharmacodynamic tolerance. It is important to note that some investigators and clinicians personally prefer nitroprusside over intravenous nitroglycerin for virtually all forms of acute/severe CHF.

Intravenous nitroglycerin is commonly added to dobutamine or dopamine infusions for the purpose of providing additional preload and/or afterload reduction.[119,188] Dobutamine or dopamine are not infrequently added to ongoing nitroglycerin infusions to further augment ventricular performance, stroke volume, cardiac output, and systemic blood pressure.[119]

Dupuis and colleagues[34] have shown that a 72-hr infusion of nitroglycerin can evoke sustained clinical benefit in patients with severe end-stage heart failure, a benefit lasting well beyond the discontinuation of the infusion. The mechanism for the sustained improvement is likely related to nitrate-induced augmentation of subendocardial perfusion.[32,34] The role of this form of intervention has yet to be defined, but may provide a therapeutic option in the management of patients with severe, end-stage CHF refractory to all combinations of orally administered medications and who are not eligible for cardiac transplantation or are entering the long waiting period for such.

Chronic Nitrate Therapy (Table 24.2)

As sole vasodilator therapy, two established heart failure laboratories have shown that 30 to 40 mg of isosorbide dinitrate administered orally every 6 hr for 12 weeks to heart failure patients improves clinical status, exercise capacity, and central hemodynamics compared to blinded, parallel-placebo control.[163,175] However, chronic administration at this dose was accompanied by the development of pharmacodynamic tolerance in the systemic arterial-arteriolar responses.[163] The favorable venous and pulmonary vascular effects persisted during chronic administration, suggesting that the improvement in clinical status and exercise capacity during chronic nitrate therapy is likely linked to drug-induced chronic reduction in ventricular filling pressures or preload and/or to long-term improvement of right heart hemodynamics (secondary to reduction of right heart afterload).

Kulick and colleagues[189] have observed that certain subsets of heart failure patients are hemodynamically resistant to orally administered isosorbide dinitrate, even at very high doses. Twelve of 50 (24%) heart failure patients failed to respond hemodynamically to 120 mg. This patient subset appeared to have a higher mean right atrial pressure compared to responders (14 ± 5 vs. 10 ± 36 mm Hg) at pretreatment baseline.

Long-term treatment data from blinded, control studies are not yet available for other nitrate preparations (e.g., nitroglycerin ointment).

Unless a patient cannot tolerate converting enzyme inhibitors or hydralazine, nitrates are not commonly used as sole vasodilator therapy. Nitrates usually are combined with hydralazine, and the combination prescribed as chronic preload-afterload reduction therapy for chronic CHF.[6,68,190–192] The hydralazine-isosorbide dinitrate combination, when added to chronic digoxin and diuretic therapy, was shown by the V-HeFT trial to improve survival in moderate heart failure (functional Class II and III) over that achieved when chronic placebo or prazosin therapy was added to digoxin and diuretics.[6] Despite this favorable effect on survival, the hydralazine-nitrate combination is not generally employed as first-line therapy in CHF. This combination is used most often in the place of converting enzyme inhibitors for patients whose symptoms are refractory to converting enzyme inhibitors or who are experiencing intolerable side effects to converting enzyme inhibitors. The hydralazine-nitrate combination also is used to supplement therapy for patients still symptomatic on digoxin, diuretics, and converting enzyme inhibitors, a situation most commonly encountered in very advanced, end-stage CHF.

Nitrates have been studied hemodynamically in combination with other vasodilating agents (e.g., minoxidil, nifedipine) and converting enzyme inhibitors, generally achieving hemodynamic responses superior to those of each drug alone.[193–195] The clinical efficacy of these particular combinations has not been examined with long-term controlled trials.

Certain heart failure subgroups may benefit greatly from nitrate administration, and should be targeted for this form of therapy. Heart failure resulting from severe occlusive coronary artery disease or symptoms directly related to episodic or chronic myocardial ischemia (such as intermittent pulmonary edema, paroxysmal nocturnal dyspnea, and angina) tend to respond favorably to chronic nitrate therapy. Patients with metabolic or ischemic forms of reversible diastolic dysfunction deserve a trial of nitrate therapy. Nitrates are particularly effective in controlling predictably timed heart failure symptoms. For example, some patients notice dyspnea only at work, whereas others experience only paroxysmal nocturnal dyspnea; 1 to 2 in of nitroglycerin ointment topically or 30 to 40 mg isosorbide dinitrate orally at the beginning of the work shift or at bedtime, respectively, can be quite effective in controlling their disruptive symptoms.

Administration

Sublingual Nitroglycerin

Sublingual nitroglycerin, effective as acute nitrate therapy, is administered in 0.3-mg to 0.6-mg doses every 5 to 10 min as needed to lower elevated ventricular filling pressures and to reduce moderate to severe resting dyspnea. The onset of action is 3 to 6 min and the effect can last 15 to 30 min. Nitroglycerin spray can be employed in a similar fashion.

Sublingual nitroglycerin is useful in controlling severe heart failure symptoms and elevated ventricular filling pressures until nitroglycerin can be infused intravenously and/or an effective diuresis is achieved. The authors have found that patients themselves frequently can avert episodic exacerbations of heart failure (e.g., pulmonary edema) at home by taking sublingual or spray nitroglycerin at the earliest recognizable point in the exacerbation; even if not totally effective, the patient usually can call his physician or get to an emergency room in a far less compromised condition.

Intravenous Nitroglycerin

Similar to most intravenously administered cardioactive drugs, nitroglycerin is started at a low dose (0.2 μg/kg/min) and titrated upward as needed to achieve the desired clinical and hemodynamic end-points. Hemodynamic effects are detectable within 3 to 6 min, and responses plateau by 10 to 15 min. The dose during chronic administration invariably must be advanced to overcome pharmacodynamic tolerance.

Isosorbide Dinitrate, Orally

Chronic nitrate therapy is attainable with isosorbide dinitrate, administered orally at 30 mg or more every 6 to 8 hr. Side effects may require doses to be lowered to 10 to 20 mg during the initial phases of therapy. Hemodynamic responses occur by 15 min, peak at 30 to 60 min, and dissipate by 5 to 6 hr. The development of tolerance can be averted by shifting dosing to every 8 hr or dropping one of the every 6-hr doses per day. As noted above, isosorbide dinitrate is frequently administered in combination with hydralazine.

Topical Nitroglycerin

Nitroglycerin ointment is an inexpensive means of delivering chronic nitrate therapy.[152,196,197] The dose for the 2% ointment (1 in = 12.5 mg) ranges from $\frac{1}{2}$ to 3 in every 8 to 12 hr. A hemodynamic effect becomes apparent by 1 hr, peaks at 2 to 5 hr, and wanes by 6 to 10 hr. A declining blood concentration or nitrate-free interval generally is required to prevent the development of pharmacodynamic tolerance to nitroglycerin ointment.

The 24-hr transdermal-nitroglycerin patch delivery systems are an expensive means of administering chronic nitrate therapy.[152,173,198,199] Doses of ≥ 60 cm^2 generally are required to attain even low serum nitroglycerin levels and mild hemodynamic effects in CHF. Pharmacodynamic tolerance becomes apparent at 12 to 18 hr after placement of the patch.[198]

Other Preparations

The response/time course of sublingual isosorbide dinitrate is similar to that of sublingual nitroglycerin.[174,184] The response/time course of chewable isosorbide dinitrate resides between that of sublingual nitroglycerin and oral isosorbide dinitrate.[169,200] The dose response and hemodynamic effects of intravenously administered

isosorbide dinitrate are virtually identical to those of intravenous nitroglycerin[61]; however, the intravenous preparation of isosorbide dinitrate is not yet commercially available.

Isosorbide-5-mononitrate is a major metabolite of isosorbide dinitrate, but has a considerably longer half-life. Preliminary studies on the intravenous and oral preparations of isosorbide-5-mononitrate in human heart failure indicate a favorable hemodynamic profile.[201–203]

Potential Adverse Effects and Toxicity

As a group, the nitrates are relatively safe to administer. The vast majority of side effects are readily reversed with downward adjustment or discontinuation of dosing. Systemic hypotension, headaches, and flushing are the most commonly noted adverse effects. Rebound hemodynamic deterioration after discontinuation of intravenous nitroglycerin is far less common and problematic than after nitroprusside withdrawal.[61]

In contrast to nitroprusside, intravenously administered nitroglycerin does not significantly lower systemic arterial oxygen content.[61,130] Sublingual nitroglycerin was observed to lower systemic arterial pO$_2$ in non-failure patients with angina.[204] In 10 patients with heart failure, Pierpont and colleagues[205] found that mean arterial pO$_2$ tended to fall (75.1 $\pm$ 3.7 to 69.8 $\pm$ 3.5 mm Hg, but not statistically significant) when 20 to 30 mg of chewable isosorbide dinitrate was added 2 hr after the ingestion of 100 mg hydralazine; whether these data are relevant to standard chronic dosing of hydralazine-isosorbide dinitrate in heart failure remains to be determined.

Significant methemoglobinemia is an unusual complication of standard nitrate administration.[206–208] Mild methemoglobinemia occurs only after prolonged (> 5–7 days) high-dose nitroglycerin infusions and rarely impairs oxygen delivery or evokes symptoms.[207,208] Patients with congenital deficiency of NADH-methemoglobin reductase are likely to be more susceptible to the development of elevated methemoglobin levels during nitrate therapy.[209]

Pharmacodynamic Resistance

In a report by Magrini and Niarchos,[210] clinical and hemodynamic responsiveness to sublingual nitroglycerin at the high doses of 1.6 to 2.4 mg was blunted in patients with elevated right atrial pressures and massive peripheral edema. Diuretic therapy with removal of edema and reduction of the elevated ventricular filling pressures converted the nitrate nonresponders to responders. Orally administered isosorbide dinitrate at doses as high as 120 mg fail to evoke significant hemodynamic responses in about 20% to 25% of heart failure patients; this subgroup was found by Kulick et al.[189] to have higher mean right atrial pressures. Armstrong and colleagues[148] noted that intravenous nitroglycerin at doses as high as 400 μg/min was ineffective in lowering mean pulmonary artery pressure by 25% in about 30% of the heart failure patients they investigated.

The mechanism(s) for the pharmacodynamic resistance to nitroglycerin has not been elucidated. Elevated right atrial pressure appears to be a recurring finding in nonresponders.[148,189,210-212] Elevated right atrial pressure also may be a determinant of the effectiveness of other drugs (e.g., hydralazine) used in the treatment of heart failure.[211]

Pharmacodynamic Tolerance

Nitrates are prototypic of the pharmacologic phenomenon of tolerance.[163,198,212-221] Tolerance represents a loss of drug response over time despite drug concentrations maintained at or above initial levels.

Continuous infusions or repeated dosing of nitrates are invariably associated with some loss of hemodynamic responsiveness.[163,198,212,215-221] Tolerance can be seen as early as 4 to 8 hr of an intravenous infusion[61,218] and within 12 hr after the application of a 24-hr transdermal nitroglycerin patch.[198,219,220]

Loss of responsiveness to nitrates does not uniformly involve all hemodynamic parameters or clinical indicators.[61,163,220,221-224] Chronic dosing (12 weeks) of isosorbide dinitrate at 40 mg orally every 6 hr resulted in loss of systemic arterial-arteriolar responsiveness with retention of nitrate-effect on the systemic venous and pulmonary vasculature.[163] The major side effects, namely headaches and hypotension, disappeared with repeated dosing, and overall clinical status and exercise capacity improved.[163]

The mechanisms for nitrate-evoked tolerance have not been fully elucidated, but are likely to be multifactorial.[212,215-221,225-227] A shift of extracellular fluid to the intravascular space and neurohormonal and/or renin activation probably are important in the development of tolerance to intravenously administered nitrates.[212,221] Stimulation of guanylate cyclase by nitrates appears to depend on the availability of sulfhydryl groups for conversion of the nitrate to an S-nitrosothiol.[141,142,225] Thus, sulfhydryl depletion may be an additional mechanism for the development of tolerance. This consideration is supported by reports showing that the administration of sulfhydryl contributors or repletors (e.g., N-acetylcysteine, methionine) concomitant with nitrates enhances the nitrate effect and blunts the development of nitrate tolerance.[228,229] Unfortunately, studies are also available indicating that this approach is ineffective in preventing pharmacodynamic tolerance to nitrates.[221,230]

TABLE 24.3. Strategies to prevent the development of nitrate tolerance in CHF.

1. Titrate dose only to the clinically or hemodynamically effective levels needed (i.e., avoid excessive dosing and hypotension)
2. Prevent fluid retention and expansion of intravascular volume (diuretics)
3. Allow a substantial reduction in serum nitrate concentrations (dose-free interval or widely spaced dosing)
4. Time-target the symptoms responsive to nitrate therapy
5. Other considerations to circumvent nitrate tolerance, directed at a few patients or yet to be proven effective in heart failure:
   a. Increase of dose (a short-term solution for some patients)
   b. Sulfhydryl contributors (N-acetylcysteine, methionine)
   c. Control neurohormonal or renin-aldosterone activation (e.g., captopril)
   d. Unique compounds (e.g., S-nitrosocaptopril)

Interestingly, the converting enzyme inhibitor, captopril, is capable of contributing a sulfhydryl group and retarding neurohormonal responses in heart failure. Angiotensin-converting enzyme (ACE) inhibitors appear to retard the development of nitrate tolerance in normal persons.[230a] However, Dupuis et al.[231] and Dakak et al.[232] found that captopril was not effective in preventing the development of tolerance to intravenously administered nitroglycerin in heart failure. Preliminary animal studies indicate that the chronic administration of a rather unique molecule, S-nitrosocaptopril, maintains hemodynamic responsiveness to this compound.[233,234]

Certain strategies can be employed to circumvent the problem of nitrate tolerance (Table 24.3). If only a brief or temporary solution to tolerance is needed, most patients will respond initially to a significant increase in dose or infusion rate. Four major therapeutic strategies are important in preventing or reversing nitrate tolerance. First, excessive nitrate dosing with associated undesirable responses (e.g., hypotension) must be avoided. Second, nitrate-induced fluid retention and intravascular volume expansion should be controlled with appropriate diuretic intervention. Prevention of neurohormonal and renin-aldosterone activation may be important in this regard, but the precise means for achieving such (e.g., converting enzyme inhibition, α-adrenergic blockade) have not yet been determined. Third, the dosing schedule must be adjusted to allow nitrate plasma levels to decrease considerably or approach zero every 16 to 24 hr. Fourth (and extension of the last consideration), the clinician, recognizing that he may have a 12- to 16-hr period of nitrate therapy to work with per day, should individually time-target the nitrate for each patient. Many patients clearly need the nitrate effect most at specific times of the day or night (e.g., at night for orthopnea or paroxysmal nocturnal dyspnea).

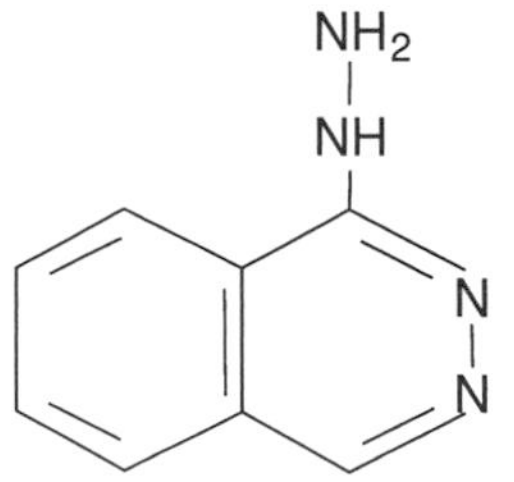

FIGURE 24.13. The molecular structure of hydralazine.

Direct-Acting, Orally Administered Vasodilators

This general category of compounds consists of a variety of "direct-acting" agents whose cellular mechanism of action is not well defined and which cannot be appropriately placed in another major drug group; as such, this particular drug grouping represents somewhat of a "wastebasket" category. Nevertheless, this category contains very important agents (e.g., hydralazine, flosequinan) currently used in the treatment of heart failure.

Hydralazine

Hydralazine, a hydrazinophthalazine (Fig. 24.13) and a potent dilator of arteriolar smooth muscle, was introduced as an antihypertensive agent about 40 years ago. Its vascular effects have earned a role in the management of CHF.

Basic Pharmacology, Metabolism, and Pharmacokinetics

The mechanisms whereby hydralazine mediates its "direct" effects are not clearly understood. A modulating effect on intracellular calcium kinetics is likely, and a hydralazine-induced elevation of cyclic adenosine monophosphate (cAMP) or cGMP have been proposed.[235,236] Hydralazine's mechanism(s) of action may not all be "direct" either. Hydralazine-induced alterations in sympathetic nervous system tone, release of prostenoids, and inhibition of thromboxane A_2 biosynthesis also have been suggested.[237–239]

Hydralazine is rapidly and almost totally absorbed from the gastrointestinal tract with peak plasma concentrations occurring 30 to 60 min after ingestion.[235,240–242] Hydralazine undergoes significant first-pass metabolism by the liver, accounting for a bioavailability of 10% to 35%.[235,240] More than 90% of administered hydralazine is cleared by the liver, and the remainder via renal excretion. Chronic administration of high doses can saturate the first-pass effect and exceed drug clearance, greatly raising bioavailability and plasma concentrations.[240] The hydralazine molecule is metabolized via acetylation, oxidative reactions, ring-hydroxy-

lation, and glucuronide-conjugation.[235,240] Genetic "slow acetylators" achieve higher plasma concentrations and shift much of the metabolism of hydralazine from acetylation to primary oxidative reactions and hydroxylation.[235,240,241] Eighty to 90% of circulating hydralazine is protein bound. Elimination half-life is 0.5 to 2.0 hr and clearance can range from 30 to 150 ml/min/kg.

Whether CHF influences the pharmacokinetics of hydralazine has not been convincingly resolved. Hanson and colleagues[242] noted that a single orally administered 50-mg dose of hydralazine attained a significantly higher "area under the concentration curve" in chronic heart failure patients than that noted for the same dose in acetylator-matched patients with essential hypertension. A decreased hepatic clearance rate for hydralazine in heart failure is the suggested mechanism. In contrast, another laboratory found that CHF had little effect on hydralazine's bioavailability, half-life, and clearance compared to populations without heart failure.[240,241]

Cardiovascular Pharmacology in CHF

Central Hemodynamic Effects

The hemodynamic effects of hydralazine have now been extensively investigated in humans with CHF.[63,65,243–259] Hydralazine, a potent arteriolar vasodilator, decreases systemic and pulmonic vascular resistances (Fig. 24.14). The resultant fall in ventricular afterload (right and left heart) evokes an overall improvement in ventricular performance with a resultant augmentation of stroke volume, stroke work, and cardiac output (Fig. 24.14). As with most other vasodilators in heart failure, the augmented stroke volume averts the development of significant systemic hypotension and reflex tachycardia. Hemodynamic effects in human heart failure generally become apparent by 20 min, peak at 60 to 120 min, and wane from 6 to 8 hr after oral dosing.

Studies from our laboratories have shown that chronic afterload reduction in heart failure with hydralazine, with or without concomitant nitrate administration, is accompanied by regression of myocardial cell hypertrophy.[54]

It has now been well demonstrated in human heart failure that hydralazine also elicits a positive inotropic response (Fig. 24.15).[80,259] This property, in large part, explains (a) the greater enhancement in ventricular performance after a hydralazine dose in heart failure compared to that of most other vasodilating agents and converting enzyme inhibitors,[247,249,259] and (b) the infrequent occurrence of hypotension with hydralazine therapy in heart failure of all degrees of severity. The inotropic effects of hydralazine (a vasodilator with positive inotropic properties) have made this agent the drug of choice for withdrawing dobutamine (a positive

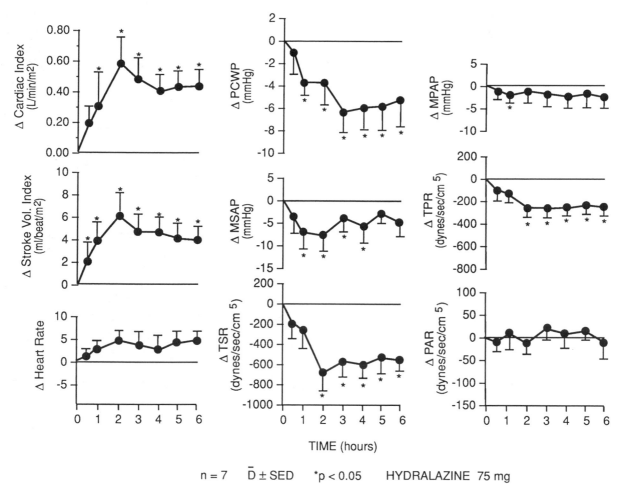

n = 7   D̄ ± SED   *p < 0.05   HYDRALAZINE 75 mg

FIGURE 24.14. Central hemodynamic response to orally administered hydralazine (75 mg) in 7 patients with severe CHF. Abbreviations: D ± SED = change (Δ) ± standard error; MPAP = mean pulmonic arterial pressure; MSAP = mean systemic arterial pressure; PAR = pulmonary arteriolar resistance; PCWP = pulmonary capillary wedge pressure; TPR = total pulmonary vascular resistance; TSR = Total systemic vascular resistance; vol = volume. Adapted, with permission, from ref. 65. Copyright by the American Heart Association.

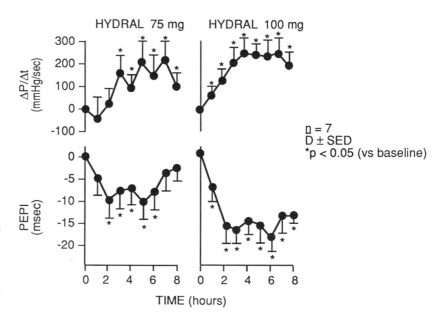

FIGURE 24.15. Hydralazine-induced changes in the inotropic parameters, ▲P/▲t (isovolumic developed pressure/isovolumic contraction time) and PEPI (preejection period index), in 7 patients with severe CHF. D ± SED = change (Δ) ± standard error. Adapted, with permission, from ref. 259.

inotropic agent with vasodilating properties) from dobutamine-dependent, end-stage heart failure patients.[260] Enhancement of sympathetic nervous system tone appears to be the mechanism explaining much of hydralazine's positive inotropic properties, although direct myocardial stimulation has not been convincingly excluded.[261,262]

A common misconception is that hydralazine has no effect on ventricular preload. Most laboratories experienced in the human hemodynamic investigations have reported modest to mild reductions in ventricular filling pressure with hydralazine even in the absence of detectable valvular regurgitation.[65,245,246,248–252] However, the amount of preload reduction is insufficient for most patients with moderate to severe CHF and, thus, requires the concomitant administration of another compound with substantial preload-reducing properties, generally nitrates and occasionally converting enzyme inhibitors.

Hydralazine's powerful arteriolar vasodilating effects make it one of the drugs of choice to decrease the amount of valvular regurgitation across any incompetent heart valve[42,59,263–266] and the degree of left to right shunting of atrial and ventricular septal defects.[267–269] In these conditions, hydralazine can lower ventricular filling pressures considerably despite its modest venodilating preload-reducing capabilities.[267–269]

Myocardial Energetics and Coronary Blood Flow

In contrast to most vasodilating agents and converting enzyme inhibitors, hydralazine, because of its positive inotropic effects, can increase myocardial oxygen consumption to a mild degree (Fig. 24.16)[270–272] For heart failure patients without occlusive coronary artery dis-

ease (e.g., nonischemic DCM), the rise in myocardial oxygen consumption is invariably accompanied by a still greater rise in coronary blood flow and oxygen delivery to myocardium.[270,272] For patients with occlusive coronary artery disease, the rise in myocardial oxygen demands with hydralazine may not be matched in all regions of the ventricular wall with an adequate increase in coronary blood flow and myocardial perfusion. For this reason, most clinicians do not administer sizable doses of hydralazine to patients with occlusive coronary artery disease without concomitant nitrate therapy.

Regional Blood Flow

Hydralazine significantly increases blood flow to limb musculocutaneous structures in patients with heart failure; the increase is dose-related, generally proportional to the rise in cardiac output, and maintained with chronic administration (see Fig. 24.17).[63,65,273] The augmentation of limb flow at rest may not be accompanied by an increase in nutritional flow to working muscle during exercise.[256,257,274,275]

Hepatic-splanchnic blood flow tends to increase during hydralazine therapy in heart failure, although the change is less than the concomitant elevation in cardiac output.[63,65,273]

Hydralazine is one of the few drugs used in heart failure management that is capable of substantially reducing renal vascular resistance and increasing renal blood flow.[60,63,65,101,243,276–278] This favorable response was described in hypertensive patients 40 years ago,[276] and in human heart failure about 25 years ago.[243] The rise in renal blood flow is dose-related and proportional to the elevation in cardiac output, and persists during chronic therapy.[63,273]

Hydralazine's effects on the remaining renal function parameters are far less dramatic than its influence on renal blood flow. Glomerular filtration rate, cation (Na^+ and K^+) excretion, and water clearance either do not change or increase only modestly (Fig. 24.18).[243,276–278] Except for patients with severe heart failure secondary to marked valvular insufficiency, the authors have not commonly witnessed a clinically apparent diuretic effect by simply initiating hydralazine therapy. It has been suggested that hydralazine may enhance the renal clearance of digoxin and furosemide.[279,280]

Exercise Hemodynamics

Most of the favorable central hemodynamic responses noted after hydralazine in the heart failure patient at rest persist as the patient exercises.[249,253–258,274,275] With initial dosing, this transfer of favorable hemodynamic effects generally does not achieve an increase in exercise capacity. This may, in part, be explained by the inability of hydralazine to enhance nutritional

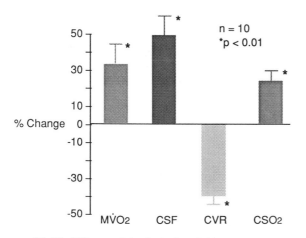

FIGURE 24.16. Effects of hydralazine 75 mg orally on myocardial oxygen consumption ($M\dot{V}O_2$), myocardial blood flow (coronary sinus flow, CSF), coronary vascular resistance (CVR), and coronary sinus oxygen content (CSO_2) in 10 patients with nonischemic DCM and CHF studied in our laboratories.

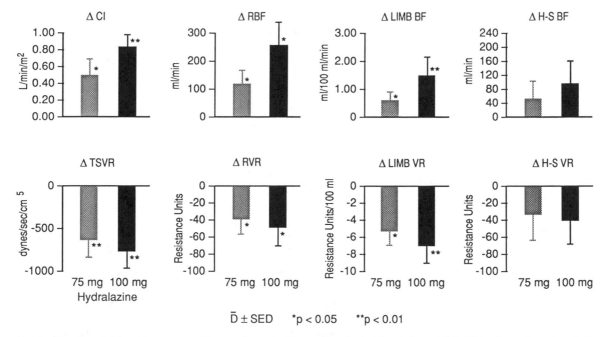

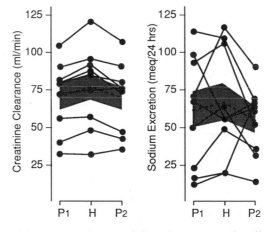

FIGURE 24.17. Regional hemodynamic effects of oral 75- and 100-mg doses of hydralazine in severe heart failure. Abbreviations: BF = blood flow; CI = cardiac index; D ± SED = change (Δ) ± standard error; H-S BF = hepatic- splanchnic blood flow; H-S VR = hepatic-splanchnic vascular resistance; RBF = renal blood flow; RVR = renal vascular resistance; VR = vascular resistance. Adapted, with permission, from ref. 63.

blood flow of working skeletal muscle during exercise.[256,257,274,275,281]

Clinical Application

Vasodilator Therapy with Hydralazine Alone

Several uncontrolled studies have indicated that long-term hydralazine therapy may be effective as sole vasodilator therapy in CHF[54,244,246,249,250,253,254,273,282]; this applies to both persistence of favorable hemodynamic effects and improvement of clinical status with repeated dosing over weeks to months. Two small, placebo-controlled trials arrived at rather conflicting results. In the report by Franciosa and colleagues,[283] 16 patients were randomized to hydralazine (200 mg daily) and 16 to placebo; after 26 weeks, no differences were noted between the two groups in clinical status, ejection fraction, or exercise duration. The results of another small (n = 27), placebo-controlled study reported by Conradson et al.[284] showed that hydralazine (mean dose of 150 mg daily) favorably affected exercise capacity over 1 yr of treatment. Basically, hydralazine alone as chronic vasodilator therapy has not been adequately studied in human heart failure and, thus, statements regarding long-term effectiveness of this agent as sole vasodilator therapy cannot be convincingly rendered.

Although not supported by blinded, controlled trials, hydralazine as a sole vasodilator appears to be effective in three clinical situations: (a) as chronic afterload-reduction therapy for valvular regurgitation, (b) as a

FIGURE 24.18. Values for creatinine clearance and sodium excretion during a prehydralazine placebo period (P_1), hydralazine treatment period (H), and a posthydralazine placebo period (P_2) in patients with moderately severe CHF. Hydralazine induced a mild, but statistically significant, increase in creatinine clearance and a slight, but insignificant, numerical rise in mean sodium excretion. Adapted, with permission, from ref. 277. Copyright by the American Heart Association.

means of withdrawing dobutamine from dobutamine-dependent patients, and (c) as an option in "tailored" or hemodynamically directed and targeted vasodilator therapy.

Afterload-Reduction in Valvular Insufficiency. In heart failure complicated by significant mitral regurgitation, hydralazine, by reducing systemic vascular resistance and ventricular afterload, decreases the degree of regurgitation and ventricular systolic and diastolic volume, and increases forward stroke volume.[42,66,263,265] Similar favorable responses were observed in patients with chronic aortic valvular regurgitation.[44,45,263,264,266]

Withdrawal of Dobutamine from Dobutamine-Dependent Patients. More than 60% of patients with severe heart failure who are hemodynamically and clinically dependent on continuous dobutamine administration can be withdrawn using hydralazine support.[260] Hydralazine is administered in incremental doses, starting at 25 mg orally every 4 to 6 hr, while the dobutamine dose is gradually lowered.

"Tailored" Vasodilator Therapy. Stevenson et al.[66] have employed hydralazine as one of the therapeutic options in "tailored" medical therapy directed at improving the hemodynamic and clinical status of end-stage heart failure patients, many referred for cardiac transplantation. Optimal hemodynamic responses are achieved initially with nitroprusside, and are then pursued with orally administered agents, one of which is hydralazine.

Hydralazine-Nitrate Combination

For most patients with CHF, hydralazine alone does not provide optimal "unloading," since its ability to drop ventricular filling pressures and preload in the absence of valvular regurgitation usually is less than needed. For this reason, nitrates, in the form of isosorbide dinitrate orally or nitroglycerin ointment topically, are added to hydralazine. Numerous studies have now shown that this combination evokes a hemodynamic response more favorable than that of each drug alone.[65,253,261,274,285–290] Hydralazine-nitrate combination effects a greater reduction in systemic vascular resistance and afterload and a greater increase in stroke volume and cardiac output than nitrates alone, and a greater reduction in ventricular filling pressures than hydralazine alone.

The regional blood flow profile of hydralazine-nitrate combination is the same as that of hydralazine alone.[65] Nitrates' propensity to reduce renal blood flow appears to be negated by concomitant hydralazine administration.

The favorable hemodynamic responses of hydralazine-nitrate combination in heart failure patients at rest are sustained during exercise.[274,287,290] Although initial dosing with the combination generally does not augment exercise capacity, an improvement of exercise capacity is suggested from chronic dosing studies.[68a,291]

A reasonably large, multicenter trial (referred to as the "V-HeFT trial") demonstrated that the long-term oral administration of combination hydralazine-isosorbide dinitrate, when added to chronic digitalis-diuretic therapy, improved survival in patients with moderate CHF (functional class II and III, New York Heart association) above that achieved with placebo or the α_1-adrenergic blocker, prazosin.[6] A number of issues regarding this trial have raised concern and provocative inquiry. The hydralazine-nitrate treatment group had a high dropout rate for side effects, raising the concern of a modified treatment population. It is unknown which drug of the combination provided the survival factor—hydralazine, the nitrate, or both. The clinical and hemodynamic predictors of the improved survival remain elusive, although hydralazine-nitrate therapy appeared to be associated with an increase in ejection fraction and exercise capacity.[6,291] Nevertheless, the V-HeFT trial is the first valid study to convincingly show that: (a) it is possible to influence survival favorably in chronic CHF, (b) chronic vasodilator therapy can improve survival in this population, and (c) the vasodilator therapy accomplishing such was the hydralazine-isosorbide dinitrate combination.

The results of the V-HeFT II trial indicate that long-term converting enzyme inhibitor therapy (enalapril) achieves a slightly more favorable effect on survival, but with less improvement in ejection fraction and exercise capacity than chronic hydralazine-nitrate therapy in patients with symptomatic heart failure.[68a]

Other Hydralazine Preparations and Combinations

Intravenous Hydralazine. The central hemodynamic profile of intravenous hydralazine is similar to that attained with oral administration.[243,276,292] The effective intravenous doses are considerably lower (range: 5–30 mg) than the oral doses, and the onset of action is 3 to 10 min for intravenous hydralazine versus 30 to 60 min for the oral preparation. Although useful in clinical research protocols, the intravenous preparation of hydralazine currently has a very limited to no role in clinical medicine and therapeutics. All of the therapeutic objectives of intravenous hydralazine can be more quickly, predictably, and reliably achieved with other agents (e.g., nitroprusside, dobutamine, amrinone).

Combinations. Although not tested with controlled trials, hydralazine has augmented hemodynamic and clinical responses of nonnitrate agents (e.g., converting enzyme inhibitors).[293,294] It is not uncommon for patients with severe, end-stage CHF to be managed optimally with a low to moderate dose of each of a converting enzyme inhibitor, hydralazine, and occasionally, a nitrate.

Congeners. The hydralazine molecule has been modified in an attempt to eliminate the fast-versus-slow acetylator variable and the risk of drug-induced systemic lupus erythematosus (SLE), while maintaining the favorable hemodynamic profile of the hydralazine molecule. Examples of such congeners include endralazine and dihydralazine.[295-297] The development of these agents for general clinical use in heart failure has perhaps been tempered somewhat by the clinical development and widespread use of the converting enzyme inhibitors.

Administration

The oral dose range of hydralazine in CHF is wide, ranging from 25 to 200 mg every 6 to 8 hr. The usual dose is 75 to 100 mg every 6 to 8 hr, often combined with $\frac{1}{2}$ to 2 in of 2% nitroglycerin ointment every 8 hr or oral isosorbide dinitrate 20 to 40 mg every 6 to 8 hr. An occasional patient may require a dose exceeding 200 mg every 6 hr.

Potential Undesirable Properties and Effects

Hydralazine also is susceptible to the pharmacologic phenomena of drug resistance and tolerance. Patients with a high mean right atrial pressure (>10 mm Hg) appear to be hemodynamically more resistant to oral hydralazine[211]; some of these patients require an oral dose of 600 to 800 mg or intravenously administered hydralazine to effect a hemodynamic response. The results of a short-term (15–24 days) study suggest that heart failure patients with a left ventricular minor axis diastolic dimension <60 mm appear to have a less favorable clinical course during hydralazine therapy than those with larger ventricular dimensions.[298]

Pharmacodynamic tolerance to hydralazine may occur during chronic administration, although the prevalence and predisposing factors for the development of this problem have not been established.[273,282-284,299,300] Interestingly, the sudden withdrawal of hydralazine has been reported to precipitate severe CHF in isolated instances.[301]

From the standpoint of side effects, hydralazine is generally less well tolerated than most other major vasodilating drugs or converting enzyme inhibitors. Thirty-six of 186 (19.4%) patients treated with combination hydralazine-nitrate in the V-HeFT trial experienced one or more side effects to this therapy,[6] many presumably related to the hydralazine part of the combination. Headache and dizziness were the predominant side effects with the combination (also attributable to nitrates). Seven patients (of 36) complained of gastrointestinal symptoms and six experienced arthralgias or a SLE-like illness. A rash developed in three patients.

In contrast to chronic hydralazine therapy for systemic hypertension, the problems of drug-induced arthralgias, rheumatoid manifestations, and SLE are relatively uncommon in CHF, irrespective of the acetylator-type status. Only 6 of 186 (3.2%) hydralazine-nitrate–treated patients in the V-HeFT trial had arthralgia or

lupus-like manifestations.[6] In more than 200 patients with heart failure followed on hydralazine therapy, one of the authors (CVL) has witnessed only two lupus-like reactions ($<1\%$). One patient experienced a macular rash and arthralgias and the other, arthralgias, pleuritis, and pericarditis; these complications were readily controlled with antiinflammatory medication and abated within 3 weeks after the discontinuation of hydralazine.

As a potent arteriolar-dilator, hydralazine is capable of evoking systemic hypotension. However, this is a rather uncommon problem with proper patient and dose selection. Since the hypotension may not become apparent until the patient assumes an upright position,[302] it is generally recommended that postural blood pressure and heart rate recordings be obtained at 1 and 2 hr after initial hydralazine dosing. Cutaneous flushing is not uncommon during hydralazine administration.

Although effective in reducing the severity of valvular regurgitation, hydralazine must be used with caution in patients whose heart failure is complicated by stenotic valvular disease[303]; any fall in vascular resistance may not be accompanied by an adequate rise in stroke volume and cardiac output. Greenberg and Massie[303a] found that when mild to moderate aortic stenosis is accompanied by a depressed stroke volume and cardiac output and an elevated systemic vascular resistance, afterload reduction therapy (hydralazine or prazosin) over 24 hr evokes favorable hemodynamic responses.

Hydralazine can evoke symptoms and signs of myocardial ischemia and cause infarction in heart failure patients with occlusive coronary artery disease, and in the authors' experience, in patients with marked myocardial hypertrophy and normal epicardial coronary arteries. Twelve of 52 (23%) heart failure patients with occlusive coronary artery disease experienced 16 ischemic events (angina in 12, infarction in 4) during initial hydralazine administration.[304] These events often are not preceded by significant hypotension or tachycardia, suggesting that hydralazine's positive inotropic effects and its tendency to enhance sympathetic nervous system tone are potentially threatening properties (which increase myocardial oxygen consumption) in patients with significantly occluded coronary arteries (inability to increase oxygen supply).

Hypotension and tachycardia, occasionally evoked by hydralazine, would further exacerbate myocardial ischemic events. Although not proven in this clinical setting, adding nitrates to hydralazine therapy for heart failure patients with occlusive coronary artery disease theoretically can be supported.

Select patients may experience an increase in heart rate with hydralazine; patients with lower ventricular filling pressures (<15 mm Hg) and those receiving an excessive dose are particularly susceptible to this undesirable effect. Hydralazine enhances atrioventricular (AV) node conduction[305] and, thus, can accelerate the ventricular rate in atrial fibrillation-flutter. In the absence of provoked ischemia, hypotension, and tachycardia, hydralazine does not appear to elicit serious ventricular arrhythmias.[306,307] Interestingly, the hydralazine-nitrate combination of the V-HeFT trial was superior to placebo or prazosin in reducing cardiovascular mortality in heart failure patients with ≥ 3 successive ventricular ectopic beats.[307]

Systemic arterial oxygen tension and content remains unaltered or increases slightly during initial hydralazine dosing.[205,308]

Minoxidil

Minoxidil is a potent direct-acting arterial-arteriolar vasodilator. Its central hemodynamic effects in heart failure are similar to those of hydralazine.[194,309-314] Minoxidil reduces systemic and pulmonic vascular resistance and ventricular afterload with consequent augmentation of stroke volume and cardiac output. Changes in ventricular diastolic filling pressures are modest. These favorable hemodynamic properties also occur during exercise, and tend to persist with chronic administration.[310-314]

Despite the favorable hemodynamic responses to minoxidil during initial and chronic dosing, these responses may not be accompanied by improvement in clinical status or exercise capacity. A blinded, placebo-controlled trial in chronic heart failure patients by Franciosa et al.[314] demonstrated that minoxidil therapy over 3 months augmented ejection fraction significantly (26.6% ± 17.7 to 42.7% ± 22.3), but did not increase exercise duration or maximal oxygen consumption. Patients receiving minoxidil clinically fared less well and experienced significantly more adverse effects than patients receiving placebo. All of the minoxidil-treated patients required increased diuretic dosage.

Reported adverse effects of chronic minoxidil therapy in human heart failure include weight gain, exacerbation of peripheral edema, or increased diuretic requirements in virtually all patients, deterioration of heart fail-

ure, hypotension, tachycardia, ventricular arrhythmias, angina pectoris, myocardial infarction, pericarditis, and hypertrichosis. Minoxidil elevates plasma renin activity and norepinephrine concentrations in heart failure.[313]

Although select heart failure patients may respond favorably to chronic minoxidil therapy,[194,311] the role of this agent in the standard treatment of heart failure is little to none. Chronic administration in heart failure should be restricted to patients who cannot tolerate converting enzyme inhibitors or hydralazine and whose symptoms cannot be controlled on nitrates, digitalis, and diuretics alone. Minoxidil may then be considered on a trial basis. The dose ranges from 5 to 30 mg orally, and is generally administered every 12 hr.

Flosequinan

Flosequinan (BTS 49465), a 7-fluorinated quinoline (Fig. 24.19), is a unique orally active cardiovascular agent that possesses direct arterial and venous dilating properties.[315] Since its synthesis in 1979 and initial administration to man in 1982, this "balanced" vasodilator has shown promise as a drug that could have an important impact on the pharmacologic management of CHF.

Basic Pharmacology, Metabolism, and Pharmacokinetics

Studies utilizing both animals and humans have identified flosequinan as a "direct" arterial and venous dilator.[315,316] When administered to healthy volunteers, flosequinan elicits reductions in forearm vascular resistance and venous tone, which coincide with its systemic hypotensive effect.[315] Flosequinan also reverses hypoxic pulmonary vasoconstriction in dogs and a small study in hypertensive patients demonstrated a reduction in renal vascular resistance after 5 months of therapy with flosequinan.[317,318] In addition to these systemic and regional vasodilatory effects, flosequinan recently has been shown to exhibit positive inotropic properties in vitro and in vivo, and this may add to its overall

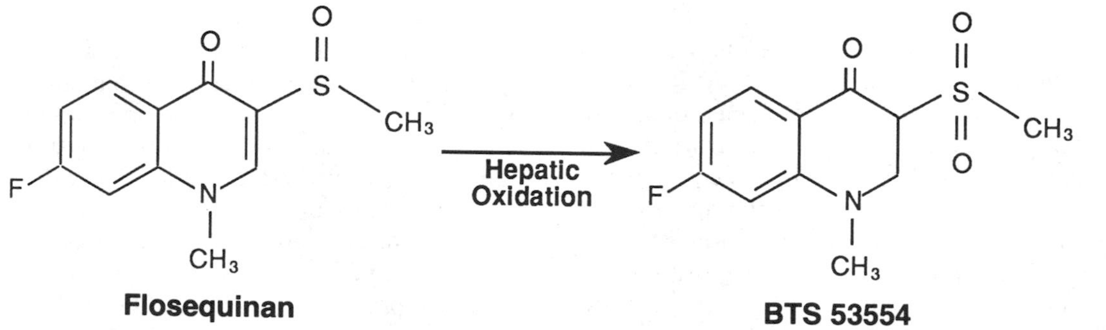

FIGURE 24.19. Molecular structure of flosequinan (BTS 49465) and its active sulfone metabolite (BTS 53554).

hemodynamic effectiveness.[319–321] Despite a significant amount of clinical testing, however, much more remains to be learned regarding the basic pharmacology of this drug. It has not been shown to interact with known vascular receptors (α- or β-adrenoreceptors, dopaminergic, or 5-hydroxytryptamine receptors) however, an effect on intracellular calcium handling has been suggested.[322] Further investigation at the cellular level will be required to define the precise mode of action of flosequinan.

Flosequinan is absorbed rapidly from the gastrointestinal tract, and reaches peak plasma concentrations 30 to 90 min after ingestion.[323] The parent compound is cleared from the systemic circulation with a half-life of 1.6 hr by hepatic oxidation to the pharmacologically active sulfone metabolite (BTS 53554) (Fig. 24.19).[323,324] This metabolite reaches peak plasma levels within 6 to 8 hr and is eliminated via renal excretion with a plasma half-life of 38 hr.[323,324] These pharmacokinetic properties support a once-daily oral dosing regimen.

The degree of hepatic and/or renal dysfunction commonly observed in patients with severe CHF could significantly alter the pharmacokinetics of flosequinan and its active metabolite. A preliminary report by Packer et al.[325] suggests that continuously elevated trough levels of flosequinan or its metabolite achieves few additional hemodynamic benefits, and potentially may increase adverse effects. It is therefore probable that downward adjustments in the dosing of flosequinan would be required in patients with hepatic or renal disease.

Cardiovascular Pharmacology in CHF

Central Hemodynamic Effects

Flosequinan favorably alters central hemodynamics in patients with acute and chronic CHF.[326–328] The balanced vasodilating effect of a single oral dose of 100 mg consistently evokes significant reductions in systemic and pulmonary vascular resistances with concomitant reductions in left and right ventricular filling pressures. These changes in ventricular loading are associated with improved left ventricular performance as manifested by augmented stroke volume and cardiac output. As a result, significant hypotension and reflex tachycardia are not commonly observed. Improvement in central hemodynamics has been observed up to 24 hr after a single dose of flosequinan, thus supporting the concept of a once-daily dosing regimen.[328,329]

The hemodynamic response to repeated administration of flosequinan has been shown to parallel the first-dose response.[330–332] During short-term therapy with flosequinan (3–8 days), there is no evidence that hemodynamic tolerance develops. In fact, further hemodynamic improvement may occur as a result of the cumulative plasma level and vasodilator effect of the active metabolite.[331,332] This continued hemodynamic

efficacy may be related in part to the finding that unlike other arterial vasodilators, flosequinan minimally activates neurohormonal systems during short-term therapy.[316,323,329,332]

There is recent evidence supporting a direct positive inotropic effect of flosequinan and its metabolite in CHF. Results from studies employing an acute heart failure animal model (propranolol-induced) have identified marked increases in myocardial contractility after flosequinan administration.[319–321] It remains to be determined, however, whether the positive inotropic effect of flosequinan is clinically important or apparent at the vasodilatory doses commonly used in humans. Studies from our laboratories have not identified significant changes in left ventricular contractile function with acute or chronic flosequinan therapy.[326,333] Conversely, Corin et al.[334] have reported that 100 mg of flosequinan given orally significantly increases peak rate of rise in left ventricular pressure (dP/dt) over that attributable to its vasodilatory effects in patients with CHF.[334] Certainly, further investigation will be required to ascertain the clinical significance of this finding.

Regional Blood Flow

Our laboratory has shown that 100 mg of flosequinan does not significantly increase blood flow to upper limb, renal, or hepatic-splanchnic vascular regions in patients with moderately severe CHF.[326] During chronic flosequinan therapy, however, Cowley et al.[329] reported an improvement in resting forearm blood flow in heart failure patients. This also was associated with a significant augmentation in calf blood flow immediately after submaximal exercise. Interestingly, patients exhibiting this response had significantly better exercise tolerance than placebo controls.[329]

Clinical Application

Several placebo-controlled, randomized studies have tested the clinical utility of flosequinan for treating chronic CHF.[324,333,335–338,338a,338b] Results have consistently shown that the addition of flosequinan to digoxin and diuretics, with or without concomitant converting enzyme inhibitor therapy, for 4 to 12 weeks significantly improves symptoms and exercise capacity compared to placebo. During chronic therapy, flosequinan increases oxygen consumption at peak exercise and the anaerobic threshold.[335,336]

The beneficial effect of flosequinan on symptoms and exercise capacity in chronic CHF may not be associated with an improvement in survival. At the time of this writing, enrollment in a multicenter trial (PROFILE) designed to assess the effect of flosequinan on survival during background therapy with digitalis, diuretics, and converting enzyme inhibitors has been terminated (unpublished data). This was necessary because of preliminary data showing an increased risk of death in patients randomized to flosequinan (100 mg daily) compared to the placebo. Although no trend was observed in patients receiving flosequinan at 75 mg per day, this group was small and recommendations regarding dosing at this level must await further data analysis.

At the present time, flosequinan, at a dose of 50–75 mg once a day, should only be considered for those patients with severe CHF who remain symptomatic despite treatment with digitalis, diuretics, and converting enzyme inhibitors. The most frequently recognized adverse effects include those related to vasodilation (headache, flushing, postural hypotension, tachycardia, and palpitations). A sustained increase in heart rate has been noted during chronic therapy.[333,337]

Nicorandil

Nicorandil, a nicotinamide derivative, is a newly developed drug that exhibits systemic and coronary vasodilating properties.[339] Experimental and clinical investigations in animals, normal volunteers, and patients with hypertension and ischemic heart disease have reported that nicorandil significantly reduces preload and afterload while augmenting cardiac output and coronary blood flow.[339–344] Nicorandil has no effect on the cardiac conduction system, and exhibits negative inotropic properties only at very high doses. These findings suggest that nicorandil may induce desirable hemodynamic effects in patients with CHF.

Nicorandil evokes vasodilation by at least two mechanisms.[340,341,345] Its nicotinamide moiety increases membrane potassium conductance, resulting in hyperpolarization of vascular smooth muscle membranes, thus preventing activation of voltage-dependent calcium channels. Therefore, the vasodilating effect of nicorandil is similar in part to that of calcium channel antagonists. The nicorandil molecule also contains a terminal nitro group that enhances vasodilation by generating intracellular cGMP. Unlike other nitrovasodilators, tolerance to nicorandil has not been demonstrated in vitro or in animals.[339,345] It remains to be determined, however, whether tolerance is a factor in humans during chronic administration.

In animals and normal volunteers, nicorandil is absorbed rapidly from the gastrointestinal tract, and reaches peak plasma levels at 60 min after oral administration.[339,343] The site of metabolic conversion to an inactive metabolite is primarily the liver, although several different metabolic pathways may exist in humans.[339] Nicorandil has a biphasic elimination profile. The half-life of the rapid phase is 0.6 hr, and that of the slower second phase is approximately 13.6 hr.[339]

Multiple clinical investigations have assessed the efficacy of nicorandil in the treatment of ischemic heart disease[342,346–352]; however, few clinical trials have evaluated its hemodynamic effects in patients with CHF.[353–355] Results from a preliminary investigation by Solal et al.[353] and a double-blind, placebo-controlled study from our laboratories[354] are in agreement with respect to acute central hemodynamic effects of nicorandil in patients with moderate to severe chronic CHF. Consistent with a balanced vasodilating effect, a single dose of nicorandil (usually > 40 mg) reduced systemic and pulmonary resistances and right and left heart filling pressures. These changes were associated with a concomitant increase in cardiac output and minimal alterations in heart rate and systemic arterial pressure. Interestingly, the duration of action of nicorandil in these studies was short, with nearly all hemodynamic parameters returning to near baseline within 3 to 4 hr.[353,354] Tice et al.[354] showed that the loss of hemodynamic effect occurred in concert with a rapid plasma clearance of nicorandil as determined by serial measurements of plasma drug concentration. Galie et al.[355] reported similar favorable acute hemodynamic changes after nicorandil (40–60 mg) in patients with mild to moderate heart failure; however, the duration of the hemodynamic effect in their study lasted 6 to 8 hr. In addition, a nicorandil-induced reduction in pulmonary capillary wedge pressure was observed during exercise. Nicorandil did not alter forearm blood flow or venous capacitance, and an increase in plasma renin activity was seen after dosing with 40 to 60 mg.[355]

The most common adverse effects of first-dose nicorandil therapy in human heart failure are headaches, flushing, and symptomatic orthostatic hypotension.[354,355] These symptoms are typically evident 30 to 60 min after an oral dose.

Although the acute hemodynamic effects of nicorandil appear favorable in human heart failure, a great deal remains to be learned regarding this drug's efficacy during long-term treatment. Furthermore, it will be imperative to explore the factors governing patient variability with respect to drug dose and duration of effect.

Dipyridamole

Dipyridamole is a potent coronary vasodilator with peripheral vasodilating effects when given in large doses.[356–358] Favorable central hemodynamic effects have been observed after the administration of intravenous dipyridamole (30–80 mg) in human heart failure.[356] These effects are brief (less than 90 min), and all qualitatively and quantitatively similar to hemodynamic changes induced by oral hydralazine (100 mg). In contrast, oral dipyridamole (in single doses as high as 300 mg) induces inconsistent and modest hemodynamic effects in patients with severe heart failure. Parker et al.[356] reported that only one of eight patients exhibited a decrease in peripheral resistance after a 150-mg dose, and only two additional patients had significant peripheral vasodilation after 300 mg. These effects persisted for only 3 to 4 hr. Thus, because of the inconsistency of response, large-dose requirement, and brief duration of hemodynamic effect after oral dipyridamole, it is unlikely that this drug will be of benefit in treating chronic CHF. Although significant hemodynamic improvement may be observed after intravenous dipyridamole, a continuous infusion would be required to maintain this effect.

Calcium Channel Blocking Drugs

The calcium channel blocking agents have proved efficacious in the management of ischemic heart disease and systemic hypertension.[359-362] In that these compounds exert potent systemic and coronary vasodilator effects, there has been considerable interest over the past 10 years in their use as vasodilators in treating human heart failure.[362] Since intracellular calcium flux is an important determinant of vasoconstriction, calcium channel blockade would seem to be a rational approach for reducing systemic vascular resistance and aortic impedance and improving hemodynamics in this condition.[363] Thus far, these agents have undergone extensive clinical evaluation, and at the present time, their role in the management of chronic CHF remains uncertain.

The calcium antagonists currently are divided into three classes based on their chemical structure.[364,365] The dihydropyridines, typified by nifedipine, are the largest group. The other first generation calcium blockers include verapamil and diltiazem, which are members of the phenylalkylamine and benzothiazepine classes, respectively. All calcium channel blockers inhibit the slow inward calcium current through the voltage-dependent calcium channel in vascular smooth muscle and myocardium. This results in a decrease in calcium availability to contractile proteins in these tissues.[366] As a result, these drugs preferentially dilate arterioles and can reduce ventricular contractility.

Significant differences exist between classes regarding vasodilator potency, degree of negative inotropy, and effect on cardiac conduction. In general, nifedipine can be considered the most potent vasodilator, whereas verapamil exhibits the greatest negative inotropic effect. Both verapamil and diltiazem slow heart rate and AV conduction whereas nifedipine can increase heart rate via reflex mechanisms.[366] Importantly, the overall hemodynamic profile of each calcium channel blocker must be considered not only in light of its direct effects on the vasculature and myocardium, but also with respect to the propensity to activate neurohumoral mechanisms.[362] For example, the negligible net effect of

nifedipine on contractility in vivo is dependent on an intact sympathetic nervous system. During β-adrenergic blockade, nifedipine reduces ventricular contractility to a degree similar to verapamil.[367,368] This has important implications in the treatment of CHF where sympathetic tone is markedly enhanced and cardiovascular reflexes impaired.[362,369]

The acute hemodynamic effects of calcium channel blockers in human heart failure have been well defined.[64,195,370-373] Nifedipine, because it represents the most potent vasodilator of the first generation drugs, has been studied most extensively. When administered orally or intravenously to patients with heart failure, it lowers systemic vascular resistance and arterial pressure while increasing stroke volume and cardiac output. Since nifedipine has little effect on venous capacitance vessels, it induces only modest changes in right and left ventricular filling pressures.[64,374] As a result of improved stroke volume and cardiac output, heart rate usually is unchanged despite some drop in mean arterial pressure.

Our laboratories reported an improvement in exercise hemodynamics after initial dose nifedipine in heart failure patients.[64] This favorable hemodynamic effect was not accompanied by enhanced exercise capacity. Nifedipine does not appear to improve blood flow significantly to a specific vascular region, but there may be preferential dilatation of limb vasculature.[64] Nifedipine decreases renal vascular resistance without significantly altering renal blood flow or glomerular filtration rate.[64,278] Acute reversible renal dysfunction has been described after initiation of nifedipine therapy in patients with chronic renal insufficiency.[375] All calcium channel blockers significantly dilate the coronary vascular bed.[376]

Significant adverse hemodynamic and clinical events have been reported during nifedipine therapy in heart failure.[64,377-379] In patients with severe left ventricular dysfunction, the negative inotropic action of nifedipine can approximate that seen with verapamil.[377,378]

The acute hemodynamic effects of diltiazem in human heart failure are similar to those described with nifedipine.[380] It should be noted, however, that diltiazem has the propensity to precipitate significant bradycardia or AV block in patients with underlying conduction system disease.[380]

Verapamil, because of its marked negative inotropic effect, may induce clinical and hemodynamic deterioration in patients with impaired systolic function, and therefore has a limited role in the management of heart failure.

The second generation calcium channel blockers (e.g., nicardipine, nitrendipine, nisoldipine, felodipine, isradipine) are similar to nifedipine with respect to their hemodynamic profile in CHF. Because of their relative "vasoselectivity", they purportedly are less likely to depress ventricular systolic function.[381–383] Although these drugs generally are well tolerated acutely,[381–387] a favorable hemodynamic response may not be accompanied by an improvement in clinical status or exercise capacity.[386,387] Clinical deterioration, possibly related to activation of neurohormonal mechanisms, has been described during chronic therapy with some second generation calcium blockers.[381,388,389] Conversely, there is recent evidence that two of these calcium channel blockers, felodipine and amlodipine, decrease plasma levels of norepinephrine, and thus may improve symptoms and exercise capacity in CHF[390–392]; long-term felodipine is a current treatment limb of V-HeFT III, and amlodipine is being studied in the PRAISE trial.

Results from two recent studies have added significantly to our current understanding of the chronic effects of calcium channel blockade in patients with poor left ventricular systolic function. A secondary analysis of the Multicenter Diltiazem Postinfarction Trial (MDPIT) evaluated the effect of chronic diltiazem therapy in postmyocardial infarction patients with baseline left ventricular dysfunction.[393] The findings indicate that patients with significant impairment in ventricular contractility postinfarct are at increased risk for subsequent development of CHF when treated with diltiazem. Among those patients with baseline left ventricular ejection fractions <40%, late heart failure developed in 12% receiving placebo and 21% taking diltiazem. The authors concluded that diltiazem should be administered with caution to patients with postinfarction left ventricular dysfunction.

Elkayam et al.[394] evaluated the effects of nifedipine alone or in combination with isosorbide dinitrate in a controlled trial involving 28 patients with chronic CHF. These investigators found that treatment with nifedipine (whether alone or in combination with nitrates) resulted in a significantly higher incidence of heart failure deterioration than during treatment with nitrates alone.[392,394] No patients required hospitalization during therapy with nitrates. However, 24% of nifedipine-treated patients and 26% percent of those receiving nifedipine and nitrates required hospitalization because of worsening heart failure. Although patients experiencing clinical deterioration could not be predicted by baseline ejection fraction or exercise capacity, a significant reduction in diastolic blood pressure was evident in both groups receiving nifedipine. It is possible that this reduction in blood pressure contributed to worsening heart failure by reducing coronary blood flow and/or activating neurohumoral responses.

A substantial percentage of patients presenting with CHF will have normal ventricular contractility and markedly abnormal diastolic function. These patients may benefit from calcium channel blockade. In a study by Setaro et al.,[395] verapamil significantly improved exercise capacity and ventricular peak filling rate in patients with preserved systolic function and impaired diastolic filling. Although it is uncertain whether calcium channel blockers uniformly improve ventricular diastolic properties, they also may augment ventricular filling via alterations in loading conditions and enhanced sympathetic activity.[396,397] However, it is important to note that Nishimura and colleagues[397a] recently reported a rise in mean left ventricular end-diastolic pressure and the mean time constant of relaxation following intravenous verapamil in 20 patients with diastolic dysfunction secondary to coronary artery disease and normal systolic function (ejection fraction >40%).

Currently, calcium channel blockers cannot be recommended as first-line vasodilators for patients with heart failure and impaired systolic function. Their direct negative inotropic effects, together with their capacity to activate neurohormonal systems, may lead to clinical deterioration. Whether second or third generation calcium antagonists will be beneficial in heart failure remains to be determined.

Agents that Vasodilate via Inhibition/Interruption of Sympathetic Nervous System Activity

In response to cardiac failure, the sympathetic nervous system is activated to increase and maintain cardiac output and systemic blood pressure. As previously discussed, the activation of this system also evokes an unfavorable increase in ventricular afterload and preload via norepinephrine and renin release and stimulation of postjunctional α-adrenergic receptors.[398,399] Drugs have been developed to interrupt the sympathetic nervous system at various levels and a number of these agents have been investigated in the clinical setting of CHF.[398–400]

Central and Peripheral Presynaptic α-Adrenergic Receptor Agonism

Stimulation of α_2-adrenergic receptors within the central nervous system (CNS) reduces sympathetic outflow and peripheral sympathetic nervous system tone, and presynaptic agonism of the α_2 receptor at the peripheral nerve junction inhibits norepinephrine release.[398] Clonidine and quanabenz are examples of such agents. α-Methyldopa acts similarly after it is converted to methylnorepinephrine.

Intravenous (0.15 mg) or initial oral (0.2 and 0.4 mg) administration of clonidine significantly decreases systemic and pulmonic arterial pressures and ventricular filling pressures.[401–404] The reduction in central sympathetic outflow after clonidine results in a negative chronotropic and inotropic response in patients with heart failure.[402] As a result, stroke volume and cardiac output change little with clonidine, despite a fall in systemic arterial pressure and ventricular afterload. Calculated systemic vascular resistance only decreases modestly after clonidine dosing in heart failure. Limb vascular resistance falls slightly without an augmentation of limb blood flow.[403] Renal and hepatic-splanchnic blood flow and vascular resistance are not altered by clonidine in heart failure.[403] The results of a small trial of chronic clonidine therapy in heart failure are not impressive.[404] A hypertensive response and exacerbation of heart failure can follow clonidine withdrawal in patients with ventricular dysfunction.[405]

The hemodynamic effects of quanabenz in heart failure are similar to those noted for clonidine.[406] In contrast to most other forms of vasodilation, vasodilation via central sympathetic inhibition (e.g., quanabenz) can depress plasma norepinephrine concentrations (less norepinephrine release), but may not affect plasma renin activity.[406] No long-term trials of quanabenz are available, but the results are not likely to differ much from those noted with chronic clonidine administration.

Intravenously or orally administered α-methyldopa also reduces ventricular filling, systemic and pulmonary arterial pressures, and heart rate with modest effects on cardiac output and vascular resistances.[407,408] A blinded, placebo-controlled trial by Kirlin and colleagues[407] failed to demonstrate a significant impact of long-term α-methyldopa therapy on the clinical status and exercise capacity of a small (n = 14) heart failure population.

α_1-Adrenergic Receptor Blocking Agents

With respect to the use of α_1 blockers in the treatment of heart failure, few interventions in heart failure have made a more dramatic entry followed by an early, equally rapid exit. First-dose prazosin in CHF was noted to reduce significantly ventricular filling pressures and vascular resistances and increase stroke volume and cardiac output.[409–412] These ideally favorable, "balanced" responses (preload *and* afterload reduction) led many to refer to prazosin as the "oral nitroprusside." The development of pharmacodynamic tolerance after only 2 to 5 doses, reported almost simultaneously from several established laboratories, rang the death knell for prazosin as a vasodilating drug in heart failure.[413–416] This profound limitation has now been applied generally to all α_1-blocking agents despite little blinded, placebo-controlled, chronic-dosing data to support such for most of the nonprazosin agents. There currently is little general use of α_1-adrenergic blockade in the management of CHF and still less activity in the clinical investigation of this group of drugs. It is nevertheless important to present information on α_1 blockade in heart failure because the clinical studies involved have taught us a considerable amount about the pathophysiology and pharmacophysiology of heart failure, and about the limitations of our investigative techniques.

Prazosin

Prazosin, a quinazoline derivative, has variable bioavailability (40–70%) to oral administration.[417] Prazosin is highly protein-bound (90–97%) and more than 90% is metabolized by the liver (*O*-demethylation) and excreted in the bile.[417] The distribution and clearance follows a two-compartment model with a mean elimination half-life in normal persons of 2.5 hr.[417] Plasma clearance of prazosin is reduced in heart failure with a plasma half-life in this condition of 5 to 7 hr.[417–420] In heart failure, time to peak concentration is about 2 hr and, in general, a linear relationship exists between dose, mean peak concentration, and mean area under the curve.[418]

Initial oral doses ($\geq$ 1 mg) of prazosin elicit a balanced, "nitroprusside-like" effect (reduction of both preload and afterload) on central hemodynamics in CHF.[63,259,271,400,409–416,421–428] First-dose prazosin significantly drops systemic and pulmonic vascular resistances and ventricular filling pressures, while increasing stroke volume and cardiac output. Although systemic arterial pressure may fall modestly, heart rate changes little or may decrease slightly. These favorable hemodynamic effects also are noted during exercise.[429]

First-dose prazosin in heart failure at oral doses of 2 to 5 mg preferentially reduces hepatic-splanchnic vascular resistance and augments hepatic-splanchnic blood flow.[63] As the dose increases from 5 to 10 mg, hepatic-splanchnic blood flow falls and limb flow rises, probably representing an example of systemic-regional "steal." Renal vascular resistance and blood flow are not altered by prazosin.[63]

Attenuation of the hemodynamic effects of prazosin in heart failure is partially present after the second oral dose and is virtually complete by the third to fifth dose.[413–416] The early impressions that tolerance develops in only $\leq$ 40% of patients receiving this drug chronically[430] and that hemodynamic attenuation does not occur during exercise[431] are not supported by most other well designed studies.[413–416,432,433] The development of pharmacodynamic tolerance also occurs for the regional hemodynamic effects of prazosin during repeated administration in heart failure.[63]

The hemodynamic attenuation is accompanied by a lack of improvement in clinical status and exercise capacity during chronic prazosin dosing in chronic CHF. The apparent cardiovascular and clinical benefits noted during chronic prazosin administration in small, unblinded, or uncontrolled trials[410,412,422,425,427,428,430,434–437] have not been substantiated by trials employing more rigorous testing and better study design.[6,424,432,433,438,439] Long-term prazosin administration, when added to chronic digitalis and diuretic therapy, did not improve survival in the sizable V-HeFT heart failure population over that achieved with long-term placebo.[6]

The precise mechanisms involved in the development of pharmacodynamic tolerance to repeated prazosin dosing in heart failure have not been elucidated fully and probably are multifactoral. A change in bioavailability is an unlikely explanation, because peak plasma prazosin levels with repeated dosing are higher than those after the first dose.[413,415] Prazosin tends to evoke a significant increase in plasma norepinephrine, and in some studies, a rise in plasma renin activity as well[425,433,434,440-445]; each is capable of reversing the favorable hemodynamic responses to prazosin. Although diuretic requirements usually increase (or weight gain occurs) during long-term prazosin therapy, spironolactone administration or furosemide-induced diuresis has not consistently prevented or reversed the development of tolerance.[414,428,433,434,439,443,444] Prazosin does not adversely affect intrinsic renal function in heart failure.[445]

Other α_1-Adrenergic Blocking Agents

A number of other quinazoline derivatives have been studied in human CHF including terazosin, trimazosin, and doxazosin.[446-452] The hemodynamic responses of these agents are similar to those of prazosin with the exception that the newer agents have a longer duration of action: 8 to 24 hr compared to 6 to 8 hr for prazosin. Preliminary studies have suggested that clinical status and exercise tolerance can be improved during the chronic administration of these compounds; however, most of the studies were small, uncontrolled, or nonblinded.[446,450,451] In a double-blind, placebo-controlled trial on 73 patients with chronic heart failure, DiBianco et al.[452] found that chronic doxazosin therapy effected a modest improvement of symptoms, general activity tolerance, and ventricular ectopy. From a historical perspective, the documented effectiveness and general availability of the converting enzyme inhibitors, coupled with the demonstration of pharmacodynamic tolerance to prazosin and the failure of prazosin to improve survival of heart failure patients, removed the enthusiasm and effort from further investigation of α_1 blockade in heart failure.

Indoramin, a member of the benzamidopiperidylethylindole group of compounds elicits α_1-adrenergic blockade and hemodynamic responses at rest and during exercise similar to those of prazosin.[453-455] Chronic administration achieves little improvement in rest or exercise hemodynamics and no improvement over placebo in clinical status or exercise capacity.[456,457]

Nonspecific α-Adrenergic Receptor Blocking Agents

α-Adrenergic vasoconstriction in heart failure is mediated by both α_1 and α_2 postsynaptic (junctional and extrajunctional) adrenergic receptors.[398,458] Agents that block both α_1 and α_2 receptors therefore should be effective vasodilating agents. Phentolamine is the nonspecific α-blocking drug studied most commonly in the clinical setting of CHF.[2,3,79,459-470] Many of the very earliest reports of afterload-preload reduction in the management of CHF involved the use of phentolamine as the vasodilating agent.[2,3,459-463]

Intravenously and orally administered phentolamine, at respective doses of 10 to 30 μg/kg/min and 25 to 50 mg every 6 hr, significantly reduces systemic vascular resistance with resultant augmentation of stroke volume and cardiac output. Systemic blood pressure may fall to a variable degree and heart rate remains unchanged or rises slightly. The phentolamine-induced reduction in systemic vascular resistance does not appear to be accompanied by an increase in nutritional blood flow to limb musculature at rest or during exercise.[471,472] Although somewhat less dramatic than its arterial-arteriolar dilating effects, phentolamine also lowers ventricular filling pressures and pulmonary vascular resistance. Its relatively modest effects on pulmonary vasculature perhaps accounts for the absence of arterial desaturation after proper phentolamine dosing.[469]

Phentolamine has been shown to effectively reduce excessive afterload and preload in acute heart failure and pulmonary edema.[2,3,460,462,464] This agent has been particularly effective in patients whose ventricular dysfunction and CHF is complicated by systemic hypertension or valvular (aortic or mitral) regurgitation.[461,470] Chronic administration in chronic heart failure may have a favorable effect on clinical status and activity/exercise tolerance[468]; however, this finding has not been adequately tested with a blinded, placebo-controlled study.

Phenoxybenzamine, another nonspecific α-adrenergic blocking agent, has been employed effectively in the management of the hypertensive events and heart failure surrounding pheochromocytoma.[473]

The failure of nonspecific α-adrenergic blockade, specifically phentolamine and phenoxybenzamine, to have a significant impact on the current management of heart failure is related to several factors. In one author's (CVL) personal, unpublished experience, individual hemodynamic responses to phentolamine are highly variable. Its predominant effects on systemic arterial-arteriolar vessels can evoke myocardial ischemia and angina, particularly if sympathetic reflexes are activated.[468] Concomitant nitrate administration usually is required to deliver a more "balanced" preload-afterload effect in most patients with CHF. In the setting of acute heart failure, phentolamine or phenoxybenzamine offer little to no advantage over nitroprusside or nitroglycerin, and in chronic CHF, no benefit over converting enzyme inhibition or hydralazine.

Combined β- and α-Adrenergic Blockade

Labetalol nonspecifically blocks β-adrenergic receptors (both β_1 and β_2 adrenoreceptors) and specifically blocks α_1 receptors. The rationale for studying this compound in heart failure resides in applying the presumed "protective" effects of β-adrenergic blockade and employing the vasodilatation of α_1 blockade to hemodynamically counter, via afterload reduction, any myocardial depression evoked by β-adrenergic blockade.

Labetalol's β-blockade effects are considerably more potent than its α-blocking properties.[474] Nevertheless, labetalol has been effective and relatively safe as an antihypertensive agent at standard antihypertensive doses (200–1600 mg/day) in patients with hypertension and left ventricular dysfunction.[475] An occasional patient may experience an exacerbation of heart failure in this setting.[475,476] Based on the authors' experience in managing hypertension in patients with heart failure and on the knowledge gained from the β-blockade heart failure trials, exacerbation of heart failure with labetalol is less likely when lower doses (25–100 mg/day) are administered initially, followed by a very gradual advancement of the dose.

In a small (n = 12) but blinded and placebo-controlled, crossover trial, Leung and colleagues[477] concluded that labetalol, at a mean daily dose of 275 mg, favorably influenced clinical status and exercise performance in patients with chronic heart failure.

Carvediolol, a new combined β-α-adrenergic blocking agent, was found to improve hemodynamics, exercise capacity, and clinical status in a small population (n = 12) of patients with heart failure during an 8-week, open-label, uncontrolled study.[478] A number of carvedilol trials are currently being performed in larger CHF populations.

Other Sympatholytic-Vasodilating Compounds

Most of the remaining sympatholytic-vasodilating agents are interesting primarily from a historical perspective. Hexamethonium, a ganglionic blocking agent, and guanethidine, a drug that blocks norepinephrine release and reuptake, were employed more than 25 years ago to demonstrate that much of the pathophysiology and clinical manifestations of CHF were related to systemic vasoconstriction.[1,479] Trimethaphan, another ganglionic blocking drug, also reduces systemic vascular tone and ventricular filling pressures in heart failure.[480]

Other Vasodilators

Many other compounds, because of their vasodilating properties, have important roles in the pathophysiology and potentially in the therapeutics of CHF. These include a number of endogenous substances (e.g., atrial natriuretic factor, prostaglandins, prostacyclin, endothelium-derived relaxation factor), β_2-adrenergic agonists (e.g., pirbuterol, terbutaline), endogenous and exogenous dopaminergic agents (e.g., dopamine, dopexamine, ibopamine, bromocriptine), "vasodilating" β-adrenergic blocking drugs (e.g., bucindolol), phosphodiesterase inhibitors (e.g., milrinone, enoximone), renin, angiotensin, and vasopressin antagonists, inhibitors of norepinephrine synthesis (e.g., α-methyltyrosine), and others. These substances and compounds are discussed elsewhere in this book.

The Practical Application of Vasodilator Therapy in Heart Failure

Various vasodilators, especially nitroprusside, nitrates, and hydralazine, have earned a major role in the management of a number of heart failure conditions. The most common current applications of vasodilator therapy are listed in Table 24.4. It is important to note that these clinical applications are not absolute indications for vasodilator therapy, but merely represent clinical situations that often benefit from proper vasodilator administration. The details of proper administration of each vasodilator are presented in the sections of this chapter specifically addressing each agent.

Acute Intervention

Intravenously administered nitroglycerin is an effective means of acutely reducing the excessively elevated ventricular filling pressures and vascular resistances and associated symptoms present in acute heart failure, acute pulmonary edema, acute severe valvular regurgitation, severely decompensated chronic CHF, and similar clinical conditions. Nitroglycerin infusions are started at 0.2 to 0.3 μg/kg/min, and advanced every 10 to 15 min as needed to achieve the desired clinical and hemodynamic end-points (Table 24.5). Infusions lasting longer than 6 hr generally will require gradual dose incrementation to offset the development of pharmacodynamic tolerance or a switch to nitroprusside to maintain the desired reduction of afterload and preload.

Sublingual tablets or lingual aerosol spray of nitroglycerin is an effective, temporary means of acutely reducing preload-afterload, until nitroglycerin or nitroprusside can be infused intravenously. This form of intervention (lingual, sublingual nitroglycerin) is particularly useful in the very earliest stages of managing

TABLE 24.4. Clinical application of vasodilator therapy in the setting of heart failure.

Acute intervention (nitroprusside; sublingual tablets, lingual, aerosol, and intravenous nitroglycerin)
— Acute heart failure
— Cardiogenic pulmonary edema
— Acute ischemic myocardium—heart failure syndromes (e.g., papillary muscle dysfunction, ischemic diastolic dysfunction)
— Acute/severe valvular regurgitation (aortic or mitral)
— Rupture of interventricular septum or ventricular free wall
— Additional preload-afterload reduction when added to other cardioactive agents (e.g., dopamine, dobutamine)
— Acute or severe decompensation of chronic CHF
— Stabilizing the chronic CHF patient through major diagnostic or surgical procedures
— Withdrawal from cardiopulmonary bypass and during early postoperative phase of cardiac surgery

Chronic vasodilator therapy with drugs other than converting enzyme inhibitors (e.g., hydralazine, nitrates, combination hydralazine-nitrates, flosequinan, calcium channel blocking agents)
— Chronic afterload-preload reduction in heart failure patients intolerant of or refractory to converting enzyme inhibitors (consider hydralazine-nitrate combination, flosequinan)
— Hemodynamically directed and targeted vasodilator therapy[66]
— Time- or activity-targeted vasodilator therapy (e.g., bedtime nitrates for orthopnea or paroxysmal nocturnal dyspnea)
— Heart failure caused or complicated by aortic and/or mitral valvular regurgitation (consider hydralazine)
— Heart failure complicated by myocardial ischemia, angina, and angina-equivalent syndromes (consider nitrates)
— Dobutamine withdrawal from dobutamine-dependent patients (consider hydralazine)
— Diastolic-dysfunction heart failure (consider nitrates, Ca^{2+} channel blocking agents)
— Potential augmentation of survival (consider hydralazine-nitrate combination)

TABLE 24.5. General clinical and hemodynamic endpoints for acute vasodilator therapy in acute, severe CHF.

Reduce pulmonary congestion and dyspnea
Improve peripheral perfusion and organ function
Decrease left ventricular filling pressure to ≤15–18 mm Hg
Increase cardiac output to adequate levels of oxygen delivery (DO_2)
Without drug-induced clinical deterioration, significant systemic hypotension, tachycardia, or other clinically significant adverse effects

severe acute cardiogenic pulmonary edema (i.e., administered within the first 0–3 min of seeing the patient). Certain chronic heart failure patients can be trained to safely self-administer sublingual/lingual nitroglycerin to avert recurrent episodes of acute heart failure and pulmonary edema, or at least to allow a more comfortable trip to the emergency department.

Nitroprusside should be considered instead of nitroglycerin if: (a) more aggressive afterload-reduction is needed (e.g., severe low-output failure and pulmonary edema secondary to rupture of a papillary muscle), (b)

a nitroglycerin infusion up to reasonably high doses has not been effective in improving the decompensated hemodynamic and clinical condition, and (c) if nitroglycerin's hemodynamic effectiveness and clinical benefit wane during a continuous infusion (>4–6 hr) because of the development of pharmacodynamic tolerance. In the first situation, nitroprusside is generally the initial drug of choice, and in the latter two conditions, the patient would be best served by switching the afterload-preload reduction therapy as needed from nitroglycerin to nitroprusside.

Nitroprusside infusions usually are started at 0.05 to 0.10 μg/kg/min and advanced every 8 to 10 min as needed to attain the desired clinical and hemodynamic end-points (Table 24.5).

Nitroglycerin and nitroprusside usually are employed as short-term supportive intervention—supportive until the patient's compromised cardiovascular condition abates, definitive intervention is performed (e.g., mitral valve repair or replacement for severe mitral regurgitation), or the needed reduction in afterload-preload can be achieved effectively and safely with orally administered agents (e.g., converting enzyme inhibitors, hydralazine-nitrate combination). Nitroglycerin and nitroprusside thus can be viewed as a form of "pharmacologic bridge" to definitive intervention or recovery.

The end-points of acute vasodilator therapy (Table 24.5) can vary somewhat within any heart failure population, but generally the clinical end-points are a reduction of pulmonary congestion and dyspnea and an improvement of peripheral perfusion and organ function (e.g., improve renal function, raise urine output) without evoking other forms of clinical deterioration or undesirable effects. Reasonable hemodynamic end-points include a reduction in left ventricular filling pressure to ≤ 15 to 18 mm Hg and an increase in cardiac output to levels of adequate systemic oxygen delivery (DO_2) (generally, a cardiac index >2.5 L/min/m²) without evoking significant systemic hypotension (≤ 90/70 depending on baseline systemic blood pressure) or troublesome tachycardia. Although not absolutely necessary in all patients with acute heart failure, the placement of monitoring catheters (flow-directed, triple-lumen, thermodilution pulmonary artery catheter and systemic arterial catheter) by experienced personnel greatly facilitates the most efficient, effective, and safe administration of acute vasodilator therapy.

Nitroglycerin or nitroprusside infusions, via afterload and preload reduction, augment the hemodynamic effects of other cardiovascular interventions, such as dopamine and dobutamine. These combinations are commonly employed in low-output CHF to optimize hemodynamics.[119]

More specific and detailed information concerning nitroprusside and nitroglycerin infusions in heart failure is discussed earlier in this chapter.

Chronic Vasodilator Therapy

Overview

At the present time, the nonconverting enzyme inhibitor (CEI) forms of chronic vasodilator therapy most commonly employed in heart failure are nitrates, hydralazine, or a combination of these. Other agents may be considered in certain conditions such as calcium channel blocking drugs for heart failure complicated by hypertension (systemic and/or pulmonic) or reversible metabolic diastolic dysfunction. Other clinically effective vasodilating agents hopefully will be developed and become available for clinical use in the near future. The vasodilator flosequinan was recently approved for use in chronic heart failure however, its specific role in the treatment of CHF remains to be determined in light of the preliminary findings from PROFILE that 100 mg daily increases mortality. Incidentally, nitrates, hydralazine, and most other non-CEI vasodilators have not yet been approved by the Food and Drug Administration for use in the treatment of heart failure; this, of course, does not obviate the need, effectiveness, and importance of this group of drugs in managing individual patients with chronic heart failure.

The clinical conditions and situations for which chronic vasodilator therapy might be considered are presented in Table 24.4.

General Role and Application

Current information and widespread clinical experience do *not* justify the routine use of non-CEI vasodilators in place of or in addition to converting enzyme–inhibiting agents (e.g., captopril, enalapril). At the present time, first-line drug therapy for chronic CHF is digitalis, diuretics, and converting enzyme inhibition. In a general chronic heart failure population, long-term non-CEI vasodilator therapy, usually in the form of hydralazine-nitrate combination, or flosequinan, is recommended for the following types of heart failure patients: (a) patients whose symptoms are refractory to or incompletely controlled by chronic CEI, digitalis, and diuretic therapy, (b) patients who are intolerant of properly administered CEI therapy (e.g., severe hypotension, serious side effects), and (c) patients whose heart failure is complicated by clinical conditions particularly responsive to specific vasodilators (e.g., hydralazine for valvular insufficiency, nitrates for myocardial ischemia, angina, and angina-equivalent syndromes).

For heart failure patients who are intolerant of CEI therapy or who remain symptomatic on optimal CEI therapy, the hydralazine-nitrate combination may offer clinical benefit in terms of symptom relief and survival. For most heart failure patients, the combination can be started on an outpatient basis using low doses initially, and gradually advancing dosage over the ensuing weeks. Hydralazine and nitrates usually can be started simultaneously in the heart failure patients who have an adequate systemic blood pressure (> 110–120 mm Hg systolic) and clinical evidence of elevated ventricular filling pressures. Nitrates alone or hydralazine with nitrates is recommended as non-CEI vasodilator therapy for patients with ischemic myocardial disease (i.e., rarely hydralazine alone). For most of the remaining patients, the authors initiate hydralazine therapy, follow the clinical course, and superimpose nitrates as needed to effect further reduction in elevated ventricular filling pressures, venous pressures, and congestion; this stepwise approach is employed to avert significant systemic hypotension that can occur in some heart failure patients initially treated with both hydralazine and nitrates.

In patients who clinically are relatively "stable," and considering the clinical scenarios mentioned above, the authors start hydralazine at 25 mg orally every 6 to 8 hr and/or 2% nitroglycerin ointment at 0.5 in topically every 6 to 12 hr (or isosorbide dinitrate orally at 20 mg every 6 hr), whether administered alone or as a combination. A sitting (or supine) and standing systemic blood pressure and heart rate are recorded at baseline and 30, 60, and 120 min after initial dosing and with each major incrementation of dose. The average maintenance dose of hydralazine ranges from 50 to 100 mg orally every 6 hr, nitroglycerin ointment 1 to 2 in topically every 8 hr (if administered every 6 hr with hydralazine, one application should be deleted daily to avoid nitrate tolerance), and isosorbide dinitrate 20 to 40 mg orally every 6 hr (if nitrate tolerance becomes suspect, skipping a dose every 24 hr will reinstate responsiveness). Flosequinan may be used at 50–75 mg daily. At the present time, advancement of the dose beyond 75 mg is not recommended.

Use of Multiple "Unloading" Agents

A considerable number of heart failure patients, mostly those in severe advanced stages, cannot tolerate more than modest doses of CEI (e.g., 6.25 mg captopril, 2.5 mg enalapril) because of baseline and/or CEI-induced systemic hypotension (systolic pressure <80–90 mm Hg). It is not uncommon for these patients to respond symptomatically best to low-dose CEI (e.g., ≤6.2 mg captopril every 8–12 hr) and low-dose vasodilators (25–50 mg hydralazine every 6–8 hr ± nitroglycerin ointment 0.5–1 in every 8 hr) in addition to digoxin and judicious diuretic therapy. In this subgroup, as in all patients with heart failure, an effort is made to facilitate patient compliance by avoiding drug-related adverse effects (via the aforementioned dosing schedules) and by adjusting the timing of drug administration for patient convenience (e.g., avoid an every 6- *and* an every 8-hr dosing schedule in the same patient).

Hemodynamically Directed and Targeted Vasodilator Therapy

Heart failure patients who remain markedly symptomatic despite what appears to be the "optimal" therapeutic plan often benefit from a hemodynamically monitored pharmacodynamic study.[66,481] In such a "vasodilator study", hemodynamic data derived from indwelling catheters (triple-lumen thermodilution pulmonary artery catheter, and system arterial catheter) are employed to arrive at cardioactive and vasodilating agents that provide the maximally beneficial hemodynamic responses. The clinical experience of our laboratory in this setting is similar to that reported by Stevenson and colleagues[66]; a substantial number of "end-stage" heart failure patients, many referred while supported by intravenous infusions of dobutamine or dopamine for cardiac transplantation or "experimental inotropes," can be placed on clinically effective cardioactive vasodilator agents based on the data derived from skilled hemodynamic assessment. Many of these patients can be discharged and managed reasonably on an outpatient basis, and many can be diverted or removed safely from the transplant "waiting list" (a reasonable quest in view of the limited number of heart donors).[66]

Time- and Activity-Targeted Vasodilator Therapy

Vasodilators, particularly nitrates, often are useful as specific time- or activity-targeted therapy. Some patients develop heart failure symptoms only at certain times of the day or with certain activities. Vasodilators can be directed to pretreat and, thus, prevent these time- or activity-related symptoms. For example, 1 to 4 in of 2% nitroglycerin ointment at bedtime can be very effective in averting paroxysmal nocturnal dyspnea or orthopnea in a heart failure patient consistently disturbed by these problems. (More aggressive diuretic therapy at bedtime also may be effective in this specific example, but requires frequent interruptions of sleep to void.)

Chronic Vasodilator Therapy Directed at Specific Cardiac Conditions

Certain cardiac conditions causing or exacerbating heart failure may improve with a specific vasodilator. Aortic and mitral valvular regurgitation can decrease markedly with the afterload reduction of hydralazine. Nitrates often are clinically effective in heart failure patients, whose symptoms are attributable to or exacerbated by myocardial ischemia and the ischemia syndromes (e.g., ischemia-induced diastolic dysfunction, ischemia-induced papillary muscle dysfunction with mitral regurgitation). Heart failure symptoms secondary to metabolic or ischemic diastolic dysfunction deserve a trial of nitrates and/or calcium channel blockade.

Dobutamine Withdrawal

Withdrawing dobutamine from dobutamine-dependent (hemodynamically and clinically) heart failure patients remains a major challenge in clinical medicine. Of the various agents studied by the authors (orally administered phosphodiesterase inhibitors, converting enzyme inhibitors, β_2-adrenergic agonists, and hydralazine), hydralazine has been by far the most effective agent for this purpose.[260] Apparently, the orally administrable vasodilator with positive inotropic effects, namely, hydralazine, provides a reasonable hemodynamic substitute for intravenously delivered dobutamine, a positive inotropic drug with vasodilating properties. Our laboratory has been able to "wean" dobutamine successfully from more than 60% of patients who were unequivocally dobutamine-dependent. After an initial attempt at a slow withdrawal (over 1–3 days) of dobutamine has failed (in the face of adequate ventricular filling pressures and after discontinuing hypotension-evoking drugs), hydralazine is started at a dose of 25 mg orally every 4 to 6 hr and gradually increased using systemic blood pressure, heart rate, and adverse effects as a guide while the dobutamine dose is gradually withdrawn. This exchange usually takes 2 to 6 days, and results in a maintenance oral hydralazine dose in the range of 50 to 400 mg every 4 to 6 hr. Once dobutamine is withdrawn completely and systemic blood pressure is stabilized ($\geq 100/70$ mm Hg) on hydralazine, the addition of nitrates or a converting enzyme inhibitor at low initial doses can be attempted cautiously if these agents are deemed necessary for optimal therapeutic support.

The Use of Chronic Vasodilator Therapy to Reduce Mortality in Heart Failure

In view of the findings of the V-HeFT trial,[6] the question of whether the hydralazine-nitrate combination should ever be administered solely to improve survival remains controversial, especially for CHF patients, intolerant of CEI, with untreated, "asymptomatic" left ventricular dysfunction or ventricular dysfunction well-compensated, on digoxin and diuretics.

Potential Adverse Effects of Vasodilator Therapy in CHF

The major adverse or undesirable effects that can occur during non-CEI vasodilator therapy are presented in Table 24.6.

The most common adverse effect of vasodilator therapy in general is systemic hypotension. As a general rule, this effect is not a problem unless marked in degree ($\leq 80/60$ mm Hg) or accompanied by organ hypoperfusion. Specific organ hypoperfusion can cause azotemia and varying degrees of renal failure, myo-

TABLE 24.6. Potential adverse or undesirable effects of vasodilators.

Vasodilators in general
Systemic hypotension
Vasodilatory shock
Myocardial ischemia
  Angina, angina-equivalent conditions
  Myocardial infarction and associated complications (e.g.,
    cardiogenic shock, death)
Activation of the sympathetic nervous system with catecholamine
  release
  Positive chronotropy and inotropy, rise in myocardial oxygen
    consumption, renin release
Activation of the renin-angiotensin-aldosterone axis
Nonosmotic stimulation of vasopressin release
Fluid volume retention
Weight gain
Edema
Expanded intravascular volume
Maldistribution of cardiac output
  Derangement of regional blood flow
Systemic arterial O_2 desaturation via pulmonic V/Q mismatch
Pharmacodynamic tolerance

*Specific major vasodilators (in addition to the adverse effects already
  listed above)*
Nitroprusside
  "Rebound" hemodynamic effects and clinical deterioration after
    discontinuation
  Methemoglobinemia
  Cyanide and thiocyanate toxicity
  Myocardial ischemia via "coronary steal"
Nitrates
  Skin flushing
  Headaches
  Nearsyncope/syncope, lightheadedness
  Visual disturbances, myopia
  Nitrate-induced bradycardia
Hydralazine
  Headache
  Nearsyncope/syncope, lightheadedness
  Anxiety, tremor
  Gastrointestinal symptoms, dysgeusia
  Skin flushing
  Arthralgias, "SLE-like" illness
  Positive inotropy, palpitations, angina
Calcium channel blocking agents
  Negative inotropy with exacerbation of ventricular dysfunction
  Deterioration of heart failure
  Gastrointestinal symptoms, constipation
  fatigue, malaise
  Nearsyncope/syncope, lightheadedness
Flosequinan
  Positive chronotropy
  Headache
  Skin flushing
  Nearsyncope, lightheadedness
  Gastrointestinal symptoms

cardial ischemia-infarction, confusion, poor mentation, and nearsyncope/syncope, and symptoms/signs of dysfunction of other regions and organ systems. In the vast majority of heart failure patients, proper patient, drug, and dose selection averts the development of clinically significant systemic hypotension; the issues of patient selection, choice of vasodilator, and dosing are presented in the sections of this chapter discussing individual vasodilator drugs.

Systemic hypotension is but one of the factors that can result in myocardial ischemia-infarction during vasodilator therapy in heart failure patients; other contributing factors include high-grade occlusive coronary artery disease, myocardial hypertrophy, reflex activation of the sympathetic nervous system, and drugs with positive inotropic effects (e.g., hydralazine).

Table 24.6 also presents the most common, potential adverse effects that are rather unique to each major vasodilator. A more detailed account of these adverse effects and others are available in the discussion of each agent in this chapter.

With individual exceptions, vasodilators generally are not employed in patients with significantly stenotic valvular disease. For aortic outflow stenosis, a rise in the transobstructive pressure gradient and a substantial fall in systemic blood pressure can be expected. A rise in the transmitral pressure gradient and pulmonary capillary wedge pressure and systemic hypotension can follow vasodilator administration in patients with mitral stenosis. On the other hand, cautiously administered vasodilator therapy should be considered for patients whose hemodynamic decompensation, low cardiac output, markedly increased vascular resistances, and elevated ventricular filling pressures are primarily attributable to ventricular dysfunction rather than valvular stenosis. Because vasodilators can markedly increase the left ventricular outflow pressure gradient in hypertrophic obstructive cardiomyopathy, most of these agents should be avoided in this condition; certain vasodilating drugs that may improve ventricular compliance (e.g., calcium channel blocking drugs) may be the exceptions to this general rule.

References

1. Burch GE. Evidence for increased venous tone in chronic congestive heart failure. *Arch Intern Med.* 1956;98:750–766.
2. Gould L, Zahir M, Ettinger S. Phentolamine and cardiovascular performance. *Br Heart J.* 1969;31:154–162.
3. Majid PA, Sharma B, Taylor SH. Phentolamine for vasodilator treatment of severe heart failure. *Lancet.* 1971;2:719.
4. Franciosa JA, Guiha NH, Limas CJ, Rodriguera E, Cohn JN. Improved left ventricular function during nitroprusside infusion in acute myocardial infarction. *Lancet.* 1972;1:650–654.
5. Cohn JN, Franciosa JA. Vasodilator therapy of cardiac failure. *N Engl J Med.* 1977;297:27–31, 254–258.
6. Cohn JN, Archibald DG, Ziesche S, et al. Effect of vasodilator therapy on mortality in chronic congestive

heart failure: results of a Veterans Administration Cooperative Study. *N Engl J Med.* 1986;314:1547–1552.

7. The CONSENSUS trial study group. Effects of enalapril on mortality in severe congestive heart failure: results of the Cooperative North Scandinavian Enalapril Survival Study (CONSENSUS). *N Engl J Med.* 1987;316: 1429–1435.

8. Lewis RP. Digitalis. In: Leier CV, ed. *Cardiotonic Drugs*. New York/Basel: Marcel Dekker; 1986:85–150.

9. Imperial ES, Levy MN, Zieske H Jr. Outflow resistance as an independent determinant of cardiac performance. *Circ Res.* 1961;9:1148–1155.

10. Sonnenblick EH, Downing SE. Afterload as a primary determinant of ventricular performance. *Am J Physiol.* 1963;204:604–610.

11. Mason DT. Afterload reduction and cardiac performance: physiologic basis of systemic vasodilators as a new approach in treatment of congestive heart failure. *Am J Med.* 1978;65:106–125.

12. Pepine CJ, Nichols WW, Curry RC, Conti CR. Aortic input impedance in heart failure. *Circulation.* 1978;58: 460–465.

13. Finkelstein SM, Cohn JN, Collins VR, Carlyle PF, Shelley WJ. Vascular hemodynamic impedance in congestive heart failure. *Am J Cardiol.* 1985;55:423–427.

14. Laskey WK, Kussmaul WG. Arterial wave reflection in heart failure. *Circulation.* 1987;75:711–722.

15. Starling EH. *Linacre Lecture on the Law of the Heart.* London: Longmans; 1918.

16. Gaasch WH, Levine HJ, Quinones MA, Alexander JK. Left ventricular compliance: mechanisms and clinical implications. *Am J Cardiol.* 1976;38:645–653.

17. Lewis BS, Gotsman MS. Current concepts of left ventricular relaxation and compliance. *Am Heart J.* 1980;99:101–112.

18. Dougherty AH, Naccarelli GV, Gray EL, Hicks CH, Goldstein RA. Congestive heart failure with normal systolic function. *Am J Cardiol.* 1984;54:778–782.

19. Soufer R, Wohlgelernter D, Vita NA, et al. Intact systolic left ventricular function in clinical congestive heart failure. *Am J Cardiol.* 1985;55:1032–1036.

20. Barry WH, Brooker J, Alderman EH, Harrison DC. Changes in diastolic stiffness and tone of the left ventricle during angina pectoris. *Circulation.* 1974;49:255–263.

21. Mann T, Brodie BR, Grossman W, McLaurin LP. Effects of angina on the left ventricular pressure-volume relationship. *Circulation.* 1977;55:761–766.

22. Bonow RO, Bacharach SL, Green MV, et al. Impaired left ventricular diastolic filling in patients with coronary artery disease: assessment with radionuclide angiography. *Circulation.* 1981;64:315–323.

23. Grossman W, McLaurin LP, Stefadouros MA. Left ventricular stiffness associated with chronic pressure and volume overload in man. *Circ Res.* 1974;35:793–800.

24. Fouad FM, Slominski JM, Tarazi RC. Left ventricular diastolic function in hypertension: relation to left ventricular mass and systolic function. *J Am Coll Cardiol.* 1984;3:1500–1506.

25. Hanrath P, Mathey DG, Siegert R. Left ventricular relaxation and filling pattern in different forms of left ven-

tricular hypertrophy. An Echocardiographic study. *Am J Cardiol.* 1980;45:15–23.

26. Schwartz F, Flameng W, Schaper J, Hehrlein F. Correlation between myocardial structure and diastolic properties of the heart in chronic aortic valve disease: effects of corrective surgery. *Am J Cardiol.* 1978;42:895–903.

27. Smith VE, White WB. Improved left ventricular filling accompanies reduced ventricular mass during therapy of essential hypertension. *J Am Coll Cardiol.* 1986; 8:1449–1454.

28. Unverferth DV, Baker PB, Arn AR, Magorien RD, Fetters JK, Leier CV. Aging of the human myocardium: a histologic study based upon endomyocardial biopsy. *Gerontology.* 1986;32:241–251.

29. Taylor RR, Covell JW, Sonnenblick EH, Ross J Jr. Dependence of ventricular distensibility on filling of the opposite ventricle. *Am J Physiol.* 1967;203:711–718.

30. Bemis CE, Serur JR, Borkenhagen D, Sonnenblick EH, Urschel CW. Influence of right ventricular filling pressure on left ventricular pressure and dimension. *Circ Res.* 1974;34:498–504.

31. Watanabe J, Levine MJ, Bellotto F, Johnson RG, Grossman W. The effects of coronary sinus pressure on left ventricular diastolic distensibility. *Circ Res.* 1990;67:923–932.

32. Unverferth DV, Magorien RD, Lewis RP, Leier CV. The role of subendocardial ischemia in perpetuating myocardial failure in patients with nonischemic congestive cardiomyopathy. *Am Heart J.* 1983;105:176–179.

33. DeMarco T, Chatterjee K, Rouleau JL, Parmley WW. Abnormal coronary hemodynamics and myocardial energetics in patients with chronic heart failure caused by ischemic heart disease and dilated cardiomyopathy. *Am Heart J,* 1988;115:809–815.

34. Dupuis J, Lalonde G, Lebeau R, Bichet D, Rouleau JL. Sustained beneficial effect of a seventy-two hour intravenous infusion of nitroglycerin in patients with severe chronic congestive heart failure. *Am Heart J.* 1990;120:625–637.

35. Unverferth DV, Magorien RD, Altschuld R, Kolibash AJ, Lewis RP, Leier CV. The hemodynamic and metabolic advantages gained by a three-day infusion of dobutamine in patients with congestive cardiomyopathy. *Am Heart J.* 1983;106:29–34.

36. Strauss RH, Stevenson LW, Dadourian BA, Child JS. Predictability of mitral regurgitation detected by Doppler echocardiography in patients referred for cardiac transplantation. *Am J Cardiol.* 1987;59:892–894.

37. Keren G, Katz S, Strom J, Sonnenblick EH, LeJemtel TH. Dynamic mitral regurgitation, an important determinant of the hemodynamic response to load alterations and inotropic therapy in severe heart failure. *Circulation.* 1989;80:306–313.

38. Keren G, Katz S, Gage J, Strom J, Sonnenblick EH, LeJemtel TH. Effect of isometric exercise on cardiac performance and mitral regurgitation in patients with severe congestive heart failure. *Am Heart J.* 1989; 118:973–979.

39. Goodman DJ, Rossen RM, Holloway EL, Alderman

EL, Harrison DC. Effect of nitroprusside on left ventricular dynamics in mitral regurgitation. *Circulation.* 1974;50:1025–1032.

40. Harshaw CW, Grossman W, Munro AB, McLaurin LP. Reduced systemic vascular resistance as therapy for severe mitral regurgitation of valvular origin. *Ann Intern Med.* 1975;83:312–316.

41. Weiland DS, Konstam MA, Salem DN, et al. Contribution of reduced mitral regurgitation volume to vasodilator effect in severe left ventricular failure secondary to coronary artery disease or idiopathic dilated cardiomyopathy. *Am J Cardiol.* 1986;58:1046–1050.

42. Stevenson LW, Bellil D, Grover-McKay M, et al. Effects of afterload reduction (diuretics and vasodilators) on left ventricular volume and mitral regurgitation in severe congestive heart failure secondary to ischemic or idiopathic dilated cardiomyopathy. *Am J Cardiol.* 1987;60:654–658.

43. Delius W, Enghoff E. Studies of the central and peripheral hemodynamic effects of amyl nitrate in patients with aortic insufficiency. *Circulation.* 1970;42:787–796.

44. Miller R, Vismara L, DeMaria A, Salel AF, Mason DT. Afterload reduction therapy with nitroprusside in severe aortic regurgitation: improved cardiac performance and reduced regurgitant volume. *Am J Cardiol.* 1976;38:564–567.

45. Greenberg B, Massie B, Cheitlin M, et al. Long-term vasodilator therapy of chronic aortic insufficiency. *Circulation.* 1988;78:92–103.

46. Herman MV, Gorlin R. Implications of left ventricular asynergy. *Am J Cardiol.* 1969;23:538–547.

47. Roberts CS, Maclean D, Maroko PR, Kloner RA. Early and late remodeling of the left ventricle after acute myocardial infarction. *Am J Cardiol.* 1984;54:407–410.

48. McKay RG, Pfeffer MA, Pasternak RC, et al. Left ventricular remodeling following myocardial infarction: a corollary to infarct expansion. *Circulation.* 1986;74:693–702.

49. Pfeffer MA, Lamas GA, Vaughn DE, Parisi AF, Braunwald E. Effect of captopril on progressive ventricular dilatation after anterior myocardial infarction. *N Engl J Med.* 1988;319:80–86.

49a. Pfeffer MA, Braunwald E, Moye' LA, et al. Effect of captopril on mortality and morbidity in patients with left ventricular dysfunction after myocardial infarction. *N Engl J Med.* 1992;327:669–677.

49b. McDonald KM, Francis GS, Matthews J, et al. Long-term oral nitrate therapy prevents chronic ventricular remodeling in the dog. *J Am Coll Cardiol.* 1993;21:514–522.

49c. Konstam MA, Rousseau MF, Kronenberg MW, et al. Effects of the angiotensin converting enzyme inhibitor enalapril on the long-term progression of left ventricular dysfunction in patients with heart failure. *Circulation.* 1992;86:431–438.

50. Rowlands DB, Glovert DR, Ireland MA, Glover DR, McLeay RAB, Watson RDS. Assessment of left ventricular mass and its response to antihypertensive treatment. *Lancet.* 1982;1:467–470.

51. Fouad FM, Nakashima Y, Tarazi RC, Salcedo EE. Reversal of left ventricular hypertrophy with methyldopa. *Am J Cardiol.* 1982;49:795–801.

52. Pardis IP, Kotler MN, Ren JF. Development and regression of left ventricular hypertrophy. *J Am Coll Cardiol.* 1984;3:1309–1320.

53. Schmieder RE, Messerli FH, Sturgill D, Garavaglia GE, Nunez BD. Cardiac performance after reduction of myocardial hypertrophy. *Am J Med.* 1989;87:22–27.

54. Unverferth DV, Mehegan JP, Magorien RD, Unverferth BJ, Leier CV. Regression of myocardial cellular hypertrophy with vasodilator therapy in chronic congestive heart failure associated with idiopathic dilated cardiomyopathy. *Am J Cardiol.* 1983;51:1392–1398.

55. Nadal-Ginard B, Mahdavi V. Molecular basis of cardiac performance: plasticity of the myocardium generated through protein isoform switches. *J Clin Invest.* 1989;84:1693–1700.

56. Messerli FH. Clinical determinants and consequences of left ventricular hypertrophy. *Am J Med.* 1983;75(Suppl 3A):51–56.

57. Kannel WB, Gordon T, Offut D. Left ventricular hypertrophy by electrocardiogram: prevalence, incidence, and mortality in the Framingham Study. *Ann Intern Med.* 1969;71:89–105.

58. Hammer DF, Altschuld RA, Leier CV, Unverferth DV. Improvement of myocardial ATP in heart failure patients treated with hydralazine and isosorbide dinitrate. *Circulation.* 1986;74:II-309. Abstract.

59. Hamilton MA, Stevenson LW, Child JS, Moriguchi JD, Woo M. Acute reduction of atrial overload during vasodilator and diuretic therapy in advanced congestive heart failure. *Am J Cardiol.* 1990;65:1209–1212.

60. Leier CV. Regional blood flow responses to vasodilators and inotropes in congestive heart failure. *Am J Cardiol.* 1990;62:86E–93E.

61. Leier CV, Bambach D, Thompson MJ, Cattaneo SM, Goldberg RJ, Unverferth DV. Central and regional hemodynamic effects of intravenous isosorbide dinitrate, nitroglycerin, and nitroprusside in patients with congestive heart failure. *Am J Cardiol.* 1981;48:1115–1123.

62. Cogan JJ, Humphreys MH, Carlson CJ, Benowitz NL, Rapaport E. Acute vasodilator therapy increases renal clearance of digoxin in patients with congestive heart failure. *Circulation.* 1980;64:973–976.

63. Magorien RD, Triffon DW, Desch CE, Bay WH, Unverferth DV, Leier CV. Prazosin and hydralazine in congestive heart failure: regional hemodynamic effects in relation to dose. *Ann Intern Med.* 1981;95:5–13.

64. Leier CV, Patrick TJ, Hermiller JB, et al. Nifedipine in congestive heart failure: effects on resting and exercise hemodynamics and regional blood flow. *Am Heart J.* 1984;108:1461–1468.

65. Leier CV, Magorien RD, Desch CE, Thompson MJ, Unverferth DV. Hydralazine and isosorbide dinitrate: comparative central and regional hemodynamic effects when administered alone or in combination. *Circulation.* 1981;63:102–109.

66. Stevenson LW, Dracup KA, Tillisch JH. Efficacy of medical therapy tailored for severe congestive heart

failure in patients transferred for urgent cardiac transplantation. *Am J Cardiol.* 1989;63:461–464.

67. Evans RW, Manninen DL, Garrison LP, Maier AM. Donor availability as the primary determinant of the future of heart transplantation. *JAMA.* 1986;255:1982–1988.

68. Ghali JK, Cooper R, Ford E. Trends in hospitalization rates for heart failure in the United States, 1973–1986. *Arch Intern Med.* 1990;150:769–773.

68a. Cohn JN, Johnson G, Ziesche S, et al. A comparison of enalapril with hydralazine-isosorbide dinitrate in the treatment of chronic congestive heart failure. *N Engl J Med.* 1991;325:303–310.

69. Palmer RF, Lasseter KC. Sodium nitroprusside. *N Engl J Med.* 1975;292:294–297.

70. Cohn JN, Burke LP. Nitroprusside. *Ann Intern Med.* 1979;91:752–757.

71. Blaschke TF, Melmon KL. Antihypertensive agents and the drug therapy of hypertension. In Gilman AF, Goodman LS, Gilman A, eds. *Goodman and Gilman's the Pharmacologic Basis of Therapeutics.* 6th ed. New York: Macmillan; 1980;805–806.

72. Tsai SC, Adamik R, Manganiello VC, Moss J. Effects of nitroprusside and nitroglycerin on cGMP content and PGI_2 formation in aorta and vena cava. *Biochem Pharmacol.* 1989;38:61–65.

73. Schulz V. Clinical pharmacokinetics of nitroprusside, cyanide, thiosulphate and thiocyanate. *Clin Pharmacokinet.* 1984;9:239–251.

74. Page IH, Corcoran AC, Dustan HP, Koppanyi T. Cardiovascular actions of sodium nitroprusside in animals and hypertensive patients. *Circulation.* 1955;11:188–198.

75. Schlant RC, Tsagaris TS, Robertson RJ. Studies on the acute cardiovascular effects of intravenous sodium nitroprusside. *Am J Cardiol.* 1962;9:51–59.

76. Guiha NH, Cohn JN, Mikulic E, Franciosa JA, Limas CJ. Treatment of refractory heart failure with infusion of nitroprusside. *N Engl J Med.* 1974;291:587–592.

77. Cohn JN, Mathew KJ, Franciosa JA, Snow JA. Chronic vasodilator therapy in the management of cardiogenic shock and intractable left ventricular failure. *Ann Intern Med.* 1974;81:777–780.

78. Chatterjee K, Swan HJ, Kaushik US, Jobin G, Magnusson P. Effects of vasodilator therapy in acute myocardial infarction on short-term and late prognosis. *Circulation.* 1976;53:797–802.

79. Miller RR, Vismara LA, Williams DO, Amsterdam EA, Mason DT. Pharmacological mechanisms for left ventricular unloading in clinical congestive heart failure. *Circ Res.* 1976;39:127–133.

80. Leier CV, Magorien RD, Boudoulas H, Lewis RP, Bambach D, Unverferth DV. The effect of vasodilator therapy on systolic and diastolic time intervals in congestive heart failure. *Chest.* 1982;81:723–729.

81. Franciosa JA, Silverstein SR. Hemodynamic effects of nitroprusside and furosemide in left ventricular failure. *Clin Pharmacol Ther.* 1982;32:62–69.

82. Packer M, Meller J, Medina N, Yushak M. Quantitative differences in the hemodynamic effects of captopril and nitroprusside in severe chronic heart failure. *Am J Cardiol.* 1983;51:183–188.

83. Pepine CJ, Nichols WW, Curry RC Jr, Conti CR. Aortic input impedance during nitroprusside infusion. *J Clin Invest.* 1979;64:643–654.

84. Merillon JP, Fontenier G, Lerallut JF, et al. Aortic input impedance in heart failure: comparison with normal subjects and its changes during vasodilator therapy. *Eur Heart J.* 1984;5:447–455.

85. Yin FC, Guzman PA, Brin KP, et al. Effect of nitroprusside on hydraulic vascular loads on the right and left ventricle of patients with heart failure. *Circulation.* 1983;67:1330–1339.

86. Konstam MA, Weiland DS, Conlon TP, et al. Hemodynamic correlates of left ventricular versus right ventricular radionuclide volumetric responses to vasodilator therapy in congestive heart failure secondary to ischemic or dilated cardiomyopathy. *Am J Cardiol.* 1987;59:1131–1137.

87. Konstam MA, Salem DN, Isner JM, et al. Vasodilator effect on right ventricular function in congestive heart failure and pulmonary hypertension: end-systolic pressure-volume relation. *Am J Cardiol.* 1984;54:132–136.

88. Brodie BR, Grossman W, Mann T, McLaurin LP. Effects of sodium nitroprusside on left ventricular diastolic pressure-volume relations. *J Clin Invest.* 1977;59:59–68.

89. Herrmann HC, Ruddy TD, Dec GW, Strauss HW, Boucher CA, Fifer MA. Diastolic function in patients with severe heart failure: comparison of the effects of enoximone and nitroprusside. *Circulation.* 1987;75:1214–1221.

90. Masuyama T, St. Goar FG, Alderman EL, Popp RL. Effects of nitroprusside on transmitral flow velocity patterns in extreme heart failure: a combined hemodynamic and Doppler echocardiographic study of varying loading conditions. *J Am Coll Cardiol.* 1990;16:1175–1185.

91. Lavine SJ, Campbell CA, Held AC, Johnson V. Effect of inotropic and vasodilator therapy on left ventricular diastolic filling in dogs with severe left ventricular dysfunction. *J Am Coll Cardiol.* 1990;15:1165–1172.

92. Olivari MT, Levine TB, Cohn JN. Abnormal neurohumoral response to nitroprusside infusion in congestive heart failure. *J Am Coll Cardiol.* 1983;2:411–417.

93. Miller RR, Vismara LA, Zelis R, Amsterdam EA, Mason DT. Clinical use of sodium nitroprusside in chronic ischemic heart disease. *Circulation.* 1975;51:328–336.

94. Hasenfuss G, Holubarsch C, Heiss W, et al. Myocardial energetics in patients with dilated cardiomyopathy. *Circulation.* 1989;80:51–64.

95. Powers ER, Reison DS, Berke A, Weiss MB, Cannon PJ. The effect of nitroprusside on coronary and systemic hemodynamics in patients with severe congestive heart failure. *Circulation.* 1982;66:II-211. Abstract.

96. Chatterjee K, Parmley WW, Ganz W, et al. Hemodynamic and metabolic responses to vasodilator therapy in acute myocardial infarction. *Circulation.* 1973;48:1183–1193.

97. Miller RR, Awan NA, Mason DT. Nitroprusside therapy in acute and chronic coronary heart disease. *Am J Med.* 1978;65:167–172.

98. Awan NA, Miller RR, Vera Z, Amsterdam EA, Mason DT. Reduction of ST segment elevation with infusion of nitroprusside in patients with acute myocardial infarction. *Am J Cardiol.* 1976;38:435–439.

99. Chiariello M, Gold HK, Leinbach RC, Davis MA, Maroko PR. Comparison between the effects of nitroprusside and nitroglycerin on ischemic injury during acute myocardial infarction. *Circulation.* 1976;54:766–773.

100. Mann T, Cohn PF, Holman BL, Green LH, Markis JE, Phillips DA. Effect of nitroprusside on regional myocardial blood flow in coronary artery disease. *Circulation.* 1978;57:732–738.

101. Cogan JJ, Humphreys MH, Carlson CJ, Rapaport E. Renal effects of nitroprusside and hydralazine in patients with congestive heart failure. *Circulation.* 1980;61:316–323.

102. Francis GS, Olivari MT, Goldsmith SR, Levine TB, Pierpont G, Cohn JN. The acute response of plasma norepinephrine, renin activity, and arginine vasopressin to short-term nitroprusside and nitroprusside withdrawal in congestive heart failure. *Am Heart J.* 1983;106:1315–1320.

103. Stone JG, Hoar PF, Faltas AN, et al. Comparison of intraoperative nitroprusside unloading in mitral and aortic regurgitation. *J Thorac Cardiovasc Surg.* 1979;78:103–109.

104. Lukes SA, Romero CA, Resnekov L. Hemodynamic effects of sodium nitroprusside in 21 subjects with congestive heart failure. *Br Heart J.* 1979;41:187–191.

105. Miller RR, Awan NA, Joye JA, et al. Combined dopamine and nitroprusside therapy in congestive heart failure. *Circulation.* 1977;55:881–884.

106. Stemple DR, Kleiman JH, Harrison DC. Combined nitroprusside-dopamine therapy in severe chronic congestive heart failure. Dose-related hemodynamic advantages over single drug infusions. *Am J Cardiol.* 1978;42:267–275.

107. Nadjmabad MH, Aftandelian E, Kashani IA, Rastan H, Bastanfar M. Simultaneous dopamine and nitroprusside therapy following open heart surgery. *Jpn Heart J.* 1980;21:325–333.

108. Keung EC, Ribner HS, Schwartz W, Sonnenblick EH, LeJemtel TH. Effects of combined dopamine and nitroprusside therapy in patients with severe pump failure and hypotension complicating acute myocardial infarction. *J Cardiovasc Pharmacol.* 1980;2:113–119.

109. Artman M, Graham TP. Guidelines for vasodilator therapy of congestive heart failure in infants and children. *Am Heart J.* 1987;113:994–1005.

110. Beekman RH, Rocchini AP, Dick M, Crowley DC, Rosenthal A. Vasodilator therapy in children: acute and chronic effects in children with left ventricular dysfunction or mitral regurgitation. *Pediatrics.* 1984;73:43–51.

111. Beekman RH, Rossini AP, Rosenthal A. Hemodynamic effects of nitroprusside in infants with a large ventricular septal defect. *Circulation.* 1981;64:553–558.

112. Subramanyam R, Tandon R, Shrivastava S. Hemodynamic effects of sodium nitroprusside in patients with ventricular septal defect. *Eur J Pediatr.* 1982;138:307–310.

113. Addonizio LJ, Gersony WM, Robbins RC, et al. Elevated pulmonary vascular resistance and cardiac transplantation. *Circulation.* 1987;76:V52–V55.

114. Aroney CN, Hermann HC, Semigran MJ, Dec GW, Boucher CA, Fifer MA. Linearity of left ventricular end-systolic pressure-volume relation in patients with severe heart failure. *J Am Coll Cardiol.* 1989;14:127–134.

115. Flaherty JT. Comparison of intravenous nitroglycerin and sodium nitroprusside in acute myocardial infarction. *Am J Med.* 1983;74(6B):53–60.

116. Cohn JN, Franciosa JA, Francis GS, et al. Effect of short-term infusion of sodium nitroprusside on mortality rate in acute myocardial infarction complicated by left ventricular failure: results of a veterans administration cooperative study. *N Engl J Med.* 1982;306:1129–1135.

117. Durrer JD, Lie KI, Van Capelle FJ, Durrer D. Effect of sodium nitroprusside on mortality in acute myocardial infarction. *N Engl J Med.* 1982;306:1121–1128.

118. Simkus GJ, Fitchett DH. Radial artery pressure measurements may be a poor guide to the beneficial effects of nitroprusside on left ventricular systolic pressure in congestive heart failure. *Am J Cardiol.* 1990;66:323–326.

119. Leier CV. Acute inotropic support: intravenously administered positive inotropic drugs. In: Leier CV, ed. *Cardiotonic Drugs.* New York: Marcel Dekker; 1986; 49–84.

120. Vesey CJ, Cole PV, Simpson PJ. Cyanide and thiocyanate concentrations following sodium nitroprusside infusion in man. *Br J Anaesth.* 1976;48:651–660.

121. Vesey CJ, Cole PV, Linnell JC, Wilson J. Some metabolic effects of sodium nitroprusside in man. *Br Med J.* 1974;2:140–142.

122. duCailar J, Mathieu-Daude JC, Kienlen J, Chardon P. Blood and urinary cyanide concentrations during long-term sodium nitroprusside infusions. *Anesthesiology.* 1979;51:363–364.

123. Vesey CJ, Cole PV. Blood cyanide and thiocyanate concentrations produced by long-term therapy with sodium nitroprusside. *Br J Anaesth.* 1985;57:148–155.

124. Norris JC, Hume AS. In vivo release of cyanide from sodium nitroprusside. *Br J Anaesth.* 1987;59:236–239.

125. Vesey CJ, Krapez JR, Cole PV. The effects of sodium nitroprusside and cyanide on haemoglobin function. *J Pharm Pharmacol.* 1980;32:256–261.

126. Spiegel HE, Kucera V. Some aspects of sodium nitroprusside reaction with human erythrocytes. *Clin Chem.* 1977;23:2329–2331.

127. duCailar J, Mathieu-Daude JC, Deschodt J, Lamarche Y, Castel C. Nitroprusside, its metabolites, and red cell function. *Can Anaesth Soc J.* 1978;25:92–105.

128. Mehta P, Mehta J, Miale TD. Nitroprusside lowers platelet count. [Letter] *N Engl J Med.* 1978;299:1134.

129. Mehta J, Mehta P. Platelet function studies in heart disease. Enhanced platelet aggregate formation activity in congestive heart failure: inhibition by sodium nitroprusside. *Circulation.* 1979;60:497–503.

130. Mookerjee S, Keighley JF, Warner RA, Bowser MA, Obeid AI. Hemodynamic, ventilatory and blood gas changes during infusion of nitroferricyanide: studies in patients with congestive heart failure. *Chest.* 1977;72:273–278.

131. Pierpont G, Hale KA, Franciosa JA, Cohn JN. Effects of vasodilators on pulmonary hemodynamics and gas exchange in left ventricular failure. *Am Heart J.* 1980;99:208–216.

132. Bencowitz HZ, LeWinter MM, Wagner PD. Effect of sodium nitroprusside on ventilation-perfusion mismatching in heart failure. *J Am Coll Cardiol.* 1984;4:918–922.

133. Reid GM, Muther RS. Nitroprusside-induced acute azotemia. *Am J Nephrol.* 1987;7:313–315.

134. Packer M, Miller J, Medina N, Gorlin R, Herman MV. Rebound hemodynamic events after the abrupt withdrawal of nitroprusside in patients with severe chronic heart failure. *N Engl J Med.* 1979;301:1193–1197.

135. Cottrell JE, Illner P, Kittay MJ, Steele JM, Lowenstein J, Turndorf H. Rebound hypertension after sodium nitroprusside-induced hypotension. *Clin Pharmacol Ther.* 1980;27:32–36.

136. Packer M, Meller J, Medina N, Yushak M, Gorlin R. Determinants of drug response in severe chronic heart failure: activation of vasoconstrictive forces during vasodilator therapy. *Circulation.* 1981;64:506–514.

137. Nourok DG, Glassock KJ, Soloman DH, Maxwell MH. Hypothyroidism following prolonged sodium nitroprusside therapy. *Am J Med Sci.* 1964;248:129–138.

138. Packer M. New perspectives on therapeutic application of nitrates as vasodilator agents for severe chronic heart failure. *Am J Med.* 1983;74(6B):61–72.

139. Cohn JN. Nitrates for congestive heart failure. *Am J Cardiol.* 1985;56:19A–23A.

140. Cohn JN. Role of nitrates in congestive heart failure. *Am J Cardiol.* 1987;60:39H–43H.

141. Needleman P, Jakschik B, Johnson EM. Sulfhydryl requirement for relaxation of vascular smooth muscle. *J Pharmacol Exp Ther.* 1973;187:324–331.

142. Ignarro LJ, Lippton H, Edwards JC, Baricos WH, Kadowitz PJ, Gruetter CA. Mechanism of vascular smooth muscle relaxation by organic nitrates, nitrites, nitroprusside and nitric oxide: evidence for the involvement of S-nitrosothiols as active intermediates. *J Pharmacol Exp Ther.* 1981;218:739–749.

143. Levin RI, Jaffe EA, Weksler BB, Tack-Goldman K. Nitroglycerin stimulates synthesis of prostacyclin by cultured human endothelial cells. *J Clin Invest.* 1981;67:762–769.

144. DeCaterina R, Dorso CR, Tack-Goldman K, Weksler BB. Nitrates and endothelial prostacyclin production: studies in vitro. *Circulation.* 1985;71:176–182.

145. Morcillio E, Reid PR, Dubin N, Ghodgaonkar R, Pitt B. Myocardial prostaglandin E release by nitroglycerin and modification by indomethacin. *Am J Cardiol.* 1980;45:53–57.

146. Armstrong PW, Moffat JA, Marks GS. Arterial-venous nitroglycerin gradient during intravenous infusion in man. *Circulation.* 1982;66:1273–1276.

147. Fung HL. Pharmacokinetic determinants of nitrate action. *Am J Med.* 1984;76(Suppl 6A):22–26.

148. Armstrong PW, Armstrong JA, Marks GS. Pharmacokinetic-hemodynamic studies of intravenous nitroglycerin in congestive heart failure. *Circulation.* 1980;62:160–166.

149. Armstrong PW, Armstrong JA, Marks GS. Blood levels after sublingual nitroglycerin. *Circulation.* 1979;59:585–589.

150. Fung HL. Pharmacokinetics and pharmacodynamics of isosorbide dinitrate. *Am Heart J.* 1985;110:213–216.

151. Moe G, Armstrong PW. Influence of skin site on bioavailability of nitroglycerin ointment in congestive heart failure. *Am J Med,* 1986;81:765–770.

152. Armstrong PW. Pharmacokinetic-hemodynamic studies of transdermal nitroglycerin in congestive heart failure. *J Am Coll Cardiol.* 1987;9:420–425.

153. Fung HL, Ruggirello D, Stone JA, Parker JO. Effects of disease, route of administration, cigarette smoking, food intake on the pharmacokinetics and circulatory effects of isosorbide dinitrate. *Z Kardiol.* 1983;72(Suppl 3):5–10.

154. Thadani U, Whitsett T. Relationship of pharmacokinetic and pharmacodynamic properties of organic nitrates. *Clin Pharmacokinet.* 1988;15:32–43.

155. Franciosa JA, Blank RC, Cohn JN. Nitrate effects on cardiac output and left ventricular outflow resistance in chronic congestive heart failure. *Am J Med.* 1978;64:207–213.

156. Mason DT, Braunwald E. The effects of nitroglycerin and amyl nitrite on arteriolar and venous tone in the human forearm. *Circulation.* 1965;32:755–765.

157. Ferrer MI, Bradley SE, Wheeler HO, et al. Some effects of nitroglycerin upon the splanchnic, pulmonary, and systemic circulations. *Circulation.* 1966;33:357–373.

158. Gold HK, Leinbach RC, Sanders CA. Use of sublingual nitroglycerin in congestive failure following acute myocardial infarction. *Circulation.* 1972;46:839–845.

159. Franciosa JA, Mikulic E, Cohn JN, Jose E, Fabie A. Hemodynamic effects of orally administered isosorbide dinitrate in patients with congestive heart failure. *Circulation.* 1974;50:1020–1024.

160. Mantle JA, Russell RO, Moraski RE, Rackley CE. Isosorbide dinitrate for the relief of severe heart failure after myocardial infarction. *Am J Cardiol.* 1976;37:263–268.

161. Gomes JAC, Carambas CR, Moran HE, et al. The effect of isosorbide dinitrate on left ventricular size, wall stress, and left ventricular function in chronic refractory heart failure. *Am J Med.* 1978;65:794–802.

162. Gray R, Chatterjee K, Ganz W, Forrester JS, Swan HJ. Hemodynamic and metabolic effects of isosorbide dinitrate in chronic congestive heart failure. *Am Heart J.* 1975;90:346–352.

163. Leier CV, Huss P, Magorien RD, Unverferth DV. Improved exercise capacity and differing arterial and venous tolerance during chronic isosorbide dinitrate. *Circulation.* 1983;67:817–822.

164. Konstam MA, Salem DN, Isner JM, et al. Vasodilator effect on right ventricular function in congestive heart failure and pulmonary hypertension: end-systolic pressure-volume relation. *Am J Cardiol.* 1984;54:132–136.

165. Packer M, Medina N, Yushak M, Lee WH. Comparative effects of captopril and isosorbide dinitrate on pulmonary arteriolar resistance and right ventricular function in patients with severe left ventricular failure. *Am Heart J.* 1985;109:1293–1299.

166. Kingma I, Smiseth OA, Belenkie I, et al. A mechanism for the nitroglycerin-induced downward shift of left ven-

tricular diastolic pressure-diameter relation. *Am J Cardiol.* 1986;57:673–677.

167. Elkayam U, Roth A, Kumar A, et al. Hemodynamic and volumetric effects of venodilation with nitroglycerin in chronic mitral regurgitation. *Am J Cardiol.* 1987; 60:1106–1111.

168. Williams DO, Bommer WJ, Miller RR, Amsterdam EA, Mason DT. Hemodynamic assessment of oral peripheral vasodilator therapy in chronic congestive heart failure. Prolonged effectiveness of isosorbide dinitrate. *Am J Cardiol.* 1977;39:84–90.

169. Figueras J, Taylor WR, Ogawa T, Forrester JS, Singh BN, Swan HJC. Comparative hemodynamic and peripheral vasodilator effects of oral and chewable isosorbide dinitrate in patients with refractory congestive cardiac failure. *Br Heart J.* 1979;41:317–324.

170. Lavine SJ, Campbell CA, Held AC, Johnson V. Effect of nitroglycerin-induced reduction of left ventricular filling pressure on diastolic filling in acute dilated heart failure. *J Am Coll Cardiol.* 1989;14:233–241.

171. Ludbrook PR, Byrne JD, Kurnik PB, McKnight RC. Influence of reduction of preload and afterload by nitroglycerin on left ventricular diastolic pressure-volume relation and relaxation in man. *Circulation.* 1977;56:937–943.

172. Amende I, Simon R, Hood WP, Lichtlen PR. Effects of nitroglycerin on left ventricular diastolic properties in man. *Z Kardiol.* 1983;72(Suppl 3):62–65.

173. Olivari MT, Carlyle PF, Levine TB, Cohn JN. Hemodynamic and hormonal response to transdermal nitroglycerin in normal subjects and in patients with congestive heart failure. *J Am Coll Cardiol.* 1983;2:872–878.

174. Franciosa JA, Cohn JN. Effect of isosorbide dinitrate on response to submaximal and maximal exercise in patients with congestive heart failure. *Am J Cardiol.* 1979; 43:1009–1014.

175. Franciosa JA, Goldsmith SR, Cohn JN. Contrasting immediate and long-term effect of isosorbide dinitrate on exercise capacity in congestive heart failure. *Am J Med.* 1980;69:559–566.

176. Stephens J, Camm J, Spurrell R. Improvement in exercise hemodynamics by isosorbide dinitrate in patients with severe congestive cardiac failure secondary to ischemic heart disease. *Br Heart J.* 1978;40:832–837.

177. Wilson JR, Ferraro N. Effect of isosorbide dinitrate on submaximal exercise capacity of patients with chronic left ventricular failure. *Chest.* 1982;82:701–704.

178. Wilson JR, Untereker W, Hirshfeld J. Effects of isosorbide dinitrate and hydralazine on regional metabolic responses to arm exercise in patients with heart failure. *Am J Cardiol.* 1981;48:934–938.

179. Wilson JR, Ferraro N. Circulatory improvement after hydralazine or isosorbide dinitrate administration in patients with heart failure. Effect on metabolic responses to submaximal exercise. *Am J Med.* 1981;71:627–633.

180. Hoelzer M, Schaal SF, Leier CV. Electrophysiologic and antiarrhythmic effects of nitroglycerin in man. *J Cardiovasc Pharmacol.* 1981;3:917–923.

181. Flaherty JT, Reid PR, Kelly DT, Taylor DR, Weisfeldt ML, Pitt B. Intravenous nitroglycerin in acute myocardial infarction. *Circulation.* 1975;51:132–139.

182. Armstrong PW, Walker DC, Burton JR, Parker JO. Vasodilator therapy in acute myocardial infarction: a comparison of sodium nitroprusside and nitroglycerin. *Circulation.* 1975;52:1118–1122.

183. Flaherty JT, Come PC, Baird MG, et al. Effects of intravenous nitroglycerin on left ventricular function and ST segment changes in acute myocardial infarction. *Br Heart J.* 1976;38:612–621.

184. Baxter RH, Tait CM, McGuinness JB. Vasodilator therapy in acute myocardial infarction: use of sublingual isosorbide dinitrate. *Br Heart J.* 1977;39:1067–1070.

185. Bussmann WD, Schupp D. Effect of sublingual nitroglycerin in emergency treatment of severe pulmonary edema. *Am J Cardiol.* 1978;41:931–936.

186. Bussmann WD, Barthe G, Klepzig H, Kaltenbach M. Controlled study of intravenous nitroglycerin treatment for two days in patients with recent myocardial infarction. *Clin Cardiol.* 1980;3:399–405.

187. Cintron GB, Glasser SP, Weston BA, et al. Effect of intravenous isosorbide dinitrate versus nitroglycerin on elevated pulmonary arterial wedge pressure during acute myocardial infarction. *Am J Cardiol.* 1988;61:21–25.

188. Stephens J, Dymond D, Spurrell R. Enhancement by isosorbide dinitrate of hemodynamic effects of dopamine in chronic congestive heart failure. *Br Heart J.* 1978; 40:838–844.

189. Kulick D, Roth A, McIntosh N, Rahimtoola SH, Elkayam U. Resistance to isosorbide dinitrate in patients with severe chronic heart failure: incidence and attempt at hemodynamic prediction. *J Am Coll Cardiol.* 1988;12:1023–1028.

190. Massie B, Chatterjee K, Werner J, Greenberg B, Hart R, Parmley WW. Hemodynamic advantage of combined administration of hydralazine orally and nitrates nonparenterally in the vasodilator therapy of chronic heart failure. *Am J Cardiol.* 1977;40:794–801.

191. Walsh WF, Greenberg BH. Results of long-term vasodilator therapy in patients with refractory congestive heart failure. *Circulation.* 1981;64:499–505.

192. Massie BM, Kramer B, Shen E, Haughom F. Vasodilator treatment with isosorbide dinitrate and hydralazine in chronic heart failure. *Br Heart J.* 1981;45:376–384.

193. Halon DA, Rosenfeld T, Hardoff R, Lewis BS. Advantage of combined therapy with captopril and nitrates in severe congestive heart failure. *Isr J Med Sci.* 1988;24:664–670.

194. Chatterjee K, Drew D, Parmley WW, Klausner SC, Polansky J, Zacherle B. Combination vasodilator therapy for severe chronic congestive heart failure. *Ann Intern Med.* 1976;85:467–470.

195. Kubo SH, Fox SC, Prida XE, Cody RJ. Combined hemodynamic effects of nifedipine and nitroglycerin in congestive heart failure. *Am Heart J.* 1985;110:1032–1034.

196. Meister SG, Engel TR, Guiha N, et al. Sustained hemodynamic action of nitroglycerin ointment. *Br Heart J.* 1976;38:1031–1036.

197. Taylor WR, Forrester JS, Magnusson P, Takano T, Chatterjee K, Swan HJC. Hemodynamic effects of nitroglycerin ointment in congestive heart failure. *Am J Cardiol.* 1976;38:469–473.

198. Jordan RA, Seth L, Henry A, Wilen MM, Franciosa JA. Dose requirements and hemodynamic effects of transdermal nitroglycerin compared with placebo in patients with congestive heart failure. *Circulation*. 1985;71:980–986.

199. Sharpe N, Coxon R, Webster M, Luke R. Hemodynamic effects of intermittent transdermal nitroglycerin in chronic congestive heart failure. *Am J Cardiol*. 1987;59:895–899.

200. Mikulic E, Franciosa JA, Cohn JN. Comparative hemodynamic effects of chewable isosorbide dinitrate and nitroglycerin in patients with congestive heart failure. *Circulation*. 1975;52:477–482.

201. Gammage MD, Murray RG, Littler WA. Isosorbide-5-mononitrate in the treatment of acute left ventricular failure following acute myocardial infarction. *Eur J Clin Pharmacol*. 1986;29:639–643.

202. Schneeweiss A. Comparative evaluation of isosorbide-5-mononitrate and nitroglycerin in chronic congestive heart failure. *Am J Cardiol*. 1988;61:19E–21E.

203. Debbas N, Woodings D, Marks C, et al. Dose-ranging study of isosorbide-5-mononitrate in chronic congestive heart failure treated with diuretics and angiotensin-converting enzyme inhibitor. *Am J Cardiol*. 1988;61:28E–30E.

204. Mookerjee S, Fuleihan D, Warner RA, Vardan S, Obeid AI. Effects of sublingual nitroglycerin on resting pulmonary gas exchange and hemodynamics in man. *Circulation*. 1978;57:106–110.

205. Pierpont G, Hale KA, Franciosa JA, Cohn JN. Effects of vasodilators on pulmonary hemodynamics and gas exchange in left ventricular failure. *Am Heart J*. 1980;99:208–216.

206. Saxon SA, Silverman ME. Effects of continuous infusion of intravenous nitroglycerin on methemoglobin levels. *Am J Cardiol*. 1985;56:461–464.

207. Kaplan KJ, Taber M, Teagarden JR, Parker M, Davidson R. Association of methemoglobinemia and intravenous nitroglycerin administration. *Am J Cardiol*. 1985;55:181–183.

208. Gibson GR, Hunter JB, Raabe DS, Manjoney DL, Ittleman FP. Methemoglobin produced by high-dose intravenous nitroglycerin. *Ann Intern Med*. 1982;96:615–616.

209. Jaffee ER. Methaemoglobinemia. *Clin Haematol*. 1981;10:99–122.

210. Magrini F, Niarchos AP. Ineffectiveness of sublingual nitroglycerin in acute left ventricular failure in the presence of massive peripheral edema. *Am J Cardiol*. 1980;45:841–847.

211. Packer M, Meller J, Medina N, Gorlin R, Herman MV. Dose requirements of hydralazine in patients with severe chronic congestive heart failure. *Am J Cardiol*. 1980;45:655–660.

212. Packer M, Medina N, Yushak M, Lee WH. Hemodynamic factors limiting the response to transdermal nitroglycerin in severe chronic congestive heart failure. *Am J Cardiol*. 1986;57:260–267.

213. Stewart DD. *Remarkable Tolerance to Nitroglycerin*. Philadelphia: Polyclinic; 1988.

214. Myers HB, Austin VT. Nitrate toleration. *J Pharmacol Exp Ther*. 1929;36:226–230.

215. Abrams J. Nitrate tolerance and dependence. *Am Heart J*. 1980;99:113–123.

216. Leier CV. Nitrate tolerance. *Am Heart J*. 1985;110:224–232.

217. Armstrong PW, Moffet JA. Tolerance to organic nitrates: clinical and experimental perspectives. *Am J Med*. 1983;74(Suppl 6B):73–84.

218. Elkayam U, Kulick D, McIntosh N, Roth A, Hsueh W, Rahimtoola SH. Incidence of early tolerance to hemodynamic effects of continuous infusion of nitroglycerin in patients with coronary artery disease and heart failure. *Circulation*. 1987;76:577–584.

219. Jordan RA, Seth L, Casebolt P, Hayes MJ, Wilen MM, Franciosa J. Rapidly developing tolerance to transdermal nitroglycerin in congestive heart failure. *Ann Intern Med*. 1986;104:295–298.

220. Roth A, Kulick D, Freidenberger L, Hong R, Rahimtoola SH, Elkayam U. Early tolerance to hemodynamic effects of high dose transdermal nitroglycerin in responders with severe chronic heart failure. *J Am Coll Cardiol*. 1987;9:858–864.

221. Dupuis J, Lalonde G, Lemieux R, Rouleau JL. Tolerance to intravenous nitroglycerin in patients with congestive heart failure: role of increased intravascular volume, neurohormonal activation, and lack of prevention with N-acetylcysteine. *J Am Coll Cardiol*. 1990;16:923–931.

222. Franciosa JA, Cohn JN. Sustained hemodynamic effects without tolerance during long-term isosorbide dinitrate treatment of chronic left ventricular failure. *Am J Cardiol*. 1980;45:648–654.

223. Rajfer SI, Demma FJ, Goldberg LI. Sustained beneficial hemodynamic responses to large doses of transdermal nitroglycerin in congestive heart failure and comparison with intravenous nitroglycerin. *Am J Cardiol*. 1984;54:120–125.

224. Natarajan D, Khurana TR, Karhade V, Nigam PD. Sustained hemodynamic effects with therapeutic doses of intravenous nitroglycerin in congestive heart failure. *Am J Cardiol*. 1988;62:319–321.

225. Needleman P, Johnson EM. Mechanism of tolerance development to organic nitrates. *J Pharmacol Exp Ther*. 1973;184:709–715.

226. Mulsch A, Busse R, Bassenge E. Clinical tolerance to nitroglycerin is due to impaired biotransformation of nitroglycerin and biological counterregulation, not to desensitization of guanylate cyclase. *Z Kardiol*. 1989;78(Suppl 2):22–25.

227. Packer M. What causes tolerance to nitroglycerin? The 100 year old mystery continues. *J Am Coll Cardiol*. 1990;16:932–935.

228. Packer M, Lee WH, Kessler PD, Gottlieb SS, Medina N, Yushak M. Prevention and reversal of nitrate tolerance in patients with congestive heart failure. *N Engl J Med*. 1987;317:799–804.

229. Levy WS, Katz RJ, Wasserman AG. Methionine restores the venodilative response to nitroglycerin after the development of tolerance. *J Am Coll Cardiol*. 1991;17:474–479.

230. Parker JO, Farrell B, Lahey KA, Rose BF. Nitrate tolerance: the lack of effect of n-acetylcysteine. *Circulation.* 1987;76:572–576.

230a. Katz RJ, Levy WS, Buff L, Wasserman AG. Prevention of nitrate tolerance with angiotensin converting enzyme inhibitors. *Circulation.* 1991;83:1271–1277.

231. Dupuis J, Lalonde G, Bichet D, Rouleau J. Captopril does not prevent nitroglycerin tolerance in heart failure. *Can J Cardiol.* 1990;6:281–286.

232. Dakak N, Makhoul N, Flugelman MY, et al. Failure of captopril to prevent nitrate tolerance in congestive heart failure secondary to coronary artery disease. *Am J Cardiol.* 1990;66:608–613.

233. Cooke JP, Andon N, Loscalzo J. S-nitrosocaptopril: effects on vascular reactivity. *J Pharmacol Exp Ther.* 1989;249:730–734.

234. Cooke JP, Andon N, Loscalzo J, Dzau VJ. S-Nitrosocaptopril: a novel nitrovasodilator resistant to nitrate tolerance. *Circulation.* 1989;80:II-559 (Abstract).

235. Rudd P, Blaschke TF. Antihypertensive agents and the drug therapy of hypertension. In: Gilman AG, Goodman LS, Rall TW, Murad F, eds. *Goodman and Gilman's the Pharmacologic Basis of Therapeutics.* 7th ed. New York: MacMillan; 1985:784–805.

236. McLean AJ, Barron K, duSouich P, et al. Interaction of hydralazine and hydrazone derivatives with contractile mechanisms in rabbit aortic smooth muscle. *J Pharmacol Exp Ther.* 1978;205:418–425.

237. Haeusler G, Gerold M. Increased levels of prostaglandin-like material in canine blood during arterial hypotension produced by hydralazine, dihydralazine and minoxidil. *Arch Pharmacol (Naunyn-Schmiedeberg).* 1979;310:155–167.

238. Greenwald JE, Wong LK, Rao M, Bianchine JR, Panganamala RV. A study of three vasodilating agents as selective inhibitors of thromboxane A$_2$ biosynthesis. *Biochem Biophys Res Commun.* 1978;84:1112–1118.

239. Worcel M, Saiag B, Chevillard C. An unexpected mode of action for hydralazine. *Trends Pharmacol Sci.* 1980;1:136–138.

240. Crawford MH, Ludden TM, Kennedy GT. Determinants of systemic availability of oral hydralazine in heart failure. *Clin Pharmacol Ther.* 1985;38:538–543.

241. Mulrow JP, Crawford MH. Clinical pharmacokinetics and therapeutic use of hydralazine in congestive heart failure. *Clin Pharmacokinet.* 1989;16:86–89.

242. Hanson A, Johansson BW, Wernersson B, Wahlander LA. Pharmacokinetics of hydralazine in chronic heart failure. *Eur J Clin Pharmacol.* 1983;25:467–473.

243. Judson WE, Hollander W, Wilkins RW. The effects of intravenous apresoline (hydralazine) on cardiovascular and renal function in patients with and without congestive heart failure. *Circulation.* 1968;13:664–674.

244. Chatterjee K, Parmley WW, Massie B, et al. Oral hydralazine therapy for chronic heart failure. *Circulation.* 1976;54:879–884.

245. Franciosa JA, Pierpont G, Cohn JN. Hemodynamic improvement after oral hydralazine in left ventricular failure. *Ann Intern Med.* 1977;86:388–393.

246. Fitchett DH, Neto JAM, Oakley CM, Goodwin JF. Hydralazine in the management of left ventricular failure. *Am J Cardiol.* 1979;44:303–309.

247. Chatterjee K, Ports TA, Arnold S, Brundage B, Parmley WW. Comparison of hemodynamic effects of oral hydralazine and prazosin hydrochloride in patients with chronic congestive heart failure. *Br Heart J.* 1979;42:657–663.

248. Packer M, Meller J, Medina N, Gorlin R, Herman MV. Hemodynamic evaluation of hydralazine dosage in refractory heart failure. *Clin Pharmacol Ther.* 1980;27:337–346.

249. Hindman MC, Slosky DA, Peter RH, Newman GE, Jones RH, Wallace AG. Rest and exercise hemodynamic effects of oral hydralazine in patients with coronary artery disease and left ventricular dysfunction. *Circulation.* 1980;61:751–758.

250. Artman M, Parrish MD, Appleton S, Boucek RJ, Graham TP. Hemodynamic effects of hydralazine in infants with idiopathic dilated cardiomyopathy and congestive heart failure. *Am Heart J.* 1987;113:144–150.

251. Ueda K, Sakai M, Matsushita S, Kuwajima I, Murakami M. Effect of orally administered hydralazine on neurohumoral factors and hemodynamic response in aged patients and chronic congestive heart failure. *Jpn Heart J.* 1983;24:711–721.

252. Ribner HS, Zucker MJ, Stasior C, Talentowski D, Stadnicki R, Lesch M. Vasodilators as first-line therapy for congestive heart failure: a comparative hemodynamic study of hydralazine, digoxin, and their combination. *Am Heart J.* 1987;114:91–96.

253. Chatterjee K, Massie B, Rubin S, Gelberg H, Brundage BH, Ports TA. Long-term outpatient vasodilator therapy of congestive heart failure. Consideration of agents at rest and during exercise. *Am J Med.* 1978;65:134–145.

254. Rubin SA, Chatterjee K, Ports JA, Gelberg HJ, Brundage BH, Parmley WW. Influence of short-term oral hydralazine therapy on exercise hemodynamics in patients with severe chronic heart failure. *Am J Cardiol.* 1979;44:1183–1189.

255. Ginks WR, Redwood DR. Hemodynamic effects of hydralazine at rest and during exercise in patients with chronic heart failure. *Br Heart J.* 1980;44:259–264.

256. Rubin SA, Chatterjee K, Parmley WW. Metabolic assessment of exercise in chronic heart failure patients treated with short term vasodilators. *Circulation.* 1980;61:543–548.

257. Wilson JR, Ferraro N. Circulatory improvement after hydralazine or isosorbide dinitrate administration in patients with heart failure: effect on metabolic responses to submaximal exercise. *Am J Med.* 1981;71:627–633.

258. Broudy DR, Greenberg BH, Siemienczuk D, Reinhart S, Morris C, Demots H. Static exercise with congestive heart failure and the response to vasodilating drugs. *Am J Cardiol.* 1987;59:100–104.

259. Leier CV, Desch CE, Magorien RD, et al. Positive inotropic effects of hydralazine in human subjects: comparison with prazosin in the setting of congestive heart failure. *Am J Cardiol.* 1980;46:1039–1044.

260. Binkley PF, Starling RC, Hammer DF, Leier CV. Usefulness of hydralazine to withdraw from dobutamine in

severe congestive heart failure. *Am J Cardiol*. 1991;69: 1103–1106.

261. Daly P, Rouleau JL, Cousineau D, Burgess JH, Chatterjee K. Effects of captopril and a combination of hydralazine and isosorbide dinitrate on myocardial sympathetic tone in patients with severe heart failure. *Br Heart J*. 1986;56:152–157.

262. Elkayam U, Roth A, Hsueh W, Weber L, Freidenberger L, Rahimtoola SH. Neurohumoral consequences of vasodilator therapy with hydralazine and nifedipine in severe congestive heart failure. *Am Heart J*. 1986; 111:1130–1138.

263. Slosky DA, Hindman MC, Peter RH, Wallace AG. Effects of oral hydralazine on rest and exercise hemodynamics in patients with aortic or mitral regurgitation and left ventricular dysfunction. *Clin Cardiol*. 1981;4:162–167.

264. McKay CR, Nana M, Kawanishi DT, et al. Importance of internal controls, statistical methods, and side effects in short-term trials of vasodilators: a study of hydralazine kinetics in patients with aortic regurgitation. *Circulation*. 1985;72:865–872.

265. Stevenson LW, Brunker RC, Belil D, et al. Afterload reduction with vasodilators and diuretics decreases mitral regurgitation during upright exercise in advanced heart failure. *J Am Coll Cardiol*. 1990;15:174–180.

266. Dumesnil JG, Tran K, Dagenais GR. Beneficial long-term effects of hydralazine in aortic regurgitation. *Arch Intern Med*. 1990;150:757–760.

267. Kolibash AJ, Magorien RD, Robinson JL, Leier CV. Hemodynamic effects of vasodilator therapy in severe left heart failure combined with large atrial septal defects. *Am J Med*. 1982;73:439–444.

268. Beekman RH, Rocchini AP, Rosenthal A. Hemodynamic effects of hydralazine in infants with large ventricular septal defect. *Circulation*. 1982;65:523–528.

269. Artman M, Parrish MD, Boerth RC, Boucek RJ, Graham TP. Short-term hemodynamic effects of hydralazine in infants with complete atrioventricular canal defects. *Circulation*. 1984;69:949–954.

270. Magorien RD, Brown GP, Unverferth DV, et al. Effects of hydralazine on coronary blood flow and myocardial energetics in congestive heart failure. *Circulation*. 1982;65:528–533.

271. Rouleau JL, Chatterjee K, Benge W, Parmley WW, Hiramatsu B. Alterations in left ventricular function and coronary hemodynamics with captopril, hydralazine, and prazosin in chronic ischemic heart failure, a comparative study. *Circulation*. 1982;65:671–678.

272. Magorien RD, Unverferth DV, Brown GP, Leier CV. Dobutamine and hydralazine: comparative influences of positive inotropy and vasodilation on coronary blood flow and myocardial energetics in nonischemic congestive heart failure. *J Am Coll Cardiol*. 1983;1:499–505.

273. Magorien RD, Unverferth DV, Leier CV. Hydralazine therapy in chronic congestive heart failure: Sustained central and regional hemodynamic responses. *Am J Med*. 1984;77:267–274.

274. Wilson JR, Untereker W, HIrshfeld J. Effects of isosorbide dinitrate and hydralazine on regional metabolic re-

sponses to arm exercise in patients with heart failure. *Am J Cardiol*. 1981;48:934–938.

275. Wilson JR, Martin JL, Ferraro N, Lueber KT. Effect of hydralazine on perfusion and metabolism in the leg during upright bicycle exercise in patients with heart failure. *Circulation*. 1983;68:425–432.

276. Wilkinson EL, Backman H, Hecht HH. Cardiovascular and renal adjustments to a hypotensive agent. *J Clin Invest*. 1952;31:872–878.

277. Pierpont GL, Brown DC, Franciosa JA, Cohn JN. Effect of hydralazine on renal failure in patients with congestive heart failure. *Circulation*. 1980;61:323–327.

278. Elkayam U, Weber L, Campese VM, Massry SG, Rahimtoola SH. Renal hemodynamics effects of vasodilation with nifedipine and hydralazine in patients with heart failure. *J Am Coll Cardiol*. 1984;4:1261–1267.

279. Cogan JJ, Humphreys MH, Carlson CJ, Benowitz NL, Rapaport E. Acute vasodilator therapy increases renal clearance of digoxin in patients with congestive heart failure. *Circulation*. 1981;64:973–976.

280. Nomura A, Yasuda H, Katoh K, Akimoto T, Miyazaki K, Arita T. Hydralazine and furosemide kinetics. *Clin Pharmacol Ther*. 1982;32:303–306.

281. Wilson JR, Hoyt RW, Ferraro N, Janicki JS, Weber KT. Effect of hydralazine on nutritive flow to working canine gracilis skeletal muscle. *J Am Coll Cardiol*. 1984;4:529–534.

282. Chatterjee K, Ports TA, Brundage BH, Massie B, Holly AN, Parmley WW. Oral hydralazine in chronic heart failure: sustained beneficial hemodynamic effects. *Ann Intern Med*. 1980;92:600–604.

283. Franciosa JA, Weber KT, Levine TB, et al. Hydralazine in the long-term treatment of chronic heart failure: Lack of difference from placebo. *Am Heart J*. 1982;104:587–594.

284. Conradson TB, Ryden L, Ahlmark G, et al. Clinical efficacy of hydralazine in chronic heart failure: one year double-blind placebo-controlled study. *Am Heart J*. 1984;108:1001–1006.

285. Pierpont GL, Cohn JN, Franciosa JA. Combined oral hydralazine-nitrate therapy in left ventricular failure. *Chest*. 1978;73:8–13.

286. Mehta J, Pepine CJ, Conti CR. Hemodynamic effects of hydralazine and of hydralazine plus glyceryl trinitrate paste in heart failure. *Br Heart J*. 1978;40:845–850.

287. Franciosa JA, Cohn JN. Immediate effects of hydralazine-isosorbide dinitrate combination on exercise capacity and exercise hemodynamics in patients with left ventricular failure. *Circulation*. 1979;59:1085–1091.

288. Nelson GI, Ahuja RC, Silke B, Hussain M, Taylor SH. Arteriolar or venous dilatation in left ventricular failure following acute myocardial infarction: a hemodynamic trial of hydralazine and isosorbide dinitrate. *J Cardiovasc Pharmacol*. 1983;5:574–579.

289. Massie B, Chatterjee K, Werner J, Greenberg B, Hart R, Parmley WW. Hemodynamic advantage of combined administration of hydralazine orally and nitrates nonparenterally in the vasodilator therapy of chronic heart failure. *Am J Cardiol*. 1977;40:794–801.

290. Massie BM, Kramer B, Shen E, Haughom F. Vasodila-

tor treatment with isosorbide dinitrate and hydralazine in chronic heart failure. *Br Heart J*. 1981;45:376–384.

291. Cohn JN, Archibald D, Johnson G, and VA cooperative study group. Effects of vasodilator therapy on peak exercise oxygen consumption in heart failure: V-HeFT. *Circulation*. 1987;76:IV-443. Abstract.

292. Wilson JR, St. John Sutton M, Schwartz JS, Ferraro N, Reichele N. Determinants of circulatory response to intravenous hydralazine in congestive heart failure. *Am J Cardiol*. 1983;52:299–303.

293. Massie BM, Packer M, Hanlon JT, Combs DT. Hemodynamic responses to combined therapy with captopril and hydralazine in patients with severe heart failure. *J Am Coll Cardiol*. 1983;2:338–344.

294. Drexler H, Lollgen H, Just H. Short- and long-term effects of hydralazine and combined hydralazine-prenalterol therapy in severe chronic congestive heart failure. *Klin Wochenschr*. 1981;59:647–654.

295. Morand P, Lavigne G, Masson D, Latour F, Alison D. Treatment of severe chronic cardiac insufficiency with dihydralazine: short-and median-term results. *Arch Mal Coeur*. 1979;72:268–275.

296. Quyyumi AA, Wagstaff D, Evans TR. Acute hemodynamic effects of endralazine: a new vasodilator for chronic refractory congestive heart failure. *Am J Cardiol*. 1983;51:1353–1357.

297. Quyyumi AA, Wagstaff D, Evans TR. Long-term effects of endralazine, a new arteriolar vasodilator at rest and during exercise capacity in chronic congestive heart failure. *Am J Cardiol*. 1984;54:1020–1024.

298. Packer M, Meller J, Medina N, Gorlin R, Herman MV. Importance of left ventricular chamber size in determining the response to hydralazine in severe heart failure. *N Engl J Med*. 1980;303:250–255.

299. Elkayam U, Mathus M, Frishman W, LeJemtel T, Strom J, Sonnenblick EH. Dynamic responses to continuous use of prazosin and hydralazine in patients with refractory heart failure. *Clin Pharmacol Ther*. 1981;30:23–30.

300. Packer M, Meller J, Medina N, Yushak M, Gorlin R. Hemodynamic characterization of tolerance to long-term hydralazine therapy in chronic heart failure. *N Engl J Med*. 1982;306:57–62.

301. Black JR, Mehta J. Precipitation of heart failure following a sudden withdrawal of hydralazine. *Chest*. 1979;75:724–725.

302. Massie B, Kramer B, Haughom F. Postural hypotension and tachycardia during hydralazine-isosorbide dinitrate therapy for chronic heart failure. *Circulation*. 1981;63:658–664.

303. Gould L, Patel S, Gomes GI, Reddy CV. Paradoxical response to the vasodilators. *Angiology*. 1982;33:125–130.

303a. Greenberg BH, Massie BM. Beneficial effects of afterload reduction therapy in patients with congestive heart failure and moderate aortic stenosis. *Circulation*. 1980;61:1212–1216.

304. Packer M, Meller J, Medina N, Yushak M, Gorlin R. Provocation of myocardial ischemic events during initiation of vasodilator therapy for severe chronic heart failure: clinical and hemodynamic evaluation of 52 con-

secutive patients with ischemic cardiomyopathy. *Am J Cardiol*. 1981;48:939–946.

305. Gould L, Reddy CVR, Zen B, Singh BK, Becker WH. Electrophysiologic properties of hydralazine in man. *PACE*. 1980;3:548–554.

306. Heer KR, Davies J, MacArthur CG. The effect of hydralazine on arrhythmias in congestive cardiomyopathy. *Int J Cardiol*. 1981;1:117–121.

307. Fletcher R, Johnson G, Cohn JN, and V-HeFT cooperative study group. Vasodilator improvement of mortality in CHF is dependent on the presence of ventricular arrhythmia. *Circulation*. 1988;78:II-347. Abstract.

308. Rubin SA, Brown HV, Swan HJ. Arterial oxygenation and arterial oxygen transport in chronic myocardial failure at rest, during exercise and after hydralazine treatment. *Circulation*. 1982;66:143–148.

309. Franciosa JA, Cohn JN. Effects of minoxidil on hemodynamics in patients with congestive heart failure. *Circulation*. 1981;63:652–657.

310. Nathan M, Rubin SA, Siemienczuk D, Swan HJC. Effects of acute and chronic minoxidil administration on rest and exercise hemodynamics and clinical status in patients with severe, chronic heart failure. *Am J Cardiol*. 1982;50:960–966.

311. Packer M, Meller J, Medina N, Yushak M. Sustained effectiveness of minoxidil in heart failure after development of tolerance to other vasodilator drugs. *Am J Cardiol*. 1981;48:375–379.

312. McKay CR, Chatterjee K, Ports TA, Holly AN, Parmley WW. Minoxidil therapy in chronic congestive heart failure. *Am Heart J*. 1982;104:575–580.

313. Markham RV, Gilmore A, Pettinger WA, Brater DC, Corbett JR, Firth BG. Central and regional hemodynamic effects and neurohumoral consequences of minoxidil in severe congestive heart failure and comparison to hydralazine and nitroprusside. *Am J Cardiol*. 1983;52:774–781.

314. Franciosa JA, Jordan RA, Wilen MM, Leddy CL. Minoxidil in patients with chronic left heart failure: contrasting hemodynamic and clinical effects in a controlled trial. *Circulation*. 1984;70:63–68.

315. Cowley AJ, Wynne RD, Hampton FR. The effects of BTS 49465 on blood pressure and peripheral arteriolar and venous tone in normal volunteers. *J Hypertens*. 1984;2(Suppl 3):547–549.

316. Sim MF, Yates DB, Parkinson R, Cooling MJ. Cardiovascular effects of the novel arteriovenous dilator agent, flosequinan in conscious dogs and cats. *Br J Pharmacol*. 1988;94:371–380.

317. Smith JG, Kinasewitz GT. Effect of BTS 49465 on hypoxic pulmonary vasoconstriction. *J Cardiovasc Pharmacol*. 1986;8:878–884.

318. Dupont AG, De Meirleir K, Van Der Niepen P, Six RO. Renal haemodynamic and blood pressure lowering effects of flosequinan. *Br J Clin Pharmacol*. 1988;25:149–150.

319. Greenberg S, Touhey B, Paul S. Effect of flosequinan (BTS 49465) on myocardial oxygen consumption. *Am Heart J*. 1990;119:1355–1366.

320. Flaotico R, Haertlein BJ, Lakas-Weiss CS, Salata JJ,

Tobia AJ. Positive inotropic and hemodynamic properties of flosequinan, a new vasodilator, and a sulfone metabolite. *J Cardiovasc Pharmacol.* 1989;14:412–418.

321. Greenberg S, Touhey B. Positive inotropy contributes to the hemodynamic mechanism of action of flosequinan (BTS 49465) in the intact dog. *J Cardiovasc Pharmacol.* 1990;15:900–910.

322. Yates DB. Pharmacology of Flosequinan. *Am Heart J.* 1991;121:974–983.

323. Wynne RD, Crampton EL, Hind ID. The pharmacokinetics and haemodynamics of BTS 49465 and its major metabolite in healthy volunteers. *Eur J Clin Pharmacol.* 1985;28:659–664.

324. Kerth P, Frisk-Holmberg M, Meyer P. Antihypertensive activity and pharmacokinetics of flosequinan and its major metabolite in healthy volunteers after repeated dosing. *J Hypertens.* 1986;4(Suppl 6):S128–130.

325. Packer M, Kessler PD, Porter RS, Medina N, Yushak M, Gottlieb SS. Do plasma levels of flosequinan correlate with its hemodynamic effects in severe chronic heart failure? *J Am Coll Cardiol.* 1988;11:42A. (Abstract.)

326. Haas GJ, Binkley PF, Carpenter JA, Leier CV. Central and regional hemodynamic effects of flosequinan for congestive heart failure. *Am J Cardiol.* 1989;63:1354–1359.

327. Schneeweiss A, Wynne RD, Marmor A. Effect of flosequinan in patients with acute-onset heart failure complicating acute myocardial infarction. *Crit Care Med.* 1989;17:879–881.

328. Kessler PD, Packer M. Hemodynamic effects of BTS 49465, a new long- acting systemic vasodilator drug, in patients with severe congestive heart failure. *Am Heart J.* 1987;113:137–143.

329. Cowley AJ, Wynne RD, Stainer K, Fullwood L, Rowley JM, Hampton JR. Flosequinan in heart failure: acute haemodynamic and longer term symptomatic effects. *Br Med J.* 1988;297:169–173.

330. Schneeweiss A, Plich M, Green T, Wynne RD, Marmor A. Efficacy and safety of flosequinan, given over 3 days, evaluated by continuous hemodynamic monitoring. *Cardiology.* 1989;76:201–205.

331. Kessler PD, Packer M, Medina N, Yushak M. Cumulative hemodynamic response to short-term treatment with flosequinan (BTS 49465), a new direct-acting vasodilator drug, in severe chronic congestive heart failure. *J Cardiovasc Pharmacol.* 1988;12:6–11.

332. Riegger G, Kahles H, Wagner A, Kromer EP, Elsner D, Kochsiek K. Exercise capacity, hemodynamic, and neurohumoral changes following acute and chronic administration of flosequinan in chronic congestive heart failure. *Cardiovasc Drugs Ther.* 1990;4:1395–1402.

333. Haas GJ, Binkley PE, Leier CV. Chronic vasodilator therapy with flosequinan in congestive heart failure. *Clin Cardiol.* 1990;13:414–420.

334. Corin WJ, Monrad ES, Strom JA, Giustino S, Sonnenblick ES, LeJemtel T. Flosequinan: a vasodilator with positive inotropic activity. *Am Heart J.* 1991;121:537–540.

335. Elborn JS, Riley M, Stanford CF, Nicholls DP. The effects of flosequinan on submaximal exercise in patients with chronic cardiac failure. *Br J Clin Pharmacol.* 1990;29:519–524.

336. Elborn JS, Stanford CF, Nicholls DP. Effect of flosequinan on exercise capacity and symptoms in severe heart failure. *Br Heart J.* 1989;61:331–335.

337. Pinsky DJ, Wilson PB, Ahern D, Kukin ML, Gottlieb SS, Packer M. Flosequinan improves symptoms and exercise tolerance in heart failure: Results of a placebo-controlled trial. *Circulation.* 1990;82:III-322. Abstract.

338. Packer M, Narahara KA, Elkayam U, et al. Randomized, multicenter, double-blind, placebo-controlled study of the efficacy of flosequinan, a new, long-acting vasodilator drug, in patients with chronic heart failure. *Circulation.* 1990;82:III-323. Abstract.

338a. Massie BM, Berk MR, Brozena S, et al. Can further benefit be achieved by adding a vasodilator to triple therapy in CHF: results of the flosequinan-ACE inhibitor trial (FACET)? *Circulation.* 1992;86:I-645 (Abstract).

338b. Packer M, Pitt B. Efficacy of flosequinan in patients with heart failure who are withdrawn from therapy with converting-enzyme inhibitors: a double-blind controlled study. *Circulation.* 1992;86:I-644 (Abstract).

339. Sakai K, Nakano H, Nagano H, Uchida Y. Nicorandil. In: Scriabine A, ed. *New Drugs Annual: Cardiovascular Drugs.* New York: Raven Press; 1983:227–242.

340. Sumimoto K, Domae M, Yamanaka K, et al. Actions of nicorandil on vascular smooth muscles. *J Cardiovasc Pharmacol.* 1987;10(Suppl 8):566–575.

341. Taira N. Similarity and dissimilarity in the mode and mechanism of action between nicorandil and classical nitrates: an overview. *J Cardiovasc Pharmacol.* 1987;10(Suppl 8):51–59.

342. Kambara H, Tamaki S, Nakamura Y, Kawai C. Effect of intravenous administration of nicorandil on cardiovascular hemodynamics and left ventricular function. *Am J Cardiol.* 1989;63:56J–60J.

343. Belz GG, Matthews JH, Beck A, Wagner G, Schneider B. Hemodynamic effects of nicorandil, isosorbide dinitrate, and dihydralazine in healthy volunteers. *J Cardiovasc Pharmacol.* 1985;7:1107–1112.

344. Levenson J, Bouthier J, Chau NP, Roland E, Simon AC. Effects of nicorandil on arterial and venous vessels of the forearm in systemic hypertension. *Am J Cardiol.* 1989;63:40J–43J.

345. Kukovetz WR, Holzmann S. Cyclic GMP in nicorandil-induced vasodilatation and tolerance development. *J Cardiovasc Pharmacol.* 1987;10(Suppl 8):S25–S30.

346. Sieke B, Satya VP, Ali MS, Goldhammer E, Taylor SH. Effects of nicorandil on left ventricular hemodynamics and volume at rest and during exercise-induced angina pectoris. *Am J Cardiol.* 1989;63:49J–55J.

347. Gross G, Pieper G, Farber NE, Warltier D, Hardman H. Effects of nicorandil on coronary circulation and myocardial ischemia. *Am J Cardiol.* 1989;63:11J–17J.

348. Lamping KA, Christensen CW, Pelc LR, Warltier DC, Gross GJ. Effects of nicorandil and nifedipine on protection of ischemic myocardium. *J Cardiovasc Pharmacol.* 1984;6:536–542.

349. Pieper GM, Gross GJ. Salutary action of nicorandil, a new antianginal drug, on myocardial metabolism during

ischemia and on postischemic function in a canine preparation of brief, repetitive coronary artery occlusions: comparison with isosorbide dinitrate. *Circulation.* 1987; 76:916–928.

350. Lamping KA, Warltier DC, Hardman HF, Gross GJ. Effects of nicorandil, a new antianginal agent, and nifedipine on collateral blood flow in a chronic coronary occlusion model. *J Pharmacol Exp Ther.* 1984;229:359–363.

351. Kobayashi K, Hakuta T. Effects of nicorandil on coronary hemodynamics in ischemic heart disease: comparison with nitroglycerin, nifedipine and propranolol. *J Cardiovasc Pharmacol.* 1987;(Suppl 8):S109–S115.

352. Kinoshita M, Nishikawa S, Sawamura N, et al. Comparative efficacy of high dose versus low-dose nicorandil therapy for chronic stable angina pectoris. *Am J Cardiol.* 1986;56:733–738.

353. Solal AC, Jaeger P, Bouthier J, Juliard JM, Dahan M, Gourgon R. Hemodynamic action of nicorandil in chronic congestive heart failure. *Am J Cardiol.* 1989;63:44J–48J.

354. Tice FD, Binkley PF, Cody RJ, et al. Hemodynamic effects of oral nicorandil in congestive heart failure. *Am J Cardiol.* 1990;65:1361–1367.

355. Galie N, Varani E, Maiello L, et al. Usefulness of nicorandil in congestive heart failure. *Am J Cardiol.* 1990;65:343–348.

356. Packer M, Gorlin R, Meller J, Medina N. Central hemodynamic effects of dipyridamole in severe heart failure: comparison with hydralazine. *Clin Pharmacol Ther.* 1982;32:54–61.

357. Bousvarous GA, Campbell JE, McGregor M. Haemodynamic effects of dipyridamole at rest and during exercise in healthy subjects. *Br Heart J.* 1966;28:331–334.

358. Wendt WE, Sundermeyer JF, DenBakker PB, Bing RJ. The relationship between coronary blood flow, myocardial oxygen consumption and cardiac work as influenced by Persantin. *Am J Cardiol.* 1962;9:449–454.

359. Strauss WE, Parisi AF. Combined use of calcium channel and beta-adrenergic blockers for the treatment of chronic stable angina. Rationale, efficacy and adverse effects. *Ann Intern Med.* 1989;109:570–581.

360. Ellrodt G, Chew CYC, Singh BN. Therapeutic implications of slow-channel blockade in cardiocirculatory disorders. *Circulation.* 1980;62:669–679.

361. Bidiville J, Nussberger J, Waeber G, Porchet M, Waeber B, Brunner HR. Individual responses to converting enzyme inhibitors and calcium antagonists. *Hypertension.* 1988;11:166–173.

362. Packer M, Kessler PD, Lee WH. Calcium-channel blockade in the management of severe chronic congestive heart failure: a bridge too far. *Circulation.* 1987;75(Suppl V):56–64.

363. Cody RJ, Riew KD, Kubo SH. Reversal of calcium-mediated vasoconstrictor component in patients with congestive heart failure. *Clin Pharmacol Ther.* 1989; 46:291–296.

364. Dollery CT. Clinical pharmacology of calcium antagonists. *Am J Hypertens.* 1991;4:88s–95s.

365. McAllister RG. Clinical pharmacology of slow channel blocking agents. *Prog Cardiovasc Dis.* 1982;25:83–102.

366. Weiner DA. Calcium channel blockers. *Med Clin North Am.* 1988;72:83–114.

367. Nakaya H, Schwartz A, Millard RW. Reflex chronotropic and inotropic effects of calcium channel blocking agents in conscious dogs. *Circ Res.* 1983;52:302–311.

368. Urquhart J, Patterson RE, Bacharach SL, et al. Comparative effects of verapamil, diltiazem, and nifedipine on hemodynamics and left ventricular function during acute myocardial ischemia in dogs. *Circulation.* 1984;69:382–390.

369. Levine TB, Francis GS, Goldsmith SR, Cohn JN. The neurohumoral and hemodynamic response to orthostatic tilt in patients with congestive heart failure. *Circulation.* 1983;5:1070–1075.

370. Colucci WS, Fifer MA, Lorell BH, Wynne J. Calcium channel blockers in congestive heart failure: theoretic considerations and clinical experience. *Am J Med.* 1985;78(Suppl 2B):9–17.

371. Klugmann S, Salvi A, Camerini F. Haemodynamic effects of nifedipine in heart failure. *Br Heart J.* 1980;43:440–446.

372. Kurnik PB, Tiefenbrunn AJ, Ludbrook PA. The dependence of the cardiac effects of nifedipine on the responses of the peripheral vascular system. *Circulation.* 1984;69:963–972.

373. Ludbrook PA, Tiefenbrunn AJ, Reed FR, Sobel BE. Acute hemodynamic responses to sublingual nifedipine: dependence on left ventricular function. *Circulation.* 1982;65:489–498.

374. Gascho JA, Apollo WP. Effects of nifedipine on the venodilatory response to nitroglycerine. *Am J Cardiol.* 1990;65:99–102.

375. Diamond JR, Cheung JY, Fang LST. Nifedipine-induced renal dysfunction. Alterations in renal hemodynamics. *Am J Med.* 1984;77:905–909.

376. Cohn PF. Effects of calcium channel blockers on the coronary circulation. *Am J Hypertens.* 1990;3:299s–304s.

377. Elkayam U, Weber L, McKay C, Rahimtoola S. Spectrum of acute hemodynamic effects of nifedipine in severe congestive heart failure. *Am J Cardiol.* 1985; 56:560–566.

378. Packer M, Lee WH, Medina N, Yushak M, Bernstein JL, Kessler PD. Prognostic importance of the immediate hemodynamic response to nifedipine in patients with severe left ventricular dysfunction. *J Am Coll Cardiol.* 1987;10:1303–1311.

379. Packer M, Medina N, Yushah M. Adverse hemodynamic and clinical effects of calcium channel blockade in pulmonary hypertension secondary to obliterative pulmonary vascular disease. *J Am Coll Cardiol.* 1984;4:890–901.

380. Walsh RW, Porter CB, Starling MR, O'Rourke RA. Beneficial hemodynamic effects of intravenous and oral diltiazem in severe congestive heart failure. *J Am Coll Cardiol.* 1984;3:1044–1050.

381. Packer M. Second generation calcium channel blockers in the treatment of chronic heart failure: are they any better than their predecessors? *J Am Coll Cardiol.* 1989;14:1339–1342.

382. Nienaber CA, Spielmann RP, Aschenberg W, Fehr A, Clausen A. Comparison of the acute hemodynamic

response to intravenous nisoldipine (Bay K 5552) and intravenous nifedipine for left ventricular dysfunction secondary to myocardial infarction. *Am J Cardiol.* 1987;60:836–841.

383. Lewis BS, Shefer A, Merdler A, Flugelman MY, Hardoff R, Halon DA. Effect of the second-generation calcium channel blocker nisoldipine on left ventricular contractility in cardiac failure. *Am Heart J.* 1988;115:1238–1244.

384. Klowski W, Erne P, Pfisterer M, Mueller J, Buehler FR, Burkart F. Arterial vasodilator, systemic and coronary hemodynamic effects of nisoldipine in congestive heart failure secondary to ischemic or dilated cardiomyopathy. *Am J Cardiol.* 1987;59:1118–1125.

385. Erlemeier HH, Kupper W. Acute haemodynamic and neurohumoral effects of intravenous nisoldipine in patients with severe congestive heart failure. *Eur J Clin Pharmacol.* 1990;38:11–15.

386. Tan LB, Murray RG, Littler WA. Felodipine in patients with chronic heart failure: discrepant hemodynamic and clinical effects. *Br Heart J.* 1987;58:112–118.

387. Maisch B, Hofman J, Borst U, Drude L, Herzum M, Kocksiek K. Nisoldipine in dilated cardiomyopathy. *Circulation.* 1988;78(Suppl II):II-618. Abstract.

388. Barjon JN, Rouleau JL, Bichet D, Juneau C, De Champlain J. Chronic renal and neurohumoral effects of the calcium entry blocker nisoldipine in patients with congestive heart failure. *J Am Coll Cardiol.* 1987;9:622–630.

389. Schofer J, Hobuss M, Aschenberg W, Tews A. Acute and long-term haemodynamic and neurohumoral response to nisoldipine vs captopril in patients with heart failure: A randomized double-blind study. *Eur Heart J.* 1990;11:712–721.

390. Kassis E, Amtorp O. Long-term clinical, hemodynamic, angiographic, and neurohumoral responses to vasodilation with felodipine in patients with chronic congestive heart failure. *J Cardiovasc Pharmacol.* 1990;15:347–352.

391. Dunselman PH, Kuntze CEE, van Bruggen A, et al. Efficacy of felodipine in congestive heart failure. *Eur Heart J.* 1989;10:354–364.

392. Packer M. Calcium channel blockers in chronic heart failure. The risks of "physiologically rational" therapy. *Circulation.* 1990;82:2254–2257.

393. Goldstein RE, Boccuzzi SJ, Cruess D, Nattel S, the Adverse Experience Committee, and the Multicenter Diltiazem Postinfarction Research Group. Diltiazem increases late-onset congestive heart failure in postinfarction patients with early reduction in ejection fraction. *Circulation.* 1991;83:52–60.

394. Elkayam U, Amin J, Aniekumar M, Vasquez J, Weber L, Rahimtoola SH. A prospective, randomized, double-blind crossover study to compare the efficacy and safety of chronic nifedipine therapy with that of isosorbide dinitrate and their combination in the treatment of chronic congestive heart failure. *Circulation.* 1990;82:1954–1961.

395. Setaro JF, Zaret BL, Schulman DS, Black HR, Soufer R. Usefulness of verapamil for congestive heart failure associated with abnormal left ventricular diastolic filling and normal left ventricular systolic performance. *Am J Cardiol.* 1990;66:981–986.

396. Walsh RA, O'Rourke RA. Direct and indirect effects of

calcium entry blocking agents on isovolumic left ventricular relaxation in conscious dogs. *J Clin Invest.* 1985;75:1426–1434.

397. Lewis BS, Shefer A, Flugelman MY, Merdler A, Halon DA, Hardoff R. Effect of the second-generation calcium channel blocking drug nisoldipine on diastolic left ventricular dysfunction in heart failure. *Am Heart J.* 1989;118:505–511.

398. Leier CV, Binkley PF, Cody RJ. Alpha-adrenergic component of the sympathetic nervous system in congestive heart failure. *Circulation.* 1990;82(Suppl I):68–76.

399. Giles TD, Sander GE, Thomas MG, Quiroz AC. Alpha-adrenergic mechanisms in the pathophysiology of left ventricular heart failure—an analysis of their role in systolic and diastolic dysfunction. *J Mol Cell Cardiol.* 1986;18(Suppl 5):33–43.

400. Good AP, Unverferth DV, Leier CV. Hemodynamic responses to different levels of alpha-adrenergic interruption in congestive heart failure. *Cardiovasc Drugs Ther.* 1988;1:529–534.

401. Giles TD, Iteld BJ, Mautner RK, Rognoni PA, Dillenkoffer RL. Short-term effects of intravenous clonidine in congestive heart failure. *Clin Pharmacol Ther.* 1981;30:724–728.

402. Hermiller JB, Magorien RD, Leithe ME, Unverferth DV, Leier CV. Clonidine in congestive heart failure: a vasodilator with negative inotropic effects. *Am J Cardiol.* 1983;51:791–795.

403. Magorien RD, Hermiller JB, Unverferth DV, Leier CV. Regional hemodynamic effects of clonidine in congestive heart failure. *J Cardiovasc Pharmacol.* 1985;7:91–96.

404. Giles TD, Thomas MG, Quiroz A, Rice JC, Planche W, Sander GE. Acute and short-term effects of clonidine in heart failure. *Angiology.* 1987;38:537–548.

405. Van der Geest S, Van Dijk RB, Donker AJ. Clonidine withdrawal syndrome in a patient with heart failure. *Crit Care Med.* 1985;13:444–445.

406. Olivari MT, Levine TB, Cohn JN. Acute hemodynamic and hormonal effects of central versus peripheral sympathetic inhibition in patients with congestive heart failure. *J Cardiovasc Pharmacol.* 1986;8:973–977.

407. Kirlin PC, Das S, Grekin R, et al. Sympathetic inhibition with methyldopa in heart failure. *J Cardiovasc Pharmacol.* 1986;8:1092–1100.

408. Manolis AS, Varriole P, Nobile J. Short-term hemodynamic effects of intravenous methyldopa in patients with heart failure. *Pharmacotherapy.* 1987;7:216–222.

409. Miller RR, Awan NA, Maxwell KS, Mason DT. Sustained reduction of cardiac impedance and preload in congestive heart failure with the antihypertensive vasodilator prazosin. *N Engl J Med.* 1977;297:303–307.

410. Awan NA, Miller RR, DeMaria AN, Maxwell KS, Neumann A, Mason DT. Efficacy of ambulatory systemic therapy with oral prazosin in chronic refractory heart failure. *Circulation.* 1977;56:346–354.

411. Awan NA, Miller RR, Mason DT. Comparison of effects of nitroprusside and prazosin on left ventricular function and the peripheral circulation in chronic refractory congestive heart failure. *Circulation.* 1978;57:152–159.

412. Awan NA, Miller RR, Miller MP, Specht K, Vera Z,

Mason DT. Clinical pharmacology and therapeutic application of prazosin in acute and chronic refractory congestive heart failure. Balanced, systemic venous and arterial dilation improving pulmonary congestion and cardiac output. *Am J Med.* 1978;65:146–154.

413. Desch CE, Magorien RD, Triffon DW, Blanford MF, Unverferth DV, Leier CV. Development of pharmacodynamic tolerance to prazosin in congestive heart failure. *Am J Cardiol.* 1979;44:1178–1182.

414. Parker M, Miller J, Gorlin R, Herman MV. Hemodynamic and clinical tachyphylaxis to prazosin-mediated afterload reduction in severe chronic congestive heart failure. *Circulation.* 1979;59:531–539.

415. Arnold SB, Williams RL, Ports TA, et al. Attenuation of prazosin effect on cardiac output in chronic heart failure. *Ann Intern Med.* 1979;91:345–349.

416. Elkayam U, Lejemtel TH, Mathur M, et al. Marked early attenuation of hemodynamic effects of oral prazosin therapy in chronic congestive heart failure. *Am J Cardiol.* 1979;44:540–545.

417. Jaillon P. Clinical pharmacokinetics of prazosin. *Clin Pharmacokinet.* 1980;5:365–376.

418. Silke B, Lakhani ZM, Taylor SH. Pharmacokinetic and pharmacodynamic studies with prazosin in chronic heart failure. *J Cardiovasc Pharmacol.* 1981;3:329–335.

419. Baughman RA, Arnold S, Benet LZ, Lin ET, Chatterjee K, Williams RL. Altered prazosin pharmacokinetics in congestive heart failure. *Eur J Clin Pharmacol.* 1980;17:425–428.

420. Jaillon P, Rubin P, Yee YG, et al. Influence of congestive heart failure on prazosin kinetics. *Clin Pharmacol Ther.* 1979;25:790–794.

421. Mehta J, Iacoma M, Feldman RL, Pepine CJ, Conti CR. Comparative hemodynamic effects of intravenous nitroprusside and oral prazosin in refractory heart failure. *Am J Cardiol.* 1978;41:925–930.

422. Reuben SR, Kuan P, Gale EV, Wilde PM. Hemodynamic effects of prazosin in CHF. *Acta Med Scand.* 1981;210(Suppl):145–148.

423. Parmley WW, Chatterjee K, Arnold S, et al. Hemodynamic effects of prazosin in chronic heart failure. *Am Heart J.* 1981;102:622–625.

424. Von der Lippe G, Olim OJ, Lund-Johansen P. Acute hemodynamic and long-term clinical effects of prazosin in the treatment of chronic congestive heart failure. *Acta Med Scand.* 1981;210:213–216.

425. Hayashi H, Sassa H, Oba M, et al. Acute and chronic cardiocirculatory effects of oral prazosin in chronic refractory heart failure. *Jpn Heart J.* 1980;21:827–836.

426. Packer M, Meller J, Gorlin R, Herman MV. Differences in hemodynamic effects of nitroprusside and prazosin in severe chronic congestive heart failure: evidence for a direct negative chronotropic effect of prazosin. *Am J Cardiol.* 1979;44:310–317.

427. Stein L, Foster RR, Friedman AW, Statza J, McHenry PL. Acute and chronic hemodynamic effects of prazosin in left ventricular failure. *Br Heart J.* 1981;45:186–192.

428. Rouleau JL, Warnica JW, Burgess JH. Prazosin and congestive heart failure: short- and long-term therapy. *Am J Med.* 1981;71:147–152.

429. Chatterjee K, Rubin SA, Ports TA, Parmley WW. Influence of oral prazosin therapy on exercise hemodynamics in patients with severe chronic heart failure. *Am J Med.* 1981;71:140–146.

430. Awan NA, Lee G, DeMaria AN, Mason DT. Ambulatory prazosin treatment of chronic congestive heart failure: development of late tolerance reversible by higher dosage and interrupted substitution therapy. *Am Heart J.* 1981;101:541–547.

431. Rubin SA, Chatterjee K, Gelberg HJ, Ports TA, Brundage BH, Parmley WW. Paradox of improved exercise but not resting hemodynamics with short-term prazosin in chronic heart failure. *Am J Cardiol.* 1979;43:810–815.

432. Higginbotham MB, Morris KG, Bramlet DA, Coleman RE, Cobb FR. Long-term ambulatory therapy with prazosin versus placebo for chronic heart failure: relation between clinical response and left ventricular function at rest and during exercise. *Am J Cardiol.* 1983;52:782–788.

433. Markham RV, Corbett JR, Gilmore A, Pettinger WA, Firth BG. Efficacy of prazosin in the management of chronic congestive heart failure: a 6 month randomized, double-blind, placebo-controlled study. *Am J Cardiol.* 1983;51:1346–1352.

434. Colucci WS, Wynne J, Holman EL, Braunwald E. Long-term therapy of heart failure with prazosin: a randomized double blind trial. *Am J Cardiol.* 1980;45:337–344.

435. Bartel O, Burkart F, Buhler FR. Sustained effectiveness of chronic prazosin therapy in severe chronic congestive heart failure. *Am Heart J.* 1981;101:529–533.

436. Feldman RC, Ball RM, Winchester MA, Jaillon P, Kates RE, Harrison DC. Beneficial hemodynamic response to chronic prazosin therapy in congestive heart failure. *Am Heart J.* 1981;101:534–540.

437. Goldman SA, Johnson LL, Escala E, Cannon PJ, Weiss MB. Improved exercise ejection fraction with long-term prazosin therapy in patients with heart failure. *Am J Med.* 1980;68:36–42.

438. Packer M, Medina N, Yushak M. Comparative hemodynamic and clinical effects of long-term treatment with prazosin and captopril for severe chronic congestive heart failure secondary to coronary artery disease and idiopathic dilated cardiomyopathy. *Am J Cardiol.* 1986;57:1323–1327.

439. Reifort N, Moritz AD, Nady M, Kaltenbach M, Bussmann WD. Lack of symptomatic and long-term hemodynamic effects of prazosin in chronic heart failure. Double-blind, randomized study over one year. *Z Kardiol.* 1985;74:205–212.

440. Stein L, Henry DP, Weinberger MH. Increase in plasma norepinephrine during prazosin therapy for chronic congestive heart failure. *Am J Med.* 1981;70:825–832.

441. Ogasawara B, Ogawa K, Hayashi H, Sassa H. Plasma renin activity and plasma concentrations of norepinephrine and cyclic nucleotides in heart failure after prazosin. *Clin Pharmacol Ther.* 1981;29:464–471.

442. Colucci WS, Williams GH, Braunwald E. Clinical, hemodynamic, and neuroendocrine effects of chronic prazosin therapy for congestive heart failure. *Am Heart J.* 1981;102:615–621.

443. Riegger GAJ, Haeske W, Kraus C, Kromer EP, Koch-

siek K. Contribution of the renin-angiotensin-aldosterone system to development of tolerance and fluid retention in chronic congestive heart failure during prazosin treatment. *Am J Cardiol.* 1987;59:906–910.

444. Packer M, Medina N, Yushak M. Role of the renin-angiotensin system in the development of hemodynamic and clinical tolerance to long-term prazosin therapy in patients with severe chronic heart failure. *J Am Coll Cardiol.* 1986;7:671–680.

445. Pierpont GL, Franciosa JA, Cohn JN. Effect of prazosin on renal function in congestive heart failure. *Clin Pharmacol Ther.* 1980;28:335–339.

446. Leier CV, Patterson SE, Huss P, Parrish D, Unverferth DV. The hemodynamic and clinical responses to terazosin, a new alpha blocking agent, in congestive heart failure. *Am J Med Sci.* 1986;292:128–135.

447. Magorien RD, Sinnathamby S, Leier CV, Boudoulas H, Unverferth DV. Rest and exercise cardiovascular effects of terazosin in congestive heart failure. *Am J Cardiol.* 1990;65:638–643.

448. Franciosa JA, Cohn JN. Hemodynamic effects of trimazosin in patients with left ventricular failure. *Clin Pharmacol Ther.* 1978;23:11–18.

449. Awan NA, Hermanovich J, Whitcomb C, Skinner P, Mason DT. Cardiocirculatory effects of afterload reduction with oral trimazosin in severe chronic congestive heart failure. *Am J Cardiol.* 1979;44:126–131.

450. Weber KT, Kinasewitz GT, West JS, Janicki JS, Reichek N, Fishman AP. Long-term vasodilator therapy with trimazosin in chronic cardiac failure. *N Engl J Med.* 1980;303:242–250.

451. Aronow WS, Greenfield RS, Alimadadian H, Danahy DT. Effect of the vasodilator trimazosin versus placebo on exercise performance in chronic left ventricular failure. *Am J Cardiol.* 1977;40:789–793.

452. DiBianco R, Parker JO, Chakko S, et al. Doxazosin for the treatment of chronic congestive heart failure: results of a randomized double-blind and placebo-controlled study. *Am Heart J.* 1991;121:372–380.

453. Olivari MT, Garberg VR, Selby T, Cohn JN, Levine TB. Acute hemodynamic and hormonal response to indoramin in congestive heart failure. *Clin Pharmacol Ther.* 1984;36:297–301.

454. Leier CV, Majetich N, Binkley PF, Unverferth DV. Hemodynamic responses to indoramin at rest and during exercise in congestive heart failure. *Pharmacotherapy.* 1987;7:61–68.

455. Silke B, Nelson GI, Verma SP, et al. Hemodynamic dose-response effects of intravenous indoramin in acute heart failure complicating myocardial infarction. *J Cardiovasc Pharmacol.* 1986;8(Suppl 2):S102–S106.

456. Leier CV, Binkley PF, Randolph PH, Unverferth DV. Long-term indoramin therapy in congestive heart failure: a double-blind, randomized, parallel placebo-controlled trial. *J Am Coll Cardiol.* 1987;9:426–432.

457. Seth L, Galie N, Casebolt P, Gimenez H, Malloy M, Franciosa JA. Indoramin in heart failure: possible adverse effects on hemodynamics and exercise capacity. *Clin Pharmacol Ther.* 1986;40:567–574.

458. Kubo SH, Rector TS, Heifetz SM, Cohn JN. Alpha 2-receptor–mediated vasoconstriction in patients with congestive heart failure. *Circulation.* 1989;80:1660–1667.

459. Gould L, Zahir M, Shariff M, Giuliani M. Phentolamine use in congestive heart failure. *Jpn Heart J.* 1970;11:17–25.

460. Gould L, Zahir M, Shariff M, Giuliani M. Phentolamine use in pulmonary edema: preliminary report. *Jpn Heart J.* 1970;11:141–148.

461. Kelly DT, Delgado CE, Taylor DR, Pitt B, Ross RS. Use of phentolamine in acute myocardial infarction associated with hypertension and left ventricular failure. *Circulation.* 1973;47:729–735.

462. Gardaz JP, Reynaert M, Grimbert F, Enrico JF, Perret C. Phentolamine in the treatment of left heart failure in the acute stage of myocardial infarct. *Schweiz Med Wochenschr.* 1974;104:1588–1589.

463. Perret CL, Gardaz JP, Reynaert M, Grimbert F, Enrico JF. Phentolamine for vasodilator therapy in left ventricular failure complicating acute myocardial infarction: hemodynamic study. *Br Heart J.* 1975;37:640–646.

464. Henning RJ, Shubin H, Weil MH. Afterload reduction with phentolamine in patients with acute pulmonary edema. *Am J Med.* 1977;63:568–573.

465. Stern MA, Gohlke HK, Loeb HS, Croke RP, Gunnar RM. Hemodynamic effects of intravenous phentolamine in low output failure: dose-response relationships. *Circulation.* 1978;58:157–163.

466. Gould LA, Reddy CV. Oral therapy with phentolamine in chronic congestive heart failure. *Chest.* 1979;75:487–491.

467. Schreiber R, Maier PT, Gunnar RM, Loeb HS. Hemodynamic improvement following a single dose of oral phentolamine administration in patients with chronic low output cardiac failure. *Chest.* 1979;76:571–575.

468. Georgopoulos AJ, Valasidis A, Siourthas D. Treatment of chronic heart failure with slow release phentolamine. *Eur J Clin Pharmacol.* 1978;13:325–329.

469. Renard M, Verhoeven A, Liebens I, Bernard R. Blood gas and hemodynamic changes induced by the treatment of pulmonary congestion with vasodilators in the acute phase of myocardial infarction. *Acta Cardiol.* 1986;41:111–121.

470. Gould L, Reddy CV, Patel S, Gomes GI, Becker WH. Noninvasive assessment of load reduction in chronic congestive heart failure patients. *Angiology.* 1981;32:552–560.

471. LeJemtel TH, Maskin CS, Lucido D, Chadwick BJ. Failure to augment maximal limb blood flow in response to one-leg versus two-leg exercise in patients with severe heart failure. *Circulation.* 1986;74:245–251.

472. Wilson JR, Frey MJ, Mancini DM, Ferraro N, Jones R. Sympathetic vasoconstriction during exercise in ambulatory patients with left ventricular failure. *Circulation.* 1989;79:1021–1027.

473. Stenstrom G, Holmberg S. Cardiomyopathy in pheochromocytoma. *Eur Heart J.* 1985;6:539–544.

474. Wallin JD, O'Neill WM. Labetalol: current research and therapeutic status. *Arch Intern Med.* 1983;143:485–490.

475. Johnson LL, Cubbon J, Escala E, et al. Hemodynamic effects of labetalol in patients with combined hypertension and left ventricular failure. *J Cardiovasc Pharmacol.* 1988;12:350–356.

476. Frais MA, Bayley TJ. Left ventricular failure with labetalol. *Postgrad Med J.* 1979;55:567–568.

477. Leung WH, Lau CP, Wong CK, Cheng CH, Tai YT, Lim SP. Improvement in exercise performance and hemodynamics by labetalol in patients with idiopathic dilated cardiomyopathy. *Am Heart J*. 1990;119:884–890.

478. Gupta PD, Broadhurst P, Raftery EB, Lahiri A. Value of carvedilol in congestive heart failure secondary to coronary artery disease. *Am J Cardiol*. 1990;66:1118–1123.

479. Burch GE, Leon-Galindo J, Cronvich JA. "New" treatment for chronic intractable congestive heart failure. *Am Heart J*. 1976;91:735–746.

480. Korewicki J, Kraska T, Opolski G, Ostrzycki A. Vasodilator drugs in patients with chronic ischemic heart failure. *Cor Vasa*. 1985;27:329–336.

481. Haas GJ, Leier CV. Invasive cardiovascular testing in chronic congestive heart failure. *Crit Care Med*. 1990;18:S1–S4.

25
Beta-Adrenergic Receptor Agonists and Antagonists in Heart Failure

Ray E. Hershberger

Over the past 20 years a great deal of knowledge has accumulated regarding β-adrenergic receptor function and physiology in heart failure. This knowledge includes a greater understanding of the neurohumoral activation in heart failure and the increased levels of endogenous β-adrenergic receptor ligands such as norepinephrine, which has been reviewed in Chapter 5. Additionally, a great deal of experimental evidence has been collected regarding the use of β-adrenergic receptor agonists and antagonists in heart failure. However, the fundamental pathophysiological event or events that trigger heart muscle to fail still is not understood.

The rational clinical use of β-adrenergic receptor agonists and antagonists in patients with heart failure depends on knowledge of agents active at β-adrenergic receptors, β-adrenergic receptor structure and function, and postreceptor signal transduction pathways in the heart and vascular systems of patients with heart failure. Such knowledge will enhance the understanding and interpretation of a great deal of clinical data. This chapter attempts to bridge basic and clinical investigation of the β-adrenergic receptor system in human heart failure. It has been written to provide clinicians with an overview of concepts and understandings that reflect the rapid expansion of basic knowledge regarding β-adrenergic receptor structure and function. This overview will provide a backdrop for a comprehensive review of the clinical uses of β-adrenergic receptor agonists and antagonists in patients with heart failure. A secondary goal is to focus research issues for basic investigators less familiar with the clinical issues of the β-adrenergic receptor pathways in human heart failure. Several excellent reviews[1-3] recently have appeared.

Molecular and Cellular Concepts: Receptors, Drugs, and Signal Transduction

The rational use of β-adrenergic agonists and antagonists in patients with heart failure requires an understanding of the mechanisms of how such drugs and neurotransmitters exert their effects. The use of such agents also requires a knowledge of the target tissues in the heart failure condition, and in particular in alterations associated with heart failure that may affect responses to these agents. Over the past 10 years a great deal of progress has been made in understanding how β-adrenergic agonists and antagonists exert their effects, both in model systems and in clinical practice. It is now appreciated that such agents work primarily via interactions with cell surface structures called receptors, which in turn activate, or in the case of antagonists, inhibit, activation of signaling pathways.

Receptors

Receptors are cellular structures that are the site of interaction for any chemical agent.[4] One major class, the cell surface receptors, reside in the membrane bilayer of virtually all living cells and enable a wide variety of hormones and neurotransmitters to communicate with internal cellular systems. The naturally occurring sympathetic amines represent a family of such neurotransmitters and are widely distributed through all mammalian organ systems. The principal endogenous catecholamine neurotransmitters are dopamine,

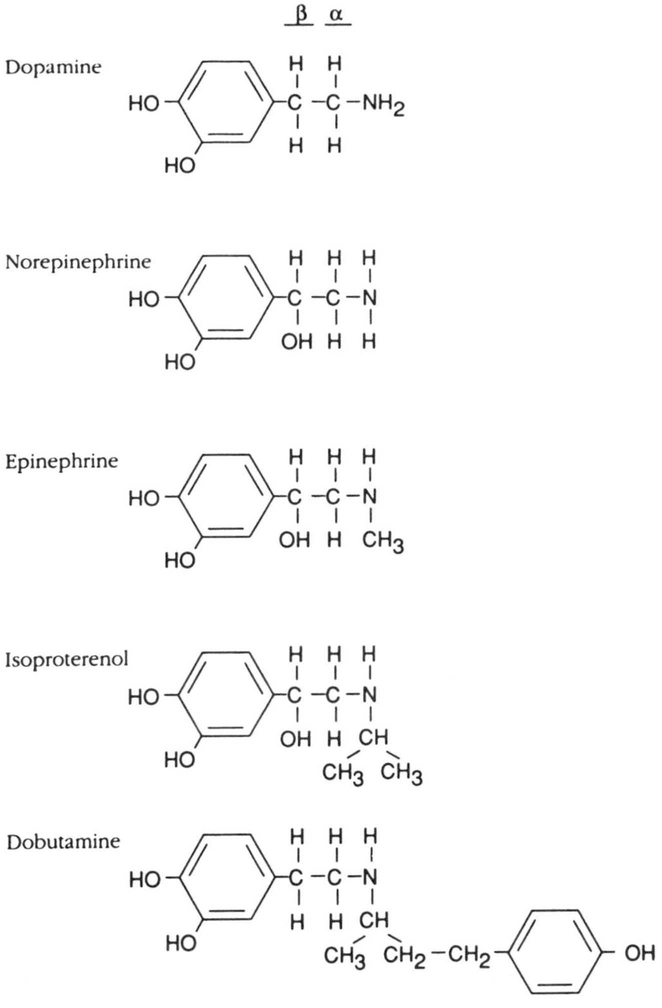

FIGURE 25.1. The chemical structures of the endogenous sympathomimetic amines dopamine, norepinephrine, and epinephrine. The chemical structure consists of a benzene ring and an ethylamine side chain, with substitutions possible on both. The -OH groups on the benzene ring provide the catecholamine identity. Isoproterenol, a β-selective synthetic catecholamine, has the bulky $CH(CH_3)_2$ amino group substitution. Dobutamine has a further bulky aromatic substitution on the amine group. See ref. 5 for additional details. Reprinted, with permission, from ref. 168.

norepinephrine, and epinephrine, of which the latter two are the primary endogenous catecholamines important in cardiovascular function outside of the central nervous system[5] (Fig. 25.1). Catecholamines communicate with intracellular systems via adrenergic receptors.

The adrenergic receptors were classified by Alquist in 1948 into α and β receptors based on vasoconstrictive and vasodilator responses to different agonists, respectively, with the rank order of potency of agonists (epinephrine ≥ norepinephrine ≫ isoproterenol vs. isoproterenol > epinephrine ≥ norepinephrine, α vs. β, respectively).[6] α-adrenergic receptors are of significance primarily in the peripheral vasculature in human heart failure because they are represented in low density in the human heart[7] and have little if any direct chronotropic or inotropic effect.[8,9] The initial classification of α receptors has taken on considerable complexity, with at least two subtypes of both α_1 and α_2 receptors present in a variety of tissues (see ref. 10 for review). The potential contributions of α-adrenergic receptors in heart failure will not be reviewed further in this chapter, but recent reports and reviews are available.[7,9,11-19]

Lands et al. in 1967 further divided β-adrenergic receptors into cardiac (β_1) and smooth muscle, lung, and other sites (β_2) based on differing agonist rank order of potency.[20,21] These subtypes have remained an extremely useful classification of β-adrenergic receptors, and remain the primary members of the β-adrenergic receptor subfamily. Both receptor subtypes are important in human heart failure and are the subject of this review. The cDNA (complementary DNA, or gene that encodes) for a third human β-adrenergic receptor subtype, termed the β_3-adrenergic receptor, has been identified[22] and exhibits atypical behavior with greater sensitivity to norepinephrine and greater resistance to blockade with propranolol.[23] Its role in cardiac physiology is unknown.

The β-adrenergic receptor molecular and amino acid sequences were identified for the hamster β_2-adrenergic[24] and avian β-adrenergic[25] receptors in 1986, and subsequently the human β_2- and β_1-adrenergic receptors in 1987.[26,27] These receptors are members of the G protein–coupled super family of cell surface receptors.[28] This superfamily takes its name because of the characteristic interaction, or coupling, to G proteins, the guanine nucleotide binding proteins that in turn interact with other intracellular signaling systems such as adenylyl cyclase. The G protein–coupled receptor superfamily is characterized by similar topography, most notably by seven transmembrane spanning domains (Fig. 25.2) This topography has been modeled as helical cylinders[29] (Fig. 25.3) with the agonist binding pocket comprised of the juxtaposition of transmembrane domains, a model based on extensive experiments utilizing site-directed mutagenesis and other methods.[28-30]

Drugs Active at Receptors: Agonists and Antagonists

Agents that interact with receptors can be categorized as agonists or antagonists. An agonist is a drug, hormone, or neurotransmitter that activates a receptor to promote the chemical and physiological changes associated with that receptor.[4] Receptor activation implies specificity of activation and also implies a change in the rate of some physiological process. As such, agonists do not cause de novo effects, but only modulate functions or processes already present, but present at a much

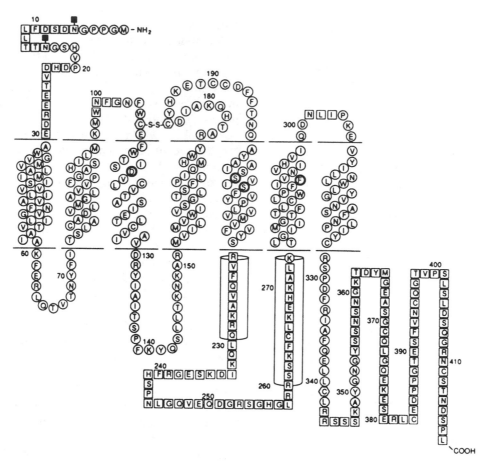

FIGURE 25.2. The primary structure and model for the β-adrenergic receptor. The amino acid sequence has been shown and organized for the seven transmembrane domains. The extracellular surface is at the top of the figure. The Asp113 [aspartic acid (D) position 113] in the third transmembrane region, when replaced with asparagine or glutamine, dramatically affected ligand binding, and probably represents an essential amino acid in the ligand binding pocket (see Fig. 25.3). This aspartic acid is conserved in all other G protein-coupled receptors that bind biogenic amines. Similarly, the serines (S) 204 and 207 in the fifth transmembrane segment, and the phenylalanine (F) 290 in the sixth transmembrane segment, also decreased agonist binding. These residues are shown in bold. Studies such as these form the basis for additional model prediction (Fig. 25.3). The amino acids in squares could be deleted without affecting agonist binding. Reprinted, with permission, from ref. 29.

lower rate.[4] In contrast, antagonists are compounds that interact with receptors to block the action of an agonist—drug, hormone, or neurotransmitter—and by this blocking action antagonists mediate their effects. Antagonists are classified into two general types, competitive and noncompetitive. Competitive antagonists follow mass-action laws and permit drug dissociation with increasing concentration of agonist, whereas noncompetitive antagonists can be thought to bind irreversibly and thereby do not permit receptor activation by agonist even with very high agonist concentrations.[4] One of the fundamental questions of molecular pharmacology is the precise difference in structure of agonists versus antagonists that allow for high affinity binding with activation in the case of agonists versus high affinity binding that does not cause receptor activation in the case of antagonists.

An agonist binds to specific areas of the receptor transmembrane domains (as proposed in Fig. 25.3). This binding causes a change in the receptor conformation to activate G proteins, as reviewed in greater detail below. An antagonist will recognize and bind specifically to the same receptor, but is thought to be unable to cause the required conformational change in receptor structure and hence the intracellular signaling system cannot be activated.

The equilibrium for an inactive versus activated receptor has been illustrated (Fig. 25.4). Three possibilities for drug interaction exist. In the first situation, a drug binds to the receptor but does not affect the basal or resting relationship of active versus inactive receptor. Such an effect would be consistent with an antagonist, because as it binds it blocks the ability of an agonist to occupy and activate that receptor. In the second case,

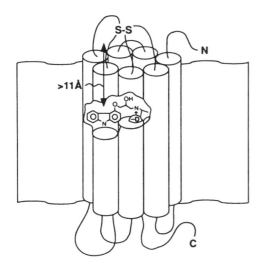

FIGURE 25.3. A model for the three-dimensional structure of the β-adrenergic receptor. The seven transmembrane regions are shown as cylinders, a model based on mutagenesis experiments described in Fig. 25.2. The position of Asp113 in the third transmembrane domain is shown by the "D." See reference for additional details. Reprinted, with permission, from ref. 29.

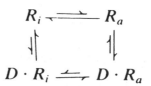

FIGURE 25.4. This is a model of receptor (R) and drug (D) interaction. In this model, the receptor can exist in two conformations, the active (R_a) or the inactive (R_i) states. The inactive and active states are in equilibrium, and the inactive state will predominate when no agonist is present. If a drug binds with a greater affinity for the active conformation, then it will act as an agonist and activate the receptor. In contrast, if the drug has a relatively greater affinity to bind to the inactive state of the receptor, then the receptor will remain relatively more inactive, and the drug functions as an antagonist. The equilibrium between the active and inactive states is a function of the relative affinities of the drug for the active vs. inactive conformations. Furthermore, the degree or extent of activation or inactivation determines the magnitude of effect. A similar argument holds for antagonists. An antagonist is a drug that binds to a receptor and does not alter the resting R_a ↔ Ra_i equilibrium, but its presence and binding to the receptor prevents an agent that could activate the receptor (partial or full agonist) from shifting the equilibrium to the active state. Similarly, an antagonist with a small degree of agonist effect (termed intrinsic sympathomimetic activity, or ISA for β-antagonists—see Fig. 25.5) would tend to push the equilibrium further to the active conformation relative to a full antagonist. Reprinted, with permission, from ref. 4.

another drug binds to the receptor and shifts the equilibrium to the activated state, and thus behaves as an agonist. If the drug promotes complete receptor activation, it would be considered a full agonist. A drug that promotes an intermediate state of receptor activation versus inactivation is called a partial agonist. It should be noted that a partial agonist at higher concentrations occupies receptors to function as an antagonist relative to lower concentrations of a full agonist, because to displace the partial agonist and increase the receptor activation, greater concentrations of full agonist are required. The third situation is primarily theoretical, where a drug actually shifts the receptor inactive/active equilibrium in the resting state even further to the inactive state. Such agents are uncommon, and have been termed inverse agonists or super-antagonists.[4] However, if the basal relationship favors the inactive receptor state, identification and separation of super-antagonists from antagonists can be difficult. Only a few β-blockers of this type have been synthesized, and no super-antagonists are available for clinical use.

These concepts underlie the idea that even though an antagonist is present in patients with heart failure, during times of stress (such as exercise) when catecholamine concentration may increase acutely, the antagonist can be displaced and the β-adrenergic receptor can be activated by agonist, even though an antagonist is present. Additionally, if chronic antagonist exposure can prevent or reverse receptor desensitization and downregulation, then receptor activation during stress can promote more complete receptor pathway activation if

the concentration of receptors is a determinant for overall pathway activation (see Fig. 25.6), later.

The term "intrinsic sympathomimetic activity," or ISA, has been used with increasing frequency in the descriptions of β-adrenergic receptor antagonists. In light of the above description, intrinsic sympathomimetic activity represents an agent with more antagonist properties than agonist, but some properties of each (Fig. 25.5).

Receptor reserve is another important concept to understand the effects of drugs that act via β-adrenergic receptors in patients with heart failure. Simply stated, receptor reserve is present when only a portion of receptors need to be activated by agonist to achieve the maximal effect of that receptor pathway.[31,32] This is in contrast to a system with no receptor reserve, where any loss of receptors will lead to a diminished total pathway activation. In a system with receptor reserve (also termed spare receptors) loss of receptors will tend to shift a dose response curve to the right with no loss of efficacy (maximal effect), whereas with no receptor reserve loss of receptors will not shift a dose response curve but will decrease the maximal effect of the system[31,32] (Fig. 25.6).

The binding affinity of a drug for a receptor and the

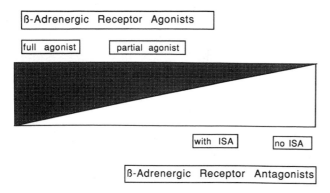

FIGURE 25.5. This figure depicts the relationships of β-adrenergic receptor agonists and antagonists. The dark hatched area to the left represents a full agonist. Partial agonists are those compounds with less than full agonist effects, and are shown as a decrease in the dark-hatched area. β-receptor antagonists are represented by the open area, with a full antagonist represented to the right of the figure. Intrinsic sympathomimetic activity (*ISA*) describes a property of antagonists where some agonist property is present.

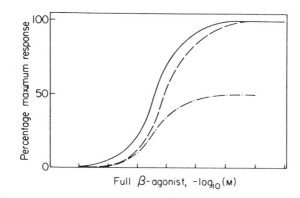

FIGURE 25.6. This is a theoretical dose response curve for activation of a β-receptor pathway. The horizontal axis gives increasing concentration of β-agonist, and the vertical axis gives the percent of maximal pathway response for the receptor. The solid line (—) gives the pathway response (e.g.; contractile response) with 100% of receptors and a full agonist. The dashed curve (--) gives the response of the same receptor system with a competitive antagonist present, which occupies 50% of the receptors. This same curve would be present after loss of 50% of receptors in a system with receptor reserve (spare receptors). In contrast, the stippled curve (—·—·—·) represents the response in a system without receptor reserve where 50% of receptors (and hence 50% of response) has been lost. Reprinted, with permission, from ref. 184.

concentration of drug will determine the fractional receptor occupancy when mass action and equilibrium conditions are met.[4,31,32] Therefore, greater concentrations of drug are necessary to achieve an equivalent receptor occupancy if that drug has a lower binding affinity.

The intrinsic activity or efficacy of a drug is a measure of activation of a receptor signaling system.[4,31,32] For a full agonist, the intrinsic activity or efficacy would be 100% versus a partial response from a partial agonist, or no response (0% efficacy) from an antagonist. The intrinsic activity or efficacy of a drug can be quantitated for any receptor/effector system. However, such a measure of intrinsic activity gives no insight into the structural features of a drug to explain its efficacy. The structural variation within a family of drugs that provides the spectrum of efficacy from agonists to antagonists remains one of the most intensely investigated areas of molecular pharmacology, and includes attempts to understand both drug and receptor secondary and tertiary structures, and the critical receptor binding domains that promote receptor activation.

Signal Transduction: G Proteins and Effector Systems

β-Adrenergic receptors are members of the superfamily of G protein–coupled receptors, which were named because they couple to guanine nucleotide binding proteins, or G proteins.[33–39] The G proteins, in turn, couple the receptor-initiated signal to other intracellular signaling systems, such as adenylyl cyclase for β-adrenergic receptors. The characteristic seven-transmembrane topology of such receptors is undoubtedly essential for G-protein interaction. G proteins can be divided by their action into two major roles—activation or inhibition—of intracellular signaling systems, and two main types of G proteins promote stimulation or inhibition of second messenger systems via G_s or G_i, respectively. Additionally, multiple other related subtypes of G proteins have been identified. β-adrenergic receptors interact with the stimulatory G protein, G_s, which then interacts with the membrane-bound adenylyl cyclase enzyme to catalyze the production of cyclic adenosine monophosphate (cAMP), the intracellular "second messenger" (Fig. 25.7). cAMP interacts with cAMP-dependent protein kinase A (protein kinase A, or PKA). In cardiac tissue, PKA in turn phosphorylates additional intracellular proteins to increase intracellular calcium via several mechanisms to increase the chronotropic and inotropic state of the heart. The β-receptor/G_s complex also has been shown to couple directly to calcium channels in reconstituted systems.[40] However, more recently this coupling was not identified in a more physiologic system.[41]

The G-protein complex is comprised of α, β and γ subunits, which are heterotrimeric proteins made from independent gene products. The β and γ subunits, aside from minor variations, appear to be similar between G-protein complexes, and are approximately 30 kDa and 12 kDa in size. The α subunit is larger and exists in several forms. The stimulatory G protein, αG_s, exists in two forms of 45 and 52 kDa, and the inhibitory G pro-

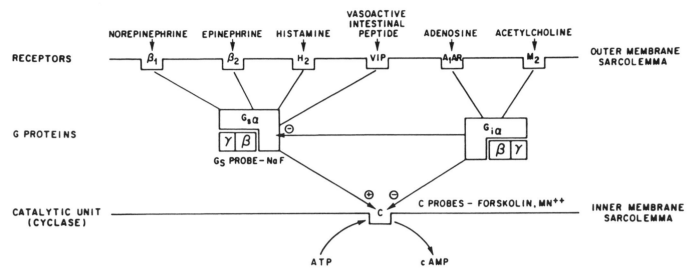

FIGURE 25.7. A schematic representation of the sarcolemmal membrane of human cardiac tissue with several of the receptors, G proteins, and adenylyl cyclase shown. These receptors are characteristic G protein–coupled receptors with seven transmembrane spanning domains (see Figs. 25.2, 25.3). The endogenous agonist is shown above each receptor. The G proteins G_s and G_i are shown, including the α, β, and γ subunits. When stimulatory receptors such as β-adrenergic receptors are activated by binding of agonist, the receptor activates G_s, which in turn activates adenylyl cyclase (C) to catalyze the conversion of ATP to cAMP. cAMP activates cAMP-dependent protein kinase (PKA), which phosphorylates additional intracellular proteins to increase intracellular calcium and increase the inotropic response in cardiac tissue. Not shown in this schematic is direct coupling of G proteins to channels (see text for discussion). Reprinted, with permission, from ref. 1. Copyright 1990 by the American Heart Association.

tein, αG_i, exists in at least three forms, from 39 to 41 kDa. Additional G proteins include two αG_o (other) species of approximately 40 kDa that couple receptors to the inhibition of adenylyl cyclase, and the activation and inhibition of certain ion channels.[33,36] Multiple other αG_x proteins recently have been identified[33,36]; their roles for receptor effector coupling are incompletely characterized. Several extensive reviews are available.[33–39]

Adenylyl cyclase is a membrane-bound enzyme that converts adenosine triphosphate (ATP) to cAMP, the nucleotide intracellular second messenger. The cDNA for adenylyl cyclase recently has been obtained.[42] More recently, multiple forms of adenylyl cyclase have been identified, including types that respond not only to α subunits but also $\beta\gamma$ subunits.[43] The significance of these observations for cardiovascular physiology and pharmacology is unknown at this time. Receptor/G protein/adenylyl cyclase cycling has been proposed as follows. Agonist binding to the β-adrenergic receptor catalyzes the activation of the stimulatory G protein, $G_{s\alpha}$ (Fig. 25.8). The activated (agonist-occupied) receptor catalyzes the dissociation of the guanine nucleotide guanosine diphosphate (GDP) and the association of guanosine triphosphate (GTP) with the G-protein complex. $G_{s\alpha}$.GTP dissociates from the agonist/receptor complex and activates adenylyl cyclase. The intrinsic GTPase activity of $G_{s\alpha}$ eventually degrades the GTP to GDP, which causes dissociation and inactivation of $G_{s\alpha}$, which then reassociates with the $\beta\gamma$ complex. The rate-limiting steps are at the receptor-catalyzed activation when GDP dissociates in favor of GTP association, and when GTP is degraded to GDP.

The stoichiometry of receptor/effector activation has not been clearly established for most receptor systems. The β-adrenergic receptor system probably has been the most intensively investigated for any receptor coupled to adenylyl cyclase. Data obtained in model systems indicate an excess of G protein relative to receptor,[44] with a β-adrenergic receptor able to activate multiple stimulatory G-protein complexes. When measured directly with forskolin binding in the murine S49 cell line, adenylyl cyclase was present at an approximately 10-fold lower concentration than was $G_{s\alpha}$. These preliminary data suggest that after receptors, the adenylyl cyclase enzyme may be the limiting feature of a receptor/G protein/adenylyl cyclase system rather than G proteins.

The preferential coupling of receptor or receptor subtypes to selected subtypes of G proteins has been postulated as a general mechanism to enhance the specificity of receptor signaling systems. This idea is especially attractive to help explain differential coupling of multiple receptor subtypes to various effector systems. In favor of this idea is recent evidence that indicates that two receptors coupled to inhibition of adenylyl cyclase via G_o were coupled specifically and discretely via G_{o1} versus G_{o2}.[45] A great deal of additional complexity and specificity in signaling pathways will likely be identified in the next several years.

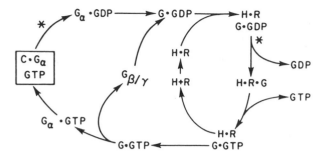

FIGURE 25.8. The receptor/$G_s\alpha$ activation cycle, where the * indicates the rate-limiting steps for the cycle. H is hormone or neurotransmitter, R is receptor, G is G protein, *GTP* is guanosine triphosphate, an endogenous guanine nucleotide whose association with $G_s\alpha$ is necessary for downstream activation of adenylyl cyclase. The endogenous GTPase activity of $G_s\alpha$ hydrolyzes GTP to GDP, of which the $G_s\alpha$/GDP complex then favors dissociation from adenylyl cyclase and reassociation to the β/γ complex, the inactive form of G protein. The presence of hormone or neurotransmitter catalyzes the dissociation of GDP in favor of GTP, the active G protein, and the cycle begins again. Reprinted, with permission, from ref. 1. Copyright 1990 by the American Heart Association.

Mechanisms of Receptor Desensitization

A great deal of progress has been made recently to determine the mechanisms of receptor desensitization. The β-adrenergic receptor/adenylyl cyclase system has been extensively investigated (for reviews see refs 28, 46–50). General mechanisms of desensitization include regulation of cell surface receptor density and regulation of receptor/G protein interaction. Homologous desensitization of a receptor occurs when exposed to its agonist. Receptor density regulation appears to be controlled by changes in the receptor degradation rate and in posttranslational regulation of receptor expression.[28,51,53]

In the β-adrenergic receptor/adenylyl cyclase system, agonist-induced desensitization results from three general processes, which include uncoupling, sequestration, and downregulation. Uncoupling occurs rapidly over seconds to minutes, and is accomplished by receptor phosphorylation by at least two receptor kinases, cAMP-dependent PKA and the β-adrenergic receptor kinase (βARK).[28,51,54,55] Receptor sequestration also is a rapid, agonist-dependent process, but it is unclear whether the receptor is physically internalized away from the cell membrane or continues to reside in the membrane but is unable to recognize agonist secondary to conformational change.[28] The precise mechanism of receptor sequestration is not known.[56]

Downregulation is the third general mechanism of receptor desensitization.[54] Downregulation is defined as loss of receptor binding sites anywhere in the cell and results in diminished signal transduction. In contrast to uncoupling and sequestration, this process occurs over minutes to hours, and is clinically relevant for the use of β-adrenergic receptor agonists. Data from experimental systems indicate that agonist-induced β-adrenergic receptor downregulation occurs from two general mechanisms. First, receptor synthesis is decreased as receptor messenger RNA stability is diminished, a form of post-translational control.[51–53] It has been postulated that control of receptor messenger RNA stability may reside in the 3' untranslated region of the receptor gene[54]; however, specific mechanisms have not been clearly defined.[54] The production of receptor mRNA (control at the level of transcription) plays little if any role in the downregulation of receptor density, at least in carefully studied experimental systems, except for upregulation in experimental systems where β-adrenergic receptor transcriptional rate could be increased over hours with hormonal therapy.[57] Also, more recently β-adrenergic receptor agonists have been shown to increase transcriptional rate in the initial seconds to few minutes of agonist stimulation,[58] but this agonist-induced effect appears to be transient.[54,59] The second mechanism of receptor downregulation is related to increased receptor degradation. The mechanisms of the increased rate of receptor degradation are not well understood, but may result from receptor phosphorylation by PKA or possibly by other cAMP-independent mechanisms.[28,51,52]

Cardiovascular Pharmacology of β-Adrenergic Receptors

The sympathetic nervous system in heart failure has been reviewed elsewhere in this book. Activation of the sympathetic nervous system in heart failure has a broad range of hemodynamic and metabolic effects. One principal effect observed is that of increased peripheral catecholamine release, among other neurotransmitters. The effects of the sympathetic nervous system on β-adrenergic receptors are mediated via the endogenous catecholamines norepinephrine and epinephrine. Norepinephrine resides in the nerve terminals of sympathetic neurons of the autonomic nervous system, and epinephrine outside of the central nervous system is synthesized and released from the adrenal gland. Dopamine, another endogenous sympathomimetic amine found predominantly in the central nervous system, exerts its direct effects via dopamine receptor activation. The cardiovascular effects of peripheral or exogenously administered dopamine result from its ability to stimulate norepinephrine release from sympathetic nerves. The action of a neurotransmitter to stimulate release of a second neurotransmitter to cause a physiological effect is termed an indirect effect.[60–62] The direct effects of dopamine at β_1-adrenergic receptors are as a weak partial agonist.[60-62] Both epinephrine and norepinephrine are direct agonists at α- and β_1-adrenergic receptors; epinephrine is a full agonist at β_2-adrenergic receptors whereas norepinephrine is a weaker β_2 agonist.[5]

In the heart failure condition, endogenous catecholamines activate adrenergic receptors in several tissues, including β-adrenergic receptors in the kidney, to stimulate increased renin release, and α-adrenergic receptors in the peripheral vasculature to cause vasoconstriction. Endogenous catecholamines also activate cardiac β-adrenergic receptors, which increase heart rate and contractility and cause other potentially adverse cardiac effects such as arrhythmias.

The physiological effects of norepinephrine and epinephrine on the heart include inotropic, chronotropic, and lusitropic effects.[5] Both β_1- and β_2-adrenergic receptors are coupled to contraction in human ventricular myocardium, as reviewed in detail below. Additionally, both β_1- and β_2-adrenergic receptors are coupled to chronotropic responsiveness, with greater chronotropic responsiveness from β_2 receptors.[63,64] Although epinephrine and norepinephrine are agonists at both α- and β-adrenergic receptors, α-adrenergic receptors probably play little or no role for inotropic control in human heart.[7,8] α-adrenergic receptor-mediated contractile responses were absent when human ventricular myocardium was examined directly.[9] Human ventricular myocardium, unlike that of smaller animal species, is functionally a β-adrenergic organ, with 75% to 80% of β-adrenergic receptors β_1 subtype (approximately 75 fmol/mg protein) and 20% to 25% (approximately 20 fmol/mg protein) of β_2 subtype in nonfailing ventricle (Fig. 25.9). In contrast, α-adrenergic receptors are present in much lower concentration in human ventricular myocardium of approximately 12 to 15 fmol/mg protein.[7] This is in marked contrast to rat heart, which has approximately a two fold greater concentration of α-adrenergic receptors compared to β-adrenergic receptors.[65,66]

Direct pharmacologic studies have shown that norepinephrine has an approximately 10-fold greater affinity for the human cardiac β_1-adrenergic receptor than the β_2-adrenergic receptor.[7,65] As such, the β_1-adrenergic receptor can be functionally considered a norepinephrine receptor. Previous studies have indicated that the β_1-adrenergic receptor resides in proximity to sympathetic neurons where the local concentrations of norepinephrine may be increased in the synaptic cleft.[67] In contrast, the β_2-adrenergic receptor is an epinephrine-preferring receptor, and the β_2-adrenergic receptor appears to be situated independent of sympathetic nerve terminals. As epinephrine is a circulating hormone, the epinephrine-preferring β_2-adrenergic receptor may be more responsive to circulating catecholamines.

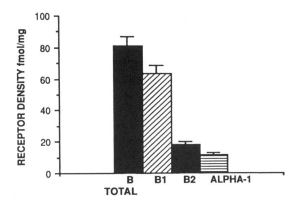

FIGURE 25.9. Total β-, β_1-, β_2-, and α_1-adrenergic receptor densities in membranes prepared from 18 nonfailing human left ventricles. Reprinted, with permission, from ref. 1. Copyright 1990 by the American Heart Association.

β-Adrenergic Receptor Pathways in Human Heart Failure

The most important observation of β-adrenergic receptor physiology seen in patients with end-stage heart failure is the markedly subsensitive inotropic response of ventricular myocardium to β-adrenergic receptor agonists. Cardiac catecholamine subsensitivity has been observed in a variety of experiments with whole animal or cardiac preparations over the past three decades, but until recently data from failing human heart were not available. The implications for this observation regarding the more fundamental causes of heart failure are still incompletely understood, as discussed in the β-blocker section below. However, the observation of β-agonist subsensitivity has important implications for heart failure treatment strategies.

Subsensitive Inotropic Response to β-Agonists: Ex Vivo Experiments

The first direct (ex vivo) demonstration of diminished inotropic response to β-adrenergic receptor agonists in failing human ventricular myocardium was in 1982.[68] These experiments were made possible by the availability of fresh, functional cardiac tissue at the Stanford University heart transplant program. In myocardium obtained from end-stage failing hearts removed from patients undergoing cardiac transplantation, Bristow and colleagues exposed right and left ventricular trabeculae in tissue bath to isoproterenol, and observed that the contractile response was substantially reduced compared to trabeculae removed from nonfailing control hearts.[68]

The β-agonist subsensitivity in failing heart was associated with a decrease in β-adrenergic receptor density.[68] In crude membrane preparations taken from the ventricles of patients with end-stage heart failure primarily from idiopathic dilated cardiomyopathy (IDC), β-adrenergic receptor density was diminished by approximately 50% when compared to nonfailing ventricles. This decrease in β-adrenergic receptor density in failing versus nonfailing heart was present whether receptor density was normalized to membrane protein concentrations, to quantity of whole heart used for preparations, or to the quantity of myosin, a measure of contractile proteins.

The physiological and functional evaluation of receptor down- (or up-) regulation in any experimental system requires complete knowledge of the entire pathway to understand the potential physiological effects of the receptor changes. In the case of the superfamily of G protein–coupled receptors, which are coupled to activation of adenylyl cyclase, regulation at the receptor, G-protein, or catalytic unit of adenylyl cyclase could be present. Additionally, it is also possible that pathway regulation could occur distal to adenylyl cyclase, including at the level of cAMP-dependent phosphodiesterase, the cAMP-dependent PKA, or one of several additional points beyond this, including a change in quantity or sensitivity of calcium available at the contractile apparatus.

To determine if the decrease in β-adrenergic receptor density was related to the diminished inotropic responses identified in failing human heart in tissue bath, the β-adrenergic receptor pathway was examined more carefully in vitro by measuring the increase in adenylyl cyclase activity with β-adrenergic receptor activation.[68] If the β-adrenergic receptor pathway in human heart had receptor reserve, a common finding in some receptor/effector systems where only a fraction of receptors are needed to activate fully the effector pathway, then a 50% reduction in β-adrenergic receptor density may not have been the cause of the decreased response to isoproterenol. However, in failing heart, adenylyl cyclase activation was decreased with isoproterenol. Several points regarding this system deserve comment. First, the β_1- versus β_2-adrenergic receptor coupling to adenylyl cyclase (discussed in the following section) was not examined in this initial report. Second, in this initial examination, function of stimulatory G proteins and catalytic adenylyl cyclase did not appear to be altered in heart failure.[68] That is, the stimulation in failing and nonfailing heart by one other $G_{s\alpha}$-coupled receptor, the H_2-histamine receptor, was not different and fluoride, a direct activator of $G_{s\alpha}$, gave similar adenylyl cyclase responses in failing and nonfailing heart. Multiple additional examinations have substantiated these initial observations and are summarized below. To rule out a difference beyond the receptor/adenylyl cyclase complex at the contractile apparatus, the contraction responses of failing and nonfailing ventricular myocardium to a saturating concentration of calcium were examined.[69] Calcium added to ventricular myocardium in a tissue bath at pharmacologic concentrations will act beyond the receptor/adenylyl cyclase complex at the contractile apparatus to provide a more direct measure of contractile unit function. No difference was present in the contractile responses to calcium of nonfailing and failing trabeculae. These data suggested that, at least for the maximal developed force response, the contractile apparatus was not different in failing heart compared to nonfailing heart. Together, these data indicated that the decreased density of β-adrenergic receptors was related to the β-adrenergic agonist subsensitivity in patients with heart failure.

β_1- and β_2-Adrenergic Receptor Subtypes in Human Ventricular Myocardium

Evaluation of β_1- versus β_2-adrenergic receptor regulation was the next question to be addressed. In 1982, β-adrenergic receptor subtypes were examined initially in nonfailing human atria, and β_1- and β_2-adrenergic receptor fractions were found to be similar.[70] In contrast, in ventricular tissue from autopsy specimens β_1/β_2-adrenergic receptor fractions in atria and ventricles were .74/.26 and .86/.14, respectively.[71] Additional questions regarding β-adrenergic receptor coupling[72–74] and G-protein function[73,75] also have been investigated, and more definitive tissue bath experiments with calcium and other agents that act beyond the receptor were performed. This initial work ex vivo also stimulated in vivo experiments that evaluated more directly the inotropic responses to β-adrenergic agonists in patients with heart failure.

In 1986, Bristow and colleagues reported that the diminished β-adrenergic receptor density observed in failing ventricular myocardium resulted from a reduction in β_1-adrenergic receptor density, with no change in β_2-adrenergic receptor density.[74] The studies were performed with cardiac tissue removed from the ventricles of 12 patients with IDC undergoing cardiac transplantation for end-stage heart failure. In nonfailing ventricular myocardium removed from 12 control ventricles, β_1-adrenergic receptor density accounted for approximately 80% of total β-adrenergic receptors, whereas β_2-adrenergic receptors accounted for approximately 20%. Total β-adrenergic receptor density in left ventricular myocardium was 88 versus 43 fmol/mg, nonfailing versus failing. The β-adrenergic receptor subtype percentage changed from approximately 80:20 to 60:40, β_1:β_2 respectively.[74] In failing ventricular myocardium, β_1-adrenergic receptor density was decreased from approximately 67 to 26 fmol/mg, with no statistically significant change in β_2-adrenergic receptor density (21 vs. 17 fmol/mg).

Similar cardiac β-adrenergic receptor subtype changes from a larger series of heart failure patients are

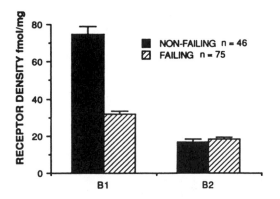

FIGURE 25.10. β_1- and β_2-adrenergic subtype densities in membranes prepared from failing and nonfailing human left and right ventricles. Values are ±SEM, with $p < .0001$ for β_1, and $p = \text{NS}$ for β_2. Reprinted, with permission, from ref. 1. Copyright 1990 by the American Heart Association.

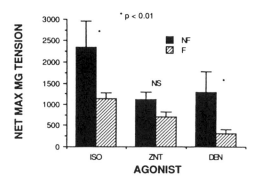

FIGURE 25.11. Contractile responses of nonfailing (NF) or failing (F) right ventricular trabeculae in tissue bath are shown to the nonselective agonist isoproterenol (ISO), or the β_2-agonist zinterol (ZNT), and the β_1-agonist denopamine (DEN). The marked subsensitivity of the denopamine response is consistent with the substantial downregulation of the β_1-adrenergic receptor (see Fig. 25.10). The responses shown are maximal responses less basal responses. Reprinted, with permission, from ref. 1. Copyright 1990 by the American Heart Association.

shown graphically (Fig. 25.10). To determine if the diminished β_1-adrenergic receptor density was associated with a functional defect in the β_1-adrenergic receptor pathway, the contractile responses of failing and nonfailing ventricular myocardium were examined in tissue bath with β_1- and β_2-adrenergic selective agonists.[74] As previously observed,[68] the contractile responses again were diminished with the nonselective β-adrenergic receptor agonist isoproterenol. Consistent with diminished β_1-adrenergic receptor density, contractile responses to the highly selective β_1 agonist denopamine also were reduced markedly by more than 90% of the control nonfailing responses, consistent with a weak β_1-adrenergic partial agonist in a markedly downregulated system[74] (Fig. 25.11). The responses to the β_2-adrenergic selective agonist zinterol also were decreased approximately 30%, a nonstatistically significant decrease (Fig. 25.11). These data indicated that the β_1-adrenergic receptor that stimulated contraction was markedly subsensitive to nonselective and β_1-adrenergic selective agonists in failing heart, and that the β_2-adrenergic receptor pathway was mildly uncoupled from contraction.[74]

Further investigation of the β_1- and β_2-adrenergic receptor coupling to adenylyl cyclase demonstrated that the β_2-adrenergic receptor is coupled more tightly compared to the β_1-adrenergic receptor[73] and most of the decrease in the adenylyl cyclase activity in preparations of failing human heart is related to "uncoupling" of the β_2-adrenergic receptor.[73]

Subsensitive Inotropic Responses to β_2-Adrenergic Agonists: In Vivo Experiments

The next series of experiments was performed in patients and was reported in 1986.[76] These experiments evaluated the degree of heart failure and the degree of

β-agonist subsensitivity relative to β-adrenergic receptor downregulation. Two groups of patients with mild to moderate or severe heart failure secondary to IDC were compared to a third group with no heart failure. β-adrenergic receptor density was measured in right ventricular endomyocardium from milligram quantities of tissue removed at right ventricular cardiac biopsy. In this patient population with IDC, similar degrees of right and left ventricular failure were present. The β-adrenergic receptor pathway was evaluated by measuring the inotropic response to increasing concentrations of intravenously infused dobutamine, a β-adrenergic receptor agonist. A micromanometer-tipped catheter was placed into the left ventricle and dp/dt was measured to indicate changes in ventricular contractility. β-adrenergic receptor densities were evaluated in three patient groups: Group I with normal cardiac function, and Groups II and III with mild to moderate and severe heart failure, respectively (Fig. 25.12). Group I consisted of seven patients with normal hemodynamics and a mean ejection fraction of .59; Group II consisted of 10 patients with a mean pulmonary artery wedge pressure of 12 mm Hg, a cardiac index of 2.4 L/min/m², and a mean ejection fraction of .38; and Group III consisted of 19 patients with a right atrial pressure of 11 mm Hg, a mean pulmonary artery wedge pressure of 25 mm Hg, a cardiac index of 2.1 L/min/m², and a mean ejection fraction of .17. β-adrenergic receptor density was decreased with increasing severity of heart failure, regardless of the methods to normalize receptor density. Nonfailing heart contained 147 fmol/mg β receptors, with values of 92 fmol/mg and 69 fmol/mg in Groups II and III, respectively, values that were 63% and 47% of control, respectively. For the functional evaluation with

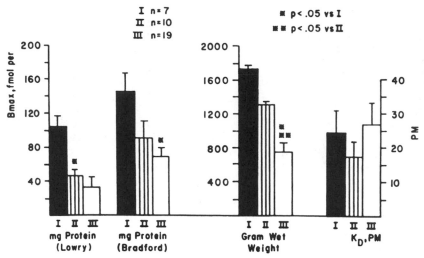

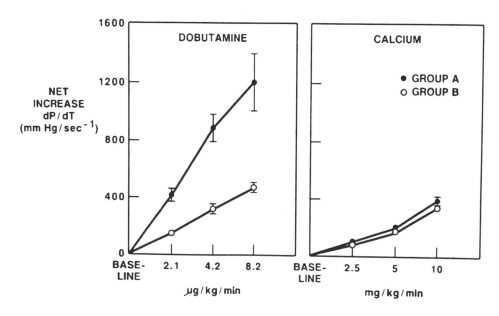

FIGURE 25.12. Progressive downregulation of myocardial β-adrenergic receptor density with progressive heart failure. β-adrenergic receptor densities were measured from right ventricular endomyocardial biopsies from three groups of patients, Group I subjects with no heart failure and left ventricular ejection fractions >0.50, Group II subjects with mild to moderate cardiac dysfunction and LV ejection fractions 0.25 to 0.50, and Group III subjects with severe ventricular dysfunction and LV ejection fractions <0.25. Receptor densities were measured by ^{125}iodocyanopindolol (*ICYP*) radioli-

gand binding methods, and maximal receptor binding (B$_{max}$) normalized to three different measurements. Receptors were normalized to protein concentrations by two methods (Lowry, Bradford), and the third normalization was to tissue weight, a direct measurement of endomyocardial biopsy specimen weight. All three normalizations gave similar results between groups. The ICYP binding dissociation constant (K$_D$) was not different between groups. Reprinted, with permission, from ref. 76. Copyright 1986 by the American Heart Association.

dobutamine infusion, patients were divided into two groups: those with ejection fractions (EF) >0.40 and <0.30. With dobutamine, the net increase in dp/dt in the EF >0.40 group was substantially greater than in the EF >0.30 group (Fig. 25.13). Although no load-independent measure of dp/dt was obtained, the small hemodynamic changes observed would be unlikely to explain the substantial differences in dp/dt observed be-

tween these groups. The inotropic reserve of the contractile apparatus was evaluated with a calcium gluconate infusion, a direct inotrope independent of receptor activation or cAMP levels. The change in dp/dt with calcium infusion was similar in both groups (Fig. 25.13), which indicated that at least pharmacologically for the development of dp/dt, the contractile reserve in failing heart was similar to that of nonfailing heart. Taken

FIGURE 25.13. Net increase in the peak positive dp/dt in two groups of heart failure patients to dobutamine infusion of 2.1, 4.2, and 8.2 μg/kg/min in the left panel, and during calcium gluconate infusion of 2.5, 5, and 10 mg/kg/min in the right panel; group A (*solid circles*) had ejection fractions >0.40, and group B had ejection fractions <0.30. Reprinted, with permission, from ref. 76. Copyright 1986 by the American Heart Association.

together, these data indicated that the diminished β-adrenergic receptor density was progressive with advancing heart failure, and that the inotropic response to β agonists also was diminished in heart failure patients. Additionally, when taken with the β-adrenergic receptor density data,[74] these observations indicated that the catecholamine subsensitivity was related to downregulation of the β_1-adrenergic receptor.

In a study designed specifically to examine the tissue bath contractile responses of failing versus nonfailing human ventricular myocardium, Feldman and co-workers[77] demonstrated that peak isometric tension generated when calcium was added to the failing heart in tissue bath was similar to control, nonfailing tissue (Fig. 25.14). Although the time course of contraction and the rate of relaxation were markedly prolonged in the failing tissue, observations that suggest that calcium handling may be abnormal in myocardium from heart failure patients (see ref. 78 for review), the maximal isometric tension was unchanged. This observation substantiated the conclusion that no obvious or large intrinsic defect for overall force development was present at the contractile apparatus in failing ventricular myocardium. Additionally, using the diterpene agent forskolin, a direct activator of adenylyl cyclase and therefore independent of receptor activation and acetylstrophanthidin, a cardiotonic steroid that increases contraction by

mechanisms unrelated to adenylyl cyclase activation, these investigators again observed that failing heart could generate overall maximal tension responses not different from nonfailing tissue (Fig. 25.15). In additional experiments, the use of phosphodiesterase inhibitors milrinone, caffeine, and isomethylbutylxanthine were minimally effective when used as individual agents. However, with a minimally effective concentration of forskolin present to activate adenylyl cyclase directly and increase cAMP production, the contraction responses exceeded nonfailing control responses. Taken together, these experiments confirmed that deficient production of cAMP was related to a defective receptor or receptor/G protein/adenylyl cyclase coupling.[77] Additional data have confirmed that the overall magnitude of calcium responses in tissue bath are similar in failing and nonfailing heart.[79,80] Finally, the idea that β-agonists combined with phosphodiesterase inhibition may give additive inotropic effects had been proposed in preliminary reports, but this was the first functional demonstration in isolated human cardiac tissue.[77] Similar experiments in vivo have demonstrated the additive effects of dobutamine and amrinone in patients with severe heart failure.[81]

The definitive experiment that demonstrated inotropic subsensitivity with β-agonists in the failing human heart in vivo was performed by Colucci and co-workers.[82,83] To avoid systemic effects that might change loading conditions, dobutamine was infused directly into the left main coronary artery of patients with normal cardiac function or with advanced heart failure. Left ventricular dp/dt was measured with a micromanometer-tipped catheter placed into the left ventricle, and a dobutamine dose response curve was performed for each patient. Eight patients with no heart failure and with normal cardiac function served as controls. The heart failure groups consisted of 8 patients with IDC, and 16 with ischemic cardiomyopathy, with EFS of 0.15 and 0.31 for the two etiologies, respectively. All heart failure patients were New York Heart Association (NYHA) Class III–IV. Dobutamine dose response curves were markedly subsensitive in heart failure patients and gave approximately 60% of the response observed in nonfailing control patients, even though the maximal dobutamine infusion rate was 4 times higher (Fig. 25.16). The dose response curve (Fig. 25.16) suggested a near maximal response in heart failure patients, as the top of the curve tended to approach a plateau. In contrast, even though a substantially greater effect was seen in nonfailing patients with a fourfold lower dobutamine infusion rate, there was little indication that the top of the dose response curve was achieved. The dose response curve was abbreviated to the 50 μg/min infusion rate in patients with normal hearts secondary to palpitations and other minor adverse events. The systemic effects of the dobutamine

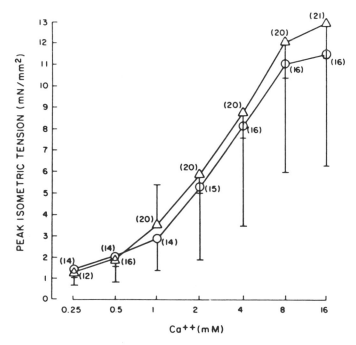

FIGURE 25.14. The contractile responses to increasing concentrations of calcium for trabeculae removed from control (*open circles*) and failing (*open triangles*) hearts. The number of trabeculae are given at each concentration, and data are ±SEM. Reprinted, with permission, from ref. 77. Copyright 1987 by the American Heart Association.

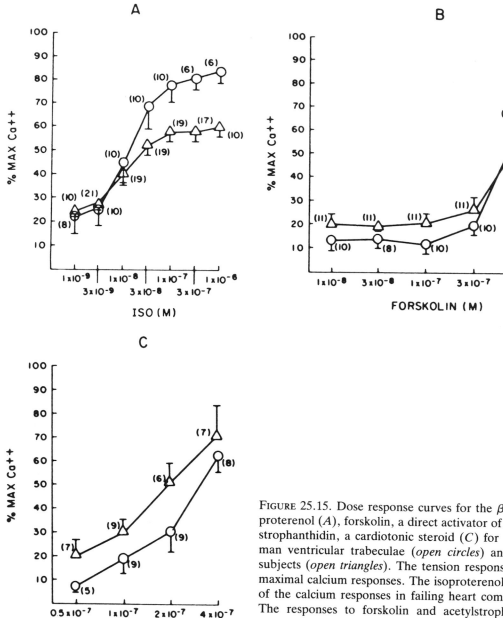

FIGURE 25.15. Dose response curves for the β-adrenergic receptor agonist iso-proterenol (*A*), forskolin, a direct activator of adenylyl cyclase (*B*), and acetyl-strophanthidin, a cardiotonic steroid (*C*) for tension responses in control human ventricular trabeculae (*open circles*) and trabeculae from heart failure subjects (*open triangles*). The tension responses were expressed as percent of maximal calcium responses. The isoproterenol responses were reduced to 60% of the calcium responses in failing heart compared to 85% in control hearts. The responses to forskolin and acetylstrophanthidin were similar in both groups. Reprinted, with permission, from ref. 77. Copyright by the American Heart Association.

infusion were minimal, and the method was essentially load-independent. In summary, this study definitively demonstrated β-adrenergic receptor pathway inotropic subsensitivity in patients with moderately severe to severe heart failure.[82]

In summary, both in vivo experiments and tissue bath experiments from multiple laboratories have conclusively demonstrated β-agonist inotropic subsensitivity in the failing human heart. Although the precise mechanism or inciting circumstances that lead to this β-agonist subsensitivity are still not clear, it is apparent that the reduced inotropic response to β-agonists is one of the most important fundamental defects of the heart failure

condition. The above experiments have demonstrated that the chronically failing human heart is subsensitive to β-agonists, and the markedly downregulated β_1-adrenergic receptor is one likely explanation for this subsensitivity.

Are Mechanisms in Addition to Decreased β_1 Receptor Density Present to Explain the Subsensitive Inotropic Response to β-Agonists in the Chronically Failing Human Heart?

In a pharmacological system with no receptor reserve, downregulation of a receptor by 50% is sufficient to ex-

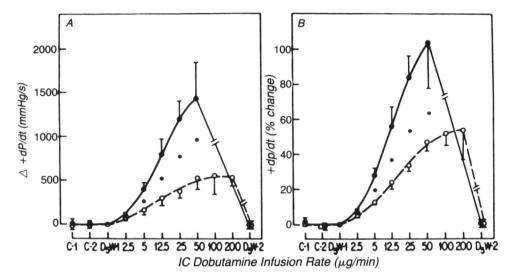

FIGURE 25.16. The dose response curves for intracoronary dobutamine are shown for left ventricular dp/dt in patients without (*closed circles*) and with (*open circles*) heart failure. Panel A gives the change in dp/dt, and panel B expresses the same data from panel A as a percent increase over the dp/dt measured at baseline. Baseline dp/dt measurements were 1445 ± 87 and 886 ± 97 mm Hg/s in control and heart failure patients, respectively. The asterisks indicate $p < .01$ for control vs. heart failure dose responsiveness. Reprinted, with permission, from ref. 82.

plain a subsensitivity response of approximately 50%. For the subsensitivity response to β agonists in the failing human heart, the downregulation of the β_1-adrenergic receptor is sufficient to explain the diminished responses to β agonists. However, until recently, formal experiments had not been performed in human cardiac tissue to evaluate for the presence of β-adrenergic receptor reserve. It is possible that other conditions could affect the β-adrenergic receptor transduction pathway in addition to the observed downregulation of the β_1 receptor, such as receptor uncoupling from a variety of posttranslational modifications or altered states of the G proteins that couple β-adrenergic receptors to adenylyl cyclase. Additionally, if receptor reserve would be present for the β-adrenergic receptor pathways, then the diminished inotropic responses could be related to factors other than the decreased receptor density.

The usual approach to evaluate for receptor reserve is to label receptors of interest with a noncompetitive antagonist that binds irreversibly. By using several increasing concentrations of irreversible antagonist, greater percentages of the receptor population can be functionally inactivated. The percentage of remaining receptors can be quantitated by radioligand binding, and the activation of the effector pathway can be evaluated for this remaining receptor population. In the case of no receptor reserve, a 50% reduction in receptor density should give a 50% reduction in pathway activation. In contrast, with a fivefold receptor reserve, more than 80% of receptors would need to be inactivated by a noncompetitive antagonist before a decrement in receptor/effector activation would be observed.

However, with loss of receptors in a system with receptor reserve, the dose response curve will tend to shift to the right (see Fig. 25.6).

Evaluation of β-adrenergic receptor reserve in human ventricular myocardium is complicated by the presence of two receptor subtypes, β_1 and β_2 which have differential coupling of each receptor subtype with the β_2-adrenergic receptor subtype much more "tightly" coupled to adenylyl cyclase activation.[73] However, with the irreversible antagonist bromoacetylalprenolol (BAAM), preliminary data indicate that no detectable receptor reserve is present for β-adrenergic receptors in human ventricular myocardium.[84] Indirect evidence also supports this, where functional dose response curves to β-agonist either in membrane preparations for adenylyl cyclase activation[73] or in patients[82] have not indicated that dose response curves are right-shifted with diminished maximal effect (see Figs. 25.6, 25.15, 25.16).

The β_2-adrenergic receptor is unchanged in density in the failing human heart,[1,74] although the adenylyl cyclase data and the muscle contraction data from tissue bath studies indicate that some mild uncoupling has occurred.[1,74] Because the magnitude of the β_2-adrenergic receptor-coupled response is relatively low, the decrease in contraction in tissue bath has not been statistically significant, although it is in general agreement with an approximate 30% reduction in adenylyl cyclase activation.[73] The magnitude of reduction for both contraction and adenylyl cyclase activation is still much less than for the β_1-adrenergic receptor. Because β_2-adrenergic receptor density has not changed, the mechanism for this uncoupling is not clear. It is possible that the β_2-adrenergic receptor has undergone some posttranslational modification in the heart failure condition. An alternative explanation is a change in quantity or function of the G protein that couples to the β_2-adrenergic receptor in the heart failure condition. As summarized in greater detail below, no quantitative or qualitative changes in αG_s have been detected in myocardium from heart failure patients, but αG_i was increased approximately 35%. It is plausible to associate the uncoupled β_2-adrenergic receptor with the increase in αG_i,[74] but no direct experimental data are available to support this contention.

G Proteins in Failing Ventricular Myocardium

The role of G proteins in failing and nonfailing human ventricular myocardium has been examined carefully[75,85,86] and has been reviewed recently.[34,38,39] In short, αG_i is increased in failing ventricular myocardium by approximately 35% when measured by ADP-ribosylation, with similar degrees of increase in both idiopathic and ischemic cardiomyopathy.[87] In contrast, αG_s is not changed in quantity. Adenylyl cyclase responses with in vitro experimental conditions designed to evaluate G-protein function are consistent with increased inhibitory G protein and no change in the stimulatory G protein.[75,87] αG_i exists in three major forms, denoted αG_{i1}, αG_{i2} and αG_{i3}, of which the latter is the predominant type of inhibitory G protein in human ventricular myocardium.[88] Receptors coupled to inhibition of adenylyl cyclase are present in human ventricular myocardium, and include the A_1 adenosine receptor[89-91] and the M_2 muscarinic,[92-94] neither of which has been shown to have enhanced coupling to adenylyl cyclase inhibition[89,92] or to increased negative inotropic responses in tissue bath.[90-92,94] The functional significance for inotropic control in failing heart of this increased αG_i is not known.

The β-Adrenergic Receptor/G Protein/Adenylyl Cyclase System in Ischemic Cardiomyopathy

Recent data indicate that the β-adrenergic receptor downregulation may have subtle but important differences in ischemic cardiomyopathy from that observed in the myocardium of patients with IDC,[87] and as discussed below in the section on β-blocker use in patients with heart failure, these differences may be important for treatment outcome.

In general, the overall findings of the β-adrenergic receptor system in patients with ischemic cardiomyopathy were similar to those of IDC.[87] Total β-adrenergic receptor density was decreased secondary to a decrease in β_1-adrenergic receptor density, and β_2-adrenergic receptor density was not changed. However, the magnitude of β_1-adrenergic receptor downregulation was less

in ischemic cardiomyopathy. In an overall analysis of combined right and left ventricles, total β-adrenergic receptor density was 28% greater with ischemic etiology compared to idiopathic (74.0 ± 47 vs. 49.1 ± 1.9 vs. 63.4 ± 2.9; 7 nonfailing patients, 14 chambers vs. 26 IDC patients, 52 chambers, vs. 28 ischemic cardiomyopathic subjects, 55 chambers, respectively, all in fmol/mg protein). Similar to the idiopathic group, the downregulation of β-adrenergic receptors was secondary to loss of only β_1-adrenergic receptors, with no change in β_2-adrenergic receptor density; however, the degree of β_1-adrenergic receptor downregulation was less with ischemic than with idiopathic etiology (54.8 ± 4.5 vs. 32.2 ± 1.7 vs. 42.0 ± 2.5, in the same numbers of patients nonfailing vs. idiopathic vs. ischemic patients, respectively, all in fmol/mg protein).

G-protein content and function, at least as measured by toxin-catalyzed ADP-ribosylation and post–receptor-stimulated adenylyl cyclase activities, indicate similar findings in ventricular myocardium from patients with idiopathic and ischemic cardiomyopathy: G_i is increased in both etiologies by the same degree, with no significant change in G_s.[87]

Responses to β-adrenergic receptor stimulation, whether examined by muscle contraction or by adenylyl cyclase, were subsensitive with both etiologies, but even though β_1-adrenergic receptors demonstrated less downregulation with ischemic etiology, the degree of β-adrenergic receptor uncoupling was greater.[87] The reason for this relatively greater uncoupling of β_1-adrenergic receptors in ischemic cardiomyopathy was not clear, but could reside in the G-protein coupling unit or some other as yet undefined difference. Additionally, even though the degree of sympathetic neurotransmitter depletion was similar in idiopathic and ischemic groups, sympathetic denervation of noninfarcted muscle is known to occur after myocardial infarction.[95] It is possible that the decrease in sympathetic neurotransmitters may be related to denervation rather than to the heart failure condition itself, as seen with the idiopathic etiology. This contention is supported by the lack of association between the β_1-adrenergic receptor downregulation in ischemic etiology and tissue norepinephrine even though this relationship was highly significant with idiopathic etiology.[87] It is possible that other features of the ischemic cardiomyopathy etiology may have contributed to the observed differences, such as chronic low grade ischemia of ventricular myocardium that may be responsible for the greater degree of β_1 receptor uncoupling.

Subsensitive Chronotropic Responses to β Agonists

The exercise physiology of heart failure patients has been described elsewhere and will not be reviewed in this chapter. However, the blunted heart rate response, at least in part, appears to be related to desensitization of an atrial β-adrenergic receptor pathway coupled to chronotropic control. In a study with age-matched non-failing control patients and patients with differing degrees of heart failure, the heart rate response to exercise was reduced even though in these experiments circulating norepinephrine was significantly increased.[96] Additionally, the heart rate responses from increasing concentrations of infused isoproterenol gave markedly blunted responses in heart failure patients.

Peripheral Vascular Responses to β Agonists

In contrast to the blunted chronotropic responses identified in heart failure patients, the peripheral vasodilatory effects of β-agonists were not changed in heart failure patients.[97] The forearm vasodilatation potential with nitroprusside and with isoproterenol was preserved, which indicated that B-adrenergic receptor desensitization did not occur in the limb vessels of heart failure patients.

Clinical Approaches to Heart Failure Management: β-Adrenergic Receptor-Active Agents

Heart failure encompasses a range of impaired cardiac function from multiple etiologies. The use of β-adrenergic receptor agents in heart failure, either agon-

ists or antagonists, must take into account the nature and extent of cardiac dysfunction. For this discussion, heart failure will be divided into two general categories: moderate and severe (advanced) heart failure (Fig. 25.17).

The only consensus for the appropriate use of any β-adrenergic receptor agent (agonist or antagonist) would be that of an infused β agonist such as dobutamine for acute circulatory support of the patient with advanced heart failure (Fig. 25.17), especially in those settings where β-agonist infusions may constitute a short- or intermediate-term medical bridge to cardiac transplantation. With advanced heart failure, β agonists may be used in concert with phosphodiesterase inhibitors, a treatment approach that may be pharmacologically[98] and clinically[81,82,98,99] additive to the effects of β-agonists. Most of these patients will be hospitalized, and many will be in intensive care units for invasive hemodynamic monitoring. In this setting, many patients will have continuous electrocardiographic monitoring, which enhances the safety profile of intravenous β agonists by reducing the risk of unattended life-threatening arrhythmias. Also, some patients with advanced heart failure who are not candidates for cardiac transplantation may require intermittent β-agonist infusions at some point in their clinical course to provide acute symptomatic relief from congestive and low-output states. Such intermittent use has been associated with prolonged benefit that may last for days or weeks,[100] although the mechanisms of this prolonged benefit are not well understood.[101] Additionally, the skillful use of

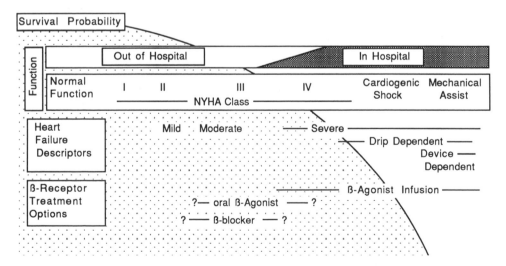

FIGURE 25.17. The degree of heart failure by New York Heart Association functional classification (NYHA Class), the general probability of death and hospitalization vs. function, and various drug interventions that have been or are currently approved or under investigation. Various clinical descriptors of heart failure are given. Oral β-agonists [shown to acceler-ate mortality at least in one study (see text) and not currently undergoing drug development], and β-blockers (currently experimental) are flanked by questions marks. The survival probability is shown as a stippled backdrop and emphasizes the increased mortality risk as heart function deteriorates.

diuretics and vasodilators is essential to optimal symptom relief. Vasodilators such as angiotensin-converting enzyme inhibitors or other direct-acting agents have been discussed elsewhere.

The role, if any, for β-adrenergic receptor active agents for out-of-hospital patients with all classes of heart failure is unsettled, both for agonists and antagonists. Most clinicians and researchers would accept that the basic problem in heart failure is a failing heart. This is not to discount the profound influences of the peripheral vasculature to complicate the heart failure condition, and the contributions of other organs such as the kidney to perpetuate the heart failure condition. Probably the best support for the contention that the basic problem of heart failure is a failing heart comes from the immediate, nearly complete reversal of the heart failure syndrome with cardiac transplantation and restoration of normal cardiac output. The working clinical hypothesis has been that if the fundamental problem of heart failure is a failing heart, then measures to improve cardiac function may improve heart failure symptoms and also decrease mortality. One of the most fascinating aspects of heart failure research over the past 10 years has been the simultaneous evaluation of both β-adrenergic receptor agonists and antagonists to treat the heart failure condition. Seldom do we see the development and evaluation of treatment strategies that are so antithetical to each other.

As reviewed in the section that follows, extensive efforts have been made to evaluate β agonists for oral use to improve symptoms and prolong life in patients with heart failure. At the same time, growing support for the opposite approach, the use of β-adrenergic receptor antagonists (β-blockers) in heart failure, has been receiving increasing emphasis and is supported by an enlarging body of clinical and basic research. Certain fundamental questions remain with both approaches to treatment, and the background and current status of each of these approaches to heart failure treatment will be reviewed.

Use of β-Adrenergic Receptor Agonist in Heart Failure

In contrast to the widely accepted use of intravenous β agonists such as dobutamine for advanced heart failure, the appropriate indications, if any, are unknown for oral β agonists in the treatment of heart failure. This section reviews clinical trials of β agonists used in clinically stable outpatients; no studies have shown clear benefits. As discussed in greater detail in the section on β-blockers for heart failure, and as illustrated in Figure 25.17, β agonists and β antagonists have been used in research protocols for the same patient populations and for similar degrees of heart failure. However, at this time neither class of drugs can be considered standard or accepted therapy for heart failure, and both oral β agonists and β antagonists remain experimental. Thus, the fundamental questions of the adrenergic pathophysiology of heart failure remain with us—what are the appropriate uses of β-adrenergic receptor active agents—including agonists and antagonists—in heart failure.

The evaluation of risk/benefit ratios is a primary issue for β agonist use in heart failure. There is no doubt that patients with advanced heart failure who decompensate may face certain death without intravenous inotropes. In this setting, inotropes are life-saving, particularly as a medical bridge-to-cardiac transplantation. If β-agonist infusions are indicated for some patients with advanced heart failure, then it might be argued that an efficacious, orally administered, partial agonist might be a useful therapeutic option to replace the intravenously administered agents already available, even if such an agent would only be used for a small, select group of patients, even possibly restricted to drug administration within a hospital setting. However, few data are available with oral β-agonist inotropic agents in the sickest patients, where the risk/benefit ratio may be most favorable for their use.

Most clinical research protocols in the early to mid-1980s administered oral β agonists to predominantly stable outpatients with mild to moderate heart failure[102–109] (Table 25.1). The clinical outcomes have been variable regarding symptomatic improvement. More recently, a larger trial performed in sicker patients, primarily NYHA Class III–IV, did not show benefit with a partial β agonist,[109] and rather indicated an adverse survival effect. There is little doubt that as clinical heart failure progresses, the overall probability of survival drops off sharply (Fig. 25.17). In the very high mortality group the use of infused β agonists or β agonists combined with aggressive vasodilator therapy may be lifesaving. Even though the use of β agonists undoubtedly adds some risk (e.g., from arrhythmias), the risk/benefit ratio would clearly favor the use of such agents. When patients are less ill than advanced Class IV, the risk/benefit ratios change, and it is not clear at what point with regard to cardiac function the use of β agonists no longer has a favorable risk/benefit ratio. Even if an orally active sympathomimetic agent could meet basic criteria for use—safety, efficacy, and an acceptable side effect profile—it is possible, and based on current clinical trials, more likely probable, that if a patient can be safely removed from intravenous β agonists then additional β agonists of any kind may only be injurious. It is also possible that there may be no indication for oral sympathomimetics for any degree of heart failure treatment out of hospital, and that the use of such agents may decrease survival.

TABLE 25.1. β-Adrenergic agonist double-blinded, randomized clinical trials in heart failure.

Agent: Author, yr, ref #	Study duration, design	No. of patients	HF etiology	NYHA	Total dose/day	Heart rate	Exercise duration	ECHO	Cardiac index	Ejection fraction	Study Conclusion	Comments
Prenalterol: (β₁ selective, partial agonist)												
Currie, 1984[102]	2-wk crossover	8	5 IDC 3 Ischemia	II–III	200	↑	No change		↑ Acutely ↓ 2 wks	0.25 No change	No benefit	2 points withdrawn w/ ↑ HF No ACE Inhibitors
Dahlstrom, 1984[103]	4-wk crossover	10	Ischemia	III–IV	100–200	↓ w/ exercise	No change	No change			No benefit	HR ex. ↓ on drug. No ACE inhibitors
Roubin, 1984[104]	2-wk crossover	11	6 IDC 11 Ischemia	II–III	50–100	Exercise max ↓	No change		No change	0.24	No benefit	No ACE inhibitors
Lambertz, 1984[105]	3 mos double-blind 3 mos open-label all patients	16	11 IDC 5 Ischemia	III–IV No change	40–120	↑ at 1 wk, 3 and 6 months	No change	↑ Initially, no change 3, 6 mos	↑ at 1 wk No change 3, 6 mos	0.20, ↑ at 1 wk (.27) No change at 3, 6 mos	No benefit	Effects not sustained with long-term use. No ACE inhibitors
Glover, 1985[106]	6 mos	37	Ischemia	III	40–5 pts 100–15 pts 200–17 pts	Exercise max ↓	↑ Exercise compared to baseline		↑ Acutely No change at 6 mos	0.27 No change at 6 mos	Beneficial	2 deaths in placebo and prenalterol groups, improved clinical scores. No ACE inhibitors
Pirbuterol: (β₂ selective, partial agonist)												
Weber, 1982[107]	7 wks	12	10 valvular	III–IV	60 mg	No change	No change	No change			No benefit	Adverse effects: nervousness and tremolousness. No ACE inhibitors
Xamoterol: (β₁ selective, weak partial agonist; or β₁ antagonist with prominent ISA)												
German/Austrian Study Group, 1988[108]	3 mos	433	74% not specified	I—25% II—63% III—12%	400	No change at rest, ↓ w/exercise	↑ From 263 to 299	No change	No change	No change	Improved exercise	On ACE inhibitors
Severe Heart Failure Study Group, 1990[109]	13 wks	516	Ischemia—60% IDC—30%	III—75% IV—25%	400	↓ Rest ↑ Exercise	No change	No change	No change	Baseline 0.25	Accelerated mortality w/drug	No change in plasma NE in either group. On ACE inhibitors

HF = heart failure; IDC = idiopathic dilated cardiomyopathy; ACE = angiotensin-converting enzyme; NE = novepinephrine.

Oral β Agonists

In the past 10 years many clinical studies have been performed with oral β agonists. These trials have been based on the clinical hypothesis that if a fundamental defect of heart failure was the diminished inotropic state of the myocardium, then judicious use of inotropes might improve heart failure symptoms, quality of life, and possibly survival. However, the experience with orally active β agonists in outpatients with stable heart failure has not shown a beneficial survival effect or consistent improvement in symptoms.

Randomized, double-blinded, placebo-controlled trials of β agonists in patients with heart failure have been summarized in Table 25.1 (see refs.110–112 for exhaustive reviews). In the early 1980s, several new drugs were available for clinical testing, including partial agonists with β_1 or β_2 subtype selectivity (Table 25.2).

Prenaterol

Five double-blinded, placebo-controlled studies were performed with prenalterol, a β_1-selective weak partial agonist[102–106] (Table 25.1). At higher doses and with acute exposure the agonist properties are observed, such as tachycardia, increased cardiac output, and decrease in left ventricular filling pressures. Prenalterol acutely activates the renin-angiotensin-aldosterone system, and increases insulin release.[113] However, with chronic use exercise tachycardia was blunted in most but not all reports,[102,105] consistent with an antagonist effect (Table 25.1). Because of the relatively small numbers of patients tested, and the duration of testing in 2 to 4 weeks in three of the five studies, it is not possible to draw firm conclusions about the agonist versus antagonist effects of this agent. Additionally, most patients studied had ischemic cardiomyopathy, and as reviewed below, ischemic cardiomyopathy may have subtle but important differences compared to IDC with regard to efficacy of β antagonists.[114] The same may be true with β agonists.

It is probably more than coincidence that the only study to suggest a beneficial effect was performed in the largest patient population (37 patients), and the study remained double-blinded for the entire 6-month period.[106] Additionally, this patient group may have been more homogeneous, as all were NYHA Class III patients with ischemic cardiomyopathy and an average EF of 0.27. Two patients died in each group: two from sudden death in the placebo group and one from sudden death and one from progressive heart failure in the prenalterol group. Five patients were withdrawn: three in the placebo group (two from increased angina, one from acute onset diabetes mellitus) and two in the prenalterol group (one from progressive heart failure and one acute myocardial infarction). Exercise time was increased at 6 months in the prenalterol group compared with its own baseline, but not compared to the placebo group. The clinical score, a measure of patient well-being, was increased in the prenalterol group versus placebo. This study differs from later studies in that patients were taking digoxin and diuretics but not angiotensin-converting enzyme inhibitors. No plasma catecholamine measurements were performed, and therefore the impact of prenalterol on neurohumoral activation cannot be evaluated. Prenalterol clinical trials were terminated in 1984 because toxicology studies in animals suggested adverse effects.[106] Other uncontrolled trials of prenalterol are available.[113,115–117]

Pirbuterol and Other β_2-Selective Agonists

Pirbuterol is an orally active β_2-selective agonist.[118] In a randomized, placebo-controlled trial for 7 weeks in 12 patients, most with cardiomyopathy from valvular disease, pirbuterol did not provide benefit and was complicated with nervousness and tremulousness, adverse effects presumably related to β_2-agonist properties. There were no objective improvements to suggest efficacy[107] (Table 25.1). Additional uncontrolled trials of pirbuterol[119–121] and other β_2-agonists including salbutamol[122,123] and terbutaline[124] have been performed, but efficacy cannot be evaluated because of the uncontrolled nature of these studies.

Xamoterol

More recently, large clinical trials have been performed with xamoterol, a β_1-selective drug that can be de-

TABLE 25.2. β-Adrenergic selectivity and agonist/antagonist properties of selected agents.

	Nonselective	β_1 selective	β_2 selective
Full agonist	Isoproterenol		
	Dobutamine		
		Denopamine[†]	Salbutamol
			Pirubuterol
			Terbutaline
	Pindolol	Prenalterol	
	Practolol	Xamoterol	
	Carvedilol*	Alprenolol	
	Bucindolol*‡		
	Oxprenolol		
Full antagonist	Timolol	Acebutol	
	Nadolol	Esmolol	
	Propranolol	Atenolol	
		Metoprolol	
		Betaxolol[†]	

* α-adrenergic receptor antagonist properties (labetolol ≫ carvedodol > bucindolol).
† Highly β_1 selective.
‡ Bucindolol has minimal intrinsic sympathomimetic activity in certain experimental systems,[217,218] but not in human ventricular myocardium.[215]

scribed as a weak partial agonist or a β-blocker with prominent intrinsic sympathomimetic activity[125–132] (Table 25.2). Two large clinical trials have been published[108,109] (Table 25.1). In 1988, a randomized, double-blinded, placebo-controlled efficacy trial was reported in 433 patients, of which most were NYHA Class I–II. The study indicated that over a 3-month period, the primary endpoint of exercise time increased. There were only two deaths, one each in the placebo and xamoterol arms.[108]

In a more recent clinical trial, xamoterol accelerated mortality in a much sicker Class III–IV patient population.[109] The results are summarized in Table 25.1. The study was designed as an efficacy trial, with exercise as the primary end-point. All patients were taking diuretics and angiotensin-converting enzyme inhibitors. Doses of xamoterol between groups were comparable. The patient groups were well balanced for age, sex, etiology, NYHA Class, resting heart rate, presence of atrial fibrillation, blood pressure, exercise capacity (351 vs. 360 s, by exercise bicycle, 10 W baseline +10 W/min increase), left ventricular function measured by cardiothoracic ratio (0.59 vs. 0.58), left ventricular end-diastolic dimension (67 vs. 68), fractional shortening (16% vs. 15%), and ejection fraction (24% vs. 26%, placebo vs. xamoterol groups, respectively). No difference was present between groups for exercise duration, the primary end-point.

More patients dropped out of the xamoterol group than placebo (19% vs. 12%), and of the withdrawals on drug approximately three fourths were from cardiovascular changes. Although the study was not designed as a mortality trial, it was stopped prematurely by the safety monitoring committee because by an intention-to-treat analysis: a 9.2% (32 patients) versus 3.7% (6 patients) mortality rate was present in the xamoterol-treated group, with a hazard ratio of 2.54 (95% confidence limits of 1.04–6.18). Twelve patients had stopped taking xamoterol (and one patient on placebo) 9 days or more before death. The causes of death included progression of heart failure, sudden unexpected death, and other causes. Seventeen (4.8%) of 32 deaths in the xamoterol group were from progression of heart failure versus 2 (1.2%) in the placebo group; 13 sudden deaths (3.7%, xamoterol) versus 3 (1.8%, placebo), and other causes 2 (0.6%, xamoterol) versus 1 (0.6%, placebo). In summary, in patients who died, xamoterol was associated with a fourfold increased progression of heart failure, and a twofold higher incidence of sudden or unexpected death.

Summary of Oral β Agonist

In summary, the available evidence indicates that oral β-adrenergic agonists given chronically to heart failure patients may reduce survival. The mechanisms for re-

duced survival are not known. However, β agonists have been associated with adverse events, such as worsening of arrhythmias and electrolyte abnormalities such as hypokalemia,[133,134] both of which may contribute to decreased survival.

Additionally, the use of oral β agonists in outpatients may not be effective. One potential explanation relates to agonist-induced subsensitivity of the receptor pathway. This was proposed in 1981 for the β_2 agonist pirbuterol to explain its lack of sustained effect.[119] Acutely, pirbuterol increased cardiac index and ejection fraction, but at 1-month values were not different from baseline. The studies performed were not load-independent and therefore could not evaluate a tachyphylaxis to cardiac versus peripheral β_2-adrenergic receptor-mediated vasodilator effects. However, lymphocyte β-adrenergic receptor densities were measured and were decreased substantially at 1 month. Although myocardial β-adrenergic receptor density was not measured, heart rate, blood pressure, and cardiac size did not change. Myocardial adrenergic receptor pathways may have been desensitized, which contributed to the loss of clinical effect.

Other Agents

This review has been limited to double-blinded, placebo-controlled trials of sympathomimetic agents administered to heart failure patients. Exhaustive reviews that include uncontrolled trials are available elsewhere.[110–112] Such agents include the orally absorbed precursor to dopamine, levodopa, which has inotropic effects,[135] but its use has been limited by side effects.[136] Other dopamine-like agents with prominent β-agonist effects include propyl butyl dopamine,[137] ibopamine,[138,139] butopamine,[140] and dopexamine, reviewed below. A highly selective direct-acting β_1 partial agonist TA-064,[141] and other highly selective β_2 agonists such as terbutaline,[124] also have been examined in experimental settings, but none are used clinically at the present time, nor are these agents approved for use in heart failure treatment.

Intravenous β Agonists in Heart Failure

Clinical Use of Intravenous β Agonists in Heart Failure

The knowledge of receptor downregulation and post-receptor signal transduction systems in failing human ventricular myocardium provides invaluable insight for the rational use of intravenous β agonists in heart failure patients. First and most importantly, β-adrenergic receptor agonists are the most powerful, clinically useful means to augment contractility in the failing human heart even though the β_1-adrenergic receptor pathway is markedly downregulated and the β_2-adrenergic receptor pathway is mildly uncoupled, as described in detail above. Additionally, the use of a nonselective β-adrenergic receptor agent is required for optimal response because the ratio of $\beta_1:\beta_2$-adrenergic receptors in failing heart is approximately 60%:40%. Furthermore, the effects of β-adrenergic receptor agonists to stimulate adenylyl cyclase and thereby increase cAMP in the end-stage severely failing heart can be markedly potentiated by the addition of phosphodiesterase inhibitors, which will provide an additive inotropic effect.[81,98] This is reviewed in greater detail in the chapter that follows. Finally, direct versus indirect β agonists are preferred for long-term hemodynamic support in patients with advanced heart failure.[80]

Direct-acting agonists are full or partial agonists that bind directly to β-adrenergic receptors to cause receptor activation. Indirect-acting agents have a primary mechanism of action of releasing catecholamines that in turn activate β-adrenergic receptors.[5,60-62] Dopamine and dopexamine are both indirect agents with their primary mechanism of action to release norepinephrine from cardiac nerves.[5,60-62] Dopexamine also is a potent blocker of the norepinephrine uptake$_1$ system,[142] Dopamine[60,61,80,143] and dopexamine[144-148] also are weak direct-acting partial β agonists, and these combined indirect and direct properties give the pharmacologic profile. Norepinephrine tissue stores are diminished in the failing human heart, and an inotropic agent whose mechanism of action relies primarily on indirect effects will predictably be less useful in patients with advanced heart muscle disease than in patients with mild heart failure.[80]

In general, most β agonists are used to improve the inotropic state of the heart in hospitalized patients who have either acute or chronic cardiac dysfunction. A variety of conditions may lead to acute cardiac dysfunction, including myocardial ischemia or myocardial infarction, anesthesia, cardiopulmonary bypass, or complications of other injuries, diseases, or treatments that may temporarily cause myocardial dysfunction. For chronic heart failure, β agonists are used in patients with advanced, Class IV heart failure when lesser forms of therapy are inadequate, or in patients with chronic Class II–III heart failure with an acute metabolic or hemodynamic imposition that threatens to provoke advanced heart failure, for example, during the peripartum or perioperative periods, or during severe systemic or febrile responses to infection or allergy.

Endogenous Catecholamines

The endogenous catecholamines with either direct or indirect β-adrenergic receptor agonist effects include epinephrine, norepinephrine, and dopamine. The endogenous catecholamines have been reviewed elsewhere, and will be reviewed here only relative to their use as inotropes in heart failure. Their structure, synthesis, and general effects have been extensively reviewed.[5,110] The synthetic sympathomimetic dobutamine has more desirable hemodynamic effects than the three endogenous catecholamines, all of which are commonly available for intravenous infusion. Another synthetic sympathomimetic related to dopamine, dopexamine,[144-148] has received attention recently,[143,149-154] but because of its indirect mechanism of action, it is not likely to be useful for treatment of advanced heart failure.[80]

The pharmacokinetic profiles of the endogenous and synthetic agents are similar, and all are suitable for intravenous use.[155] The plasma half-life is short, from 2 to 3 min, and for this reason no loading doses are required. Steady-state plasma levels can be achieved within 10 to 15 min. Also, should side effects occur and necessitate a dose reduction, plasma levels will fall quickly. The responses to these agents are predictable. For dobutamine the effects are linear with plasma levels, and plasma levels are related directly to infusion rate.[156]

Epinephrine

Epinephrine is a powerful α- and mixed β_1- and β_2-adrenergic receptor agonist with complex effects from its mixed actions (see ref. 5 for review). It is a powerful inotrope with direct agonist effects on β_1- and β_2-adrenergic receptors in cardiac muscle. Epinephrine also has potent agonist effects at α-adrenergic receptor, which promotes peripheral vasoconstriction, especially when larger doses are given by intravenous bolus injection, but the equally or more powerful β_2 agonist effects promote vasodilation. With a very small dose of epinephrine given by constant infusion (0.1 μg/kg), the blood pressure may fall because of the more potent β_2-adrenergic receptor effects. With higher infusion doses, relatively greater α-adrenergic–mediated vasoconstriction will be observed. Heart rate will increase, but the inotropic effect is much more prominent. In contrast to the newer synthetic agents, cardiac work and oxygen consumption are increased substantially. Additionally, epinephrine is proarrhythmic. Metabolic effects include hyperglycemia and elevated lactate levels. It should be noted that epinephrine administered to a patient receiving β-blockers will give primarily an α-adrenergic response, and the hypertensive effects (pure α-adrenergic with β_2-adrenergic receptor effects blocked) can be extremely severe.

Even though epinephrine may be the most powerful agonist at β-adrenergic receptors, it is used infrequently for inotropic support in chronic heart failure except in situations resistant to the more usual treatments because of its arrhythmic potential, adverse oxygen consumption, and metabolic effects. At higher doses epinephrine causes direct toxicity of vascular and cardiac muscle (see section below on myocardial catecholamine toxicity). In cardiogenic shock or cardiac resuscitation in the setting of severe heart failure, a carefully titrated epinephrine infusion may be life-saving for a few minutes to a few hours until mechanical assistance or other support measures can be instituted. The one setting in which an epinephrine infusion is routinely indicated is the acutely failing but otherwise normal heart unresponsive to other less powerful β agonists. This setting is represented by the postcardiopulmonary bypass period, or the immediate postcardiac transplant setting, when a newly transplanted heart may suffer contractile dysfunction from the process of preservation and reimplantation, including hypothermic injury, ischemia, reperfusion injury, and possible acute immunologic insult.

Norepinephrine

Norepinephrine release, circulating levels, and prognostic significance for the heart failure condition have been reviewed elsewhere. As an endogenous catecholamine, norepinephrine has prominent α- and β_1-adrenergic agonist effects, but much less β_2 agonist effect relative to epinephrine. The prominent cardiovascular effects of norepinephrine in normal persons is to increase total peripheral resistance, with either no change or a decrease in cardiac output.[5] Similar effects are present in patients with heart failure. As such, norepinephrine has little indication in the management of heart failure except when a powerful peripheral vasoconstrictor agent is required.

Dopamine

Dopamine is the third endogenous catecholamine and in human physiology is primarily a central neurotransmitter. It is the immediate precursor of epinephrine and norepinephrine. Dopamine is degraded by monoamine oxidase (MAO) and catechol-O-methyltransferase (COMT), and is therefore ineffective orally.[5] It is administered as a continuous intravenous infusion when used clinically for inotropic support.[136] Its cardiovascular effects are mediated via direct activation of dopaminergic receptors in the kidney and splanchnic beds,[136,155,157] weak partial agonist effects at β_1-adrenergic receptors directly, and release of norepinephrine from sympathetic nerve terminals. This latter property is particularly important for its cardiac actions, as the release of endogenous norepinephrine appears to be its primary effect in cardiac tissue.[5,60-62] In low doses (<2 μg/kg/min IV) the activation of D_1 vascular dopamine receptors predominate, with vasodilatation especially important in the renal vascular bed to enhance glomerular filtration rate, renal blood flow,

and sodium excretion.[136] This property makes dopamine useful to increase splanchnic and renal blood flow in low-output states such as heart failure. With intermediate doses (2–10 μg/kg/min), cardiac effects are observed from β_1-adrenergic receptor activation, primarily from norepinephrine release. At higher infusion rates (5–20 μg/kg/min), dopamine stimulated norepinephrine release activates α-adrenergic receptors to give vasoconstriction, although pressor effects can be seen in some patients with lower doses.

The inotropic effects of dopamine result primarily from its indirect effects. As such, its use in advanced heart failure is limited presumably from the neurotransmitter depletion present in the failing heart.[80] In the management of patients with minimal or mild heart failure, dopamine may give similar effects to dobutamine except for a greater tendency to increase heart rate and a tendency to increase systemic vascular resistance (SVR) and ventricular filling pressures at medium and higher doses.[158,159] At low doses (1–2 μg/kg/min), dopamine interacts with renal dopamine receptors to promote renal artery dilatation and to enhance renal blood flow.

Synthetic Sympathomimetics: Indirect-Acting Agents

Dopexamine

Dopexamine is a synthetic sympathomimetic closely related to dopamine,[144-148] with an indirect mechanism of action. In failing ventricular myocardium the response to dopexamine in isolated tissue is similar to dopamine.[144-148] This agent has undergone extensive evaluation in patients with heart failure.[143,149-154] In patients with advanced heart failure, a dopexamine infusion rapidly loses efficacy at an average of 36 hr, but as quickly as 12 hr in patients with advanced heart failure.[80] The cardiovascular effects of dopexamine may be rapidly attenuated in chronic heart failure presumably related to its indirect mechanism of action and progressive cardiac norepinephrine depletion.[80]

Synthetic Sympathomimetics: Direct-Acting Agents

Dobutamine

Dobutamine is a direct-acting synthetic sympathomimetic agent,[160] that is administered intravenously. It has proved to be an extremely useful agent to support cardiac function in patients with moderate to severe heart failure. Its pharmacology is complex, as the dobutamine molecule is asymmetric and the overall effects are secondary to the combined effects of a racemic mixture of enantiomers.[161] These characteristics provide the basis for understanding its actions in clinical use.

The pharmacology of the (−) and (+) isomers of dobutamine has been elucidated, as reviewed by Ruffo-lo and Messick.[162] Dobutamine may have some minimal $\beta_1 > \beta_2$ selectivity.[62,161-163] The isomers of dobutamine have the ability to bind α- and β-adrenergic receptors, with both agonist and antagonist properties. The (+) isomer is a 10-fold more potent β-adrenergic receptor agonist with approximately 2 times greater activity (efficacy) than the (−) isomer, evaluated by contractility experiments in cat papillary muscle. The dose response curve for the racemic mixture was approximately two fold to the right of the (+) isomer. The chronotropic effects of both isomers are similar to the contractility responses. For α-adrenergic receptor effects, the (−) isomer was observed to provide a potent partial α-adrenergic receptor contractile response in rat aorta. The (+) isomer bound α receptors with similar affinity as the (−) isomer but had no agonist activity, and therefore functioned as a similarly potent α-receptor competitive antagonist. In summary, the clinically available racemic mixture provides direct β-adrenergic receptor activation primarily from the (+) isomer, with minimal effect from the (−) isomer. The α-receptor agonist effects from the (−) isomer are largely blocked by the (+) isomer to give minimal or no α-adrenergic agonist effects.

Dobutamine has been investigated extensively in humans.[155,156,158,159,164-168] Dobutamine has prominent inotropic effects and increases cardiac contractility via direct receptor activation[166] with only minimal increases in heart rate, but the exact biochemical basis for these favorable actions are not completely understood. In a direct examination of the β_1- versus β_2-adrenergic receptor selectivity of dobutamine, dobutamine was observed to have several-fold higher binding affinity for β_1- versus β_2-adrenergic receptors.[163] However, additional studies have indicated a nonselective β-agonist profile.[62,162,169] In animal tissues and experimental preparations designed to elucidate β-adrenergic receptor subtype specificities, dobutamine had an intrinsic activity of 0.7 to 1.0 that of isoproterenol at both β_1- and β_2-adrenergic receptors.[161,166] In human ventricular myocardium dobutamine had an intrinsic activity of 0.5.[170]

The inotropic effects of dobutamine have been partially attributed to α-adrenergic receptor activation,[162,171,172] especially in the setting of desensitization of β-adrenergic receptors.[171,172] However, studies of cardiac contractility utilizing α-adrenergic agonists in rodent heart may give different results from those observed in human or other large animal hearts. In rat heart, the α-adrenergic receptor density is twice that of β-adrenergic receptor density and rat heart functions as an α-adrenergic receptor organ. In contrast, the adrenergic inotropic responsiveness of the human heart is almost entirely from β-adrenergic receptor activation

(see above and Fig. 25.9). In a preliminary report utilizing the direct intracoronary infusion technique,[173] a small but significant increase in dp/dt was observed by the (−) isomer of dobutamine in human patients. This isomer has potent α-adrenergic receptor agonist effects, and this response was blocked by the nonselective α-receptor antagonist phentolamine. The positive inotropic effect of the racemic mixture of dobutamine could not be blocked with phentolamine in previous studies,[174] which indicates that the potent α-adrenergic antagonist properties of the (+) isomer in the racemic mixture of dobutamine (the drug available for clinical use) probably blocks any inotropic effects observed with the (−) dobutamine isomer. Additionally, as reviewed above, direct examination did not demonstrate α-adrenergic receptor-mediated contractile responses in human ventricular myocardium.[9] Together, these findings indicate that if an α-adrenergic receptor is coupled to contractility in the human heart, the response is very small.

Dobutamine is superior to dopamine for use in patients with heart failure.[158,159,175] In 1978, Leier and coworkers demonstrated that prolonged infusions (24 hr) of dobutamine but not dopamine increased cardiac output and peripheral blood flow.[158] In patients with advanced heart failure given dopamine and dobutamine in a cross-over trial, dobutamine decreased systemic and pulmonary artery resistance and pulmonary capillary wedge pressure, while the increase in cardiac output was maintained with no change in heart rate. In contrast, dopamine increased cardiac output at a low dose (4 μg/kg/min), but gave no additional beneficial effects at higher doses, as heart rate and pulmonary artery wedge pressure increased, both undesirable effects for long-term inotropic support. In summary, dobutamine is a useful direct β agonist for inotropic support of the failing human heart.

Recent work has demonstrated that dobutamine favorably changes aortic impedance to facilitate ventricular vascular coupling.[176] This has been more dramatically demonstrated by Binkley and colleagues by an increase in cardiac output in calves with artificial hearts, which is probably secondary to modulation of venous and arterial vessels.[177]

Dobutamine usually is used acutely for periods of hours to a few days to support patients with exacerbations of chronic heart failure or to support individuals with impaired cardiac function who have deteriorated from additional cardiac demands such as recurrent myocardial infarction, fever, anemia, infection, labor and delivery, trauma, etc. If the condition that precipitated worsening heart failure is temporary and reversible and cardiac function improves, the dobutamine support can be withdrawn. However, in chronically progressive heart failure, many patients enter a phase where they become resistant to the usual heart failure medical regimen of diuretics and vasodilators. Despite outpatient administration of intravenous loop diuretics, these patients eventually will present to the clinic or hospital in worsening symptomatic heart failure and will require inotropic support. Frequently a dobutamine infusion for 3 to 5 days will be extremely beneficial to relieve symptoms and to improve the heart failure condition, and may provide a period of days to weeks of continued stability and improvement in heart failure symptoms. Unfortunately, a subset of these patients can be removed from the dobutamine infusion only with great difficulty. The usual approach is to attempt to replace inotropic support with vasodilators, and after some angiotensin-converting enzyme (ACE) inhibitor is in place, hydralazine is the vasodilator of choice.[155] To wean a dobutamine infusion in patients with end-stage and refractory heart failure, dobutamine withdrawal frequently requires knowledge of right and left ventricular filling pressures by continuous hemodynamic monitoring. Occasionally patients cannot be weaned safely from dobutamine and in this group of patients continuous or intermittent, outpatient dobutamine therapy has been used[178,179] via long-term, indwelling central venous catheters. Based on the data of oral partial β agonists reviewed above, it is quite possible that continuous use may accelerate mortality. However, the safety and efficacy of this form of inotropic treatment is unknown because appropriately controlled mortality trials have not been conducted. Therefore, outpatient dobutamine therapy should be undertaken only as a last resort in a patient fully informed to the potential life-threatening nature of this treatment.

β-Adrenergic Receptor Antagonists in the Treatment of Heart Failure

The use of β-adrenergic receptor antagonists in the treatment of heart failure was initially proposed in 1975 by the heart failure group in Goteborg, Sweden. Since that time, a number of clinical trials (Table 25.3) have been performed after initially favorable responses with uncontrolled trials.[180,181] Like β agonists, treatment with β antagonists is experimental, and the use of β antagonists in heart failure patients with moderate or severe cardiac dysfunction can lead to acute cardiac decompensation or even death.[182] For this reason, experimental protocols with β antagonists have used very small initial doses of drug, and the dose has been increased over a period of weeks to months. However, some patients will be intolerant of even extremely small doses of β-adrenergic receptor antagonist; such intolerance illustrates the critical nature of sympathetic activation to preserve cardiac function, especially in advanced heart failure.

As reviewed above, the general rationale for the use of β-adrenergic receptor agonists in heart failure in the early to mid-1980s was relatively straightforward—if a primary defect in the failing heart is diminished contractility, then an augmentation of contractility with a β agonist might improve cardiac function, improve quality of life, and possibly diminish mortality. Unfortunately, the clinical trials to date have not indicated favorable long-term effects, as summarized in Table 25.1. In contrast to β-agonist use, the rationale for the use of β-adrenergic receptor antagonists, also known as β-blockers, is not as intuitively obvious, and the causes for the favorable short-term effects that have been observed are incompletely understood.

Rationale for β-Blocker Use in Heart Failure

Other chapters have reviewed in detail the neurohumoral activation in patients with heart failure, and in particular the increase in sympathetic drive. This is evident by increased levels of circulating norepinephrine in patients with heart failure both in peripheral venous blood as well as in the venous drainage to the heart, which can be evaluated by measuring norepinephrine content in coronary sinus blood. Coronary sinus norepinephrine has been observed to increase as left ventricular function deteriorates, and β-adrenergic receptor density in myocardium obtained at right ventricular endomyocardial biopsy was further downregulated with advanced heart failure (Fig. 25.18).

What might be the cause of improved cardiac function with the use of β-blockers in heart failure? This question has been the subject of intense investigation and review.[1,3,183,184] The simplest analysis would suggest that the decreased inotropic state of the failing heart is related to decreased myocardial β_1-adrenergic receptor density, which results from chronic overstimulation by excess norepinephrine exposure from cardiac sympathetic neurons. In this setting, a β-adrenergic receptor antagonist blocks the effects of norepinephrine at the receptor to interrupt the signal to downregulate β_1-adrenergic receptors. With decreased agonist occupancy, β-adrenergic receptor pathway sensitivity may be restored and β_1-adrenergic receptor density may upregulate. With increased β-adrenergic receptor density, the actions of the endogenous catecholamines, norepinephrine and epinephrine, could more effectively augment cardiac function in periods of stress or exercise. This latter point is not intuitively obvious—that β-adrenergic receptor sensitivity can be increased in the failing human heart even though a β-blocker is present in therapeutic concentrations. However, in a system with no receptor reserve, the only means to resensitize such a system that has been downregulated at the receptor level is to increase receptor density. Even with a competitive antagonist present (which is the case for all commercially available β-blockers), if the levels of endogenous agonist (norepinephrine, epinephrine) in-

TABLE 25.3. β-Adrenergic receptor antagonist clinical trials in heart failure.

Author, yr	Study design — Study duration, design	Patient population — Number of patients; NYHA	HF etiology	Agent total dose/day	Results — Heart rate	Results — NYHA
Waagstein, 1975[180]	5.4 mos (mean), range 2–12, uncontrolled	7	Viral CM-6	*Practolol (β_1, ISA) 100–800 mg *Alprenolol (NS, mod ISA) 100 mg	↓ (98 to 69)	
Swedberg, 1980[181]	22.3 mos (mean), range 6–62, uncontrolled	28 (5 pts first reported in Waagstein, 1975), (4 additional pts died within 2 mos); II–1, III–19, IV–8	IDC	Metoprolol (17) 50–200 Alprenolol (7) 75–200 practolol (2) 200 propranolol (2) 80–120		
Engelmeier, 1985[205]	12 mos randomized double-blind, placebo-controlled crossover	25 mean NYHA = 2.4; I–5, II–10, III–7, IV–1	IDC	Metoprolol 100	↓ (94 to 69) in metoprolol group; no change (92 to 92) in placebo	Improved in metoprolol group, no change in placebo group
Anderson, 1985[206]	23 mos mean (range 1–38 mos.) randomized double-blind, placebo-controlled	50, mean NYHA 2.8 vs. 2.7 placebo vs. metoprolol	IDC	Metoprolol avg = 61 mg. range 50–100	Nonsignificant ↓ (85 to 75) in metoprolol group. No change in placebo (85 to 84)	Improved in metoprolol group
Heilbrunn, 1989[207]	6 mos uncontrolled	16, I–5, II–7, III–3	IDC	Metoprolol avg 105 (75–150)	↓ (94 to 69)	
Waagstein, 1989[209]	Uncontrolled 15.9 (mean)	33	IDC	Metoprolol 75–200		Mean NYHA 3.8 to 1.8
Gilbert, 1990[211]	3 mos randomized double-blind, placebo-controlled	23, II–10, III–13	IDC	Bucindolol 170 (25–200) (NS β antagonist, no ISA α antagonist)	↓ (86 to 75)	Improved
Ikram, 1981[204]	1 mo randomized double-blind placebo-controlled crossover	17; II–7, III–10	12 alcoholic 5 idiopathic	Acebutolol (β_1, ISA) 400 mg	↓ (90 to 70)	No change
Currie, 1984[185]	1 mo randomized double-blind placebo-controlled crossover	10; all III	Idiopathic	Metoprolol 130 avg, range 100–200	↓ with β-B (82 to 61); no change with placebo	No change
Anderson, 1991[222]	23 mos (17–30) long-term follow-up to study of Gilbert, 1990	20	Idiopathic	Bucindolol 176 mg (25–200)	↓ with β-B	Improved
Woodley, 1991[114]	3 mos randomized double-blind, placebo-controlled stratified for Ischemic vs. idiopathic	49; II–18, III–32	27 Ischemic, 22 idiopathic	Bucindolol 170–180	Ischemic (83 to 70), IDC (86 to 75)	↑ IDC β-B only (2.4 to 1.5), no change in ischemic or IDC placebo groups
Nemanich, 1990[210]	2 mos uncontrolled	10; II–6, III–4	4 idiopathic 6 ischemic	Metoprolol 100	Resting HR ↓ (87 to 62), peak exercise HR 133 to 105	
Eichorn, 1990[212]	3 mos uncontrolled	15; I–1, II–7, III–5, IV–2	12 idiopathic 3 ischemic	Bucindolol 200	↓ (82 to 73)	
Anderson, 1991[219]	mean 14 mos uncontrolled	21; II–5, III–12, IV–4	13 idiopathic 6 ischemic 2 other	Metoprolol 127 mg avg (75–200)	↓ (90 to 74)	Improved (3 to 2.3)
Leung, 1990[214]	8-wk randomized double-blind placebo-controlled crossover	12; II–3, III–5, IV–4	Idiopathic	Labetolol mean 275 (range 100–400)		↑ 3.2 to 2.2 with ↑-B; no change in placebo
Pollock, 1990[213]	3 mos randomized double-blind placebo-controlled	19; II–1, III–14, IV–4	7 ischemic 12 idiopathic	Bucindolol 200	No change (90 to 82)	
Packer, 1996[1]	4 Stratified programs of protocols; open-label challenge dose; 6–12 mos randomized, double-blind, placebo-controlled	1,094; II-582, III-480, IV-32	521 ischemic, 570 nonischemic dilated cardiomyopathy, 3 unknown	carvedilol, up to 25 mg twice daily for patients under 85 kg or 50 mg twice daily for heavier patients; mean 45 ± 27 mg	↓ (by 12.6 ± 12.8)	Significant reduction in risk of death from progressive heart failure; worsening heart failure as an adverse reaction during treatment. Less frequent than with placebo

*Practolol is a nonselective β-blocker with 0.1–0.5 the potency of metoprolol and prominent intrinsic sympathomimetic activity (ISA). Alprenolol is β_1 selective with similar potency to metoprolol but with prominent ISA. Acebutolol a β_1 selective with 0.1–0.5 the potency of metoprolol and mild (+) sympathomimetic effects (see Table 2 and ref. 223)

HF = heart failure; IDC = idiopathic dilated cardiomyopathy; NYHA = New York Heart Association; ISA = intrinsic sympathomimetic activity; RV = right ventricle; β-B = beta-blocker; pts = patients; β-AR = beta-adrenergic receptor; EF = ejection fraction; NE = norepinephrine.

Results					Comments
Exercise duration/ Capacity	Cardiac index	Ejection fraction	Plasma catecholamines	Study conclusion	
Improved				Cardiac function improved	First series of case reports
		↑ (0.32–0.42)		Improved cardiac function	10 pts died in follow-up, 3 pts died on alprenolol and 2 on practolol
Improved in metoprolol group (2 to 1.5)		↑ (0.13–0.18) in metoprolol group; no change in placebo (0.18–0.21)		Improved functional class and exercise tolerance with metoprolol	3 pts died (2 placebo, 1 metoprolol)
No change		0.27, 0.29 at baseline, placebo vs. drug		Trend to improved survival	3 patients died (actual treatment), 8 patients died (control) $p = .12$
	Nonsignificant ↑ (2.8–3.2)	↑ (0.26–0.39)		Improved response to catecholamine infusion	β-AR density in RV increased from 39 to 80 fmol/mg; dobutamine dp/dt ↑ 74%
	↑ (2.2–2.6)	↑ (0.24–0.42) (↑ again after withdrawal and readministration 0.23–0.33)		Beneficial clinical and hemodynamic effects	↑ β-AR density (30.3 to 49.0 fmol/mg), withdrawal of β-blocker caused deterioration in 6/34 with sudden death in 3 pts. 7 pts died within 3 months; 5 intolerant of 5 mg; 2 died in dose titration after pulmonary embolus
No change	↑ (2.2–2.5)	↑ (0.26–0.35)	Plasma norepinephrine decreased (423 to 202) in β-B group; no change in placebo	Improved resting cardiac function	Entry required tolerance to 12.5 mg q 12 h for 2–3 doses (1/24 pts excluded)
Decreased		No change		No improvement	No dose uptitration
No change	No change (2.5 vs. 2.4)	No change (0.27 baseline, 0.31 metoprolol, 0.28 placebo)		No improvement	
No change		↑ (.25–.35)		Patients improved long term	Long-term follow-up study; all patients survived
No change in any groups	↑ Only in β-B IDC (2.2–2.5)	↑ IDC β-B (0.26 to 0.35); no change in ischemic or IDC placebo groups	↓ Plasma NE in IDC β-B group only (461 to 211)	Improvement in idiopathic group but not ischemic group with bucindolol	At entry, the EF in ischemic group was significantly less (0.20) than the IDC group (0.25). The ischemic group also had less exercise capacity and higher diuretic doses
↑ (7.7–9.1 min)		β (0.15–0.25)	↓ NE (613 to 303) ↓ Epi 71 to 40)	Patients improved	2 pts intolerant and withdrawn
	↑ Cardiac output (5.0–5.8 l/min) ↓ LVEDP (19–15 mm Hg)	↑ (0.23–0.29)		Diastolic relaxation improved, contractile function improved even though myocardial oxygen consumption was unchanged	↑ stroke volume (64 to 82 ml) ↑ dp/dt
↑ supine bicycle work (104–130 w)	↑ (2.1–2.5) ↑ exercise (3.8–4.6)	↑ (0.21–0.32)	↓ NE (arterial) (3.72 to 2.19); no change in Epi.	Improvement in IDC group; no change in ischemic group	4 pts intolerant to test done (5 mg bid × 2 days)
↑ (580–683 s); no change in placebo	No change			Improved rest and exercise tolerance	
↑ (445–530 s)	↑ (4.0 to 4.7)	↑ (0.19 to 0.23) in β-B group; no change in placebo		Effective	
				Significantly reduced risk of death and hospitalization for cardiovascular causes in patients with chronic heart failure who are receiving treatment with diuretics, an angiotensin-converting-enzyme inhibitor and/or digoxin	

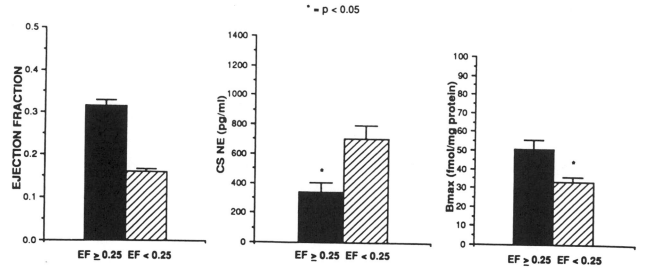

FIGURE 25.18. Data from 47 subjects with idiopathic dilated cardiomyopathy divided into mild to moderate left ventricular dysfunction [ejection fraction (*EF*) ≥0.25 and advanced left ventricular dysfunction EF <0.25]. The left panel gives ejection fractions for both groups, the middle panel the coronary sinus (*CS*) norepinephrine (*NE*) levels, and the right panel gives β-adrenergic receptor density (B_{max}) of right ventricular endomyocardial biopsy specimens. All values are ±SEM. Reprinted, with permission, from ref. 1. Copyright 1990 by the American Heart Association.

crease acutely with exercise or other stress, the antagonist will be competitively displaced by a higher concentration of agonist. With increased receptor density the maximal inotropic sensitivity of the β-adrenergic receptor system is restored, because the maximal effect of the system is proportional to receptor density (see Fig. 25.6). As reviewed below and summarized in Table 25.3, this hypothesis has experimental data to support it. In patients with heart failure from IDC, cardiac β-adrenergic receptors will upregulate with some types of β-blockers.

A second analysis is not as straightforward as the first, but also has experimental data to support it. This hypothesis suggests that actions of β antagonists that are independent of receptor upregulation may play an important if not primary role for the improved cardiac and clinical status. Several actions are possible, and include a direct cardioprotective effect to prevent continued catecholamine toxicity (reviewed below), and indirect protective effects such as from free radical formation, beneficial effects on neurohumoral activation such as a decrease in the activation of the renin-angiotensin system,[185] or other favorable effects such as vascular or antiarrhythmic effects.[186,187] With this analysis, the β-adrenergic receptor upregulation may be a marker of an improved overall heart failure condition.

These analyses are not mutually exclusive. The first analysis above is an interpretation based on the known receptor pharmacology. The second analysis implies that decreased β-adrenergic receptor density and elevated circulating catecholamines may only be markers of the heart failure condition, and that upregulation of β-adrenergic receptors with β-blocker use likewise may be only a general or nonspecific marker of improvement in the heart failure condition. This contention underlies persistent questions in heart failure research—what are the fundamentally important mechanisms for how the human heart fails, and what are the mechanisms for how the failing heart improves with β-blockade. Additional issues of β-blockade in heart failure include the time course and magnitude of clinical improvement relative to receptor upregulation.

Myocardial Catecholamine Toxicity

Myocardial catecholamine toxicity has been investigated over the past three decades. It is known that high concentrations of catecholamines can induce myocardial injury in animals secondary to a catecholamine infusion[188–190] or pheochromocytoma,[191,192] as well as in humans with pheochromocytoma.[193,194] Myocarditis has been observed at autopsy in patients with pheochromocytoma and elevated catecholamine concentrations.[193–195] The exact mechanisms of myocardial injury are still incompletely understood, but both receptor-mediated and direct mechanisms of toxicity have been postulated. Theories advanced for mechanisms of direct injury include local hypoxia[196] and ischemic damage from vasoconstriction,[192,197–200] and toxicity from catecholamine metabolites.[192,201,202] For receptor-mediated causes, both α-[188,190,192,193] and β-adrenergic[190,192,203] receptor-mediated toxicity has been postulated, as toxicity in these experiments could be reduced or eliminated with either α- or β-blockade.

Clinical Trials of β-Blockers in Heart Failure Patients

Long-term clinical trials (weeks to months) of β-blockers in heart failure are summarized in Table 25.3. The initial report of β-blocker use in heart failure was from the Göteborg, Sweden, group in 1975.[180] Their trial was prompted by the beneficial use of β antagonists in patients with acute myocardial infarction with left ventricular dysfunction. Alprenonolol was used for the first patient, and practolol in the remaining six patients. All patients had tachycardia and were Class III patients. Clinical improvement was noted over a period of 2 to 12 months (Table 25.3). A second larger, uncontrolled series containing an additional 23 patients was reported in 1980, and again suggested that β-blockade improved cardiac function in patients with heart failure[181] (Table 25.3).

Two randomized, double-blinded, placebo-controlled trials with a crossover design were reported by Ikram and Fitzpatrick in 1981[204] and by Currie et al. in 1984[185] in 17 and 10 patients, respectively. Neither study identified clinical improvement. Features that may have precluded a positive result included the relatively shorter study duration (1 month) and the use of an agent with mild ISA.[204] The second study by Currie and co-workers was a double-blinded, placebo-controlled study and used an average of 130 mg/day of metoprolol, but the study size (five patients in each group) and the duration (1 month) may have been inadequate to observe a positive result should one have occurred.

In 1985, the first positive β-blocker study in heart failure, conducted with a randomized, double-blinded, placebo-controlled design, was reported by Englemeier and colleagues.[205] It was performed in 25 patients with IDC. Patients were randomized to metoprolol or placebo, and were followed for 12 months. Placebo-treated patients ultimately were crossed over to active drug. Most patients were NYHA functional Class II or III. The study indicated that functional class, ejection fraction, and exercise duration improved in the β-blocker group (Table 25.3).

In 1985, a second randomized trial with metoprolol was reported from Anderson and co-workers,[206] and has been the largest series to date. The study, designed as a mortality trial, enrolled 50 patients with a follow-up time of 1 to 38 months. By an intention-to-treat analysis there was no difference in outcome, but by actual treatment, three β-blocker versus eight control patients died, with a trend to statistical significance (Table 25.3).

In 1989, Heilbrunn and co-workers reported the hemodynamic response to catecholamine stimulation before and after 6 months of metoprolol administration in an uncontrolled trial conducted in 14 patients[207] (Table 25.3). This was the first attempt to examine the hypothesis that improved cardiac function with long-

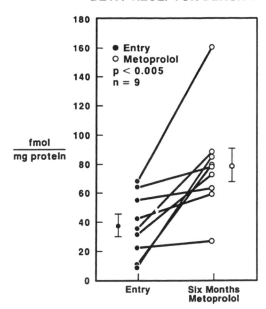

BETA-RECEPTOR DENSITY

FIGURE 25.19. Right ventricular endomyocardial β-adrenergic receptor density at baseline (*entry*) and after 6 months of metoprolol therapy (6 months metoprolol) for nine patients. Data are mean+SEM. Reprinted, with permission, from ref. 207. Copyright 1989 by the American Association.

term β-blockade may be associated with improvement in cardiac β-adrenergic receptor density (upregulation), and with improved hemodynamic responses to catecholamines. In this study, myocardial β-adrenergic receptor density and hemodynamics at rest and with a dobutamine infusion were compared before and at the completion of 6 months of metoprolol treatment. The patient cohort consisted of patients with IDC and NYHA Class I, II, and III heart failure symptoms who were given an average daily dose of 105 mg of metoprolol (range 75–150).

This study provided new and exciting results. At the 6-month end-point, heart rate had decreased from 94 to 69 bpm, left ventricular EF had increased substantially from 0.26 to 0.39 (Fig. 25.19), and myocardial β-adrenergic receptor density had doubled, from 39 to 80 fmol/mg (Fig. 25.20). The hemodynamic responses to dobutamine also were significantly improved (Fig. 25.21). Thus, catecholamine sensitivity was restored, β-adrenergic receptors were upregulated, and ventricular function was improved in the setting of metoprolol administration. It is likely that metoprolol caused the upregulation of β-adrenergic receptors, and it would be tempting to conclude that the upregulation of β-adrenergic receptors was a primary cause for the observed clinical improvement. However, as discussed above, it is also possible that the increase in β-adrenergic receptors was a more general marker for an improved heart failure state, which may imply that the

EJECTION FRACTION

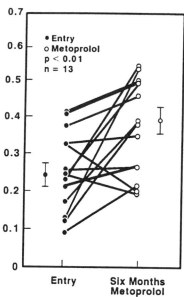

FIGURE 25.20. The ejection fraction determined at angiography at baseline (*entry*) and after 6 months of metoprolol therapy for 13 patients. Data are mean ±SEM. Reprinted, with permission, from ref. 207. Copyright 1989 by the American Heart Association.

RESPONSE TO DOBUTAMINE
PERCENT CHANGE LV dP/dt

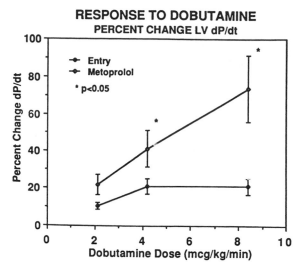

FIGURE 25.21. The responses to dobutamine infusion for left ventricular dp/dt in the same group of patients (n = 8) as Figs. 25.19 and 25.20. At baseline (*entry*), the change in dp/dt was flat, but substantially and significantly increased with 6 months of metoprolol therapy. Data are mean ±SEM. Reprinted, with permission, from ref. 207. Copyright 1989 by the American Heart Association.

important actions of β-blockers may be something in addition to receptor blockade. Additionally, it would seem to be unlikely that spontaneous regression of the heart failure condition would have occurred in these patients without metoprolol, but without a randomized control group the study design does not allow for this conclusion.

A recent preliminary report indicated that in patients with IDC treated with carvediolol, the EF improved without β-adrenergic receptor upregulation.[208] In a different group treated with metoprolol, EF improved and myocardial β-adrenergic receptors upregulated to a similar degree. These data suggest that functional improvement (EF) may be dissociated from changes in β-adrenergic receptor density.[208] In the Heilbrunn study,[207] the improvement in cardiac function observed with β-blockade may have been related to metoprolol, but the mechanism or mechanisms that contributed to this improvement are not known. Additional studies will be required to determine these mechanisms.

In 1989, Waagstein and co-workers reported an uncontrolled trial of the effects of short- and long-term metoprolol administration, withdrawal, and readministration in 33 patients with IDC[209] (Table 25.3). The study group excluded patients treated for arrhythmias. Advanced heart failure was present in most patients— 16 NYHA Class IV, 15 Class III, and only 2 patients with Class II symptoms, and all patients had been hos-

pitalized for heart failure. Only two patients were receiving ACE inhibitors, two hydralazine, and one nitroglycerin, and all vasodilator therapy had been initiated before entry into the metoprolol trial. The sickest patients may not have been stabilized completely before metoprolol challenge. The reports notes that efforts were made to "obtain a hemodynamically stable condition during conventional treatment before initiation of β-blockers, but this was accomplished in only 5 of the 16 patients of functional Class IV." Seven of the 33 patients died within 3 months, and the remaining 26 survived longer than 6 months. Of the seven patients who died, all were Class IV, and all died of progressive heart failure. When compared to the Class IV patients who survived, they appeared to be the sicker patients. Five of the seven could not tolerate oral metoprolol 5 mg bid, and the remaining two patients tolerated 5 mg bid but both died of massive pulmonary embolism during dose uptitration. Of the surviving 26 patients, the average EF had increased from 0.25 to 0.41. After metoprolol administration for a mean of 16 months, 24 of 26 patients had metoprolol withdrawn and 8 of 24 remained clinically stable without deterioration. The remaining 16 deteriorated, and 4 patients died. The four patients who died had all been Class III patients, three who had improved to Class II, and one patient to Class I. The EFs of the remaining 12 patients had decreased to 0.23 over an average of 8 months. These patients were rechallenged with metoprolol, and similar beneficial changes occurred; for example, EF increased from

0.23 to 0.33. β-adrenergic receptor densities were measured in a subgroup of nine patients at baseline with a mean EF of 0.21, which increased to 0.30 with chronic treatment. β-adrenergic receptor densities were 30.3 fmol/mg at baseline versus 49.0 fmol/mg with chronic treatment.

This is an interesting and important trial that was designed for longitudinal follow-up through β-blocker challenge, withdrawal, and rechallenge. The study did not contain a placebo group, and therefore the study was not able to evaluate the degree of spontaneous improvement that might have occurred in some of these patients. Additionally, the study was not blinded. However, the fascinating observation was that the withdrawal of metoprolol caused regression of cardiac function in most patients, and reinstitution of drug to those who survived metoprolol withdrawal again was associated with clinical improvement. Taken together, the data indicate that a beneficial effect associated with metoprolol was present, at least in those patients who survived the initial (3-month) challenge, but the mechanism or mechanisms of these beneficial effects have not been determined. Additionally, the mechanism of deterioration upon withdrawal of β-blockade was not elucidated. Finally, as noted below, the overall effects on survival for β-blockers are unknown.

In 1990, five additional heart failure studies were published that evaluated the use of metoprolol,[210] bucindolol,[211-213] and labetalol[214] in patients with heart failure (Table 25.3). Bucindolol is a nonselective β-blocker with mild to moderate peripheral vasodilatory activity[215,216] and no evidence of ISA in human cardiac tissue,[215] even though very weak ISA has been observed in nonhuman experimental preparations.[217,218] The vasodilatory activity is thought to be secondary to α-adrenergic receptor antagonist effects.[215] Labetalol is similar to bucindolol, except that the α-adrenergic antagonist effects are much more pronounced, and labetalol has much more prominent vasodilator effects. In contrast to bucindolol and labetalol, metoprolol is a pure antagonist and has no vasodilatory actions.

Gilbert and co-workers randomized 23 patients with IDC to bucindolol or placebo[211] (Table 25.3). Patients improved in functional class, ejection fraction, and cardiac index, and plasma norepinephrine decreased in the group who received bucindolol. No changes occurred in the placebo group. Bucindolol was well tolerated in Class II and III patients, and the only patient excluded from the study because of initial open-label drug challenge was a patient with advanced Class IV heart failure. Pollock and co-workers used bucindolol in a similar design,[213] but combined 7 patients with ischemic cardiomyopathy and 12 patients with IDC. Bucindolol improved resting and exercise cardiac function (Table 25.3). Leung and co-workes[214] randomized 12 patients

with IDC to placebo or labetalol for 8 weeks, and showed an improvement in functional class and improved resting and exercise capacity (Table 25.3).

β-Blockers for Ischemic Versus Idiopathic Cardiomyopathy

In 1991, Woodley and co-workers reported their experience with bucindolol in patients with ischemic cardiomyopathy compared to IDC[114] (Table 25.3). This has been the only prospectively designed study to stratify the response to β-blockade by etiology of heart failure. Forty-nine patients were randomized and were stratified between ischemic cardiomyopathy (n = 27) and IDC (n = 22) in a double-blinded, placebo-controlled trial. The groups were reasonably matched, except that the ischemic group was overall the sicker group at study entry. The EF in the ischemic group was significantly less than the IDC group (0.20 vs. 0.24), and the ischemic group had reduced exercise capacity and increased average daily doses of diuretics. Both treatment groups were given similar total average daily doses of bucindolol. Beneficial effects in the ischemic group given bucindolol did not achieve statistical significance, although the absolute change was similar but of smaller magnitude compared to the idiopathic group. When both groups were combined together, significant improvements in ejection fraction, stroke volume index, pulmonary artery wedge pressure, and stroke work index were observed. However, step-wise regression analysis confirmed that the favorable changes observed with the combined groups were secondary to the idiopathic group. This study indicated that the responses of ischemic cardiomyopathy to metoprolol were generally similar but quantitatively less compared to IDC.

Unresolved Issues with β-Blocker Use in Heart Failure

Despite considerable progress, fundamental issues regarding the potential use of β-blockers in heart failure remain to be resolved. The single most important question to be resolved is the mortality effect in heart failure patients. This and other issues are as follows.

Do β-Blockers Provide Survival Benefits in Patients with Heart Failure?

Undoubtedly the single most important question is whether β-blockers prolong life in patients with heart failure. This question must be resolved with an appropriately sized mortality trial with adequate duration to settle the issue. As illustrated in Table 25.3, several smaller randomized, blinded, placebo-controlled trials have demonstrated encouraging improvement in functional capacity in heart failure patients, primarily with

IDC. However, the only trial with survival as a primary end-point[219] (Table 25.3) was inconclusive because of inadequate size. One large international trial, the Metoprolol in Dilated Cardiomyopathy (MDC), reported an increase in left ventricular ejection fraction, and a reduction in the combined endpoint of death or need for transplantation. All of this lacter effect was attributable to the reduction in need for transplantation, however, with no difference in mortality.[219a]

In 1996, the results of the U.S. Carvedilol Heart Failure Trials Program,[219b] four concurrent clinical trials of efficacy and safety, were summarized as evidence of a survival benefit with carvedilol in patients with chronic heart failure. Overall, this program randomized 1,094 patients with chronic heart failure in a double-blind, placebo-controlled stratified program. Patients with ejection fractions ≤ 0.35 were assigned to one of four treatment protocols (mild, moderate to severe, and severe heart failure as well as a dose-ranging study) on the basis of their baseline exercise capacity. Background therapy with diuretics, an angiotensin-converting-enzyme inhibitor (if tolerated) and/or digoxin was kept constant, and patients were followed for six months (12 months for patients with mild heart failure). In an intent-to-treat analysis of-all-cause mortality, 7.8% of the placebo group died as opposed to only 3.2% in the carvedilol group; the reduction in risk attributable to carvedilol was 65% (95% confidence interval: 39% to 80%; $p < 0.001$). This finding represents an effect that led the Data Safety Monitoring Board to recommend early termination of the program. The beneficial effect of carvedilol on survival was consistent in all evaluated subgroups (age, sex, cause of heart failure, ejection fraction, exercise tolerance, systolic blood pressure, heart rate or protocol assignment) and was reflected in a decrease in the risk of death from progressive heart failure as well as in the risk of sudden death. In addition, as compared to placebo, carvedilol therapy was accompanied by a 27% reduction in the risk of hospitalization for cardiovascular causes as well as a 38% reduction in the combined risk of hospitalization or death in a time-to-first event analysis (24.6% versus 15.8%, $p < 0.001$).

It is unclear whether the beneficial effects of carvedilol represent solely a beta-blocker class effect or are in part due to some more unique properties of the drug. The ancillary vasodilator effects (alpha blockage) of carvedilol may enable more heart failure patients to tolerate higher doses and therefore more complete beta receptor blockade. Alternatively, a unique ancillary effect of carvedilol, described in experimental models, is its ability to inhibit the generation of oxygen free radicals. Through this antioxidant effect, it is conceivable that carvedilol could reduce direct cellular activation (stimulation of adhesion molecules, inflammatory cytokines and iNOS) as well as cellular toxicity and induced cell death (apoptosis).[219c]

Which β-Blockers Are Best Suited for Use in Heart Failure?

Metoprolol, a β_1-selective antagonist, has been used most extensively for β-blockade in heart failure. Several other drugs also have been used, including those with β_1 and nonselective properties. More recent experience has been obtained with bucindolol, a nonselective β-antagonist that appears to give results similar to metoprolol. The issue of β_1 versus nonselective β-blockers has not been tested in heart failure treatment.

A second unresolved issue is the role of β-blockers with vasodilator properties. Several β-blockers with vasodilator effects have recently been investigated (Table 25.2). Bucindolol, carvediolol, and labetalol all have peripheral vasodilatory activities that apparently result from α_1-antagonist properties.[215,220,221] Bucindolol has approximately a 30- to 100-fold β-blocker versus α-blocker selectivity. In contrast, for β- versus α-adrenergic receptor antagonism, carvediolol is approximately 10- to 30-fold selective, and labetalol two to fourfold selective. These properties may provide an explanation for the vasodilator profile of labetalol $\geqslant$ carvediolol $>$ bucindolol.[215] It has been suggested that the mild vasodilatory properties may enhance successful drug initiation and up-titration, but experiments have not been done that directly compare β-blockers with vasodilator effects versus those agents that do not have this property.

A third issue is one of quantity—how much β-blocker is enough? Is it better to titrate the dose to maximally tolerated levels, or are smaller doses more effective? Can some physiologic measurement, such as heart rate, provide an indication of adequate β-blockade? The dosage of metoprolol, the most commonly used agent, has varied approximately twofold between studies.

What Is the Best Strategy to Initiate β-Blockers in Patients with Heart Failure?

Most studies have used extremely small doses of β-blocker with gradually increasing doses over several weeks. First doses of β-blockers frequently have been given in the hospital setting, many times during the inhospital phase of a clinical protocol. β-blockers decrease sympathetic drive, a potentially lethal pharmacologic strategy if used in excess with a failing heart that requires high levels of adrenergic stimulation. The safety and monitoring measures required for acute administration and uptitration of β-blockers will require careful consideration.

Are There Certain Clinical Characteristics of Patients with Heart Failure that Predict Success with β-Blockers, such as Idiopathic Dilated Cardiomyopathy Versus Ischemic Cardiomyopathy?

A recent major trial has indicated that important differences in response to β-blockade may be present between patients with IDC and ischemic cardiomyopathy.[114] Idiopathic versus ischemic cardiomyopathy is undoubtedly one of the most important questions regarding clinical characteristics for the general applicability of β-blockers in heart failure. The only carefully performed comparison was a randomized, placebo-controlled, double-blinded trial with bucindolol.[114] The IDC group had an unmistakable response to bucindolol versus the idiopathic cohort who received placebo, but the treated ischemic group gave little indication of a favorable response either to its own baseline or to its randomized placebo-treated ischemic group (see Table 25.3, and discussion above). As reviewed in the receptor section above, the degree of cardiac β_1-adrenergic receptor downregulation is less prominent in ischemic cardiomyopathy versus IDC, even with similar degrees of functional impairment. The reasons for this are not clear, but may relate to different pathophysiological mechanisms of cardiac dysfunction[87] between these two forms of heart muscle disease—myocyte loss from infarction and scarring in ischemic cardiomyopathy versus myocyte hypertrophy and dysfunction from unknown cause or causes in IDC.

Other issues of potential importance include the degree of illness of a heart failure patient and the immediate and short-term risks of β-blocker use versus the potential for long-term benefit. Such issues can be clarified only with large prospectively randomized mortality trials. Other issues include age- or sex-related differences in responses to β-blocker treatment, the effects of other concomitant therapy, or special considerations for the use of β-blockers in heart failure patients with atrial fibrillation.

Are There Clinical Characteristics that Predict Those Heart Failure Patients Who Will Not Benefit from β-Blockers?

There are no clinical or laboratory findings that indicate when a patient is too sick to attempt β-blockade other than progressive Class IV heart failure or those patients who require intravenous β agonists. Because of concern about the potential adverse effects of β-blockers with advanced heart failure, most studies have been performed in stable Class II–III patients with IDC. However, the most favorable responses to β-blockers may occur in those sickest patients (the late Class III) who are still capable of safely starting and uptitrating β-blockers. The degree of illness can vary greatly between early and late Class III heart failure. The advanced Class III/early Class IV group, the sickest group that β-blockers might be considered, is undoubtedly the most difficult to initiate β-blocker therapy. This group requires the closest supervision, at times within the hospital setting, for initial drug administration. However,

this group also may have greater potential for benefit. The ability to identify clinical features that predict those too ill to achieve benefit will be possible only when large studies with sufficient clinical data are completed. The mid- or late Class IV heart failure group cannot tolerate any degree of β-blockade, and intravenous β agonists frequently will be the drug of choice.

What Is the Optimal Management for Patients on β-Blockers Who Have Progressive Heart Failure?

In a recent prospectively designed trial reviewed above, metoprolol withdrawal caused clinical deterioration in most of the patients who had had a favorable response.[209] It has been suggested that patients with advanced heart failure may deteriorate rapidly when β-blockers are withdrawn. However, if β-blockade is shown to be indicated for heart failure treatment, and assuming β-blockade is not curative therapy and that the heart failure condition eventually will progress, the indications for withdrawal of β-blockade will need to be determined.

Summary and Conclusions

A great deal of progress has been made in the last 10 years to understand the role of β-adrenergic agonists and antagonists in the treatment of chronic heart failure. However, fundamental clinical questions remain to be answered and make this area of heart failure research a particularly exciting area. Continued basic research in receptor structure, mechanisms of transmembrane signaling, and the various intracellular components of signal transduction systems will be required. These overall efforts will allow greater understanding of drug effects, the basis for new therapeutic strategies, and new insight into mechanisms of disease.

Acknowledgment. The expert secretarial assistance of Gail Manickam is gratefully acknowledged.

References

1. Bristow MR, Hershberger RE, Port JD, et al. β-adrenergic pathways in nonfailing and failing human ventricular myocardium. *Circulation.* 1990;82(Suppl 1): 12–25.
2. Homcy CJ, Vatner SF, Vatner DE. β-adrenergic receptor regulation in the heart in pathophysiologic states: abnormal adrenergic responsiveness in cardiac disease. *Annu Rev Physiol.* 1991;53:137–159.
3. Packer M. Pathophysiological mechanisms underlying the effects of β-adrenergic agonists and antagonists on functional capacity and survival in chronic heart failure. *Circulation.* 1990;82(Suppl 1):77–88.
4. Ross EM, Gilman AG. Pharmacodynamics: mechanisms

of drug action and the relationship between drug concentration and effect. In: Goodman Gilman A, Goodman LS, Rall TW, Murad F, eds. *The Pharmacological Basis of Therapeutics*. New York: Macmillan; 1985:35–48.

5. Weiner N. Norepinephrine, epinephrine, and the sympathomimetic amines. In: Goodman Gilman A, Goodman LS, Rall TW, Murad F, eds. *The Pharmacological Basic of Therapeutics*. New York: Macmillan; 1985:145–180.

6. Ahlquist RP. A study of adrenotropic receptors. *Am J Physiol*. 1948;153:586–600.

7. Bristow MR, Minobe W, Rasmussen R, Hershberger RE, Hoffman BB. α_1-adrenergic receptors in the non-failing and failing human heart. *J Pharmacol Exp Ther*. 1988;247:1039–1045.

8. Landzberg JS, Parker JD, Gauthier DF, Colucci WS. Effects of myocardial α_1-adrenergic receptor stimulation and blockade on contractility in humans. *Circulation*. 1991;84:1608–1614.

9. Gristwood R, Ginsburg R, Zera P. Are alpha-adrenoceptors coupled to contraction in human heart? *Circulation*. 1986;74(Suppl II):374.

10. Harrison JK, Pearson WR, Lynch KR. Molecular characterization of α_1- and β_2-adrenoceptors. *TIPS*. 1991;12:62–67.

11. Michel MC, Brodde OE, Insel PA. Peripheral adrenergic receptors in hypertension. *Hypertension*. 1990;16:107–120.

12. Vago T, Bevilacqua M, Norbiato G, et al. Identification of α_1-adrenergic receptors on sarcolemma from normal subjects and patients with idiopathic dilated cardiomyopathy: characteristics and linkage to GTP-binding protein. *Circ Res*. 1989;64:474–481.

13. van Zwieten PA. Interaction between α- and β-adrenoceptor-mediated cardiovascular effects. *J Cardiovasc Pharmacol*. 1986;8(Suppl 4):S21–S28.

14. Benfey RG. Function of myocardial α-adrenoceptors. *Life Sci*. 1990;46:743–757.

15. Bohm M, Diet F, Feiler G, Kemkes B, Erdmann E. α-Adrenoceptors and α-adrenoceptor-mediated positive inotropic effects in failing human myocardium. *J Cardiovasc Pharmacol*. 1988;12:357–364.

16. Bruckner R, Meyer W, Mugge A, Schmitz W, Scholz H. α-Adrenoceptor-mediated positive inotropic effect of phenylephrine in isolated human ventricular myocardium. *Eur J Pharmacol*. 1984;99:345–347.

17. Schmitz W, Scholz H, Erdmann E. Effects of α- and β-adrenergic agonists, phosphodiesterase inhibitors and adenosine on isolated human heart muscle preparations. *Trends Pharmacol Sci*. 1987;8:447–450.

18. Jakob H, Nawrath H, Rupp J. Adrenoceptor-mediated changes of action potential and force of contraction in human isolated ventricular heart muscle. *Br J Pharmacol*. 1988;94:584–590.

19. Endoh M, Hiramoto T, Ishihata A, Takanashi M, Inui J. Myocardial α_1-adrenoceptors mediate positive inotropic effect and changes in phosphatidylinositol metabolism: species differences in receptor distribution and the intracellular coupling process in mammalian ventricular myocardium. *Circ Res*. 1991;68:1179–1190.

20. Lands AM, Arnold A, McAuliff JP, Luduena FP, Brown TG Jr. Differentiation of receptor systems activated by sympathomimetic amines. *Nature*. 1967;214:597–598.

21. Lands AM, Luduena FP, Buzzo HJ. Differentiation of receptors responsive to isoproternol. *Life Sci*. 1967;6:2241–2249.

22. Emorine LJ, Marullo S, Briend-Sutren MM, et al. Molecular characterization of the human β_3-adrenergic receptor. *Science*. 1989;245:1118–1121.

23. Zaagsma J, Nahorski SR. Is the adipocyte β-adrenoceptor a prototype for the recently cloned atypical β_3-adrenoceptor. *TIPS*. 1990;11:3–7.

24. Dixon RAF, Kobilka BK, Strader DJ, et al. Cloning of the gene and cDNA for mammalian β-adrenergic receptor and homology with rhodopsin. *Nature*. 1986;321:75–79.

25. Yarden Y, Rodriguez H, Wong SK-F, et al. The avian β-adrenergic receptor: primary structure and membrane topology. *Proc Natl Acad Sci USA*. 1986;83:6795–6799.

26. Kobilka BK, Frielle T, Dohlman HG, et al. Delineation of the intronless nature of the genes for the human and hamster β_2-adrenergic receptor and their putative promoter regions. *J Biol Chem*. 1987;262:7321–7327.

27. Frielle T, Collins S, Daniel KW, Caron MG, Lefkowitz RJ, Kobilka BK. Cloning of the cDNA for the human β_1-adrenergic receptor. *Proc Natl Acad Sci USA*. 1987;84:7920–7924.

28. O'Dowd BF, Lefkowitz RJ, Caron MG. Structure of the adrenergic and related receptors. *Annu Rev Neurosci*. 1989;12:67–83.

29. Tota MR, Candelore MR, Dixon RAF, Strader CD. Biophysical and genetic analysis of the ligand-binding site of the β-adrenoceptor. *TIPS*. 1991;12:4–6.

30. Wong SK-F, Slaughter C, Ruoho AE, Ross EM. The catecholamine binding site of the β-adrenergic receptor is formed by juxtaposed membrane-spanning domains. *J Biol Chem*. 1988;263:7925–7928.

31. Kenakin TP. The classification of drugs and drug receptors in isolated tissues. *Pharmacol Rev*. 1984;36:165–221.

32. Ruffolo RR Jr. Important concepts of receptor theory. *J Auton Pharma*. 1982;2:277–295.

33. Birnbaumer L, Abramowitz J, Brown AM. Receptor-effector coupling by G proteins. *Biochim Biophys Acta*. 1990;90:163–224.

34. Fleming JW, Wisler PL, Watanabe AM. Signal transduction by G proteins in cardiac tissues. *Circulation*. 1992;85:420–433.

35. Robishaw JD, Foster KA. Role of G proteins in the regulation of the cardiovascular system. *Annu Rev Physiol*. 1989;51:229–244.

36. Brown AM, Birnbaumer L. Ionic channels and their regulation by G protein subunits. *Annu Rev Physiol*. 1990;52:197–213.

37. Gilman AG. G proteins and regulation of adenylyl cyclase. *JAMA*. 1989;262:1819–1825.

38. Feldman AM. Experimental issues in assessment of G protein function in cardiac disease. *Circulation*. 1991;84:1852–1861.

39. Holmer SR, Homcy CJ. G proteins in the heart: a redundant and diverse transmembrane signaling network. *Circulation*. 1991;84:1891–1902.

40. Yatani A, Brown AM. Rapid beta-adrenergic modula-

tion of calcium channel currents by a fast G protein pathway. *Science.* 1989;245:71–74.

41. Hartzell HC, Mery P-F, Fischmeister R, Szabo G. Sympathetic regulation of cardiac calcium current is due exclusively to cAMP-dependent phosphorylation. *Nature.* 1991;351:573–576.

42. Krupinski J, Coussen F, Bakalyar HA, et al. Adenylyl cyclase amino acid sequence: possible channel- or transporter-like structure. *Science.* 1989;244:1558–1564.

43. Tang WJ, Gilman AG. Type-specific regulation of adenylyl cyclase by G protein βγ subunits. *Science.* 1991;254:1500–1503.

44. Alousi AA, Jasper JR, Insel PA, Motulsky HJ. Stoichiometry of receptor-G$_s$-adenylate cyclase interactions. *FASEB J.* 1991;5:2300–2303.

45. Kleuss C, Hescheler J, Ewel C, Rosenthal W, Schultz G, Wittig B. Assignment of G-protein subtypes to specific receptors inducing inhibition of calcium currents. *Nature.* 1991;353:43–48.

46. Benovic JL, Bouvier M, Caron MG, Lefkowitz RJ. Regulation of adenyl cyclase-coupled β-adrenergic receptors. *Annu Rev Cell Biol.* 1988;4:405–428.

47. Collins S, Bolanowski MA, Caron MG, Lefkowitz RJ. Genetic regulation of β-adrenergic receptors. *Annu Rev Physiol.* 1989;51:203–215.

48. Lefkowitz, RJ, Hausdorff WP, Caron MG. Role of phosphorylation in desensitization of the β-adrenoceptor. *TIPS.* 1990;11:190–194.

49. Lefkowitz RJ, Caron MG. Models for the study of receptors coupled to guanine nucleotide regulatory proteins. *J Biol Chem.* 1988;263:4993–4996.

50. Malbon CC, Hadcock JR, Rapiejko PJ, Ros M, Wang HY, Watkins DC. Regulation of transmembrane signalling elements: transcriptional, post-transcriptional and post-translational controls. *Biochem Soc Symp.* 1990; 56:155–164.

51. Campbell PT, Hnatowich M, O'Dowd BF, Caron MG, Lefkowitz RJ, Hausdorff WP. Mutations of the human β$_2$-adrenergic receptor that impair coupling to Gs interfere with receptor down-regulation but not sequestration. *Mol Pharm.* 1991;39:192–198.

52. Collins S, Altschmied J, Herbsman O, Caron MG, Mellon PL, Lefkowitz RJ. A cAMP response element in the β$_2$-adrenergic receptor gene confers transcriptional autoregulation by cAMP. *J Biol Chem.* 1990;265:19330–19335.

53. Bouvier M, Hnatowich M, Collins S, et al. Expression of a human cDNA encoding the β$_2$-adrenergic receptor in Chinese hamster fibroblasts (CHW): functionality and regulation of the expressed receptors. *Mol Pharm.* 1988;33:133–139.

54. Clark RB, Friedman J, Dixon RAF, Strader CD. Identification of a specific site required for rapid heterologous desensitization of the β-adrenergic receptor by cAMP-dependent protein kinase. *Mol Pharm.* 1989; 36:343–348.

55. Bouvier M, Collins S, O'Dowd BF, et al. Two distinct pathways for cAMP-mediated down-regulation of the β$_2$-adrenergic receptor. *J Biol Chem.* 1989;264:16786–16792.

56. Lefkowitz RJ, Hausdorff WP, Caron MG. Role of phosphorylation in desensitization of the β-adrenoceptor.

TIPS. 1990;2:190–194.

57. Hadcock JR, Wang H, Malbon CC. Agonist-induced destabilization of β-adrenergic receptor mRNA. *J Biol Chem.* 1989;264:19928–19933.

58. Collins S, Caron MG, Lefkowitz RJ. Regulation of adrenergic receptor responsiveness through modulation of receptor gene expression. *Annu Rev Physiol.* 1991;53:497–508.

59. Hadcock JR, Malbon CC. Down-regulation of β-adrenergic receptors: agonist-induced reduction in receptor mRNA levels. *Proc Natl Acad Sci USA.* 1988;85:5021–5025.

60. Mugelli A, Ledda F, Mantelli L, Torrini M, Maccioni T. Studies on the positive inotropic effect of dopamine in the guinea-pig heart. *Naunyn-Schmiedeberg's Arch Pharmacol.* 1977;301:49–55.

61. Brodde O-E, Inui J, Motomura S, Schümann H-J. The mode of direct action of dopamine on the rabbit heart. *J Card Pharm.* 1980;2:567–582.

62. Ruffolo RR Jr, Messick K, Horng JS. Interactions of three inotropic agents, ASL-7022, dobutamine and dopamine, with α- and β-adrenoceptors in vitro. *Naunyn-Schmiedeberg's Arch Pharmacol.* 1984;326:317–326.

63. Brodde O-E, Daul A, Wellstein A, Palm D, Michel MC, Beckeringh JJ. Differentiation of β$_1$- and β$_2$-adrenoceptor-mediated effects in humans. *Am J Physiol.* 1988;254(*Heart Circ Physiol* 23):H199–H206.

64. Carlsson E, Dahlöf CG, Hedberg A, Persson H, Tångstrand B. Differentiation of cardiac chronotropic and inotropic effects of β-adrenoceptor agonists. *Naunyn-Schmiedeberg's Arch Pharmacol.* 1977;300:101–105.

65. Bristow MR, Sandoval AB, Gilbert EM, Deisher T, Minobe W, Rasmussen R. Myocardial α- and β-adrenergic receptors in heart failure: is cardiac-derived norepinephrine the regulatory signal? *Eur Heart J.* 1988;9(Suppl H):35–40.

66. Mukherjee A, Haghani Z, Brady J, et al. Differences in myocardial α- and β-adrenergic receptor numbers in different species. *Am J Physiol.* 1983;245(*Heart Circ Physiol* 14):H957–H961.

67. Bryan LJ, Cole JJ, O'Donnell SR, Wanstall JC. A study designed to explore the hypothesis that *Beta*-1 adrenoceptors are "innervated" receptors and *Beta*-2 adrenoceptors are "hormonal receptors". *J Pharm Exp Ther.* 1981;216:395–400.

68. Bristow MR, Ginsburg R, Minobe W, et al. Decreased catecholamine sensitivity and β-adrenergic-receptor density in failing human hearts. *N Engl J Med.* 1982;307:205–211.

69. Ginsburg R, Bristow MR, Billingham ME, Stinson EB, Schroeder JS, Harrison DC. A study of the normal and failing isolated human heart: decreased response of failing heart to isoproterenol. *Am Heart J.* 1983;106:535–540.

70. Robberecht P, Delhaye M, Taton G, et al. The human heart *beta*-adrenergic receptors. *Mol Pharm* 1983;24: 169–173.

71. Stiles GL, Taylor S, Lefkowitz RJ. Human cardiac beta-adrenergic receptors: subtype heterogeneity delineated by direct radioligand binding. *Life Sci.* 1983;33:467–473.

72. Kaumann AJ, Lemoine H. β$_2$-adrenoceptor-mediated

positive inotropic effect of adrenaline in human ventricular myocardium. *Naunyn-Schmiedeberg's Arch Pharmacol.* 1987;335:403–411.

73. Bristow MR, Hershberger RE, Port JD, Rasmussen R. β_1 and β_2 adrenergic receptor mediated adenylate cyclase stimulation in nonfailing and failing human ventricular myocardium. *Mol Pharm.* 1989;35:295–303.

74. Bristow MR, Ginsburg R, Umans V, et al. β_1- and β_2-adrenergic-receptor subpopulations in nonfailing and failing human ventricular myocardium: coupling of both receptor subtypes to muscle contraction and selective β_1-receptor down-regulation in heart failure. *Circ Res.* 1986;59:297–309.

75. Feldman AM, Cates AE, Veazey WB, et al. Increase of the Mr 40,000 pertussis toxin substrate in the failing human heart. *J Clin Invest.* 1988;82:189–197.

76. Fowler MB, Laser JA, Hopkins GL, Minobe W, Bristow MR. Assessment of the β-adrenergic receptor pathway in the intact failing human heart: progressive receptor down-regulation and subsensitivity to agonist response. *Circulation.* 1986;74:1290–1302.

77. Feldman MD, Copelas L, Gwathmey JK, et al. Deficient production of cyclic AMP: pharmacologic evidence of an important cause of contractile dysfunction in patients with end-stage heart failure. *Circulation.* 1987;75:331–339.

78. Morgan JP. Abnormal intracellular modulation of calcium as a major cause of cardiac contractile dysfunction. *N Engl J Med.* 1991;325:625–632.

79. Hershberger RE, Anderson FL, Bristow MR. Vasoactive intestinal peptide receptor in failing human ventricular myocardium exhibits increased affinity and decreased density. *Circ Res* 1989;65:283–294.

80. Port JD, Gilbert EM, Larrabee P, et al. Neurotransmitter depletion compromises the ability of indirect acting amines to provide inotropic support in the failing human heart. *Circulation.* 1990;81:929–938.

81. Gage J, Rutman H, Lucido D, LeJemtel TH. Additive effects of dobutamine and amrinone on myocardial contractility and ventricular performance in patients with severe heart failure. *Circulation.* 1986;74:367–373.

82. Colucci WS, Denniss AR, Leatherman GF, et al. Intracoronary infusion of dobutamine to patients with and without severe congestive heart failure. *J Clin Invest.* 1988;81:1103–1110.

83. Colucci WS, Leatherman GF, Ludmer PL, Gauthier DF. β-adrenergic inotropic responsiveness of patients with heart failure: studies with intracoronary dobutamine infusion. *Clrc Res.* 1987;61 (Suppl 1):82–86.

84. Port JD, Bristow MR. Lack of spare β-adrenergic receptors in the human heart. *FASEB J.* 1988;2:A602.

85. Neumann J, Schmintz W, Scholz H, Meyerinck L, Doring V, Kalmar P. Increase in myocardial G_i-proteins in heart failure. *Lancet.* 1988;2:936–937.

86. Böhm M, Giershik P, Jakobs KH, Schnable P, Kemkes B, Erdmannt E. Localization of a "postreceptor" defect in human dilated cardiomyopathy. *Am J Cardiol.* 1989;64:812–814.

87. Bristow MR, Anderson FL, Port JD, et al. Differences in β-adrenergic neuroeffector mechanisms in ischemic versus idiopathic dilated cardiomyopathy. *Circulation.* 1991;84:1024–1039.

88. Feldman AM, Ray PE, Silan CM, Mercer JA, Minobe W, Bristow MR. Selective gene expression in failing human heart. *Circulation.* 1991;83:1866–1872.

89. Hershberger RE, Feldman AM, Bristow MR. The A_1 adenosine receptor pathway in failing and nonfailing human heart. *Circulation.* 1991;83:1343–1351.

90. Böhm M, Meyer W, Mügge A, Schmitz W, Scholz H. Functional evidence for the existence of adenosine receptors in the human heart. *Eur J Pharm.* 1985;116:323–326.

91. Böhm M, Pieske B, Ungerer M, Erdmann E. Characterization of A_1 adenosine receptor in atrial and ventricular myocardium from diseased human hearts. *Circ Res.* 1989;65:1201–1211.

92. Hershberger RE, Kimball JA, Meixell, GE, et al. The M_2 muscarinic receptor in failing and nonfailing human ventricular myocardium mediates a negative inotropic response through inhibition of adenylate cyclase, and a positive inotropic response through stimulation of phosphoinositide hydrolysis. In press.

93. Delhaye M, DeSmet JM, Taton G, et al. A comparison between muiscarinic receptor occupancy, adenylate cyclase inhibition, and inotropic response in human heart. *Naunyn-Schmiedeberg's Arch Pharmacol.* 1984;325:170–175.

94. Böhm M, Gierschik P, Jakobs K, et al. Increase of $G_i\alpha$ in human hearts with dilated but not ischemic cardiomyopathy. *Circulation.* 1990;82:1249–1265.

95. Barber MJ, Mueller TM, Felten HD, Zipes DP. Transmural myocardial infarction in the dog produces sympathectomy in noninfarcted myocardium. *Circulation.* 1983;67:787–796.

96. Colucci WS, Ribeiro JP, Rocco MB, et al. Imparied chronotropic response to exercise in patients with congestive heart failure. *Circulation.* 1989;80:314–323.

97. Creager MA, Quigg RJ, Ren CJ, Roddy MA, Colucci WS. Limb vascular responsiveness to β-adrenergic receptor stimulation in patients with congestive heart failure. *Circulation.* 1991;83:1873–1879.

98. Gilbert EM, Hershberger RE, O'Connell JB, Renlund DG, Bristow MR. Additivity of the effects of enoximone and dobutamine in the failing human heart. Submitted.

99. Lee HR, Hershberger RE, Port JD, et al. Low-dose enoximone in subjects awaiting cardiac transplantation. *J Thorac Cardiovasc Surg.* 1991;102:246–258.

100. Unverferth et al. Long term benefit of dobutamine in patients. *Am Heart J.* 1980;100:622–630.

101. Leier CV, Huss P, Lewis RP, et al. Drug induced conditioning in congestive heart failure. *Circulation.* 1982;65:1382–1387.

102. Currie PJ, Kelly MJ, Middlebrook K, et al. Acute intravenous and sustained oral treatment with the beta$_1$ agonist prenalterol in patients with chronic severe cardiac failure. *Br Heart J.* 1984;51:530–538.

103. Dahlström ULF, Areskog M, Wranne B, Karlsson E. Prenalterol as long-term therapy for chronic congestive heart failure. *Acta Med Scand.* 1984; 216:199–207.

104. Roubin GS, Choong CYP, Devenish-Meares S, et al. β-adrenergic stimulation of the failing ventricle: a double-blind, randomized trial of sustained oral therapy with prenalterol. *Circulation.* 1984;69:955–962.

105. Lambertz H, Meyer J, Erbel R. Long-term hemodyna-

mic effects of prenalterol in patients with severe congestive heart failure. *Circulation*. 1984;69:298–305.

106. Glover DR, Wathen CG, Murray RG, Petch MC, Muir AL, Littler WA. Are the clinical benefits of oral prenalterol in ischaemic heart failure due to beta blockade? *Br Heart J*. 1985;53:208–215.

107. Weber KT, Andrews V, Janicki JS, Likoff M, Reichek N. Pirbuterol, an oral beta-adrenergic receptor agonist, in the treatment of chronic cardiac failure. *Circulation*. 1982;66:1262–1267.

108. The German and Austrian Xamoterol Study Group. Double-blind placebo-controlled comparison of digoxin and xamoterol in chronic heart failure. *Lancet*. 1988;1:489–493.

109. The Xamoterol in Severe Heart Failure Study Group. Xamoterol in severe heart failure. *Lancet*. 1990;336:1–6.

110. Farah AE, Alousi AA, Schwarz RP Jr. Positive inotropic agents. *Annu Rev Pharmacol Toxicol*. 1984;24:275–328.

111. Colucci WS, Wright RF, Braunwald E. New positive inotropic agents in the treatment of congestive heart failure. *N Engl J Med*. 1986;314:290–299 (Part 1 of 2).

112. Colucci WS, Wright RF, Braunwald E. New positive inotropic agents in the treatment of congestive heart failure. *N Engl J Med*. 1986;314:349–358 (Part 2 of 2).

113. Fitzpatrick D, Ikram H, Nicholls MG, Espiner EA. Hemodynamic, hormonal and electrolyte responses to prenalterol infusion in heart failure. *Circulation*. 1983;67:613–619.

114. Woodley SL, Gilbert EM, Anderson JL, et al. β-blockade with bucindolol in heart failure caused by ischemic versus idiopathic dilated cardiomyopathy. *Circulation*. 1991;84:2426–2441.

115. Waagstein F, Reiz S, Ariniego R, Hjalmarson A. Clinical results with prenalterol in patients with heart failure. *Am Heart J*. 1981;102:548–554.

116. Kirlin PC, Walton JA Jr, Brymer JF, Beauman G, Pitt B. Hemodynamic and myocardial metabolic effects of the β-agonist prenalterol in ischemic left ventricular dysfunction. *J Cardiol Pharm*. 1984;6:852–858.

117. Wirtzfeld A, Klein G, Bibra HV, Sauer E. Prenalterol: a partial beta₁-adrenoceptor agonist or a beta-blocker with intrinsic activity? *Int J Clin Pharm*. 1985;23:20–27.

118. Sharma B, Hoback J, Francis GS, et al. Pirbuterol: a new oral sympathomimetic amine for the treatment of congestive heart failure. *Am Heart J*. 1981;102:533–541.

119. Colucci WS, Alexander RW, Williams GH, et al. Decreased lymphocyte beta-adrenergic-receptor density in patients with heart failure and tolerance to the beta-adrenergic agonist pirbuterol. *N Engl J Med*. 1981;305:185–190.

120. Dawson JR, Canepa-Anson R, Kuan P, Reuben SR, Poole-Wilson PA, Sutton GC. Symptoms, haemodynamics, and exercise capacity during long term treatment of chronic heart failure. *Br Heart J*. 1983;50:282–289.

121. Canepa-Anson R, Dawson JR, Kuan P, et al. Differences between acute and long-term metabolic and endocrine effects of oral β-adrenoceptor agonist therapy with pirbuterol for cardiac failure. *Br J Clin Pharm*. 1987;23:173–181.

122. Sharma B, Goodwin JF. Beneficial effect of salbutamol on cardiac function in severe congestive cardiomyopathy. *Circulation*. 1978;58:449–460.

123. Mettauer B, Rouleau JL, Burgess JH. Detrimental arrhythmogenic and sustained beneficial hemodynamic effects of oral salbutamol in patients with chronic congestive heart failure. *Am Heart J*. 1985;109:840–847.

124. Wang RYC, Tse TF, Yu DYC, Lee PK, Chow MSS. Beneficial hemodynamic effects of intravenous terbutaline in patients with severe heart failure. *Am Heart J*. 1982;104:1016–1021.

125. Molajo AO, Bennett DH. Effect of xamoterol (ICI 118587), a new beta₁ adrenoceptor partial agonist, on resting haemodynamic variables and exercise tolerance in patients with left ventricular dysfunction. *Br Heart J*. 1985;54:17–21.

126. Marlow HF. Xamoterol, a β₁-adrenoceptor partial agonist: review of the clinical efficacy in heart failure. *Br J Clin Pharm*. 1989;28:23S–30S.

127. Bhatia SJS, Swedberg K, Chatterjee K. Acute hemodynamic and metabolic effects of ICI 118,587 (Corwin), a selective partial beta₁ agonist, in patients with dilated cardiomyopathy. *Am Heart J*. 1986;111:692–696.

128. Schwinger RHG, Böhm M, Erdmann E. The effect of xamoterol in failing human myocardium. *Eur Heart J*. 1990;11:323–327.

129. Hadfield SE, Slee S-J, Snow HM. The cardiovascular pharmacology of xamoterol, cicloprolol, prenalterol and pindolol in the anaesthetised dog. *Br J Clin Pharm*. 1989;28:78S–81S.

130. Brodde O-E, Daul A, Michel-Reher M, et al. Agonist-induced desensitization of β-adrenoceptor function in humans. *Circulation*. 1990;81:914–921.

131. Hicks PE, Cavero I, Manoury P, Lefevre-Borg F, Langer SZ. Comparative analysis of *Beta*-1 adrenoceptor agonist and antagonist potency and selectivity of cicloprolol, xamoterol and pindolol. *J Pharm Exp Ther*. 1987;242:1025–1034.

132. Lemoine H, Bilski A, Kaumann AJ. Xamoterol activates β₁- but not β₂-adrenoceptors in mammalian myocardium: comparison of its affinity for β₁- and β₂-adrenoceptors coupled to the adenylate cyclase in feline and human ventricle with positive inotropic effects. *J Cardiol Pharm*. 1989;13:105–117.

133. Brown MJ, Brown DC, Murphy MB. Hypokalemia from beta₂-receptor stimulation bycirculating epinephrine. *N Engl J Med*. 1983;309:1414–1419.

134. Vincent HH, Boomsma F, Man in't Veld AJ, Derkx FHM, Wenting GJ, Schalekamp MADH. Effects of selective and nonselective β-agonists on plasma potassium and norepinephrine. *J Cardiol Pharm*. 1984;6:107–114.

135. Rajfer SI, Anton AH, Rossen JD, Goldberg LI. Beneficial hemodynamic effects of oral levodopa in heart failure: relation to the generation of dopamine. *N Engl J Med*. 1984;310:1357–1362.

136. Goldberg LI, Rajfer SI. Dopamine receptors: applications in clinical cardiology. *Circulation*. 1985;72:245–248.

137. Fennell WH, Taylor AA, Young JB, et al. Propylbutyldopamine: hemodynamic effects in conscious dogs, normal human volunteers and patients with heart failure. *Circulation*. 1983;67:829–836.

138. Dei Cas L, Manca C, Bernardini B, Vasini G, Visioli O. Noninvasive evaluation of the effects of oral ibopamine

(SB 7505) on cardiac and renal function in patients with congestive heart failure. *J Cardiovasc Pharmacol.* 1982;4:436–440.

139. Dei Cas L, Bolognesi R, Cucchini F, Fappani A, Riva S, Visioli O. Hemodynamic effects of ibopamine in patients with idiopathic congestive cardiomyopathy. *J Cardiovasc Pharmacol.* 1983;5:249–253.

140. Thompson MJ, Huss P, Unverferth DV, Fasola A, Leier CV. Hemodynamic effects of intravenous butopamine in congestive heart failure. *Clin Pharmacol Ther.* 1980;28:324–334.

141. Kino M, Hirota Y, Yamamoto S, et al. Cardiovascular effects of a newly synthesized cardiotonic agent (TA-064) on normal and diseased hearts. *Am J Cardiol.* 1983;51:802–810.

142. Mitchell PD, Smith GW, Wells E, West PA. Inhibition of Uptake$_1$ by dopexamine hydrochloride (*in vitro*). *Br J Pharmacol.* 1987;92:265–270.

143. Leier CV, Binkley PF, Carpenter J, Randolph PH, Unverferth DV. Cardiovascular pharmacology of dopexamine in low output congestive heart failure. *Am J Cardiol.* 1988;62:94–99.

144. Bass AS, Kohli JD, Lubbers N, Goldberg LI. Mechanisms mediating the positive inotropic and chronotropic changes induced by dopexamine in the anesthetized dog. *J Pharm Exp Ther.* 1987;242:940–944.

145. Smith GW, Hall JC, Farmer JB, Simpson WT. The cardiovascular actions of dopexamine hydrochloride, an agonist at dopamine receptors and β_2-adrenoceptors in the dog. *J Pharm Pharmacol.* 1987;39:636–641.

146. Brown RA, Dixon J, Farmer JB, et al. Dopexamine: a novel agonist at peripheral dopamine receptors and β_2-adrenoceptors. *Br J Pharmaol.* 1985;85:599–608.

147. Brown RA, Farmer JB, Hall JC, Humphries RG, O'Connor SE, Smith GW. The effects of dopexamine on the cardiovascular system of the dog. *Br J Pharmacol.* 1985;85:609–619.

148. Jaski BE, Wijns W, Foulds R, Serruys PW. The haemodynamic and myocardial effects of dopexamine: a new β_2-adrenoceptor and dopaminergic agonist. *Br J Clin Pharmacol.* 1986;21:393–400.

149. DeMarco T, Kwasman M, Lau D, Chatterjee K. Dopexamine hydrochloride in chronic congestive heart failure with improved cardiac performance without increased metabolic cost. *Am J Cardiol.* 1988;62:57C–62C.

150. Colardyn FA, Vandenbogaerde JF. Use of dopexamine hydrochloride in intensive care patients with low-output left ventricular heart failure. *Am J Cardiol.* 1988;62:68C–72C.

151. Tan L-B, Littler WA, Murray RG. Beneficial haemodynamic effects of intravenous dopexamine in patients with low-output heart failure. *J Cardiovasc Pharmacol.* 1987;10:280–286.

152. Bayliss J, Thomas L, Poole-Wilson P. Acute hemodynamic and neuroendocrine effects of dopexamine, a new vasodilator for the treatment of heart failure: comparison with dobutamine, captopril, and nitrate. *J Cardiovasc Pharmacol.* 1987;9:551–554.

153. Dawson JR, Thompson DS, Signy M, et al. Acute haemodynamic and metabolic effects of dopexamine, a new dopaminergic receptor agonist in patients with chronic heart failure. *Br Heart J.* 1985;54:313–20.

154. Gollub SB, Emmot WW, Johnson DE. Hemodynamic effects of dopexamine hydrochloride infusions of 48 to 72 hours' duration for severe congestive heart failure. *Am J Cardiol.* 1988;62:83C–88C.

155. Leier CV, Binkley PF. Acute positive inotropic intervention: the catecholamines. *Am Heart J.* 1991;121:1866–1870.

156. Leier CV, Unverferth DV, Kates RE. The relationship between plasma dobutamine concentrations and cardiovascular responses in cardiac failure. *Am J Med.* 1979;66:238–242.

157. Leier CV. Regional blood flow responses to vasodilators and inotropes in congestive heart failure. *Am J Cardiol.* 1988;62:86E–93E.

158. Leier CV, Heban PT, Huss P, Bush CA, Lewis RP. Comparative systemic and regional hemodynamic effects of dopamine and dobutamine in patients with cardiomyopathic heart failure. *Circulation.* 1978;58:466–475.

159. Loeb HS, Bredakis J, Gunnar RM. Superiority of dobutamine over dopamine for augmentation of cardiac output in patients with chronic low output cardiac failure. *Circulation.* 1977;55:375–381.

160. Tuttle RR, Mills J. Development of a new catecholamine to selectively increase cardiac contractility. *Circ Res.* 1975;36:185–196.

161. Ruffolo RR Jr, Spradlin TA, Pollock GD, Waddell JE, Murphy PJ. *Alpha* and *beta* adrenergic effects of the stereoisomers of dobutamine. *J Pharm Exp Ther.* 1981;219:447–452.

162. Ruffolo RR Jr, Messick K. Effects of dopamine, (±)-dobutamine and the (+)- and (−)-enentiomers of dobutamine on cardiac function in pithed rats. *J Pharm Exp Ther.* 1985;235:558–565.

163. Williams RS, Bishop T. Selectivity of dobutamine for adrenergic receptor subtypes. *J Clin Invest.* 1981;6:1703–1711.

164. Leier CV, Webel J, Bush CA. The cardiovascular effects of the continuous infusion of dobutamine in patients with severe cardiac failure. *Circulation.* 1977;56:468–472.

165. Unverferth DV, Blanford M, Kates RE, Leier CV. Tolerance to dobutamine after a 72 hour continuous infusion. *Am J Med.* 1980;69:262–266.

166. Leier CV, Unverferth DV. Drugs five years later: dobutamine. *Ann Intern Med.* 1983;99:490–496.

167. Sundram P, Reddy HK, McElroy PA, Janicki JS, Weber KT. Myocardial energetics and efficiency in patients with idiopathic cardiomyopathy: response to dobutamine and amrinone. *Am Heart J.* 1990;119:891–898.

168. Chatterjee K. *Dobutamine.* New York: NCM Publishers; 1989.

169. Maccarrone C, Malta E, Raper C. β-adrenoceptor selectivity of dobutamine: *in vivo* and *in vitro* studies. *J Cardiovasc Pharmacol.* 1984;6:132–141.

170. Wollmering MM, Wiechmann RJ, Port JD, Hershberger RE, Focaccio A, Bristow MR. Dobutamine is a partial agonist with an intrinsic activity of 0.5 in human myocardium. *J Am Coll Cardiol.* 1991;17:283A.

171. Hayes JS, Bowling N, Pollock GD. Effects of *beta* adrenoceptor down-regulation on the cardiovascular responses to the stereoisomers of dobutamine. *J Pharm Exp Ther.* 1985;235:58–65.

172. Hayes JS, Bowling N. Role of the *alpha* agonist activity of dobutamine in mediating cardiac output: effects of prolonged isoproterenol infusion. *J Pharm Exp Ther*. 1987;241:861–869.

173. Landzberg JS, Parker JD, Gauthier DF, Colucci WS. Does the levo isomer of dobutamine exert a positive inotropic effect in man via stimulation of α-adrenergic receptors? *Circulation*. 1991;84(suppl II):242.

174. Colucci WS, Denniss AR, Quigg R, Leatherman GF, Rocco MB, Gauthier DF. Lack of positive inotropic effect of alpha-adrenergic receptor stimulation by dobutamine in patients with congestive heart failure. *Circulation*. 1987;76(Suppl IV):IV-71.

175. Benotti JR, McCue JE, Alpert JS. Comparative vasoactive therapy for heart failure. *Am J Cardiol*. 1985;56:19B–24B.

176. Binkley PF, Van Fossen DB, Nunziata E, Unverferth DV, Leier CV. Influence of positive inotropic therapy on pulsatile hydraulic load and ventricular-vascular coupling in congestive heart failure. *J Am Coll Cardiol*. 1990;15:1127–1135.

177. Binkley PF, Murray KD, Watson KM, Myerowitz PD, Leier CV. Dobutamine increase cardiac output of the total artificial heart: implications for vascular contribution of inotropic agents to augment ventricular function. *Circulation*. 1991;84:1210–1215.

178. David S, Zaks JM. Arrhythmias associated with intermittent outpatient dobutamine infusion. *J Vasc Dis*. 1986;37:86–91.

179. Krell MJ, Kline EM, Bates ER, et al. Intermittent, ambulatory dobutamine infusions in patients with severe congestive heart failure. *Am Heart J*. 1986;112:787–791.

180. Waagstein R, Hjalmarson Ä, Varnauskas E, Wallentin I. Effect of chronic beta-adrenergic receptor blockade in congestive cardiomyopathy. *Br Heart J*. 1975;37:1022–1036.

181. Swedberg K, Hjalmarson A, Waagstein F, Wallentin I. Beneficial effects of long-term beta-blockade in congestive cardiomyopathy. *Br Heart J*. 1980;44:117–133.

182. Stephen SA. Unwanted effects of propranolol. *Am J Cardiol*. 1966;18:463–472.

183. Bristow MR. The adrenergic nervous system in heart failure. *N Eng J Med*. 1984,311:850–851.

184. Bristow MR, Kantrowitz NE, Ginsburg R, Fowler MB. β-adrenergic function in heart muscle disease and heart failure. *J Mol Cell Cardiol*. 1985;17(Suppl 2):41–52.

185. Currie PJ, Kelly MJ, McKenzie A, et al. Oral beta-adrenergic blockade with metoprolol in chronic severe dilated cardiomyopathy. *J Am Coll Cardiol*. 1984;3:203–209.

186. Pratt C, Lichstein E. Ventricular antiarrhythmic effects of beta adrenergic blocking drugs: a review of mechanism and clinical studies. *J Clin Pharmacol*. 1982;22:335–347.

187. Woosley RL, Kornauser D, Smith R, et al. Suppression of chronic ventricular arrhythmias with propranolol. *Circulation*. 1980;60:819–827.

188. Downing SE, Lee JC. Contribution of α-adrenoceptor activation to the pathogenesis of norepinephrine cardiomyopathy. *Circ Res*. 1983;52:471–478.

189. Tanaka M, Tsuchihashi Y, Katsume H, Ijichi H, Ibata Y. Comparison of cardiac lesions induced in rats by isoproterenol and by repeated stress of restraint and water immersion with special reference to etiology of cardiomyopathy. *Jpn Circ J*. 1980;44:971–980.

190. Blaiklock RG, Hirsh EM, Dapson S, Paino B, Lehr D. Epinephrine induced myocardial necrosis: effects of aminophylline and adrenergic blockade. *Res Comm Chem Path Pharm*. 1981;34:179–192.

191. Snavely MD, Mahan LC, O'Connor DT, Insel PA. Selective down-regulation of adrenergic receptor subtypes in tissues from rats with pheochromocytoma. *Endocrinology*. 1983;113:354–361.

192. Rosenbaum JS, Ginsburg R, Billingham ME, Hoffman BB. Effects of adrenergic receptor antagonists on cardiac morphological and functional alterations in rats harboring pheochromocytoma. *J Pharm Exp Ther*. 1987;241:354–360.

193. Van Vliet PD, Burchell HB, Titus JL. Focal myocarditis associated with pheochromocytoma. *N Engl J Med*. 1966;274:1102–1108.

194. Kline IK. Myocardial alterations associated with pheochromocytomas. *Am J Pathol*. 1961;38:539–551.

195. Schaffer MS, Zuberbuhler P, Wilson G, Rose V, Duncan WJ, Rowe RD. Catecholamine cardiomyopathy: an unusual presentation of pheochromocytoma in children. *J Pediatrics*. 1981;99:276–279.

196. Raab W. Neurogenic multifocal destruction of myocardial tissue (pathogenic mechanism and its prevention). *Rev Can Biol*. 1963;22:217–239.

197. Simons M, Evans Downing S. Coronary vasoconstriction and catecholamine cardiomyopathy. *Am Heart J*. 1985;109:297–304.

198. Kahn DS, Rona G, Chappel Cl. Isoproterenol-induced cardiac necrosis. *Ann NY Acad Sci*. 1969;156:285–293.

199. Ferrans VJ, Hibbs RG, Black WC, Weilbaecher DG. Isoproterenol-induced myocardial necrosis: a histochemical and electron microscopic study. *Am Heart J*. 1964;68:71–90.

200. Rona G, Chappel CI, Balazs T, Gaudry R. An infact-like myocardial lesion and other toxic manifestations produced by isoproterenol in the rat. *Arc Pathol*. 1959;67:443–455.

201. Yates JC, Beamish RE, Dhalla NS. Ventricular dysfunction and necrosis produced by adrenochrome metabolite of epinephrine: relation to pathogenesis of catecholamine cardiomyopathy. *Am Heart J*. 1981;102:210–221.

202. Muller E. Histochemical studies on the experimental heart infarction in the rat. *Naunyn-Schmiedeberg's Arch Pharmacol*. 1966;254:439–447.

203. Mann DL, Kent RL, Parsons B, Cooper G. Adrenergic effects on the biology of the adult mammalian cardiocyte. *Circulation*. 1992;85:790–804.

204. Ikram H, Fitzpatrick D. Double-blind trial of chronic oral beta blockade in congestive cardiomyopathy. *Lancet*. 1981;1:490–492.

205. Engelmeier RS, O'Connell JB, Walsh R, Rad N, Scanlon PJ, Gunnar RM. Improvement in symptoms and exercise tolerance by metoprolol in patients with dilated cardiomyopathy: a double-blind, randomized, placebo-controlled trial. *Circulation*. 1985;72:536–546.

206. Anderson JL, Lutz JR, Gilbert EM, et al. A randomized trial of low-dose beta-blockade therapy for idiopathic dilated cardiomyopathy. *Am J Cardiol*. 1985;55:471–475.

207. Heilbrunn SM, Shah P, Bristow MR, Valantine HA, Ginsburg R, Fowler MB. Increased β-receptor density and improved hemodynamic response to catecholamine stimulation during long-term metoprolol therapy in heart failure from dilated cardiomyopathy. *Circulation*. 1989; 79:483–490.

208. Gilbert EM, Olsen SL, Mealey P, Volkman K, Larrabee P, Bristow MR. Is β-receptor up-regulation necessary for improved LV function in dilated cardiomyopathy? *Circulation*. 1991;84(Suppl II):469.

209. Waagstein F, Caidahl K, Wallentin I, Bergh CH, Hjalmarson Å. Long-term β-blockade in dilated cardiomyopathy. *Circulation*. 1989;80:551–563.

210. Nemanich JW, Veith RC, Abrass IB, Stratton JR. Effects of metoprolol on rest and exercise cardiac function and plasma catecholamines in chronic congestive heart failure secondary to ischemic or idiopathic cardiomyopathy. *Am J Cardiol*. 1990;66:843–848.

211. Gilbert EM, Anderson JL, Deitchman D, et al. Long-term β-blocker vasodilator therapy improves cardiac function in idiopathic dilated cardiomyopathy: a double-blind, randomized study of bucindolol versus placebo. *Am J Med*. 1990;88:223–229.

212. Eichhorn EJ, Bedotto JB, Malloy CR, et al. Effect of β-adrenergic blockade on myocardial function and energetics in congestive heart failure. *Circulation*. 1990,82:473–483.

213. Pollock SG, Lystash J, Tedesco C, Craddock G, Smucker ML. Usefulness of bucindolol in congestive heart failure. *Am J Cardiol*. 1990;66:603–607.

214. Leung WH, Lau CP, Wong CK, Cheng CH, Tai YT, Lim SP. Improvement in exercise performance and hemodynamics by labetalol in patients with idiopathic dilated cardiomyopathy. *Am Heart J*. 1990;119:884–890.

215. Hershberger RE, Wynn JR, Sundberg L, Bristow MR. Mechanism of action of bucindolol in human ventricular myocardium. *J Cardiovasc Pharmacol*. 1990;15:959–967.

216. Deitchman D, Perhach JL, Snyder RW. β-adrenoceptor and cardiovascular effects of MJ 13105 (bucindolol) in anesthetized dogs and rats. *Eur J Pharmacol*. 1980; 61:263–277.

217. Leff AR, Garrity ER, Munoz NM, et al. Selectivity of the intrinsic sympathomimetic activity of the β-adrenergic blocking drug bucindolol. *J Cardiovasc Pharmacol*. 1984;6:859–866.

218. Stanton HC, Dungan KW. In vitro effects of beta adrenoceptor agonists and antagonists on the rat ovarian suspensory ligament. *J Pharmacol Exp Ther*. 1986;239:591–596.

219. Andersson B, Blomstrom-Lundqvist C, Hedner T, Waagstein F. Exercise hemodynamics and myocardial metabolism during long-term beta-adrenergic blockade in severe heart failure. *J Am Coll Cardiol*. 1991;18:1059–1066.

219a. Waagstein F, Bristow MR, Swedberg K, Camerini F, Fowler MB, Silver MA, Gilbert EM, Johnson MR, Goss FG, Hjalmarson A, for the Metroprolol in Dilated Cardiomyopathy (MDC) Trial Study Group. Beneficial effects of metoprolol in idiopathic dilated cardiomyopathy. Lancet 1993;342:1331–46.

219b. Packer M, Bristow MR, Cohn JN, Colucci WS, Fowler MB, Gilbert EM. The effect of carvedilol on morbidity and mortality in patients with chronic heart failure. N Engl J Med 1996;334:1349–38.

219c. Feuerstein GZ, Ruffolo RR. Carvedilol: preclinical profile and rationale for its use in hypertension, coronary syndromes and congestive heart failure. CVR&R October 1996:27–38.

220. Sponer G, Strein K. Müller-Beckman B, Tartsch W. Studies on the mode of vasodilating action of carvedilol. *J Cardiovasc Pharmacol*. 1987;10(Suppl 11):S42–48.

221. Rimele TJ, Aarhus LL, Lorenz RR, Rooke TW, Vanhoutte PM. Pharmacology of bucindolol in isolated canine vascular smooth muscle. *J Pharmacol Exp Ther*. 1984;231:317–325.

222. Anderson JL, Gilbert EM, O'Connell JB, et al. Long-term (2 year) beneficial effects of beta-adrenergic blockade with bucindolol in patients with idiopathic dilated cardiomyopathy. *J Am Coll Cardiol*. 1991;17:1373–1381.

223. Weiner N. Drugs that inhibit adrenergic nerves and block adrenergic receptors. In: Goodman Gilman A, Goodman LS, Rall TW, Murad F, eds. *The Pharmacological Basis of Therapeutics*. New York: Macmillan 1985:181–214.

26
Phosphodiesterase Inhibitors in Heart Failure: An Overview

Barry F. Uretsky

The introduction into clinical medicine of amrinone, the first intravenously and orally active phosphodiesterase inhibitor, was heralded as a potentially important advance in the treatment of heart failure.[1] Simultaneously, fears regarding the use of this and other agents in this class were raised.[2] To some extent both these expectations and fears have been realized in clinical studies completed over the past 14 years. The common feature of agents in this class is the inhibition, particularly in the myocardium and peripheral vasculature, of a cyclic adenosine monophosphate (cAMP)-specific phosphodiesterase. Despite a major difference in chemical structure, agents in this class are more similar than disparate in their hemodynamic and clinical effects. This chapter discusses characteristics of the class and describes some unique characteristics of individual agents. Specific features are discussed for the intravenous bipyridines amrinone and milrinone, which are currently commercially available and in clinical use in many parts of the world and the imidazalone enoximone, which is in clinical use in Europe. Because it is unlikely that the oral forms of these compounds will be clinically employed in the near future, only an overview of completed clinical trials on the oral compounds are reviewed.

Mechanism of the Inotropic and Vasodilating Effects of Phosphodiesterase Inhibitors

It has been proposed that the generation of increased levels of cAMP by inhibition of its breakdown to 5'-AMP by a specific cAMP phosphodiesterase inhibitor subtype is the mechanism by which phosphodiesterase inhibitors produce their inotropic effect.[3–18] Studies have demonstrated a correlation between the concentration of intracellular cAMP after phosphodiesterase inhibition and the myocardial contractile state.[3–18,20] In myocardial cells cAMP has actions that enhance both contraction and relaxation. cAMP phosphorylates a sarcolemmal protein kinase that increases calcium conductance through the calcium channel. Increased calcium uptake by the sarcoplasmic reticulum is enhanced by cAMP phosphorylation of protein components in this structure. These two actions summate to increase calcium availability during electrical depolarization.

The concentration of intracellular calcium is a major determinant of the strength of contraction of the individual myocyte. Intracellular calcium concentration increases both by extracellular calcium passing through the calcium channel during electrical depolarization and by release of much larger stores of calcium from the sarcoplasmic reticulum, probably as a secondary effect of increased intracellular calcium concentration during depolarization ("calcium-triggered calcium release"). cAMP also decreases the affinity of calcium for the regulatory protein troponin, in particular the subunit troponin I.[16] This action in effect increases the speed of actin-myosin uncoupling, which in an intact ventricle may lead to an increase in the rate of active relaxation.

Increasing cAMP concentration in the smooth muscle of the vasculature, particularly the arterioles, results in smooth muscle relaxation.[21–23] This effect appears to be related to lowering of intracellular calcium. It has been proposed that cAMP phosphorylates a calcium-dependent adenosine triphosphatase (ATPase) in the sarcoplasmic reticulum, which in turn increases calcium sequestration in this organelle. This sequestered calcium is then extruded extracellularly by an unknown mechanism. cAMP also phosphorylates myosin kinase, thereby decreasing its affinity to bind with calcium and the regulatory protein calmodulin.[19] This complex is required to activate myosin to crosslink with actin for smooth muscle contraction. Recent data also suggest that cAMP activates cyclic guanosine monophosphate (cGMP)-dependent protein kinases that decrease intracellular calcium concentration.[24]

cAMP as a Potential Cell Poison

It has been suggested, based on experimental data, that excessive concentrations of intracellular cAMP are toxic to the myocardial cell and may stimulate clinically relevant arrhythmias.[25–29] Based on current data, this statement must be considered as a hypothesis. Abnormalities induced by increased levels of cAMP may be related more to increasing intracellular calcium or phosphorylation of proteins that produce unwanted effects rather than the direct effects of cAMP itself. Stated another way, if increased intracellular calcium is the culprit, then all positive inotropic drugs rather than only drugs that increase cAMP may be implicated in disrupting cell homeostasis and producing deleterious effects.[30]

Limitations of Intracellular cAMP in Myopathic Cells

Beta agonists and phosphodiesterase inhibitors show diminished inotropic effects in isolated human myopathic tissue whereas calcium and digitalis compounds demonstrate increases in developed tension comparable to normal tissue.[2,31–35] Developed tension with phosphodiesterase inhibitors can be increased by agents that stimulate adenylate cyclase, such as forskolin.[31] With addition of various phosphodiesterase inhibitors after stimulating adenylate cyclase, concentrations of intracellular cAMP are similar in normal and diseased hearts.[4] Thus, the decreased efficacy of phosphodiesterase inhibitors in failing myocardium appears to be secondary to a deficiency in cAMP generation, which in turn may be related to the phenomenon of beta receptor "downregulation" in heart failure and/or an increased activity of the adenylate cyclase–linked inhibitor G protein.[36] As a result of a decrease in maximal cAMP stimulation with phosphodiesterase inhibition alone, the maximal inotropic response in human heart failure is less than expected. In fact, in some studies, the inotropic effects of at least one phosphodiesterase inhibitor, amrinone, were so unimpressive that the authors attributed the entire hemodynamic effect to peripheral vasodilation.[37–39,48]

Positive Inotropic Effects of Phosphodiesterase Inhibitors

The positive inotropic effects of phosphodiesterase inhibitors have been amply demonstrated in isolated muscle strips, isolated heart, and whole animal preparations in both normal and heart failure models.[41–46,48] There are differences in the sensitivity of inotropy among different species; the rat is particularly resistant to the positive inotropic effect of phosphodiesterase inhibitors.[43,47] In humans positive inotropy has been demonstrated by increases in peak left ventricular positive dp/dt, a shift to the left of the end-systolic pressure/volume relationship, and noninvasively by a shift of the end-systolic pressure/dimension relationship.[1,49–55] The magnitude of the positive inotropic effect is diminished significantly in heart failure patients compared to normals, which in turn may be related in part to the relative decrease in cAMP production in myocardial cells.[31]

Improvement in the contractile state with phosphodiesterase inhibitors is dose-related.[46,51,56,57] The difference in phosphodiesterase inhibitor effect probably is related to the amount of cAMP-specific phosphodiesterase present in the myocardium of different species.[47] Humans appear to be moderately sensitive to the effects of phosphodiesterase inhibitors.

Positive Lusitropic Effects of Phosphodiesterase Inhibitors

An increase in contractile state with an inotropic agent does not necessarily mean that ventricular relaxation (lusitropy) will be enhanced. In experimental studies there are multiple examples of divergence between effects on contraction and relaxation. For example, with an experimental agent that causes increased calcium entry through the calcium channel during depolarization, the contractile state is increased but relaxation is unchanged.[58] In muscle strip and isolated heart preparations, phosphodiesterase inhibitors enhance the rate of relaxation probably through their effects on tropinin I.[12,42] In human studies, measurement of intrinsic diastolic properties including relaxation are somewhat problematic. With this limitation in mind, it has been shown that phosphodiesterase inhibitors do, in fact, increase the rate of ventricular relaxation (using the time constant of relaxation measured invasively) and the peak filling rate (derived from radionuclide ventriculography).[59–61]

Vasodilation by Phosphodiesterase Inhibitors

In isolated arterial strips application of phosphodiesterase inhibitors produces vasorelaxation.[23,62] In animal preparations, in normal humans, and in patients with heart failure, arterial vasodilation has been demonstrated.[53,63,64] Similar to the inotropic effects, vascular effects of phosphodiesterase inhibitors are dose-related. It has been suggested based on lowering of right atrial pressure in animal and human studies that phosphodiesterase inhibitors produce venodilation. Studies of milrinone injected intraarterially in heart failure patients suggest the possibility of some degree of venodilation.[67] At present, data do not allow differentiation of a primary effect from a secondary effect due to reflex sympathetic withdrawal. In isolated aortic strips application of digoxin before milrinone attenuates vasodilation.[65] A similar attenuation of milrinone-induced vasodilation has been observed in patients with heart failure.[66]

Electrophysiologic Effects of Phosphodiesterase Inhibitors

By acting directly on cells of the sinus node, phosphodiesterase inhibitors will increase the spontaneous rate of sinus node firing.[68,69] In animal and human studies, this effect is dose related, and may take on clinical significance at the upper end of the dosing scale.[57,70] Acute oral dosing in heart failure patients has demonstrated a dose-related increase in heart rate, which was not observed in one long-term controlled trial of an oral phosphodiesterase inhibitor.[57,71] Phosphodiesterase inhibitors will modestly enhance both normal atrioventricular (AV) nodal conduction[68,72,73] and conduction in depressed canine Purkinje fibers.[68] The effect of phosphodiesterase inhibition on other electrophysiological properties in normal animals and man is rather modest.

Addition of amrinone to individual myocytes produces an increase in spontaneous ectopy.[74] Programmed electrical stimulation in heart failure patients using phosphodiesterase inhibitors has suggested in some studies that arrhythmia inducibility is enhanced whereas in others it has not.[72–76] Lynch et al. have demonstrated in an animal model that phosphodiesterase inhibitors will facilitate the development of refractory ventricular fibrillation after an acute ischemic insult despite an inability to induce sustained ventricular arrhythmias in the preischemic state.[83] Uncontrolled clinical experience and controlled clinical trials in heart failure patients have suggested an increase in ambient ventricular arrhythmias with both intravenous and oral preparations.[72,73,77–81]

Hemodynamic Effects of Phosphodiesterase Inhibitors in Heart Failure

The hemodynamic effects of phosphodiesterase inhibitors in animal models of heart failure and humans with heart failure can be predicted by their inotropic, chronotropic, and vasodilating actions. It has been difficult to determine precisely the percentage of the hemodynamic effect that is caused by the positive inotropic as opposed to the vasodilating actions of the drug, and it is likely to be different in individual patients.

Cardiac output increases, primarily because of an increase in stroke volume, but also in most clinical studies because of some increase in heart rate.[1,51,53,55,56,83–85] Left and right ventricular filling pressures decrease as does the pulmonary artery pressure. Left ventricular stroke work increases and mean arterial pressure usually decreases. Intravenous and oral forms of these compounds have qualitatively similar hemodynamic effects.[85] Differences in maximal effects between dosage forms are likely due to pharmacokinetic issues such as absorption rates, peak blood levels, etc. For example, in one study of intravenous enoximone using approximately 6 mg/kg, the peak increase in cardiac output was 76%.[56] The same group of investigators used 6 mg/kg orally and found only a 28% peak increase in cardiac output and also found that 3 mg/kg produced the same degree of improvement and comparable blood levels.[86] These findings suggest a limitation in absorption of enoximone. Another group of investigators found that when oral enoximone was given in repetitive hourly doses the peak cardiac output from oral dosing equaled that obtained by intravenous dosing.[85] The major determinant of the hemodynamic effects of these agents appears to be the amount of phosphodiesterase inhibitor reaching the effector sites. The hemodynamic effects of phosphodiesterase inhibitors appear sustained in most but not all studies, both with prolonged (48 hr) intravenous infusion and long-term (6–12 weeks) oral dosing.[80,86,87,91,92,94–96]

Hormonal Effects of Phosphodiesterase Inhibitors

The effects of phosphodiesterase inhibitors on neurohormonal activation in most studies are not striking.[99–101,106] Beta agonists stimulate renin release; this response may be mediated by increased intracellular concentrations of cAMP.[97,98] In man, phosphodiesterase inhibitors appear to increase renin secretion in some studies but not in others,[99–101] an increase in plasma renin activity is particularly evident when phosphodiesterase inhibitor decreases systemic arterial (renal perfusion) pressure, a well known stimulus for renin release.[99] Sympathetic nervous system activity as judged by plasma norepinephrine does not appear to be consistently affected, nor does arginine vasopressin secretion.[99,100] Atrial natriuretic peptide decreases, probably related to atrial unloading.[100–102]

Response of Regional Blood Flow to Phosphodiesterase Inhibitors

In normal rats, milrinone at low doses increases blood flow to brain and myocardium, and at higher doses to liver, to a lesser extent to muscle, and to a slight but not significant degree to the kidneys.[53] As pointed out by Drexler et al., the improvements seen in regional flow at high doses may be difficult to achieve clinically because of the decrease in systemic pressure that may occur at doses that improve these regional flows.[64] In a model of right ventricular failure, Liang et al. showed that milrinone increases myocardial, renal, and splanchnic blood flow.[103] Interestingly, skeletal muscle blood flow fell in this study, which the investigators attributed to a substantial decrease in systemic arterial pressure and secondary activation of the sympathetic nervous system.[103] In patients with heart failure, milrinone and enoximone have been shown to increase blood flow preferentially to the periphery, particularly the skeletal muscles.[104-106] Renal and liver blood flows remain unchanged with enoximone.[93,104]

Myocardial Oxygen Consumption with Phosphodiesterase Inhibitors

A concern with the use of any positive inotropic agent is its effect on myocardial oxygen consumption (MV02). With the possible exception of the "calcium-sensitizing" group of inotropic agents,[107] all other classes should increase MV02 in individual myocytes. In the intact animal or human, predicting the effect of any positive inotropic agent is more difficult because of its often opposing effects on the determinants of MV02. Phosphodiesterase inhibitors may increase oxygen consumption secondary to their positive inotropic effects and an increase in heart rate or decrease it by virtue of their unloading effects and/or reflex withdrawal of neurohumoral activation.

In an animal model of acute ischemic heart failure, amrinone was shown to improve hemodynamics while decreasing MV02.[108] There are some conflicting data on the effect of phosphodiesterase inhibitors on MV02 in heart failure patients. Groups of heart failure patients given various phosphodiesterase inhibitors have shown a small decrease, no change, or slight to moderate increase in MV02.[64,109-113] In individual patients the balance may be unfavorable and MV02 may rise.[110,113] In fact, in susceptible individuals myocardial ischemia may develop.[36,89] As high as 10% to 20% of patients may be adversely affected. Based on these data, it is suggested that the lowest hemodynamically effective dose be utilized to minimize the possibility of the development of myocardial ischemia. Hasenfuss et al. have shown that

in patients with idiopathic dilated cardiomyopathy and congestive heart failure, MV02 decreases with enoximone.[115] Compared to the pure vasodilator nitroprusside, however, the slope of MV02 versus systolic stress time integral is less steep with enoximone, suggesting the energy cost from positive inotropy.

An interesting, and not altogether intuitive, result has been found utilizing the phosphodiesterase inhibitor enoximone in patients with angina pectoris. In a study by Thormann et al., the threshold for pacing-induced angina pectoris actually increased.[11] Although the mechanism for this response is unknown, it may be a result of the unloading effects of enoximone.

Comparison to Other Agents in Heart Failure

Intravenous phosphodiesterase inhibitors have been compared to other intravenous agents in the treatment of heart failure. It is important to qualify comparisons by describing the method by which drugs are compared. If the question is "Which drug is more effective in decreasing the pulmonary wedge pressure?", the question should be qualified to ask, for example, which drug is more effective at the *same* cardiac output, blood pressure, etc. It might be expected that in comparison to agents with predominant inotropic activity such as dobutamine, phosphodiesterase inhibitors may decrease the systemic arterial pressure and ventricular filling pressures to a greater extent at comparable increases in cardiac output. Several investigators have confirmed these expected findings.[99,114,117] With a predominant unloading agent such as nitroprusside, one might expect that at identical decreases in pulmonary wedge pressure the cardiac output or stroke work (from the inotropic effect of the phosphodiesterase inhibitor) might be greater with phosphodiesterase inhibitors. This prediction also has been confirmed.[51,118]

Phosphodiesterase Inhibitors in Combination with Other Intravenous Agents

Phosphodiesterase inhibitors have been studied in combination with other agents in patients with severe but relatively compensated heart failure and in patients whose clinical status approximates what one might observe in patients actually requiring these agents in clinical practice.[119-122] Both amrinone and enoximone have been shown to have additive hemodynamic effects to dobutamine.[119-122] Experimental data suggest that this potentiation decreases with worsening heart failure.[148] Additionally, the combination of amrinone to dobutamine has additive effects on renin secretion.[63] Phosphodiesterase inhibitors have been used with nitroprusside in patients with severe heart failure.[112] This combination must be used cautiously in view of the vasodilating aspect of both drugs, which together may provoke clinically significant hypotension.

Support of the Failing Circulation with Intravenous Phosphodiesterase Inhibitors

These agents are indicated for the short-term support of the failing circulation. All should be given under electrocardiographic monitoring. Their use, as is the case with dobutamine, has not been established as long-term intravenous therapy in an out-of-hospital setting.[123] Such use may be considered in an individual patient who is refractory to oral agents but data are lacking at present to justify this approach, which, based on published data on dobutamine and oral milrinone, may increase the risk of sudden death.[25,123,151] It is also important to note that all three phosphodiesterase inhibitors have a relatively long half-life in heart failure patients.[124] Thus, if an individual patient has an adverse effect (e.g., hypotension), reversal may require some time (i.e., minutes to hours).

Amrinone

Amrinone and its congener, milrinone, are bipyridines. Amrinone is the only intravenous phosphodiesterase inhibitor with wide clinical experience. Amrinone has been shown to produce salutary hemodynamic effects in decompensated patients with chronic heart failure due to systolic dysfunction and in acute heart failure after bypass surgery.[125-127] It has also been used as a "bridge" (i.e, stabilizing factor) to heart transplantation.[122-128] Data on the use of any phosphodiesterase inhibitor including amrinone after myocardial infarction are limited.

The effect of all phosphodiesterase inhibitors including amrinone appear to be sustained for at least 48 hr (i.e., no obvious "tachyphylaxis"), a phenomenon that has been described with pure beta agonists.[80,129]

The adverse effects of intravenous amrinone include liver function abnormalities, fever, and nausea.[88] Probably the side effect of greatest concern with short-term use is the development of thrombocytopenia.[88] The exact incidence of this complication in the group of patients who actually receive this agent is unknown. It has been reported to be in the range of 7% in a large company-sponsored study,[88] but it is the impression of this author that the incidence is higher.

Amrinone has a rather long elimination half-life in

normals ($T\frac{1}{2}$ = 2.5 hr) and much longer (3–15 hr) in heart failure patients.[90] Dosing requires a bolus (usually 0.5–0.75 mg/kg) and continuous infusion (2.5–20 μg/kg/min). Possible drug accumulation over time may increase hemodynamic effects, particularly the potential for increased vasodilation producing hypotension.

Milrinone

Milrinone, although similar to amrinone, has the real advantage over amrinone of rarely being associated with thrombocytopenia. It tends to produce less of a decrease in systemic arterial pressure. The onset of action is rapid and sustained over a 48-hr infusion.[73,80] As with amrinone, prolonged infusion is associated with a slight but definite increase in heart rate of approximately 10%.[80] The elimination half-life is 48 min normals and 108 min in patients with moderate to severe congestive heart failure (CHF).[90] The usual dosing regimen includes a bolus (50 μg/kg) followed by infusion (0.375–1.0 μg/kg/min). Most frequent or concerning side effects include headache and occasional provocation of a serious arrhythmia.

Enoximone

Enoximone is an imidazolone derivative. Its half-life in heart failure patients and that of an active sulfoxide derivative are rather long (approximately 4.3 hr).[91] In some studies it has been used as multiple pulse dosing (e.g., 10.5 mg/kg) spaced at intervals based on hemodynamic effects whereas in other studies it has been used as a bolus (0.5–1.5 mg/kg) followed by an infusion (0.25–0.10 μg/kg/min).[93,122,125,127] Infusion at a rate 5 μg/kg/min may produce progressive changes in hemodynamics, suggesting elimination mechanisms are saturable. As with milrinone, provocation of serious arrhythmia is uncommon but does occur occasionally.

"Atypical" Phosphodiesterase Inhibitors

Pimobendan

Pimobendan is a phosphodiesterase inhibitor but it also possesses the interesting property of sensitizing the contractile apparatus to intracellular calcium; that is, for any given intracellular calcium concentration, the force of concentration is enhanced with pimobendan.[107,130,131] A recent clinical trial suggested that exercise capacity in patients with moderate to severe heart failure could be enhanced with pimobendan.[132] Because of concerns related to phosphodiesterase inhibitors in general, the pharmaceutical company that has developed pimobendan has halted further evaluation of this agent at the time of this writing.

Vesnarinone (OPC-8212)

Vesnarinone (OPC-8212) has phosphodiesterase inhibitor activity[133] and has been described as a member of this class of agents,[25] but some of its hemodynamic and electrophysiologic properties suggest that its main mechanism of action may be different. Unlike typical phosphodiesterase inhibitors, vesnarinone does not increase heart rate or produce marked vasodilation. In addition, vesnarinone, in contrast to "classic" phosphodiesterase inhibitors, prolongs the action potential. Vesnarinone increases intracellular sodium concentration, activating the sodium-calcium exchange mechanism, eventuating in increased intracellular calcium concentration.[134] Vesnarinone also increases the slow inward calcium current leading to increased intracellular calcium concentration.[135] Vesnarinone at high doses (approximately 6 mg/kg) has demonstrated salutary acute hemodynamic effects including an increase in cardiac output.[136] However, in doses (60 mg) found to be effective in clinical trials (see below), an impressive *lack* of hemodynamic effect has been observed acutely and at 28 days of vesnarinone use.[137] The major adverse effect of vesnarinone is a reversible form of agranulocytosis in 1% to 3% of patients. This serious adverse occurrence requires a careful strategy for leukocyte surveillance (e.g., leukocyte monitoring weekly), particularly during the first 6 months of therapy, as all reported cases have occurred during this period.

A large, multicenter, randomized, placebo-controlled trial on vesnarinone has been reported recently in preliminary form.[138] A total of 564 New York Heart Association (NYHA), functional class III or IV patients with severe ventricular dysfunction were randomized to 60 mg or 120 mg of vesnarinone or placebo. The "high-dose" vesnarinone arm (120 mg) was discontinued prematurely because of a strong trend to early and increased mortality. On the other hand, the 60-mg arm demonstrated a significant and marked improvement (50% reduction) in the combined end-point of all-cause mortality and need for inhospital intravenous inotropic therapy. In addition, there was a 62% decrease in all-cause mortality (Fig. 26.1).

The decrease in mortality with the 60-mg OPC-8212 dose is the largest reported over a 6-month period for any therapeutic agent studied in heart failure. The mechanism by which this improvement is effected is unclear. The trend toward higher mortality in the 120-mg dose suggests that either vesnarinone has a narrow therapeutic toxic ratio or that doses lower than 60 mg also may be effective. As these data are published in full-length form, a more thorough understanding of the place of OPC-8212 in the treatment of heart failure should be forthcoming.

Should Phosphodiesterase Inhibitors Be Primary Therapy to Support the Failing Circulation?

The most popular positive inotropic agent in use today to support the failing circulation is dobutamine. It has the advantage compared to other catecholamines of producing less positive chronotropic effect and less primary effect on the periphery. Its very short half-life makes it ideal for titration and predictability of hemodynamic effects after a short infusion period. On the other hand, continued stimulation of beta receptors produces a decreasing effect over time (down-regulation).[129]

Based on current knowledge, should any phosphodiesterase inhibitor be recommended to replace dobutamine as primary therapy?[139] On the positive side is the lack of hemodynamic attenuation with phosphodiesterase inhibitors observed in several studies. The effect on myocardial oxygen consumption *may* be less marked than dobutamine. On the other hand, the vasodilating effect with its potential attendant decrease in systemic arterial pressure may be difficult to manage in an individual patient. This effect may be particularly troublesome because of the relatively long half-life of these agents. Theoretically, the effects of these agents may be blunted by a decrease in available cAMP, which may require further enhancement by adenylate cyclase stimulation. Additionally, amrinone in particular has the troubling side effect of thrombocytopenia. The use of milrinone or enoximone probably will eliminate this problem.

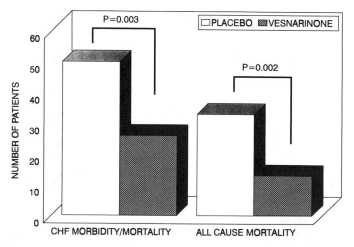

FIGURE 26.1. Data from the double-blind, randomized trial comparing vesnarinone to placebo. The primary endpoints morbidity (requirement for intravenous inotropic therapy) plus all cause mortality were reduced by 50% in patients receiving 60 mg of vesnarinone compared to placebo at 6 months. Mortality alone from all causes was also significantly reduced (62%) in the vesnarinone group.

Clearly, controlled comparative studies are required to recommend either dobutamine or a phosphodiesterase inhibitor as first-line therapy. End-points of these studies will require clinical, rather than hemodynamic, end-points. Only when such data are available can any particular drug be recommended as first-line therapy.

Use of Phosphodiesterase Inhibitors After Myocardial Infarction: Experimental Studies

Ventricular remodeling occurs after the damage produced by myocardial infarction.[140] It has been suggested that modification of this process will retard the development of heart failure and improve survival.[140] Milrinone has been used in a rat model of myocardial infarction and has been shown to decrease ventricular dilation and improve survival.[141,142]

Similar results have been the basis of large scale human trials on the efficacy of converting enzyme inhibitors in this setting. It should be emphasized, however, that in the rat positive inotropy from milrinone is quite trivial, if present at all. The major effect in this species is vasodilation. Thus, the mechanism for the observed experimental results with milrinone may have been related to ventricular unloading rather than positive inotropy. Since positive inotropy does occur in humans, the results in patients may be different from those observed in the rat. Published studies in patients with chronic heart failure described below suggest caution in embarking on any human studies in this regard.

Long-Term Treatment of Congestive Heart Failure with Oral Phosphodiesterase Inhibitors

End-points utilized to determine clinical efficacy of phosphodiesterase inhibitors have included hemodynamics, symptoms, exercise capacity, medical interventions including hospitalizations and increases in diuretic use, and survival. The availability of controlled clinical trials supersedes the results of multiple uncontrolled observations. In contrast to angiotensin-converting enzyme (ACE) inhibitors, first-dose administration of phosphodiesterase inhibitors may improve acute exercise performance compared to placebo.[143-145] On the other hand, two placebo-controlled, randomized trials on oral amrinone failed to demonstrate long-term (3 month) improvement in either symptoms or exercise tolerance.[146,147] This negative result was thought to be due in part to the inability to administer in many patients the full dose of amrinone because of adverse side effects. On the other hand, the second generation

bipyridine milrinone was shown in one study to be more effective than placebo and equally as effective as digoxin in improving exercise tolerance.[81] In this study, withdrawals in the milrinone-treated were more frequent than in the digoxin-treated groups.[81] Furthermore, there was a strong trend ($p = .064$) toward increased mortality in milrinone-treated versus non–milrinone-treated patients.[81] In a multicenter trial of the phosphodiesterase inhibitor enoximone, a trend toward improvement in maximal oxygen consumption during exercise occurred at 4 weeks of therapy; this improvement was not apparent by 16 weeks.[149] Unexpectedly, using either intention-to-treat or actual treatment analysis, mortality was higher with enoximone than placebo.[149] In a trial on the phosphodiesterase inhibitor imazodan, mortality was higher with the active agent than with placebo.[150] To date, the major trial to show improved exercise tolerance with a phosphodiesterase inhibitor was the digoxin-milrinone trial.[81] In this trial digoxin was not used as background therapy as it was in all the other trials of phosphodiesterase inhibitors. In fact, in the milrinone plus digoxin group, effect on exercise tolerance was no better than in the digoxin group alone. When milrinone was substituted for digoxin, a higher percentage of patients clinically deteriorated than in the group continued on digoxin. These data suggest that if phosphodiesterase inhibitors are effective in improving exercise capacity and symptoms, their effect is slight and may be most apparent when digoxin is not used as part of the therapeutic regimen.

None of the above-noted studies was designed as a mortality study. The PROMISE (Prospective Milrinone Survival Evaluation) trial was specifically designed to evaluate the effect of milrinone on survival in patients with severe (NYHA III–IV) heart failure taking diuretics and/or digoxin and/or ACE inhibitors[25] (Fig. 26.2). The milrinone group demonstrated an excess 28% mortality compared to placebo.[25] The effect was particularly prominent in NYHA class IV patients. In addition, withdrawal of study drug was more frequent in the milrinone- than the placebo-treated group. The increase in deaths was related to a higher incidence of sudden cardiac death in the milrinone group.[151]

Mechanism of Worsened Survival with Classic Phosphodiesterase Inhibitors

The above data strongly suggest that classic phosphodiesterase inhibitors dosed to have an acute hemodynamic effect and given long-term worsen survival in patients with moderate to severe heart failure. In the PROMISE trial this effect appeared to be due to an increased risk of sudden death.[151] In the smaller studies with milrinone, enoximone, and imazodan, the increased mortality was not as clearly related to arrhyth-

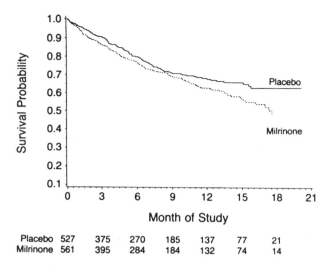

FIGURE 26.2. The excess in mortality in the group assigned to milrinone as compared to placebo in the PROMISE trial (see text). Reprinted, with permission, ref. 25. Copyright 1991 by the New England Journal of Medicine.

mogenicity. Lynch et al. have demonstrated in a canine model of sudden coronary occlusion that pretreatment with phosphodiesterase inhibitors promotes ventricular fibrillation.[83] Thus, patients on chronic phosphodiesterase inhibitors may be at higher risk to develop fatal cardiac arrhythmias when a negative cardiac perturbation occurs (e.g., myocardial ischemia, hypokalemia, increased myocardial wall stress from an increase in peripheral resistance, etc.). It has also been suggested that phosphodiesterase inhibitors may accelerate myocyte death by upsetting the balance between energy production and utilization.[2] Experimental data remain limited on this point.[140] It is possible that malignant arrhythmias and sudden death seen in the PROMISE trial reflect, in fact, cell "burnout" or accelerated myocyte decline rather than a sudden arrhythmia in a relatively stable cellular environment.

The effects on mortality of agents with "some" phosphodiesterase inhibition (e.g. vesnarinone and flosequinan) but with other cellular mechanisms may be more difficult to predict and ultimately may be a function of dose used (note the increased mortality rate with 120 mg and the decreased mortality rate with 60 mg of vesnarinone in the multicenter vesnarinone study described above).

The Issue of Proper Dose

Whenever a new drug is being evaluated, the proper dose must be determined. An example of the problems in determining the proper dose may be found with the digitalis glycosides. The positive inotropic effect is linear until a plateau is reached. It is probable that the inotropic effect of digitalis is more pronounced in hu-

mans at blood levels generally considered toxic. If digitalis were being developed today as a new drug and the dose range chosen were above the doses used today, it is likely that although exercise capacity and symptoms may have shown improvement, mortality also may have worsened, with increased mortality due primarily to arrhythmic events.

The basis for choosing the appropriate test dose with phosphodiesterase inhibitors has been their effect on central hemodynamics. In the multicenter enoximone trial, the dose was chosen specifically to be at the middle to the lower end of the hemodynamic continuum.[149] Exercise improvement was observed at that dose. By design there was an increase in enoximone dose between 30 and 160 days; exercise improvement was no longer apparent. A similar result was found in a controlled trial of imazodan and a second enoximone trial.[71,150] These data are not convincing that doses of phosphodiesterase inhibitors at the high end (i.e., near maximal hemodynamic effect) are superior to lower doses. This observation may also hold for vesnarinone but because of the multiplicity of cellular effects, the lower dose may have been beneficial by activating one mechanism and detrimental at the higher dose because of activation of another mechanism, namely, phosphodiesterase inhibition.

It is therefore entirely possible that the effective and safe dose range for phosphodiesterase inhibitors is below the range tested in controlled trials reporting a negative outcome. If the goal of phosphodiesterase inhibition is to improve symptoms and exercise tolerance, more cAMP may be needed during exercise but not necessarily at rest. At very low doses, phosphodiesterase inhibitors may be able to increase cAMP during exercise only when beta stimulation increases the generation of cAMP. Thus, the situation may be more "physiologic"; that is, an increase in myocardial cAMP concentration during exercise but not at rest. This hypothesis is testable, but the challenge will be to test it safely.

Summary

Phosphodiesterase inhibitors are used in our practice to sustain the patient with decompensated heart failure. At present we typically employ amrinone or milrinone when catecholamines, particularly dobutamine, do not produce adequate hemodynamic and clinical responses. Controlled trials and, to a lesser extent, clinical experience will determine whether a phosphodiesterase inhibitor, a beta agonist, or a combination of both will be preferred as initial therapy to support the failing circulation. Classic oral phosphodiesterase inhibitors have failed to demonstrate efficacy in groups of heart failure patients in well controlled trials. We are unconvinced that they are truly effective and at this time recommend caution, not only in their occasional use for individual "responders," but also in the development of future clinical studies on agents in this class.

On the other hand, certain agents with phosphodiesterase inhibitory activity but also with other cellular mechanisms (e.g., vesnarinone) appear to offer clinical benefit above that expected with diuretics, ACE inhibitors, and digoxin. Further understanding of the mechanisms that effect improvement in these "atypical" phosphodiesterase inhibitors are clearly required to determine if phosphodiesterase inhibition is part of the reason for their efficacy or part of their limitations.

Acknowledgement. I would like to extend my gratitude for the expertise and diligence provided by Mrs. Rhonda Oliver in preparing this chapter.

References

1. Benotti JR, Grossman W, Braunwald E, Davolos DD, Alousi AA. Hemodynamic assessment of amrinone: a new inotropic agent. *N Engl J Med.* 1978;299:1373–1377.

2. Katz A. A new inotropic drug: its promise and a caution. *New Engl J Med.* 1978;299:1409–1410.

3. Adelstein RS, Pato MD, Conti MA. The role of phosphorylation in regulating contractile proteins. In: Dumont JE, Greengard P, Robinson GA, eds. *Advances in Cyclic Nucleotide Research.* vol. 14. New York: Raven Press; 1981:361–373.

4. Schmitz W, von der Leyen H, Meyer W, Neumann J, Scholz H. Phosphodiesterase inhibition and positive inotropic effects. *J Cardiovas Pharmacol.* 1989;14(Suppl 3):S11–S14.

5. Drummond GI, Severson DL. Cyclic nucleotides and cardiac function. In: *Brief Reviews from Circulation Research 1980, Monograph 69.* Dallas: American Heart Association; 1980:8–16.

6. Endoh M, Yamashita S, Taira N. Positive inotropic effect of amrinone in relation to cyclic nucleotide metabolism in the canine ventricular muscle. *J Pharmacol Exp Ther.* 1982;221:775–783.

7. Honerjager P, Schafer-Korting M, Reiter M. Involvement of cyclic AMP in the direct inotropic action of amrinone. *Arch Pharmacol.* 1981;318:112–120.

8. Kukovetz WR, Poch G, Wurm A. Quantitative relations between cyclic AMP and contraction as affected by stimulators of adenylate cyclase and inhibitors of phosphodiesterase. In: Drummond GI, Greengard P, Robinson GA, eds. *Advances in Cyclic Nucleotide Research.* vol. 5. New York: Raven Press; 1975:395–414.

9. England PJ, Gristwood RW, Leigh BK, Owen DAA, Reeves ML. Specific inhibition of type III phosphodiesterase activity: comparison with positive inotropic potency. *Br J Pharmacol.* 1985;86:631P–637P.

10. Gristwood RW, English TAH, Wallwork J, Sampford KA, Owen DAA. Analysis of responses to a selective phosphodiesterase III inhibitor SK&F 94120 on isolated myocardium including human ventricular myocardium from "end-stage" failure patients. *J Cardiovas Pharm.* 1987;9:719–727.

11. Tsien RW. Cyclic AMP and contractile activity in heart. In: Greengard P, Robinson GA, eds. *Advances in Cyclic Nucleotide Research.* vol. 8. New York: Raven Press; 1977:363–420.

12. Katz AM. Cyclic adenosine monophosphate effects on the myocardium: a man who blows hot and cold with one breath. *J Am Coll Cardiol.* 1983;2:143–149.

13. Katz AM. Role of the contractile proteins and sarcoplasmic reticulum in the response of the heart to catecholamines: an historical review. In: Greengard P, Robinson GA, eds. *Advances in Cyclic Nucleotide Research.* New York: Raven Press; 1979:303–349.

14. Katz AM, Tada M, Kirchberger MA. Control of calcium transport in the myocardium by the cyclic-AMP-protein kinase system. In: Drummond GI, Greengard P, Robinson GA, eds. *Advances in Cyclic Nucleotide Research.* vol. 5. New York: Raven Press; 1975:453–472.

15. Scholz H. Inotropic drugs and their mechanisms of action. *J Am Coll Cardiol.* 1984;4:389–397.

16. Kariya T, Wille LJ, Dage RC. Biochemical studies on the mechanism of cardiotonic activity of MDL 17,043. *J Cardiovascular Pharmacol.* 1982;4:509–514.

17. England PJ, Pask HT, Mills D. Cyclic-AMP-dependent phosphorylation of cardiac contractile proteins. In: Greengard P ed. *Advances in Cyclic Nucleotide and Protein Phosphorylation Research.* vol. 17. New York: Raven Press; 1984:383–391.

18. Kariya T, Dage RC. Tissue distribution and selective inhibition of subtypes of high affinity cAMP phosphodiesterase. *Biochemical Pharmacol.* 1988;37:3267–3270.

19. Adelstein RS, Sellers JR, Conti MA, Pato MD, de Lanerolle P. Regulation of smooth muscle contractile proteins by calmodulin and cyclic AMP. *Fed Proc.* 1982;41:2873–2878.

20. Olson EM, Kim D, Smith TW, Marsh JD. Mechanism of the positive inotropic effect of milrinone in cultured embryonic chick ventricular cells. *J Mol Cell Cardiol.* 1987;19:95–104.

21. Movsesian MA. Calcium-physiology in smooth muscle. *Prog Cardiovasc Dis.* 1982;25:211–224.

22. Morgan JP, Gwathmey JK, DeFeo TT, Morgan KG. The effects of amrinone and related drugs on intracellular calcium in isolated mammalian cardiac and vascular smooth muscle. *Circulation.* 1986;73 (Suppl III):65–76.

23. Kauffman RF, Schenck KW, Utterback BG, Crow VG, Cohen ML. In vitro vascular relaxation by new inotropic agents: relationship to phosphodiesterase inhibition and cyclic nucleotides. *J Pharmacol Exp Ther.* 1987;242:864–872.

24. Lincoln TM, Cornwell TL, Taylor AE. cGMP-dependent protein kinase mediates the reduction of calcium by cAMP in vascular smooth muscle cells. *Am J Physiol.* 1990;258:C399–C407.

25. Packer M, Carver JR, Rodeheffer RJ, et al. Effect of oral milrinone on mortality in severe chronic heart failure. *N Engl J Med.* 1991;325:1468–1475.

26. Lee JC, Downing SE. Cyclic AMP and the pathogenesis

of myocardial injury. *Res Common Chem Pathol Pharmacol.* 1980;27:305–318.

27. Martorana PA. The role of cyclic AMP in isoprenaline-induced cardiac necroses in the rat. *J Pharm Pharmacol.* 1971;23:200–203.

28. Ebbesen P. Myocardial degeneration in mice treated with dibutyryl cyclic AMP and/or theophylline. *Virchows Archr.* 1976;372:89–95.

29. Lubbe WF, Podzuweit TH, Daries PS, Opie LH. The role of cyclic adenosine monophosphate in adrenergic effects on ventricular vulnerability to fibrillation in the isolated perfused rat heart. *J Clin Invest.* 1978;61:1260–1269.

30. Katz AM. Energetics and the failing heart. *Hosp Prac.* 1991;78–90.

31. Feldman MD, Copelas L, Gwathmey JK, et al. Deficient production of cyclic AMP: pharmacologic evidence of an important cause of contractile dysfunction in patients with end-stage heart failure. *Circulation.* 1987;75:331–339.

32. Schmitz W, Scholz H, Erdmann E. Effects of alpha- and beta-adrenergic agonists, phosphodiesterase inhibitor and adenosine on isolated human heart muscle preparations. *Trends Pharmacol Sci.* 1987;8:447–450.

33. Erdmann E. The effectiveness of inotropic agents in isolated cardiac preparations from the human heart. *Klin Wochenschr.* 1988;66:1–6.

34. Wilmshurst PT, Walker JM, Fry CH, et al. Inotropic and vasodilator effects of amrinone on isolated human tissue. *Cardiovasc Res.* 1984;18:302–309.

35. Firth BG, Ratner AV, Grassman ED, Winniford MD, Nicod P, Hillis LD. Assessment of the inotropic and vasodilator effects of amrinone versus isoproterenol. *Am J Cardiol.* 1984;54:1331–1336.

36. Bristow MR, Ginsburg R, Minobe W, et al. Decreased catecholamine sensitivity and beta-adrenergic-receptor density in failing human hearts. *N Engl J Med.* 1982;307:205–211.

37. Wilmshurst PT, Thompson DS, Juul SM, Jenkins BS, Coltart DJ, Webb-Peploe MM. Comparison of the effects of amrinone and sodium nitroprusside on haemodynamics, contractility, and myocardial metabolism in patients with cardiac failure due to coronary artery disease and dilated cardiomyopathy. *Br Heart J.* 1982;52:38–48.

38. Thormann J, Kramer W, Kindler M, Kremer P, Schlepper M. Assessment of the effective components of amrinone by continuous analysis of the pressure/volume relationship. *Z Kardiol.* 1987;76:530–540.

39. Wilmshurst PT, Thompson DS, Jenkins BS, Coltart DJ, Webb-Peploe MM. Haemodynamic effects of intravenous amrinone in patients with impaired left ventricular function. *Br Heart J.* 1983;49:77–82.

40. Grose R, Strain J, Greenberg M, LeJemtel TH. Systemic and coronary effects of intravenous milrinone and dobutamine in congestive heart failure. *J Am Coll Cardiol.* 1986;7:1107–113.

41. Alousi AA, Johnson DC. Pharmacology of the bipyridines: amrinone and milrinone. *Circulation.* 1986;73:III 10–24.

42. Alousi AA, Stankus GP, Stuart JC, Walton LH. Characterization of the cardiotonic effects of milrinone, a new and potent cardiac bipyridine, on isolated tissues from several animal species. *J Cardiovasc Pharmacol.* 1983; 5:804–811.

43. Alousi AA, Canter JM, Montenaro MJ, Fort DJ, Ferrari RA. Cardiotonic activity of milrinone, a new and potent cardiac bipyridine, on the normal and failing heart of experimental animals. *J Cardiovasc Pharmacol.* 1983;5: 792–803.

44. Roebel LE, Lucas RW, Hodgeman RJ, Burke SM, Woodward JK. Selective inotropic activity of RMI 17,043 in anesthetized and conscious dogs. *Fed Proc.* 1982;41:1316.

45. Roebel LE, Dage RC, Cheng HC, Woodward JK. Characterization of the cardiovascular activities of a new cardiotonic agent: MDL 17,043 (1,3-dihydro-4-methyl-5-[4-(methylthio)-benzoyl]-2H-imidazol-2-one). *J Cardiovasc Pharmacol.* 1982;4:721–729.

46. Dage RC, Roebel LE, Hsieh CP, Weiner DL, Woodward JK. Cardiovascular properties of a new cardiotonic agent: MDL 27,043, (1,3-dihydro-4-methyl-5-[4-methylthio)-benzoyl]-2H-imidazol-2-one). *J Cardiovasc Pharmacol.* 1982;4:500–508.

47. Weishaar RE, Kobylarz-Singer DC, Steffen RP, Kaplan HR. Subclasses of cyclic AMP-specific phosphodiesterase in left ventricular muscle and their involvement in regulating myocardial contractility. *Circ Res.* 1987;61: 539–547.

48. Wilmshurst PT, Walker JM, Fry CH, et al. Inotropic and vasodilator effects of amrinone on isolated human tissue. *Cardiovasc Res.* 1984;18:302–309.

49. Herrmann HC, Ruddy TD, Dec GW, Strauss HW, Boucher CA, Fifer MA. Inotropic effect of enoximone in patients with severe heart failure: demonstration by left ventricular end-systolic pressure-volume analysis. *J Am Coll Cardiol.* 1987;9:1117–1123.

50. Borow KM, Come PC, Neumann A, Baim DS, Braunwald E, Grossman W. Physiologic assessment of the inotropic, vasodilator and afterload reducing effects of milrinone in subjects without cardiac disease. *Am J Cardiol.* 1985;55:1204–1209.

51. Jaski BE, Fifer MA, Wright RF, Braunwald E, Colucci WS. Positive inotropic and vasodilator actions of milrinone in patients with severe congestive heart failure. *J Clin Invest.* 1985;75:643–649.

52. Crawford MH, Richards KL, Sodums MT, Kennedy GT. Positive inotropic and vasodilator effects of MDL 17,043 in patients with reduced left ventricular performance. *Am J Cardiol.* 1984;53:1051–1053.

53. Strain J, Grose R, Maskin CS, LeJemtel TH. Effects of a new cardiotonic agent, MDL 17043, on myocardial contractility and left ventricular performance in congestive heart failure. *Am Heart J.* 1985;110:91–96.

54. Ludmer PL, Wright RF, Arnold MO, Ganz P, Braunwald E, Colucci WS. Separation of the direct myocardial and vasodilator actions of milrinone administered by an intracoronary infusion technique. *Circulation.* 1986;73: 130–137.

55. Baim DS, McDowell AV, Cherniles J, et al. Evaluation

of a new bipyridine inotropic agent-milrinone-in patients with severe congestive heart failure. *N Engl J Med.* 1983;309:748–756.

56. Uretsky BF, Generalovich T, Reddy PS, Spangenberg RB, Follansbee WP. The acute hemodynamic effects of a new agent, MDL 17,043, in the treatment of congestive heart failure. *Circulation.* 1983;67:823–828.

57. Murali S, Uretsky BF, Betschart AR, Tokarczyk TR, Kolesar JA, Reddy PS. Differential hemodynamic effects of oral enoximone in severe congestive heart failure. *Am J Cardiol.* 1990;65:515–519.

58. Endoh M, Yanagisawa T, Taira N, Blinks JR. Effects of new inotropic agents on cyclic nucleotide metabolism and calcium transients in canine ventricular muscle. *Circulation.* 1986;73(Suppl III):III-117–133.

59. Binkley PF, Shaffer PB, Ryan JM, Leier CV. Augmentation of diastolic function with phosphodiesterase inhibition in congestive heart failure. *J Lab Clin Med.* 1989;114:266–271.

60. Monrad ES, McKay RG, Baim DS, et al. Improvement in indexes of diastolic performance in patients with congestive heart failure treated with milrinone. *Circulation.* 1984;70:1030–1037.

61. Piscione F, Jaski BE, Wenting GJ, Serruys PW. Effect of a single oral dose of milrinone on left ventricular diastolic performance in the failing human heart. *J Am Coll Cardiol.* 1987;10:1294–1302.

62. Harris AL, Grant AM, Silver PJ, Evans DB, Alousi AA. Differential vasorelaxant effects of milrinone and amrinone on contractile responses of canine coronary, cerebral, and renal arteries. *J Cardiovasc Pharmacol.* 1989;13:238–244.

63. Cody RJ, Muller FB, Kubo SH, Rutman H, Leonard D. Identification of the direct vasodilator effect of milrinone with an isolated limb preparation in patients with chronic congestive heart failure. *Circulation.* 1986;73:124–129.

64. Drexler H, Hoing S, Faude F, Wollschlager H, Just H. Central and regional vascular hemodynamics following intravenous milrinone in the conscious rat: comparison with dobutamine. *J Cardiovasc Pharmacol.* 1987;9:563–569.

65. Harris AL, Silver PJ, Lemp BM, Evans DB. The vasorelaxant effects of milrinone and other vasodilators are attenuated by ouabain. *Eur J Pharmacol.* 1988;145:133–139.

66. Jondeau G, Klapholz M, Katz SD, et al. Control of arteriolar resistance in heart failure: partial attenuation of specific phosphodiesterase inhibitor-mediated vasodilation by digitalis glycosides. *Circulation.* 1922;85:54–60.

67. Arnold JMO, Ludmer PL, Wright RF, Ganz P, Braunwald E, Colucci WS. Role of reflex sympathetic withdrawal in the hemodynamic response to an increased inotropic state in patients with severe heart failure. *J Am Coll Cardiol* 1986;8:413–418.

68. Davidenko J, Antzelevitch C. The effects of milrinone on action potential characteristics, conduction, automaticity, and reflected re-entry in isolated myocardial fibers. *J Cardiovasc Pharm.* 1985;7:341–349.

69. Kodama I, Kondo N, Shibata S. Electrical and mechan-

ical effects of amrinone on isolated guinea pig ventricular muscle. *J Cardiovasc Pharmacol* 1983;5:903–912.

70. Pop T, Treese N, Cremer GMJ, Haegele KD, Meyer J. Electrophysiological effects of intravenous MDL 17043. *Int J Cardiol.* 1986;12:223–232.

71. Narahara K and the Western Enoximone Study Group. Oral enoximone therapy in chronic heart failure: a placebo-controlled randomized trial. *Am Heart J.* 1991;121:1471–1479.

72. Naccarelli GV, Gray EL, Dougherty AH, Hanna JE, Goldstein RA. Amrinone: acute electrophysiologic and hemodynamic effects in patients with congestive heart failure. *Am J Cardiol.* 1984;54:600–604.

73. Goldstein RA, Geraci SA, Gray EL, Rinkenberger RL, Dougherty AH, Naccarelli GV. Electrophysiologic effects of milrinone in patients with congestive heart failure. *Am J Cardiol.* 1986;57:624–628.

74. Hohnloser SH, Zehender M, Geibel A, Meinertz T, Just H. Electrophysiologic effects of enoximone in patients with congestive heart failure. *J Cardiovasc Pharmacol.* 1989;14(Suppl 1):S29–S32.

75. Malecot CO, Arlock P, Katzung BG. Amrinone effects on electromechanical coupling and depolarization induced automaticity in ventricular muscle of guinea pigs and ferrets. *J Pharmacol Exp Ther.* 1985;232:10–19.

76. Miles WM, Heger JJ, Minardo JD, Klein LS, Prystowsky EN, Zipes DP. The electrophysiologic effects of enoximone in patients with pre-existing ventricular tachyarrhythmias. *Am Heart J.* 1989;117:112–121.

77. Anderson JL, Askins JC, Gilbert EM, Menlove RL, Lutz JR. Occurrence of ventricular arrhythmias in patients receiving acute and chronic infusions of milrinone. *Am Heart J.* 1986;111:466–474.

78. Ludmer PL, Baim DS, Antman EM, et al. Effects of milrinone on complex ventricular arrhythmias in congestive heart failure secondary to ischemic or idiopathic dilated cardiomyopathy. *Am J Cardiol.* 1987;59:1351–1355.

79. Holmes JR, Kubo SH, Cody RJ, Kligfield P. Milrinone in congestive heart failure: observations on ambulatory ventricular arrhythmias. *Am Heart J.* 1985;110:800–806.

80. Pflugfelder PW, O'Neill BJ, Ogilvie RI, et al. A Canadian multicenter study of a 48 h infusion of milrinone in patients with severe heart failure. *Can J Cardiol.* 1991;7:5–10.

81. DiBianco R, Shabetai R, Kostuk W, et al. A comparison of oral milrinone, digoxin, and their combination in the treatment of patients with chronic heart failure. *N Engl J Med.* 1989;320:677–683.

82. Klein NA, Siskind SJ, Frishman WH, Sonnenblick EH, LeJemtel TH. Hemodynamic comparison of intravenous amrinone and dobutamine in patients with chronic congestive heart failure. *Am J Cardiol.* 1981;48:170–175.

83. Lynch JJ Jr, Uprichard ACG, Frye JW, Driscoll EM, Kitzen JM, Lucchesi BR. Effects of the positive inotropic agents milrinone and pimobendan on the development of lethal ischemic arrhythmias in conscious dogs with recent myocardial infarction. *J Cardiovasc Pharmacol.* 1989;14:585–597.

84. Anderson JL, Baim DS, Fein SA, et al. Efficacy and

safety of sustained (48 hour) intravenous infusion of milrinone in patients with severe congestive heart failure: a multicenter study. *J Am Coll Cardiol.* 1987;9:711–722.

85. Kereiakes D, Chatterjee K, Parmley WW, et al. Intravenous and oral MDL 17,043 (a new inotrope-vasodilator agent) in congestive heart failure: hemodynamic and clinical evaluation in 38 patients. *J Am Coll Cardiol.* 1984;4:884–889.

86. Uretsky BF, Generalovich T, Verbalis JG, Valdes AM, Reddy PS. MDL 17,043 therapy in severe congestive heart failure: characterization of the early and late hemodynamic, pharmacokinetic, hormonal, and clinical response. *J Am Coll Cardiol.* 1985;5:1414–1421.

87. Khalife K, Zannad F, Brunotte F, et al. Placebo-controlled study of oral enoximone in congestive heart failure with initial and final intravenous hemodynamic evaluation. *Am J Cardiol.* 1987;60:75C–79C.

88. INOCOR I.V. (Amrinone) National Experience Trial (I-NET), 1987.

89. Ferry DR, Kennedy GT, O'Rourke RA, Crawford MH. Hemodynamic effects of prolonged intravenous therapy with enoximone in patients with severe congestive heart failure. *J Cardiovasc Pharmacol.* 1988;11:115–122.

90. DiBianco R. The bipyridine derivatives. In: Leier C, ed. *Cardiotonic Drugs.* New York: Marcel Dekker; 1991: 255–304.

91. Maskin CS, Sinoway L, Chadwick B, Sonnenblick EH, LeJemtel TH. Sustained hemodynamic and clinical effects of a new cardiotonic agent, WIN 47203, in patients with severe congestive heart failure. *Circulation.* 1983;67:1065–1070.

92. Sinoway LS, Maskin CS, Chadwick B, Forman R, Sonnenblick EH, LeJemtel TH. Long-term therapy with a new cardiotonic agent, WIN 47203: drug-dependent improvement in cardiac performance and progression of the underlying disease. *J Am Coll Cardiol.* 1983;2:327–331.

93. Smith NA, Kates RE, Lebsack C, et al. Clinical pharmacology of intravenous enoximone: pharmacodynamics and pharmakokinetics in patients with heart failure. *Am Heart J.* 1991;122:755–762.

94. Biddle TL, Benotti JR, Creager MA, et al. Comparison of intravenous milrinone and dobutamine for congestive heart failure secondary to either ischemic or dilated cardiomyopathy. *Am J Cardiol.* 1987;59:1345–1350.

95. Maisel AS, Wright CM, Carter SM, Ziegler M, Motulsky HJ. Tachyphylaxis with amrinone therapy: association with sequestration and down-regulation of lymphocyte beta-adrenergic receptors. *Ann Intern Med.* 1989; 110:195–201.

96. Rubin SA, Tabak L. MDL 17,043: short- and long-term cardiopulmonary and clinical effects in patients with heart failure. *J Am Coll Cardiol.* 1985;5:1422–1427.

97. Keeton TK, Campbell WB. The pharmacologic alteration of renin release. *Pharmacol Rev.* 1981;31:81–227.

98. Churchill PC, Churchill NC. Isoproterenol-stimulated renin secretion in the rat: second messenger roles of Ca and cyclic AMP. *Life Sci.* 1982;30:1313–1319.

99. Uretsky BF, Verbalis JG, Generalovich T, Valdes AM, Reddy PS. Comparative hemodynamic and hormonal response of enoximone and dobutamine in severe congestive heart failure. *Am J Cardiol.* 1986;58:110–116.

100. Jafri SM, Reddy BR, Budzinski D, Goldberg AD, Pilla A, Levine TB. Acute neurohormonal and hemodynamic response to a new peak III phosphodiesterase inhibitor (ICI 153, 110) in patients with chronic heart failure. *J Cardiovasc Pharmacol.* 1990;16:360–366.

101. Uretsky BF, Valdes AM, Reddy PS. Positive inotropic therapy for short-term support and long-term management of congestive heart failure: the hemodynamic and clinical efficacy of MDL 17,043. *Circulation.* 1986; 73(Suppl III):III-219–III-229.

102. Murali S, Uretsky BF, Valdes AM, Kolesar JA, Reddy PS. The acute hemodynamic and hormonal effects of CI-930, a new phosphodiesterase inhibitor, in patients with severe congestive heart failure. *Am J Cardiol.* 1987;59:1356–1360.

103. Liang C-S, Thomas A, Imai N, Stone CK, Kawashima S, Hood WB Jr. Effects of milrinone on systemic hemodynamics and regional circulations in dogs with congestive heart failure: comparison with dobutamine. *J Cardiovasc Pharmacol.* 1987;10:509–516.

104. LeJemtel TH, Maskin CS, Mancini D, Sinoway L, Feld H, Chadwick B. Systemic and regional hemodynamic effects of captopril and milrinone administered alone and concomitantly in patients with heart failure. *Circulation.* 1985;72:364–369.

105. Leier CV, Lima JJ, Meiler SEL, Unverferth DV. Central and regional hemodynamic effects of oral enoximone in congestive heart failure: a double-blind, placebo-controlled study. *Am Heart J.* 1988;115:1051–1059.

106. Cody RJ, Kubo SH, Covit AB, et al. Regional blood flow and neurohormonal responses to milrinone in congestive heart failure. *Clin Pharmacol Ther.* 1986;39:128–135.

107. Ruegg JC. Effects of new inotropic agents on calcium sensitivity on contractile proteins. *Circulation.* 1986; 73(Suppl III):III-78–III-84.

108. Jentzer JH, LeJemtel TH, Sonnenblick EH, Kirk ES. Beneficial effect of amrinone on myocardial oxygen consumption during acute left ventricular failure in dogs. *Am J Cardiol.* 1981;48:75–83.

109. Benotti JR, Grossman W, Braunwald E, Carabello BA. Effects of amrinone on myocardial energy metabolism and hemodynamics in patients with severe congestive heart failure due to coronary artery disease. *Circulation.* 1980;62:28–34.

110. Martin JL, Likoff MJ, Janicki JS, Laskey WK, Hirshfeld JW, Weber KT. Myocardial energetics and clinical response to the cardiotonic agent MDL 17,043 in advanced heart failure. *J Am Coll Cardiol.* 1984;4:875–883.

111. Monrad ES, Baim DS, Smith HS, Lanoue A, Braunwald E, Grossman W. Effects of milrinone on coronary hemodynamics and myocardial energetics in patients with congestive heart failure. Acute effects on left ventricular systolic function and myocardial metabolism. *Circulation.* 1985;71:972–979.

112. Timmis AD, Smyth P, Monaghan M, et al. Milrinone in heart failure. Acute effects on left ventricular systolic function and myocardial metabolism. *Br Heart J.* 1985;54:36–41.

113. Viquerat CE, Kereiakes D, Morris L, et al. Alterations in left ventricular function, coronary hemodynamics and myocardial catecholamine balance with MDL 17,043, a new inotropic vasodilator agent, in patients with severe heart failure. *J Am Coll Cardiol*. 1985;5:326–332.

114. Amin DK, Shah PK, Shellock FG, et al. Comparative hemodynamic effects of intravenous dobutamine and MDL-17,043, a new cardioactive drug, in severe congestive heart failure. *Am Heart J*. 1985;109:91–98.

115. Hasenfuss G, Holubarsch C, Heiss HW, et al. Myocardial energetics in patients with dilated cardiomyopathy. Influence of nitroprusside and enoximone. *Circulation*. 1989;80:51–64.

116. Thormann J, Kremer P, Mitrovic V, Neuzner J, Bahawar H, Schlepper M. Effects of enoximone in coronary artery disease: increased pump function, improved ventricular wall motion, and abolition of pacing-induced myocardial ischemia. *J Appl Cardiol*. 1989;4:31–45.

117. Colucci WS, Wright RF, Jaski BE, Fifer MA, Braunwald E. Milrinone and dobutamine in severe heart failure: differing hemodynamic effects and individual patient responsiveness. *Circulation*. 1986;73(Suppl III):III-175–III-183.

118. Amin DK, Shah PK, Hulse S, Shellock F. Comparative acute hemodynamic effects of intravenous sodium nitroprusside and MDL-17,043, a new inotropic drug with vasodilator effects, in refractory congestive heart failure. *Am Heart J*. 1985;109:1006–1012.

119. Uretsky BF, Lawless CE, Verbalis JG, Valdes AM, Kolesar JA, Reddy PS. Combined therapy with dobutamine and amrinone in severe heart failure. *Chest*. 1987;92:657–662.

120. Gage J, Rutman H, Lucido D, LeJemtel TH. Additive effects of dobutamine and amrinone on myocardial contractility and ventricular performance in patients with severe heart failure. *Circulation*. 1986;74:367–313.

121. Vincent JL, Leon M, Berre J, Melot C, Kahn RJ. Addition of phosphodiesterase inhibitors to adrenergic agents in acutely ill patients. *Int J Cardiol*. 1990;28:S7–S11.

122. Loisance D, Dubois Rande JL, Deleuze PH, et al. Pharmacological bridge to cardiac transplantation. *Eur J Cardiothorac Surg*. 1989;3:196–202.

123. Dies F, Krell MJ, Whitlow P, et al. Intermittent dobutamine in ambulatory outpatients with chronic cardiac failure. *Circulation*. 1986;74(Suppl II):II-38. Abstract.

124. Alousi AA, Fabian RJ, Baker JF, Stroshane RM. Milrinone. In: Scriabine A, ed. *New Drugs Annual: Cardiovascular Drugs*. vol 3. New York: Raven Press; 1985:245–283.

125. Boldt J, Kling D, Schuhmann E, Dapper F, Hempelmann G. Hamodynamische effekte des nuven phosphodiesterasehemmers enoximone bei kardiochirugischen patienten. *Anesthetist*. 1989;38:238–244.

126. Boldt J. Dieterich HA, Hemelmann G. Comparison of haemodynamic efficacy of enoximone and dobutamine in coronary surgery patients. *Br J Clin Pract*. 1989;(Suppl 64):41–45.

127. Gonzalez M, Desager J-P, Jacquemart J-L, Chenu P, Muller T, Installe E. Efficacy of enoximone in the management of refractory low-output states following cardiac surgery. *J Cardiothorac Anest*. 1988;2:409–418.

128. Bolling SF, Deeb GM, Crowley DC, Badellino MM, Bove EL. Prolonged amrinone therapy prior to orthotopic cardiac transplantation in patients with pulmonary hypertension. *Transpl Proc*. 1988;20(Suppl 1):753–756.

129. Unverferth DV, Blanford M, Kates RE, Leier CV. Tolerance to dobutamine after a 72 hour infusion. *Am J Med*. 1980;69:262–267.

130. Endoh M, Shibasaki T, Satoh H, Norota I, Ishihata A. Different mechanisms involved in the positive inotropic effects of benzimidazole derivative UD-CG115BS (pimobendan) and its demethylated metabolite UD-CG212C1 in canine ventricular myocardium. *J Cardiovasc Pharmacol*. 1991;17:365–375.

131. Fujino K, Sperelakis N, Solaro RJ. Sensitization of dog and guinea pig heart myofilaments to calcium activation and the inotropic effect of pimobendan: comparison with milrinone. *Circ Res*. 1988;63:911–922.

132. Kubo SH, Gollub S, Bourge R, et al. Beneficial effects of pimobendan on exercise tolerance and quality of life in patients with heart failure. *Circulation*. 1992;85:942–949.

133. Endoh M, Yanagisawa T, Taira N, Blinks JR. Effects of new inotropic agents on cyclic nucleotide metabolism and calcium transients in canine ventricular muscle. *Circulation*. 73(Suppl III):III-117–III-133.

134. Feldman AM, Baughman KL, Lee WK, et al. Usefulness of OPC-8212, a quinolinone derivative, for chronic congestive heart failure in patients with ischemic heart disease or idiopathic dilated cardiomyopathy. *Am J Cardiol*. 1991;68:1203–1210.

135. Iijima T, Taira N. Membrane current changes responsible for the positive inotropic effect of OPC-8212, a new positive inotropic agent, in single ventricular cells of the guinea pig heart. *J Pharm Exp Ther*. 1987;260:657–661.

136. Asanoi H, Sasayama S, Iuchi K, Kameyama T. Acute hemodynamic effects of a new inotropic agent (OPC-8212) in patients with congestive heart failure. *J Am Coll Cardiol*. 1987;9:865–871.

137. Kubo SH, Rector TS, Strobeck JE, Cohn JN. OPC-8212 in the treatment of congestive heart failure: results of a pilot study. *Cardiovasc Drugs Ther*. 1988;2:653–660.

138. Feldman AM, Bristow MR, Parmley WW, et al. Results of a multi-center study of OPC-8212 in chronic congestive heart failure. *Circulation*. 1992;86(Suppl I):I-374.

139. Franciosa JA. Intravenous amrinone: an advance or a wrong step? *Ann Intern Med*. 1985;102:399–400.

140. Pfeffer MA, Pfeffer JM, Steinberg C, Finn P. Survival after an experimental myocardial infarction: beneficial effects of long term therapy with captopril. *Circulation*. 1985;72:406–412.

141. et CS, Ludden CT, Stabilito II, Emmert SE, Heyse JF. Beneficial effects of milrinone and enalapril on long term survival of rats with healed myocardial infarction. *Eur J Pharmacol*. 1988;147:29–37.

142. Jain P, Brown EJ Jr, Langenback EG, et al. Effects of milrinone or left ventricular remodeling after acute myocardial infarction. *Circulation*. 1991;84:796–804.

143. White HD, Ribeiro JP, Hartley LH, Colucci WS. Immediate effects of milrinone on metabolic and sympathetic responses to exercise in severe congestive heart failure. *Am J Cardiol* 1985;56:93–98.

144. Siskind SJ, Sonnenblick EH, Forman R, Scheuer J, LeJemtel TH. Acute substantial benefit of inotropic therapy with amrinone on exercise hemodynamics and metabolism in severe congestive heart failure. *Circulation*. 1981;64:966–973.

145. Itoh H, Taniguehi K, Doi M, Koike A, Sakuma A. Effects of enoximone on exercise tolerance in patients with mild to moderate heart failure. *Am J Cardiol*. 1991;68:360–364.

146. DiBianco R, Shabetai R, Silverman BD, et al. Oral amrinone for the treatment of chronic congestive heart failure: results of a multicenter randomized double-blind and placebo-controlled withdrawal study. *J Am Coll Cardiol*. 198;4:855–866.

147. Massie B, Bourassa M, DiBianco R, et al. Long-term oral administration of amrinone for congestive heart failure: lack of efficacy in a multi-center controlled trial. *Circulation*. 1985;71:963–971.

148. Buser PT, Auffermann W, Wu ST, Jasmin G, Parmley WW, Wikman-Coffelt J. Dobutamine potentiates amrinone's beneficial effects in moderate but not in advanced heart failure. *Circ Res*. 1990;66:747–753.

149. Uretsky BF, Jessup M, Konstam MA, et al. Multicenter trial of oral enoximone in patients with moderate to moderately severe congestive heart failure. *Circulation*. 1990;82:774–780.

150. Goldberg AD, Nicklas J, Goldstein S, for the Imazodan Research Group. Effectiveness of imazodan for treatment of chronic congestive heart failure. *Am J Cardiol*. 1991;68:631–636.

151. Packer M, Francis GS, Abrams J, et al. Oral milrinone increases the risk of sudden risk of sudden death in severe chronic heart failure: the PROMISE trial. *Circulation*. 1991;(Suppl II):310.

Part V
Therapeutic Approach in
Acute Congestive Heart Failure

27
Hemodynamic Monitoring, Pharmacologic Therapy, and Arrhythmia Management in Acute Congestive Heart Failure

Jean-Louis Vincent

Acute heart failure represents an imbalance between the oxygen supply to the tissues and their oxygen requirements. In many patients, acute heart failure represents only a reduction in cardiac output, while the oxygen demand of the tissues remains normal. However, the oxygen consumption can be elevated sometimes in acutely ill cardiac patients.[1] The increased release of various immunological mediators of sepsis can be involved in this process.[2] Simple reference to a cardiac output to evaluate the cardiac function has to be reassessed in view of recent findings indicating that the myocardial contractility can be depressed even when cardiac output is normal or elevated. Therefore, the therapy of the patient with severe heart failure should be based on close monitoring of the cardiac function in relation to the needs of the tissues.[1,3] The symptoms related to the vascular congestion also commonly require a therapeutic intervention aimed at the reduction in cardiac filling pressures. However, preload cannot be reduced excessively in order for the cardiac output and the oxygen delivery to be maintained.

Invasive monitoring frequently is required in the management of severe heart failure, especially when the response to conventional therapy is unsatisfactory. It can help to define better the underlying pathophysiologic alterations and to orient therapy. Invasive hemodynamic monitoring also can clarify the role of specific alterations such as tamponade, valvular regurgitation, septal rupture, or right ventricular infarction.

By taking these elements into account, pharmacologic therapy will aim at the restoration of hemodynamic variables within the range of not necessarily normal values but optimal values. This therapy will be based not only on inotropic support to increase contractility but also on vasodilating therapy to reduce ventricular afterload and on fluid administration whenever required to maintain a sufficient ventricular preload.

The third part of this chapter reviews the management of serious arrhythmias in the patient with acute congestive heart failure (CHF). This important therapeutic aspect has been modified considerably with the introduction of amiodarone into our therapeutic armementarium.

Hemodynamic Monitoring

Invasive hemodynamic monitoring using the flow-directed pulmonary artery (PA) catheter allows the collection of two important types of parameters: first the cardiac filling pressures and in particular the pulmonary artery wedge pressure (also called pulmonary artery balloon-occluded pressure) and second, the determination of the cardiac output together with the withdrawal of mixed venous samples necessary to its interpretation.[4,5]

Measurement of PA Wedge Pressure

Heart failure usually is characterized by a low cardiac output associated with elevated cardiac filling pressures, which are in turn responsible for the development of cardiogenic pulmonary edema. Hence, classical therapy of CHF usually includes fluid and salt restriction together with the administration of diuretics. However, PA wedge pressure (PWP) is not necessarily elevated in patients with acute heart failure. First, the pulmonary edema is not always associated with a high hydrostatic pressure (i.e., it is not always hemodynamic in nature). Noncardiac factors such as sepsis, aspiration, trauma, etc. can be incriminated in the development of a non-hemodynamic type of pulmonary edema leading to the adult respiratory distress syndrome (ARDS). Second, cardiogenic pulmonary edema can be associated with a normal or only mildly elevated PWP at time of the measurement. Indeed, the formation of hemodynamic pulmonary edema is associated with the extravasation of water outside the pulmonary capillaries, resulting in

TABLE 27.1. Most typical hemodynamic patterns of the most common causes of low cardiac output.

	Right atrial pressure	Pulmonary artery pressure	Pulmonary artery balloon-occluded pressure	Cardiac index
LV failure	Normal	Elevated	Elevated	Reduced
Mitral stenosis	Normal	Elevated	Elevated	Normal or reduced
RV failure (RV infarction)	Elevated	Normal	Normal	Reduced
Pulmonary embolism, respiratory failure	Elevated	Elevated	Normal	Reduced
Tamponade	Elevated	Elevated (diastolic more than systolic)	Elevated	Reduced
Hypovolemia	Normal or reduced	Normal or reduced	Normal or reduced	Reduced

LV = left ventricular; RV = right ventricular.

a reduction in plasma volume.[6] By allowing the simultaneous measurements of PWP together with right atrial pressure (identical to the central venous press), the PA catheter allows to define relative degrees of failure of the two ventricles and thus to apply the most appropriate therapy to optimize ventricular preload (Table 27.1).

The PWP is normally about 3 to 5 mm Hg higher than the right atrial pressure. This left to right-sided pressure gradient can increase in the presence of left ventricular (LV) failure or decrease (and sometimes become negative) in the presence of right ventricular (RV) failure related to a loss in RV contractility (like in RV myocardial infarction) or in the presence of an increased RV afterload due to an increment in PA pressures (like in long-standing chronic lung disease or pulmonary vascular disease). It should be emphasized that according to the Frank-Starling relationship it is the degree of stretching of the myocardial fiber or by extension the end-diastolic volume that determines the degree of myocardial shortening. As shown by Calvin and co-workers,[7] the pressure/volume relationship of both ventricles can be altered in the critically ill patient. Bedside measurements of RV volumes have become available using the thermodilution technique.[8] However, the superiority of measurements of ventricular volumes rather than pressures in the management of the acutely ill patient has not been demonstrated.

The interpretation of PWP has two facets.

First, it represents the filling pressure of the LV, in the absence of an obstruction between the tip of the catheter and the LV. Such obstructions could be an excessive increase in airway pressure that could exceed the microvascular pressure. However, this phenomenon is uncommon in the absence of significant hypovolemia or application of high airway pressure during mechanical ventilation. The use of high levels of positive end-expiratory pressure (PEEP) has been critically reexamined recently and is now felt to be seldom required in patients with acute heart failure. The presence of

mitral valve disease represents another situation associated with a discrepancy between the PWP and the LV end-diastolic pressure. However, it usually can be recognized easily at the bedside by the use of echo-Doppler techniques. In most conditions, PWP correlates well with the end-diastolic LV pressure.[5]

Second, the PWP reflects the hydrostatic pressure in the lung capillaries. Hemodynamic pulmonary edema is related primarily to an increase in the hydrostatic pressure in the lung microvasculature, although a reduction in the plasma colloid osmotic pressure can increase the egress of fluids associated with an increase in hydrostatic pressures. Therefore, some authors have recommended the use of the colloid osmotic pressure–PWP gradient to assess the risk of development of hemodynamic pulmonary edema.[9] Incidentally, the term "hemodynamic" pulmonary edema has replaced the term "cardiogenic" because an increase in PWP can be related to heart failure, hypervolemia, or both. For example, a hemodynamic pulmonary edema can be found in an oliguric patient with terminal renal failure but with a normal cardiac function.

The therapy of the acutely ill often is based on the balance between these two elements. On the one hand, one would often like to increase PWP as a LV filling pressure, in order to maximize stroke volume by the Frank-Starling mechanism. On the other hand, one would like to decrease the PWP as a pulmonary hydrostatic pressure, in order to minimize the formation of pulmonary edema. Some investigators[10] reported that in patients with dilated heart failure, filling pressure can be maintained in the normal range without compromise of cardiac output. In acutely ill patients, PWP sometimes must be maintained at higher levels. Although the normal PWP is 7 to 10 mm Hg, a PWP of 15 to 18 mm HG often may be required to optimize stroke volume in acute myocardial infarction.[11] In patients with severe heart failure, some degree of hemodynamic pulmonary edema sometimes must be tolerated to maintain stroke volume by increasing ventricular preload.

Determination of the Cardiac Output

Together with the arterial oxygen content, cardiac output is the major determinant of the oxygen delivery to the tissues. It is therefore essential to approximate its value in the patient with acute heart failure, not only to confirm its low value, but to quantitate the degree of hemodynamic impairment and to evaluate objectively the response to therapy. There are various methods to determine cardiac output. The method based on the Fick principle, calculating cardiac output by dividing the oxygen consumption by the arteriovenous oxygen difference, has served as a reference. However, it is invasive and the determination of the oxygen uptake is subject to many technical problems. Determination of the production of carbon dioxide (CO_2), based on the indirect application of the Fick principle, is totally noninvasive, because the arterial CO_2 is considered as similar to the end-tidal CO_2, while the mixed venous CO_2 can be determined by rapid respiration into a bag until the CO_2 levels reach an equilibrium.[12] Unfortunately, this technique requires a relatively unaltered pulmonary function, so that it is not easily applicable in the acutely ill patient. The thermodilution technique, initially described by Fegler in 1954[13] but applied to the pulmonary artery catheter by Ganz and colleagues in 1971,[14] is simple, accurate, and easily repeated. The thermodilution technique is based on the Stewart-Hamilton principle using the dilution of a thermal indicator (i.e., the injection of a solution at a colder temperature than the body). The first method based on this principle was the indocyanine green dilution technique, which was relatively complex, time-consuming, and required the removal of blood. For the thermodilution technique, the modern techniques of injection and temperature measurement close to the site of injection have reduced the approximations of the measurement to less than 10%.[5]

Noninvasive techniques of course would be very valuable. For their application in the acutely ill patient, they should be accessible and easily repeated at the bedside. Hence, determinations based on radionuclide techniques or nuclear magnetic resonance cannot be considered in the acutely ill. Two potentially interesting methods are based on the electrical bioimpedance and on the echo-Doppler techniques.

Electrical Bioimpedance

In electrical bioimpedance, the thorax is considered as a homogeneous cylinder (Kubicec's formula) or a trunked cone (Sramek's formula), whose base is the thorax circumference at the xyphoid appendix level. An electrical current of low amplitude and high frequency is applied on electrodes placed on the upper and lower parts of the thorax. The measurement of cardiac output is based on the reduction in impedance related to the pulsatile changes in aortic flow. The technique is quite attracting, as it allows a simple, continuous, beat-to-beat analysis of the aortic blood flow. Unfortunately, the thorax is far from homogeneous, especially in the critically ill patient. In addition to underlying anatomic deformation, the presence of valvular disease, the development of pulmonary edema or lung infection, and even the use of mechanical ventilation can limit the validity of the measurement.[15] The presence of any metallic material such as a pacemaker in the thorax also invalidates the measurement. Therefore, correlations between cardiac output determinations by bioimpedance and thermodilution have yielded relatively poor results in acutely ill patients.[15–17] Additional information including a thoracic fluid index to evaluate the degree of pulmonary edema and some bioimpedance-derived indexes of contractility have been suggested, but these derived parameters are inaccurate.[18] Some authors, however, reported more accurate correlations between bioimpedance and thermodilution measurements in the child,[19] so that its use in the pediatric intensive care unit could be useful, especially when one takes into account the difficulties related to invasive hemodynamic monitoring in the child.

Echo-Doppler Techniques

Technological developments have allowed the use of echo-Doppler techniques in almost every intensive care unit (ICU) not only to visualize the intracardiac structures but also to monitor cardiac output. Unfortunately, measurements of cardiac output using the suprasternal approach have yielded inconsistent results. Good approximations have been observed in less severely ill patients. Some investigators have emphasized that this technique could track changes in cardiac output rather than give accurate actual values.[20] Comparing the measurements obtained by pulsed Doppler and by thermodilution in acutely ill patients has been rather disappointing. To limit some technical shortcomings, some authors proposed the use of dual beam concentric Doppler,[21] in which one beam explores the surface area of the aorta while the other, narrower, explores a more defined aortic area. Even though the technique alleviated the need to combine the Doppler measurement of flow velocity to the echocardiographic determination of the aortic diameter, the positioning of the probe remains difficult, so that the quality of the results highly rely on the operator's capabilities.[22] In a recent study, however, Niclou et al.[23] did not observe any significant influence of the operator's experience on the precision of the technique, but nevertheless concluded that the technique is "difficult if not impossible in many intensive care scenarios."[23]

The quality of transthoracic echocardiographic images often is limited not only by anatomic abnormalities, but also by the presence of dressings, drains, or the use of mechanical ventilation. Transesophageal Doppler techniques can avoid many of these problems due to transthoracic passage of the ultrasound waves. Tolerance of the technique is not a major problem in many critically ill patients with impaired consciousness related either to their underlying disease or to sedative therapy. Transesophageal techniques could even be used for continuous monitoring over prolonged periods of time, as in the operating room. Simpler esophageal probes have been suggested for this purpose,[24,25] but recent studies have not confirmed the validity of these measurements.[26] In patients during surgery, Muhuideen et al.[27] reported a poor correlation between esophageal Doppler techniques and the thermodilution technique. The esophageal Doppler technique recognized increases in cardiac output only when they exceeded 15%, but often missed the reductions in cardiac output. Some investigators have coupled a smaller Doppler probe to an endotracheal tube in mechanically ventilated patients, but this technique also has been found unreliable.[28] Furthermore, the time required to position the endotracheal tube averaged 10 min.[28]

Interpretation of a Cardiac Output Value

The cardiac output must adapt constantly to the oxygen requirements of the cells. Oxygen demand can be supranormal even in patients with acute-like chronic[29] heart failure. Resting energy expenditure has been found to be markedly greater in patients with chronic heart failure than in matched control subjects.[29] Increased work of breathing, higher catecholamines levels, increased sympathetic stimulation, increased immunological response,[2] development of tachycardia, and intercurrent infections can all contribute to this increase in cellular oxygen demand.

Oxygen consumption ($\dot{V}O_2$) cannot be determined routinely because such measurement requires sophisticated equipment and is subject to technical limitations. The technique is particularly difficult and uncomfortable in spontaneously breathing patients. The use of the pulmonary artery catheter allows access to mixed venous blood samples and the ability to determine its oxygen content. Although the $\dot{V}O_2$ value can be obtained by the application of the Fick equation, this is seldom necessary, as the interpretation of the mixed venous blood saturation ($S\overline{v}O_2$) alone usually is sufficient. By rearranging the Fick equation, $\dot{V}O_2 = CO \cdot (CaO_2 - C\overline{v}O_2)$, in which CaO_2 and $C\overline{v}O_2$ represent the O_2 contents of the arterial and the mixed venous blood, respectively.

As the O_2 content of the blood is primarily depends on the amount of O_2 bound to hemoglobin (Hb), one can simplify the relation by neglecting the dissolved O_2:

1) $\dot{V}O_2 = CO \cdot Hb(SaO_2 - SvO_2)$, where SaO_2 = arterial saturation

2) $CO \cdot Hb \cdot S\overline{v}O_2 = CO \cdot Hb \cdot SaO_2 - \dot{V}O_2$

3) $SvO_2 = SaO_2 - \dfrac{\dot{V}O_2}{CO \cdot Hb}$

Thus, once anemia and hypoxemia have been excluded or, when present, corrected, SvO_2 directly reflects the relationship between cardiac output and $\dot{V}O_2$. A reduction in SvO_2 below its normal value of 70% usually reflects an imbalance between the oxygen demand and the oxygen supply to the tissues. Admittedly, the arterial partial pressure of oxygen (PaO_2) can vary from about 60 to 120 mm Hg, so that the corresponding SaO_2 can vary from 90% to 98% in acutely ill patients. Therefore, oxygen extraction usually is preferred to more simple measurements of SvO_2.

Oxygen extraction can be simplified as $CaO_2 - C\overline{v}O_2/CaO_2 = SaO_2 - S\overline{v}O_2/SaO_2$, in which CaO_2 and $C\overline{v}O_2$ represent the oxygen contents of the arterial and the mixed venous blood, respectively. The relationship between cardiac output and oxygen extraction allows one to quantitate the degree of acute heart failure and to appreciate the response to therapy.[3] Curvilinear isopleths can represent various degrees of $\dot{V}O_2$, calculated by entering a hemoglobin level into the Fick equation (Fig. 27.1). The more severe the degree of heart failure, the greater the shift down and to the right (i.e., to lower cardiac index and higher degree of O_2 extraction).

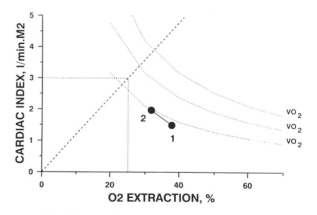

Figure 27.1. Diagram based on the relation between cardiac index and oxygen extraction serving to interpret the severity of heart failure. The line of reference (interrupted) passes through normal values for cardiac index (3 l/min/M³) and oxygen extraction (25%). The greater the severity of the heart failure, the larger the shift down and to the right. The curves (interrupted) represent serial $\dot{V}O_2$ isopleths. This example concerns a 64-year-old patient with severe heart failure after coronary surgery. When the doses of adrenergic agents were increased (from 1 to 2), the increase in cardiac index was associated with a shift toward the line of reference without significant change in $\dot{V}O_2$.

This analysis should have two important limitations. First, the ultimate goal is not always to restore a normal hemodynamic status. Some patients can tolerate very low cardiac output and high O_2 extraction ratios.[30] In some patients an increase in cardiac output is simply impossible to achieve. Second, the extraction capabilities are largely unknown in patients. Some patients with heart failure can have extremely high extraction ratios,[30] but these could become altered if an infection develops. Blood lactate levels can serve as a useful guide to detect the development of anaerobic metabolism when tissue hypoxia has occurred.[31] Blood lactate levels have been long recognized as a useful prognostic factor in acute heart failure related or not to myocardial infarction.[32,33]

Benefits and Risks of Pulmonary Artery Catheterization

Invasive hemodynamic monitoring is not required in every patient with acute heart failure. For instance, the patient with hemodynamic pulmonary edema responding rapidly to standard therapy or the patient with hopeless terminal disease probably will not benefit from this intervention. The risks related to the PA catheterization cannot be neglected (Table 27.2). However, the patient who does not improve readily with therapy or the patient whose underlying hemodynamic status is uncertain are likely to benefit from a goal-oriented therapy based on invasive parameters. The evaluation of the hemodynamic status by clinical means often is misleading and well recognized in critically ill patients.[4,5,34] A recent study by Chakko et al.[35] stressed that even in patients with chronic heart failure referred for evaluation for heart transplantation, physical and radiographic findings had poor predictive value in identifying patients with markedly elevated PWP.

Invasive hemodynamic monitoring can help to recognize the presence of RV myocardial infarction by a larger elevation of the RV filling pressure. Analysis of pressure waveform and determinations of the oxygen saturation in the right side of the heart can contribute to the diagnosis of various complications such as ventricular septal defect, mitral regurgitation, or free wall rupture.[5] However, the wide availability of the echo-Doppler techniques has largely obviated the need of invasive studies to reach these diagnoses.

Treatment of Acute Heart Failure

The primary goal of therapy of acute heart failure is the restoration of adequate diffusion of oxygen (DO_2) to the tissues. As DO_2 is determined primarily by the arterial oxygen content and the cardiac output, these two elements will be considered in rapid succession.

Oxygen should be administered immediately in the hypoxemic patient. Oxygen administration should not be delayed until the initial blood gases are obtained, because the interpretation of the PaO_2 is still possible if the inspired oxygen concentration (FiO_2) is known. Acutely ill patients with anemia should be transfused. When there is risk of cellular hypoxia, hemoglobin level should be restored to at least 10 g/dl (or hematocrit to 30%).

Cardiac output can be increased by acting on one or several of its four determinants: contractility, preload, afterload, and heart rate.

Contractility

Although various classes of inotropic agents are available today (Fig. 27.2), adrenergic agents remain the mainstay in the management of acute heart failure (Table 27.3). Some studies, however, indicated that patients with severe heart failure related or not to acute myocardial infarction could still benefit from digitalis glycosides.[36]

In acute heart failure, dobutamine has become the treatment of choice, as it exerts strong inotropic but limited chronotropic and no vasoconstrictive effect. Dobutamine induces less tachycardia than isoprotere-

TABLE 27.2. Risks associated with the use of the PA catheter.

1. Complications related to insertion: pneumothorax, nerve lesions, hematoma
2. Catheter-knotting in the right-sided structures
3. Arrhythmias: ventricular ectopic beats, ventricular tachycardia and fibrillation, complete AV block
4. Endocardial lesions
5. Pulmonary artery thrombosis and infarction
6. Catheter-related infection
7. Pulmonary artery rupture

PA = pulmonary artery; AV = arteriovenous.

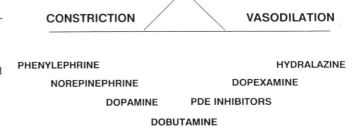

FIGURE 27.2. List of inotropic agents according to their peripheral vascular effects.

TABLE 27.3. Doses and effects of the most commonly used adrenergic agents.

Agent	Dose	Primary goal of therapy
Dobutamine	1–20 μg/kg/min	Increase cardiac output
Dopamine	2–20 μg/kg/min	Increase arterial pressure
Norepinephrine	5–50 μg/min	Increase arterial pressure if dopamine ineffective
Adrenaline	2–20 μg/min	Increase cardiac output and arterial pressure if dobutamine ineffective
Dopexamine	1–5 μg/kg/min	Increase cardiac output and splanchnic blood flow (adjunctive therapy)

nol, so that the risk of myocardial ischemia is reduced. Changes in arterial pressure usually are modest with dobutamine. However, sometimes a significant increase in arterial pressure can be associated with a prompt cardiac output response. On the contrary, a reduction in arterial pressure during dobutamine infusion should raise the possibility of underlying hypovolemia.

The use of dopamine has been limited to severe cases of cardiovascular collapse, imposing the use of a vasopressor to restore a minimal tissue perfusion pressure. By its vasoconstricting effects, dopamine tends to increase LV afterload and the cardiac filling pressures. Even though low doses of dopamine (below 5 μg/kg/min) do not have vasoconstrictive properties in normal individuals, the clinical response sometimes differs in acutely ill patients. Altered metabolism of dopamine and downregulation of the beta-adrenergic receptors could contribute to this different response. Although the dopaminergic effects of dopamine may increase the urine output, protective effects of dopamine on the renal function have not been demonstrated conclusively.[37] Nevertheless, dopamine can be useful in restoring minimal coronary perfusion pressure. In some patients with severe pulmonary hypertension, higher levels of arterial pressure are required to maintain RV function. Indeed, the coronary blood supply to the RV, taking place during both diastole and systole, is determined by the pressure gradient between the aorta and the right ventricle. Norepinephrine (Levophed) might be required in the most severe cases. In any case, these vasoconstrictors should be used for a minimum period of time and weaned off as soon as feasible. Epinephrine is also sometimes used in the most severe cases.

Dopexamine is a new synthetic catecholamine that combines beta-2 and dopaminergic properties. With this pharmacological profile, dopexamine associates vasodilating and inotropic properties. In acutely ill patients with cardiorespiratory failure, dopexamine administration increases cardiac index by combined increases in stroke volume and heart rate.[38] In patients with heart failure, dopexamine administration has been shown also to increase urine and water excretion.[39,40] As dopexamine has significant tachycardic effects, doses usually are limited to a maximum of 5 μg/kg/min.

Phosphodiesterase (PDE) inhibitors such as milrinone or enoximone represent another group of "inodilating" agents that do not, however, stimulate the adrenergic receptors. Some PDE inhibitors have been reported to increase the affinity of myocardial fibers for calcium.[41] Interestingly, they usually do not increase the myocardial oxygen requirements, probably because the effects of the increase in myocardial contractility are offset by the reduction in ventricular afterload. Used alone, these agents have greater vasodilating properties than dobutamine.[42] These differences usually result in a larger reduction in cardiac filling pressures and also in arterial pressure with PDE inhibitors than with dobutamine.[43] The major drawback of these agents in the acutely ill patient is their long half-life, which complicates their titration. When hypotension occurs, it can persist for sometimes several hours.

The major interest of the PDE inhibitors in acutely ill patients lies in their combination with adrenergic agents.[44] Even in patients with cardiogenic shock, small doses of enoximone can consistently increase cardiac output without any significant effect on arterial pressure[45] (Fig. 27.3). In view of these pharmacological properties, we favor the use of repeated boluses of small doses of PDE inhibitors to the commonly used alternative of a constant infusion.[46]

Preload

In chronic heart failure, the pulmonary vascular congestion secondary to LV failure is frequently the source of respiratory symptoms, and is treated as such by sodium restriction and diuretic therapy. In some patients with coronary insufficiency, the reduction in ventricular stress that can result from diuretic therapy can improve ventricular function. In contrast, the positioning of the cardiac function on the flat portion of the Frank-Starling relationship makes any beneficial effect from volume therapy highly hypothetical. The situation might be quite different in acute heart failure, in which volume overload may be minimal or absent. Acute heart failure is commonly due to an ischemic event that is associated with a reduction in ventricular compliance, so that a higher ventricular end-diastolic pressure might be required to maintain a sufficient ventricular preload in the presence of an acute myocardial depression.[11] As it was stressed earlier, the preload corresponds to the degree of stretch of the myocardial sarcomere rather than to the end-diastolic pressure. Myocardial ischemia-like vasoconstriction are conditions where the ventricular pressure/volume relation can be altered in such a way that a higher end-diastolic pressure is required to maintain a sufficient end-diastolic volume.[7,11] Patients

FIGURE 27.3. Effects on mean arterial pressure and cardiac index of the addition of enoximone (0.5 mg/kg once or twice) to dobutamine therapy in patients with cardiogenic shock. The open circles represent a patient after cardiac transplantation. Reprinted, with permission, from ref. 45.

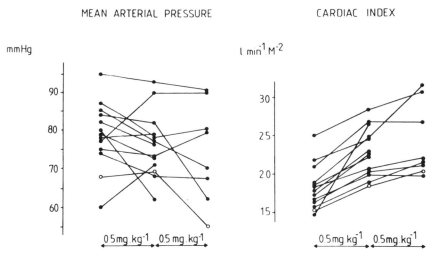

with acute pulmonary edema have been found to have a decreased plasma volume secondary to the egress of fluids into the interstitial spaces.[6] In these patients who sometimes present with hypotension, diuretic therapy might further compromise their hemodynamic status.[47] As an alternative, the use of vasoconstrictors also can be hazardous by increasing myocardial oxygen requirements and by inducing peripheral vasoconstriction. In heart failure secondary to acute myocardial infarction, fluid infusion occasionally can be the treatment of choice, provided that it is performed according to a fluid challenge technique, under strict control of the cardiac filling pressures.[48] Recommendations for fluid challenge technique can be found elsewhere.[49] It should be emphasized that therapeutic agents can alter cardiac filling pressures. In particular, vasoconstrictor agents like dopamine tend to increase PWP, in contrast to dobutamine, which usually maintains or reduces PWP (Fig. 27.4). In summary, diuretics should be used cautiously in hemodynamically unstable patients be-

cause they can limit cardiac output and lead to failure of other organs. In case of doubt, invasive monitoring should be used to monitor PWP, cardiac output, and the oxygen-derived variables.

Afterload

The administration of peripheral vasodilators to reduce ventricular afterload has represented a major improvement in the management of heart failure. However, the use of pure vasodilators in the critically ill often is limited by the risk of reduction in arterial pressure. Although various vasodilating agents are currently available (Table 27.4), intravenous agents with a short half-life are preferred in these patients. Nitroglycerin (or dinitrate isosorbide) and sodium nitroprusside are the most popular agents. Nitroglycerin usually is preferred in the presence of severe coronary heart disease (for its effects on the coronary distribution of blood flow) or elevated cardiac filling pressures (for its more predominant effects on preload), whereas nitroprusside is preferred in the presence of arterial hypertension. The development of profound hypotension with these agents should raise the possibility of a reduction in preload compatible with underlying hypovolemia or a right ventricular myocardial infarction.

As they combine vasodilating and negative inotropic properties, calcium entry blockers should be avoided in the treatment of patients with acute heart failure. In the presence of severe pulmonary hypertension, prostaglandin E_1 (PGE_1) probably represents the vasodilating agent of choice. Prostacyclin (PGI_2) has similar effects. In patients after cardiac transplantation, a combination of PGE_1, with vasopressors like norepinephrine, can be very beneficial.[50]

Nonpharmacological support to reduce LV afterload can consist of an increase in the intrathoracic pressure by the use of mechanical ventilation or simply by the application of a continuous positive airway pressure

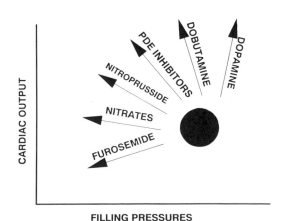

FIGURE 27.4. Effects of some commonly used agents on the relationship between cardiac output and cardiac filling pressures.

TABLE 27.4. Most commonly used vasodilating agents with their usual dose, duration of effects, and predominant cardiovascular effects.

	Dose	Duration of effects	Predominant vascular effect	Inotropic effect
Intravenous				
Sodium nitroprusside	20–250 μg/min	2–3 min	Balanced	None
Nitroglycerin	10–200 μg/min	3–5 min	Venous > arterial	None
Prostaglandin E$_1$	40–120 ng/kg/min	3–5 min	Pulmonary > systemic	None
Hydralazine	10–40 mg	4–6 hr	Arterial > venous	Positive (slight)
Oral				
Isosorbide dinitrate	10–40 mg	6–8 hr	Venous > arterial	None
Prazocine	2–4 mg	6–8 hr	Balanced	None
Hydralazine	25–100 mg	6–10 hr	Arterial > venous	Positive (slight)
Minoxidil	10–30 mg	8–12 hr	Arterial > venous	None
Nifedipine	5–20 mg	3–6 hr	Arterial > venous	Negative

(CPAP) by a facial mask.[51] During systole, the higher pressures around the heart reduce the pressure gradient for the ejection of blood. At first sight, the application of the positive pleural pressure should be limited to the systolic part of the cardiac cycle to avoid any impeding effects of the higher intrathoracic pressure on venous return.[52] However, a higher pleural pressure can reduce LV afterload also during diastole by reducing the thoracic aortic blood volume, which in turn decreases the systolic intracardiac pressure.[53] This can explain the observations by Pinsky et al,[52] that pressure changes induced by high frequency jet ventilation were almost as effective during diastole than during systole. Therefore, patients with transient episodes of worsening heart failure (like in hemodynamic pulmonary edema) can improve markedly by the application of CPAP by mask.[51]

In the presence of cardiogenic shock associated with hemodynamic pulmonary edema, the use of mechanical ventilation often results in a dramatic improvement that is sometimes wrongly attributed by the nonspecialist to a direct effect of the higher intrathoracic pressure on the edema formation. On the contrary, experimental studies show that the application of positive airway pressure might increase the extravascular lung water. The beneficial effects of mechanical ventilation can be related to both an increase in DO$_2$ and a reduction in the O$_2$ requirements. DO$_2$ is ameliorated by the improvement in gas exchange and the improvement in cardiac function associated with the reduction in LV afterload. The reduction in VO$_2$ is related to the relieving effect on the work of breathing and the resting of the respiratory muscles.[54] Other nonpharmacological options to sustain cardiac function is presented in other chapters of this book.

Heart Rate

Except in profound bradycardia, manipulation of heart rate is not effective in increasing cardiac output, be-

cause the increase in heart rate is associated with a corresponding reduction in stroke volume. When heart rate is significantly reduced in the presence of heart failure, the administration of isoproterenol is sometimes preferred to the external electrical stimulation to benefit from the additional beta-adrenergic–mediated increase in myocardial contractility.

Management of Arrhythmias

The discussion of the various therapeutic options in the management of serious arrhythmias should be preceded by some general comments pertinent to all forms of acute dysrhythmias associated with heart failure. Treatment can aim at the restoration of the hemodynamic stability as well as at the prevention of more severe arrhythmias. Therefore, the need for aggressive management of cardiac arrhythmias should be dictated not only by the severity of the arrhythmia but also by the clinical context. Underlying precipitating factors should be corrected, such as mechanical contact (catheter-induced ventricular arrhythmias), potassium disturbances, or hypoxemia. Treatment should be profiled not only for efficacy but also for safety. However, in the management of serious arrhythmias, a limited incidence of side effects can be accepted as the price to pay for rapid efficacy.

Many new agents have been developed this last decade for management of chronic arrhythmias, but few have represented a real progress in the management of acute arrythmias. Although a parenteral form has been developed for most of these new agents, few medications have been developed especially for rapid intravenous administration. The exception to this rule has been the development of amiodarone, which combines excellent activity against both supraventricular and ventricular arrhythmias and remarkable hemodynamic tolerance. As amiodarone represents a real breakthrough in the management of serious arrhythmias in the intensive care unit, we will also briefly review the main characteristics of this agent. More extended reviews can be found elsewhere.[55–57]

Management of Supraventricular Tachycardia

Narrow QRS Tachycardias

Rapid supraventricular arrhythmias can be the source of hemodynamic compromise and require rapid therapeutic intervention. Although vagotonic maneuvers should be tried first, they are seldom effective in the acutely ill patient. If the supraventricular tachycardia is poorly tolerated, immediate QRS-synchronized cardioversion should be performed. Energy levels of 100 J usually are sufficient. As the cells of the AV node are calcium-dependent, the calcium entry blocker verapamil usually is effective in all types of narrow QRS tachycardia: atrial tachycardia, intra-AV nodal reentry tachycardia, and reciprocal tachycardia associated with accessory pathways. Verapamil should be administered as a slow bolus of 5 to 10 mg over 2 min. The negative inotropic effects of verapamil sometimes can result in clinical deterioration, so that digitalis might be preferred initially in patients with myocardial failure.

In the acutely ill patient, supraventricular tachycardias often are due to a true atrial tachycardia, and verapamil will only transiently slow down the ventricular response. If treatment is required, amiodarone generally represents an effective and safe mode of therapy, with a much lesser myocardial depressant effect than verapamil.[58]

Atrial Flutter and Fibrillation

Calcium entry blockers, beta-blocking agents, and digoxin have been largely used in these situations but they are poorly effective and, when they are, have a short duration of action. These agents can be effective for the control of the ventricular response. Intravenous administration of amiodarone rapidly slows the ventricular response and restores a normal sinus rhythm in most cases.[55–58] A recent randomized, controlled study confirmed that amiodarone is more effective than verapamil in the conversion of paroxysmal atrial fibrillation to sinus rhythm; the conversion rate was 71% with amiodarone.[59]

Atrial fibrillation can occur in the context of an accessory pathway with anterograde conduction. A sometimes very rapid ventricular rate can present as an irregular polymorphic tachycardia with a substantial number of broad QRS complexes, reflecting the depolarization pathway over the AV node, the accessory pathway, or both. In the presence of hemodynamic instability, cardioversion is the treatment of choice. In stable situations, medical treatment might be preferred; however, antiarrhythmic agents depressing the AV node should be avoided, as these could accelerate the ventricular response through the accessory pathway. Instead of a calcium entry blocker, digoxin, or even amiodarone, preference should be given to an agent having predominant effects on the accessory pathway. Class 1c drugs such as flecainide or propafenone are the agents of choice.[60,61] They must be administered prudently, however, because they exert strong negative inotropic effects. Doses of 1 to 2 mg/kg should be administered as a slow bolus over 5 to 10 min. Alternatively, a slow intravenous infusion could be administered over 1 hr or more.

Management of Ventricular Arrhythmias

Poorly tolerated ventricular arrhythmias require immediate cardioversion. If the cardiovascular status remains stable, medical therapy can be attempted. Differential diagnosis between ventricular tachycardia and supraventricular tachycardia with aberration is sometimes difficult. Nevertheless, in an acute setting, all tachycardias with broad QRS complexes should be considered as ventricular tachycardia, unless proven otherwise. Lidocaine still represents the drug of choice in the short-term, emergency management of serious ventricular arrhythmias, as it is rapidly effective and well tolerated. Lidocaine is particularly effective in the prevention of ventricular arrhythmias; it is probably also effective in stopping the ventricular tachycardia. If lidocaine is ineffective, bretylium or amiodarone should be added. The use of bretylium should be limited to CPR.[62] Some studies reported that amiodarone might be superior to bretylium in life-threatening arrhythmias.[63] Amiodarone is preferred for prolonged administration over several days. When lidocaine cannot control the ventricular arrhythmia, the addition of other types of antiarrhythmic agents, such as mexiletine, tocainamide, or procainamide, is of little protection. The potential benefit could be outweighed by the potential toxicity of a polypharmaceutical approach. A class 1c agent would represent a more logical choice, but the negative inotropic effects of these agents and their possible proarrhythmic action must be taken into account.[61]

Amiodarone

Amiodarone is a benzofuran derivative, which was first introduced in Belgium in 1967 as an antianginal agent. As weak alpha- and beta-adrenergic–inhibiting properties, amiodarone has smooth muscle relaxant properties and coronary vasodilating effects. Nevertheless, its antianginal properties were found as relatively weak while its antiarrhythmic properties were discovered only subsequently.

Amiodarone prolongs the action potential duration and refractoriness of all cardiac tissues, slows the sinus node discharge rate, reduces the conduction through the AV node, and suppresses atrial, junctional, and ventricular ectopy. These unique effects, in part attributed to an alteration in potassium channel currents, justified its placement into the class III of the Vaughan-Williams classification.

With oral administration, the absorption is slow, incomplete, and variable and the bioavailability is less than 50%. Peak blood levels are obtained only 3 to 7 hr after a single dose, but clearance from plasma is low so that persistence in the blood can be observed up to 1 month after a single oral dose. Therefore, intravenous administration is preferred in the acutely ill patient, even though oral therapy can be started concurrently.

Slow intravenous or oral administration of the drug does not produce any significant hemodynamic change, even in patients with poor myocardial function.[64–66] A reduction in heart rate is an almost universal finding. Mild negative inotropic effects are compensated by slight vasodilating effects. Therefore, amiodarone is not contraindicated in patients with acute heart failure. Amiodarone is also well tolerated in the presence of ischemic heart disease.[67] In an experimental study on dogs, DeBoer et al.[68] observed that amiodarone reduced the infarct size presumably by reducing the myocardial oxygen requirements related to the combined reductions in heart rate, contractility, and afterload.

The rapid administration of amiodarone is associated with a fall in arterial pressure and an increase in heart rate, but these effects are primarily due to the vehicle. Therefore, amiodarone probably should be administered as a short-term infusion rather than a direct bolus. However, some investigators administered amiodarone as a rapid bolus over 1 min.[69] At the other extreme, some studies have used a continuous infusion of 5 to 10 mg/kg over the first 12 hr. The usual recommended dose is 300 mg (diluted in 5% dextrose) over 20 min (possibly repeated), followed by a constant infusion of 900 to 1500 mg/24 hr. Remme et al.[70] recently reported that the administration of 5 mg/kg of amiodarone over 5 min was not only well tolerated but improved the cardiac pump function in patients with impaired LV function. There was, however, a tendency to increase the left-sided filling pressures. In these conditions, the electrophysiological effects of amiodarone were sometimes observed as soon as 5 min after the intravenous infusion.[71] To avoid phlebitis, the drug should be administered via a central line.

As an alternative, a rapid oral loading of amiodarone also has been suggested.[72] Some investigators[72,73] observed that an oral loading protocol of 2 to 4 g/day can result in arrhythmias suppression within 24 to 48 hr. A recent study of 16 patients[74] reported the good clini-

cal tolerance of a high oral dose loading consisting of 50 mg/kg/day for 3 days, then 30 mg/kg/day for 2 days, followed by maintenance therapy of 600 to 800 mg/day. In any case, the onset of action of amiodarone seems longer with oral than with intravenous loading as described above.

The metabolism of amiodarone takes place primarily in the liver, and the only identified metabolite is desethylamiodarone. Amiodarone is not eliminated by hemodialysis.

Various studies have emphasized the remarkable efficacy and the excellent tolerance of amiodarone in the emergency management of severe ventricular arrhythmias.[57,64,66,67,75,76] Ochi et al.[67] recently studied the effects of intravenous amiodarone in 22 critically ill patients with coronary artery disease and recurrent life-threatening ventricular tachyarrhythmias refractory to conventional antiarrhythmic therapy. In the 24 hr preceding the administration of amiodarone, patients had 2.4 episodes of life-threatening arrhythmias requiring a mean of four cardioversions, despite medical therapy with a mean of 3.7 antiarrhythmic agents. Arrhythmias were controlled in one half of the patients within 24 hr and in two thirds in the second 24 hr. Other studies have stressed the good tolerance to intravenous amiodarone, even in patients with severe heart failure requiring adrenergic therapy.[64]

Amiodarone administration is associated with a substantial list of side effects, which, however, usually occur during chronic therapy (Table 27.5). The high iodine content (37%) of amiodarone accounts for the thyroid abnormalities, especially in the elderly patient. Amiodarone inhibits the peripheral conversion of T4 to T3, producing an increase in reverse T3. This should be

TABLE 27.5. Secondary effects of amiodarone.

Type of effect	Relative incidence (%)
Cardiac	
Bradycardia	2–10
Worsening of heart failure	1–8
Gastrointestinal	
Nausea, anorexia	5–10
Abnormal liver tests	10–25
Pulmonary	2–10
Thyroid abnormalities	1–7
Dermatologic	
Photosensitivity	20–50
Blue skin	2–6
Ophthalmologic	
Corneal deposits	>60
Blurred vision	2–7
Neurologic	
Weakness/fatigue	2–8
Tremor	2–20
Neuropathy	1–10
Sleep disturbances	5–10

compensated by an increase in thyroid-releasing hormone (TRH) and thyroid-stimulating hormone (TSH). Therefore, amiodarone therapy is associated with hypo- more often than hyperthyroidism. The most severe complication of amiodarone therapy is the development of interstitial pneumonitis, characterized by dyspnea, dry cough, low grade fever, and a bilateral chest infiltrate that is sometimes mistaken for a pulmonary edema.[77] Gallium scanning can assist in the diagnosis. Pulmonary toxicity can be seldom related to a hypersensitivity reaction. It is important to emphasize that the administration of lower doses of amiodarone can be well tolerated and still be effective. A recent double-blinded study by Nicklas et al.[78] indicates that an oral dose of 400 mg/day for 4 weeks followed by a dose of 200 mg/day can significantly suppress spontaneous ventricular ectopy in patients with severe heart failure. This treatment was safe and side effects were absent.

Conclusion

Treatment of acute heart failure should be based on rational manipulations of contractility, afterload, preload, and sometimes heart rate to maintain cardiac output and oxygen delivery and to satisfy the tissue's oxygen demand. Frequently, the clinical assessment does not provide sufficient information about the elements so that therapy must be guided by invasive hemodynamic monitoring. Arrhythmias can represent other important problems that require prompt intervention to correct their cause, to control their consequences, and to prevent their life-threatening complications.

References

1. Resnik H, Friedman B. Studies on the mechanism of the increased oxygen consumption in patients with cardiac disease. *J Clin Invest*. 1935;14:551–562.
2. Levine B, Kalman J, Mayer L, et al. Elevated circulating levels of tumor necrosis factor in severe chronic heart failure. *N Engl J Med*. 1990:323:236–241.
3. Vincent JL. Advances in the concepts of intensive care. *Am Heart J*. 1991;121:1859–1865.
4. Vincent JL. The pulmonary artery catheter: twenty years of use. *Clin Intens Care*. 1991;1(6):244–248.
5. European Society of Intensive Care Medicine. Expert panel. The use of the pulmonary artery catheter. *Intens Care Med*. 1991;17:I–VIII.
6. Da Luz PL, Weil MH, Liu VY, et al. Plasma volume prior to and following volume loading during shock complicating acute myocardial infarction. *Circulation*. 1974; XLIX:98–105.
7. Calvin JE, Driedger AA, Sibbald WJ. Does the pulmonary capillary wedge pressure predict left ventricular preload in critically ill patients. *Crit Care Med*. 1981;9: 437–443.

8. Reuse C, Vincent JL, Pinsky MR. Measurements of right ventricular volumes during fluid challenge. *Chest*. 1990; 98:1450–1454.
9. Weil MH, Henning RJ, Morissette M, et al. Relationship between colloid osmotic pressure and pulmonary artery wedge pressure in patients with acute cardiorespiratory failure. *Am J Med*. 1978;64:643–649.
10. Stevenson LW, Tillisch JH. Maintenance of cardiac output with normal filling pressures in patients with dilated heart failure. *Circulation*. 1986;74:1303–1308.
11. Forrester JS, Chatterjee K, Jobin C. A new conceptual approach to the therapy of acute myocardial infarction. *Adv Cardiol*. 1975;15:111–113.
12. Powles ACP, Campbell EJM. How to be less invasive. *Am J Med*. 1979;67:98–104.
13. Fegler GA. Measurement of cardiac output in anesthetized animals by a thermodilution method. *Q J Exp Physiol*. 1954;39:153–164.
14. Ganz W, Donoso R, Marcus HS, et al. A new technique for measurement of cardiac output by thermodilution in man. *Am J Cardiol*. 1971;27:392–395.
15. Preiser JC, Daper A, Parquier JN, et al. Transthoracic electrical bioimpedance versus thermodilution technique for cardiac output measurement during mechanical ventilation. *Intens Care Med*. 1989;15:221–223.
16. Donovan KD, Dobb GJ, Woods WPD, et al. Comparison of transthoracic electrical impedance and thermodilution methods for measuring cardiac output. *Crit Care Med*. 1986;14:1038–1044.
17. Spinale FG, Smith AC, Crawford FA. Relationship of bioimpedance to thermodilution and echocardiographic measurements of cardiac function. *Crit Care Med*. 1990;18:414–418.
18. Miles DS, Gotshall RW, Quinones JD, et al. Impedance cardiography fails to measure accurately left ventricular ejection fraction. *Crit Care Med*. 1990;18:221–228.
19. Mickell JJ, Lucking SE, Chaten FC, et al. Trending of impedance-monitored cardiac variables: method and statistical power analysis of 100 control studies in pediatric intensive care unit. *Crit Care Med*. 1990;18:645–650.
20. Rose JS, Nanna M, Rahimtoola SH, et al. Accuracy of determination of changes in cardiac output by transcutaneous continuous-wave doppler computer. *Am J Cardiol*. 1984;54:1099–1101.
21. Looyenga DS, Liebson PR, Bone RC, et al. Determination of cardiac output in critically ill patients by dual beam Doppler echocardiography. *J Am Coll Cardiol*. 1989;13:340–347.
22. Wong DH, Mahutte CK. Two-beam pulsed Doppler cardiac output measurement: reproducibility and agreement with thermodilution. *Crit Care Med*. 1990;18:433–437.
23. Niclou R, Teague SM, Lee R. Clinical evaluation of a diameter sensing Doppler cardiac output meter. *Crit Care Med*. 1990;18:428–432.
24. Freund PR. Transesophageal Doppler scanning versus thermodilution during general anesthesia. *Am J Surg*. 1987;153:490–494.
25. Singer M, Clarke J, Bennett ED. Continuous hemodynamic monitoring by esophageal Doppler. *Crit Care Med*. 1989;17:447–452.
26. Kamal GD, Symreng T, Starr J. Inconsistent esophageal

Doppler cardiac output during acute blood loss. *Anesthesiology*. 1990;72:95–99.

27. Muhiudeen IA, Kuecherer HF, Lee E, et al. Intraoperative estimation of cardiac output by transesophageal pulsed Doppler echocardiography. *Anesthesiology*. 1991;74:9–14.

28. Siegel LC, Fitzgerald DC, Engstrom RH. Simultaneous intraoperative measurement of cardiac output by thermodilution and transtracheal Doppler. *Anesthesiology*. 1991;74:664–669.

29. Riley M, Elborn JS, McKane WR et al. Resting energy expenditure in chronic cardiac failure. *Clin Sci*. 1991;80:633–639.

30. Schlichtig R, Cowden VL, Chaitman BR. Tolerance of unusually low mixed venous oxygen saturation adaptations in the chronic low cardiac output syndrome. *Am J Med*. 1986;80:813–818.

31. Vincent JL. The value of blood lactate monitoring in clinical practice. In: Gutierrez G, Vincent JL, eds. *Tissue Oxygen Utilization. Update in Intensive Care and Emergency Medicine*. vol. 12. Berlin, Heidelberg, New York: Springer-Verlag; 1991:260–268.

32. Weil MW, Afifi AA. Experimental and clinical studies on lactate and pyruvate as indicators of acute circulatory failure. *Circulation*. 1970;16:989–1001.

33. Mavric Z, Zaputovic L, Zagar D, et al. Usefulness of blood lactate as a predictor of shock development in acute myocardial infarction. *Am J Cardiol*. 1991;67:565–568.

34. Connors AF Jr, McCaffree DR, Gray BA. Evaluation of right-heart catheterization in the critically ill patient without acute myocardial infarction. *N Engl J Med*. 1983;308:263–267.

35. Chakko S, Woska D, Martinez H, et al. Clinical, radiographic, and hemodynamic correlations in chronic congestive heart failure: conflicting results may lead to inappropriate care. *Am J Med*. 1991;90:353–359.

36. Rackow EC, Packman MI, Weil MH. Hemodynamic effects of digoxin during acute cardiac failure: a comparison in patients with and without acute myocardial infarction. *Crit Care Med*. 1987;15:1001–1005.

37. Vincent JL. Do we need a dopaminergic agent in the management of the critically ill? *J of Autonom Pharmacol*. 1990;10(Suppl 1):123–127.

38. Vincent JL, Reuse C, Kahn RJ. Administration of dopexamine, a new adrenergic agent, in cardiorespiratory failure. *Chest*. 1989;96:1233–1236.

39. Leier CV, Binkley PF, Carpenter J, et al. Cardiovascular pharmacology of dopexamine in low output congestive heart failure. *Am J Cardiol*. 1988;62:94–99.

40. Baumann G, Felix SB, Filcek SAL. Usefulness of dopexamine hydrochloride versus dobutamine in chronic congestive heart failure and effects on hemodynamics and urine output. *Am J Cardiol*. 1990;65:748–754.

41. Fujino K, Sperelakis N, Solaro RJ. Sensitization of dog and guinea pig heart myofilaments to Ca^{2+} activation and the inotropic effect of pimobendan: comparison with milrinone. *Circ Res*. 1988;63:911–922.

42. Marcus RH, Raw K, Patel J, et al. Comparison of intravenous amrinone and dobutamine in congestive heart failure due to idiopathic dilated cardiomyopathy. *Am J Cardiol*. 1990;66:1107–1112.

43. Uretsky BF, Generalovich T, Verbalis JG, et al. Comparative hemodynamic and hormonal response to enoximone and dobutamine in severe congestive heart failure. *Am J Cardiol*. 1986;58:110–116.

44. Gage J, Rutman H, Lucido D, et al. Additive effects of dobutamine and amrinone on myocardial contractility and ventricular performance in patients with severe heart failure. *Circulation*. 1986;74:367–373.

45. Vincent JL, Carlier E, Berré J, et al. Administration of enoximone in cardiogenic shock. *Am J Cardiol*. 1988;62:419–423.

46. Vincent JL, Léon M, Berré J, et al. Addition of enoximone to adrenergic agents for the management of severe heart failure. *Crit Care Med*. 1992;20:1102–1106.

47. Hoffman MJ, Greenfield LJ, Sugerman JH, et al. Unsuspected right ventricular dysfunction in shock and sepsis. *Ann Surg*. 1983;198:307–319.

48. Figueras J, Weil MH. Hypovolemia and hypotension complicating management of acute cardiogenic pulmonary edema. *Am J Cardiol*. 1979;44:1349–1355.

49. Vincent JL. Fluids for resuscitation. *Br J Anaesth*. 1991:67:185–193.

50. Vincent JL, Carlier E, Goldstein J, et al. PGE1 infusion for pulmonary hypertension after cardiac transplantation. *J Thorac Cardiovasc Surg*. 1992;103:33–39.

51. Rasanen J, Heikkila J, Downs J, et al. Continuous positive airway pressure by face mask in acute cardiogenic pulmonary edema. *Am J Cardiol*. 1985;55:296–300.

52. Pinsky MR, Matuschak GM, Bernardi L, et al. Hemodynamic effects of cardiac cycle-specific increases in intrathoracic pressure. *J Appl Physiol*. 1986;60:604–612.

53. Fessler HE, Brower RG, Wise RA, et al. Mechanism of reduced LV afterload by systolic and diastolic positive pleural pressure. *J Appl Physiol*. 1988;65(3):1244–1250.

54. Aubier M, Viires N, Syllie G, et al. Respiratory muscle contribution to lactic acidosis in low cardiac output. *Am Rev Respir Dis*. 1982;126:648–652.

55. Mason JW. Amiodarone. *N Engl J Med*. 1987;316:455–466.

56. Michelson EL, Dreifus LS. Newer antiarrhythmic drugs. *Med Clin of North Am*. 1988;72:275–319.

57. Kadish A, Morady F. The use of intravenous amiodarone in the acute therapy of life-threatening tachyarrhythmias. *Prog Cardiovasc Dis*. 1989;31:281–294.

58. Gomes JAC, Kang PS, Hariman RJ, et al. Electrophysiologic effects and mechanisms of termination of supraventricular tachycardia by intravenous amiodarone. *Am Heart J*. 1984;107:214.

59. Noc M, Stajer S, Horvat M. Intravenous amiodarone versus verapamil for acute conversion of paroscsysmal atrial fibrillation to sinus rhythm. *Am J Cardiol*. 1991;65:679–680.

60. Hammill SC, McLaran CJ, Wood DL, et al. Double-blind study of intravenous propafenone for paroxysmal supraventricular reentrant tachycardia. *J Am Coll Cardiol*. 1987;9:1364–1368.

61. Funck-Brentano C, Kroemer HK, Lee JT, et al. Propafenone. *N Engl J Med*. 1990;322:518–525.

62. Vachiery JL, Reuse C, Blécic S, et al. Bretylium tosylate versus lidocaine in experimental cardiac arrest. *Am J Emerg Med*. 1990;8(6):492–495.

63. Rosalion A, Snow NJ, Horrigan TP, et al. Amiodarone versus bretylium for suppression of reperfusion arrhythmias in dogs. *Ann Thorac Surg*. 1991;51:84–85.

64. Leak D. Intravenous amiodarone in the treatment of refractory life-threatening cardiac arrhythmias in the critically ill patient. *Am Heart J*. 1986;111:456–462.

65. Sheldon RS, Mitchell LB, Duff HJ, et al. Right and left ventricular function during chronic amiodarone therapy. *Am J Cardiol*. 1988;62:736–740.

66. Schwartz A, Shen E, Morady F, et al. Hemodynamic effects of intravenous amiodarone in patients with depressed left ventricular function and recurrent ventricular tachycardia. *Am Heart J*. 1983;106:848–855.

67. Ochi RP, Goldenberg IF, Almquist A, et al. Intravenous amiodarone for the rapid treatment of life-threatening ventricular arrhythmias in critically ill patients with coronary artery disease. *Am J Cardiol*. 1989;64:599–603.

68. DeBoer LWV, Nosta JJ, Kloner RA, et al. Studies of amiodarone during experimental myocardial infarction: beneficial effects on hemodynamics and infarct size. *Circulation*. 1982;65:508–512.

69. Wellens HJJ, Brugada P, Abdollah H, et al. A comparison of the electrophysiologic effects of intravenous and oral amiodarone in the same patient. *Circulation*. 1984;69:120–124.

70. Remme WJ, Kruyssen HACM, Look MP, et al. Hemodynamic effects and tolerability of intravenous amiodarone in patients with impaired left ventricular function. *Am Heart J*. 1991;122:96–103.

71. Morady F, Di Carlo LA, Krol RB, et al. Acute and chronic effects of amiodarone on ventricular refractoriness, intraventricular condition and ventricular tachycardia induction. *Am Coll Cardiol*. 1986;7:148–156.

72. Escoubet B, Coumel P, Poirier JM, et al. Suppression of arrhythmias within hours after a single oral dose of amiodarone and relation to plasma and myocardial concentrations. *Am J Cardiol*. 1985;55:696–702.

73. Mostow ND, Vrobel TR, Noon D, et al. Rapid suppresion of complex ventricular arrhythmias with high dose oral amiodarone. *Circulation*. 1986;73:1231–1238.

74. Evans SJL, Myers M, Zaher C, et al. High dose oral amiodarone loading: electrophysiologic effects and clinical tolerance. *J Am Coll Cardiol*. 1992;19:169–173.

75. Alves LE, Rose EP, Cahill TB. Intravenous amiodarone in the treatment of refractory arrhythmids. *Crit Care Med*. 1985;13:750–752.

76. Helmy I, Herre JM, Gee G, et al. Use of intravenous amiodarone for emergency treatment of life-threatening ventricular arrhythmias. *J Am Coll Cardiol*. 1988;12:1015–1022.

77. Gleadhill IC, Wise RA, Schonfeld SA, et al. Serial lung function testing in patients treated with amiodarone: a prospective study. *Am J Med*. 1989;86:4–10.

78. Niklas JM, McKenna WJ, Stewart RA, et al. Prospective, double-blind, placebo-controlled trial of low-dose amiodarone in patients with severe heart failure and arrhythmias. *Crit Care Med*. 1985;13:750–752.

28
Intraaortic Balloon Pumping in Congestive Heart Failure

Adrian Kantrowitz, Raul R. Cardona, John Au, and Paul S. Freed

Today, almost a quarter century since its first trial in patients, the intraaortic balloon pump is the most commonly used cardiac assist device.[1] Indeed, intraaortic balloon pumping (IABP) has become standard in coronary care and cardiac surgery facilities, where it has established its role in the management of acute left ventricular (LV) dysfunction. In this chapter, we outline the theoretical concept of diastolic augmentation and summarize early experimental studies that supported the concept and enabled advances toward clinical implementations of cardiac assistance based on this principle. We then discuss the hemodynamic effects of IABP. A critical review of knowledge as to the determinants of the efficacy of IABP follows, setting the stage for consideration of the capabilities and limitations of currently available IABP apparatus. Next, we turn to clinical aspects, setting out IABP indications and contraindications, the technique of balloon catheter insertion, and other details of clinical management, with special emphasis on the insufficiently appreciated nuances of IABP timing. We then describe the clinical responses to IABP in LV failure and shock and in association with cardiac surgical procedures. Since IABP was first attempted, the complications detected in conjunction with its use have been defined with considerable precision, as we go on to indicate. Finally, we comment on new directions in mechanical support of the failing heart: the prospect of automated control of IABP, recently strengthened, we feel, as a result of the initial clinical trial of our closed-loop system; IABP in pediatric patients; pulmonary artery balloon counterpulsation; skeletal muscle counterpulsation; valved left ventricular assist devices (LVADs); and the avalvular permanent IABP. Because the literature on balloon pumping is now voluminous, the approach we have taken is selective, allowing us to examine key issues in sufficient detail to provide grounding for the interested clinician.

The extensive laboratory and clinical studies undertaken since balloon pumping entered the clinical setting have amplified insight into its physiologic actions and therapeutic benefits. This work has confirmed the conclusions that the method is readily applied by trained personnel and that it provides substantial hemodynamic benefits in acute cardiac failure, as well as in other conditions. These studies also have deepened our understanding of the many determinants of effective balloon pumping whose mastery is essential for the clinician who works with this technique.

History: From Theoretical Principle to Clinical Practice

In 1953, a novel way of increasing the blood supply to ischemic myocardium was proposed by Kantrowitz and Kantrowitz.[2] In experiments in which the arrival of the arterial pressure pulse at the coronary artery was delayed by interposing a length of rubber tubing, they demonstrated that coronary artery blood flow can be significantly augmented (Figs. 28.1, 28.2). Subsequently, the concept of diastolic augmentation underlying this observation was applied in harnessing the motor power of the diaphragm to create an auxiliary ventricle.[3] A hemidiaphragm was wrapped around the distal portion of the thoracic aorta and stimulated during diastole, resulting in increased diastolic arterial pressure. This work was presented at the 1960 meeting of the American Society of Artificial Internal Organs. In discussing it, Sarnoff, who with colleagues had recently defined the myocardial tension-time index,[4] agreed that diastolic augmentation of LV function might support the myocardium by maintaining or increasing cardiac output while simultaneously decreasing myocardial oxygen consumption.[5] Despite the appeal of using skeletal muscle as an auxiliary ventricle, the problem of muscle fatigue did not yield to the techniques available in that era and we turned to mechanical approaches.

Seeking to develop an assist device capable of provid-

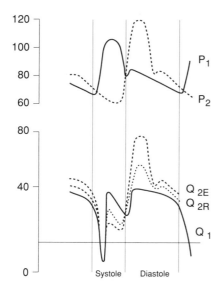

FIGURE 28.1. Concept of diastolic augmentation. Heavy lines indicate normal aortic pressure (P_1) and phasic coronary flow (Q_1). Dashed and dotted lines indicate predicted flows when the anterior descending coronary artery is perfused with pulse pressure out of phase with myocardial systole. P_2 represents delayed coronary pressure; Q_{2R}, calculated flow in presumed rigid coronary system; Q_{2E}, calculated flow in presumed elastic coronary system. Reprinted with permission from reference 2.

ing long-term support of the chronically failing heart, our laboratory designed a succession of valveless mechanical auxiliary ventricles, culminating in a U-shaped unit that spanned the transected aortic arch. After a several-year effort in the animal laboratory was completed, in 1966, this device was implanted in two patients with far-advanced chronic congestive heart failure (CHF).[6] Both patients succumbed, one on the first postoperative day. The other survived 13 days, during which striking hemodynamic benefits were demonstrated, including prompt and decisive relief of episodes of pulmonary edema. Further clinical use was nonetheless suspended because of the inability to control thromboembolization associated with the U-shaped configuration. Our laboratory then began to explore the possibilities of implanting a mechanical auxiliary ventricle in the aorta or in its wall. As will become evident, both possibilities have been fruitful.

Elsewhere, other workers had begun to apply the concept of "counterpulsation." Harken and colleagues at the Harvard Surgical Research Laboratory hypothesized that by aspirating a bolus of blood from the arterial side of the circulation during systole and returning it in diastole, the heart's "pressure work" (and, consequently, oxygen consumption) could be lowered while maintaining perfusion.[7] The "arterial counterpulsator" was built by Birtwell, and its hemodynamic effects convincingly demonstrated by several workers in 1961.[8–10] Although this system could not remove and return sufficient blood rapidly enough to achieve significant

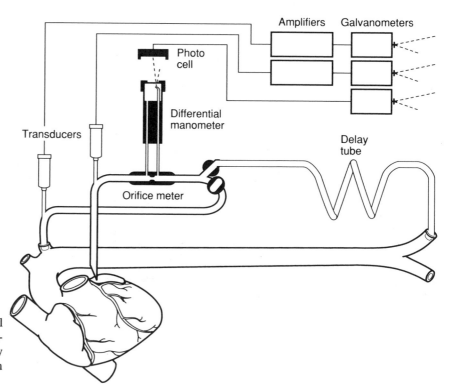

FIGURE 28.2. Schematic of experimental pressure pulse delay circuit used to demonstrate feasibility of augmenting coronary blood flow. Reprinted with permission from reference 2.

hemodynamic effects without evoking undue hemolysis, it was used clinically with modest success.[11]

Applying the physiologic principle of diastolic augmentation, Clauss and co-workers,[12] and independently, Moulopoulos et al.,[13] then described an intraaortic counterpulsating device, that is, an inflatable chamber placed inside the aorta. This approach eliminated the necessity of cannulating a peripheral artery with a large-bore catheter and avoided damage to formed blood elements by high flow velocities. Both groups, however, used carbon dioxide to inflate latex balloons, which occluded the aorta, compromising the potential benefits. Neither group reported further work on balloon pumping after 1962.

To return to 1966, with several years' documentation of the beneficial hemodynamic responses to diastolic augmentation in experimentally induced cardiac failure, our laboratory began development of a temporary LVAD that could be deployed within the aorta, and soon afterward, of a permanent system, as discussed below. For temporary use, we designed and fabricated a nondistensible, polyurethane balloon as a pumping chamber (Fig. 28.3). The balloon could be introduced into the aorta via the femoral artery without the need for thoracic surgery (Fig. 28.4). Helium (which has 1/20th the density of CO_2 and therefore affords more rapid inflation and deflation of the balloon) was chosen as the driving gas (Fig. 28.5). The results of canine experiments were published in 1967.[14] The first successful clinical use of IABP, giving evidence that it could reverse pharmacologically refractory cardiogenic shock after acute myocardial infarction, was reported in 1968.[15]

After an initial series of patients further confirmed the clinical value of the balloon pump, we organized a cooperative study in which nine centers followed a common protocol. The findings in 87 patients documented the technique's physiologic efficacy and relative free-

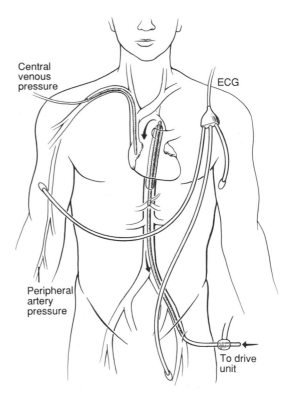

FIGURE 28.4. Schematic of IABP positioned in a patient. Reprinted with permission from reference 15.

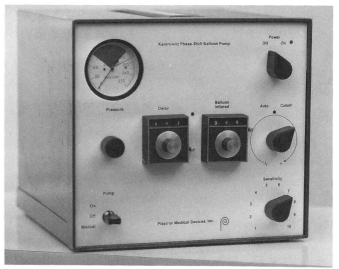

FIGURE 28.5. Early control unit for IABP used in initial patients.

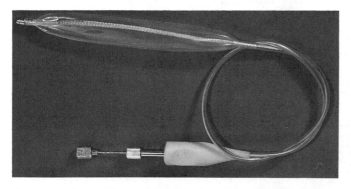

FIGURE 28.3. IABP used in initial patients (1967). It was fabricated of polyurethane and exposed to transmembrane pressures of 50 mm Hg during operation but could withstand 300 mm Hg without undergoing elastic deformation. Markedly higher pressures were required to burst the balloon.

dom from adverse effects in cardiogenic shock refractory to standard medical therapy.[16] Other groups soon began to report clinical experiences with IABP.[17,18] By 1975 hundreds of patients were being treated annually for a set of indications enlarged to include perioperative support for cardiac surgery. In 1979, the Datascope Corporation introduced the percutaneous balloon pump, which offered an alternative to surgical insertion.[19] Cardiologists qualified in the Seldinger technique could now carry out the procedure, and the use of IABP expanded. Currently, worldwide, at least 75,000 patients per year undergo IABP.

Hemodynamic Effects of IABP in Acute Congestive Heart Failure

For purposes of this discussion, we define CHF as the pathophysiological state that results when the circulation cannot meet tissue metabolic needs. (See discussion of the pathophysiology of CHF elsewhere in this book.) Most patients in *acute* CHF refractory to medical treatment present with low central aortic blood pressure and elevated preload as reflected by elevated central venous pressure, pulmonary capillary wedge pressure, and LV end-diastolic pressure. Cardiac output and peripheral perfusion are decreased.[20]

In recent years, effective pharmacologic regimens have been developed for acute CHF and its variants, as discussed elsewhere in this book. The experience of the last 25 years, however, has made it clear that there is a subset of patients in acute CHF who can survive only if their heart function is augmented by external energy, the equivalent of providing additional functioning heart muscle. In such patients, IABP, as a temporary form of mechanical cardiac assistance, is performed with these goals:

1. to improve the balance of myocardial O_2 demand and supply (by reducing LV afterload and increasing coronary artery perfusion pressure)
2. to maintain perfusion of vital structures (by increasing cardiac output)
3. through these actions, to shift the circulation toward a stable operating region, alleviating central and peripheral pathophysiological manifestations of acute CHF.

IABP meets these goals by removing volume from the central aorta before and during LV ejection—thereby mechanically reducing aortic pressure—and returning volume during diastole—thereby increasing aortic pressure. Thus, balloon counterpulsation implies inflation and deflation in synchrony with the cardiac cycle, but with pressure and flow 180° out of phase.[21]

The physiologic effects of IABP have been studied extensively in animals and humans. In animals in induced acute heart failure,[14,22] IABP brought about reduction of LV end-diastolic pressure by 40%, and of myocardial tension-time index by 20%. Cardiac output increased by 50%, coronary artery blood flow by 100%, and LV dp/dt by 25% (Fig. 28.6). Other reports indicate that IABP reduced LV peak systolic pressure from

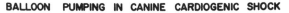

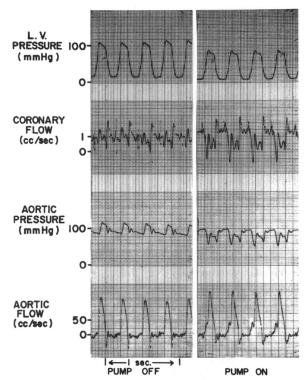

FIGURE 28.6. Recordings of hemodynamic parameters before and during IABP in an animal in induced heart failure. Reprinted with permission from reference 22.

4% to 20%,[18,23–27] mean ejection impedance from 10% to 21%,[28–29] and ejection resistance by 46%.[27]

Reduction in LV peak and end-diastolic pressures, with decline in the tension-time index, imply a decrease in myocardial wall tension, and, in turn, a diminution in myocardial O_2 consumption. At the same time, decrease in LV end-diastolic pressure is consonant with a reduction of LV volume. Since systolic ejection time is decreased, coronary perfusion increased, and myocardial wall tension reduced during IABP, myocardial oxygenation is improved. The latter hypothesis has been confirmed in clinical studies by Mueller et al.[27,30] demonstrating a shift toward normal of myocardial lactate extraction from −6% to 15% and of myocardial oxygen extraction from 79% to 61%.

In summary, balloon inflation during diastole increases diastolic pressure, coronary artery blood flow, and oxygen supply to hypoxic myocardium, thus improving contractility of the failing myocardium. With increased LV ejection, stroke volume, and cardiac output, blood flow to peripheral organs is increased. IABP effects a decrease in preload by improving mechanical contraction of the LV, which decreases LV volume (Fig. 28.7). Balloon deflation during systole decreases the work of the failing LV by reducing LV peak systolic pressure and increasing stroke volume.

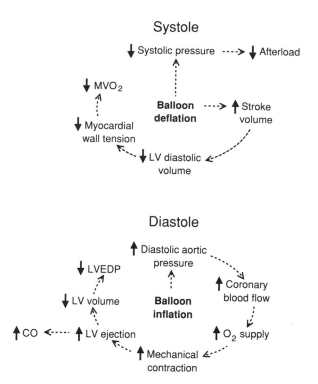

FIGURE 28.7. Hemodynamic effects of IABP. LV = left ventricular; MVO_2 = myocardial oxygen consumption; CO = cardiac output; LVEDP = left ventricular end diastolic pressure.

Determinants of IABP Efficacy

The efficacy of diastolic augmentation by means of IABP has been shown to depend on several physical and biological factors.[25,29] Physical factors include the position of the balloon pump catheter in the descending thoracic aorta, the balloon displacement volume, the balloon diameter/aortic diameter ratio, the type of gas used to inflate the balloon, and balloon timing. Biological factors comprise the heart rate and rhythm and hemodynamic variables.

Position of the Balloon Pump Catheter

The optimal location of an assist device that produces diastolic augmentation, according to several early investigators,[26,31] is as close to the aortic root as practicable; the further the assist device is from this location, the lesser the hemodynamic benefits. For the balloon pump, this means that the proximal tip of the balloon catheter should be placed about 1 cm below the origin of the left subclavian artery, where it is best accommodated.[15]

Balloon Displacement Volume

Theoretically, there is an upper boundary to the desirable stroke volume of an assist device like the balloon pump, which removes volume from the aorta during systole, namely, the LV stroke volume. If the balloon's stroke volume exceeds this limit, then deflation could cause retrograde blood flow from the coronary arteries and the vessels of the aortic arch. Feola et al.[25] studied the relationship of the volume of the inflated balloon to LV stroke volume in 20 normal dogs and 80 dogs in induced acute LV failure. They observed that IABP was maximally effective in the normal heart when the inflated balloon volume was the same as, or not more than 5 ml greater than, LV stroke volume. In dogs in induced failure, in which the inflated balloon volume was much greater than the LV stroke volume, balloon deflation produced retrograde flow from the aortic branches, particularly from the carotid arteries. Our group's view is that the stroke volume of the balloon should be approximately the same as that of the failing LV (i.e., 30–40 cc).

Balloon Diameter/Aortic Diameter Ratio

The balloon diameter usually considered appropriate for a given patient is chosen so that inflation occludes 75% to 90% of the cross-sectional area of the descending thoracic aorta.[32] Weikel et al. reported that a change in diameter from 16 to 18 mm resulted in a 33% increase in stroke volume as long as the balloon was not occlusive.[33] When the balloon diameter was 1 mm larger than the aortic diameter, however, the efficacy of assistance decreased. They measured the diameter of the thoracic aorta in 169 aortograms at two levels: the first, distal to the aortic isthmus, and the second, at the level of the diaphragm. They found that the mid-thoracic diameter varied from 16 to 30 mm, with 90% of the measurements exceeding 19 mm. The diameters of most commercially available adult balloon pump catheters are 16 to 18 mm.

Inflating Gas

Beginning with our initial reports,[14,15] we have advocated the use of helium as the shuttle gas for IABP. Helium affords faster inflation and deflation, and hence more effective diastolic augmentation for patients in acute CHF, than CO_2. Helium was not accepted universally until the mid-1980s. Speed of gas transit is critically important in patients in acute circulatory collapse. Some investigators had recommended the use of CO_2 because it is more soluble than helium in blood, therefore decreasing risks associated with gas embolism.[24,29] It must be noted that balloon leakage or rupture is rare.[34–37] Currently, because of its obvious advantages,

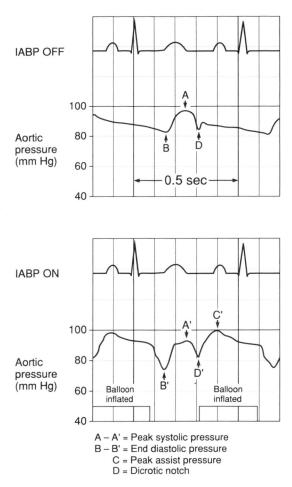

IABP OFF

Aortic pressure (mm Hg)

A

B   D

0.5 sec

IABP ON

Aortic pressure (mm Hg)

A'   C'

B'   D'

Balloon inflated

Balloon inflated

A – A' = Peak systolic pressure
B – B' = End diastolic pressure
C = Peak assist pressure
D = Dicrotic notch

FIGURE 28.8. Idealized waveforms showing timing of IABP inflation.

helium is the shuttle gas for all balloon pumps made in the U.S.[32]

Balloon Timing

Appropriate timing of balloon inflation and deflation is a necessary condition for obtaining the maximal hemodynamic benefits of diastolic augmentation. Our group's view is that (a) inflation should begin immediately after the appearance of the dicrotic notch on the central aortic blood pressure waveform, and (b) deflation should occur at the end of diastole. Under these conditions, coronary blood flow and reduction of LV afterload are both maximized. Figures 28.6 and 28.8 illustrate optimal timing. Balloon timing is discussed further below as an aspect of IABP management.

Heart Rate and Rhythm

In laboratory simulation tests, most commercially available balloon pump drive units can trigger 60 to 200 beats per minute (bpm).[32] In the clinical setting, how-

ever, with state-of-the-art equipment, triggering beyond 120 bpm results in decreased gas flow and volume, leading to small augmentation pressure and ineffective LV unloading. Diastolic augmentation and ventricular unloading are best achieved at heart rates of 80 to 120 bpm.[38] Occasional premature ventricular contractions do not appreciably reduce the benefits of assistance.

Because of the limitations of present-day IABP systems, the hemodynamic benefits of assistance are compromised in patients with tachyarrhythmias. In sinus tachycardia it has been suggested that one can improve hemodynamic benefits by assisting every second beat.[39] In our opinion, however, this further reduces an already suboptimal augmentation. It is preferable to pump on every beat, with a less than full stroke. During persistent large variations in heart rate, appropriate timing cannot be maintained without the intervention of a human operator. Atrial fibrillation with fast ventricular response exceeds even the highly trained operator's ability to maintain appropriate timing.

Hemodynamic Variables

Hemodynamic benefits of IABP are also affected by aortic blood pressure, blood volume, and systemic vascular resistance, which, in turn, influence stroke volume and pulse pressure.[40,41] Hypovolemia reduces the effectiveness of IABP by reducing the total circulating volume, venous return, and LV stroke volume. Under these conditions, the volume of blood propelled by balloon inflation is decreased, and hemodynamic benefits diminished.

Commercially Available IABP Drive Units and Catheters

To introduce the role of IABP, it may be helpful for the clinician to understand the capabilities and limitations of present-day IABP apparatus. At present, the four balloon pump systems commercially available in the U.S. are those made by Kontron Instruments, Aries Medical, Datascope, and Mansfield Cardiac Assist (Figs. 28.9, 28.10). In 1987, the Emergency Care Research Institute made a comprehensive evaluation that is still useful for understanding the capabilities and limitations of second-generation balloon pump-driving units.[32]

Drive Units

To control balloon action, the initial drive unit constructed by our group in 1966 used a fast-acting solenoid valve to admit pressurized helium from a tank to the pumping chamber. An operator, scanning the displayed electrocardiogram (ECG), manually set a time

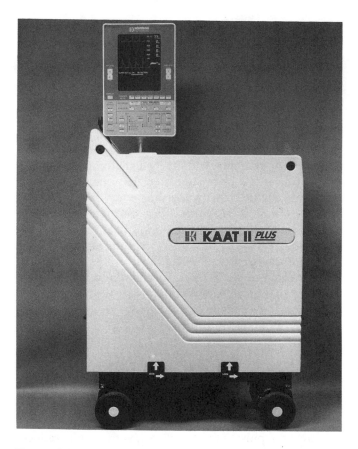

FIGURE 28.9. Kontron Instruments Model KAAT II Plus Drive Unit for Hospital and Transport Use (courtesy, Kontron Instruments, Inc.)

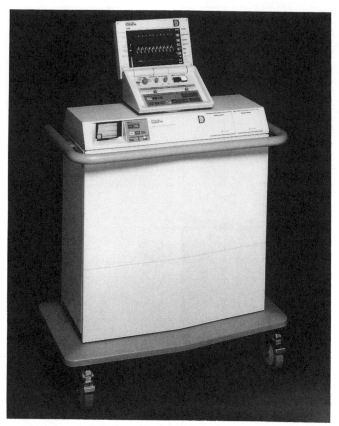

FIGURE 28.10. Datascope System 95 Drive Unit (courtesy, Datascope Corp.)

interval that extended from the occurrence of the QRS complex to aortic valve closure, as gauged from the displayed central aortic pressure waveform. The solenoid valve was opened at the end of this interval to inflate the balloon. After a second time interval, chosen to end just before cardiac systole, the helium was allowed to flow out of the balloon. This system functioned well over a broad range of heart rates and could cycle the balloon effectively even during certain arrhythmias.

Since then, balloon pump drive units have evolved considerably. Manufacturers are offering smaller and lighter second-generation drive units that facilitate interhospital and intrahospital transfer of patients during IABP assistance. These units incorporate additional safety features, alarms, and a semiautomatic mode.

In current second-generation drive units, it is recognized that the intervals from the QRS complex to mechanical events of the cardiac cycle vary from patient to patient, and, in a given patient, with the heart rate. To deal with this variability, drive units are programmed with "function" curves that represent systolic time intervals as functions of heart rate. Each function curve is based on statistical analysis of observations of systolic time intervals in large numbers of patients. The balloon

pump console operator estimates the QRS-complex-to-aortic-valve-closure interval at the patient's present heart rate and enters this into the drive unit. The unit selects the appropriate function curve containing those values from a look-up table. The function curve is constructed in such a way that given a patient's systolic time interval at one heart rate, the values of the systolic time intervals at other heart rates can be predicted. Like older drive units, newer ones deflate the balloon when a premature beat is sensed. They incorporate safety features to deal with some arrhythmias and to detect gross balloon rupture.

Nevertheless, second-generation drive units cannot deliver the maximal hemodynamic benefits of IABP when the patient has an arrhythmia or a significant change in heart rate. Under these circumstances, therefore, the timing of balloon pump inflation and deflation is essentially manual and still the responsibility of a human operator. When balloon pump timing is qualitatively assessed, there is considerable operator-to-operator, and even intraoperator, variation. Furthermore, the ability to wean the patient by gradually reducing the volume of the inflated pumping chamber is important (as discussed below), and not all driving units allow volume weaning.

Balloon Catheters

Since the introduction of the IABP catheter for clinical use in 1967,[15] catheter design, material, and instertion techniques have been advanced. Although segmented, valved, and other balloon pump designs enjoyed transient use, the original "sausage" shape still prevails, as does one or another proprietary variation of the original polyurethane material. Rather than the initial 32-cc displacement volume, 40 cc has been standard since 1978.

Originally, the balloon was inserted through a femoral arteriotomy. In 1980, percutaneous insertion (discussed below) was reported by Subramanian et al., using the Seldinger technique to introduce the balloon catheter through a 6-in sheath.[42] Readily accomplished by cardiologists, percutaneous insertion was widely adopted; however, it was found not suitable for approximately 15% of patients with iliofemoral disease. For these patients with special needs, Bemis et al. developed a longer sheath, 11 to 15 in in length.[43]

Because of the need to initiate arterial pressure monitoring more rapidly than available equipment permitted and because of difficulties encountered in inserting the balloon in patients with extreme tortuosity of the iliofemoral arteries, a central lumen concentric with, and contained within, the gas conduit was added to the catheter (Fig. 28.11). Since this lumen terminated in an opening in the catheter tip, the balloon could be introduced over a J-tip guidewire. The central lumen can be used to obtain an arterial pressure waveform for balloon timing.

Manufacturers continue to make refinements in the balloon catheter, most aimed at reducing femoral obstruction and facilitating routine introduction of the balloon.

Indications and Contraindications

Indications

Indications for IABP have evolved with increasing experience. In our view, for patients in cardiac failure or certain antecedent conditions, specific indications for IABP include:

1. postcardiotomy low cardiac output syndrome
2. pump failure after acute myocardial infarction is with or without cardiogenic shock
3. failure associated with mechanical complications of acute myocardial infarction
4. acute mitral regurgitation due to failure of native or prosthetic valve
5. failure in a patient awaiting a cardiac allograft, who therefore needs a bridge to transplantation
6. support of the failing transplanted heart

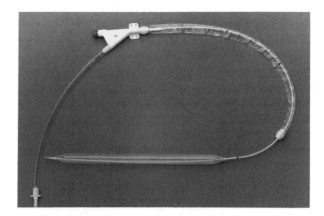

FIGURE 28.11. Modern Commercial Intraaortic Balloon Pump (courtesy, Boston Scientific Corp.)

7. unstable angina pectoris
8. ventricular arrhythmia refractory to pharmacologic therapy.

IABP also has been used in septic shock,[44,45] in cardiac arrest,[46] in high-risk cardiac patients undergoing noncardiac surgery,[47,48] and as prophylactic support in patients undergoing high-risk percutaneous transluminal coronary angioplasty. Pulmonary artery ballon counterpulsation has been reported to be beneficial in acute right ventricular failure (see below).[49]

Contraindications

IABP is contraindicated in the following conditions:

1. aortic insufficiency
2. aortic dissection.

Recently, abdominal and transesophageal echocardiography have been used to guide balloon pump insertion in aortic dissection.[50] Some workers regard the presence of a prosthetic graft in the thoracic aorta as a contraindication to IABP.[51] We believe that if the graft has been stable and functioning for a year or longer, it may be possible to perform IABP.

Clinical Management

In patients receiving IABP because of LV power failure or cardiogenic shock, hemodynamic and metabolic abnormalities due to the cardiac insult and its prior treatment must be carefully corrected. During IABP, the etiology of the acute LV failure, if not known, must be established as soon as possible to allow for prompt surgical or other intervention as appropriate. Timing of balloon inflation and deflation in relation to the events of the cardiac cycle is critically important, and is discussed separately below.

Techniques of Balloon Pump Insertion

The two principal approaches to inserting the balloon pump are the percutaneous and the direct surgical cutdown. Each has advantages and disadvantages. In either case, the balloon pump is inserted through the common femoral artery, unless use of this route is contraindicated. The femoral artery is not to be used in patients with severe local atherosclerosis, aneurysms of the thoracic or abdominal aorta, or a prosthetic graft for repair of the aorta.

The percutaneous balloon pump is inserted into the femoral artery using a modified Seldinger technique: after the J-wire is introduced into the femoral artery, the arterial wall is dilated in step-wise fashion, first with a predilator and then with a larger dilator/introducer sheath assembly. When the dilator is removed, the introducer sheath is left inside the lumen of the femoral artery, and the balloon pump is passed through it into the aorta. The entire process, in skilled hands, takes less than 15 min.[52] As noted above, a dual-lumen balloon pump can be guided into the aorta over the J-wire in patients with severe iliofemoral disease.

Surgical insertion by direct cutdown onto the common femoral artery is achieved using a "femoral conduit." The balloon pump is inserted through a 10- to 12-mm prosthetic graft sutured end to side to the common femoral artery.[53,54] This technique minimizes the risk of distal limb ischemia. Alternatively, the balloon pump is passed into the common femoral artery under direct vision through a purse-string suture.[54,55] This method, which allows rapid initiation of IABP in pulseless patients, is used only for operating room emergencies.

When the femoral artery route fails, the balloon pump has been inserted via the iliac artery, the ascending aorta,[56,57] the subclavian artery,[58,59] the brachial artery,[60] or even an aortofemoral graft.[61] Insertion via an axillary[62] or an iliac[63] artery has been advocated for patients in whom IABP is intended for chronic support, as their mobility during assistance is preserved.

Management of the Balloon Pump Patient

If not already in place, a Swan-Ganz thermodilution catheter and a radial artery line are inserted. Fluid volume and electrolyte abnormalities, as well as inadequate ventilation and disorders of cardiac rhythm, are corrected while pharmacologic treatment is given to reduce LV afterload. For details of these procedures, the reader is referred to several reports that elaborate on adjunctive management of IABP.[64–67]

As insertion of the balloon pump into the patient's vascular system begins, the balloon pump console operator sets the inflation-deflation timing delays. The balloon is advanced through the femoral and iliac arteries into the aorta. The dislodgment of a fragment of ather-omatous plaque is a genuine risk. The balloon is positioned so that the catheter tip lies about 1 cm below the origin of the left subclavian artery, as noted. When the balloon pump is activated, timing is checked and reset as appropriate. It is essential to reassess balloon timing whenever a change in the patient's heart rate is detected—even a change of only a few beats per minute. Such assessment must not be left to incompletely trained personnel.

If there are no contraindications to heparin (e.g., recent cardiac or general surgery), a 5000-unit bolus of heparin is administered intravenously at the onset of balloon pumping and every 4 hr thereafter until the balloon is removed. Alternatively, after the initial bolus, 12,000 units in 250 cc of saline solution are infused intravenously every 12 hr. The partial thromboplastin time (PTT) should be checked 6 hr after heparin administration and every day thereafter; it should be maintained at 1.5 to 2.0 times its normal value. In patients undergoing IABP after cardiac surgery, low molecular weight Dextran is given at a rate of 20 ml/hr, in a dose not to exceed 10 ml/kg/24 hr.

A chest x ray may be taken after balloon pump insertion in the intensive care unit or operating room to verify that it is positioned properly. When IABP is started in the fluoroscopy suite, the position of the balloon should be checked before the pump is turned on.

Vasopressor administration initiated prior to IABP is discontinued as soon as the central aortic pressure is high enough to prevent the inflated balloon from occluding the aorta.

The patient's hemodynamic and clinical status is monitored after the desired timing has been achieved. The parameters evaluated include heart rate, blood pressure, central venous pressure, pulmonary artery pressure, pulmonary capillary wedge pressure, cardiac output, urine output, body temperature, electrolyte concentrations, pH, pO_2, pCO_2, acid-base balance, plasma osmolarity, plasma volume, hemoglobin level, and hematocrit. A complete blood count and platelet count should be obtained daily. Transesophageal echocardiographic monitoring has been used in the management of patients who have ventricular dysfunction requiring balloon pump support after cardiac surgery.[68]

The leg through which the balloon was inserted is observed regularly for evidence of ischemia during assistance. Lower extremity, femoral, popliteal, dorsalis pedis, and posterior tibialis pulses are compared with those in the other extremity and graded on a scale of 0–4+, with 4+ being normal. The ankle/arm index also must be determined. These observations should be performed by the nursing staff once during every shift, or by the physician as necessary. A mild degree of ischemia may be well tolerated and may not dictate immediate balloon pump removal, but very close observation is indicated. When severe ischemia is detected, one has

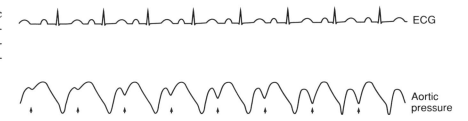

FIGURE 28.12. ECG and central aortic pressure waveforms during IABP illustrating early inflation, at left. Inflation, indicated by the arrow, is continuously delayed so that it is correct at the right.

the following options: (a) if the patient is clinically and hemodynamically stable, the balloon pump is withdrawn; (b) if the patient is unstable, or if IABP's continuation is required for any other reason, the catheter is removed and an attempt is made to insert another balloon through the contralateral femoral artery. If this fails, surgical insertion in the iliac artery may be attempted.

Management of Balloon Pump Timing

At the initiation of IABP, the central aortic blood pressure waveform with the balloon off is examined and correlated to the ECG to determine the location of the dicrotic notch. The IABP is then activated and the assisted and unassisted waveforms are compared, allowing timing corrections to be made. Inasmuch as the radial artery pressure provides a delayed and distorted record of pressure changes in the central aorta, it is more desirable to use central aortic pressure for balloon timing.

Common types of incorrect timing should be familiar to physicians, nurses, and console operators who care for IABP patients.

Early Inflation

Balloon inflation begins when the aortic valve is still open. The resultant increase in aortic pressure causes premature aortic valve closure. Early inflation also causes an increase in LV afterload and results in increased LV work. Additional consequences include incomplete ventricular emptying, decreased stroke volume, decreased cardiac output, and increased

myocardial O_2 consumption. In the presence of septal defects, early inflation can increase shunting. Early inflation is recognized by looking at the central aortic blood pressure waveform and noting that the balloon augmentation waveform is superimposed to greater or lesser degree over the LV systolic waveform, as illustrated in Fig. 28.12.

Late Inflation

Inflation begins after aortic valve closure, resulting in abbreviated, and hence suboptimal, diastolic augmentation. Late inflation can be recognized in the central aortic pressure waveform when balloon pressure begins to rise well after the appearance of the dicrotic notch, as illustrated in Fig. 28.13.

Early Deflation

Balloon deflation starts before isovolumetric contraction, reducing the duration of diastolic augmentation during ventricular diastole; LV afterload reduction may not be achieved. The central aortic blood pressure waveform exhibits a wide U-shaped segment between the peak diastolic pressure and the peak systolic pressure, as illustrated in Fig. 28.14.

Late Deflation

Balloon inflation extends into cardiac systole, obstructing LV ejection. The physiologic consequences of late deflation are increased afterload and preload, prolonged isovolumetric contraction, increased myocardial O_2 consumption, and decreased stroke volume and

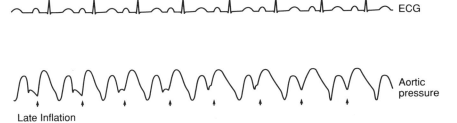

FIGURE 28.13. ECG and central aortic pressure waveforms during IABP illustrating late inflation, at left. Note time interval between dicrotic notch and balloon inflation. Inflation delay is gradually reduced, as indicated by the arrow, so that at right, timing is correct.

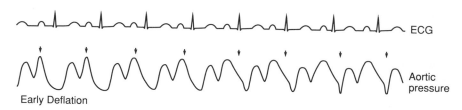

FIGURE 28.14. ECG and central aortic pressure waveforms during IABP illustrating early deflation, at left. Note wide valley following deflation. Deflation is gradually delayed so that correct timing is achieved, at extreme right.

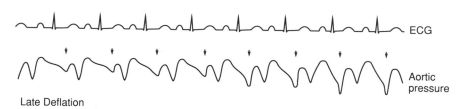

FIGURE 28.15. ECG and central aortic pressure waveforms during IABP, illustrating late deflation, at left. Note aortic pressure at end diastole is higher than pressure at the dicrotic notch. Deflation delay is gradually reduced to result in proper timing, at right.

cardiac output. Late deflation may increase shunting associated with septal defects. Its consequences can be especially severe in patients with mitral regurgitation or LV aneurysm. Figure 28.15 illustrates late deflation.

Tachyarrhythmias

As noted above, it is difficult to obtain appropriate balloon pump timing, and IABP can be more detrimental than beneficial. Some workers suggest turning the balloon pump off in this situation. In the recording shown in Fig. 28.16, the balloon pump drive unit was unable to synchronize balloon timing.

Indication to Discontinue IABP

The indication to discontinue IABP is related to the indication for balloon pump support.[69] In general, we have attempted to remove the balloon pump when the patient was hemodynamically stable. In most of our cases, if the cardiac index (CI) was >2.2 liter/min/m², pulmonary capillary pressure <18 mm Hg, and arterial pressure normal, assistance was discontinued.[70] Balloon

pumping is, of course, also halted when serious complications ensue secondary to IABP. Kyo et al.[71] have reported on the use of biplane transesophageal echocardiography (TEE) in following the cardiac status of IABP patients. They find that biplane TEE is practical in the intensive care unit (ICU) setting, allowing measurement of coronary flow, LV ejection fraction, and sequential wall motion of the ventricles. They conclude that TEE "can provide important information for patient management . . . and determination of optimal timing for discontinuation of [IABP]."

Weaning

For patients receiving IABP because of an episode of CHF, weaning is attempted after hemodynamic stability has been restored for some hours. The two methods of weaning are frequency ratio weaning and volume weaning.

In frequency ratio weaning the operator changes the ratio of assisted heart beats to the total number of heart beats from 1:1 to 1:2, 1:3, 1:4, and so on. In volume weaning, the operator gradually decreases the balloon

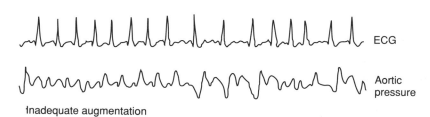

FIGURE 28.16. ECG and central aortic pressure waveforms during IABP exemplifying effects of atrial fibrillation. Drive unit is unable to synchronize balloon operation effectively to the heart.

stroke volume. As the initial step, the balloon volume is reduced by one third. If the patient's hemodynamic parameters remain stable, the balloon volume is reduced further and the patient's physiologic response observed. These steps are repeated until weaning is complete. Our preferred method is volume weaning: it is physiologic, in that as the balloon's inflation volume is reduced, the heart *gradually* takes over the circulatory load. Some manufacturers do not recommend volume weaning because they feel that the risk of clot formation within the folds of the balloon is increased. Weaning can be accomplished in as little as 1 hr. If the patient's hemodynamic status deteriorates during weaning, full-volume IABP is resumed and weaning reattempted 6 to 24 hr later.

Patients who cannot be weaned from IABP are by definition balloon-dependent. Given contemporary standards of care, the possibility of surgical treatment of the condition giving rise to the need for IABP will already have been evaluated with no correctable lesion identified. The remaining possibilities include cardiac transplantation and a permanently implanted LVAD (see below).

Balloon Pump Removal

Percutaneously placed balloon pumps generally are removed percutaneously, unless complications dictate otherwise. The balloon is deflated, and a Doppler monitor is applied on the arch vessels of the foot. (Note that heparin administration is discontinued at least 4 hr before balloon removal.) At removal, an attempt is made to flush out any thrombi that may be stripped from the balloon by the act of removal: pressure is applied to the femoral artery below the puncture site as the balloon pump is being removed, and blood is allowed to spurt for 1 to 2 s. This maneuver evacuates proximal thrombi. Pressure is then applied to the femoral artery proximal to the puncture site and backbleeding is allowed to flush out distal thrombi. Finally, the puncture site is compressed for at least 30 min to obtain hemostasis, while allowing distal flow in the femoropopliteal vessels, as demonstrated by Doppler monitoring.[72] After percutaneous balloon pump removal, patients must lie flat for at least 6 hr. The lower extremities must be observed for signs of ischemia and the ankle/arm ratio must be monitored.

Removal of surgically placed balloon pumps generally requires a second cutdown, either to oversew the prosthetic graft or to repair the femoral artery. Many surgeons perform a concomitant embolectomy to retrieve any thrombotic material that may be dislodged at the time of balloon pump removal. This may be one of the reasons for the lesser vascular complication rate after surgical insertion.[52] Recently, a different method for closed removal of surgically placed balloon pumps

was proposed by Opie.[73] A purse-string suture is placed around the arterial puncture site. The suture is left long and passed through a tourniquet. After removal of the balloon pump, the suture is at first tightened and then released; it is removed about 20 hr later.

Clinical Responses to IABP

Severe Left Ventricular Failure, Cardiogenic Shock

In our initial clinical experience, IABP was restricted to patients in pharmacologically refractory cardiogenic shock after acute myocardial infarction, as noted above. Our findings indicated that shock was reversed during assistance in more than 80% of patients.[64] More than half of the patients recovered from the episode of acute circulatory decompensation, maintaining homeostasis after termination of balloon pumping. In the cooperative study of 87 similar patients reported in 1973 by Scheidt et al.,[16] the survival rate was 17%, almost identical to the 16% rate reported in 1972 by Dunkman et al.[74] In 1977, our group reported the results of IABP alone in 386 patients in cardiogenic shock: 113 (29%) did not improve; 87 (22.5%) became balloon pump–dependent; 94 (24%) improved but died in the hospital; and 92 (24%) improved and were discharged from the hospital.[75] In reports of other groups, the overall survival rate ranges from 15% to 38%.[67,76–78] The variability in outcomes undoubtedly reflects such elements as differences in philosophy as to when to undertake assisted circulation and alternative ways of conducting IABP and its adjunctive management.

The overall survival rate of patients in severe refractory heart failure without shock secondary to myocardial infarction who undergo IABP without surgery ranges between 25% and 68%.[79,80] Using Myocardial Infarction Research Unit (MIRU) criteria, Hagemeijer et al. reported 25 patients in class III or class IV LV failure after recent myocardial infarction who were treated with IABP alone.[65] Three patients (12%) did not improve and died during pumping. Two patients (8%) who had improved died during attempted weaning. In 20 patients, IABP was successful in restoring circulatory stabilization. Of these, 6 (24%) died within 3 months. Fourteen (56%) survived longer than 3 months. These patients all received IABP for as long as 24 days. Twelve were in functional class II, and six returned to their occupations (class I). Seven of 10 patients who received balloon pump support for more than 10 days were included among the long-term survivors. Hagemeijer's results suggest that prolonged support with IABP may restore myocardial metabolism in the absence of surgical or other interventions.

Freed et al. of our group reported prolonged use of

IABP (>20 days) in 27 patients.[70] Twelve had prior histories of CHF (44%). Of 15 in the series who did not undergo a cardiac surgical procedure during or after IABP (55% of the entire series), 7 survived (47%) and were discharged from the hospital, and 8 died (53%). Seven patients with histories of CHF who were assisted for 23 to 66 days (average, 33 days) were discharged alive from the hospital. All died within 6 months (one after a cerebrovascular accident and six of CHF). After undergoing prolonged IABP support and experiencing substantial improvement in cardiac function, these patients survived for months despite the fact that they were no longer receiving balloon pump support.

Although thrombolysis, coronary angioplasty, coronary artery bypass grafting, and other interventions probably are contributing to prevention of cardiogenic shock after myocardial infarction, IABP remains a staple of management once shock or its immediate precursors arise. The data reported by Freed et al. suggest as well that IABP may have a role in chronic CHF and point to the possibility that when a definitive surgical procedure is not an option for such patients, a permanent form of IABP might be useful, as discussed below.

IABP as an Adjunct to Cardiac Surgery

Preoperative IABP

IABP may be initiated preoperatively in patients in cardiogenic shock[81-83] and in high-risk cardiac and noncardiac surgical patients with severe impairment of LV function.[47,48] The frequency of its use on an elective basis depends on the institution and its patient population; the criteria for prophylactic IABP are not universally accepted. Bolooki regards patients who have a preoperative ejection fraction of <30%, an LVEDP of >22 mm Hg, a CI of <1.8 L/min/m², and who are expected to undergo ischemic arrest prolonged to more than 3 hr as candidates for elective IABP.[38] Fuhrman et al. concluded that patients with a preoperative CI of <2.0 L/min/m², systemic vascular resistance (SVR) of >1800 dynes/s/cm⁻⁵, and LV minute work index of <3.0 kg m/min/m² should be considered potential balloon pump candidates.[84] However, preoperative IABP in such patients has not been shown to be more advantageous than postoperative IABP,[85] except in the case of cardiogenic shock.[86] Kirklin in the discussion after Bolooki et al.'s paper on clinical and hemodynamic criteria for IABP characterized elective IABP as unnecessary,[87] and D'Agostino and Baldwin[51] and Golding et al.[88] considered it controversial. Early survival rates of more than 90% have been reported for cases in which preoperative IABP was performed.[87,89]

In large part, however, these excellent results reflect patient selection (e.g., Bolooki[87] excluded patients with

preoperative cardiogenic shock) and cannot be directly compared with results of intra- or postoperative IABP. When patients in preoperative cardiogenic shock were included, early survival was no better than that associated with intra- or postoperative IABP.[90]

Postcardiotomy Low Cardiac Output Syndrome

A major indication for IABP is postcardiotomy low cardiac output syndrome (LOS). Initially suggested by our group in 1968,[15] and subsequently reported by Buckley et al.[91] and others,[92,93] this use of IABP is of demonstrated efficacy.[35,90,94] Numerous factors are involved in the development of LOS. Aside from technical misadventures, probably the most important is imperfect myocardial preservation.[95] Acute myocardial failure of this type is frequently reversible. Recent insights into postischemic myocardial dysfunction, or "stunned myocardium,"[96] are refining the pathophysiological basis for the use of IABP in this condition. "Stunned myocardium" has been shown to be deficient in high-energy phosphates and adenine nucleotides,[97,98] and exhibits a massive increase in O_2 consumption for any given level of tension it develops.[99] IABP, by increasing diastolic coronary artery flow and reducing LV afterload, alters the balance of myocardial O_2 supply and demand in the postischemic situation.[100,101]

The incidence of LOS requiring IABP is 2% to 7%,[89,90,94,102,103] a range that has remained relatively constant even though the characteristics of the cardiac surgery patient population have been changing.[38] Proposed criteria for the use of IABP after cardiac surgery include (a) failure to wean the patient from cardiopulmonary bypass after 30 to 45 min at flow rates >500 ml/min, as well as (b) hypotension (<65 mm Hg mean arterial pressure) and low cardiac index (<1.8 L/min/m²) with high left atrial/pulmonary capillary wedge pressures (>25 mm Hg) despite inotropic support.[38,93] IABP is used intraoperatively in 60% to 80% of patients who cannot be weaned from cardiopulmonary bypass and postoperatively in 15% to 30%.[90,94,102]

Of patients who require IABP for LOS, 50% to 80% are weaned from balloon support and 10% succumb after balloon removal.[93,94,102] Early survival rates are consistently reported as 40% to 70%,[38,89,94,102,103] a sharp contrast to mortality rates in excess of 90% in cases in which IABP is not used.[104] Early survival rates have been found to be inversely correlated to the time delay between the end of the operation and the onset of balloon pump assist.[38,88] Thus, once the need for IABP is recognized, its prompt initiation is of paramount urgency.

Favorable prognostic indicators for postcardiotomy IABP support include early recovery of cardiac function,[105] a preoperative LV ejection fraction of >50%, and a preoperative LVEDP of <13 mm Hg.[106]

Adverse preoperative factors related to early mortality include female sex, New York Heart Association functional class (NYHA) III or IV, and renal failure or chronic LV failure.[107] Norman et al.[103] classified survivors and nonsurvivors of postcardiotomy IABP in three classes according to the CI and SVR at optimal preload levels (PCWP, 15–18 mm Hg): Class A—CI >2.1 L/min/m² with SVR <2100 dynes/s/cm⁻⁵; Class B—CI <2.1 L/min/m² but >1.2 L/min/m² with SVR <2100 dynes/s/cm⁻⁵; Class C—CI <2.1 L/min/m² with SVR >2100 dynes/s/cm⁻⁵ or CI <1.2 L/min/m² regardless of SVR. All patients who were in Class A survived; 80% of patients in Class B survived. All patients who remained in Class C for 12 hr or more after operation with balloon pump support died. They concluded that the postcardiotomy balloon pump–supported patients who remain in Class C for 12 hr or more are at the highest risk and are candidates for LVADs.[103]

Data on long-term survival after postcardiotomy IABP are scant. Bolooki[38] reported a survival rate of 43%, and Lefemine et al., one of 47%.[89] Neither author defined "long-term survival." Hedenmark reported a survival rate of 51% after a mean follow-up of 23 months.[105] However, the range of follow-up was not stated. Golding et al. reported a 2-yr cardiac actuarial survival of patients discharged alive from the hospital of 96%.[88] Only 69% of that study population had IABP for postcardiotomy support. For these patients, a survival rate of 63% after a mean follow-up of 18 months (range 6–40 months) can be calculated from their data. More representative of the real picture are the results of Kuchar et al. and Lund et al., who reported 5-yr actuarial survival rates of 25% and 22%, respectively, in all postcardiotomy balloon pump patients.[107,108]

Functional outcomes in survivors of postcardiotomy balloon pump support have been assessed by Davies et al.[109] In 23 such patients studied at a mean of 23 months, resting LV ejection fraction remained unchanged from preoperative values in 9, whereas in the remaining 14 patients, it increased by >10% in 4 and fell by >10% in 10. Twelve of the 23 patients were in NYHA functional class I (preoperatively, none), 9 were in class II (1), and 2 in class III (10). Twenty-one of the 23 patients had improved by at least one functional class. These results are in accord with those of Kuchar et al.[108]

Bridge to Transplantation

Cardiac transplantation is now an accepted treatment for end-stage heart disease. One-year survival by more than 85% is being achieved routinely.[110] The number of donor hearts available appears to be leveling at under 2000 per year. At the same time, the number of patients accepted for transplantation has increased, consequently extending the period of waiting for a donor organ. Because, as a rule, candidates survive only a few months, an increasing number are being supported with mechanical circulatory assist devices as a bridge to transplantation.[111] An important question, from the standpoint of resource allocation, is whether the survival of such patients is comparable to that of those not requiring mechanical assistance. Available data suggest that whereas their perioperative mortality may be higher,[111] overall medium-term survival is the same.[112,113]

The use of IABP as a bridge to transplantation is well documented.[111–114] Depending on the institution, IABP is the modality employed in 40% to 90% of patients requiring mechanical assistance. Some clinicians prefer the percutaneous route for such patients, as it may be associated with a smaller incidence of major infectious complications.[52,112] The duration of balloon pump support in most instances has ranged from 1.5 to 27 days, although support for as long as 327 days has been reported.[115] Most workers regard IABP as the assisted circulation modality of choice in such patients, followed by parallel-flow LVADs, which in some cases have been implanted for months (as discussed elsewhere in this book). Some of the considerations applying to choice of mechanical assist technique have been discussed by Kantrowitz of our group.[116]

Complications of IABP

With the large experience accumulated worldwide during the 24 years of clinical use of IABP, its risks have been defined with some precision. The overall incidence of IABP complications ranges between 14% and 45%.[34,35,89,117–119] The incidence of major and minor complications ranges between 4% and 9% and 22% and 41%, respectively. Balloon pump support has contributed as a direct cause of death in less than 1% of cases.[34,35]

The most common complications observed after successful initiation of IABP are vascular—9% to 22%—and infectious—1% to 22%,[34,35,89,117–122] followed by failure to place the balloon pump—5% to 11.7%[34,35,52,118] and bleeding—4% to 10%.[34,35,56]

Complications Related to Insertion Technique

The incidence of failure to insert the balloon pump through the femoral artery has been reported to be as low as 3%[80] and as high as 30%.[89] The true incidence is probably between 5% and 12%,[34,52,54,123,124] with no difference in failure rates between the percutaneous and the surgical techniques.[52,80]

Several nonrandomized studies have compared the percutaneous and surgical techniques. Most have demonstrated that the rate of vascular and overall complications is higher for the percutaneous technique,[34,54,80,90,122,124] although other results have been reported.[125,126] Gottlieb, in a multivariate risk factor analysis of vascular complications of IABP in 206 patients, found that a history of preexisting peripheral vascular disease and the percutaneous approach were the major risk factors.[119] Duration of balloon pump support did not increase the incidence of vascular complications. These findings imply that vascular complications are related to initial balloon pump placement rather than to the prolonged presence of the balloon pump in the vascular system.[34,127] From a randomized study, our group (Goldberg et al.[52]) concluded that although the percutaneous technique affords more rapid initiation of IABP than the surgical technique (13 versus 31 min), it is associated with a higher incidence of vascular complications (22% vs. 4%). Interestingly, some data suggest that the so-called open puncture surgical technique, which we do not recommend, may lead to a higher complication rate than the "femoral conduit" surgical technique.[54]

Vascular Complications

Vascular complications include loss of distal pulse, pain in the leg, thrombosis, emboli, ischemic neuropathy, delayed vascular complications (arterial stenosis, claudication, ischemic foot ulcer, foot drop), amputation, aortic dissection, iliac artery laceration, and false aneurysm. Sex, among other factors, has been associated with a differential incidence of vascular complications, women having a higher risk (32%) than men (18%).[34] Some investigators have proposed that this difference may be due to sex-linked differences in the caliber of the arteries[119]; others report that more women than men have diabetes and systemic hypertension, both predisposing factors to vascular complications.[34,125,128] Wasfie et al. reported from our laboratory that vascular complications occurred in 34% of insulin-dependent diabetics, 18% of other diabetics, and 14% of nondiabetic patients.[129]

Our group also reported that patients with a history of systemic hypertension had more frequent vascular complications (27%) than others (20%).[34] As noted above, Goldberg et al. reported that percutaneous insertion is associated with a higher incidence of vascular complications (22%) than is surgical insertion (4%),[52] a finding others also have made.[42,90,119,128,130]

Other investigators have found that the incidence of complications increases directly with the duration of IABP.[117,131] Factors that do not increase the incidence of vascular complications are patient's age, hemodynamic status, and emergency as opposed to elective insertion.[119,125] Differences in the hospital location in which IABP was initiated do not explain variations in the frequency of vascular complications.[34]

Infectious Complications

Infectious complications include local infection, graft infection, bacteremia, and fever. We[34] related their rates of occurrence to the location of IABP initiation: coronary care unit, 26%; surgical intensive care unit, 23%; catheterization laboratory, 17%; and operating room, 12%. These findings can in part be explained by differences in the degree of asepsis typical of each location. Freed et al., also of our group, reported that infectious complications were more frequent in patients on prolonged support (20–71 days)—67%—than in those assisted for less than 20 days—25%.[70] The rate of fever and bacteremia increased significantly in patients on prolonged support, but the rate of local infection did not.[34,70] Bacteremia has been detected more frequently after surgical than percutaneous insertion.[52,119,132] Band and Maki considered the presence of monitoring lines as an additional factor in the incidence of fever and bacteremia.[133] In the report of McEnany et al., the rate of local infection was 3.2%, and only four of their patients required surgery to remove the prosthetic graft.[35] In obese and diabetic patients, the incidence of infection was as high as 37%.[125,129,130]

Other Complications

Among the complications reported by McEnany et al., excessive wound bleeding occurred in 21 patients (4%), 18 of whom required surgical exploration.[35] Three patients had disseminated intravascular coagulation associated with multisystem failure and sepsis. Seven patients had detectable gastrointestinal or genitourinary bleeding while receiving heparin-Dextran; the bleeding episodes stopped when heparin was discontinued.[35]

Some less common complications include balloon pump rupture, perforation, entrapment,[134,135] gas embolism,[136–138] small bowel infarction,[139] late paraplegia probably associated with dissection of the aorta,[140] and neurologic abnormalities in the leg.[141]

Recent Developments and New Directions

IABP in Pediatric Patients

The first reported use of the balloon pump in children after open heart surgery appeared in 1980.[142] In a series of 14 children (age, $1\frac{1}{2}$–18 years, weight, 8–52 kg) in whom this procedure was attempted, successful augmentation was achieved in 8. Balloon sizes ranged from 7 to 12F and balloon volumes, from 9 to 30 ml. Severe leg ischemia, thought to be related to the large balloon catheter, necessitated termination of IABP support in two patients. Renal failure occurred in two other patients as a result of obstruction of the renal arteries by the overly long pumping chamber. Difficulty in synchronizing balloon action to the higher heart rates of the patients also was a problem: as would be expected, augmentation was poor or unobtainable above a rate of 140 bpm. The elasticity of the aorta in young children also was thought to contribute to the poor augmentation. Even so, there were seven immediate and five long-term survivors. However, no child under the age of 5 yr survived. Since then, balloon pumps with catheter diameters as small as 3.5F and volumes as low as 1 ml have been manufactured. Such small balloon volumes have enabled successful support in infants as small as 2 kg at heart rates up to 200 bpm.[143–146]

The use of IABP in pediatric patients nevertheless remains limited. Most cases involve patients in refractory LOS. Published results indicate an immediate survival of 50% to 67% and a long-term survival of 25% to 33% (as in the report by Pollock et al.), outcomes that are comparable to the results in adults with LOS.[142] The interested reader is referred to Veasy's detailed account of current indications, technique, and management of pediatric IABP.[144]

Pulmonary Artery Balloon Counterpulsation

Counterpulsation of the pulmonary artery by various methods has been shown to increase pulmonary blood flow and decrease right ventricular preload and afterload in open-chest animal models of right ventricular failure.[147–151] The first clinical use of pulmonary artery balloon counterpulsation was reported by Miller et al. in 1980.[152] Using commercially available cardiovascular supplies, pulmonary artery balloon counterpulsation was achieved by means of a 35-ml balloon pump placed within a 20-mm tubular Dacron graft anastomosed end to side to the main pulmonary artery. "Good" pulmonary artery diastolic augmentation was obtained, and the system enabled cardiopulmonary bypass to be discontinued in a patient who probably would not have survived. The patient subsequently died of refractory ventricular fibrillation. Other workers have reported pulmonary artery balloon counterpulsation using the same technique,[153–155] or a modification in which the balloon pump was placed partly in the pulmonary artery and partly in the graft.[156] Of seven such cases reported, all were weaned from cardiopulmonary bypass, but only two survived long term. Noteworthy is the fact that both survivors had predominant right ventricular failure; it is known that when biventricular assistance is required for LOS, the outlook is extremely poor.[157]

Experimental evidence from animal models of profound biventricular failure suggests that pulmonary artery balloon counterpulsation in association with left heart bypass cannot restore systemic perfusion to normal.[147,158] On the basis of this and current clinical data, pulmonary artery balloon counterpulsation may be expected to provide adequate support in mild to moderate isolated right ventricular failure, but right heart bypass probably should be employed for profound right ventricular or biventricular failure. Current efforts are directed at producing a dedicated intrapulmonary artery balloon,[156] or improving the efficiency of pulmonary artery counterpulsation by the use of valveless pulsatile assist devices with stroke volumes of up to 100 ml.[158,159]

Closed-Loop, Fully Automated IABP

Ideally, the balloon pump should provide maximum assistance on each heart beat. This can be accomplished at present only if the patient has a regular rhythm and a well trained operator is available. In the presence of significant arrhythmia, even a well trained operator must make compromises that reduce the effectiveness of assistance.

A computerized system that could automatically respond to the changing hemodynamic status of the pa-

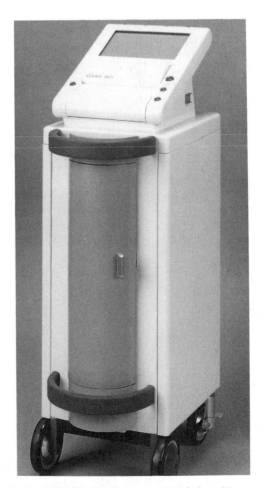

FIGURE 28.17. AISIN/L.VAD prototype of closed loop, totally automatic IABP drive unit (courtesy, Aisin Human Systems Co., Ltd.).

tient as well as arrhythmias, beat by beat, has long been sought.[160–162] With the Aisin Seiki Company of Japan and academic collaborators, we are developing a third-generation IABP (Fig. 28.17) that automatically makes and implements timing decisions for balloon inflation and deflation on a beat-by-beat basis. The reconfigured balloon pump incorporates an aortic pressure sensor and ECG electrodes to detect physiological signals, affording continuous optimization of diastolic augmentation without operator intervention.

Studies in a large series of dogs in sinus rhythm and a variety of experimentally induced arrhythmias demonstrate that this system is capable of correctly responding, among others, to tachycardia (to over 200 bpm) and rapid atrial fibrillation (Figs. 28.18, 28.19).[163] An initial trial in 11 patients confirmed the feasibility of the system for use in the clinical setting.[164,165] Safety and efficacy of the system are being investigated further in a multicenter trial.

Skeletal-Muscle Counterpulsation

The use of skeletal muscle to assist the failing circulation was first proposed by Kantrowitz and McKinnon in 1959. As noted above, by wrapping a hemidiaphragm around the descending thoracic aorta, significant diastolic augmentation was achieved, but further development was impeded by early muscle fatigue (Fig. 28.20).[3] Recently, the demonstration of the feasibility of using chronic low-frequency electrical stimulation to trans-

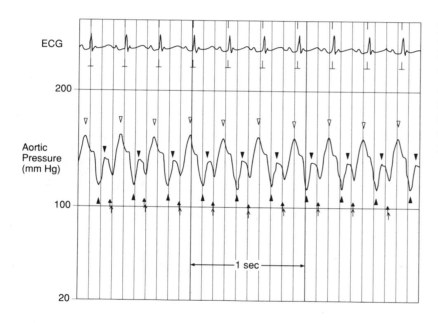

FIGURE 28.18. Tracings obtained during experimental use of the closed-loop, fully automatic IABP in a dog at a heart rate of 197 bpm. The symbols indicate features of the waveforms as detected by the drive unit. Note that full augmentation was obtained even at this rate. (Paper speed 50 mm/s); ▲ = end diastole; ▼ = peak systole; ▽ = peak assist pressure; ↑ = dicrotic notch; ⇡ = IABP inflation.

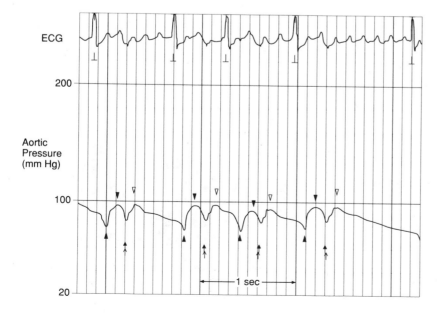

FIGURE 28.19. Tracings obtained during experimental use of the closed-loop, fully automatic IABP in a dog in atrial flutter. Note that the timing of augmentation is adjusted automatically on each beat even though R-R intervals vary widely (paper speed 50 mm/s).

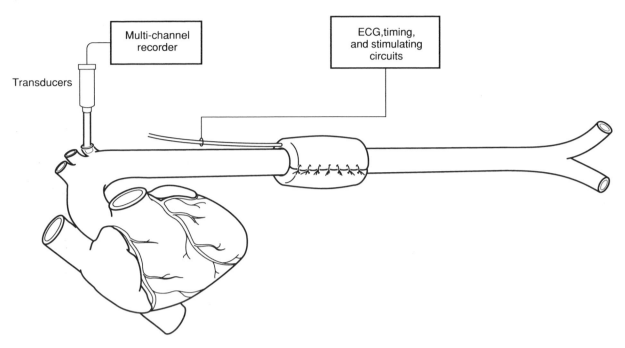

Transducers

Multi-channel
recorder

ECG, timing,
and stimulating
circuits

FIGURE 28.20. Diagram of experimental preparation for skeletal-muscle counterpulsation. Reprinted with permission from reference 3.

form skeletal muscle into fatigue-resistant fibers, and the advent of implantable synchronized burst electrical stimulators, have renewed interest in using skeletal muscle for cardiac assistance. Current research centers on two major approaches: (a) in latissimus dorsi dynamic cardiomyoplasty, the conditioned latissimus dorsi muscle flap is wrapped around the heart and stimulated in systole to assist cardiac action;[166,167] (b) diastolic LV assistance is achieved by using skeletal muscle to power an extraaortic ventricle,[168] a paraaortic counterpulsator,[169] or a dynamic "aortomyoplasty."[170]

Other Counterpulsation Devices

The development and use of various mechanical LVADs in recent years have defined a group of patients in whom total support of the left heart in profound refractory cardiac failure can produce significant long-term survival.[171] Some of these systems, for example, the Pierce-Donachy pulsatile sac-type device, or the Thermedics Model 10 LVAD, are capable of pumping in the synchronized counterpulsation mode, with flows of up to 2.9 L/min/m².[172] In contrast to the IABP, these LVADs utilize valved conduits to achieve unidirectional flow and have much larger stroke volumes. However, their use involves cannulation of the left atrium or LV for arterial inflow and of the aorta for arterial return, and hemorrhage is a major problem in up to 90% of patients. Recently, some workers have revived the permanently implanted, valveless auxiliary ventricle, or arterial counterpulsator, in an attempt to circumvent

some of the technical problems associated with the aforementioned LVADs. In their current fabrication, stroke volumes range up to 100 ml. Not surprisingly, these systems have been shown to be hemodynamically superior to IABP in animal failure models.[173,174] Implantation of these devices still requires cannulation of the abdominal aorta or the subclavian artery, and their clinical role has not been established.

Permanent In-Series Left Ventricular Assist

As described above, the demonstration of the efficacy of the balloon pump for temporary use renewed our laboratory's determination to develop an in-series technique for long-term use.[175] A "permanent balloon pump," having a larger stroke volume (60 cc) than the stroke volume of the balloon pump and designed for implantation in the wall of the thoracic aorta, has been brought to the point where clinical trial is appealing. The current configuration takes advantage of new technology so that the driving apparatus weighs less than 5 pounds and can be readily accommodated in a vest.

The permanent in-series LV assist system consists of three major parts: the implanted blood pump, the percutaneous access device, which allows reliable long-term transcutaneous passage of a gas conduit and electrical leads, and the external pneumatic drive unit (Figs. 28.21, 28.22). The blood pump comprises a fusiform pumping bladder whose intravascular surface possesses documented hemocompatibility.[69,176] The pumping bladder is valveless and minimally alters the topography

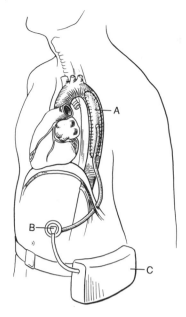

FIGURE 28.21. The permanent in-series LV assist system has two implantable components. **A**, The blood pump, which can be used intermittently, and **B**, the percutaneous access device. The patient can detach the connector to **C**, the external drive unit when the blood pump is passive.

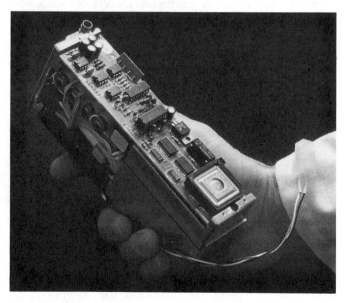

FIGURE 28.22. Drive unit for permanent in-series LVAD, which can be vest mounted or attached to a belt.

of the aorta. Consequently, it can be deactivated for extended periods of time without putting the patient at risk.

Laboratory studies of the initial system (then designated the dynamic aortic patch) confirmed that it replicates the hemodynamic effects of IABP, to the extent that the response to IABP predicts the hemodynamic effects of permanent balloon pumping—an important

clinical consideration in evaluating the risk/benefit ratios of alternative LVADs for chronic CHF. Life tests of the permanently implanted apparatus, cycling continuously, indicated that the system is highly reliable for as long as 7 yr. No adverse effects on the hemostatic mechanisms have been observed in extended animal experiments.[177,178]

During the 1970s, clinical investigations were undertaken in three male patients with advanced chronic CHF in whom pharmacologic management had become ineffective.[179,180] One patient lived 96 days after implantation of the permanent balloon pump. After the operation the patient was no longer bedridden. Catheterization demonstrated substantial amelioration of cardiac function, which corresponded to a remarkable clinical improvement in the patient's exercise tolerance. Although the patient died of an infection and its complications, the permanent balloon pump functioned effectively until the end. Since then, significant progress has been made in preventing infection by improving the percutaneous access device[181–183] and pumping chamber. The system's documented hemodynamic efficacy in chronic CHF, relative simplicity, and capability for intermittent operation promise that a substantial segment of the chronic CHF population may benefit from its use.

Comments

IABP has affected the lives of nearly a million individuals in acute CHF. By reason of that impact as well as its simplicity, efficacy, and low risk, it has become the de facto standard against which other mechanical cardiac assist devices for temporary use are judged. As more and more types of cardiac assist devices are being developed, a comment on the role of the ideal of simplicity in the design of both apparatus and technique may be in order. In the instance of IABP, the goal was to hold complexity of clinical use to the minimum, consistent with maximal hemodynamic efficacy and safety; the same philosophy has been followed in developing the permanent balloon pump.

Numerous variations on the design of the original balloon pump chamber have been proposed, tested, and discarded. The modification allowing percutaneous insertion represents a milestone in balloon pump catheter development. But the pumping chamber is, to this day, a polyurethane "sausage"—essentially unchanged since its advent in the wards of Maimonides Hospital in Brooklyn on June 29, 1967.

This is not to suggest that IABP design, technique, and apparatus are "frozen." On the contrary, it would be desirable, as an example, to reduce the caliber of the balloon catheter without reducing the speed of helium shuttling. This improvement would go far toward reducing the frequency of vascular complications of IABP.

For patients in right ventricular heart failure, it would be important to develop a truly satisfactory blood pump for counterpulsation in the pulmonary artery.

A completely safe and effective totally automated balloon pump system would strengthen the clinical usefulness of IABP. More effective diastolic augmentation could be provided to patients with the most severe cardiac arrhythmias. More consistent diastolic augmentation could be provided to those in normal sinus rhythm. Balloon pump capability could find its way to coronary care units in community hospitals, where the myocardial infarction patient is frequently first brought. Moreover, manpower costs for IABP utilization could lessen. As noted above, our own laboratory is collaborating in the development of such a third generation totally automatic balloon pump system, which has shown its feasibility in an initial clinical trial.

But perhaps the most intriguing possibility on the horizon is the permanent configuration of the IABP, which demonstrates promise for the treatment of chronic CHF. By implanting the balloon pump into the aortic wall, it is transformed into an "on demand" system with advantages of simplicity, reliability, "wearability," and convenience of use, relative to other long-term blood pumps. To be sure, clinical investigation is needed to confirm that the current design of this externally powered, implanted, in-series LVAD can be used with freedom from infection. But with its role in chronic CHF defined in clinical trials, the permanent balloon pump may come to rival in importance the temporary use first attempted clinically more than two decades ago.

Acknowledgments. The authors thank Michael Meyer, Carlos Rios, M.D., Ana Miriam Lopez, M.D., Kevin Gage, Niki E. Kantrowitz, M.D., Jean Rosensaft, Dennis Keller, and Beverly Stella for assistance in the preparation and review of this chapter. The research described was supported in large part by USPHS National Heart Lung and Blood Institute and National Institute of Diabetes and Digestive and Kidney Disease (NIDDKD) grants and contracts: HF9063, HE3023, H-5977, HE06510, HE11173, HL13737, HL34250, PH-43-66-7, HV-8-2821, and DK36778, as well as grants from the David and Minnie Berk Foundation, the John A. Hartford Foundation, Inc., and the Education Corporation of Sinai Hospital, Detroit, Michigan.

References

1. ACC/AHA Task Force. Guidelines and indications for coronary artery bypass surgery. A report of the American College of Cardiology/American Heart Association Task Force on assessment of diagnostic and therapeutic cardiovascular procedures (Subcommittee on Coronary Artery Bypass Graft Surgery). Kirklin JW, Subcommittee Chairman, Fisch C, Task Force Chairman, Beller GA, DeSanctis RW, Dodge HT, Kennedy JW, Reeves TJ, Weinberg SL. *J Am Coll Cardiol.* 1991;17:543–589.

2. Kantrowitz A, Kantrowitz A. Experimental augmentation of coronary flow by retardation of the arterial pressure pulse. *Surgery.* 1953;34:678–687.

3. Kantrowitz A, McKinnon WMP. The experimental use of the diaphragm as an auxiliary myocardium. *Surg Forum.* 1959;IX:265–267.

4. Sarnoff SJ, Braunwald E, Welch GH, Jr, Case RB, Stainsby WN, Macruz R. Hemodynamic determinants of oxygen consumption of the heart with special reference to the tension-time-index. *Am J Physiol.* 1958;192:148–156.

5. Sarnoff SJ, in discussion: Kantrowitz A. Functioning autogenous muscle used experimentally as an auxiliary ventricle. *Trans Am Soc Artif Intern Organs.* 1960; VI:305–310.

6. Kantrowitz A, Akutsu T, Chaptal PA, Krakauer J, Kantrowitz AR, Jones RT. A clinical experience with an implanted mechanical auxiliary ventricle. *JAMA.* 1966;197:525–529.

7. Harken DE. Counterpulsation: foundation and future, with a tribute to William Clifford Birtwell (1916–1978). In: Unger F, ed. Assisted Circulation. New York: Springer-Verlag, 1979:20–23.

8. Clauss RH, Birtwell WC, Albertal G, et al. Assisted circulation. I. The arterial counterpulsator. *J Thorac Cardiovasc Surg.* 1961;41:447–458.

9. Watkins DH, Duchesne ER. Postsystolic myocardial augmentation. I. Developmental considerations and technique. *AMA Arch Surg.* 1961;82:839–855.

10. Willman VL, Cooper T, Riberi A, Hanlon CR. Cardiac assistance by diastolic augmentation: hemodynamic evaluation in dogs with complete heart block. *Trans Am Soc Artif Intern Organs.* 1961;VII:198–201.

11. Soroff HS, Birtwell WC, Giron F, et al. Treatment of power failure by means of mechanical assistance. *Circulation.* 1969;39–40(Suppl IV):IV-292–314.

12. Clauss RH, Missier P, Reed GE, Tice D. Assisted circulation by counter-pulsation with an intra-aortic balloon. Methods and effects. In: *Digest, 15th Annual Conference on Engineering in Medicine and Biology.* vol 4. Chicago: Northwestern University; 1962:44.

13. Moulopoulos SD, Topaz SR, Kolff WJ. Extracorporeal assistance to the circulation and intraaortic balloon pumping. *Trans Am Soc Artif Intern Organs.* 1962; VIII:85–89.

14. Schilt W, Freed PS, Khalil G, Kantrowitz A. Temporary non-surgical intraarterial cardiac assistance. *Trans Am Soc Artif Intern Organs.* 1967;XIII:322–327.

15. Kantrowitz A, Tjønneland S, Freed PS, Phillips SJ, Butner AN. Sherman JL Jr. Initial clinical experience with intraaortic balloon pumping in cardiogenic shock. *JAMA.* 1968;203:135–140.

16. Scheidt S, Wilner G, Mueller H, et al. Intraaortic balloon pumping in cardiogenic shock. Report of a cooperative clinical trial. *N Engl J Med.* 1973;288:979–984.

17. Bregman D, Kripke DC, Goetz RH. The effect of syn-

chronous unidirectional intraaortic balloon pumping on hemodynamics and coronary blood flow in cardiogenic shock. *Trans Am Soc Artif Intern Organs*. 1970; XVI:439–449.

18. Buckley MJ, Leinbach RC, Kastor JA, et al. Hemodynamic evaluation of intraaortic balloon pumping in man. *Circulation*. 1970;41–42(Suppl II):II-130–136.

19. Wolvek S. The evolution of the intra-aortic balloon: the Datascope contribution. *J Biomat Appl*. 1989;3:527–543.

20. McElkoy PA, Shroff SG, Weber KT. Pathophysiology of the failing heart. *Cardiol Clin*. 1989;7:25–37.

21. Jaron D, Tomecek J, Freed PS, Welkowitz W, Fich S, Kantrowitz A. Measurement of ventricular load phase angle as an operating criterion for in series assist devices: hemodynamic studies utilizing intra-aortic balloon pumping. *Trans Am Soc Artif Intern Organs*. 1970;XVI:466–471.

22. Kantrowitz A, Krakauer JS, Zorzi G, et al. Current status of intraaortic balloon pump and initial clinical experience with aortic patch mechanical auxiliary ventricle. *Transplant Proc*. 1971;3:1459–1472

23. Tyberg JV, Keon WJ, Sonnenblick EH, Urschel CW. Effectiveness of intra-aortic balloon counterpulsation in the experimental low output state. *Am Heart J*. 1970;80:89–95.

24. Bregman D, Goetz RH. Clinical experience wtih a new cardiac assist device. The dual-chambered intra-aortic balloon assist. *J Thorac Cardiovasc Surg*. 1971;62:577–591.

25. Feola M, Adachi M, Akers WW, Ross JN Jr, Wieting DW, Kennedy JH. Intraaortic balloon pumping in the experimental animal. Effects and problems. *Am J Cardiol*. 1971;27:129–136.

26. Brown BG, Goldfarb D, Topaz SR, Gott VL. Diastolic augmentation by intra-aortic balloon. Circulatory hemodynamics and treatment of severe, acute left ventricular failure in dogs. *J Thorac Cardiovasc Surg*. 1967;53:789–804.

27. Mueller H, Ayres SM, Giannelli S, Conklin EF, Mazzara JT, Grace WJ. Effect of isoproterenol, *l*-norepinephrine, and intraaortic counterpulsation on hemodynamics and myocardial metabolism in shock following acute myocardial infarction. *Circulation*. 1972; XLV:335–351.

28. Urschel CW, Eber L, Forrester J, Matloff J, Carpenter R, Sonnenblick E. Alteration of mechanical performance of the ventricle by intraaortic balloon counterpulsation. *Am J Cardiol*. 1970;25:546–551.

29. Weber KT, Janicki JS, Walker AA. Intra-aortic balloon pumping: an analysis of several variables affecting balloon performance. *Trans Am Soc Artif Intern Organs*. 1972:XVIII:486–492.

30. Mueller H, Ayres SM, Conklin EF, et al. The effects of intraaortic counterpulsation on cardiac performance and metabolism in shock associated with acute myocardial infarction. *J Clin Invest*. 1971;50:1885–1900.

31. Nosé Y, Schamaun M, Kantrowitz A. Experimental use of an electronically controlled prosthesis as an auxiliary left ventricle. *Trans Am Soc Artif Intern Organs*. 1963:IX:269–274.

32. ECRI (Emergency Care Research Institute). Health De-

vices. Intraaortic balloon pumps. Plymouth Meeting, PA, 1987;16:135–176.

33. Weikel AM, Jones RT, Dinsmore R, Petschek HE. Size limits and pumping effectiveness of intraaortic balloons. *Ann Thorac Surg*. 1971;12:45–53.

34. Kantrowitz A, Wasfie T, Freed PS, Rubenfire M, Wajszczuk W, Schork MA. Intraaortic balloon pumping. 1967 through 1982: analysis of complications in 733 patients. *Am J Cardiol*. 1986;57:976–983.

35. McEnany MT, Kay HR, Buckley MJ, et al. Clinical experience with intraaortic balloon pump support in 728 patients. *Circulation*. 1978;58(Suppl I):I-124–132.

36. Mayerhofer KE, Billhardt RA, Codini MA. Delayed abrasion perforation of two intraaortic balloons. *Am Heart J*. 1984;108:1361–1363.

37. Rajani R, Keon WJ, Bédard P. Rupture of an intra-aortic balloon: a case report. *J Thorac Cardiovasc Surg*. 1980;79:301–302.

38. Bolooki H, ed. *Clinical Application of Intra-aortic Balloon Pumping*. New York: Futura Publishing Company; 1984.

39. Satler LF, Rackley CE. Assessment of adequate circulatory assist during intra-aortic balloon counterpulsation. In: Rackley CE, Brest AN, eds. *Advances in Critical Care Cardiology*. Philadelphia: FA Davis Co; 1986:141–149.

40. Weber KT, Janicki JS. Intraaortic balloon counterpulsation. A review of physiological principles, clinical results, and device safety. *Ann Thorac Surg*. 1974;17:602–636.

41. Schottler M, Schaefer J, Schwarzkopf HJ, Wysocki R. Experimentally induced change of arterial mean and aortic opening pressure by controlled variation of diastolic augmentation. *Basic Res Cardiol*. 1974;69:597–607.

42. Subramanian VA, Goldstein JE, Sos TA, McCabe JC, Hoover EA, Gay WA Jr. Preliminary clinical experience with percutaneous intraaortic balloon pumping. *Circulation*. 1980;62:I-123–129.

43. Bemis CE, Mundth ED, Mintz GS, et al. Comparison of techniques for intraaortic balloon insertion. *Am J Cardiol*. 1981;47:417. Abstract.

44. Berger RL, Saini VK, Long W, Hechtman H, Hood W Jr. The use of diastolic augmentation with the intra-aortic balloon in human septic shock with associated coronary artery disease. *Surgery*. 1973;74:4:601–606.

45. Mercer D, Doris P, Salerno TA. Intra-aortic balloon counterpulsation in septic shock. *Can J Surg*. 1981; 24:6:643–645.

46. Bregman D, Nichols AB, Weiss MB, Powers ER, Martin EC, Casarella WJ. Percutaneous intra-aortic balloon insertion. *Am J Cardiol*. 1980;46:261–64.

47. Grotz RL, Yeston NS. Intra-aortic balloon counterpulsation in high-risk cardiac patients undergoing noncardiac surgery. *Surgery*. 1989;106:1–5.

48. Georgen RF, Dietrick JA, Pifarre R, Scanlon PJ, Prinz RA. Placement of intra-aortic balloon pump allows definitive biliary surgery in patients with severe cardiac disease. *Surgery*. 1989;106:808–814.

49. Spence PA, Weisel RD, Easdown J, Jabr AK, Yap V, Salerno TA. The hemodynamic effects and mechanism of action of pulmonary artery balloon counterpulsation

in the treatment of right ventricular failure during left heart bypass. *Ann Thorac Surg.* 1985;39:329–335.

50. Nakatani S, Beppu S, Tanaka N, Andoh M, Miyatake K, Nimura Y. Application of abdominal and transesophageal echocardiography as a guide for insertion of intraaortic balloon pump in aortic dissection. *Am J Cardiol.* 1989;64:1082–1083.

51. D'Agostino RS, Baldwin JC. Intra-aortic balloon counterpulsation: present status. *Comp Ther.* 1986;12 47–54.

52. Goldberg MJ, Rubenfire M, Kantrowitz A, et al. Intraaortic balloon pump insertion: a randomized study comparing percutaneous and surgical techniques. *J Am Coll Cardiol.* 1987;9:515–523.

53. Kantrowitz A, Phillips SJ, Butner AN, Tjonneland S, Haller JD. Technique of femoral artery cannulation for phase-shift balloon pumping. *J Thorac Cardiovasc Surg.* 1968;56:219–220.

54. Di Lello F, Mullen DC, Flemma RJ, Anderson AJJ, Kleinman LH, Werner PH. Results of intraaortic balloon pumping after cardiac surgery: experience with the Percor balloon catheter. *Ann Thorac Surg.* 1988;46 442–446

55. Zada F, McCabe JC, Subramanian VA. Simplified technique for intra-aortic balloon insertion. *Ann Thorac Surg.* 1980;29 573–574.

56. Snow N, Horrigan TP. Ascending aortic IABP complications. [Letter]. *Ann Thorac Surg.* 1986;42:229.

57. Krause AH Jr, Bigelow JC, Page US. Transthoracic intraaortic balloon cannulation to avoid repeat sternotomy for removal. *Ann Thorac Surg.* 1976;21:562–565.

58. Mayer JH. Subclavian artery approach for insertion of intra-aortic balloon. *J Thorac Cardiovasc Surg.* 1978;76:61–63.

59. Rubenstein RB, Karhade NV. Supraclavicular subclavian technique of intra-aortic balloon insertion. *J Vasc Surg.* 1984;1:577–578.

60. Cascade PN, Rubenfire M, Kantrowitz A. Radiographic aspects of the phase-shift balloon pump. *Radiology.* 1972;103:299–302.

61. Shahian DM, Jewell ER. Intraaortic balloon pump placement through Dacron aortofemoral grafts. *J Vasc Surg.* 1988;7:795–797.

62. McBride LR, Miller LW, Naunheim KS, Pennington DG. Axillary artery insertion of an intraaortic balloon pump. *Ann Thorac Surg.* 1989;48:874–875.

63. Gaul G, Blazek G, Deutsch M, et al. Chronic use of an intra-aortic balloon pump in congestive cardiomyopathy. In: Unger F, ed. *Assisted Circulation 2.* New York: Springer-Verlag; 1984:28–37.

64. Krakauer JS, Rosenbaum A, Freed PS, Jaron D, Kantrowitz A. Clinical management ancillary to phase-shift balloon pumping in cardiogenic shock. *Am J Cardiol.* 1971;27:123–128.

65. Hagemeijer F, Laird JD, Haalebos MMP, Hugenholtz PG. Effectiveness of intraaortic balloon pumping without cardiac surgery for patients with severe heart failure secondary to a recent myocardial infarction. *Am J Cardiol.* 1977;40:951–956.

66. Perret C. Management of severe heart failure. *Acta Anaesth Belg.* 1988(Suppl 2);39:103–108.

67. Sturm JT, Fuhrman TM, Igo SR, et al. Quantitative indices of intra-aortic balloon pump (IABP) dependence during post-infarction cardiogenic shock. *Artificial Organs.* 1980;4:8–12.

68. Drexler M, Mayer E, Oelert H, Erbel R, Meyer J. Transesophageal echocardiographic monitoring during positive inotropic drug intervention and balloon pumping. In: Ergel R, Khandheria BK, Brennecke R, et al., eds. *Transesophageal Echocardiography. A New Window to the Heart.* Berlin: Springer-Verlag; 1989:218–220.

69. Kantrowitz A. Intra-aortic balloon pumping: clinical aspects and prospects. In: Unger F, ed. *Assisted Circulation III.* Berlin: Springer-Verlag; 1989:52–73.

70. Freed PS, Wasfie T, Zado B, Kantrowitz A. Intraaortic balloon pumping for prolonged circulatory support. *Am J Cardiol.* 1988;61:554–557.

71. Kyo S, Matsumura M, Takamoto S, Neya K, Omoto R. Transesophageal Doppler echo monitoring of cardiac function during assist circulation. In: Ergel R, Khandheria BK, Brennecke R, et al., eds. *Transesophageal Echocardiography. A New Window to the Heart.* Berlin: Springer-Verlag; 1989:221–228.

72. Rodigas PC, Finnegan JO. Technique for removal of percutaneously placed intraaortic balloons. *Ann Thorac Surg.* 1985;40:80–81.

73. Opie JC. Hemorrhage control after removal of surgically implanted intraaortic balloon pump. *Ann Thorac Surg.* 1990;49:326–327.

74. Dunkman WB, Leinback RC, Buckley MJ, et al. Clinical and hemodynamic results of intraaortic balloon pumping and surgery for cardiogenic shock. *Circulation.* 1972;46:465–477.

75. Kantrowitz A. The physiologic bases of in-series cardiac assistance and the clinical application of intra-aortic devices. In: Davila JC, ed. *2nd Henry Ford Hospital International Symposium on Cardiac Surgery.* New York: Appleton-Century-Crofts; 1977;640–643.

76. O'Rourke MF, Chang VP, Windsor HM, et al. Acute severe cardiac failure complicating myocardial infarction. Experience with 100 patients referred for consideration of mechanical left ventricular assistance. *Br Heart J.* 1975;36:169–181.

77. Sanfelippo PM, Baker NH, Ewy GH, et al. Experience with intraaortic balloon counterpulsation. *Ann Thorac Surg.* 1986;41:36–41.

78. Goldberger M, Tabak SW, Prediman SK. Clinical experience with intra-aortic balloon counterpulsation in 112 consecutive patients. *Am Heart J.* 1986;111:497–502.

79. O'Rourke MF, Sammel N, Chang VP. Arterial counterpulsation in severe refractory heart failure complicating acute myocardial infarction. *Br Heart J.* 1979;41:308–316.

80. Lorente P, Gourgon R, Beaufils P, et al. Multivariate statistical evaluation of intraaortic counterpulsation in pump failure complicating acute myocardial infarction. *Am J Cardiol.* 1980;46:124–134.

81. Mundth ED, Buckley MJ, Leinbach RC, et al. Myocardial revascularisation for the treatment of cardiogenic shock complicating acute myocardial infarction. *Surgery.* 1971;70:78–85.

82. Mundth ED, Buckley MJ, Daggett WM, Sanders CA,

Austen WG. Surgery for complications of acute myocardial infarction. *Circulation*. 1972;45:1279–1291.

83. Bolooki H. Emergency cardiac procedures in patients in cardiogenic shock due to complications of coronary artery disease. *Circulation*. 1989;79(Suppl I):I-137–148.

84. Fuhrman TM, Sturm JT, Holub DA, et al. Right and left ventricular hemodynamic indices as predictors of the need for and outcome of postcardiotomy mechanical (intra-aortic balloon pump) support. *Trans Am Soc Artif Intern Organs*. 1979;XXV:171–175.

85. Mundth ED. Preoperative intraaortic balloon pump assistance. *Ann Thorac Surg*. 1976;22:603–604.

86. Craver JM, Kaplan JA, Jones EL, Kopchak J, Hatcher CR. What role should the intra-aortic balloon have in cardiac surgery? *Ann Surg*. 1979;189:769–776.

87. Bolooki H, Williams W, Thurer RJ, et al. Clinical and hemodynamic criteria for use of the intra-aortic balloon pump in patients requiring cardiac surgery. *J Thorac Cardiovasc Surg*. 1976;72:756–768.

88. Golding LAR, Loop FD, Peter M, Cosgrove DM, Taylor PC, Phillips DF. Late survival following use of intraaortic balloon pump in revascularization operations. *Ann Thorac Surg*. 1980;30:48–51.

89. Lefemine AA, Kosowsky B, Madoff I, Black H, Lewis M. Results and complications of intraaortic balloon pumping in surgical and medical patients. *Am J Cardiol*. 1977;40:416–420.

90. Pennington DG, Swartz M, Codd JE, Merjavy JP, Kaiser GC. Intraaortic balloon pumping in cardiac surgical patients: a nine-year experience. *Ann Thorac Surg*. 1983;36:125–131.

91. Buckley MJ, Craver JM, Gold HK, Mundth ED, Daggett WM, Austen WG. Intra-aortic balloon pump assist for cardiogenic shock after cardiopulmonary bypass. *Circulation*. 1973;47–48(Suppl III):III-90–94.

92. Parker FB Jr, Neville JF, Hanson EL, Webb WR. Intraaortic balloon counterpulsation and cardiac surgery. *Ann Thorac Surg*. 1974;17:144–151.

93. Bregman D, Parodi EN, Edie RN, Bowman FO, Reemtsma K, Malm JR. Intraoperative unidirectional intraaortic balloon pumping in the management of left ventricular power failure. *J Thorac Cardiovasc Surg*. 1975;70:1010–1023.

94. McGee NG, Zillgitt SL, Trono R, et al. Retrospective analyses of the need for mechanical circulatory support (intraaortic balloon pump/abdominal left ventricular assist device or partial artificial heart) after cardiopulmonary bypass. A 44 month study of 14,168 patients. *Am J Cardiol*. 1980;46:135–142.

95. Maloney JV Jr, Nelson RL. Myocardial preservation during cardiopulmonary bypass An overview. *J Thorac Cardiovasc Surg*. 1975;70:1040–1050.

96. Braunwald E. The stunned myocardium: newer insights into mechanism and clinical implications. [Letter.] *J Thorac Cardiovasc Surg*. 1990;100:310–311.

97. DeBoer LWV, Ingwall JS, Kloner RA, Braunwald E. Prolonged derangements of canine myocardial purine metabolism after a brief coronary artery occlusion not associated with anatomic evidence of necrosis. *Proc Natl Acad Sci USA*. 1980;77:5471–5475.

98. Reimer KA, Hill ML, Jennings RB. Prolonged depletion of ATP and of the adenine nucleotide pool due to delayed resynthesis of adenine nucleotides following reversible myocardial ischemic injury in dogs. *J Mol Cell Cardio*. 1981;13:229–239.

99. Bavaria JE, Furukawa F, Kreiner G, et al. Myocardial oxygen utilization after reversible global ischemia. *J Thorac Cardiovasc Surg*. 1990;100:210–220.

100. Soroff HS, Levine HJ, Sachs BF, Birtwell WC, Deterline RA Jr. Assisted circulation. II. Effect of counterpulsation on left ventricular oxygen consumption and hemodynamics. *Circulation*. 1963;27:722–731.

101. Gill CC, Wechsler AS, Newman GE, Oldham HN Jr. Augmentation and redistribution of myocardial blood flow during acute ischemia by intraaortic balloon pumping. *Ann Thorac Surg*. 1973;16:445–453.

102. Sturm JT, McGee MG, Fuhrman TM, et al. Treatment of postoperative low output syndrome with intraaortic balloon pumping: experience with 419 patients. *Am J Cardiol*. 1980;45:1033–1036.

103. Norman JC, Cooley DA, Igo SR, et al. Prognostic indices for survival during postcardiotomy intra-aortic balloon pumping. Methods of scoring and classification, with implications for left ventricular assist device utilization. *J Thorac Cardiovasc Surg*. 1977;74:709–720.

104. Najafi H, Henson D, Dye WS, et al. Left ventricular hemorrhagic necrosis. *Ann Thorac Surg*. 1969;7:550–561.

105. Hedenmark J, Ahn H, Henze A, Nystrom SO, Svedjeholm R, Tyden H. Intra-aortic balloon counterpulsation with special reference to determinants of survival. *Scand J Thor Cardiovasc Surg*. 1989;23:57–62.

106. Corral CH, Vaughn CC. Intraaortic balloon counterpulsation: an eleven-year review and analysis of determinants of survival. *Texas Heart Inst J*. 1986;13:39–44.

107. Lund O, Johansen G, Allermand H, et al. Intraaortic balloon pumping in the treatment of low cardiac output following open heart surgery—immediate results and long-term prognosis. *Thorac Cardiovasc Surg*. 1988;36:332–337.

108. Kuchar DL, Campbell TJ, O'Rourke MF. Long-term swvival after counterpulsation for medically refractory heart failure complicating myocardial infarction and cardiac swgery. *Eur Heart J*. 1987;8:490–502.

109. Davies RA, Laks H, Wackers FJ, et al. Radionuclide assessment of left ventricular function in patients requiring intraoperative balloon pump assistance. *Ann Thorac Surg*. 1982;33:123–131.

110. Kaye MP. The registry of the International Society for Heart Transplantation: Fourth official report—1987. *J Heart Transplant*. 1987;6:63–67.

111. Oaks TE, Wisman CB, Pae WE, Pennock JL, Bwg J, Pierce WS. Results of mechanical circulatory assistance before heart transplantation. *J Heart Transplant*. 1989;8:113–115.

112. Hardesty RL, Griffith BP, Trento A, Thompson ME, Ferson PF, Bahnson HT. Mortally ill patients and excellent survival following cardiac transplantation. *Ann Thorac Surg*. 1986;41:126–129.

113. O'Connell JB, Renlunnd DG, Robinson JA, et al. Effect

of preoperative hemodynamic support on survival after cardiac transplantation. *Circulation.* 1988;78(Suppl III): III-78–82.

114. Reemtsma K, Drusin R, Edie R, Bregman D, Dobelle W, Hardy M. Cardiac transplantation for patients requiring mechanical circulatory support. *N Engl J Med.* 1978;298:670–671.

115. Ashar B, Turcotte LR. Analyses of longest IAB implant in human patient (327 days). *Trans Am Soc Artif Intern Organs.* 1981;XXVII:372–379.

116. Kantrowitz A. The ninth Hastings lecture. Spectrum. *Artif Organs.* 1986;10:497–510.

117. Goldman BS, Hill TJ, Rosenthal GA, Scully HE, Weisel RD, Baird RJ. Complications associated with use of the intra-aortic balloon pwmp. *Can J Surg.* 1982;25:153–156.

118. Beckman CB, Geha AS, Hammon GL, Baue AE. Results and complications of intraaortic balloon counterpulsation. *Ann Thorac Surg.* 1977;24:550–559.

119. Gottlieb SO, Brinker JA, Borkon AM, et al. Identification of patients at high risk for complications of intra-aortic balloon counterpulsation: a multivariate risk factor analysis. *Am J Cardiol.* 1984;53:1135–1139.

120. Skillman JJ, Kim D, Baim DS. Vascular complications of percutaneous femoral cardiac interventions. *Arch Surg.* 1988;123:1207–1212.

121. Iverson LIG, Herfindahl G, Ecker RR, et al. Vascular complications of intraaortic balloon cownterpulsation. *Am J Surg.* 1987;154:99–103.

122. Curtis JJ, Boland M, Bliss D, et al. Intra-aortic balloon cardiac assist: complication rates for the swgical and percutaneous insertion techniques. *Am Surg.* 1988;54:142–147.

123. Meldrum-Hanna WG, Deal CW, Ross DE. Complications of ascending aortic intraaortic balloon pump cannulation. *Ann Thorac Surg.* 1985;40:241–244.

124. Pelletier LC, Pomar JL, Bosch X, Galinanes M, Hebert Y. Complications of circulatory assistance with intra-aortic balloon pumping: a comparison of surgical and percutaneous techniques. *J Heart Transpl.* 1986;5:138–142.

125. Shahian DM, Neptune WB, Ellis FH Jr, Maggs PR. Intraaortic balloon pump morbidity: a comparative analysis of risk factors between percutaneous and surgical techniques. *Ann Thorac Surg.* 1983;36:644–653.

126. Alcan KE, Stertzer SH, Wallsh E, Franzone AJ, Bruno MS, DePasquale NN. Comparison of wire-guided percutaneous insertion and conventional surgically insertion of intra-aortic balloon pumps in 151 patients. *Am J Med.* 1983;75:24–28.

127. Isner JM, Cohen SR, Virmani R, Lawrinson W, Roberts WC. Complications of intraaortic balloon counterpulsation device: clinical and morphologic observations in 45 necropsy patients. *Am J Cardiol.* 1980;45:260–268.

128. Harvey JC, Goldstein JE, McCabe JC, Hoover El, Gay WA Jr, Subramanian VA. Complications of percutaneous intraaortic balloon pumping. *Circulation.* 1981; 64(Suppl II):II-114–117.

129. Wasfie T, Freed PS, Rubenfire M, et al. Risk associated with intraaortic balloon pumping in patients with and without diabetes mellitus. *Am J Cardio.* 1988:61:558–562.

130. Martin SR III, Moncure AC, Buckley MJ, Austen WG, Akins C, Leinback RC. Complications of percutaneous intra-aortic balloon insertion. *J Thorac Cardiovasc Surg.* 1983;85:186–190.

131. Sutorius DJ, Majewski JA, Miller SM. Vascular complications as a result of intra-aortic balloon pumping. *Am Surg.* 1979:512–516.

132. Hauser AM, Gordon S, Gangadharan, et al. Percutaneous intraaortic balloon counterpulsation. Clinical effectiveness and hazards. *Chest.* 1982;82:422–425.

133. Band JD, Maki DG. Infections caused by arterial catheters used for hemodynamic monitoring. *Am J Med.* 1979;67:735–741.

134. Stahl KD, Tortolani AJ, Nelson RL, Hall MH, Moccio CG, Parnell VA Jr. Intraaortic balloon rupture. *Trans Am Soc Artif Intern Organs.* 1988;XXXIV:496–499.

135. Milgalter E, Mosseri M, Uretzky G, Romanoff H. Intraaortic balloon entrapment: a complication of balloon perforation. *Ann Thorac Surg.* 1986;42:697–698.

136. Furman S, Vijaynagar R, Rosenbaum R, McMullen M, Escher DJ. Lethal sequelae of intra-aortic balloon rupture. *Surgery.* 1971;69:121–129.

137. Tomatis L, Nemiroff M, Riahi M, et al. Massive air embolism due to rupture of pulsatile assist device: successful treatment in the hyperbaric chamber. *Ann Thorac Surg.* 1981;32:604–608.

138. Haykal HA, Wang AM. CT diagnosis of delayed cerebral air embolism following intraaortic balloon pump catheter insertion. *Comput Radiol.* 1986;10:307–309.

139. Jarmolowski CR, Poirier RL. Small bowel infarction complicating intra-aortic balloon counterpulsation via the ascending aorta. *J Thorac Cardiovasc Surg.* 1980; 79:735–737.

140. Seifert PE, Silverman NA. Late paraplegia resulting from intraaortic balloon pump. [Letter]. *Ann Thorac Surg.* 1986;41:700.

141. Honet JC, Wajszczuk WJ, Rubenfire M, Kantrowitz A, Raikes JA. Neurological abnormalities in the leg(s) after use of intraaortic balloon pump: report of six cases. *Arch Physic Med Rehab.* 1975;56:346–352.

142. Pollock JC, Charlton MC, Williams WG, Edmonds JF, Trusler GA. Intraaortic balloon pumping in children. *Ann Thorac Surg.* 1980;29:522–528.

143. Veasy LG, Blalock RC, Orth JL, Boucek MM. Intra-aortic balloon pumping in infants and children. *Circulation.* 1983;68:1095–1100.

144. Veasy LG, Webster HF, McGough EC. Intra-aortic balloon pumping: adaptation for pediatric use. *Crit Care Clin.* 1986;2:237–249.

145. Webster H, Veasy LG. Intra-aortic balloon pumping in children. *Heart Lung.* 1985;14:548–555.

146. del Nido PJ, Swan PR, Benson LN, et al. Successful use of intraaortic balloon pumping in a 2-kilogram infant. *Ann Thorac Surg.* 1988;46:574–576.

147. Spence PA, Weisel RD, Salerno TA. Right ventricular failure. Pathophysiology and treatment. *Surg Clin North Am.* 1985;65:689–697.

148. Opravil M, Gorman AJ, Krejcie TC, Michaelis LL,

Moran JM. Pulmonary artery balloon counterpulsation for right ventricular failure: I. Experimental results. *Ann Thorac Surg.* 1984;38:242–253.

149. Kralios AC, Zwart HHJ, Moulopoulos SD, Collan R, Kwan-Gett CS, Kolff WJ. Intrapulmonary artery balloon pumping. Assistance of the right ventricle. *J Thorac Cardiovasc Surg.* 1970;60:215–232.

150. Spotnitz HM, Berman MA, Reis RL, Epstein SE. The effects of synchronized counterpulsation of the pulmonary artery on right ventricular hemodynamics. *J Thorac Cardiovasc Surg.* 1971;61:167–174.

151. de la Riviére AB, Haasler G, Malm JR, Bregman D. Mechanical assistance of the pulmonary circulation after right ventricular exclusion. *J Thorac Cardiovasc Surg.* 1983;85:809–813.

152. Miller DC, Moreno-Cabral RJ, Stinson EB, Shinn JA, Shumway NE. Pulmonary artery balloon counterpulsation for acute right ventricular failure. *J Thorac Cardiovasc Surg.* 1980;80:760–763.

153. Flege JB, Wright CB, Reisinger TJ. Successful balloon counterpulsation for right ventricular failure. *Ann Thorac Surg.* 1984;37:167–168.

154. Symbas PN, McKeown PP, Santora AH, Vlasis SE. Pulmonary artery balloon counterpulsation for treatment of intraoperative right ventricular failure. *Ann Thorac Surg.* 1985;39:437–440.

155. Gold JP, Shemin RJ, DiSesa VJ, Cohn L, Collins JJ Jr. Balloon pump support of the failing right heart. *Clin Cardiol.* 1985;8:599–602.

156. Moran JM, Opravil M, Gorman AJ, Rastegar H, Meyers SN, Michaelis LL. Pulmonary artery balloon counterpulsation for right ventricular failure: II. Clinical experience. *Ann Thorac Surg.* 1984;38:254–259.

157. Pennock JL, Pierce WS, Wisman CB, Bull AP, Waldhausen JA. Survival and complications following ventricular assist pumping for cardiogenic shock. *Ann Surg.* 1983;198:469–478.

158. Gaines WE, Pierce WS, Prophet GA, Holtzman K. Pulmonary circulatory support. A quantitative comparison of four methods. *J Thorac Cardlovasc Surg.* 1984;88:958–964.

159. Phillips SJ. Percutaneous cardiopulmonary bypass and innovations in clinical counterpulsation. *Crit Care Clin.* 1986;2:297–318.

160. Zelano JA, Li JKJ, Welkowitz. A closed-loop control scheme for intraaortic balloon pumping. *IEEE Trans Biomed Eng.* 1990;37:182–192.

161. Kuklinski WS. *Closed Loop Control of Intraaortic Balloon Pumping: Studies Using a Computer Simulation and Animal Experiments.* [Dissertation] University of Rhode Island, Kingston, 1979.

162. Moskowitz MS, Freed PS, Kantrowitz A. A system for evaluation of computer control of intraaortic balloon pumping. Proceedings of the 28th annual conference on engineering in medicine and biology. New Orleans; 1975:348.

163. Cardona RR, Rios C, Freed PS, et al. Experimental models for studies of a closed loop, fully automatic intraaortic balloon pump. Cardiovascular Science and Technology Conference, Washington, D.C, 1991–92.

164. Kantrowitz A, Freed PS, Cardona R, et al. Initial Clinical Trial of a Closed-Loop, Fully Automatic Intraaortic Balloon Pump. Abstracts 38th Annual Meeting ASAIO, Nashurlle, TN, May 7–9, 1992.

165. Kantrowitz A, Freed PS, Gardona RR, et al. Initial clinical trial of a closed-loop, fully automatic intraaortic balloon pump. *ASAIO J.* 1992;38(3):617–21.

166. Chachques JC, Grandjean PA, Schwartz K, et al. Effect of latissimus dorsi dynamic cardiomyoplasty on ventricular function. *Circulation.* 1988;78(Suppl 3):III-203–216.

167. Carpentier A, Chachques JC. Myocardial substitution with a stimulated skeletal muscle: first successful clinical case. [Letter]. *Lancet.* 1985;1:1267.

168. Acker MA, Anderson WA, Hammond RL, et al. Skeletal muscle ventricles in circulation. One to eleven weeks' experience. *J Thorac Cardiovasc Surg.* 1987; 94:163–174.

169. Li CM, Hill A, Colson M, et al. Implantable rate-responsive counterpulsation assist system. *Ann Thorac Surg.* 1990;49:356–362.

170. Chachques JC, Grandjean PA, Fischer EIC, et al. Dynamic aortomyoplasty to assist left ventricular failure. *Ann Thorac Surg.* 1990;49:225–230.

171. Miller CA, Pae WE Jr, Pierce WS. Combined registry for the clinical use of mechanical ventricular assist devices. Postcardiotomy cardiogenic shock. *Trans Am Soc Artif Intern Organs.* 1990;36:43–46.

172. Pennington DG, Bernhard WF, Golding LR, Berger RL, Khuri SF, Watson JT. Long-term follow-up of postcardiotomy patients with profound cardiogenic shock treated with ventricular assist devices. *Circulation.* 1985;72(Suppl II):II-216–226.

173. Gabbay S, Frater RWM. The extra-aortic balloon counterpulsation as an assist device. *Trans Am Soc Artif Intern Organs.* 1981;XXVII:598–603.

174. Nanas JN, Mason JW, Taenaka Y, Olsen DB. Comparison of an implanted abdominal aortic counterpulsation device with the intraaortic balloon pump in a heart failure model. *J Am Coll Cardiol.* 1986;7:1028–1035.

175. Sujansky E, Tjønneland S, Freed PS, Kantrowitz A. A dynamic aortic patch as a permanent auxiliary ventricle: experimental studies. *Surgery.* 1969;66:875–882.

176. Kantrowitz A. In-series temporary and permanent cardiac assistance. In: Kantrowitz A, ed. *ASAIO Primers in Artificial Organ. Number 3: Ventricular Assist Devices.* Philadelphia: JB Lippincott; 1988:77–96.

177. Schraut W, Kiso I, Freed PS, et al. Permanent in-series cardiac assistance with the dynamic aortic patch: blood prosthesis interaction in long term canine experiments. *Surgery.* 1976;79:193–201.

178. Baechler CA, Barnhart MI, Schraut W, Kantrowitz A. Studies on the dynamic aortic patch and the aorta in clinical trials. *Proc Scanning Electron Microscopy Symposia.* Chicago: Research Institute, 1973:443–449.

179. Kantrowitz A, Freed PS, Wasfie T, Kozlowski J, Rubenfire M. Permanent cardiac assistance in chronic congestive failure by means of mechanical auxiliary ventricle. In: Chang TMS, Bing-Lin-He, eds. *Hemoperfusion and Artificial Organs.* Beijing, China: Academic Publishers; 1983:149–169.

180. Kantrowitz A, Krakauer J, Rubenfire M, et al. Initial clinical experience with a new permanent mechanical au-

xiliary ventricle: the dynamic aortic patch. *Trans Am Soc Artif Intern Organs*. 1972;XVIII:159–167.

181. Kantrowitz A, Freed PS, Wasfie, et al. Development of percutaneous energy transmission system. Proceedings of the NHLBI Devices and Technology Branch, Contractor Meeting 1983:1–68.

182. Bar-Lev A, Freed PS, Mandell G, et al. Long-term percutaneous access device. In: *Advances in continuous ambulatory peritoneal dialysis*. Proceedings of the seven annual CAPD conference Kansas City, Missouri 1987:81–87.

183. Cardona RR, Kantrowitz A. Autologous fibroblast coating used to enhance percutaneous access device longevity. *Am Coll Surg*. 1990:29. Abstract.

29
Ventricular Assistance and Replacement

Reed D. Quinn, William S. Pierce, and Walter E. Pae

The standard methods for support of the failing heart have been discussed. The use of inotropic agents, afterload reduction, and intraaortic balloon counterpulsation are important techniques and can provide circulatory support in many patients. Occasionally, however, more aggressive measures are needed. This chapter outlines a brief historical background of ventricular assist device development, several types of pulsatile ventricular assist devices and total artificial hearts, nonpulsatile systems, some of the devices currently under development, the indications for mechanical ventricular assistance and management problems, and the bridge-to-transplantation and postoperative postcardiotomy cardiogenic shock clinical results.

Historical Background

Even before medical science had developed a clear understanding of the pathophysiology of congestive heart failure (CHF), surgeons were proposing the idea of replacing the failing heart with other forms of circulatory support. Today, severe myocardial dysfunction, which has advanced beyond response to medical management, may be managed by several different techniques (Table 29.1). This chapter discusses the development, role, and limitations of many of these techniques, but because separate chapters on cardiac transplantation and intraaortic balloon counterpulsation appear elsewhere in this text, only minimal discussion of these techniques is included here.

The surgical treatment of CHF, as well as the treatment of other cardiac anomalies, awaited and subsequently has paralleled the development of cardiopulmonary bypass techniques. Although it is difficult to identify the origin of the concept of cardiopulmonary bypass, Gibbon is generally credited with the first clinical use of this technique. In 1954, after 14 yr of laboratory research, Gibbon repaired an atrial septal defect in a young girl using cardiopulmonary bypass.[1] Although he subsequently had four clinical failures and directed his attention elsewhere, others continued his research, enabling the technique of cardiopulmonary bypass to mature and provide circulatory support for open cardiac procedures. Only 4 years after Gibbon's original success, Stuckey and associates reported using cardiopulmonary bypass to support a patient with cardiogenic shock secondary to myocardial infarction.[2] Using left atrial to femoral bypass, Spencer and associates, in 1965, successfully supported a patient for 6 hours.[3]

Akutsu and Kolff, while at the Cleveland Clinic in 1958, replaced the heart of a dog with the first mechanical ventricle.[4] The animal's survival was reported in minutes but with subsequent experimentation and experience this time was extended to hours. These early trials and minimal successes encouraged researchers to persist. Improvements in pump design, biocompatible materials, device fabrication, and control systems resulted in survivals of 100 days by the mid 1970s. Survivals of greater than 1 year are obtainable with current models.

The first clinical use of a pneumatic artificial heart was in 1969. A 47-year-old man at the Texas Heart Institute was supported for 64 hours before transplantation.[5] Although the transplant failed, the pneumatic device worked well and demonstrated the clinical feasibility of using these devices for circulatory support. Since that time, many groups have used mechanical assist devices as bridges to transplantation with improving success.[6–8] In 1985, Hill and associates reported the first long-term survival of a patient who was bridged to transplantation using mechanical ventricular assist device support.[9] In 1981, Pierce and associates, from The Pennsylvania State University, first reported their experience with the Pierce-Donachy ventricular assist device in eight patients with cardiogenic shock after cardiac

TABLE 29.1. Forms of ventricular support.

Biological
Heart transplantation
Cardiomyoplasty
Skeletal muscle–powered assist device

Mechanical (Pulsatile)
Intraaortic balloon pump
Ventricular assist devices
Artificial heart

Mechanical (Nonpulsatile)
Roller pumps
Centrifugal pumps
Hemopump

sistance, mechanical circulatory assistance will prove to be less expensive over a 5-yr period. This cost savings is mainly due to the elimination of the high cost of immunosuppressive therapy required for transplantation, and simplification of postoperative follow-up afforded by mechanical devices.

These devices, however, create new ethical and medical dilemmas that will have to be addressed. If they are implanted as temporary devices in a bridge-to-transplantation application, it intensifies the competition for already seriously limited donor organs. If implanted as a permanent life support system, a decision will have to be made on when to terminate support in otherwise critically ill patients.

operations.[10] In these eight patients, complete systemic and/or pulmonary circulatory support was maintained by the pneumatic device, and it was demonstrated that the profoundly depressed ventricular function in these postoperative patients was potentially reversible.

The first use of a total artificial heart as a permanent circulatory support device was reported by DeVries et al., at the University of Utah.[11] The patient was a 61-year-old dentist, Dr. Barney Clark, who had chronic CHF secondary to a cardiomyopathy and received the Jarvik-7 artificial heart on December 2, 1982. Dr. Clark lived 112 days and except for dysfunction of a prosthetic mitral valve that required replacement of the left ventricle of his Jarvik-7 heart on the tenth postoperative day, the device functioned well. Subsequent investigators have also used these devices for long-term circulatory support, but enthusiasm for the use of current devices as a permanent circulatory replacement has declined and awaits the development of totally implantable devices.[12]

Heart failure affects an estimated 4 million people in the United States per year and accounts for nearly 400,000 deaths. CHF is one of the only cardiovascular disorders whose prevalence is increasing. Heart transplantation, although now a clinically acceptable and successful technique, is severely limited by organ availability. In 1989, there were 1647 hearts transplanted but because of current organ donation patterns, it is not expected that this number will substantially increase. It has been estimated that as many as an additional 30,000 patients could benefit from heart transplantation. If one adds to this number patients who are not transplant candidates but could benefit from a mechanical assist device, there exists a large number of patients who could potentially benefit from this therapeutic modality. Several groups have compared the cost of mechanical circulatory support versus heart transplant. These studies suggest that even though initial hospital costs are about the same to slightly higher for mechanical as-

Intraaortic Balloon Counterpulsation

The concept of counterpulsation was first proposed by Harken in 1958.[13] By 1968, Kantrowitz et al.[14] had perfected the technique and reported the first successful clinical use. In the intraaortic counterpulsation technique, a balloon is inflated at the time of aortic valve closure, producing diastolic coronary flow augmentation, and is deflated at the onset of systole, resulting in left ventricular (LV) afterload reduction.[15–19] The development of percutaneous insertion techniques led to widespread application of the intraaortic balloon to multiple clinical settings.[20,21] The intraaortic balloon has been used in patients with postcardiotomy cardiogenic shock as postoperative support, in patients with intractable angina, and a multitude of other cardiac problems including ventricular arrhythmias, acute mitral regurgitation, or acute ventricular septal defects. Another application of the intraaortic balloon pump (IABP) has been in conjunction with nonpulsatile centrifugal pumps to provide temporary ventricular support. A detailed analysis of the indications, results, and complications of this technique is presented in Chapter 28 of this volume.

The complications from use of the intraaortic balloon stem largely from insertion of the device. Vessel perforation, limb ischemia, aortic dissection, balloon fracture, percutaneous wound problems, and delayed vascular complications can all be minimized by careful attention to insertion techniques and proper balloon removal. Intraaortic balloon counterpulsation is a proven, effective means of circulatory support.[22,23] Although it is effective, it is not a permanent solution for patients with circulatory failure. Intraaortic balloon counterpulsation is an excellent choice in patients requiring either short-term support while awaiting myocardial recovery or to facilitate and improve myocardial performance during diagnostic procedures and/or while awaiting more definitive therapy.

Biological Cardiac Assistance

There are primarily three types of biological cardiac assist techniques: (a) dynamic cardiomyoplasty, (b) the use of muscle power to activate an assist device usually as a diastolic counterpulsator, and (c) cardiac transplantation. This section of the chapter will discuss the first two of these techniques, describing their applications, indications, and limitations.

Cardiomyoplasty

Dynamic cardiomyoplasty is a surgical procedure designed to enhance cardiac performance by placing a skeletal muscle flap around the ventricle to assist or enhance ventricular contraction (Fig. 29.1). Cardiomyoplasty is a relatively new procedure and experience with it is just starting to mount. In 1990, in a review from the Carpentier group, three types of dynamic cardiomyoplasty are reported[24]:

1. *Atrial or ventricular reinforcement*: The latissimus dorsi muscle flap is wrapped around the heart to support hypokinetic areas. The atrial or ventricular hypokinesis may be secondary to acquired or congenital diseases.
2. *Ventricular substitution*: replacement of a portion of the ventricular wall. In this technique, autologous pericardium usually is harvested to create a neoendocardium and facilitate hemostatic ventricular closure. The latissimus dorsi muscle flap is then secured to the adjacent myocardium, replacing the resected cardiac muscle.
3. *Reconstructive procedure*: The procedures of reinforcement, substitution, and replacement described above are combined. This technique is useful after extensive cardiac resections for tumor, ventricular aneurysm, or echinococcal cyst.

At present, the world literature contains about 78 reported cases of cardiomyoplasty. The indications for and experience with the procedure are limited to the use of skeletal muscle for reinforcement of failing myocardium, to enhance cardiac function, for substitution of cardiac defects, and for ventricular wall reconstruction. The surgical procedure itself entails two separate incisions. Cardiopulmonary bypass is required only a if cardiac resection or intracardiac operation is anticipated. Commonly, the left latissimus dorsi muscle is chosen, mobilized from its iliac crest and paravertebral insertions, and then rotated on the thoracodorsal neurovascular pedicle, through a partial anterior second rib resection site, to the intrathoracic position. Two intramuscular pacing electrodes are implanted in the flap. A separate median sternotomy incision is performed and an intramyocardial sensing electrode is implanted so that electrical stimulation of the muscle flap can be

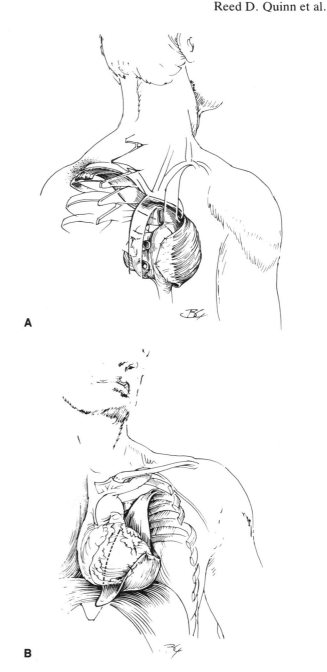

A

B

FIGURE 29.1. Cardiomyoplasty is a relatively new procedure. The figure demonstrates two applications for this procedure as the latissimus dorsi muscle flap is brought through the chest wall to reinforce (**A**) the right atrium, and (**B**) for a ventricular muscle wrap.

synchronized with ventricular depolarization. Depending on the application and surgical indications, the latissimus dorsi muscle flap is appropriately positioned on the cardiac surface. The cardiomyostimulator pulse generator is attached to the previously described electrodes, and then implanted in a subcutaneous pocket. Postoperatively, the muscle must be conditioned. Protocols vary, but traditionally a 10-day to 2-week delay before initiation of muscle flap stimulation is observed, allowing for skeletal muscle flap recovery, for skeletal-to-cardiac muscle adhesion formation, and for the development of collateral muscle flap circulation. After the initial 2-week delay, the flap is progressively stimulated, initially with single impulses and subsequently with a train of impulses. This conditioning allows the flap to develop properties of slow fatigue-resistant muscle fibers.

The goal of cardiomyoplasty is to use skeletal muscle to assist the myocardium of patients with irreversible cardiac insufficiency by improving ventricular functional contractions and by limiting cardiac dilatation.[24,25] Because ventricular volume has been identified as one of the major predictors of survival, one might hypothesize that one can improve ventricular contraction and limit cardiac dilatation, thereby reducing ventricular volume, and an improved lifestyle and survival might be expected.[26,27] The results after this new procedure have been promising. Postoperative evaluations with echocardiography, multigated studies, and hemodynamic measurements all seem to show only mild improvement in ventricular function (3–7% increase in ejection fractions) with minimal changes in ventricular compliance.[24,28] Clinically, most preoperative patients have been New York Heart Association (NYHA) Class III–IV, but surprisingly have improved postoperatively to NYHA Class I–II. This improvement is therefore difficult to explain from measured parameters.

Given the fact that the procedure is still in its infancy, many variables still must be elucidated, but some facts have been clearly established. During the surgical procedure, extreme care must be taken not to damage the muscle flap and its vascular supply. Secure adhesion of the skeletal muscle flap to the myocardium is essential. Skeletal muscle is very thrombogenic and direct blood contact will result in clot formation, so preservation of the endocardium or the use of pericardium as a blood-contacting surface is essential. Pulse-train stimulation provides better augmentation of skeletal muscle contraction than a single pulse, although best conditioning protocol has probably not yet been established. Proper alignment of the skeletal muscle fibers and hence proper functional contraction enhancement depend on muscle fiber orientation, a variable that is currently being defined. Preliminary work by Magovern et al. suggest that patients with biventricular failure and pulmonary hypertension do poorly when compared to patients with preserved right ventricular function; thus, right ventricular failure may require a different wrap configuration or may be a contraindication to cardiomyoplasty.[29] Because of the protected postoperative skeletal muscle training period (6 weeks), cardiomyoplasty cannot be used as an acute rescue for the failing ventricle.

Dynamic cardiomyoplasty is new and still a somewhat experimental procedure. It promises to be a valuable technique in the treatment of patients with end-stage ischemic cardiomyopathies, diffuse ventricular hypokinesis, ventricular aneurysms, tumors or cysts requiring partial ventricular resection, and also may be a potential aid to patients that may not be candidates for heart transplantation. Some authors have suggested that because cardiomyoplasty provides an elastic limitation to ventricular dilation, it will be useful in prevention of intrinsic arrhythmias and valvular regurgitation. As further experience is gained and current techniques improve, the indications for and results of this technique will become more evident.

Skeletal Muscle-Powered Cardiac Assist Device

The use of skeletal muscle as a diastolic counterpulsator was first reported by Kantrowitz and McKinnan in 1959.[30] In these reports, diaphragmatic muscle was used to produce counterpulsation by wrapping a muscular pedicle around the descending aorta. These experiments demonstrated that small amounts of diastolic augmentation could be achieved, but muscle weakness, muscle fatigue, and the small volume displacement by the aortic wraps limited the clinical application of this technique. Current understanding of muscle physiology, improved techniques such as pulse-train myostimulations, and improvements in conditioning protocols have renewed interest in this type of assist device. Most investigators have chosen the concept of extraaortic balloon pumps because they allow a greater counterpulsation displacement volume, they can be attached in the ascending aorta near coronary ostia allowing maximal augmentation of coronary perfusion, and they allow easier implantation with in situ muscle utilization.[31–33] These skeletal muscle ventricles usually are fashioned from several wraps of latissimus dorsi muscle, around a mandrel of known volume, producing a multilayered tube. These tubes are lined with polymer bladders (polytetrafluoroethylene, polyurethane), which form the blood-contacting surfaces. Sensing and stimulating electrodes are implanted similar to those previously described for cardiomyoplasty patients. After several weeks, a second operation connects the skeletal muscle tube to the aorta and conditioning of the skeletal muscle ventricle is begun, requiring 4 to 6 weeks for completion (Fig. 29.2).

Another biologically powered device was developed at the Cleveland Clinic by Novoa and colleagues.[33] This device is a pusher plate ventricular assist device, which has been modified so it could be muscle activated. The device has two chambers: (a) a 60-cc biolized pusher plate pump fitted with a Hexyn rubber diaphragm, and (b) a driving chamber of Hexyn rubber. A central disc attaches the two chambers and contains a Hall sensor. This sensor allows the determination of stroke volume from diaphragmatic position. The device also contains a

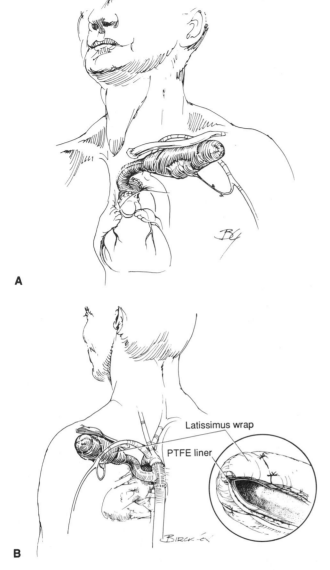

A

B

FIGURE 29.2. A diagram of an extraaortic skeletal muscle actuated balloon. The multilayer skeletal muscle ventricle is connected to (**A**) the ascending aorta, (**B**) the proximal descending aorta, and stimulated during ventricular diastole to produce maximum counterpulsation. The cut shows the polytetrafluoroethylene bladder liner.

4-mm pneumatic drive port that provides the option of connection of this device to an external drive source.

Although these devices have functioned well in exvivo and canine tests, no clinical data have been accumulated. It is believed that these devices eventually may be able to augment cardiac output as much as 10% to 20%.[34] They would offer the advantages of reduced cost, diminished infection risk, and less mechanical failure. Major design problems still must be overcome. Muscle fatiguability limits function and a minimum of 6 to 12 weeks is still needed for skeletal muscle conditioning, thus necessitating an alternate power source and

TABLE 29.2. Mechanical ventricular assist devices.

Electric motor	Roller
Novacor*[†]	Sarns[†]
Penn State[‡]	Stockert[†]
Thermedics*[†]	
Pneumatic	Centrifugal
Abiomed*[†]	Sarns/Centrimed[†]
Jarvik/Symbion	Medtronic/Biomedicus[†]
Penn State*	
Thermedics*[†]	
Thoratec*[†]	Intraventricular
Sarns/3M*[†]	Nimbus*[†]

*IDE required; [†]commercially available; [‡]experimental.

preventing their application clinically for acute myocardial rescue. Thromboembolism remains a major cause of failure in experimental models[35] and synchronization techniques incorporating appropriate counterpulsation delay generators must be developed.

Mechanical Ventricular Assistance

We have discussed mechanical and biomechanical systems that offer limited (3–20%) circulatory or ventricular functional improvement. These devices, particularly the IABP, have been and will continue to be extremely important. These devices provided the early stimulus that encouraged investigators to develop other devices capable of complete circulatory support (Table 29.2). Currently, there are a multitude of devices being developed capable of partial to complete circulatory support. Ventricular assist devices (VADs) supply partial to complete ventricular support. They are designed to assist the failing ventricle, maintain adequate circulatory pressures, and are generally applied heterotopically, leaving the patient's heart intact. The artificial heart, unlike the VADs, is designed to replace the failing heart and is placed orthotopically either as a temporary or permanent device. There are several types of VADs and artificial hearts. Some are powered pneumatically and some electrically. Some are pulsatile systems whereas others, like the centrifugal pump, offer continuous nonpulsatile flow. Currently, there are five VADs available for clinical use (Table 29.3). Three of these devices are solely pneumatically driven, one device is electrically powered, and one device can be pneumatically or electrically activated. Each of these devices has specific limitations and indications. Access to more than one of these devices may be needed so that the most efficient system can be used for each patient.[36] In this section, we will outline the pneumatic and electric VADs, centrifugal pumps, and total artificial hearts currently available and under development.

TABLE 29.3. Pulsatile ventricular assist devices currently available under IDE exemption.

Device power source	Position	SV	Maxium CO	Blood surface
ABIOMED Pneumatic	LVAD/ BVAD	80	5.0	Segmented polyurethane
Novacor Electric	LVAD only	90	9.0	Segmented polyurethane
Pierce-Donachy/ Sarns Pneumatic	LVAD/ BVAD	80	6.5	Segmented polyurethane
Thermedics Pneumatic/ Electric	LVAD only	80	9.0	Segmented polyurethane and sintered titanium
Thoratec Pneumatic	LVAD/ BVAD	80	6.5	Segmented polyurethane

LVAD = left ventricular assist device; BVAD = biventricular assist device; SV = stroke volume (ml); CO = cardiac output (l/min).

Pneumatic Ventricular Assist Devices

The Pierce-Donachy VAD, developed at The Pennsylvania State University in Hershey, Pennsylvania, has seen the widest clinical application as a ventricular assist pump and will be discussed here as the prototypic pneumatic ventricular assist (Fig. 29.3). The Pierce-Donachy device consists of a rigid polysulfone case containing a flexible diaphragm and seam-free blood sac made of segmented polyurethane. To ensure unidirectional flow, mechanical Delrin-tilting disc valves are employed in both inlet and outlet positions. Compressed air pulses are delivered through a clear polyvinyl chloride drive line from an external pneumatic drive unit. Implanted within the rigid case of the pump is a Hall effect switch. This switch is used as a control device to detect complete pump filling. The pump may be run in an automatic "full-to-empty" mode, timed to the R-wave of the electrocardiogram, or at a predetermined manual fixed rate set on the drive unit. Other parameters that can be set on the drive unit are systolic ejection duration, systolic driving pressure, and diastolic vacuum. The drive unit also contains a host of system diagnostic alarms. In clinical use, atrial or ventricular apex cannulation can be employed for device placement. Atrial cannulation is often preferred because it is technically easier and does not always require cardiopulmonary bypass (Fig. 29.4).[37,38] Because of the use of diastolic vacuum to enhance mechanical device filling, a patent foramen ovale must be searched for and closed; otherwise, a significant right-to-left shunt can result in arterial desaturation and death.[39] The outflow

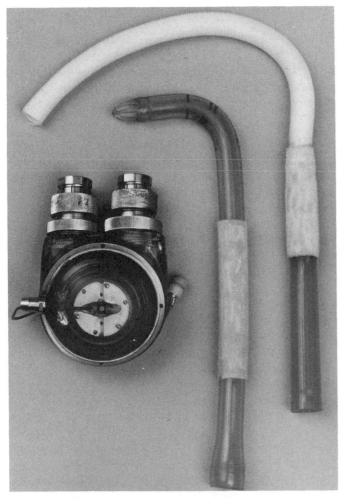

FIGURE 29.3. The Pierce-Donachy VAD developed at The Pennsylvania State University in Hershey, Pennsylvania. The photograph also shows the atrial inflow and composite aortic outflow cannulas.

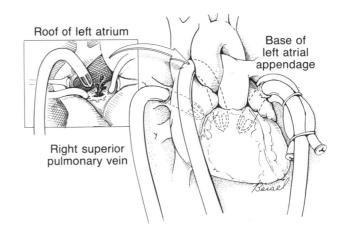

FIGURE 29.4. This figure illustrates the three possible methods of left atrial cannulation for the inlet cannula when using atrial-to-aortic LV assistance. The cannulas may be inserted through the right superior pulmonary vein, base of the left atrial appendage, or roof of the left atrium. Atrial cannulation often can be accomplished without the use of cardiopulmonary bypass.

LEFT POWER LINE EVENTS

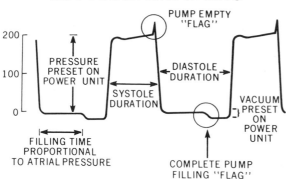

FIGURE 29.5. A pressure transducer mounted on the driveline of a LVAD gives the above idealized tracing. From these pressure tracings, complete pump filling, complete pump emptying, and systolic and diastolic durations can be determined. Changes in this standard trace can help diagnose the presence of inlet and outlet obstructions as well as other pump malfunctions.

cannula, a composite segmented polyurethane-Dacron conduit, is commonly placed in the ascending aortic arch. Both inflow and outflow cannulas exit below the costal margin and the VAD is placed paracorporeally on the abdomen. Drive line pressure tracings are monitored continuously with pressure transducers and can

provide important diagnostic information regarding pump function (Fig. 29.5).

Like many other pneumatic devices, the Pierce-Donachy VAD can be used as a single left or right assist device or as a bilateral VAD (Fig. 29.6). Because of the seamless nonthrombogenic blood sac surface, near complete blood sac washout, and high stear rates across the inlet and outlet valves, thromboembolic events have been relatively uncommon. Consequently, the use of postoperative anticoagulation therapy is controversial and ranges from intravenous low molecular weight dextran or heparin in the early postoperative period after chest tube drainage falls below 50cc/hr for 2 hr to aspirin. In high-risk patients with transmural infarction, warfarin sodium is used if extended ventricular support is required.

The Pierce-Donachy pneumatic assist device has been described in detail here; however, there are other devices as indicated in Table 29.3. Of the pneumatic devices, the Thoratec device is essentially the Pierce-Donachy pneumatic device marketed by Thoratec Laboratories Corp. of Berkley, California. The Symbion acute VAD (Symbion, Salt Lake City, UT) is patterned after the left ventricle of the Jarvik-7 total artificial heart. The Thermedics device has a titanium outer shell, with a flexible polyurethane-bonded blood contacting pusher plate. The other half of the blood-containing surface is a sintered titanium microsphere-

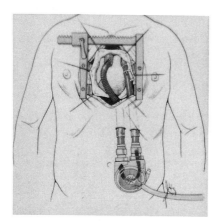
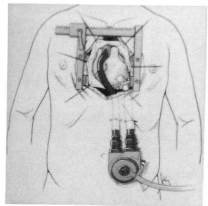
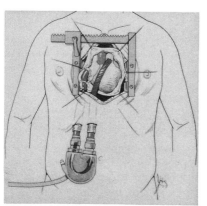
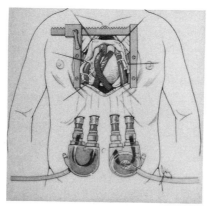

FIGURE 29.6. VADs may be utilized to provide univentricular or biventricular support. This diagram shows the Pierce-Donachy VAD employed as (clockwise from top left) left atrial to aortic LV assist, LV apical to aortic LV assist, right atrial to pulmonary artery right ventricular assist, and biventricular assistance.

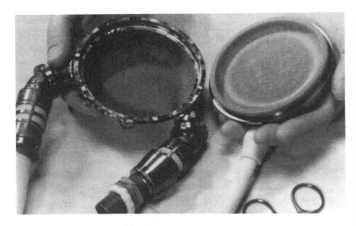

FIGURE 29.7. The Thermedics blood-contacting surfaces: half of the device has a flexible polyurethane diaphragm and the other half a sintered titanium microsphere surface.

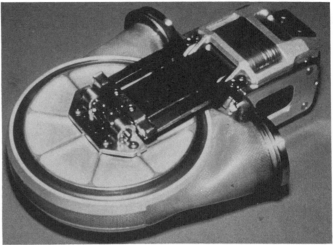

FIGURE 29.9. The NOVACOR electric VAD is a spring-coupled pulsed solenoid that compresses pusher plates together to pump blood. It has been FDA approved for the bridge-to-transplantation application.

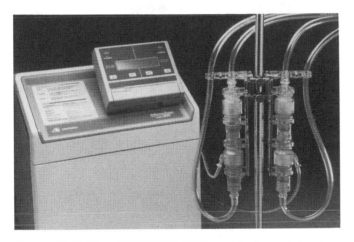

FIGURE 29.8. The ABIOMED 5000 ventricular assist system. This system is designed to be used for univentricular or biventricular pneumatic support.

surfaced inner shell (Fig. 29.7). Inlet and outlet 25-mm porcine valves are housed in a Dacron conduit and titanium cage. The pusher plate blood pump of this device may be electrically or pneumatically activated, depending on the expected length of device application. The ABIOMED Inc. system features a two-chambered assist device with trileaflet polyurethane valves (Fig. 29.8).

Electric Ventricular Assist Devices

The Novacor VAD has FDA approval for use in patients for the bridge-to-transplantation application. The Novacor device consists of a seamless, polyurethane sac that is compressed between two opposing pusher plates. A spring-coupled pulsed-solenoid energy convertor compresses the pusher plates together and pericardial tissue valves provide unidirectional flow through the de-

vice (Fig. 29.9). Because there are just a few moving parts, the system is reliable, durable, and relatively efficient. The pump is currently attached to an external power unit by a transcutaneous electrical lead.[40] However, ultimately this device will have a permanently implantable configuration; implantable electronic controls and batteries will be placed subcutaneously. Power will be transmitted transcutaneously by induction coils from an external power source. The device is implanted preperitoneally, but requires LV apical inlet cannulation. The outlet cannula can be placed in either the ascending or descending thoracic aorta. Right ventricular assist or atrial cannulation cannot be achieved.

An electric VAD is under development at Penn State. This device will be completely implantable with transcutaneous energy transfer through induction coils. Telemetric information exchange similar to current pacemaker technology for monitoring pump function and changing pump parameters will be available. The Penn State electric motor VAD contains a single blood sac housed in a rigid case. A pusher plate actuates the prosthetic ventricle when a low-speed reversing brushless DC motor translates a threaded roller screw mechanism back and forth (Fig. 29.10).

Hemopump

The Hemopump is a nonpulsatile system that is a wire-reinforced flexible indwelling catheter approximately 8 mm in diameter and 26 cm long. The system utilizes a principle similar to that of the helically inclined plane or Archimedes screw. The stainless steel disposable pump head traps and continuously propels blood by a series of spiral vanes that rotate rapidly inside a closely fitting

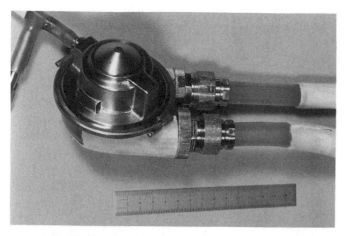

FIGURE 29.10. The Penn State electric motor VAD contains a brushless DC motor that actuates a pusher plate via a roller screw mechanism.

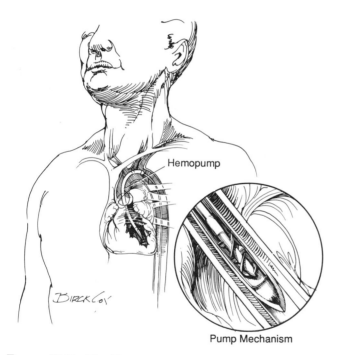

Hemopump

Pump Mechanism

FIGURE 29.11. The Hemopump is positioned high in the descending thoracic aorta, while the inflow cannula traverses the aortic valve into the LV. The cutaway shows the actual pump mechanism.

tube (Fig. 29.11). The screw is propelled by a flexible drive shaft that is magnetically coupled in the motor stator and lubricated with concentrated dextrose (40%) drip during pump use. The Hemopump may be placed either transthoracically or through femoral cannulation. In either application, an arteriotomy is made and a low porosity woven segment of vascular graft is anastomosed to the artery. The pump assembly is then passed through the graft and advanced to position the pump housing in the descending thoracic aorta. The inflow

cannula transverses the aortic arch and passes retrograde through the aortic valve into the LV. The maximum output is approximately 3 L/min. In clinical reports wide variations in plasma-free hemoglobin levels have been noted (mild to excessive hemolysis), whereas measurements of other plasma proteins (i.e., fibrinogen, fibrin split products, etc.), platelets, serum creatinine, and serum blood urea nitrogen have generally shown no adverse changes.[41,42] Several mechanical drive failures necessitating pump removal also have been reported.[42] The pump has had limited use for circulatory support after cardiogenic shock induced by myocardial infarction, or failure to wean from cardiopulmonary bypass. It has been used when short-term support of several days to less than 1 week is anticipated. A continuous heparin infusion is used to maintain clotting times $1\frac{1}{2}$ to 2 times normal.[41]

Roller Pumps

During the earlier stages of the development of mechanical circulatory assistance, the use of roller pumps was much more common. Their simplicity, availability, and low cost made them a logical choice. The disadvantages of these systems are (a) the need for full anticoagulation, (b) constant monitoring by a perfusionist, (c) increased blood and plasma protein trauma, (d) thromboembolism, and (e) tubing spaulation. The new centrifugal and mechanical assist devices have minimized or obviated many of these limitations and, thus, the use of roller pumps for circulatory assistance is diminishing.

Centrifugal Ventricular Assist Pump

Centrifugal pumps have been used for quite some time as temporary VADs in postcardiotomy cardiogenic patients and for extracorporeal blood pumps during cardiopulmonary bypass. Currently, there are two principle devices available: the Biomedicus pump and Sarns Delphin pump.

The Biomedicus pump is currently the most widely used centrifugal pump, and is a "constrained vortex" pump (Fig. 29.12). The nonocclusive pump head contains a series of three concentric cones coupled to a magnetic drive. These cones rotate to provide fluid motive energy through fluid steer stresses. An electromagnetic flow meter confirms forward flow. The Sarns Delphin pump has a similar magnetic drive, but contains a vaned nonocclusive impeller and a Doppler ultrasonic flow meter (Fig. 29.13).

Both pumps must be used with flowmeters on the outflow cannulas to verify flow. These devices are being increasingly employed as extracorporeal blood pumps for open-heart procedures; this makes the device readily available for temporary ventricular assist applica-

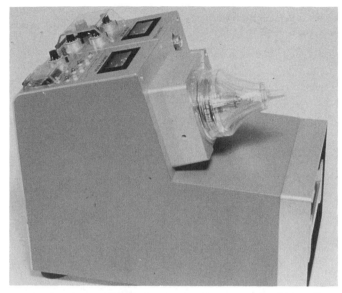

FIGURE 29.12. A "constrained vortex" pump, the Biomedicus centrifugal pump head consists of three rotating nonocclusive cones and the control console.

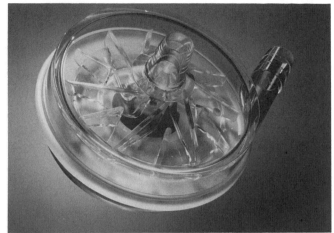

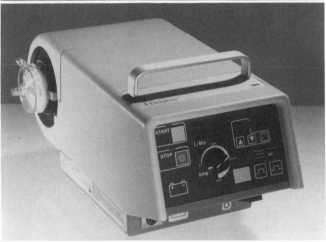

FIGURE 29.13. The Sarns Delphin pump contains a magnetically driven nonocclusive vaned impeller. The pump head and console are pictured separately.

tions. Both pumps have low rates of hemolysis, but require anticoagulation therapy, particularly at low flow rates.[44] An added advantage of this pump over its roller pump predecessors is the inability to produce high pressures in the arterial side of the cardiopulmonary bypass circuit, which could rupture the circuit or cause air embolism.

The Biomedicus pump has been coupled to percutaneously placed cardiopulmonary bypass cannulas, a membrane oxygenator, and heat exchanger to form a circuit for extracorporeal membrane oxygenation (ECMO) applications. Originally, ECMO was designed primarily for pulmonary failure caused by sepsis, trauma, or congenital abnormalities, but recently has been extended to temporary ventricular support in patients with severe cardiogenic shock.[45] Percutaneous cardiopulmonary bypass for resuscitating patients with circulatory collapse after cardiac arrest or coronary artery angioplasty has been successful.[46]

Although there are sporadic reports of prolonged (>30 days) applications of these devices, they are generally employed as temporary circulatory support devices (several days or even hours) after open-cardiac procedures, cardiac arrest, coronary artery angioplasty, or as circulatory support for septic or severely injured patients. These devices also have been used as a short-term bridge to more sophisticated long-term support systems.[47] The principle disadvantages of most of these techniques are (a) the need for anticoagulation, particularly at low flows,[48] (b) a tendency for hemolysis at high flows or with prolonged support,[44] (c) the need for continued surveillance by a cardiopulmonary perfusionist or staff member, and (d) possible damage to plasma proteins with protracted use. Because thrombus formation has been noted near the bearing housing, an area of low shear, low flow, and elevated temperature in both centrifugal pumps, many users recommend routine pump head replacement every 24 to 48 hr.[49]

Artificial Hearts

Several groups have implanted various artificial hearts primarily as devices to support the failing heart as a bridge to transplantation. Only the Symbion Jarvik-7 has been used as a permanent implant device. The two most widely used total artificial hearts, the Symbion and The Penn State University devices, are pneumatically driven. Recently, however, the Symbion device has been removed from the United States market by the FDA. The Penn State device is the only FDA-approved artificial heart and is available solely at The Pennsylvania State University Hospital (Figs. 29.14, 29.15).

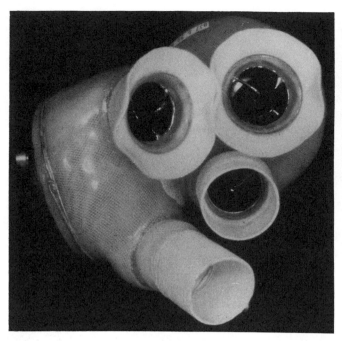

FIGURE 29.14. The Jarvik-7 artificial heart. This model was the same type used as a permanent implant in Dr. Barney Clark. The prosthetic ventricles contain Hall-Medtronic tilting disc valves. This artificial heart is currently unavailable in the United States.

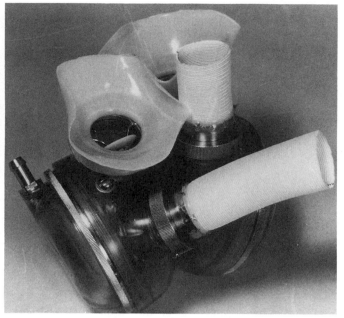

FIGURE 29.15. The Penn State University pneumatic artificial heart. The two rigid polysulfone prosthetic ventricles contain flexible segmented polyurethane blood sacs.

The Penn State Heart

The Penn State total artificial heart is a pneumatically driven device consisting of two separate rigid polysulfone ventricles. Each ventricle contains a non–blood-contacting flexible diaphragm and a compressible, segmented polyurethane blood sac. The diaphragm controls the blood sac emptying and isolates the blood from the driving gas. The pneumatic driver and control systems are in a separate, self-contained console connected to the ventricles by long (3 m) polyvinyl chloride drive lines. Pulses of compressed air actuate the diaphragm and cause emptying of the blood sacs. The filling phase of the blood sacs is either passive or enhanced by low-level vacuum. The ventricular stroke volume is 70 cc; tilting Delrin disc inlet and outlet valves provide unidirection flow. The automatic electronic control is achieved by using a feedback control system that attempts to run the pump in a full-to-empty mode. The LV rate changes automatically to maintain systemic arterial pressure within a predetermined range. This system automatically adjusts for changes in the patient's peripheral vascular resistance and prevents unwanted increases in left atrial pressure, as well as increases or decreases cardiac output based on physiologic demand. The right pump rate changes similarly to maintain left atrial pressure within a preset range. These measurements of arterial and left atrial pressures are derived in-

directly from the pneumatic drivelines, thus eliminating the need for internally implanted transducers.[49]

While the pneumatic total artificial heart has proven useful as a bridge to transplantation, infection, limited mobility, bleeding, and thromboembolic complications have severely limited quality of life and longevity of patients in whom the device has been permanently implanted.[39] Because of these limitations, the National Heart-Lung and Blood Institute has awarded contracts to four groups to develop totally implantable artificial hearts. These groups are (a) The Pennsylvania State University/Sarns 3M, (b) Cleveland Clinic/Nimbus, Inc., (c) Texas Heart Institute/ABIOMED, and (d) University of Utah. The required design specifications are delineated in Table 29.4.[51]

The Cleveland Clinic/Nimbus, Texas Heart Institute/ABIOMED, and University of Utah totally implantable systems are all based on electrohydraulic pumps (Figs. 29.16, 29.17, 29.18). For example, the University of

TABLE 29.4. Design criteria for a totally implantable artificial heart.

Sustain mean arterial pressures—100 mm Hg (peak 150 mm Hg)
Sustain mean pulmonary pressure—25 mm Hg (peak 40 mm Hg)
Maximum Cardiac output—8 L/min
Tether-free operation 5-yr operation
Biocompatible blood surfaces to avoid hemolysis, thrombosis, clots, or emboli
External rechargeable battery reserves of 10–12 hr
Internal battery back-up of 45–60 min
Operate reliably at body temperature without thermal injury

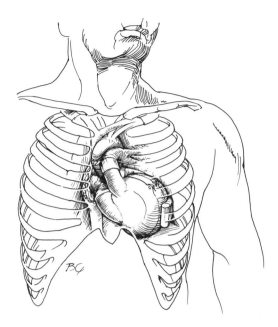

FIGURE 29.16. The E4T electric power artificial heart under development by the Cleveland Clinic and Nimbus, Inc. is pictured here in its orthotopic location. The energy transfer system, compliance chamber, and internal battery systems are not shown.

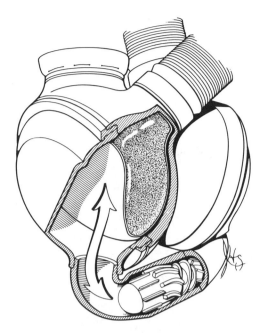

FIGURE 29.18. The proposed design for the electrohydraulic artificial heart currently under development at the University of Utah. Silicone hydraulic fluid is pumped from one ventricle to the other by reversing the direction of axial pump rotation.

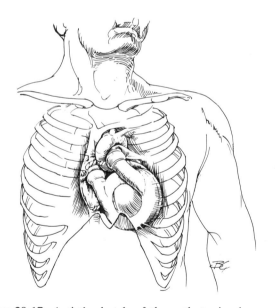

FIGURE 29.17. Artist's sketch of the orthotopic placement of the proposed ABIOMED electrohydraulic artificial heart. Not shown in this diagram would be the transcutaneous energy transfer system and external battery pack.

Utah electric hydraulic pump consists of a modification of the Jarvik-7 pneumatically powered ventricles. In this design, located between the two ventricles is a high-speed, reversing, brushless DC motor coupled to an axial flow pump. The electrohydraulic pump system is filled with silicone hydraulic fluid which is pumped from

one ventricle to the other by reversing the direction of the axial pump rotation. The electrohydraulic silicone fluid is alternately pumped between the ventricles to produce ventricular systole. The Penn State University electric heart uses two pusher plates to compress the blood sac ventricles. A low-speed, reversing, brushless DC motor with a roller screw motion translator moves the pusher plates back and forth, alternately compressing the two ventricles (Fig. 29.19).

It is expected that the energy needs of all these new completely implantable systems will be provided transcutaneously. A primary coil on the surface of the skin will be energized by either house current or a wearable battery pack. The secondary coil, inductively coupled and implanted subcutaneously, will provide the power to the electric motor. Implanted battery packs will allow internal pump function for brief periods of external power interruption. Pacemaker telemetry-like capabilities will allow physicians, engineers, and patients to monitor, alter, and evaluate pump function[52] (Fig. 29.20).

Currently, many of these systems are still under design, fabrication, and in the early stages of animal studies. The longest reported survival with these new pump systems has been achieved at The Penn State University, where the implanted electric heart supported a young Holstein calf for 222 days.[52] With continued progress, most researchers estimate that a totally implantable electric heart will be available for clinical application at the end of the 20th century.

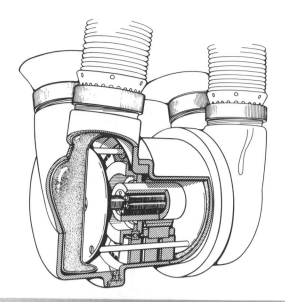

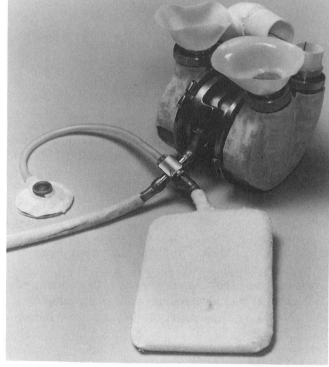

FIGURE 29.19. The electric artificial heart being developed at The Pennsylvania State University. **A:** A brushless DC motor and roller screw mechanism are positioned between the two prosthetic ventricles. **B:** The compliance chamber, percutaneous access port, and transcutaneous electric lines are shown. This heart has been used to replace the heart of a calf for more than 13 months.

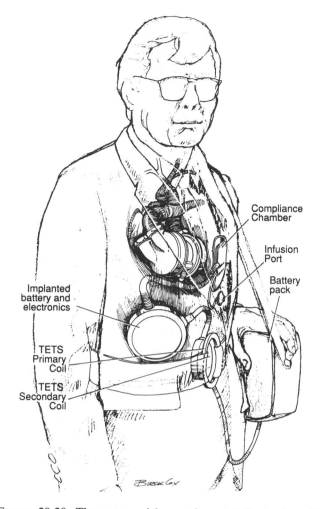

FIGURE 29.20. The proposed layout for a totally implantable electric artificial heart. The artificial heart, compliance chamber, and subcutaneous access port will be located in the thorax. The primary and secondary energy transfer cells will be located subcutaneously, on the abdomen, and will be energized by a portable battery pack.

tion of an artificial heart or ventricular assistance device, (b) "bridging" a patient to heart transplantation, and (c) postcardiotomy cardiogenic shock.[51,52]

Permanent Circulatory Assistance

The number of patients who could benefit from this type of therapy is uncertain. It is known that there is a growing disparity between the number of potential transplant candidates and the number of organs available, and it is anticipated that this gap will only increase. Even this number does not give a clear indication of the number of patients who could benefit from this therapy because it excludes those patients who, for some reason, do not meet the criteria for heart transplantation but could potentially be helped by placement of a permanent artificial heart or VAD. The limitations of this type of therapy (bleeding, infection, thromboem-

Indications for Mechanical Circulatory Assistance

The indications for initiation of mechanical circulatory assistance in a patient with CHF can be broken down into three general categories: (a) permanent implanta-

bolic complications, and immobility caused by the size of current drive systems) have severely constrained the usefulness of this technique in salvaging these critically ill patients. As indicated earlier, however, it is anticipated that within 10 years, a completely contained implantable system will be developed that will eliminate many of these restrictions. These devices will allow greater cardiac outputs, resulting in more potential reserve and will be cost effective in that they may require less intensive medical follow-up when compared to transplanted hearts.

Bridge-to-Transplantation

Currently, one of the major indications for circulatory assist devices is in the bridge-to-transplantation application. Although it is tempting to help these deteriorating patients before instituting mechanical assistance, one must be certain that these patients meet the criteria for heart transplantation. Because donor organs are a tremendously valuable resource, it is important that they be allocated to patients who have realistic hopes of complete recovery. Data to date show that with proper patient selection the results of patients bridged to transplantation compared with nonbridged patients are equivalent.[53,54]

At our institution, the minimum criteria for the institution of mechanical assist as a bridge to transplantation are that the patient must: (a) continually meet all criteria for transplantation (Table 29.5), or if organ failure exists, it must be thought to be reversible or related solely to poor cardiac function (i.e., hepatic dysfunction or renal failure), (b) remain hemodynamically unstable as evidenced by failure to respond to standard medical techniques including volume loading, pharmacological support, and intraaortic balloon counterpulsation, (c) have measured left atrial or pulmonary capillary wedge pressure greater than 25 mm Hg in the absence of mitral valve disease, (d) have systolic arterial pressure of less than 90 mm Hg, and (e) have cardiac output index less than 1.8 L/m²/min.[7,51] If the above criteria are met, then mechanical assistance may be in-

TABLE 29.5. Transplant exclusion criteria.

1. Physiologic age greater than 60 yr
2. Fixed pulmonary hypertension with PSBP > 65 mmHg or PVR > 6 Wood units
3. Severe hepatic or renal dysfunction
4. Active systemic infection
5. Behavior or psychiatric illness likely to interfere with compliance
6. Recent pulmonary infarction or abnormalities
7. Insulin-dependent diabetes mellitus with end-organ damage
8. Severe peripheral or cerebrovascular disease
9. Acute peptic ulcer disease
10. Absence of pyschosocial supports

itiated. Once the device has been placed, the patient is not listed again as a potential transplant patient until he/she meets all the criteria required of an unassisted recipient.[55]

The selection of an artificial heart versus a VAD is determined by many factors. The artificial heart will provide a greater range of cardiac output and replace the failing heart. It requires an appropriate chest diameter, IDE approval, and full systemic anticoagulation. The importance of adequate anteroposterior chest dimension cannot be overemphasized, and fit can be determined accurately by chest computerized tomography. Inadequate sternal-to-spinal dimension may result in caval-atrial compression, vena caval obstruction, and inadequate device filling with the associated complications. The VAD, although it may be limited more in the range of cardiac output and certain types require IDE approval, has minimal size restrictions, it may not always require cardiopulmonary bypass to install, has minimal risk of thromboembolism, and requires less systemic anticoagulation. It is our opinion that most patients can be supported best by single or biventricular assistance and that the artificial heart as a temporary circulatory assist device has a limited role. The results in the bridge-to-transplantation applications are clearly better for patients bridged with VADs versus those bridged with artificial hearts. Furthermore, the results of patients bridged with univentricular support and then transplanted are equal to conventional orthotopic transplantation.

Postcardiotomy Cardiogenic Shock

Despite a surgeon's best efforts at intraoperative myocardial preservation, the occurrence of refractory heart failure after cardiopulmonary bypass surgery remains a major risk factor in cardiac surgery. Patients who develop postcardiotomy cardiogenic shock currently constitute the largest group of candidates requiring mechanical circulatory support. The criteria for instituting such support are similar to those outlined above for bridge-to-transplant patients (see Table 29.6).[10] These patients have generally been unweanable from the cardiopulmonary bypass circuit despite volume loading, maximal pharmacological support, and intraaortic balloon therapy. The use of mechanical assistance is indicated in hopes that ventricular function will recover with initiation of mechanical support and subsequent ventricular unloading. Preservation of right ventricular function is an important predictor of outcome, and if right ventricular function is sufficiently depressed, it may necessitate placement of a right VAD (biventricular support). Right ventricular failure may be masked by poor LV function and become evident only after placement of a LVAD.[56] If right ventricular dysfunction fails to respond to correction of the patient's acidosis

TABLE 29.6. Minimum criteria for implementing mechanical assistance in postcardiotomy cardiogenic shock patients.

Left ventricular failure
1. Hemodynamic instability with failure to respond to volume loading, pharmacological support, and intraoperative balloon counterpulsation
2. Left atrial pressure >25 mm Hg
3. Systolic arterial pressure <90 mm Hg
4. Cardiac output index <1.8 L/min/m²

Right ventricular failure
1. Mean right atrial pressure >20 mm Hg or equal to pulmonary artery pressure in absence of tricuspid disease
2. Cardiac output index <1.8 L/min/m²
3. Left atrial pressure <15 mm Hg

and hypoxemia, to volume loading, to inotropic support, and to pharmacological reduction of pulmonary vascular resistance, biventricular support is indicated. These devices are capable of supporting systemic and pulmonary circulations and in aiding in the reversal of postcardiotomy cardiogenic shock.[10]

The choice of which device to use also may be influenced by the type and reversibility of heart failure, as well as device availability. It has been argued that the mode of operation (synchronous counterpulsatile vs. asynchronous with pulsatility) also is an important consideration. These groups state that synchronous counterpulsation should be used when myocardial injury is suspected and thus potentially reversible, whereas asynchronous pumping should be used with suspected irreversible injury to maximize cardiac output.[57] In our experience with left atrial to aortic assistance, the mode of pumping, synchronous counterpulsatile versus asynchronous, has little effect on myocardial oxygen delivery or consumption. Furthermore, recent evidence would suggest that in the postcardiotomy cardiogenic shock patients, pulsatile VADs and centrifugal nonpulsatile devices yield the same clinical results.[58]

Postoperative Management of Mechanical Assist Patients

Postoperative care of mechanical assist patients is similar to that of the postoperative cardiac patient. Regulation of the mechanical assist device in the full-to-empty mode for VADs and the automatic mode for the total artificial hearts is aimed at maintaining cardiac output index between 2.2 and 3.0 L/min/m². If the cardiac output is maintained at this level, then end-organ failure is preserved and hemolysis can be minimized. For pneumatic assist devices, lower heart rates, longer systolic durations, and reduced peak drive line pressures also result in lower levels of red cell damage.[39] Plasma hemoglobin levels are monitored, and if elevated, are treated with osmotic diuretics (mannitol 25 mg IV) and optimization of urine output (maintenance of urine output >100 cc/hr with diuretics or dopamine). In artificial hearts and VADs, cardiac output is directly related to venous return; our experience would suggest that maintenance of the left and right atrial pressures between 10 and 15 mm Hg provides optimal pump output and pulmonary function.

Asepsis

Postoperative infection after placement of a mechanical assist device is another potential major problem.[39] These patients have multiple infectious risk factors including poor nutrition, multiple transcutaneous lines, prolonged invasive monitoring, multiple surgeries, and prolonged stays in the intensive care unit. This is particularly true in the bridge-to-transplant patient who will be receiving immunosuppressive agents. This risk of infection requires special attention. Transcutaneous drive lines are equipped with velour collars to encourage tissue ingrowth, which secures the drive line and minimizes motion. The collar also provides an additional barrier to bacterial invasion. Tracts between the device and the skin should be made as long as possible. Reverse isolation rooms and daily treatment of percutaneous drive lines with alcohol, Betadine ointment, and a sterile dressing have helped to minimize the infection risk. Mechanical ventilation, invasive monitoring, and central and peripheral intravenous catheters should be discontinued as early as safely possible. When possible, enteral feedings, rather than hyperalimentation, should be instituted. With proper care, the serious infectious complications can be avoided and subsequent immunosuppression with transplantation can be successfully achieved.

Anticoagulation

Hemorrhage and thromboembolic events are of major concern. Hemorrhage in the postoperative period can result from inadequate surgical hemostasis, or more commonly is secondary to a diffuse coagulopathy resulting from hemostatic defects caused by prolonged cardiopulmonary bypass. The risk of hemorrhage is minimized by careful intraoperative hemostasis and by minimizing the cardiopulmonary bypass time. The altered platelet function, thrombocytopenia, decreased plasma proteins, fibrinolysis, and disseminated intravascular coagulation if present must be treated with the appropriate plasma products or pharmacological agents. When mediastinal drainage diminishes to less than 50 cc/hr for 2 hr, low molecular weight Dextran is begun at 20 cc/hr. After several days, an intravenous heparin infusion to maintain activated clotting times greater than 150 s can be employed as a reversible anticoagulant. If there is to be a long period of time between the initiation of mechanical support and transplantation, or if the device is placed as a permanent circulatory support system, warfarin sodium therapy should be initiated.[59] This is particularly true for recipients of artificial hearts, where because of the relatively large amount of prosthetic materials and longer atrial suture lines, risk of thromboembolism is increased.

Results of Mechanical Assistance

The database for the Combined Registry for Mechanical Circulatory Support is maintained at The Milton S. Hershey Medical Center, in Hershey, Pennsylvania. Ninety six centers contributed to the registry results as of December, 1990. A summary of these results is presented here for the bridge-to-transplantation and postcardiotomy cardiogenic shock implantations. It is interesting to note that the number of mechanical assist devices used peaked in 1988 and has declined for the last 2 yr despite an increase in the number of devices available (Table 29.7). This could possibly be related to the removal of the Symbion assist pump and artificial heart from the United States market.

A breakdown of the age versus survival for both groups of patients continues to show that patients over the age of 60 yr have a poorer prognosis than their younger counterparts (Tables 29.8, 29.9). Overall, of the postcardiotomy cardiogenic shock patients, 44.2% were weaned from mechanical support while 68.5% of the bridge-to-transplant patients were transplanted. Survival to hospital discharge also was higher in the bridge-to-transplant patients (66.4%) versus the postcardiotomy cardiogenic shock patients (22.0%).

The period of circulatory support for the various groups has been tabulated in Table 29.10. The longest period of circulatory support was 439 days in a bridge-to-transplant patient, and 40 days for a postcardiotomy cardiogenic shock patient. The duration of support for both classes of patients continues not be a significant predictor of final outcome, although experience indicates that more favorable outcomes seem to be associated with shorter periods of mechanical support.

TABLE 29.7. Number of patients undergoing mechanical assistance for bridge to transplant versus cardiogenic shock.

Year	Bridge to transplant	Postcardiotomy cardiogenic shock
1984	2	45
1985	20	71
1986	78	103
1987	107	129
1988	110	183
1989	90	132
1990	33	79

TABLE 29.8. Age versus survival for postcardiotomy cardiogenic shock.

Age of patients (yr)	No. of patients	Weaned	% Discharged
Under 39	77	34 (44.2%)	17 (22.1%)
40–49	131	58 (44.3%)	38 (29.0%)
50–59	215	108 (50.2%)	53 (24.7%)
60–69	232	94 (40.5%)	46 (19.8%)
Over 70	85	33 (38.8%)	9 (10.6%)
Total	740	327 (44.2%)	163 (22.0%)

TABLE 29.9. Age versus survival for bridge to transplant.

Age of patients (yr)	No. of patients	Transplanted	% Discharged
7–20	34	27 (79.4%)	22 (81.5%)
21–30	56	40 (71.4%)	28 (70.0%)
31–40	79	54 (68.4%)	37 (68.5%)
41–50	148	103 (69.6%)	61 (59.2%)
51–60	112	73 (65.2%)	51 (69.8%)
Over 60	19	10 (52.6%)	5 (50.0%)
Total	448	307 (68.5%)	204 (66.4%)

Table 29.11 shows the lack of any significant difference in outcome as a function of type of VAD for the postcardiotomy cardiogenic shock patients. The absence of any electric VADs in this table indicates a lack of use of this device in this class of patient (no device is currently approved by the FDA). In the bridge-to-

TABLE 29.10. Period of circulatory support (days).

	All patients	Not transplanted or not weaned	Transplanted or weaned	Transplanted or weaned and discharged
Bridge to transplant	18.0 ± 0.1	19.9 ± 4.4	17.3 ± 2.3	15.0 ± 1.7
Range	0–439	0–396	0–439	0–137
Postcardiotomy cardiogenic shock	3.4 ± 0.8	3.1 ± 0.3	4.5 ± 0.2	3.6 ± 0.3
Range	0–40	0–40	0–23	0–20

TABLE 29.11. Outcome of postcardiotomy cardiogenic shock.

	No. of patients	% Weaned	Discharged
Pneumatic	272	117 (43.0%)	57 (21.0%)
Centrifugal	559	254 (45.4%)	143 (25.6%)

TABLE 29.12. Outcome of staged cardiac transplant patients.

	No. of patients	No. of patients transplanted	Transplanted and discharged
Pneumatic	145	108 (74.5%)	86 (79.6%)
Centrifugal	65	44 (67.7%)	27 (61.4%)
Electric	51	31 (60.8%)	28 (90.3%)
TAH	189	135 (71.4%)	67 (49.6%)

TAH = total artificial heart.

TABLE 29.13. Outcome of postcardiotomy cardiogenic shock patients as a function of type of support.

VAD type	No. of patients	No. of patients weaned	Discharged
LVAD	494	254 (51.4%)	137 (27.7%)
RVAD	121	47 (38.8%)	31 (25.6%)
BVAD	350	132 (37.7%)	69 (19.7%)
Total	965	433 (44.9%)	237 (24.6%)

VAD = ventricular assist device; LVAD = left ventricular assist device; RVAD = right ventricular assist device; BVAD = biventricular assist device.

TABLE 29.14. Outcome of staged cardiac transplant patients as a function of type of support.

VAD type	No. of patients	No. of patients transplanted	Transplanted and discharged
LVAD	122	87 (71.3%)	76 (87.4%)
RVAD	4	1 (25.0%)	100 (100%)
BVAD	161	105 (65.2%)	73 (69.5%)
TAH	189	135 (71.4%)	67 (49.6%)
Total	476	328 (68.9%)	217 (66.2%)

VAD = ventricular assist device; LVAD = left ventricular assist device; RVAD = right ventricular assist device; BVAD = biventricular assist device; TAH = total artificial heart.

TABLE 29.15. Incidence of postoperative complications.

	Bridge to transplant (%)	Postcardiotomy cardiogenic shock (%)
Infection	19.4	12.6
Ventricular failure	8.52	23.3
Bleeding	34.7	38.1
Renal failure	19.4	30.6
Respiratory failure	11.8	17.6
Neurological/multisystem	7.2	11.6
Mechanical device failure	2.6	1.5

transplantation data (Table 29.12), the percentage of patients undergoing transplantation is approximately equal, but the percentage of patients transplanted and discharged is significantly poorer for those patients receiving the artificial heart. The results of postcardiotomy cardiogenic shock and the bridge-to-transplantation mechanical assist patients as a function of assist system type are presented in Tables 29.13 and 29.14. In the postcardiotomy cardiogenic shock patients, those requiring only LV support had a better survival (27.7%), whereas those patients receiving biventricular support had a poor prognosis (19.7%). Although this result continues to show a trend, it has not reached statistical significance. For the bridge-to-transplantation patients, survivals of 87.4%, 69.5%, and 49.6% were noted for LV, biventricular, and total artificial heart support, respectively, after transplantation. The difference in survival of ventricular assist group versus artificial heart patients was highly significant. There are not enough right ventricular support patients to make a meaningful conclusion in this category.

Table 29.15 compares the types of complications experienced in these two groups. The fact that many patients had more than one complication emphasizes the critical condition of these patients. The percentage of various complications is higher for the postcardiotomy cardiogenic shock patients in every area, except infection and mechanical failure. At present, the numbers of each type of device utilized are too small to afford any meaningful comparison of individual device function. Bleeding, renal failure, and infection continue to be the leading complications and continue to negatively influence patient survival.[60]

Summary and Conclusions

The future of the surgical therapy for CHF is rapidly being defined. Cardiac transplantation techniques, immunotherapy, and organ preservation techniques are improving, but this mode of therapy will likely remain donor limited. Skeletal muscle powered ventricles and cardiomyoplasty will be capable of augmenting cardiac output 10% to 15%. Although these two techniques have the advantage of using the patient's own skeletal muscle with minimal use of prosthetic materials, their limited augmentation of ventricular function and the considerable time required for skeletal muscle conditioning will limit their clinical application.

Within the next 10 yr, completely implanted permanent ventricular assist and artificial heart devices will become available. These devices will offer circulatory support for a wide range of patients who are not eligible for cardiac transplantation, who may be transplant eligible but require support because of donor unavailability, or require only univentricular support. These devices will be cost effective, becoming affordable for cardiac surgical centers. These systems will eliminate many of the restrictions currently imposed by the devices available today. Transcutaneous energy transfer systems, improved blood contacting surfaces, and use of analogous pacemaker-like monitoring technology will decrease the risk of infection and thromboembolism, while simplifying device control and monitoring. In most cases, univentricular support will be able to support the needs of most patients and has the additional advantage that the native ventricular function is preserved and could possibly support the patient in the case of device malfunction.

These results continue to emphasize the fact that these devices can be used successfully in the bridge-to-transplantation and postcardiotomy cardiogenic shock patient populations. It is important to emphasize that these devices are currently used in patients whose expected mortality would otherwise be 100%. Many researchers believe that if these devices could be applied earlier in these critically ill patients, the multiorgan system injury incurred because of hypoperfusion could be minimized and that with proper patient selection, improved outcomes could be expected. Furthermore, the results show the need for devices capable of short-, intermediate-, and longer term circulatory support. Finally, overall survival will continue to increase as patient selection, patient management, and device design are further refined.

References

1. Gibbon JH Jr. Application of a mechanical heart and lung apparatus to cardiac surgery. *Minn Med*. 1954;37:171–185.
2. Stuckey JH, Newman MN, Dennis C. The use of heart-lung machine in selected cases of acute myocardial infarction. *Surg Forum*. 1957;8:342–344.
3. Spencer FC, Eiseman B, Trinkle JK, Rossi NP. Assisted circulation for cardiac failure following intracardiac surgery with cardiopulmonary bypass. *J Thorac Cardiovasc Surg*. 1965;49:56–73.
4. Akutsu T, Kolff WJ. Permanent substitutes for valves and hearts. *Trans Am Soc Artif Intern Organs*. 1958;4:230–235.
5. Cooley DA, Liotta ID, Hallman GL, Bloodwell RD, Leachman RD, Milam JB. Orthotopic cardiac prosthesis for two-staged cardiac replacement. *Am J Cardiol*. 1969;24:723–730.
6. Griffith BP, Hardesty RL, Kormos RL, et al. Temporary use of the Jarvik-7 total artificial heart before transplantation. *N Engl J Med*. 1987;316:130–134.
7. Quinn RD, Pae WE, Pierce WS. *The Use of Mechanical Circulatory Assistance as a Bridge to Transplantation: The Penn State Experience*. Springer-Verlag of Heidelberg, in press.
8. Pennock JL, Pierce WS, Campbell DB, et al. Mechanical support of the circulation followed by cardiac transplantation. *J Thorac Cardiovasc Surg*. 1986;96:994–1004.
9. Hill JD, Farrar DJ, Hershon JS, et al. Use of prosthetic ventricle as a bridge to cardiac transplantation for postinfarction cardiogenic shock. *N Engl J Med*. 1986;314:626–628.
10. Pierce WS, Parr GVS, Myers JL, Pae WE Jr, Bull AP, Waldhausen JA. Ventricular assist pumping in patients with cardiogenic shock after cardiac operations. *N Engl J Med*. 1981;305:1606–1610.
11. DeVries WC, Anderson JL, Joyce LD, et al. Clinical use of the total artificial heart. *N Engl J Med*. 1984;310:273–278.
12. DeVries WC. The permanent artificial heart: four case reports. *JAMA*. 1988;259:849–859.
13. Harken DE. Presented at the International College of Cardiology Meeting, Brussels, Belgium, 1958.
14. Kantrowitz A, Tjonneland S, Krakauer JS, Phillips SJ, Freed PS, Butner AN. Mechanical assistance in cardiogenic shock: hemodynamic effects. *Arch Surg*. 1968;97:1000–1004.
15. Powell WJ, Daggett WM, Magro AE, et al. Effects of intra-aortic balloon counterpulsation on cardiac performance, oxygen consumption and coronary blood flow in dogs. *Circ Res*. 1970;26:753–764.
16. Buckley MJ, Leinbach RC, Kastor JA, et al. Hemodynamic evaluation of intra-aortic balloon pumping in man. *Circulation*. 1970;41(Suppl II):II130–II134.
17. Rose EA, Marrin CAS, Bregman D, Spotnitz HM. Left ventricular mechanics of counterpulsation and left heart bypass, individually and in combination. *J Thorac Cardiovasc Surg*. 1979;77:127–137.
18. Baron DW, O'Rourke MD. Long-term results of arterial counterpulsation in acute severe cardiac failure complicating myocardial infarction. *Br Heart J*. 1976;38:285–288.
19. Talpins NL, Kripke DC, Goetz RH. Counterpulsation and intra-aortic balloon pumping in cardiogenic shock: circulatory dynamics. *Arch Surg*. 1968;97:991–1000.
20. Bregman D, Casarella WJ. Percutaneous intra-aortic balloon pumping: initial clinical experiences. *Ann Thorac Surg*. 1980;29:153–155.
21. Subramanian VA, Goldstein JE, Sos TA, McCabe JC, Hoover EA, Gay WA. Preliminary clinical experience with percutaneous intra-aortic balloon pumping. *Circulation*. 1980;62(Suppl I):I123–I129.
22. Richenbacher WE, Pierce WS. Management of complications of intra-aortic balloon counterpulsation. In: Waldhausen JA, Orringer MB, eds. *Complications in Cardiothoracic Surgery*. Chicago: Mosby Year Book; 1991:97–102.
23. Pae WE Jr, Pierce WS. Intra-aortic balloon counterpulsa-

tion, ventricular assist pumping and the artificial heart. In: Baue AE, ed. *Glenn's Thoracic and Cardiovascular Surgery*. 5th ed. Norwalk, CT: Appleton & Lange; 1991:1585–1613.

24. Chachques JC, Grandjean PA, Pfeffer TA, et al. Cardiac assistance by atrial or ventricular cardiomyoplasty. *J Heart Transplant*. 1990;May/June 9(3):239–251.

25. Chagas ACP, Moreira LFP, DaLuz PL, et al. Stimulated preconditioned skeletal muscle cardiomyoplasty, an effective means of cardiac assist. *Circulation*. 1989;80(Suppl 3)(3):202–208.

26. Pfeffer MA, Pfeffer JM. Ventricular enlargement and reduced survival after myocardial infarction. *Circulation*. 1987;75(Suppl 4):93–97.

27. Fox RM, Nestico PF, Munley BJ, Hakki AH, Neuman D, Iskandvian AS. Coronary artery cardiomyopathy. Hemodynamic and prognostic implications. *Chest*. 1986;89:352–356.

28. Magovern GJ, Park SB, Kao RL, Christlieb IY, Magovern GJ Jr. Dynamic cardiomyoplasty in patients. *J Heart Transplant*. 1990;May/June 3(1):258–263.

29. Magovern JA, Furnary A, Magovern GJ, Christlieb I, Kao RL. Preliminary results with cardiomyoplasty in the United States. In: Norman JC, ed. *Cardiovascular Science and Technology: Basic and Applied II*. Oxymoron Press; 1990:34–35.

30. Kantrowitz A, McKinnan WMP. The experimental use of the diaphragm as an axillary myocardium. *Surg Forum*. 1959;9:266.

31. Acker MA, Anderson WA, Hammond RL, et al. Skeletal muscle ventricles in circulation—one to eleven weeks' experience. *J Thorac Cardiovasc Surg*. 1987;94(2):163–174.

32. Hammond RL, Bridges CR, DiMeo F, Stephenson LW. Performance of skeletal muscle ventricles: effects of ventricular chamber size. *J Heart Transpl*. 1990;9:252–257.

33. Novoa R, Jacob G, Sakakibura N, et al. Muscle-powered circulatory assist device for diastolic counterpulsator. *Trans Am Soc Artif Organs*. 1989;XXXV:408–411.

34. Neilson IR, Chiu RC-J. Skeletal muscle-powered cardiac assist using an extra-aortic balloon pump. In: Chiu RC-J, ed. *Biomechanical Cardiac Assist: Cardiomyoplasty and Muscle-Powered Devices*. Mt. Kisco, NY: Futura Publishing Company; 1986:141–150.

35. Acker MA, Anderson WA, Hammond RL, et al. Skeletal muscle ventricles in circulation: short-term studies. *J Thorac Cardiovasc Surg*. 1987;94:163–164.

36. Ott RA, Mills TC, Eugene J, Gazzumga AB. Clinical choices for circulatory assist devices. *Trans Soc Artif Intern Organs*. 1990;XXXVI:792–798.

37. Carpentier A, Perier P, Brugger JP, et al. Heterotopic artificial heart as a bridge-to-cardiac transplantation. *Lancet*. 1986;2:97–98.

38. Ganzel BL, Gray LA, Slater AD, Mavroudis C. Surgical techniques for the implantation of heterotopic prosthetic ventricles. *Ann Thorac Surg*. 1989;47:113–120.

39. Richenbacher WE, Pierce WS. Management of complications of mechanical circulatory assistance. In: Waldhausen JA, Orringer MB, eds. *Complications in Cardiothoracic Surgery*. Chicago: Mosby Year Book; 1991:103–113.

40. Portner PM, Oyer PE, Pennington G, et al. Implantable electric left ventricular assist system: bridge-to-transplantation and the future. *Ann Thorac Surg*. 1989; 47:142–150.

41. Frazier OH, Nakatani T, Duncan M, Parnis SM, Fuqua JM. Clinical experience with the Hemopump. *Trans Am Soc Artif Intern Organs*. 1989;XXXV:604–606.

42. Flameng W, Nees U, Sergeant P, Wellens F, Daenen W. Hemolytic complications during left ventricular assist using the hemopump. *J Am Coll Cardiol*. 1991; 17(2):3757A.

43. Rose DM, Laschinger J, Grossi E, Krieger KH, Cunningham JN Jr, Spencer FC. Experimental and clinical result with a simplified left heart assist device for treatment of profound left ventricular dysfunction. *World J Surg*. 1985;9:11–17.

44. Noon GP, Sekula ME, Glueck J, Coleman CL, Feldman L. Comparison of Delphin and Biomedicus pumps. *Trans Am Soc Artif Intern Organs*. 1990;36(3):616–619.

45. Pennington DG, Merjavy JP, Codd JE, Swartz MT, Miller LL, Williams GA. Extracorporeal membrane oxygenation for patients with cardiogenic shock. *Circulation*. 70(3, pt 2):I130–I137.

46. Phillip SJ, Zeft RH, Kongtahworn C, et al. Percutaneous cardiopulmonary bypass: application and indication for use. *Ann Thorac Surg*. 1989;47:121–123.

47. Joyce LD, Kiser JC, Eales F, King RM, Toninato CJ, Hansen J. Experience with the Sarns centrifugal pump as a ventricular assist device. *Trans Am Soc Artif Intern Organs*. 1990;36(3):619–623.

48. Magovern GJ, Park SB, Maher TD. Use of a centrifugal pump without anticoagulants for postoperative left ventricular assist. *World J Surg*. 1985;925–936.

49. Park SB, Liebler GA, Burkholder JA, et al. Mechanical support of the failing heart. *Ann Thorac Surg*. 1986; 42:627–631.

50. Landis DL, Pierce WS, Rosenberg G, Donachy JH, Brighton JA. Long-term in-vivo automatic electronic control of the artificial hearts. *Trans Am Soc Artif Intern Organs*. 1977;23:519–525.

51. Request for Proposal No. NHLBI-HV-86-02. Development of implantable cardiac biventricular assist and replacement devices. 1986;January:LI-6–7.

52. Rosenberg G, Snyder A, Landisu DL, Geselowitz DB, Donachy JH, Pierce WS. An electric motor-driven total artificial heart: seven months survival in the calf. *Trans Am Soc Artif Intern Organs*. 1984;30:69–74.

53. Hill, JD. Bridging to cardiac transplantation. *Ann Thorac Surg*. 1989;47:167–171.

54. Pennington DG, McBridge LR, Swartz MT. Use of the Pierce-Donachy ventricular assist device in patients with cardiogenic shock after cardiac operations. *Ann Thorac Surg*. 1989;47:130–135.

55. Copeland JO, Emery RW, Levinson MM, et al. Selection of patients for cardiac transplantation. *Circulation*. 1987;75:1–9.

56. Pierce WS. Clinical left ventricular bypass. Problems of pump inflow obstruction and right ventricular failure. *ASAIO J*. 1979;2:1–9.

57. Pantalos GM, Marks JD, Riebman JB, et al. Left ven-

tricular oxygen consumption and organ blood flow distribution during pulsatile ventricular assist. *Trans Am Soc Artif Intern Organs*. 1988;34:356–360.

58. Davis PK, Pae WE, Miller CA, Parascandola SA. Reduction of myocardial oxygen consumption during left atrial to aortic bypass: are pulsatility and synchronization important? *Surg Forum*. 1989;210:206.

59. Copeland JB, Harlear LA, Joist JH, Devries WC. Panel 3: bleeding and anticoagulation. From Circulatory Support Symposium of the Society of Thoracic Surgeons, St. Louis, Missouri, February 6–7, 1988. *Ann Thorac Surg*. 1989;47:88–95.

60. Pae WE Jr, Parascandola SA, Miller CA, Pierce WS. Results of mechanical circulatory support as a "bridge" to cardiac transplantation—combined Registry Report. In: Copper DKC, Novitzky D, eds. *The Transplantation and Replacement of Thoracic Organs*. Amsterdam: Kluwer Academic Publishers; 1990:445–452.

30
Dialysis and Hemofiltration for Congestive Heart Failure

Thomas A. Golper

The role for hemofiltration (HF) or dialysis in the management of congestive heart failure (CHF) is not clearly defined. When the patient and physician choose to be aggressive after conservative therapies have failed, hemofiltration or dialysis may be offered.

Earlier sections of this text address the pharmacologic and conservative management of CHF. If conservative therapy has failed, the clinician must ask why. Is it true resistance to therapy at the pathophysiological level or are there potentially correctable reasons for the failure of conservative therapy? For example, nonsteroidal antiinflammatory drugs impair the natriuretic effect of many diuretics and the combination should be avoided. As will be described below, HF or dialysis is associated with complications. Thus, the decision to embark down this pathway should not be made lightly.

History

Although Malinow and Korzon in 1947 first suggested extracorporeal ultrafiltration (UF) as a technique to treat uremia,[1] it was several years later at the Cleveland Clinic that this technique was applied to the removal of intractable edema.[2-4] In the meantime, Schneierson had described the use of peritoneal irrigation to treat intractable CHF.[5] Thus, the concepts of these therapies have been with us for half a century!

In 1974, Silverstein et al. described the use of pump-driven extracorporeal UF to treat volume overload in patients on chronic maintenance hemodialysis (HD).[6] In 1979, Gerhardt et al. applied a similar technique to a patient in cardiogenic shock[7] and by 1988, DiLeo et al. performed this procedure on a semichronic basis in 19 patients with chronic CHF.[8]

Simultaneously, three other techniques were evolving. One was intraoperative HD during cardiopulmonary bypass surgery, which controlled solute removal as well as that of salt and water.[9] Another involved the use of a simple hemofilter cartridge during bypass, utilized solely to control extracellular fluid volumes.[10] No diffusion component was employed. The third technique was the development of continuous arteriovenous (and hence spontaneous) hemofiltration (CAVH) as described originally by Kramer et al. in 1977.[11] This approach appeared to have distinct hemodynamic advantages and rapidly became a cornerstone in the treatment of end-stage CHF.

Principles of Ultrafiltration

When hydrostatic pressure exceeds oncotic pressure, UF (water and non–protein-bound small and middle molecular weight solutes) passes through a semipermeable membrane into the UF space (Fig. 30.1). Macromolecules, almost exclusively proteins, and cellular elements are retained. Oncotic pressure is determined by the concentration of total protein in plasma. Hydrostatic pressure is determined by the blood pressure in the filter, generated by either the patient's endogenous blood pressure or by an extracorporeal blood pump, plus the siphoning effect or suction in the UF compartment where the UF is actively drawn off. The sum of these pressures generates the pressure driving the plasma water through the membrane.

The removal of solute by UF alone is called convective transport. This represents solute following its solvent; that is, solute essentially removed passively by accompanying the solvent flow (Fig. 30.2). This is compared to the removal of solute by dialysis, which is diffusion down a concentration gradient. Small solutes move through membrane pores readily by diffusion or convection, whereas larger molecules can pass through membranes only very slowly by diffusion (Fig. 30.2A). Convection actually helps direct larger molecules through the pores, such that the transport rates for small and large molecules are equal in convective trans-

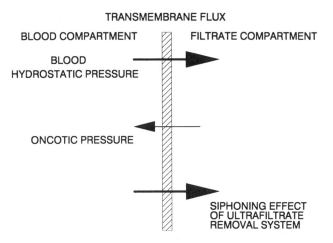

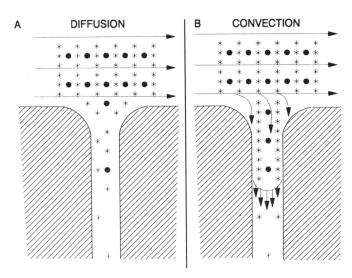

FIGURE 30.1. The relative contributions (magnitude and direction) of the pressures imposed on a hemofiltration system are displayed. Either a blood pump or systemic blood pressure generates blood side hydrostatic pressure, which is directionally opposed by the oncotic pressure of plasma proteins. The siphoning effect of the ultrafiltrate-removing device generates another hydrostatic pressure originating on the filtrate side and is additive to the total transmembrane hydrostatic pressure.

FIGURE 30.2. Diffusion (**A**) and convection (**B**) through membrane pores are diagrammed. Small molecules (*) and larger molecules (●) are shown in differing concentrations. Flows are indicated by the arrows. In A the concentration gradient determines the direction and magnitude of the thermal forces causing diffusion. In panel B mechanical forces cause convective flow of the solvent with its accompanying solutes. Note that there is a slight diffusive effect at the convective flow front within the pore.

port (Fig. 30.2B). In convective transport, the solute concentration in the UF is essentially equal to the solute concentration in the water component of the plasma on the blood side of the membrane. The sieving coefficient is the concentration of the solute in the filtrate divided by the concentration in the blood and reflects the permeability of the solute for that membrane. All membranes contain pores that have molecular size cutoffs such that molecules above that size cannot permeate that membrane even during convection. A sieving coefficient of zero states that the solute is completely rejected at the membrane (e.g., macromolecular proteins), while a sieving coefficient of unity states that the solute readily passes the membrane (e.g., sodium). Since macromolecular proteins often are too large to convect through many clinical UF membranes (except special plasmapheresis membranes), molecules bound to these proteins are also retained.[12] Drugs are the best example of this. Drugs display a sieving coefficient that resembles the fraction of the drug not bound to circulating plasma proteins.[12,13]

Ultrafiltrate can be generated from adjusting the pressures across a membrane by a variety of methods. Increasing systemic blood pressure, lowering resistance in the blood pathway, and inserting a blood pump in front of the filter are techniques of manipulating hydrostatic pressures on the blood side of the membrane. Alternatively, one could generate a suction on the filtrate side (referred to as negative pressure), literally drawing plasma water through the membrane (Fig. 30.1, bottom arrow). In peritoneal dialysis, an osmoti-

cally active substance such as glucose creates hypertonicity on the dialysate side of the membrane. This hypertonicity is the driving force for the UF of plasma water across the peritoneal membrane.

The term ultrafiltration (UF) refers to the technique wherein plasma water is removed by a filtration process as depicted in Fig. 30.3A and B. The plasma water is the dark coffee in the coffeemaker, and the level is high in A. The spigot (the filter device) is opened, filtration

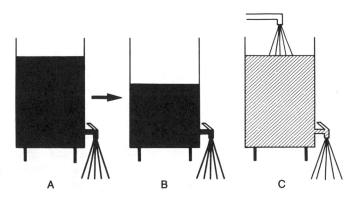

FIGURE 30.3. Coffeemaker analogy to hemofiltration treatment. The dark shading signifies an increase in body fluids. **A** is the initial fluid-overloaded condition. As the spigot is opened going from **A** to **B**, SCUF occurs. **C** represents continuous filtration with replacement of nonuremic fluid, called CAVH (courtesy of Andre A. Kaplan).

occurs, and the level of coffee drops as the plasma water component is removed, as shown in B. This plasma water component, which becomes the UF, has a sodium concentration similar to that of plasma; that is, the sieving coefficient of sodium is unity.[14,15]

The term hemofiltration (HF) generally refers to a blood-cleansing technique depicted in the coffeemaker analogy of Fig. 30.3C, wherein UF occurs, but the UF is replaced with clean fluid, thus diluting the concentration of solute in the remaining coffee. This treatment is a more complete form of renal replacement therapy. In this chapter we refer to UF and HF synonomously, although strictly speaking, they are not.

Clinical Methods in Ultrafiltration

Intermittent Hemodialysis

Background

In the mid- to late 1940's, clinical dialysis was in its infancy. The terminal events in uremia often included coma, asystole, or pulmonary edema. Thus, the treatment of uremia and CHF was to initiate chronic HD on an intermittent basis. In fact, in some patients CHF disappeared.[16] As dialysis programs multiplied, it was not uncommon for patients to present with volume overload as the major indication to initiate chronic dialysis.

Advantages

Intermittent hemodialysis (IHD; usually once to thrice weekly) is the most utilized form of chronic dialysis.[17] Widespread availability and familiarity with the technique are clearly the major advantages for this type of therapy. Further advantages include the possibility that this procedure could be done in the home setting. However, usually end-stage heart patients are not appropriate candidates for home IHD.

Disadvantages

Chronic IHD requires repeated access to the circulation. Generally this involves creation of an arteriovenous fistula with a blood flow from several hundred ml/min up to 2 L/min. This flow requires compensation by an increase in cardiac output. Consequently, the creation of these fistulae were associated with exacerbation or development of CHF in some patients.[18] Therefore, IHD by this approach may not be feasible in patients with end-stage CHF. Recently, the Quinton Permacath system has been developed that will obviate the need for an arteriovenous fistula. This double lumen silicone catheter is surgically placed into the internal jugular vein, is reasonably resistant to infection, and

may provide adequate vascular access for IHD for up to several years.[19]

The other major disadvantage to chronic IHD as a therapy for CHF is that from the hemodynamic standpoint it is the least well tolerated form of dialysis. The reason for this is discussed in depth in the section on Continuous Therapies. IHD is generally performed for 3 to 6 hr once to thrice weekly. Substantial fluid removal in such an acute situation is frequently poorly tolerated in patients with significant myocardial dysfunction.

Expectations

One IHD session can, in most circumstances, lower blood urea nitrogen (BUN) by 50%, remove 100 to 150 mEq of K^+, and remove 3 liters of ultrafiltrate. Obviously, cardiovascular status will determine the tolerance to such a degree of ultrafiltration. To accomplish these goals, the dialysis will require about 4 hr.

Peritoneal Dialysis

In the presence of CHF and/or inadequate renal perfusion, peritoneal dialysis can be a life-saving method for removing fluid and stabilizing hemodynamics. Acute peritoneal dialysis (APD) is the oldest dialysis-type dehydrating procedure and arguably the simplest to perform from a technical standpoint.[20-22] The first drainage and UF can occur within an hour of the decision to undertake APD. Furthermore, the facilities, equipment, and skills required are readily available, in contradistinction to some of the therapies discussed below. Because of these favorable factors, the complication rate is low, especially if the APD is of short duration (i.e., less than 48 hr).[23,24]

APD can be performed on an intermittent basis with repeated puncturing of the peritoneum for catheter placement. The dialysate exchange rate is rapid and the dialysis is fairly aggressive in order to keep the duration of the procedure short, which reduces the rate of complications.

Alternatively, a permanent peritoneal dialysis catheter can be placed and the PD can be performed intermittently or continuously on a chronic basis. In the hospitalized setting, the continuous form is called continuous equilibration peritoneal dialysis (CEPD),[25] whereas in the outpatient setting it is called continuous ambulatory peritoneal dialysis (CAPD). In both CEPD and CAPD, the dialysate exchange rate is slower than in APD. In CEPD usually the patient requires admission and the nursing staff performs the CEPD and in CAPD either the patient or a close family member performs the dialysis at home. Both techniques are simple and lend themselves to the slow and gentle removal of fluid. A reasonably predictable and regular amount of fluid can be removed once the system is functionally operational. Both CAPD and CEPD allow for some liberalization of the severe dietary restriction imposed on these patients. Furthermore, the electrolyte imbalances seen with aggressive diuretic therapy (e.g., hypokalemia, hyponatremia, hypochloremia, metabolic alkalosis) are encountered seldomly during chronic PD.

The osmolality of clinically available peritoneal dialysates ranges from 346 to 485 mOsm/kg, depending on the dextrose concentration. This sugar is the source of the dialysate's hypertonic activity since the electrolyte content of the dialysate generally resembles plasma water. Water diffuses down its concentration gradient from the extracellular fluid spaces, bathing the peritoneal cavity into the hypertonic peritoneal dialysate. This process begins as soon as the dialysate comes into contact with the vascular peritoneal membranes. Thus, UF occurs immediately after initiating PD and before any drainage has occurred.

Because dextrose is absorbed there is a diminished driving force for UF over time.[26–28] In addition to the absorption of dextrose, its concentration is diluted by the incoming UF. Additionally, there is the problem of utilizing the functional surface area of the peritoneal membrane. It takes time to fill the peritoneal cavity such that all the functional surface area is utilized. There is a fairly high and constant ultrafiltration rate (Q_{UF}) for about 2 hr. Thus, any exchanges of less than an hour's duration are taking advantage of this high Q_{UF}. Exchanges more rapid than hourly run the risk of leaving the peritoneal cavity partially empty and can decrease the efficiency of the system.[28]

Advantages/Disadvantages of Peritoneal Dialysis

Table 30.1 summarizes the advantages, disadvantages, and complications of PD. Despite the high rate of complications reported in the 1960s,[23] most clinicians now recognize PD as a very low-risk invasive experience. The types of complications are generally mild in nature and preventable with careful technique and experience (e.g., hypernatremia, hyperglycemia). Peritonitis, abdominal wall infection, and hydrothorax are rare in APD, but occur more frequently in CAPD. In certain circumstances of overhydration, the impaired venous return to the heart due to increased intraabdominal pressure of dialysate may be beneficial.[29] However, a serious complication of PD is respiratory compromise.[30–34] As the abdominal cavity fills with dialysate, the diaphragm elevates, reducing inspiratory capacity. This problem can be minimized by reducing dialysate volumes and increasing the exchange rate. This strategy is discussed in more detail below.

TABLE 30.1. Hemofiltration or dialysis in the management of CHF.

Advantages	Disadvantages	Complications
Peritoneal dialysis		
Technical easy	Unpredictable response	Respiratory compromise
Rapid set-up	Relative contraindications (ileus abdominal drains and prosthesis, adhesions, incisions)	Impaired venous return
Widely available		Hypernatremia
Limited training		Hyperglycemia
Low risk		Peritonitis
	Slow ultrafiltration	Abdominal wall infection
	Mild discomfort	
	Hydrothorax	
Intermittent isolated ultrafiltration		
Dialysis personnel familiarity	Requires technical expertise	Hemorrhage
Hemodynamic stability	Intermittent therapy	Air embolism
Short-duration anticoagulation	Membranes not biocompatible	Hypotension
Venovenous access	All-encompassing	
Slow continuous ultrafiltration		
Hemodynamic stability	Arterial access necessary	Bleeding
Technically easy	Continuous anticoagulation	Volume depletion
Readily available	Mild unpredictability	
Compatible membranes	Staff unfamiliarity	
Continuous venovenous hemofiltration		
Hemodynamic stability	Continuous anticoagulation	Bleeding
Compatible membranes	Extracorporeal blood pump	Air or blood leak
Predictable Q_{UF}	More expertise required	Volume depletion
No arterial access		

CHF = congestive heart failure.

The disadvantages of PD may vary depending on the clinical situation. An abnormal abdomen such as an ileus, drains, prosthetic materials (e.g., vascular graft), adhesions, or recent incisions are relative contraindications to be weighed depending on the availability of alternative therapies, as discussed herein. The discomfort associated with PD is mild and should not be a factor in decision-making. The major disadvantage of PD is that one cannot always predict in whom it may fail. Failure is almost always due to mechanical/technical problems such as the inability to drain properly. Vaamonde et al. reported inadequate drainage in 38% with about a third of those being a serious problem.[23] When the system drains properly, Q_{UF} is almost always adequate to dehydrate patients. Nonetheless, the rate of fluid removal cannot always be predicted accurately even when drainage is satisfactory.

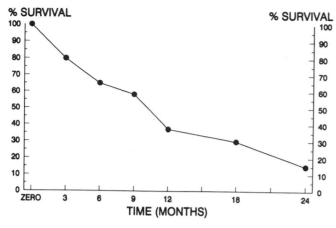

FIGURE 30.4. Survival curve in patients with severe CHF treated by peritoneal dialysis. Data represent a compilation of many studies.[35-45]

Expectations of PD in the Patient with CHF

Since Schneierson's first description of utilizing peritoneal dialysis in the management of intractable CHF,[5] the course of more than 60 patients treated this way has been described.[35-45] Most cases represent patients with New York Heart Association (NYHA) functional class III with renal failure or NYHA functional class IV where diuretics, inotropes, and vasodilators were not adequate. Overall survival by pooling these studies are approximated by Figure 30.4, which reveals a 37% 1-yr and 15% 2-yr survival. Thus, the clinician must evaluate the life expectancy benefits for each particular patient based on these data.

PD will induce physiologic changes whose direction but not magnitude can be predicted. Stablein et al. have shown that systolic BP may drop by 10 mm Hg at 1 month and by 7 mm Hg after 1 yr of CAPD.[46] Diastolic BP changes were 7 and 3 mm Hg, respectively. That CAPD lowers blood pressure (BP) better than HD in many patients is well described.[47] At least part of the mechanism for this may be an impairment in venous return to the heart secondary to the increased intra-abdominal pressure caused by the presence of peritoneal fluid.[29] This may have distinct advantages for patients with severe CHF.

However, other predictable physiologic changes may not be so advantageous. Berlyne et al. first described the pulmonary complications of PD.[34] The alveolar-arterial oxygen gradient is increased in the supine position by the presence of peritoneal dialysate.[30] Functional residual capacity decreases, mean inspiratory pressure rises, and a general pulmonary restriction occurs.[31,33] Furthermore, peritonitis, a fairly common complication of CAPD, exacerbates these pulmonary abnormalities.[31]

PD should directly help patients with CHF by inducing a net fluid loss into the dialysate. Dialysate that contains 1.5% dextrose can induce an average Q_{UF} of up to 5 mL/min. This usually requires a volume of at least 2 liters. A 2-liter 1.5% dextrose exchange over 1 hr will remove an extra 200 ml of fluid. A similar volume and duration exchange of 4.25% dextrose could generate an average Q_{UF} of 12 mL/min resulting in a net loss of greater than 600 mL/hr. The presence of ascites or residual dialysate make an hourly accounting unreliable. These figures should be averaged over 6 to 12 hr. Exchanges of 2.5% dextrose will produce intermediate results.

Technical Aspects of Acute Peritoneal Dialysis

Once the decision has been made to proceed with APD, catheter placement and initial dialysate exchange could be completed in 1 hr. Hence, UF can occur immediately. Trocar or guidewire techniques for PD catheter placement are routinely utilized in most critical care centers. Initial use of 2 liters of 4.25% dextrose dialysate may UF up to 800 mL in the first hour. Use of less hypertonic dialysate or prolongation of the dwell time of the dialysate in the peritoneum will slow the UF rate.

Effective UF requires dialysate in the peritoneum. Time can be wasted with ineffectual drainage. The fluid should flow in as quickly as the gravity feed will allow by raising the height of the feed to as high as practical. The dialysate should not be pumped or forced into the peritoneum. The "drain" time also should be as rapid as possible. Setting an upper limit to "drain" time seems appropriate, but if drainage is "apparently complete" before reaching the time limit, the next exchange should be promptly initiated. "Apparently complete" drainage occurs when the drainage stream changes from a rapid dribble to a slower dribble. If only a fraction of the initial exchange returns and the drainage was rapid even if only for a few minutes, proceed with next exchange immediately. Try draining again after 1 or 2 more liters of additional volume, depending on patient tolerance.

Since aggressive UF is planned in APD, fluid and electrolyte complications are more frequent. Besides frequent weighing and vital sign measurements, check electrolyte and glucose every 6 to 8 hr. Of all the molecules or ions moving by diffusion into the dialysate, water is the fastest and can move more quickly than Na, causing hypernatremia.[48] Hyperglycemia is a consequence of using high dextrose concentration dialysates. Measure dialysate effluent cell counts after the first exchange and twice daily thereafter. If a leukocytosis develops, it may be indicative of peritonitis. Hypokalemia can be prevented by placing appropriate amounts of KCl in the dialysate before inflow.

Permanent PD catheters are placed for CEPD or CAPD. This also can be done at the bedside under local anesthesia.[49] Patient tolerance, physician acceptance, and overall results are excellent with this approach. Since both CEPD and CAPD utilize long dwell times, UF and solute and electrolyte shifts occur more slowly and require less intense monitoring. Unlike APD, CEPD and CAPD are variations of chronic dialysis and generally require nephrologic consultation. Nonetheless, the principles of UF are identical to those described above.

Intermittent Isolated UF

Intermittent isolated UF (IIUF) is a machine-driven extracorporeal dehydrating procedure performed on dialysis equipment except that dialysate is excluded. Thus, the process is pure UF. Blood is pumped through an extracorporeal filter (usually a normal hemodialysis artificial kidney); the UF driving force is generated by the blood pump and supplemented either by suction applied to the UF compartment (negative pressure) or from resistance induced in the venous line (positive pressure). This UF process can occur in the presence or absence of dialysate in the dialysate/UF compartment. When dialysate is present, in addition to fluid and solute removal by UF (convective transport of solute), there also is solute removal by diffusion down the solute's concentration gradient. When diffusion occurs, this process is called hypotonic UF because plasma water is now hypotonic to intracellular water. In the absence of dialysate the UF process is isotonic UF, since intracellular water, plasma water, and UF are all isotonic to each other. Patients tolerate isotonic UF much better than they do hypotonic UF.[6,50–58] This is discussed in-depth in the Advantages/Disadvantages section of Continuous Therapies.

IIUF is effective in removing salt and water in overhydrated patients and in severe CHF.[6–8,59–66] The Na content of UF is equal to that of plasma water.[14,15] Many patients regain responsivity to diuretics after a series of IIUF treatments, suggesting to DiLeo et al. that "significant cardiac functional reserve was available before IIUF treatment that was uncovered and recruited" by the filtration.[8]

Advantages/Disadvantages of IIUF

Table 30.1 summarizes the advantages, disadvantages, and complications associated with IIUF. Hemodynamic stability is discussed in detail in the Advantages/Disadvantages section under Continuous Therapies. HD personnel are quite familiar with this technique.

However, the fact that dialysis personnel and equipment are required is a disadvantage limiting IIUF to certain facilities.

The short duration of therapy in IIUF limits the exposure time to systemic anticoagulation. However, the volume that must be removed in a short time is frequently large. Because of the extracorporeal blood pump, a venovenous access is adequate.

For intensive care unit (ICU)-bound patients, IIUF has the disadvantage of being intermittent, as compared to the continuous therapies discussed below. The requirement for dialysis personnel contributes to scheduling conflicts and can disrupt the continuity of care. In addition, IIUF removes fluid in one limited session per day. Thus, the extracellular fluid space may be filling and emptying in a nonphysiologic manner.

The complications of IIUF are similar to those observed in HD, but without the unique complications associated with diffusion, such as electrolyte disturbances. However, hemorrhage from anticoagulation and extracorporeal pump-related problems (e.g., air embolism) can occur. Trained dialysis personnel are required to avoid these complications.

Expectations

The only limit to Q_{UF} is the patient's hemodynamic tolerance. Tolerance is usually related to the rapidity of fluid removal. Most adult patients will tolerate a Q_{UF} of 500 to 1000 mL/hr.[64,65] During IIUF these rates are technically achievable.

Technical Aspects of IIUF

A double lumen venous dialysis catheter will generate adequate blood flow. The HD personnel connect the vascular access to the blood lines and the HD machine will functions as usual, except that dialysate is absent.

Because patient intolerance is the rate-limiting variable, it seems prudent to avoid any major therapeutic manipulations (e.g., respirator alterations) or diagnostic procedures (e.g., endoscopy) during the few hours that it takes to perform IIUF.

HD personnel or ICU nurses care for the vascular access catheters. The skin exit site must be cleaned and sterilized daily. The lumenae must be flushed (usually with heparin) to maintain their patency. Avoid using the catheters for intravenous infusions, but if absolutely necessary, crystalloids may be infused. If blood or blood products are infused through these catheters, the duration of patency will be severely compromised.

IIUF has been described in more than 100 patients in NYHA class IV CHF who had failed aggressive vasodilator, diuretic, and inotropic therapies.[6-8,59-66] After a few sessions of IIUF, in many patients diuretic responsivity was regained. In addition, ascites, peripheral ede-

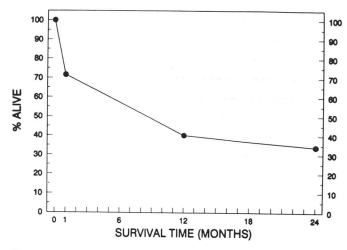

FIGURE 30.5. Survival curve in patients with severe CHF treated by CVVH.[67] Median survival is 10 months. These data represent a single center's experience with 35 patients.

ma, and respiratory compromise improve dramatically. Serum sodium normalizes while renal function (e.g., BUN, serum creatinine concentration) is unchanged. As expected, plasma volume falls and plasma oncotic pressure rises.[62] This increase in plasma oncotic pressure induces the recruitment of cell water into the extracellular space and restores the circulating volume (see below Continuous Therapies, Advantages/Disadvantages). The descriptions of the hemodynamic responses to IIUF in these patients is relatively consistent and is similar to those of chronic dialysis patients undergoing IIUF.[53–56] Most reports note that heart rate does not change and that blood pressure or systemic vascular resistance does not fall if the Q_{UF} is limited to 500 to 1000 mL/hr.[61,64–67] Cardiac output either rises[7] or is stable.[61,64,65] Pulmonary capillary wedge pressure is unchanged.[61] Right atrial pressure falls,[64,65] as does pulmonary vascular resistance.[62–64] Canaud et al. described an improved ejection fraction and a fall in the cardiothoracic index on x ray.[67] L'Abbate et al. pooled the results of several studies and concluded that of 86 patients receiving IIUF for CHF, 23 died within 2 months.[65] In the largest single-center series of Canaud et al., utilizing continuous UF in severe CHF, the survival plot is displayed in Figure 30.5.[67]

The Continuous Therapies

In 1960 Scribner et al. first suggested the use of continuous dialysis without the use of extracorporeal blood pumps.[68] Despite their pioneering efforts, the technology was simply not available for the successful performance of this treatment.

Since the mid-1960s, Henderson et al. had been studying the use of hemodiafiltration with membranes more porous than the usual HD membranes in the treatment of uremia.[69] Although their efforts were directed toward chronic intermittent HF, they were the first to suggest that this new technology also might be applied to acute circulatory congestion.[6] In 1977, Kramer et al. first applied a modification of the HF technique to anuric ICU patients.[11,70]

The simple system devised by Kramer et al. avoids the use of external blood pumps (Fig. 30.6). Using a large-bore catheter inserted into the femoral artery and the patient's own blood pressure, arterial blood is delivered to a hemofilter. Systemic blood pressure provides the driving force to achieve sufficient blood flow across the filter for UF. When hydrostatic pressure exceeds oncotic pressure, UF passes through the membrane of the filter (Fig. 30.1). UF drains by gravity through tubing into a collection bag, creating mild negative pressure in the blood chamber of the filter, further favoring UF. Since the blood cells and proteins remain in the blood chamber and are returned to the femoral vein, the filter allows efficient removal of plasma water and dissolved solutes from the vascular space while conserving blood cells and large plasma proteins.

CAVH as described by Kramer et al. was designed as a renal replacement therapy. Large volumes of uremic UF are removed and clean, nonuremic plasma water replacement solution is administered in volumes determined by the desired net fluid gains or losses. When the replacement fluid volumes are large, biochemical and clinical manifestations of uremia can be adequately controlled (Fig. 30.3C). Paganini and Nakamoto modified this procedure to remove excess fluid in the setting of diuretic-unresponsive oliguria with or without uremia.[71] During slow continuous ultrafiltration (SCUF) (Fig. 30.3B), replacement volumes are lower than with CAVH (Fig. 30.3C). The most recent advancement in this area has been the return to the use of extracorporeal blood pumps.[67,72–74] This has the major advantage of increasing blood flow to the extracorporeal device as well as obviating the need for an arteriovenous pressure gradient, allowing venovenous vascular access. Thus, arterial cannulation is avoided. This therapy is called continuous venovenous hemofiltration (CVVH).

SCUF and CVVH are ideally suited to hemodynamically unstable patients for whom PD and IIUF cannot be offered or successfully performed. Usually respiratory and abdominal status are the factors allowing PD, while hemodynamic stability (blood pressure and tolerance of rapid fluid/volume shifts) dictates the patient's acceptance of IIUF. Thus, the continuous therapies CVVH and SCUF become the recommended therapies for more critically ill hypotensive patients with CHF.

FIGURE 30.6. SCUF or CAVH using femoral artery and vein access.

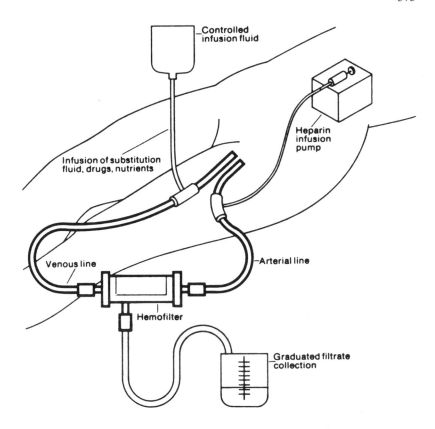

Advantages/Disadvantages

Table 30.1 lists the advantages and disadvantages of CVVH and SCUF. Technically, CVVH requires an extracorporeal blood pump and the problems inherent to it, namely, the concern that air can be pumped into a patient and that blood can be pumped out and not returned. Spontaneously driven systems like SCUF will not be vulnerable to air problems and exsanguination is limited by arterial blood flow and pressure. While the use of an extracorporeal blood pump requires more nursing expertise, the advantage gained by a constant Q_B and Q_{UF} is substantial. All continuous therapies require continuous anticoagulation, either through the endogenous disease process or by exogenous medications (see below under Technical Aspects). Volume depletion should be avoided by careful clinical management.

The avoidance of the arterial puncture is an attractive alternative. Thus, the final decision is an arterial puncture versus an extracorporeal pump. No prospective studies have compared these approaches. Kramer et al.'s initial work describing arterial punctures and catheters[75,76] and the subsequent observations of Olbricht et al. suggest that the complication rate is indeed acceptable.[77,78] There are no documented complications from the use of the extracorporeal blood pump.

The hemodynamic stability noted with isotonic UF is still not completely understood. The clinical observa-

tions of Paganini et al.[79] that severely ill patients tolerate CAVH better than HD have been corroborated by many investigators.[10,15,70,80–83] Bergstrom and associates,[52] supporting earlier work of Ing et al.,[51] noted that in patients hypotensive on HD, IIUF provided hemodynamic stability despite removal of large amounts of fluid. They attributed this to the fact that osmolarity did not change during UF. As plasma water was removed by UF, it was replaced rapidly by interstitial and cellular water. Several recent observations during HD have confirmed the importance of osmolar changes as a major causative factor in the hypotension associated with HD.[84–87] In patients studied at separate sessions with each procedure, HF, unlike HD, was characterized by either maintenance of or increases in systemic vascular resistance, leading to preservation of arterial blood pressure.[54–56] Furthermore, there appears to be autonomic dysfunction in these patients undergoing HD that is not manifested during HF.[54,55,57] Venous as well as arterial vasoconstriction helps to support cardiovascular stability during HF.[56,58] Teo et al. also speculate that convective transport removes a circulating myocardial depressant that is not removed by dialysis.[88] This speculation is discussed further below.

Recent reviews have discussed the important etiologic factors in dialysis-induced hypotension.[89–91] The major mechanism that differentiates filtration from diffusion dialysis is that the latter removes solute osmoles preferentially from the vascular space and extracellular

TABLE 30.2. Determinants of ultrafiltration rate.

Hydrostatic pressure (blood pressure, blood flow, blood access,
    ultrafiltrate column height, ultrafiltrate suction, venous clamping
    with an extracorporeal blood pump)
Oncotic pressure
Viscosity (hematocrit, protein concentration)
Length and width of blood lines and access
Filter surface area, geometry, resistance, and intrinsic membrane
    properties
Filter, lines, and access blood pathway patency

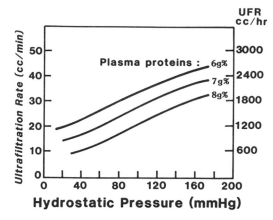

FIGURE 30.7. The effect of hydrostatic pressure and protein concentration on Q_{UF}. Modified with permission from Lauer et al.[80]

fluid. This leaves cells hypertonic to extracellular fluid, which in turn results in water movement from extracellular fluid into cells. Since dialysis also results in fluid removal across the dialyzer, extracellular fluid volume depletion and hypotension may result. In filtration, the osmolality of cells and extracellular fluid stays equal (isotonic UF). As extracellular water and solutes are removed by the filter, cellular fluids and solutes quickly replenish the extracellular fluid space.[88,92,93] The basis for maintenance of cardiovascular stability during HF relates to many factors, including minimal osmolar shifts, appropriate neurohumoral sympathetic responses, and rapid redistribution of volume. These same responses observed during HF in patients maintained on chronic HD are relevant to patients with CHF receiving CVVH, CAVH, or SCUF.[8,52–67,70–75,79–83]

Expectations

Q_{UF} depends on a variety of issues discussed below in Technical Aspects (Table 30.2). When SCUF is technically successful, Q_{UF} can vary from 0 to 20 mL/min with a practical goal of about 5 mL/min. The clinical urgency will dictate the Q_{UF}, which can be altered easily. For CVVH a Q_{UF} of 40 mL/min is readily achievable. It is important to remember that these therapies are continuous (i.e., they are functioning every minute of the day). Thus, the relatively low Q_{UF} (compared to IIUF) occurs for 24 hr, resulting in significant dehydration.

Technical Aspects of SCUF

For UF to occur there must be a transmembrane pressure (TMP) gradient from blood to the UF compartment such that plasma water is ultrafiltered (Table 30.2). The major determinants of TMP are the hydrostatic pressure of blood (induced by the systemic blood pressure or secondary to an extracorporeal blood pump), the (negative) hydrostatic pressure in the UF compartment (induced by the gravity siphon effect of the filtrate line or by a vacuum suction device), and the plasma oncotic pressure[94] (Fig. 30.1). As plasma water is ultrafiltered, blood hemoconcentrates as it passes from filter inlet to

outlet. The protein concentration rises as blood cells and proteins are retained as blood transits through the device. Thus, plasma oncotic pressure rises toward the distal end of the filter. This creates an antifiltration environment and also contributes to increased resistance (through increased viscosity) and a higher probability of filter clotting (through protein concentration and hyperviscosity). High concentrations of plasma proteins decrease ultrafiltration for the same reason, as shown in Figure 30.7. We have demonstrated that during CAVH or SCUF, the hydrostatic pressure in the blood compartment is roughly equaled by the opposing oncotic pressure.[94] Thus, the net TMP was essentially that generated by the UF compartment's siphon or vacuum suction effect. The TMP generated by the column of UF is equal to the height of the column (vertical distance from filter to UF collector) in centimeters times 0.74 mm Hg per cm of H_2O. Thus, a 40-cm column will generate a TMP of 40 cm $H_2O \times 0.74$ mm Hg/cm $H_2O = 29.6$ mm Hg. Vacuum suction can be achieved by a HD machine, portable vacuum machine, or wall suction. In these circumstances the gauges on the devices are generally accurate to within 10%.[94]

In the absence of an extracorporeal blood pump, the vascular access must guarantee an adequate arteriovenous gradient. This means the catheters must transmit the arterial pressure to the filter with minimal pressure loss to the resistance of the access itself. Large-bore percutaneous catheters require technical skills at placement.[76–78] Kramer et al.[75] designed a special catheter for CAVH that meets the requirements specified above (Vygon, Aachen FRG) and described favorable results with its use. Others have reported similar positive experiences.[78]

In vitro there is a direct relationship between pressure and flows at a given catheter length and diameter.[80,95,96] The same relationship does not always

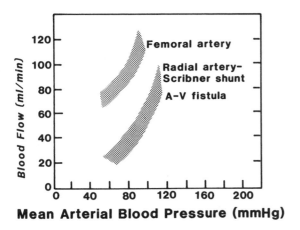

FIGURE 30.8. The effect of mean arterial pressure on Q_B. The upper shaded area represents femoral artery access; the lower shaded area represents arm vascular access. For each shaded area, the upper portions represent larger bore catheters. Modified, with permission, from Lauer A, et al.[80]

operate in vivo where the blood flows in the circuit are partially limited by the resistances of the extracorporeal circuit components.[95,96] This is shown in Figure 30.8. The upper shaded area represents the flow/pressure relationship when the femoral artery is the access site. The larger the catheter in the same blood vessel, the greater the flows at the same pressure (see below, Hagen-Poiseuille law). The lower shaded area represents the flow/pressure relationship in upper extremity accesses, the flow being better from a cannula than from a subcutaneous fistula. Ronco et al.[96] stress that since the filter itself is the major resistance in the extracorporeal circuit, the smaller catheter lumen (2 mm) does not jeopardize performance, but enhances safety. A short access of 13 gauge or larger appears to be adequate.

External shunts (e.g., Quinton-Scribner) require surgical placement and distal ligation of the artery. Furthermore, the blood flows generated by the shunts are inferior to the flows generated by the percutaneous catheters.[77,80,97] Nonetheless, in many cases adequate CAVH may be performed using this form of access. Most clinicians prefer the percutaneous access as the first choice. The external shunts may be preferable under certain circumstances, such as severe femoral vascular atherosclerosis, the presence of prosthetic femoral vascular material, the desire to maintain leg mobility, and in those situations where the hemorrhagic risk of a blind arterial puncture is unacceptable.[78]

In comparing these two modes of vascular access, the long-term complication rates (predominantly thrombosis) are equal.[78] At a given blood pressure, filtration rates are higher with the large-bore catheters because more of the arterial pressure is transmitted to the

filter[80] (Fig. 30.8). The clinician must weigh all these arguments in deciding the appropriate access for an individual patient.

There are multiple resistances in the extracorporeal circuit of CAVH including the vascular accesses, the blood lines, and the filters themselves. Pallone and Peterson have quantified these resistances.[98] The relative resistances were highest in the filter compared to the lines and vascular accesses. Nonetheless, the resistances along the entire extracorporeal circuit are additive and no component should be ignored. An approach to reduction of resistance is to alter the shape of the blood pathway. Specifically, shortening the length and increasing the radius as per the Hagen-Poiseuille law will reduce resistances in each component of the circuit.[99] This principle is exploited by various manufacturers to develop the ideal filter. Blood flow resistance usually is low with parallel plate design.[100]

Technical Aspects of CVVH

During CVVH, blood flow is guaranteed by the extracorporeal blood pump. Because of the continuous nature of CVVH, compared to IIUF, a much lower blood flow is satisfactory. Blood flow of 100 to 150 mL/min results in sufficient Q_{UF} to accomplish the immediate clinical goals. Rarely is a vacuum suction needed because there is adequate net TMP generated solely from the extracorporeal blood pump. Again because of the blood pump, the nature of the access and blood lines are less important than in SCUF. It seems sensible, however, to recommend short, wide lines whenever possible. The venovenous access could be traditional Shaldon-type dialysis catheters or double lumen catheters, which can be placed in the internal jugular, subclavian, or femoral veins.

The extracorporeal blood pump system includes a roller pump, arterial pressure sensor, air detector, and venous pressure alarms. Use of this equipment requires instruction from trained HD personnel, but many ICU nurses have become comfortable with the system.

Q_{UF} can be controlled directly by a pump on the UF line or indirectly by altering blood flow. Alternatively, venous pressure can be raised by placing a screw clamp on the venous blood line or negative pressure can be applied by vacuum suction to the UF compartment.

Anticoagulation

To ensure filter patency, blood coagulation in the extracorporeal circuit must be prevented. Under certain circumstances continuous HF can be performed without exogenous anticoagulants.[15,101] However, most of the time some form of extracorporeal anticoagulation is required. Adequate extracorporeal anticoagulation can be achieved by the infusion of heparin at 10 IU/kg/hr into the arterial blood line without significant adverse effects on systemic circulation.[102,103] However, with this same regimen in high-risk patients, Kaplan et al.[15] noted bleeding in 6 of 15 patients. Adjusting the heparin dose to achieve a 50% increase in whole blood PTT, Olbricht et al.[104] observed a 20% bleeding rate.

No set heparin dosing regimen will be universally successful. In nonuremic humans, heparin half-life varies from 45 min to 4 hr and does not correlate with weight, surface area, clotting time, or heparin dose.[105] Furthermore, as heparin doses are increased, heparin half-life may become prolonged.[106] Thus, there is great intrapatient and interpatient variability.

A loading bolus of heparin at 20 IU/kg should be administered intravenously about 2 to 3 min before allowing blood to pass into the filter. Doses for this bolus may vary depending on the clinical condition. Kramer's approach was to start with a maintenance dose of 10 IU/kg/hr and to follow the partial thromboplastin time (PTT) in both the extracorporeal circuit and the systemic circulation.[75] His goal was to keep the PTT about 90 s in the extracorporeal circuit and about 45 s in the systemic circulation. Ossenkopple and associates tried to keep the peripheral venous PTT 20 to 30 s over control.[107] At heparin infusion rates of 500 IU/h, Kramer's group had to change clotted filters at least once per day, whereas at 1,000 IU/h, very little clotting occurred.[70] With thrombocytopenia the heparin requirements will decrease.[15]

If there is clinical evidence of hemorrhage or the patient is at a high risk for bleeding, the heparin infusion rate should be reduced despite the risk of clotting the filter. In general, filter clotting is a gradual process. Should filter clotting become accelerated, one must move expeditiously to remove or replace the device to prevent extension of the clot into the blood lines or vascular accesses.

Alternative protocols for anticoagulation in CVVH and SCUF have been considered. One such alternative is the use of prostacyclin, but hypotension and other side effects were observed with the early derivatives.[108–110] Although subsequent compounds have less tendency for these adverse effects,[111] the lack of bedside monitoring for prostacyclin effect probably will preclude its use. Furthermore, the antiplatelet effect of prostacyclin is still present 2 hr after cessation of therapy,[108,109] with no known method of rapid reversal (except for platelet transfusion).

Citrate anticoagulation appears to be a reasonable alternative to heparin during conventional diffusion dialysis, where the citrate-calcium complex is removed during transit through the dialyzer.[112–114] In procedures without concurrent diffusive solute removal, citrate anticoagulation is considered experimental.[115]

Kaplan and Petrillo[116] described their results using regional heparinization during CAVH. They infused 1 mg/hr of protamine into the venous limb of the extracorporeal circuit for each 100 IU/hr of heparin administered into the arterial sleeve. Doses were adjusted to maintain the extracorporeal circuit's PTT above 150 s and the venous return blood PTT about 50 to 60 s. Complete neutralization of heparin could cause clotting in the venous access. Bronchospasm and rebound heparin effect were not noted. This was attributed to the slow infusion or protamine[117] as well as to avoidance of the build-up of unneutralized heparin.[118] This technique of regional heparinization allowed tight control of the patient's coagulation status but did not extend average filter patency.

The role of low molecular weight heparin is still undefined. It has been used in two treatments with positive results.[103,119] The variability in heparin kinetics will still be a problem with low molecular weight heparin. Schurek and Biela[120] have suggested that more adequate mixing of heparin in the arterial line may lead to a lower total dose and better local anticoagulation effect. In particular, they recommended infusing the heparin very early in the arterial circuit. There is greater radial dispersion of heparin into the blood at the arterial end of the filter when the filter is mounted with the venous end upright. A related approach is to dilute the heparin more than usual to encourage better mixing with the blood in the arterial line. In our program the heparin concentration has been reduced from 25 to 5 IU/mL. The total heparin dose is adjusted as before except that it is delivered in a more dilute saline solution.

Much of the above holds true for CVVH. The constancy of Q_B during CVVH and the higher rate of Q_B can lead to greater hemoconcentration and greater clotting risk. However, the increased Q_B also leads to less stasis of blood and this may decrease the clotting risk.

Trouble-Shooting in SCUF

It is important to observe the first few minutes of SCUF or CAVH. The initial heparin effect assures that fiber clotting has not yet occurred. If the Q_{UF} is greater than 10 mL/min, things are going well. Between 5 and 10 mL/min, it's probably going well. If the initial Q_{UF} is <5 mL/min, there are problems that must be addressed. The initial steps are listed in Table 30.3 and include a quick scan of the lines to exclude occlusion, kinking, or leaking, checking the patient's blood pressure, and noting the vertical distance between the filter and UF collector. Filter clotting is unlikely in the first few moments after initiation, so hemoconcentration is the remaining issue to evaluate. With Q_{UF} less than 5 mL/min (or <10 mL/min with systolic blood pressure >90 mm Hg), it is reasonable to evaluate the filtration fraction (Q_{UF}/plasma flow). To do that one calculates the

TABLE 30.3. Trouble shooting for decreased Q_{UF}.

Kinked lines
Fall in blood pressure
Leak
Decreased colume height (siphon effect, negative pressure)
Plasma hemo (proto) concentration
Filter clotting

plasma flow from the blood flow by the following formula[121]:

$$\text{Filtration fraction} = [1 - (Hct_{in}/Hct_{out})]/(1 - Hct_{in}),$$

where Hct_{in} and Hct_{out} refer to the Hcts in the inlet and outlet lines, respectively.

If the filtration fraction is greater than 20%, the system is working reasonably well. A filtration fraction of 35% to 40% is maximally efficient.[80] The higher the filtration fraction, the greater the risk for fiber clotting, especially when arterial protein and hematocrit concentrations are normal. This is an ideal situation to apply predilutional mode replacement fluid, namely, when the Q_{UF} is low despite a high filtration fraction. If the filtration fraction is less then 20%, the transmembrane pressure gradient favoring ultrafiltration is deficient. This could occur because the blood lines are consuming the hydrostatic pressure, the blood pressure is low, or because of inadequate negative pressure in the UF compartment. The vertical distance between filter and UF collector should be maximized, but technical limits to this approach arise. At this point, suction-assisted UF may be reasonable, as described by Kaplan et al.[122] The UF line is air seal–connected to wall suction, and gradually the suction pressure is raised to bring the Q_{UF} up to a desirable rate. Wall suction above 200 mm Hg is not recommended. The disadvantage of this approach is that the internal control to Q_{UF}, namely, blood pressure, is negated since UF will continue because of the suction. Under certain circumstances this may be a benefit. A blood leak into the UF compartment can occur, and if suction is being applied, significant blood loss may result. Routinely, no blood detection alarms are present in this system. Therefore, frequent evaluation by the ICU nurse will be necessary.

Filter clotting will decrease Q_{UF}, but this is rarely observed immediately after initiation. A later decline in Q_{UF} is the major indicator of clotting. One should go through the steps outlined above, and if clotting is suspected, one could attempt a rapid 50-mL flush of saline through the arterial sleeve (with the arterial blood line briefly occluded proximally) to observe the condition of the filter itself. Clots will appear as streaks along the filter fibers. If significant clotting has occurred to the point of limiting Q_{UF}, the filter and tubing must be changed.

Hemofiltration and the Heart in Other Settings

The UF techniques described above have been utilized to prolong survival in end-stage CHF and on occasion have served as a bridge to valve replacement surgery or transplantation.[8,67] Darup et al. were the first to describe performing hemofiltration during extracorporeal circulation.[10] Magilligan has detailed the rationale and indications for the peri- and intraoperative use of HF in the cardiac surgery patient.[123] Paganini et al. successfully utilized CAVH during intraaortic balloon pumping and/or left ventricular assist device support.[124] Coraim et al. utilized CAVH postoperatively and described improved cardiac hemodynamics, ascribing this effect to the convective removal of myocardial depressant substances.[125]

The characterization of myocardial depressant substances, especially in septic shock, is progressing.[126–128] Tumor necrosis factor (TNF) alpha is a macrophage-derived peptide cytokine that produces hemodynamic changes similar to those seen in sepsis and endotoxemia[129,130] and may be a myocardial depressant factor. In fact, patients with severe chronic heart failure[131] and after myocardial infarction[132] have elevated levels of circulating TNF.

We and others have shown that under favorable circumstances, TNF can be removed convectively (by UF).[133,134] Should TNF ultimately be one of the illusive myocardial depressants and if UF helps decrease circulating levels, this may explain the speculations of Teo et al.[88] and Coraim et al.[125] that cardiac hemodynamics are favorably altered because of the removal of some substance by UF procedures. This is an area that is receiving intense scrutiny at this time. Gomez et al. have described a septic dog model wherein left ventricular dysfunction was improved by the HF removal of a depressant substance of less than 30,000 daltons.[135]

Conclusion/Summary

CHF also may impair renal function such that correction of overhydration becomes problematic. Pharmacologic management with diuretics, inotropes, and vasoactive agents is the first step. Depending on the abdominal and respiratory status, peritoneal dialysis may be attempted as the next step. If the patient can hemodynamically tolerate IIUF (average Q_{UF} of 4–6 liters over 4–6 hr) and the technique is available, then it is the next step. If not available or if not tolerated, then either SCUF or CVVH is appropriate. CVVH requires a blood pump but avoids the arterial puncture required by SCUF. The continuous therapies seem ideally suited for unstable patients. Their only drawback is the necessity of continuous anticoagulation. Under certain circumstances this can be minimized. IIUF, SCUF, and CAPD have been shown to prolong survival and may serve as a bridge to cardiac transplantation in end-stage cardiac failure.

References

1. Malinow MR, Korzon W. An experimental method for obtaining an ultrafiltrate of the blood. *J Lab Clin Med.* 1947;32:461–471.
2. Skeggs LT, Leonards JR, Kahn JR. Removal of fluid from normal and edematous dogs by continuous ultrafiltration of blood. *Lab Invest.* 1952;1:488–494.
3. Kolff WJ, Leonards JR. Reduction of otherwise intractable edema by dialysis or filtration. *Cleve Clin Q.* 1954;21:61–71.
4. Nakamoto S. Removal of edema fluid by ultrafiltration with the disposable twin coil artificial kidney. *Cleve Clin Q.* 1961;28:10–15.
5. Schneierson SJ. Continuous peritoneal irrigation in the treatment of intractable edema of cardiac origin. *Am J Med Sci.* 1949;218:76–79.
6. Silverstein ME, Ford CA, Lysaght MJ, Henderson LW. Treatment of severe fluid overload by ultrafiltration. *N Engl J Med.* 1974;291:747–751.
7. Gerhardt RE, Abdulla AM, Mach SJ, Hudson JB. Isolated ultrafiltration in the treatment of fluid overload in cardiogenic shock. *Arch Intern Med.* 1979;139:358–359.
8. DiLeo M, Pacitti A, Bergerone S, et al. Ultrafiltration in the treatment of refractory congestive heart failure. *Clin Cardiol.* 1988;11:449–459.
9. Soffer O, MacDonnell RC, Finlayson DC, et al. Intraoperative hemodialysis during cardiopulmonary bypass in chronic renal failure. *J Thorac Cardiovasc Surg.* 1979;77:789–791.
10. Darup J, Bleese N, Kalmar P, Lutz G, Pokar H, Polonius MJ. Hemofiltration during extracorporeal circulation (ECC). *Thorac Cardiovasc Surg.* 1979;27:227–230.
11. Kramer P, Wigger W, Rieger J, Matthaei D, Scheler F. Arteriovenous haemofiltration: a new and simple method for treatment of overhydrated patients resistant to diuretics. *Klin Wochenschr.* 1977;55:1121–1122.
12. Golper TA, Wedel SK, Kaplan AA, Saad A-M, Donta ST, Paganini EP. Drug removal during continuous arteriovenous hemofiltration: theory and clinical observations. *Int J Artif Organs.* 1985;8:307–312.
13. Golper TA. Drug removal during continuous hemofiltration. *Contrib Nephrol.* 1991; 93:110–116.
14. Paganini EP, Flague J, Whitman G, Nakamoto S. Amino acid balance in patients with oliguric renal failure undergoing slow continuous ultrafiltration (SCUF). *Trans Am Soc Artif Intern Organs.* 1982;28:615–620.
15. Kaplan AA, Longnecker RE, Folkert VW. Continuous arteriovenous hemofiltration—a report of six months' experience. *Ann Intern Med.* 1984;100:358–367.
16. Bailey GL, Hampers CL, Merrill JP. Reversible cardiomyopathy in uremia. *Trans Am Soc Artif Intern Org.* 1967;13:267–270.
17. United States Renal Data System. 1990 Annual Report. NIH, NIDDK, Bethesda, MD, August 1990.
18. Anderson CB, Codd JR, Graff RA. Cardiac failure and upper extremity arteriovenous dialysis fistulas (sic). *Arch Intern Med.* 1976;136:292–297.
19. Pourchez T, Moriniere P, Fournier A, Pietri J. Use of Permacath (Quinton) catheter in uraemic patients in whom creation of conventional vascular access for haemodialysis is difficult. *Nephron.* 1989;53:297–302.
20. Frank HA, Seligman AM, Fine J. Treatment of uremia after acute renal failure by peritoneal irrigation. *JAMA.* 1976;130:703–705.
21. Odel HM, Ferris DO, Power H. Peritoneal lavage as an effective means of external excretion. *Am J Med.* 1950;9:63–77.
22. Maxwell MH, Rockney RE, Kleeman CR, Twiss MR. Peritoneal dialysis—I. Technique and application. *JAMA.* 1959;170:917–924.
23. Vaamonde CA, Michael UF, Metzger RA, Carroll KE. Complications of acute peritoneal dialysis. *J Chron Dis.* 1975;28:637–659.
24. Miller RB, Tassistro CR. Peritoneal dialysis. *N Engl J Med.* 1969;281:945–949.
25. Steiner RW. Continuous equilibrium peritoneal dialysis in acute renal failure. *Periton Dialy Intern.* 1989;9:5–7.
26. Smeby LC, Wideroe T-E, Jorstad S. Individual differences in water transport during continuous peritoneal dialysis. *ASAIO J.* 1981;4:17–27.
27. Rubin J, Nolph KD, Popovich RP, Moncrief JW, Prowant B. Drainage volume during continuous ambulatory peritoneal dialysis. *ASAIO J.* 1979;2:54–60.
28. Rubin J, Adair C, Barnes T, Bower J. Dialysate flow rate and peritoneal clearance. *Am J Kidney Dis.* 1984; 4:260–267.
29. Gotloib L, Mines M, Garmizo L, Varka I. Hemodynamic effects of increasing intrabdominal pressure in peritoneal dialysis. *Periton Dialy Bull.* 1981;1:41–43.
30. Blumberg A, Keller R, Marti HR. Oxygen affinity of erythrocytes and pulmonary gas exchange in patients on continuous ambulatory peritoneal dialysis. *Nephron.* 1984;38:248–252.
31. Taveira Da Silva AM, Davis WB, Winchester JE, Coleman DE, Weir CW. Peritonitis, dialysate infusion and lung function in continuous ambulatory peritoneal dialysis (CAPD). *Clin Nephrol.* 1985;24:79–83.
32. Epstein SW, Inouye T, Robson M, Oreopoulos DM. Effect of peritoneal dialysis fluid on ventilatory function. *Periton Dialy Bull.* 1982;2:120–122.
33. Gomez-Fernandez P, Sanchez Agudo L, Calatrava JM, et al. Respiratory muscle weakness in uremic patients under continuous ambulatory peritoneal dialysis. *Nephron.* 1984;36:219–223.
34. Berlyne GM, Lee HA, Ralston AJ, Woodcock JA. Pulmonary complications of peritoneal dialysis. *Lancet.* 1966;II:75–78.
35. Mailloux LU, Swartz CD, Onesti G, Heider C, Rameriz O, Brest AN. Peritoneal dialysis for refractory congestive heart failure. *JAMA.* 1967;199:873–878.
36. Cairns KB, Porter GA, Kloster FE, Bristow JD, Griswold HE. Clinical and hemodynamic results of peritoneal dialysis for severe cardiac failure. *Am Heart J.* 1968;76:227–234.
37. Raja RM, Krasnoff SO, Moros JG, Kramer MS, Rosen-

baum JL. Repeated peritoneal dialysis in treatment of heart failure. *JAMA*. 1970;213:2268–2269.

38. Malach M. Peritoneal dialysis for intractable heart failure in acute myocardial infarction. *Am J Cardiol*. 1972;29:61–63.

39. Shapira J, Lang R, Jutrin I, Robson M, Ravid M. Peritoneal dialysis in refractory congestive heart failure: I. Intermittent peritoneal dialysis. *Periton Dialy Bull*. 1983;3:130–132.

40. Robson M, Biro A, Knobel B, Schai G, Ravid M. Peritoneal dialysis in refractory congestive heart failure: II. Continuous ambulatory peritoneal dialysis. *Periton Dialy Bull*. 1983;3:133–134.

41. Weinrauch LA, Kaldany A, Miller DG, et al. Cardiorenal failure: treatment of refractory biventricular failure by peritoneal dialysis. *Uremia Invest*. 1984;8: 1–8.

42. Kim D, Khanna R, Wu G, Fountas P, Druck M, Oreopoulos DG. Successful use of continuous ambulatory peritoneal dialysis in refractory heart failure. *Periton Dialy Bull*. 1985;5:127–130.

43. McKinnie JJ, Bourgeois RJ, Husserl FE. Long-term therapy for heart failure with continuous ambulatory peritoneal dialysis. *Arch Intern Med*. 1985;145:1128–1129.

44. Rubin J, Ball R. Continuous ambulatory peritoneal dialysis as treatment of severe congestive heart failure in the face of chronic renal failure. *Arch Intern Med*. 1986;146:1533–1535.

45. Konig P, Geissler D, Lechleitner P, Spielberger M, Dittrich P. Improved management of congestive heart failure: use of continuous ambulatory peritoneal dialysis. *Arch Intern Med*. 1987;147:1031–1034.

46. Stablein DM, Hamburger RJ, Lindblad AS, Nolph KD, Novak JW. The effect of CAPD on hypertension control: a report of the national CAPD registry. *Periton Dialy Intern*. 1988;8:141–144.

47. Cannata JB, Isles CG, Briggs JD, Junor BJR. Comparison of blood pressure control during hemodialysis and CAPD. *Dialy Transplant*. 1986;15:674–679.

48. Gault MH, Ferguson EL, Sidhu JS, Corbin RP. Fluid and electrolyte complications of peritoneal dialysis. *Ann Intern Med*. 1971;75:253–262.

49. Ash SR, Handt AE, Bloch R. Peritoneoscopic placement of the Tenckhoff catheter: further clinical experience. *Periton Dialy Bull*. 1983;3:8–12.

50. Ing TS, Chen WT, Daugirdas JJ, Kwaan HC, Hano JE. Isolated ultrafiltration and new techniques of ultrafiltration during dialysis. *Kidney Int*. 1980;18:S77–S82.

51. Ing TS, Ashbach DL, Kanter A, Oyama JH, Armbruster KFW, Merkel FK. Fluid removal with negative-pressure hydrostatic ultrafiltration using a partial vacuum. *Nephron*. 1975;14:451–455.

52. Bergstrom J, Asaba H, Furst P, Oules R. Dialysis, ultrafiltration, and blood pressure. *Proc Eur Dialy Transplant Assoc*. 1976;13:293–305.

53. Wehle B, Asaba H, Castenfors J, et al. Haemodynamic changes during sequential ultrafiltration and dialysis. *Kidney Int*. 1979;15:411–418.

54. Quellhorst E, Schuenemann B, Hidebrand U, Falda Z. Response of the vascular system to different modification of haemofiltration and haemodialysis. *Proc Eur Dialy Transplant Assoc*. 1980;17:197–204.

55. Baldamus CA, Ernst W, Frei U, Koch KM. Sympathetic and haemodynamic response to volume removal during different forms of renal replacement therapy. *Nephron*. 1982;31:324–332.

56. Paganini EP, Fouad F, Tarazi RC, Bravo EL, Nakamoto S. Hemodynamics of isolated ultrafiltration in chronic hemodialysis patients. *Trans Am Soc Artif Intern Organs*. 1979;25:422–425.

57. Zuccelli P, Santoro A, Sturani A, Degli Esposti E, Chiarini C, Zuccala A. Effects of hemodialysis and hemofiltration on the autonomic control of circulation. *Trans Am Soc Artif Intern Organs*. 1984;30:163–167.

58. Chen WT, Chaignon M, Omvik P, Tarazi RC, Bravo EL, Nakamoto S. Hemodynamic studies in chronic hemodialysis patients with haemofiltration/ultrafiltration. *Trans Am Soc Artif Intern Organs*. 1978;24:682–686.

59. Asaba H, Bergstrom J, Furst P, Shaldon S, Wiklund S. Treatment of diuretic resistant fluid retention with ultrafiltration. *Acta Med Scand*. 1978;204:145–149.

60. Morgan SH, Mansell MA, Thompson FD. Fluid removal by haemofiltration in diuretic resistant cardiac failure. *Br Heart J*. 1985;54:218–219.

61. Simpson IA, Rae AP, Simpson K, et al. Ultrafiltration in the management of refractory congestive heart failure. *Br Heart J*. 1986;55:344–347.

62. Fauchald P, Forfang K, Amlie J. An evaluation of ultrafiltration as treatment of therapy resistant cardiac edema. *Acta Med Scand*. 1986;219:47–52.

63. Donato L, Biagini A, Contini C, et al. Treatment of end-stage congestive heart failure by extracorporeal ultrafiltration. *Am J Cardiol*. 1987;59:379–380.

64. Rimondini A, Cipolla CM, Della Bella P, et al. Hemofiltration as short-term treatment for refractory congestive heart failure. *Am J Med*. 1987;83:43–48.

65. L'Abbate A, Emdin M, Piacenti M, et al. Ultrafiltration: a rational treatment for heart failure. *Cardiology*. 1989;76:384–390.

66. Cipolla CM, Grazi S, Rimondini A, et al. Changes in circulating norepinephrine with hemofiltration in advanced congestive heart failure. *Am J Cardiol*. 1990; 66:987–994.

67. Canaud B, Cristol JP, Klouche K, et al. Slow continuous ultrafiltration: a means of unmasking myocardial functional reserve in end stage cardiac disease. *Contrib Nephrol*. 1991;93:79–85.

68. Scribner BH, Caner JEZ, Buri R, Quinton W. The technique of continuous hemodialysis. *Trans Am Soc Artif Intern Organs*. 1960;6:88–103.

69. Henderson LW, Basarab A, Michaels A, Bluemle LW. Blood purification by ultrafiltration and fluid replacement (diafiltration). *Trans Am Soc Artif Intern Organs*. 1967;13:216–226.

70. Kramer P, Kaufhold G, Grone HJ, Wigger W, Rieger D. Management of anuric intensive care patients with arteriovenous hemofiltration. *Int J Artif Organs*. 1980; 3:225–230.

71. Paganini EP, Nakamoto S. Continuous slow ultrafiltration in oliguric renal failure. *Trans Am Soc Artif Intern Organs*. 1980;26:201–204.

72. Lepape A, Bene B, Pedrix J-P, Grozel JM, Banssilon V. Double pump driven continuous veno-venous haemofiltration (CVVH). In: Sieberth HG, Mann H, eds. *Continuous Arteriovenous Haemofiltration*. Basel: Karger; 1985:53–58.

73. Canaud B, Berand JJ, Mion C. Pump assisted continuous veno-venous hemofiltration: a more flexible mode of acute uremia treatment in severely ill patients. In: La Greca G, Fabris A, Ronco C, eds. *Proc International Symposium on Continuous Arteriovenous Hemofiltration*. Milan: Wichtig Editore; 1986:185–189.

74. Favre H, Lovy M, Klohn M, Suter P. Continuous veno-venous hemofiltration. In: Paganini E, Geronemus R, eds. *Proc Third International Symposium on Acute Continuous Renal Replacement Therapy*. Ft. Lauderdale, 1987:87–93.

75. Kramer P, Buhler J, Kehr A, et al. Intensive care potential of continuous arteriovenous hemofiltration. *Trans Am Soc Artif Intern Organs*. 1982;28:28–32.

76. Grone HJ, Kramer P. Puncture and long term cannulation of the femoral artery and vein in adults. In: Kramer P, ed. *Arteriovenous Hemofiltration*. Berlin: Springer-Verlag; 1985:35–47.

77. Olbricht CJ, Schurek H-J, Stolte H, Koch KM. The influence of vascular access modes on the efficiency of CAVH. In: Sieberth H-G, Mann H, eds. *Continuous Arteriovenous Hemofiltration*. Basel: Karger; 1985:14–24.

78. Olbricht C. Vascular access for CAVH. In: Paganini E, Geronemus R, eds. *Proc Third International Symposium on Acute Continuous Renal Replacement Therapy*. Ft. Lauderdale; 1987:23–36.

79. Paganini EP, O'Hara P, Nakamoto S. Slow continuous ultrafiltration in hemodialysis resistent oliguric acute renal failure patients. *Trans Am Soc Artif Intern Organs*. 1984;30:173–177.

80. Lauer A, Sacaggi A, Ronco C, Belledonne M, Glabman S, Bosch JP. Continuous arteriovenous hemofiltration in critically ill patients. *Ann Intern Med*. 1983;99:455–460.

81. Henderson AW, Donald LL, Levin NW. Clinical use of Amicon Diafilter. *Dial Transplant*. 1983;12:523–525.

82. Synhaivsky A, Kurtz SB, Wochos DN, Schniepp J, Johnson WJ. Acute renal failure treated by slow continuous ultrafiltration: preliminary report. *Mayo Clin Proc*. 1983;58:729–733.

83. van Geelen JA, Vincent HH, Schalekamp MADH. Continuous arteriovenous haemofiltration and haemodiafiltration in acute renal failure. *Nephrol Dial Transplant*. 1988;2:181–186.

84. Henrich WL, Woodard TD, Blachley JD, Gomez-Sanchez C, Pettinger W, Cronin RE. Role of osmolality in blood pressure stability after dialysis and ultrafiltration. *Kidney Int*. 1980;18:480–488.

85. Swartz RD, Somermeyer MG, Hsu C-H. Preservation of plasma volume during hemodialysis depends on dialysate osmolality. *Am J Nephrol*. 1982;2:189–194.

86. Fleming SJ, Wilkinson JS, Greenwood RN, Aldridge C, Baker LRI, Cattell WR. Effect of dialysate composition on intercompartment fluid shift. *Kidney Int*. 1987; 32:267–273.

87. Fleming SJ, Wilkinson JS, Aldridge C, Greenwood RN, Baker LRI, Cattell WR. Blood volume changes during isolated ultrafiltration and combined ultrafiltration-dialysis. *Nephrol Dial Transplant*. 1988;3:272–276.

88. Teo KK, Basile C, Ulan RA, Hetherington MD, Kappagoda T. Effects of hemodialysis and hypertonic hemodiafiltration on cardiac function compared. *Kidney Int*. 1987;32:399–407.

89. Lazarus JM, Henderson LW, Kjellstrand CM, Weiner MW, Henrich WL, Hakim RM. Panel conference: cardiovascular instability during hemodialysis. *Trans Am Soc Artif Intern Organs*. 1982;28:656–665.

90. Henderson LW. Symptomatic hypotension during dialysis. *Kidney Int*. 1980;17:571–576.

91. Keshaviah P, Shapiro FL. A critical examination of dialysis-induced hypotension. *Am J Kidney Dis*. 1982; 2:290–301.

92. Kimura G, Irie A, Kuroda K, Kojima S, Satani M. Absence of transcellular fluid shift during haemofiltration. *Proc Euro Dial Transplant Assoc*. 1980;17:192–196.

93. Schuenemann B, Borghardt J, Falda Z, et al. Reactions of blood pressure and body spaces to hemofiltration treatment. *Trans Am Soc Artif Intern Organs*. 1978; 24:687–689.

94. Golper TA, Kaplan AA, Narasimhan N, Leone M. Transmembrane pressures generated by filtrate line suction maneuvers and predilution fluid replacement during in vitro continuous arteriovenous hemofiltration. *Intern J Artif Organs*. 1987;10:41–46.

95. Ronco C, Brendolan A, Bragantini L, et al. Studies on blood flow dynamic and ultrafiltration kinetics during continuous arteriovenous hemofiltration. Graphic Forum 4th Annual Meeting of Intern Soc Blood Purification, Osaka, Japan November 5, 1986. *Blood Purification*. 1986;4:220.

96. Ronco C, Brendolan A, Bragantini L, et al. Continuous arteriovenous hemofiltration. *Contr Nephrol*. 1985;48: 70–88.

97. Olbricht CJ, Schurek HJ, Tytul S, Miller C, Stolte H. Comparison between Scribner shunt and femoral catheters as vascular access for continuous arteriovenous hemofiltration. In: Kramer P, ed. *Arteriovenous Hemofiltration*. Berlin: Springer-Verlag; 1985:57–66.

98. Pallone TL, Peterson J. Continuous arteriovenous hemofiltration: an in-vitro simulation and mathematical model. *Kidney Int*. 1988;33:685–698.

99. Ronco C, Bosch JP, Lew S, et al. Technician and clinical evaluation of a new hemofilter for CAVH; theoretical concepts and practical application of a different flow geometry. In: LaGreca G, Fabris A, Ronco C, eds. *Proc of International Symposium on Continuous Arteriovenous Hemofiltration*. Wichtig Milan: Editore; 1986: 55–61.

100. Lindholm T, Gullberg C, Akerlund A. Laboratory and clinical experience with a new disposable parallel flow plate dialyzer. *Scand J Urol Nephrol*. 1972;(Suppl 13):4–15.

101. Smith D, Paganini EP, Suhoza K, Eisele G, Swann S, Nakamoto S. Non heparin continuous renal replacement therapy. In: Nose Y, Kjellstrand C, Ivanovich P, eds. *Progress in Artificial Organs*. Cleveland: ISAO Press; 1986:226–230.

102. Kramer P, Schrader J, Bohnsack W, Grieben G, Grone HJ, Scheler F. Continuous arteriovenous hemofiltration: a new kidney replacement therapy. *Proc Eur Dialy Transplant Assoc*. 1981;18:743–749.

103. Schrader J, Scheler F. Coagulation disorders in acute renal failure and anticoagulation during CAVH with standard heparin and with low molecular weight heparin. In: Sieberth H-G, Mann H, eds. *Continuous Arteriovenous Hemofiltration*. Basel: Karger; 1985:25–36.

104. Olbricht C, Mueller C, Schurek HJ. Treatment of acute renal failure in patients with multiple organ failure by continuous spontaneous hemofiltration. *Trans Am Soc Artif Intern Organs*. 1982;28:33–37.

105. Bull BS, Korpman RA, Huse WM, Briggs BD. Heparin therapy during extracorporeal circulation. I. Problems inherent in existing heparin protocols. *J Thorac Cardiovasc Surg*. 1975;69:674–684.

106. Bjornsson TD, Wolfram KM, Kitchell BB. Heparin kinetics determined by three assay methods. *Clin Pharmacol Ther*. 1982;31:104–113.

107. Ossenkopple GJ, van der Muellen J, Bronsveld W, et al. Continuous arteriovenous haemofiltration as an adjunctive therapy for septic shock. *Crit Care Med*. 1985;13:102–104.

108. Zusman RM, Rubin RH, Cato AE, Cocchetto DM, Crow JW. Tolkoff-Rubin N. Hemodialysis using prostacyclin instead of heparin as the sole antithrombotic agent. *N Engl J Med*. 1981;304:934–939.

109. Smith MC, Danviriyasup K, Crow JW, et al. Prostacyclin substitution for heparin in long-term hemodialysis. *Am J Med*. 1982;73:669–78.

110. Canaud B, Mion C, Arujo A, et al. Prostacyclin (epoprostenol) as the sole antithrombotic agent in postdilutional haemofiltration. *Nephron*. 1988;48:206–212.

111. Ota K, Kawaguchi H, Takahashi K, Ito K. A new prostacyclin analogue: an anticoagulant applicable to hemodialysis. *Trans Am Soc Artif Intern Organs*. 1983;12:419–424.

112. Pinnick RV, Wiegmann TB, Diederich DA. Regional citrate anticoagulation for hemodialysis in the patient at high risk for bleeding. *N Engl J Med*. 1983;308:258–261.

113. Flanigan MJ, Von Brecht J, Freeman RM, Lim VS. Reducing the hemorrhagic complications of hemodialysis: a controlled comparison of low dose heparin and citrate anticoagulation. *Am J Kidney Dis*. 1983;9:147–153.

114. Mehta RL, McDonald BR, Aguilar MM, Ward DM. Regional citrate anticoagulation for continuous arteriovenous hemodialysis in critically ill patients. *Kidney Int*. 1990;38:976–981.

115. Ahamd S, Yeo K-T, Jensen WM, et al. Citrate anticoagulation during in vivo simulation of slow hemofiltration. *Blood Purif*. 1990;170–182.

116. Kaplan AA, Petrillo R. Regional heparinization for continuous arteriovenous hemofiltration. *Trans Am Soc Artif Intern Organs*. 1987;33:312–315.

117. Milne B, Rodgers K, Cervenko F, Salerno T. Hemodynamic effects of intra-aortic administration versus intravenous administration of protamine for reversal of heparin in man. *Can Anaesth Soc J*. 1983;30:347–351.

118. Ellison N, Beatty P, Blake DR, Wurzel HA, MacVaugh H. Heparin rebound. *J Thorac Cardiovasc Surg*. 1974;67:723–729.

119. Hory B, Cachoux A, Toulemonde F. Continuous arteriovenous hemofiltration with low-molecular-weight heparin. *Nephron*. 1985;41:125.

120. Schurek HJ, Biela D. Continuous arteriovenous hemofiltration: improvement in the handling of fluid balance and heparinization. *Blood Purif*. 1983;1:189–196.

121. Bosch JP, Geronemus R, Glabman S, Lysaght M, Kalm T, Von Albertini B. High flux hemofiltration. *Artif Organs*. 1978;2:339–342.

122. Kaplan AA, Longnecker RE, Folkert VW. Suction-assisted continuous arteriovenous hemofiltration. *Trans Am Soc Artif Internal Organs*. 1983;29:408–413.

123. Magilligan DJ. Indications for ultrafiltration in the cardiac surgical patient. *J Thorac Cardiovasc Surg*. 1985;89:183–189.

124. Paganini EP, Suhoza K, Swann S, Golding L, Nakamoto S. Continuous renal replacement therapy in patients with acute renal dysfunction undergoing intraaortic balloon pump and/or left ventricular device support. *Trans Am Soc Artif Intern Organs*. 1986;32:414–417.

125. Coraim FJ, Coraim HP, Ebermann R, Stellwag FM. Acute respiratory failure after cardiac surgery: clinical experience with the application of continuous arteriovenous hemofiltration. *Crit Care Med*. 1986;14:714–718.

126. Lefer AM. Interaction between myocardial depressant factor and vasoactive mediators with ischemia and shock. *Am J Physiol*. 1987;252:R193–R205.

127. Parrillo JE, Burch C, Shelhamer JH, Parker MM, Natanson C, Schuette W. A circulating myocardial depressant substance in humans with septic shock. *J Clin Invest*. 1985;76:1539–1553.

128. Cunnion RE. Cardiac dysfunction in human septic shock. In: Parrillo JE, moderator. Septic shock in humans: advances in the understanding of pathogenesis, cardiovascular dysfunction, and therapy. *Ann Intern Med*. 1990;113:227–242.

129. Schirmer WJ, Schirmer JM, Fry DE. Recombinant human tumor necrosis factor produces hemodynamic changes characteristic of sepsis and endotoxemia. *Arch Surg*. 1989;124:445–448.

130. Suffredini AF, Fromm RE, Parker MM, et al. The cardiovascular response of normal humans to the administration of endotoxin. *N Engl J Med*. 1989;321:280–287.

131. Maury CPJ, Teppo A-M. Circulating tumour necrosis factor alpha (cachectin) in myocardial infarction. *J Intern Med*. 1989;225:333–336.

132. Levine B, Kalman J, Mayer L, Fillit HM, Packer M. Elevated circulating levels of tumor necrosis factor in severe chronic heart failure. *N Engl J Med*. 1990;323:236–241.

133. Golper TA, Jenkins R, Wright M, Klein JB. Tumor necrosis factor and hemofiltration membranes. *Intensivbehandlung*. 1990;15:119.

134. McDonald BR, Mehta RL. Transmembrane flux of IL-1B and TNF-a in patients undergoing continuous arteriovenous hemodialysis. *J Am Soc Nephrol*. 1990;1:368.

135. Gomez A, Wang R, Unruh H, et al. Hemofiltration reverses left ventricular dysfunction during sepsis in dogs. *Anesthesiology*. 1990;73:671–685.

31
Surgical Therapy for Acute Congestive Heart Failure

Eli Milgalter, Davis C. Drinkwater, and Hillel Laks

Acute left ventricular failure is an ominous state that demands immediate therapy. Without intervention, mortality of patients in cardiogenic shock (CS) exceeds 90%.[1] The three major causes of acute ventricular failure are coronary artery disease, severe valvar malfunction, and primary myocardial disease. All three causes require pharmacologic support, occasionally progressing to mechanical support devices. Emergency surgery must be considered early in those cases where the primary cause can be corrected by a surgical procedure.

Coronary Artery Disease

Acute myocardial infarction may cause heart failure in a variety of ways. Most commonly, it is caused by the extent of the infarction or the asociation of multivessel coronary artery disease. It may also be caused by the complications of acute myocardial infarction such as ventricular septal defect due to perforation of the septum, mitral regurgitation due to papillary muscle dysfunction or rupture, and rupture of the ventricular free wall (see Table 31.1).

Cardiogenic Shock

Cardiogenic shock occurs in 10% to 15% of patients after acute coronary artery occlusion, and remains the major cause of inhospital mortality after infarction.[2] Cardiogenic shock develops when more than 40% of the left ventricle is nonfunctioning[3,4] and in most cases is gradual in onset evolving 6 or more hr after a myocardial infarction. The severity of the cardiogenic shock may be assessed clinically with signs of poor perfusion, including cold skin and extremities, urine output <0.5 ml/kg/hr, metabolic acidosis, mean arterial blood pressure <60 mm Hg, and the patient may be confused or restless. Also helpful in confirming the diagnosis is the measurement by thermodilution catheter of a cardiac index <2.0 L/min/m², while the pulmonary artery wedge pressure (or left atrial pressure) is >18 mm Hg and the peripheral resistance is >1800 dyne-s/cm.

The more severe cardiogenic shock, with a left atrial pressure >18 mm Hg and a left ventricle stroke–work index of <20 g/M² (grade IV) has a 90% mortality with medical therapy alone, while the less severe grades often respond to fluid and pharmacologic management. Aggressive intervention with intraaortic balloon support followed by emergent surgery might rescue approximately 50% of the patients most adversely effected.[5,6] Any surgical intervention must precede major organ failure to salvage a significant number of patients in cardiogenic shock.

Beyersdorf and associates demonstrated that acutely ischemic muscle develops immediate dyskinesia in the area of infarction and that subsequent left ventricular power failure is moderated predominantly by the ability of the remote myocardium to compensate.[7,8] In the setting of either prior myocardial infarction or multivessel coronary artery disease, the inability of remote myocardium to maintain a state of hypercontractility may result in the gradual development of cardiogenic shock. Postinfarction left ventricle power failure represents a

TABLE 31.1. Surgical intervention for acute coronary syndromes.

Syndrome	Procedure	Operative mortality (%)
Pump failure	Revascularization	7% early operation; 31% late operation
Free wall rupture	Closure of rupture	35
Ventricular septal defect	Closure ± revascularization	25
Acute mitral insufficiency	Valve replacement and revascularization	50

severe imbalance between myocardial oxygen demand and supply, and should be considered an acute medical/surgical emergency.[9,10]

Preoperative Strategy

The need for increasing preoperative support is based on an ongoing evaluation of the patient through clinical and hemodynamic monitoring, including a Swan-Ganz and arterial catheter. The first line of therapy is pharmacologic manipulation of the preload, the contractility, and the afterload. In addition to appropriate inotropic agents, the aggressive use of vasodilators and antiarrhythmics may be instrumental in improving and maintaining an adequate cardiac output. For most patients in cardiogenic shock, the placement of an intraaortic balloon pump early in the course may stabilize the patient for both diagnostic tests and subsequent surgery and at the same time avoid some of the detrimental side effects of high-dose inotropic agents (i.e., renal vasoconstriction and arrhythmias). In patients with severe aortoiliac disease, this should be delayed until all reasonable alternate efforts have been exhausted, because of the dire consequences of significant limb ischemia.

Diagnostic Tests

A transthoracic echocardiogram should be obtained to complement or replace a left ventricle ventriculogram, assessing segmental wall motion, ejection fraction, and valvar function. If this is not adequate, a transesophageal echocardiogram may be required. Additional information about the ascending aortic calcification or intimal atherosclerosis may be obtained through the echocardiogram, aiding in the placement of arterial cannulae to avoid neurologic dysfunction due to emboli. The presence of a carotid bruit and in particular a history of transient ischemic attacks warrants a carotid duplex study. A simultaneous procedure to revascularize both coronary artery disease and affected carotids may be needed if there is bilateral >90% stenoses, or if there is >80% stenosis on the ipsilateral affected side.

Evaluation of the acutely ischemic patient should assess both the power component of the ventricle and the valvular function as it relates in particular to the mitral valve, which may have both ischemic as well as intrinsic abnormal changes. To assess myocardial viability, the presence of contraction in specific areas currently may be the best indication, reserving the use of such tests as thallium and positron emission tomography scans for the more chronic, stable patients.

The potential to recover two out of three parts of the myocardium is vital for both short- and long-term success in acute coronary revascularization. On the basis of this assessment for myocardial recovery, patients in car-

diogenic shock may be triaged to medical/interventional therapy, emergent surgical revascularization and controlled reperfusion, or finally support to transplantation, one of several therapeutic options. These include thrombolytic therapy with or without angioplasty, surgical revascularization with controlled modified reperfusion, and finally, cardiac transplantation with or without a cardiac assist device as a bridge to transplantation.

Ventricular Assist Devices

If cardiogenic shock progresses rapidly despite full support, a ventricular assist device may be required to support the circulation. This may occur in the intensive care unit or in the cardiac catheterization laboratory. The availability of the percutaneous femoral artery and vein catheters along with the Cardiac Peripheral Support (CPS) systems allow patients to be supported rapidly in the angio suite or intensive care unit. Diagnostic studies including coronary angiography and ventriculography if renal function is satisfactory may be performed expeditiously and safely with lesser supports, and the patient treated by thrombolysis, with or without Percutaneous Transluminal Coronary Angioplasty (PTCA), or taken directly to surgery.

Bridge-to-Transplantation

Patients in cardiogenic shock who are not coronary artery bypass graft candidates but who are acceptable for transplantation should be considered for a left ventricular assist device as a bridge to transplantation. Good results have been reported with this technique when carefully applied criteria are adhered to.[11]

Surgical Technique

Patients in cardiogenic shock are operated on urgently to salvage ischemic or infarcting myocardium, before end-organ dysfunction or sepsis supervenes. The placement of an intraaortic balloon pump preoperatively helps to stabilize the patient during the induction and postoperatively. For the acutely ischemic patient with cardiogenic shock, a protocol is used for reperfusion and revascularization which includes the following techniques. The left ventricle is vented through the right superior vein. Reverse saphenous vein grafts are used when available and of good quality in preference to arterial conduits because of the immediate need for adequate coronary flow in a patient who may be hypotensive. With the use of retrograde cardioplegia as described below, issues of myocardial protection and the ability to infuse cardioplegia down the vein graft is less critical and the internal mammary artery may be used in selected young patients provided it is of an adequate caliber.

TABLE 31.2. Cardioplegic solutions.

Warm Induction Blood Cardioplegia (37°C)			
Additive	Volume (ml)*	Component Mod	Concentration
Tham (0.3 mol/L)	225	pH	7.5–7.6
CPD	225	Ca^{2+}	150–250 mmol/L
D50W	40	Osmolality	380–400 mOsm
Glutamate			
Aspartate	[50]	[Substrate]	[13 mmol/L]
KCl (2 mEq/ml)	40	K$^+$	20–25 mEq/L
D5W	220		
Total	1000		

Maintenance Blood Cardioplegia			
Additive	Volume (ml)*	Component Mod	Concentration
KCl (2 MEq/ml)	15	K$^+$	8–10 mEq/L
Tham (0.3 mol/L)	225	pH	pH 7.5–7.6
CPD	50	Ca^{2+}	0.5–0.6 mmol/L
D5.25NS	550	Osmolality	340–360 mOsm

Warm Reperfusate Blood Cardioplegia (37°)			
Additive	Volume (ml)*	Component Mod	Concentration
KCl (2 mEq/ml)	15	K$^+$	8–10 mEq/L
Tham (0.3 mol/L)	225	pH	pH 7.5–7.6
CPD	225	Ca^{2+}	0.15–.25 mmol/L
Aspartate			
Glutamate	[250]	[Substrate]	[13 mmol/L]
D50W	40	Glucose	>400 mg/dl
D5W	245	Osmolality	380–400 mOsm
Total	1000		

* Blood/crystalloid 4:1.
† 4:1 dilution.
‡ 4:1 dilution.

Cardioplegia Protocol

Cardioplegia induction is achieved by warm (37°C), substrate-enriched blood cardioplegia, equally divided between antegrade and retrograde infusion at approximately 200 mL/min (Table 31.2). After a total of 4 min, cardioplegia is changed to a non–substrate-containing normothermic solution, administered retrograde at pressure less than 25 mm Hg or flows less than 125 mL/min. Cardioplegia may be infused antegrade after completion of each distal anastomosis for 1 to 2 min, or if there is visual confirmation of adequate retrograde perfusion to the area of anastomosis, the proximal attachment to the aorta may be made at this time (Table 31.2). At the end, an equally divided dose of substrate-enhanced cardioplegia is given first retrograde to deair and then antegrade, at the same time removing the retrograde cannula (Table 31.2). Regular blood is given via the retrograde cannula before unclamping the aorta and removing the retrograde cannula.

The vent is used to decompress the left ventricle until the heart is beating and ready to wean from bypass. If the proximal anastomoses are placed after the distals,

one can administer the cardioplegia antegrade, leaving the graft supplying the largest amount of viable myocardium until last to minimize the period of ischemia. The issue of saphenous vein graft versus internal thoracic artery is somewhat up to the operator, and clearly with the use of antegrade–retrograde techniques, the internal thoracic is more likely to be used, because adequate myocardial protection of a jeopardized area, particularly on the left side, is now possible.[12]

Results of Coronary Revascularization for Cardiogenic Shock

The results of coronary bypass for cardiogenic shock at UCLA have been previously reported. Among 80 patients undergoing bypass, 45 were operated on <18 hr after onset of shock with a hospital mortality of 7%, whereas the remaining 35 patients operated on >18 hr had a mortality of 31%. The results were adversely affected not only by delay in surgery but by the existence of end-organ dysfunction before surgery. (Figs. 31.1, 31.2). In those with preoperative end-organ dysfunction such as renal failure or sepsis, the mortality

FIGURE 31.1. Coronary artery bypass grafting after cardiogenic shock: Influence to time of operation (n = 80; deaths = 35). P. Wilcoxon, mean ± standard error; italic numbers indicate patients alive and well. Reprinted with permission from Allen BS, et al. *J Thorac Cardiovasc Surg*. 1989;98:691–703.

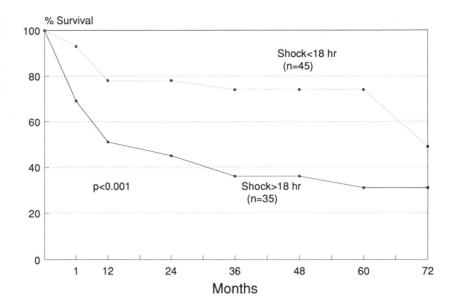

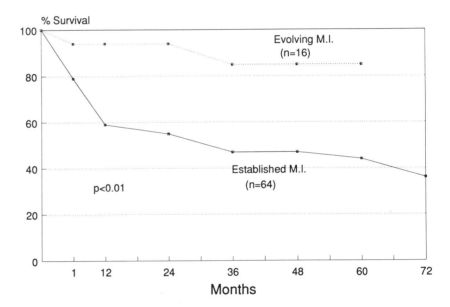

FIGURE 31.2. Influence of preoperative organ failure (n = 80; deaths = 35) on coronary artery bypass grafting after cardiogenic shock. P. Wilcoxon, mean ± standard error. Reprinted with permission from Allen BS, et al. *J Thorac Cardiovasc Surg*. 1989;98:691–703.

was 66%, whereas it was 11% in those without preoperative organ dysfunction. The late mortality was 26%, and 67% of late survivors remained physically active at 36-month mean follow-up.

Left Ventricular Free Wall Rupture

Ventricular free wall rupture may occur in 3% to 8% of patients in the first week after acute myocardial infarction, which is 3 to 4 times more common than rupture of the ventricular septum.[13–15] Clinically, the event is marked by a sudden hemodynamic collapse several days after a myocardial infarction, which either may be heralded by a sharp chest pain or, more frequently, the appearance of electromechanical dissociation. A high index of suspicion is essential for any opportunity to salvage the condition that requires direct transfer to the operating room for repair of the perforation. Although most patients succumb before reaching the operating room, of those operated, approximately 65% will survive. Important positive factors on survival include previous operation or the presence of pericardial adhesions to provide containment of the perforation.

Left Ventricle Pseudoaneurysm

The presence of a pseudoaneurysm of the left ventricle may result and should be operated on emergently regardless of size because of the propensity for both acute congestive heart failure and more seriously, free rupture.[14] Results of surgical repair of pseudoaneurysm are far better than those for rupture of the free wall or septum.[15]

Postinfarction Ventricular Septal Defect

Acute rupture of the interventricular septum occurs in 1% to 2% of acute infarctions. In general, there is less diffuse coronary artery disease with less septal collaterals and in 65% there is single-vessel coronary artery disease, involving an extensive territory of the myocardium, usually anterior.[16] Rupture and ventricular septal defect formation occurs in general around the 7th to 8th day postinfarction, although it has been reported as early as 24 hr and as late as 23 days.[17] Without intervention, 81% of patients are dead within 8 weeks, and only 7% will survive longer than one 1 yr.[18]

Sudden hemodynamic compromise associated with a new murmur several days after an acute myocardial infarction should prompt the rapid evaluation for either ventricular septal defect or mitral regurgitation papillary muscle rupture. The differential can be made at the bedside either by right heart catheterization and demonstration of a step up in the saturations between the superior vena cava and pulmonary artery, or by contrast echocardiography. Left heart catheterization is useful to delineate the coronary artery anatomy and disease, and should be performed unless the patient is deteriorating rapidly despite the use of an intraaortic balloon. Delay in surgery once cardiogenic shock or failure occurs is associated with a high mortality. Urgent surgery is the preferred method of therapy.

Preoperative Management

The diagnosis of ventricular septal defect postinfarction is an indication for operation due to the dismal results of medical therapy. Initial therapy is directed toward reducing left to right shunt and augmenting the forward flow through the use of inotropic and afterload reducing agents, and most effectively the intraaortic balloon pump. Despite this resuscitation, 50% to 60% will remain in cardiogenic shock before surgery and should be operated on as soon as possible before the onset of organ failure. More favorable results have been reported from a number of institutions when patients with postinfarction ventricular septal defect are operated on immediately, rather than waiting 4 to 6 weeks, as previously recommended.[19,20]

Surgical Management

The surgical approach is through the infarction site in the left ventricle, facilitating both infarctectomy as well as closure of the ventricular septal defect. The following principles are useful and include meticulous myocardial protection and inotropic support, complete resection of necrotic muscle, careful inspection and replacement of the mitral valve if there is papillary muscle rupture, and closure of the ventricular septal defect and the infarctectomy, with generous synthetic Dacron material lined with pericardium to prevent distortion of ventricular volumes and anatomy. Whether concomitant coronary artery bypass graft should be carried out is controversial, although most authors believe better results are obtained if significant remaining myocardium is jeopardized by existing coronary artery disease.[19] Thus, patients with multivessel coronary artery disease should undergo coronary revascularization.

A mortality rate of 25% overall can be obtained with 34% for the posterior defects, which may involve the mitral valve, and 15% for the anterior-apical ventricular septal defect. Long-term results are favorable with about 80% 5-yr survival among patients discharged from hospital and most maintained in New York Heart Association (NYHA) functional class I or II.

Acute Mitral Regurgitation After Myocardial Infarction

Acute mitral valve incompetence may occur in up to 5% of patients with acute myocardial infarction, usually localized to the circumflex or dominant right coronary artery distribution (31%). The mechanism is rupture of a papillary muscle involving the posteromedial papillary muscle in 80% of cases. Infrequently sustained mitral insufficiency is caused by ischemic dysfunction of the mitral valve.[21]

Rupture of the papillary muscle is heralded by the onset of acute pulmonary edema generally between 4 and 7 days postinfarction, but may present as cardiogenic shock. Differential diagnosis of the new-onset murmur is made by right heart catheterization showing V waves and no step-up in oxygen saturations, and by echocardiogram.[22] The diagnosis of this complication of acute myocardial infarction warrants early surgery. Placement of an intraaortic balloon pump in addition to pharmacologic support is useful preoperatively and facilitates performance of coronary angiography, which is indicated, as well as anesthetic induction, at the time of surgery. Unoperated mortality rates exceed 50% in the first 24 hr.[21]

Surgical Treatment

Optimal myocardial protection is important in the surgical management of these patients. Complete revascularization using saphenous vein grafts is important. Generally, in the presence of a ruptured papillary muscle, valve repair cannot be performed and replacement is required. Mortality rates continue to remain high in this condition (up to 50%) due largely to the presence or existence infarction in this group. The mortality is increased by the presence of cardiogenic shock preoperatively, overall decreased left ventricle function, associated lesions such as ventricular septal defect, and any significant delay before surgery.[1]

Acute Valvar Endocarditis

Acute valvar endocarditis compounded by its attendant complications of insufficiency and sepsis may cause life-threatening acute congestive heart failure. The patient in this condition requires urgent evaluation by appropriate specialists including cardiologists, surgeons, and infectious disease experts. Patients with prosthetic valves, congenital heart disease, and renal failure requiring dialysis and intravenous drug abusers represent a unique but growing subgroup at increased risk for endocarditis and its complications.[23]

Organisms

The most common infecting organisms causing endocarditis are *Staphylococcus Aureus* and *Streptococcus Veridans*; together they are responsible for 75% to 85% of infections. Other infecting organisms, predominantly of the oropharyngeal or respiratory tracts, include in order, gram negative *Pseudomonas Aeruginosa* and *Klebsiella*, and group B streptococci. While much less common, infections with these organisms have greater risks for complications such as arterial emboli and annular and splenic abscesses, and consequently require earlier intervention.[24–26]

Fungal infections from organisms such as *Candida* or *Aspergillus* also are rare in otherwise immunocompetent hosts, but extremely difficult to sterilize and usually require early surgery to eradicate.[27] Pneumococcal endocarditis occurs much less frequently since it is sensitive to penicillin; however, subpopulations of patients without spleens (postsplenectomy or asplenics with congenital heart disease) continue to remain at risk, especially if there is a lapse or absence of antibiotic prophylaxis.[28] Other rarely reported causative organisms have included brucellosis, hemophilus, gonococcus, and mycobacterium, in particular, atypical mycobacterium from contaminated porcine valves.[29–32]

Diagnosis

The patient with sudden-onset congestive heart failure with either insufficiency or rarely a stenotic murmur, fever, and chills, recent genitourinary tract manipulation, dental-oral surgery, skin infection, or history of arterial embolus is clearly endocarditis until proven otherwise. Patients also may present with a history as well as signs of intravenous drug abuse in as many as 20% to 30% of cases, depending on the patient population. A small but significant subgroup also at risk for particularly severe endocarditis that may not be responsive to antibiotic therapy are human immunodeficiency virus (HIV)-positive patients.[33]

Two-dimensional echocardiography is the mainstay for evaluating valve function, structure, and presence or absence of vegetations and abscesses.[34] Vegetations larger than 2 to 3 mm in any dimension can be visualized by M-mode technique, providing specific information concerning location, mobility, and size. Vegetations greater than 1 cm and with a pedunculated shape are at greater risk for causing emboli (26%) compared to the smaller and more sessile vegetations.[35]

Accuracy in diagnosis and delineating the anatomy is further improved with the use of transesophageal echocardiography, particularly in cases involving the mitral valve, with sensitivities improving from 75% to 100%.[36] Other tests that have been used and may provide additional information include measurements of C-reactive protein reflecting response to therapy, magnetic resonance imaging to delineate annular abscesses, and, finally, fast computerized tomography of the chest and abdomen to diagnose splenic infarcts and abscesses that can occur in up to 20% of patients.[37–39]

Native Valve Endocarditis

In most series of the general population, valves are affected in the following order of incidence: aortic 50% to 70%, mitral 25% to 35%, combined aortic-mitral 10% to 15%, and, finally, tricuspid 5%. An underlying valve abnormality may be present in up to 50% of the cases and may include a bicuspid aortic valve, subaortic stenosis (usually discrete), rheumatic mitral valve disease, and repaired valves with congenital heart disease such as partial or complete atrial ventricular canal.[40,41] Prosthetic valve infections may account for up to 33% of the patients (see section on Prosthetic Valves).

The most common indication for surgery is severe congestive heart failure and hemodynamic deterioration in up to 90%, with the remainder divided between unremitting sepsis, life-threatening arterial emboli, and intracardiac extension. The operative mortality rates vary in some series from a low of 2.5% to 18.5%, with the preponderance around 10% to 12%. Preoperative multiorgan failure was the cause of most deaths with predictors of operative mortality preoperative shock, pulmonary edema, cerebrovascular accident, as well as annular abscess, *S. aureus*, or fungal organisms. Therefore, timing of the operation before significant organ damage has occurred is vital for a satisfactory outcome. Actuarial 5-yr survival of 65% to 75% is relatively poor, considering the generally acceptable operative and hospital mortality rates achievable, and underscores the overall severity of this disease.[42–44] See Table 31.3 for

TABLE 31.3. Surgical intervention for acute endocarditis.

Site	Procedure	Operative mortality (%)
Aortic valve	Replacement	5–13
Mitral valve	Repair or replacement	5
Tricuspid valve	Replacement	7–10
Prosthetic valve	Replacement	10–15

procedures and mortality for valvular surgery in acute endocarditis.

Aortic Valve Surgery

The aortic valve has a relatively low likelihood for repair in the face of acute infection causing cuspal perforation or, frequently, virtual destruction of the valve. Other possible findings at the time of surgery include gross vegetations, single- or multiple-abscess cavities, and purulent pericarditis. One should always inspect the mitral valve to rule out involvement as typically there may be a leaflet perforation secondary to a regurgitant jet lesion. Cultures should be carefully obtained on all intraoperative specimens.

Since up to 50% of the excised valve material will grow the underlying organism in acute cases, a wide excision and debridement is indicated, in particular with associated root abscesses, followed by replacement with a homograft valve as the optimum therapy.[45,46] The aortic homografts may be placed as an isolated valve or with replacement of the root depending on the extent of root deformity and destruction. Because the risk for reinfection is virtually nil, the exclusive use of allograft and autologous material such as pericardium for the repair helps to insure a favorable result.

The presence of preoperative conduction abnormalities occurs almost exclusively with aortic valve endocarditis, and generally is an indication of annular abscesses, requiring urgent surgery.[47] Root abscesses are most commonly located in the noncoronary sinus and have been repaired with an autologous pericardial or Dacron patch and valve replacement, with a 5% to 13% mortality rate.[48,49] With extensive annular destruction, a prosthetic valve may be inserted in the ascending aorta with insertion of vein bypass grafts from the distal ascending aorta to the coronary arteries. The rare complication of sinus of Valsalva aneurysm and fistula also requires early surgical intervention.[50]

Mitral Valve Surgery

The mitral valve, because of its more redundant valve tissue and often localized disease process, generally is more amenable to valve repair for endocarditis-associated insufficiency. This decision is of course based on the extent of any premorbid valve pathology that may occur in up to 60% of patients.[51] The use of trans-esophageal echocardiography may be particularly helpful in assessing the mitral valve structure and function. The rare case of mitral stenosis secondary to endocarditis necessitates complete removal of the extensive vegetations and replacement.[52]

At the time of surgery, the findings may include, in order of frequency, chordal rupture, cuspal perforation, vegetation, and annular abscess. General principles for repair include wide excision of macroscopic disease. Autologous pericardium treated with 0.06% glutaraldehyde to provide tensile strength can be used to repair defects in the annulus from abscess erosion and to resuspend or replace the mitral valve if necessary. Using these basic principles, it is possible to repair the mitral valve in acute infections with a mortality rate of less than 5% and with satisfactory long-term functional results with mild or trace regurgitation.[53,54] In the face of extensive destruction of the valve, replacement is required.

Tricuspid Valve Surgery

Endocarditis of the tricuspid valve is found largely in patients who are intravenous drug abusers or who have indwelling central venous catheters. They may present with severe right-sided failure, but frequently can be supported with unloading therapy while attempting antibiotic sterilization.

A major indication for surgery therefore is less likely to be severe congestive heart failure, as in the left-sided lesions, but rather unresponsive sepsis and associated recurrent pulmonary emboli. If vegetations are larger than 1 cm in any diameter, antibiotic therapy alone is less likely to have a favorable outcome.[55] Preexisting valve pathology such as an Ebstein-like tricuspid valve is both more predisposed to endocarditis and would possibly require earlier intervention due to hemodynamic compromise. Overall, about 25% of tricuspid endocarditis patients will need surgery for either severe congestive heart failure or continued sepsis.[56]

Bacterial endocarditis secondary to intravenous drug abuse is a more virulent subgroup due to the heavy, and often repeated, innoculum, with wide dissemination before seeking medical care. Indeed, in a large review, the tricuspid valve alone was involved 30% of the time, right- and left-sided valves in 16%, a single left-sided valve in 41%, and both left-sided valves in 13%. The overall mortality rate in the first year after surgery is approximately 50%, while the operative mortality is 10% to 12%, thus underscoring the high rate of complications and recidivism in these patients.[57,58] If congestive heart failure alone is the indication for surgery, the success of repair using autologous pericardium or even "vegetectomy" may be possible, but significantly less often than the overall rate of 60% or greater for patients with sepsis, the main indication.[59,60]

Removal of the entire tricuspid valve may lead to severe congestive heart failure in as many as a third of the patients, which can then affect the left-sided hemodynamics through changes in geometry as well.[61] The patient already in severe acute failure therefore will require a valve replacement to restore normal cardiac function. Patients who abstain from further intravenous drug abuse, while having a slightly higher operative mortality of 7% to 10%, generally have a favorable outcome. Those who do not, unfortunately a significant number of patients, account for the overall poor prognosis of 50% survival in the first year after surgery.[62,63]

Prosthetic Valve Endocarditis

The risk of prosthetic valve endocarditis is less than 2% over the lifetime of the implanted valves. However, the higher risk of degeneration of the bioprosthetic valves places them at greater risk for infection due to turbulence on the leaflets themselves. The infection of both mechanical and bioprosthesis at the sewing ring appears equal, and commonly results in valve ring abscesses. Perivalvular leaks therefore are common presentations, the extent of which influences the degree and severity of congestive heart failure.[64,65] Earlier operations have improved the mortality rate from 30% to between 10% and 15%, and is indicated when hemodynamic instability ensues, particularly from a malfunctioning mechanical or obstructive bioprosthetic valve. Other indications for surgery previously discussed for native valve endocarditis are even stronger indications with prosthetic valve endocarditis.[66,67]

Cardiac Allograft Failure

Early Rejection

The incidence of acute congestive heart failure or power failure immediately after cardiac transplantation is rare (<3–5%) and is related to either hyperacute rejection or to acute right ventricular failure with subsequent low output.[68] The measurement of percentage reactive antibodies samples cytotoxic antibodies to a representative panel of humans and if >15%, an individual crossmatch to the donor is mandatory, and greatly lessens the risk of a hyperacute rejection occurring. In general, because of logistics of obtaining the tests, a local donor only may be considered and evaluated. Patients may be stable for minutes or hours and even days before developing severe congestive heart failure and cardiogenic shock from rejection.

The best therapy is supportive in the form of inotropes, intraaortic balloon pump, and ventricular assist devices, while the immunosuppressive regimen is administered to reverse the rejection. This includes prednisolone in 1-g boluses; OKT3, a monoclonal T3 analogue, or antithymocyte globulin. Both cytolytic agents, they have also been useful, in addition to the standard therapy of cyclosporine.[69] The risk of a repeat rejection is high with urgent retransplantation, although a donor-recipient crossmatch might better guide the decision. The use of plasmapheresis has been successful in patients who have elevated percentage reactive antibodies due to prior antigenic exposure through blood transfusions and/or childbirth.[69]

Acute Right Ventricle Failure

Right heart failure often occurs immediately after transplantation if the pulmonary vascular resistance of the recipient is unacceptably elevated relative to the donor heart. If able to compensate, a small to moderate amount of right ventricle failure is well tolerated and reversed over the ensuing 48 to 72 hr, through the use of inotropes, in particular isuprel, and PGE_1 a prostaglandin afterload reducing agent, effective on pulmonary, renal, and systemic vasculature to a lesser degree.[70] The patient with severe right heart failure, followed frequently by left heart failure secondary to geometric changes of the right ventricle and interventricular septum, as well as the poor forward flow and decreased left ventricle filling, can result in profound congestive heart failure. It is important to match the donor and recipient properly to avoid the possibility of right ventricle dysfunction, by selecting a larger donor and excellent right ventricle function for those patients with higher pulmonary vascular resistance. The need for ventricular assist devices must be individualized, but generally are not necessary to reverse the failure, if the initial acceptance has accurately assessed the recipient's pulmonary artery pressures and pulmonary vascular resistance, and if, in general, the transpulmonary gradient is <15 mm Hg.

Late Rejection

Late mortality from transplantation is from chronic rejection and the development of atherosclerosis, with a presentation usually of more chronic congestive heart failure. However, the sudden loss of a major vessel (usually without the signs of anginal pain) may present with sudden congestive heart failure, requiring pharmacologic and mechanical supports as indicated, until either a revascularization procedure is carried out successfully or the patient is retransplanted after an urgent evaluation. The chance for a successful revascularization procedure with either PTCA or coronary artery bypass graft is small, as transplant atherosclerosis affects both large and small vessels and is diffuse as well as being insidious in onset.

At any point posttransplant, a patient's acute congestive heart failure may well be due to acute fulminant rejection, usually due to noncompliance and rarely to gastrointestinal mal- or nonabsorption secondary to viral or bacterial illnesses. The blood levels of cyclosporine will help to answer that question, and indeed extremely low or nondetectable levels secondary to noncompliance represents a contraindication to retransplantation, should the rescue therapy be unsuccessful.

Conclusions

In summary, the development of acute congestive heart failure is a medical and frequently a surgical emergency. It must be dealt with rapidly to prevent major organ damage and to be successful in reversing the underlying disease and its progression regardless of the primary etiology.

References

1. Balooki H. Emergency cardiac procedures in patients in cardiogenic shock due to complications of coronary artery disease. *Circulation*. 1989;79(Suppl I):I-137–148.
2. Killip T III, Kimball JT. Treatment of myocardial infarction in a coronary care unit: a two year experience with 250 patients. *Am J Cardiol*. 1967;20:457–464.
3. Alonso DR, Scheidt S, Post M, Killip T. Pathophysiology of cardiogenic shock: quantification of myocardial necrosis, clinical, pathologic, and electrocardiographic correlations. *Circulation*. 1973;48:588–596.
4. Page DL, Caulfield JB, Kastor JA, DeSanctis R, Sanders CA. Myocardial changes associated with cardiogenic shock. *N Engl J Med*. 1971;285:133–137.
5. Balooki H. Classification of cardiogenic shock. In Balooki H, ed. *Clinical Application of Intra-aortic Balloon Pump*. Mt. Kisco, NY: Futura Publishing; 1984:159–170.
6. Guyton RA, Arcidi JM Jr, Langford DA, Morris DC, Liberman HA, Hatcher CR Jr. Emergency coronary bypass for cardiogenic shock. *Circulation*. 1987;76(Suppl V):V-22–27.
7. Beyersdorf F, Acar C, Buckberg GD, et al. Studies on prolonged regional ischemia. III. Early natural history of simulated single and multivessel disease with emphasis on remote myocardium. *J Thorac Cardiovasc Surg*. 1989; 98:368–380.
8. Beyersdorf F, Acar C, Buckberg GD, et al. Studies on prolonged acute regional ischemia. IV. Aggressive surgical treatment for intractable ventricular fibrillation after acute myocardial infarction. *J Thorac Cardiovasc Surg*. 1989;98:557–566.
9. Pennington DG. Emergency management of cardiogenic shock. *Circulation*. 1989;79(Suppl I):I-149–151.
10. Allen BS, Rosenkranz E, Buckberg GD, et al. Myocardial infarction with left ventricular power failure: a medical/surgical emergency requiring urgent revascularization with maximal protection of remote muscle. *J Thorac Cardiovasc Surg*. 1989;98:691–703.
11. Pennington DG, Golding L, Hill JD, et al. Temporary mechanical support for cardiogenic shock. *Trans Am Soc Artif Intern Organs*. 186;32:629–632.
12. Drinkwater DC, Laks H, Buckberg GD. A new simplified method of optimizing cardioplegic delivery without right heart isolation: antegrade/retrograde blood cardioplegia. *J Thorac Cardiovasc Surg*. 1990;100(1):56–64.
13. Bates RJ, Beutler S, Resnekov L, Agnostopoulos CE. Cardiac rupture-challenge in diagnosis and management. *Am J Cardiol*. 1977;40:429–437.
14. Vlodaver Z, Coe JI, Edwards JE. True and false left ventricular aneurysms: propensity for the latter to rupture. *Circulation*. 1975;51:567–572.
15. Milgalter E, Uretzky G, Levy P, Borman JB, Appelbaum A. Pseudoaneurysms of the left ventricle. *Thorac Cardiovasc Surg*. 1987;35:20–25.
16. Hill D, Lary D, Kerth W, Gerbode R. Acquired ventricular septal defects. *J Thorac Cardiovasc Surg*. 1975;70:444.
17. Kitamura S, Mendez A, Kay JH. Ventricular septal defect following myocardial infarction: experience with surgical repair through a left ventriculotomy and review of the literature. *J Thorac Cardiovasc Surg*. 1971;61:186.
18. Sanders RJ, Kern WH, Blount SG. Perforation of the interventricular septum complicating myocardial infarction. *Am Heart J*. 1956;51:736.
19. Heitmiller R, Jacobs ML, Daggett WM. Surgical management of post infarction ventricular septal rupture. *Ann Thorac Surg*. 1986;41:683.
20. Cooley DA, Belmonte BA, Zeis LB, Schnur S. Surgical repair of ruptured interventricular septum following acute myocardial infarction. *Surgery*. 1957;41:930.
21. Kirklin JW, Barratt-Boyes BG, ed. *Cardiac Surgery*. New York: John Wiley and Sons; 1986;311–319.
22. Nishimura RA, Schaff HV, Shub C, Girsh BJ, Edwards WE, Tajik AJ. Papillary muscle rupture complicating acute myocardial infarction: analysis of 17 patients. *Am J Cardiol*. 1983;51:373.
23. Zamora JL, Burdine JT, Karlberg H, Shenaq SM, Noon GP. Cardiac surgery in patients with end-stage renal disease. *Ann Thorac Surg*. 1986;42(1):113–117.
24. David TE, Bos J, Christakis GT, Brofman PR, Wong D, Feindel CM. Heart valve operations in patients with active infective endocarditis. *Ann Thorac Surg*. 1990; 49(5):701–705.
25. Komshian SV, Tablan OC, Palutke W, Reyes MP. Characteristics of left sided endocarditis caused by pseudomonas aeruginosa in the Detroit Medical Center. *Rev Infect Dis*. 1990;12(4):693–702.
26. Pringle SD, McCartney AC, Marshall DA, Cobbe SM. Infective endocarditis caused by streptococcus agalactiae. *Int J Cardiol*. 1989;24(2):179–183.
27. Kawamoto T, Nakano S, Matsudo H, Hirose H, Kawashima Y. Candida endocarditis with saddle embolism: a sucessful surgical intervention. *Ann Thorac Surg*. 1989;5:723–724.
28. Maderazo EG, Hickingbotham N, Cooper B, Murcia A. Aspergillus endocarditis: cure without surgical valve replacement. *South Med J*. 1990;83(3):351–352.
29. Powderly WG, Stanley SL, Medoff G. Pneumococcal endocarditis: report of a series and review of the literature. *Rev Infect Dis*. 1986;8(5):786–791.

30. Burstein H, Sampson MB, Kohler JP, Levitsky S. Gonococcal endocarditis during pregnancy: Simultaneous caesarian section and aortic valve surgery. *Obstet Gynecol.* 1985;66(Suppl 3):485–519.

31. al-Harthi SS. The morbidity and mortality pattern of *Brucella* endocarditis. *Int J Cardiol.* 1989;25(3):321–324.

32. Rumisek JD, Albus RA, Clarke JS. Late mycobacterium chelonel bioprosthetic valve endocarditis: activation of implanted containment. *Ann Thorac Surg.* 1985;39(3):277–279.

33. Frater RW, Sisto D, Condit D. Cardiac surgery in human immunodeficiency virus (HIV) carriers. *Eur J Cardiothorac Surg.* 1989;3(2):146–150.

34. Sheiban I, Casarotto D, Trevi G, et al. Two-dimensional echocardiography in the diagnosis of intracardiac masses: a prospective study with anatomic validation. *Cardiovasc Intervent Radiol.* 1987;10(3):157–161.

35. Jaffe WM, Morgan DE, Pearlman AS, Otto CM. Infective endocarditis, 1983–1988: echocardiographic findings and factors influencing morbidity and mortality. *J Am Coll Cardiol.* 1990;15(6):1227–1233.

36. Popp RL. Medical progress—echocardiography. *N Engl J Med.* 1990;323(3):165–172.

37. McCartney AC, Orange GV, Pringle SD, Wills G, Reece IJ. Serum C reactive protein in infective endocarditis. *J Clin Pathol.* 1988;41(1):44–48.

38. Akins EW, Limacher M, Sloan RM, Hill JA. Evaluation of an aortic annular pseudoaneurysm by MRI: comparison with echocardiography, angiography, and surgery. *Cardiovasc Intervent Radiol.* 1987;10(4):188–193.

39. Ting W, Silverman NA, Arzouman DA, Levitsky S. Splenic septic emboli in endocarditis. *Circulation.* 1990;82(Suppl 5):IV105–109.

40. Karl T, Wensley D, Stark J, De Leval M, Rees P, Taylor JFN. Infective endocarditis in children with congenital heart disease: comparison of selected features in patients with surgical correction or palliation and those without. *Br Heart J.* 1987;58:57–65.

41. Alsip SG, Blackstone EH, Kirkilin JW, Cobbs CG. Indications for cardiac surgery in patients with active infective endocarditis. *Am J Med.* 1985;78(6B):138–148.

42. Agostino RS, Miller DC, Stinson EB, et al. Valve replacement in patients with native valve endocarditis: what really determines operative outcome? *Ann Thorac Surg.* 1985;40(5):429–438.

43. Soyer R, Redonnet M, Bessou JP, Mutel P, Hubscher C, Letac B. Valve replacement in acute native valve endocarditis. *Thorac Cardiovasc Surg.* 1986;34(3):149–152.

44. Tuna IC, Orszulak TA, Schaff HV, Danielson GK. Results of homograft aortic valve replacement for active endocarditis. *Ann Thorac Surg.* 1990;49(4):619–624.

45. Zwischenberger JB, Shalaby TZ, Conti VR. Viable cryopreserved aortic homograft for aortic valve endocarditis and annular abscesses. *Ann Thorac Surg.* 1989;48(3):364–369.

46. Okita Y, Franciosi G, Matsuki D, Robles A, Ross DN. Early and late results of aortic root replacement with antibiotic-sterilized homograft. *J Thorac Cardiovasc Surg.* 1988;95(4):696–704.

47. DiNubile MJ, Calderwood SB, Steinhaus DM, Karchmer AW. Cardiac conduction abnormalities complicating native valve active infective endocarditis. *Am J Cardiol.* 1986;58(13):1213–1217.

48. David TE, Komeda M, Brofman PR. Surgical treatment of aortic root abscess. *Circulation.* 1989;80:1269–1274.

49. Fiore AC, Ivey TD, McKeown PP, Misbach GA, Allen MD, Dillard DH. Patch closure of aortic annulus mycotic aneurysms. *Ann Thorac Surg.* 1986;42:372–379.

50. Shaffer EM, Snider AR, Beekman RH, Behrendt DM, Peschiera AW. Sinus of valsalva aneurysm complicating bacterial endocarditis in an infant: diagnosis with two-dimensional and doppler echocardiography. *J Am Cardiol.* 1987;9(3):588–591.

51. Dreyfus G, Serraf A, Jebara VA, et al. Valve repair in acute endocarditis. *Ann Thorac Surg.* 1990;49(5):706–711.

52. Ghosh PK, Miller HI, Vidne BA. Mitral obstruction in bacterial endocarditis. *Br Heart J.* 1985;53(3):341–344.

53. David TE, Feindel CM. Reconstruction of the mitral annulus. *Circulation.* 1987;76(3 pt 2):III102–107.

54. Fleisher AG, David I, Mogtader A, Hutchinson JE III. Mitral valvuloplasty and repair for infective endocarditis. *J Thorac Cardiovasc Surg.* 1987;93(2):311–315.

55. Robbins MJ, Soeiro R, Frishman WH, Strom JA. Right-sided valvular endocarditis: etiology, diagnosis, and an approach to therapy. *Am Heart J.* 1986;111(1):128–135.

56. Chan P, Ogilby JD, Segal B. Tricuspid valve endocarditis. *Am Heart J.* 1989;117(5):1140–1146.

57. Dressler FA, Roberts WC. Infective endocarditis in opiate addicts: analysis of 80 cases studied at necropsy. *Am J Cardiol.* 1989;117(5):1140–1146.

58. Mammana RB, Levitsky S, Sernaque D, Beckman CB, Silverman NA. Valve replacement for left-sided endocarditis in drug addicts. *Ann Thorac Surg.* 1989;35(4):436–441.

59. Yee ES, Khonsari S. Right-sided infective endocarditis: valvuloplasty, valvectomy, or replacement. *J Cardiovasc Surg.* 1989;30(5):744–748.

60. Hughs CF, Noble N. Vegetectomy, an alternative surgical treatment for infective endocarditis of the atrioventricular valves in drug addicts. *J Thorac Cardiovasc Surg.* 1988;95(5):857–861.

61. Louie EK, Bieniarz T, Moore AM, Levitsky S. Reduced atrial contribution to left ventricular filling in patients with severe tricuspid regurgitation after tricuspid valvulectomy: a doppler echocardiographic study. *J Am Coll Cardiol.* 1990;16(7):1617–1624.

62. Stern HJ, Sisto DA, Strom JA, Soeiro R, Jones SR, Frater RW. Immediate tricuspid valve replacement for endocarditis: indications and results. *J Thorac Cardiovasc Surg.* 1986;91(2):163–167.

63. Arbulu A, Asfaw I. Management of infective endocarditis: seventeen years' experience. *Ann Thorac Surg.* 1987;43(2):144–149.

64. Lewis JF, Peniston RL, Randall OS, Spencer J, Sheller LM. Tricuspid stenosis in prosthetic valve endocarditis. Diagnosis by doppler echocardiography. *Chest.* 1987;91(2):276–277.

65. Schulte HD, Horstkotte D, Evagelopoulos N, Bircks W, Loogen F. Reoperations for malfunction of heart valve prostheses, especially with endocarditis. *Thorac Cardiovasc Surg.* 1987;35(1):16–19.

66. Rochiccioli C, Chastre J, Lecompte Y, Gandjbakhch I, Gilbert C. Prosthetic valve endocarditis: the case for prompt surgical managment. *J Thorac Cardiovasc Surg.* 1986;92(4):784–789.
67. Cowgill LD, Addonizio VP, Hopeman AR, Harken AH. A practical approach to prosthetic valve endocarditis. *Ann Thorac Surg.* 1987;43(4):450–457.
68. Armitage JM, Hardesty RL, Griffith BP. Prostaglandin E₁: an effective treatment of right heart failure after orthotopic heart transplantation. *J Heart Transplant.* 1987;6;348–351.
69. Gilbert EM, Dewitt CW, Eiswirth CC, et al. Treatment of refractory cardiac allograft rejection with OKT3 monoclonal antibody. *Am J Med.* 1987;82:202.
70. Trento A, Hardesty RL, Griffith BP, et al. Role of the antibody to vascular endothelial cells in hyperacute rejection in patients undergoing cardiac transplantation. *J Thorac Cardiovasc Surg.* 1988;95:37–41.

Part VI
Approach to Patients with Chronic Congestive Heart Failure

32
The Diagnostic Evaluation of Patients with Heart Failure

James B. Young and John A. Farmer

Sir Thomas Lewis began his seminal text, *Diseases of the Heart*, emphasizing that the central problem in patients with heart disease is recognizing and quantifying severity of heart failure as early as possible.[1] Braunwald highlighted this fact, contemporizing the point by stating ". . . More than a half century later, the situation has changed little, in that a principle complication of virtually all forms of heart disease is heart failure . . ."[2] Paul Dudley White may have only slightly overstated the issue when he noted ". . . myocardial insufficiency giving rise to congestive heart failure is the commonest of the important functional disorders of the heart."[3] Obviously, it is important to recognize this condition, although the heart failure syndrome has changed today. Now, patients with heart failure are older, have more ischemic heart disease, less valvular pathology, and are on many medications.[4]

The diagnostic evaluation of heart failure is not a simple matter of auscultating pulmonary rales and a gallop rhythm in an edematous patient complaining of dyspnea and fatigue. Furthermore, a wide spectrum of diseases can cause abnormal cardiac chamber filling or emptying. Although pathologic chamber flow dynamics are the root problem in patients with heart failure, it is their production of symptoms and physical findings that collectively create a syndrome. It is critical to remember that this syndrome has varying etiology, can be acute or chronic in presentation, and may have congestive elements that appear at occasionally unpredictable intervals. Furthermore, patients may have differing presentations based on predominance of diastolic or systolic dysfunction and selective cardiac chamber involvement (atrial vs. ventricular; right vs. left heart). Importantly, evaluation of patients with heart failure must include efforts to characterize its etiology, stage severity, and identify factors that may have precipitated clinical decompensation.

Four critical questions must be asked whenever a heart failure evaluation is planned: What caused the problem? Is the patient's prognosis poor? Can symptoms be eliminated or ameliorated? What can be done to cure or treat the underlying difficulty? Data must also be obtained to allow appropriate design of therapeutic maneuvers to prevent, cure, or treat various aspects of the heart failure syndrome. Indeed, we believe it is essential to identify patients with heart failure early in their syndrome course to have a greater chance of successfully addressing underlying diseases or, at least, to prevent further myocardial dysfunction and clinical deterioration.

The diagnostic evaluation of heart failure, therefore, is critical in differentiating this difficulty from other system malfunction, staging the syndrome severity, providing insightful prognostic information, and laying groundwork for therapeutic interventions (Fig. 32.1).

The Heart Failure Milieu

The Heart Failure Syndrome

The heart failure syndrome occurs as a milieu of symptoms and physical findings interact to create a characteristic portrait. These symptoms and findings represent a complicated intertwining of events (Fig. 32.2). The diagnostic evaluation of heart failure must take this fact into consideration since attention needs to be focused not only on underlying precipitating factors, but also on the type of ventricular dysfunction that occurs, resultant hemodynamic abnormalities, subsequent compensating mechanisms, and metabolic changes that develop.

One should review Figure 32.2 with dynamic imagination, since the heart failure milieu is constantly changing. Patients' symptoms are exacerbated or attenuated depending on fluctuation in hemodynamic abnormalities, compensating mechanisms, or success of therapeutic intervention. The representative circles in this diagram should be imagined to pulsate, and well planned

The Evaluation of Heart Failure Patients

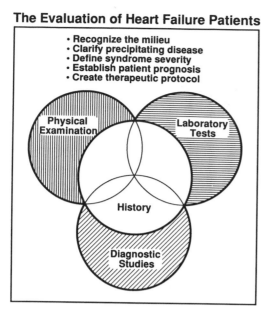

FIGURE 32.1. The purpose of the diagnostic evaluation of heart failure patients is to recognize the process, differentiate cardiac abnormalities from other system malfunction, stage the syndrome severity, provide insightful prognostic information, and lay groundwork for therapy. An evaluation will include appropriate history, physical examination, and laboratory and specialized diagnostic studies.

patient evaluations tailored to focus appropriately on each of the intertwined environments.

Heart Failure Definition

The heart failure state can be defined clinically as a condition where ventricular dysfunction (or sometimes atrial or valvular dysfunction) causes limitation in an individual's ability to perform certain physical tasks. This limitation is primarily created by syndromes of dyspnea and fatigue. From a pathophysiologic viewpoint, heart failure occurs when the metabolic demands of a patient cannot be supported by intrinsic cardiac function. Specifically, cellular respiration is impaired when nutrient delivery is compromised.

Pathophysiology

James Hope, in 1832, first proposed the concept of backward heart failure occurring due to, as Braunwald says, "damming up of blood behind one or both ventricles."[5,6] James McKenzie suggested in 1913 that the clinical symptoms of heart failure were due to the inadequate delivery of arterial blood to tissues and organs.[7] Both descriptions are directional characterizations of a state without single symptomatic vector, but do serve to emphasize that symptoms and physical findings seem mostly related to tissue congestion and

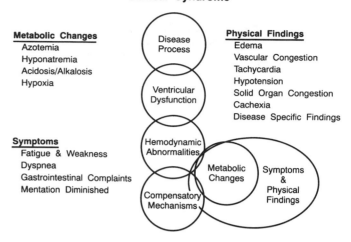

FIGURE 32.2. The heart failure milieu is characterized by an important intertwining of primary diseases producing ventricular dysfunction and subsequent hemodynamic abnormalities that eventually precipitate varying symptoms and physical findings.

organ hypoperfusion. As our diagnostic sophistication and pathophysiologic insight increase, older concepts such as "backward" and "forward" heart failure have been modified. We now realize that a subtle interplay exists between cardiac output, tissue perfusion, and volume-loading states, and that difficulties occur much earlier in the course of heart failure than was once thought. These patients require evaluation sooner rather than later.

As the severity of the precipitating disease changes, symptoms and findings can vary. It is important to remember when planning diagnostic evaluation that patients may present with acute pulmonary congestion due to severe diastolic dysfunction precipitated by hypertension and ventricular ischemia or that symptoms might have been developing slowly over several months as a heart dilates because of slow, subtle, chronic, and devastating alcohol poisoning (Fig. 32.3).

In Figure 32.3, patient 1 represents a hypothetical situation where myocardial injury is steadily progressive over time, causing gradual clinical deterioration. Patient 2 has an acute event precipitating a sudden drop in performance. Treatment improves this individual substantially and he is stable for a long period of time. Patient 3 has several sudden events, such as acute myocardial infarction, that increase significant deterioration with each episode and additive clinical deterioration. Patient 4 has a less rapid but substantial initial deterioration that, despite treatment, causes substantial impairment of clinical performance. This figure serves to remind one of the importance placed on individualized diagnostic evaluation and treatment schemes.

FIGURE 32.3. Patients can present at different points in their illness because of a variety of factors including type of initial disease process, amount of myocardial damage, and ability of the system to compensate. This figure graphically demonstrates the course of four patients. The approach to diagnosis and therapy would be expected to be different in each patient.

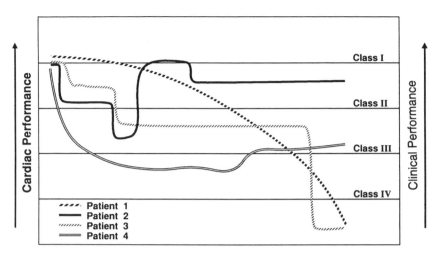

Role of History Taking and Physical Examination

Evaluation of patients with heart failure should include collecting certain historical facts, documenting pertinent physical findings, and obtaining selected laboratory and specialized diagnostic tests. Information obtained usually allows identification of the disease causing the cardiac dysfunction and staging the syndrome's severity, and facilitates prognostication. Most importantly, the data should guide therapeutic ministrations (Fig. 32.1).

The Clinical History

Gathering information that documents syndrome presentation is the first important task when heart failure symptoms are suspected or when cardiac dysfunction is discovered. Short-windedness can be a sentinel complaint. Table 32.1 lists symptoms often associated with heart failure. Elucidation of these is mandatory.

Breathlessness

Dyspnea is both a hallmark of heart failure and other pathologic conditions. Some of the many causes of dyspnea and exercise intolerance are detailed in Table 32.2. Dyspnea can be a useful marker of disease severity or therapeutic success. The sensation of difficult, labored, and uncomfortable breathing is actually related to pulmonary congestion, which decreases lung compliance and, subsequently, increases work of respiration.[8] Short-windedness may increase in severity as pulmonary congestion worsens, progressing from dyspnea on exertion, orthopnea, paroxysmal nocturnal dyspnea, or finally, dyspnea at rest. Acute pulmonary edema with a respiratory crisis may be the final point in this pathway and can be reached either suddenly, with little suggestion of prior respiratory limitation, or after progressing through each of the above-listed preceding stages.

Everyone can relate to the sensation of dyspnea. Even a healthy, vigorous, athletic individual can empathize with the description of short-windedness proffered by a heart failure patient. The distinction between the patient's complaint and an Olympic sprinter's sensation of short-windedness is simply the level of physical activity required to elicit the sensation and its persistence after exercise has been terminated. This example emphasizes one of the cardinal issues in taking a history from patients with heart failure, quantification, in some fashion, of the factors that elicit symptoms. With quantification, the syndrome's severity can be assessed and therapeutic success judged. We will repeatedly address methods that can objectively measure parameters to quantify dysfunction severity and subsequent physical limitation.

Orthopnea should be explored and quantified as well. As a patient with congestive heart failure (CHF) lies supine, intrathoracic blood volume increases and left ventricular (CHF) filling pressure rises. Subsequently, pulmonary hypertension develops. Similar in general to dyspnea, orthopnea is not specific for heart failure. It may occur in any state, causing diminished vital capacity, and can be worsened when the diaphragm is elevated as the patient reclines.

The suffocating sensation that awakens a supine patient, usually at night, is termed "paroxysmal nocturnal dyspnea" and is a symptom implying very severe heart failure. Wheezing is frequently appreciated in these patients because bronchospasm can occur with acute pulmonary congestion. The sensation is frightening and may take 30 to 60 min to resolve with the patient seated upright.

TABLE 32.1. The clinical history in heart failure.

Specific history to obtain[a]

Cardiovascular
    Angina pectoris
    Nonspecific chest pain
    Fatigue
    Weakness
    Orthostatic faintness
Pulmonary
    Dyspnea on exertion
    Orthopnea
    Paroxysmal nocturnal dyspnea
    Pleurisy
    Cough
    Hemoptysis
Gastroenterologic
    Abdominal pain
    Abdominal bloating
    Constipation
    Anorexia
    Nausea
    Vomiting
Neurologic/neuropsychiatric
    Anxiety or panic
    Depression
    Confusion
    Decreased mental acuity
Renal
    Nocturia
    Oliguria
Systemic
    Edema
    Petechiae/ecchymosis

[a] Ancillary history that elucidates concomitant cardiovascular and noncardiovascular illnesses is critical.

TABLE 32.2. Noncardiac causes of dyspnea and exercise intolerance.

Difficulty	Resulting problems
Anemia	Diminished O_2 carrying capacity with high cardiac output states
Chest wall deformity	Inadequate ventilation
Malingering	Hyperventilation or inadequate effort
Obesity	Increased workload
Peripheral vascular disease	Impaired muscle perfusion
Physical deconditioning	Ineffective systemic circulation
Pulmonary abnormalities	
Airflow limitations	Obstructed ventilation
Restrictive alveolar disease	Inadequate ventilation
Ventilation/perfusion mismatch	Impaired gas exchange

cessive mucous production.[8] Sometimes hemoptysis can occur with the cough after rupture of distended bronchial capillaries. Obviously, cough can also be caused by primary lung disease as well.

As mentioned, pulmonary congestion caused by disadvantageous hydrostatic forces in the pulmonary capillary beds produces dyspnea by increasing the work of respiration. It is important to differentiate the symptoms of breathlessness, cough, and hemoptysis due to heart failure from those symptoms caused by primary pulmonary or neurologic difficulties that can precipitate dyspnea as well. Furthermore, it is not uncommon to have two diseases with distinct pathophysiology present in the same patient, and differentiating the contribution of each to a patient's symptoms can be challenging. Pulmonary function testing may be helpful in those cases and will be discussed separately.

Cough

Cough often is associated with these syndromes of breathlessness. This sensation may be interpreted as a "dyspnea equivalent" and is generally nonproductive and occurs in settings in which one would expect to see dyspnea, such as with exertion or at night when the patient is recumbent. It has become more challenging today, however, to ascribe cough to pulmonary congestion in some patients with LF dysfunction because of the common use of angiotensin-converting enzyme (ACE) inhibitors. These agents can occasionally induce a dry, hacking, forceful cough as a side effect.[9] This problem is generally more spontaneous than the heart failure cough, which is more common during exertion or at night. In the large clinical trial, Studies of Left Ventricular Dysfunction, cough was seen in 30.2% of the placebo-treated patients and 35.0% of those on enalapril (4.8% excess). These were generally New York Heart Association (NYHA) class III or IV patients with symptomatic heart failure.[10] The tussive effect of heart failure is secondary to bronchiolar congestion with ex-

Fatigue and Weakness

Because of the low blood flow state often evident in the heart failure syndrome, another cardinal complaint patients proffer is fatigue with weakness. Those complaints are nonspecific, but in the setting of breathlessness with ventricular dysfunction, they become a critical component of a patient's history.[11] Diminished skeletal muscle perfusion undoubtedly accounts for these symptoms, but the complaints also relate to peripheral edema and electrolyte abnormalities. Simple exercise deconditioning can contribute to this problem as well.

Nocturia and Oliguria

When patients with the heart failure syndrome lie supine, a redistribution of blood flow occurs and renal perfusion increases.[12] Furthermore, with diminished global oxygen demands, peripheral vasoconstriction becomes less intense and renal perfusion transiently improves. Since many heart failure patients are volume overloaded, a nocturnal diuresis occurs and urinary frequency can develop during sleeping hours. On the other hand, when heart failure is extremely severe, patients may complain of oliguria. This complaint is, however, much less frequent than nocturia because of the difficulties most patients have quantifying their urine output versus the apparent inconvenience of rising several times at night to urinate.

Central Nervous System and Psychiatric Complaints

Any diminution in cerebral vascular blood flow can cause alteration in mental acuity. Congestive hepatopathy or cardiac cirrhosis might precipitate hepatic encephalopathy. Patients, or their close companions, may note confusion, disorientation, or memory impairment. Symptomatic complaints referable to these problems suggest very severe heart failure. Sometimes these difficulties can be precipitated or exacerbated by drugs used to treat heart failure. For example, excessive hypotension induced by vasodilators can cause confusion.

Since heart failure can produce devastating and frightening symptoms it is not surprising that patients may voice complaints of depression and anxiety. Indeed, differentiation of dyspnea secondary to heart failure from hyperventilation, anxiety neurosis, and panic attack can be challenging.

Chest Pain

Since ischemic heart disease is associated with LV dysfunction, angina pectoris can be a common complaint in patients with heart failure. As congestion develops, ventricular wall stress increases and myocardial oxygen demand rises. Ischemia therefore can be exacerbated during heart failure.[13] Also, many patients with severe pulmonary hypertension due to LV failure or mitral stenosis complain of typical exertional angina despite having normal coronary anatomy. The etiology of this pain is not entirely clear but may relate to right ventricular ischemia secondary to pulmonary hypertension.[14] These forms of chest pain are generally exertional in nature but also can occur when assuming the supine position. Referred pain in the chest or back from a distended liver or spleen can also be a problem; however, this discomfort is generally nonexertional and more sharp or pleuritic in nature. Since patients with CHF have venous stasis, peripheral venous thrombosis and subsequent pulmonary embolism can occur. Thus, the pleuritic pain of pulmonary infarction could be a component of the heart failure milieu.

Gastrointestinal Complaints

Because congestion and edema occur in the mesentery and the liver and spleen, a variety of gastrointestinal complaints are common in patients with heart failure. Right upper quadrant fullness and even pain can frequently be noted. Patients often complain of generalized abdominal bloating and fullness. Anorexia may be bothersome and relates to diminished gastric and mesenteric peristalsis engendered by bowel edema. Often, nausea and vomiting are encountered and can be due to the aforementioned edema or the effects of treatment with digitalis or dopaminergic receptor-stimulating compounds. Constipation can be a problem as well.

Faintness and Syncope

Dizziness or synocope is commonly seen in patients with heart failure and these complaints may be exacerbated by vasodilators. In the Treatment Trial of Studies of Left Ventricular Dysfunction more than 30% of patients in the placebo limb had these complaints.[10] Enalapril increased the problems by about 6%. Syncope can be due to orthostatic changes in arterial blood pressure or even exertional exacerbation of pulmonary hypertension. Also, exertional syncope is seen in patients with heart failure due to aortic stenosis, hypertrophic obstructive cardiomyopathy, and pulmonary valve stenosis. Arrhythmias can be a common component of heart failure and ventricular tachycardia or heart block also causes syncope or even sudden cardiac death.

Edema

Patients will frequently complain of peripheral edema, noting inability to wear familiar footwear and alternating exacerbation and resolution of lower extremity swelling with positional change.

Ancillary Clinical Information

In addition to complaints usually associated with heart failure as detailed above, the clinician should pursue symptoms that might suggest other specific disease entities. Obviously, there can be a great deal of overlap between heart failure symptoms and difficulties caused by other diseases. For example, hypothyroidism may cause additional complaints of lethargy and weakness, amyloidosis can create symptoms of hepatic failure, and high output states created by hyperthyroidism, anemia, or arteriovenous fistulae can produce unique symptomology. Fever is a rare complaint of patients with severe heart failure and great care must be exercised to exclude infectious problems such as endocarditis, which may cause heart failure.

Physical Examination

The second important evaluation component is the physical examination. By coupling a patient's symptoms

TABLE 32.3. Physical examination of heart failure patients.

Specific physical findings to pursue[a]

Vital signs
   Positional blood pressure
   Pulse rate, rhythm, and quality
   Respiratory rate and pattern
   Temperature
Cardiovascular
   Neck vein distention
   Abdominal-jugular neck vein reflex
   Cardiomegaly on palpitation
   Chest wall pulsatile activity
   Gallop rhythm on auscultation
   Heart murmurs (especially mitral, tricuspid, and pulmonic
     insufficiency)
   Diminished S_1 or S_2
   Friction rubs
Pulmonary
   Rales
   Rhonchi
   Friction rubs
   Wheezes
   Dullness of percussion
Abdominal
   Ascites
   Hepatosplenomegaly
   Decreased bowel sounds
Neurologic
   Mental status abnormalities
Systemic
   Edema
   Cachexia

[a]Ancillary physical examination information that elucidates concomitant cardiovascular and noncardiovascular illnesses is critical.

with the spectrum of physical abnormalities noted in the heart failure milieu, questions regarding disease etiology, syndrome severity, and appropriate therapy may be answered (Table 32.3).

General Assessment

Patients in the early stages of heart failure usually do not appear distressed. Resting dyspnea and tachycardia are not present and the blood pressure is normal or elevated. Simple tasks, though, such as undressing for the examination or ambulating in the clinic, can produce heart failure signs such as tachycardia, tachypnea, or gallop rhythm. Severe heart failure may be easy to discern with a quick visual examination of the patient when observations of jugular venous distension, cyanosis, icterus, head-bob due to tricuspid regurgitation, and cachexia are made. General nutritional status should be assessed at this time, although more formal testing of nitrogen balance may be done as an ancillary procedure. Clues to other diseases may be noted at this point with exophthalmus and goiter. One should note, however, that the hyperadrenergic state seen in some heart failure patients may cause findings similar to

hyperthyroidism! Again, the clinician must be perceptive when evaluating the relationship between the heart failure milieu and underlying precipitating diseases.

Vital Signs

Blood pressure determination is critical and should be done with the patient supine, seated, and standing to determine whether orthostatic changes occur. Extremity pressure equity should be noted. This is particularly important in patients receiving vasodilating, diuretic, or antihypertensive drugs. Heart rate determination also is essential since resting tachycardia, particularly when unassociated with hyperthyroidism or anemia, suggests severe myocardial decompensation. Likewise, the clinical diagnosis of arrhythmia is important. Irregular pulses suggesting atrial fibrillation and extrasystoles occurring in the pattern of premature ventricular contractions will need further exploration with electrocardiography, both static and ambulatory.

Pulse quality is also important, with a weak and thready pulse or pulses alternans suggesting quite severe LV dysfunction. Pulses alternans is a unique pulse beat noted in patients with regular rhythm who have alternation of strong and weak pulse pressure. The pulses are equally spaced and this is quite different from pulses bigeminus, where a weak beat follows stronger pulse volumes by a shorter time interval. This later pulse is characteristic of individuals having ventricular bigeminy. Pulses alternans can best be felt by palpating the peripheral pulses (the femoral artery being the preferred location). Pulses alternans is usually associated with an S-3 gallop and suggests extremely severe and advanced myocardial disease. A paradoxic pulse can also be felt in some patients with severe LV dysfunction. Again, by palpating peripheral pulses, particularly the femoral or brachial artery, diminution in systolic or pulse pressure can be appreciated as the patient inspires in his usual quiet, rhythmic pattern. This pulse finding is often associated with a paradoxic increase in jugular venous distension and the presence of pericardial effusion. When this constellation of finding is present, the possibility of cardiac tamponade should be considered.

As mentioned above, a low grade fever can be noted during vital sign assessment in patients with severe heart failure. Temperature elevation in these patients results from impaired heat transfer due to cutaneous vasoconstriction. The temperature associated with heart failure is generally less than 38°C, and one must always consider the possibility of infection or pulmonary infarction in the febrile heart failure patient.

Respiratory rate and pattern are important to observe during vital sign assessment. Tachypnea suggests substantive respiratory impairment and periodic respiration points toward very severe heart failure. Cheyne-Stokes breathing patterns occur because of depression in the sensitivity of respiratory centers to carbon dioxide and low flow states due to LV dysfunction.[15] This type of respiration is characterized by increasing depth of respiration with concomitant respiratory rate increase. This is then followed by sudden apnea for several seconds. Often, the patients' companions will complain of the disturbing oscillation between apnea and hyperpnea, particularly noticeable during sleep, and frequently associated with loud snoring. In some cases, obstructive sleep apnea may be present.

Pulmonary Examination

Fine, crepitent rales are frequently heard in heart failure patients when pulmonary edema fluid seeps into the alveoli. Generally, they are noted in the bases of the lungs and with worsening amounts of pulmonary edema they progress toward the apices. The absence of pulmonary rales, however, does not exclude pulmonary congestion and rales frequently are not heard in patients with chronic heart failure and long-standing congestive states. The reason for this is the development of compensatory changes in perivascular structure and in lymphatic drainage, both of which serve to prevent the accumulation of excessive fluid in the alveoli. Expiratory wheezes are frequently heard over both lung fields when severe pulmonary edema is present and may or may not be accompanied by rales. When wheezes are heard and accompanied by expectoration of frothy and blood-tinged sputum, patients have severe congestion.

Since pulmonary emboli with infarction of lung tissue is possible in the heart failure milieu, rubs may also be present and should be listened for. Rhonchi, a component of the exam in many patients with obstructive pulmonary disease, can give a clue to the presence of a concomitant complicating syndrome. Excessive bronchiolar secretions, however, can also precipitate rhonchi. This once again emphasizes the difficulty encountered in making an appropriate differential diagnosis.

The presence of percussed dullness over the posterior thorax also is important since pleural fluid accumulation can be a manifestation of the congested state. Although pleural fluid accumulation is generally bilateral, the right thorax is usually affected to a greater extent than the left. When hydrothorax is found solely on the left, another etiology for the pleural effusion must be considered. Common problems producing an isolated left pleural effusion are pulmonary malignancy and infarction of the left lung.

Elevation of Neck Veins

Systemic venous hypertension is suggested when jugular venous distension can be documented. When a patient is examined while amgulated 45° above the bed, the jugular veins normally are less than 4 cm above the sternal angle. Elevation of neck veins higher than this level,

measured with the patient breathing normally, suggests congestion. Furthermore, the pattern of pulse wave formation can give insight into cardiac pathology. When there is substantive tricuspid regurgitation, a prominent V wave with exaggerated Y descent is easily seen. The A wave, on the other hand, is more prominent than the V wave when right ventricular filling is impaired by either tricuspid valve stenosis, or as a reaction to pulmonary hypertension or pulmonic valve stenosis. Elevation of the jugular veins is normally attenuated with gentle inspiration or during exercise and this pattern may be reversed in patients with heart failure and right-sided congestion or cardiac tamponade.

Abdominal Examination

Right heart failure with peripheral venous congestion and systemic venous hypertension can cause an enlarged liver often before overt peripheral edema develops. A fullness of the abdomen may be apparent on inspection and hepatomegaly is often detected by either percussion or palpation. A congested liver is usually painful when palpated. Substantive tricuspid regurgitation causes venous transmission of right atrial V-wave pressure into the abdomen and liver with detectable late systolic hepatic pulsation. In patients with heart failure, minimal congestion, and normal neck-vein levels, insidious congestion can be detected by applying gentle pressure to the abdomen at the level of the umbilicus. A positive abdominal-jugular reflex (also called the "hepatojugular" reflex) occurs when gentle but firm, continuous compression on the abdomen causes neck veins to distend substantially. This test may be helpful in differentiating hepatomegaly due to congestive hepatopathy from hepatomegaly caused by primary liver disease. The test should not be performed with compression directly over the liver, and, holding one's breath or the Valsalva maneuver can cause a falsely positive test.

Ascites develops from long-standing venous hypertension and, chronically, impairs diaphragm drop and respiration.

Extremity Edema

Although edema is commonly present in patients with CHF, it certainly is not an essential finding and the extent may not correlate well with syndrome severity. Experience has taught us that a minimum of 5 liters of extracellular fluid volume is generally required before peripheral edema can be detected. Its presence usually suggests, therefore, that problems have been present for some time. When noted, pedal edema is usually bilateral, occurring gradually after the patient has been upright, and resolves with elevation of the dependent portion of the body. In individuals chronically bedridden, edema may first appear in the dependent sacral portion of the body. Anasarca is the development of generalized edema involving the upper as well as the lower extremities, genital region, and thoracic and abdominal walls. Heart failure patients frequently have indurated and highly pigmented lower extremities due to the effects of long-standing edema. Immobility exacerbates the collection of fluid in these patients. The location and extent of the edema as well as the ability to form pits when pressure is applied can be an important marker of therapeutic success. So-called pitting edema suggests a substantive congestive state and implies that diuretic therapy may be useful to relieve this problem.

Clinical Cardiac Findings

Cardiomegaly should be suspected in patients with heart failure and can be detected by noting a displaced apical pulse or, less easily, by percussion of the anterior left chest. A prominent pulsation can be felt in the left parasternal area when right ventricular volume or pressure overload has caused enlargement and hypertrophy of this chamber. However, the presence of mitral regurgitation with systolic filling of the posterior left atrium also can produce this finding. When the finding is caused by right ventricular pressure or volume overload, a prominent pulsation often is noted in the subxyphoid region. When cardiac dilatation is particularly severe and cardiomegaly pronounced, a double apical impulse may be detected and can represent the auscultated third heart sound (S-3 gallop).

The S-3 gallop is usually low pitched and best heard with the bell of the stethoscope placed on the heart apex while the patient is in a left, laterally recumbent position. Sometimes this sound is heard in young individuals, but in patients over 40 yr of age it should always be considered aberrant. The third heart sound is common in mitral regurgitation and may sound similar to the pericardial knock heard in patients with constrictive pericarditis. LV hypertrophy without cavity dilatation tends to attenuate the third heart sound and in these cases the S-4 gallop becomes far more prominent. The fourth heart sounds precede the normal first heart sound and tend to be higher pitched than the S-3 gallop. Both third and fourth heart sounds can be localized to the right ventricle. In this case they are exacerbated with respiration (increasing blood return to the right heart).

When heart rate increases and ventricular dysfunction is severe, a summation gallop rhythm occurs when the third and fourth sounds are superimposed, creating a loud and characteristic thump that occurs midway in the interval between the second heart sound and the first heart sound of the next cycle. S-1 is frequently diminished in intensity in the heart failure patient and, if pulmonary hypertension is present, P-2 can become very loud. The triad of a soft first heart sound, loud summation gallop, and amplified P-2 suggests severe heart failure with pulmonary hypertension.

It is also important to listen for murmurs and cardiac rubs. Not only can information be gained regarding etiology of heart disease, but the severity of LV dilation and function can frequently be assessed. As the LV cavity dilates, atrioventricular valvular insufficiency can occur with systolic regurgitant murmurs heard, generally, to the left of the sternum in the case of mitral regurgitation, and to the right in the case of tricuspid insufficiency. These murmurs tend to dissipate if successful treatment of the underlying disease can cause the ventricle to shrink in size. Often, surgery is not possible or even required in these patients. Obviously, the presence of murmurs suggesting aortic insufficiency, aortic stenosis, and mitral stenosis will be important to pursue with ancillary evaluation.

Cachexia

When heart failure has been long-standing and severe, anorexia usually is present and impaired intestinal absorption of nutrients can occur. Protein-losing enteropathy is problematic and an increase in caloric expenditure due to the excessive work of breathing combined with reduced caloric intake causes tissue mass, particularly muscle mass, to waste and "cardiac" cachexia develops. Additionally, in the severely limited heart failure patient exercise is not generally performed and, therefore, any training benefits accrued by skeletal muscles will be lost. Muscle-wasting is often most obvious in the head and neck area (particularly temporalis wasting) where facial expressions can become extremely bony. Wasting of muscles of the thenar eminence is also commonly seen in patients with advanced disease.

Ancillary Aspects of the Physical Examination

It should be apparent that all of the above-discussed physical signs sometimes seen in the setting of heart failure are neither specific nor sensitive for diagnosing the syndrome or staging its severity. Additional clinical data and laboratory or physiologic testing can help clarify ambiguous symptoms or findings that, when assessed in isolation, can be terribly confusing. A few of these are discussed.

Valsalva Maneuver

The Valsalva maneuver is an example of a simple bedside test designed to help the clinician diagnose substantive heart failure and LV dysfunction. During the holding phase, this maneuver creates an increase in intrathoracic pressure with subsequent diminution of venous return. Stroke volume falls and systemic venous pressure increases. Peripheral arterial changes normally have four phases: (a) an initial rise in systolic pressure, (b) subsequent increase in heart rate during continuation of the strain secondary to fall in venous return and diminished systolic, diastolic, and pulse pressure, (c) a sudden drop of systolic arterial pressure representing the fall in intrathoracic arterial pressure, and when inspiration resumes, (d) an overshoot of arterial pressure above control levels with wide pulse pressure and bradycardia caused by reflux inflow of blood occurring on release of the Valsalva maneuver. Phase three is seen again on release of the strain. In patients with heart failure, the baroreceptor reflex is absent and, therefore, no overshoot occurs in systolic pressure on release of the strain. Also, careful palpation of the brachial pulse in normal patients will demonstrate slowing of the pulse in phase four, a finding absent in the patient with heart failure.

Circulation Time

At one time, a rapid peripheral intravenous infusion of dehydrocholic acid (Decholin) was done to determine circulation time. This procedure is rarely done today but worth recalling. The drug produces a bitter taste when carried by arterial circulation to the mouth and this is used as an endpoint. Normally, only 9 to 16 s pass before the taste is noted. When pulmonary or systemic congestion is present in the face of diminished cardiac output, the circulation time is increased.

Venous Pressure

Venous pressure can be determined quickly in the clinic or at bedside utilizing a spinal fluid manometer hooked via short tubing to a needle inserted into a brachial vein when the patient is lying supine. Usually right atrial pressure is up to 8 cm of water and if the venous pressure is greater than 12 cm of water at rest, it is abnormal. Venous pressure can be increased further by abdominal compression or during exercise. A venous pressure of greater than 16 cm of water was utilized as a major diagnostic criteria (Table 32.4) for heart failure in the Framingham study.[16]

A compendium of symptomatology and physical findings has been used to diagnose heart failure in clinical investigations. Clinical trials, however, need to be analyzed to understand why conflicting results so often are present.[17,18] Clearly, differences in patient characteristics and the manner in which heart failure has been diagnosed plays a role in discordant outcomes. It is difficult to diagnose heart failure definitively in any patient because of the insensitivity and lack of specificity of many complaints. This should not be unduly discouraging in the individual patient. Again, an example of reproducible and sound criteria (Table 32.4) can be found in the Framingham study.[16] The Framingham study

TABLE 32.4. Clinical criteria of heart failure in Framingham study.[16]

Criteria[a]
Major Criteria
Paroxysmal nocturnal dyspnea
Neck vein distention
Rales
Cardiomegaly
Acute pulmonary edema
S-3 gallop
Increased venous pressure (>16 cm H_2O)
Hepatojugular reflex
Minor criteria
Extremity edema
Night cough
Dyspnea on exertion
Hepatomegaly
Pleural effusion
Vital capacity reduced by one third from maximum
Tachycardia (≥120)
Major or minor
Weight loss ≥4.5 kg over 5 days after treatment

[a] At least one major and two minor criteria must be concurrently detected.

suggested that specific clinical criteria could be used to diagnose heart failure. Table 32.4 summarizes these criteria and emphasizes that, for establishing a clinical diagnosis of clinical heart failure, at least one major and two minor criteria must be concurrently detected.

Laboratory Testing

Electrolytes

Table 32.5 lists the laboratory tests that should be considered. Although most patients with heart failure have

TABLE 32.5. Laboratory procedures to consider in heart failure patients[a]

Laboratory tests	
Complete blood count	Arterial blood gases
Serum electrolytes	Urinalysis
Blood urea nitrogen	Biochemistry screen
Serum creatinine	Magnesium
Liver function tests	Uric acid
Serum transaminases	Calcium
Lactic dehydrogenase	Phosphorus
Alkaline phosphatase	Serum drug levels
Bilirubin (direct and indirect)	Digoxin
Albumin	Phenytoins
Prothrombin time	Quinidine
	Procainamide
	Other antiarrhythmics

[a] Ancillary procedures that elucidate concomitant cardiovascular and noncardiovascular illnesses are critical.

normal electrolyte values, long-standing severe heart failure can produce a variety of abnormalities. Hyponatremia develops not only because of the pathophysiologic changes caused by heart failure, but also in response to therapeutic maneuvers including diuretic and ACE inhibitor therapy, especially when these are coupled with sodium restriction.[19] Furthermore, elevated circulating vasopressin also contributes to this difficulty. In the face of an increased total body sodium level with marked expansion of extracellular fluid, the hyponatremia is, essentially, dilutional. Use of thiazide diuretics seems to be particularly troublesome with respect to hyponatremia.

Possibly the most common electrolyte abnormality seen in the heart failure milieu is hypokalemia. Again, this is frequently the result of aggressive and prolonged administration of diuretic therapy but can also be produced by the increased aldosterone levels typical of heart failure.[20] Hypokalemia is exacerbated by an inability to follow a low-sodium diet. On the other hand, potassium-sparing diuretics can be particularly problematic in patients with marked reduction in renal blood flow and glomerular filtration, resulting in diminished delivery of sodium to the distal tubular exchange sites. In this setting the potassium-sparing diuretics might cause hyperkalemia. The administration of ACE inhibitors to these patients also can exacerbate potassium retention and could lead to the development of hyperkalemia.

Hepatic Function Parameters

One challenging difficulty in heart failure patients is differentiating abnormal liver function due to heart failure from that secondary to cirrhosis caused by other diseases. Although chronic CHF can certainly cause cirrhosis, the more common finding is simple congestive hepatomegaly.[21] Frequently, the serum transaminases and bilirubin will be elevated. The hyperbilirubinemia is caused by an increase in both direct and indirect fractions and jaundice may even be noted. Extremely severe or acute onset of hepatic congestion can cause rather dramatic elevations of the bilirubin (sometimes as high as 20 mg/dl). The transaminase enzymes may be increased 10- to 15-fold and there is an elevation of serum alkaline phosphatase. When the prothombin time is substantively prolonged congestive hepatopathy is, generally, severe and the prognosis grim. The major differential consideration is between the enzyme profile of heart failure and viral hepatitis. The major differentiating factor is that normalization of hepatic function rapidly occurs with successful heart failure treatment. The development of cardiac cirrhosis will produce all of the findings associated with chronic liver failure including hypoalbuminemia, hypoglycemia, ascites, and hepatic coma.

Blood Count and Sedimentation Rates

Normally, the hemoglobin and hematocrit is maintained in patients with heart failure but depending on the stage of congestion and starvation, anemia may develop. Abnormal red blood cell counts, particularly when they are low, should prompt an investigation to diagnose and explain the etiology of anemia. Indeed, anemia due to the slow, insidious, but chronic loss of blood or hemolysis frequently presents with many of the manifestations of chronic heart failure. Although the erythrocyte sedimentation rate has been said to be low in patients with CHF, recent evaluation of this simply measured parameter indicates that a low rate is correlated with severity of chronic heart failure, but proves to be of limited value during management of the syndrome.[22]

Evaluation of Renal Function

Urine analysis may demonstrate a concentrated urine when no diuretics have been given. Blood urea nitrogen is frequently elevated as are creatinine levels, and the extent of reduction in renal blood flow and glomerular filtration rate can be assessed grossly by the level of prerenal azotemia. Additional measures of renal impairment are infrequently performed in the heart failure milieu but determination of creatinine clearance may be important when attempting to quantify extent of renal function impairment.

Ancillary Diagnostic Tests

The Chest X Ray

Table 32.6 lists some of the ancillary diagnostic tests one might wish to consider when evaluating heart failure patients and Table 32.7 summarizes some of the important observations that can be made. The chest x ray can be an extraordinarily useful, not to mention relatively inexpensive, test. Not only can the size and con-

TABLE 32.6. Diagnostic procedures to consider in heart failure patients.

Specialized diagnostic tests	
Ambulatory electrocardiogram	Electrophysiologic study
Cardiac catheterization	Endomyocardial biopsy
Aortography	Exercise stress testing
Coronary angiography	Oxygen utilization
Hemodynamic assessment	Magnetic resonance imaging
Ventriculography	Position emission tomography
Chest x ray	Pulmonary function testing
Computerized tomographic scanning	Radionuclide angiogram
Echocardiogram	Scintigraphic perfusion studies
M-mode	
Pulsed Doppler	
Two-dimensional	
Electrocardiogram	

TABLE 32.7. Common ancillary diagnostic tests.

Test and important information made available
Chest x ray
Cardiothoracic ratio
Selective chamber size and shape
Pulmonary vascularity and congestion
Pleural effusions
Mass lesions or infiltrates
Mediastinal configuration
Great vessel abnormality
Electrocardiography
Rhythm
Atrial fibrillation
Ventricular arrhythmias
Heart rate
Evidence of hypertrophy
Q waves
P mitrale or pulmonale
Conduction disturbances
Digitalis effects
Metabolic changes
Echocardiography (2D/M-mode)
Chamber size and shape
Valve integrity and motion
Fractional shortening of ventricles
Mean circumferential fiber shortening
Mitral E point to septal separation
Systolic wall thickening
Wall motion analysis
Estimation of wall stress
Endomyocardial biopsy guidance
Exercise and pharmacologic stress (wall motion)
Tissue characterization
Pericardial effusion
Pericardial restriction
Pulsed Doppler echocardiography
Quantification of valve stenosis/regurgitation
Estimation of pulmonary artery pressure
Estimation of stroke volume and cardiac output
Determination of diastolic filling characteristics
Detection of shunts

figuration of the cardiac silhouette provide insight into the presence and nature of heart disease, but evidence of pulmonary congestion and pleural fluid help stage the severity of the clinical problem. Additionally, chest roentenography is useful in excluding some forms of pulmonary disease that might cause dyspnea, for instance emphysema. Cardiac enlargement manifests by an increase in the transverse diameter of the heart, particularly in relationship to the diameter of the thoracic cavity (cardiothoracic ratio >.50), is a specific but relatively insensitive indicator of increased LV volume or mass. This can be readily determined on plain x-ray films, but more precise chest x-ray voluminomitry has proved helpful in some circumstances and epidemiologic studies.[23] It should be remembered, however, that substantive LV disease may be present with a normal cardiac silhouette, but these patients generally have other abnormalities on, for example, the electrocardiogram (ECG). Indeed, a combination of certain ECG parameters and chest x-ray findings have been useful in predicting patients' LV systolic function.[24]

Enlargement of other cardiac chambers, such as the left-atrium, should be suspected when distinctive patterns of left sided cardiac contour are noted and elevation of the left main stem bronchus is seen. Right ventricular enlargement is suggested by a large anterior mediastinal silhouette noted on lateral x-ray projection. In patients who have not previously undergone cardiac surgery, obliteration of more than one third of the retrosternal air space by the cardiac silhouette is an indication that right ventricular enlargement may be present.

Intracardiac calcification can be helpful in identifying aortic or mitral valve disease in certain circumstances.

When left atrial (and subsequently pulmonary venous) pressure becomes elevated, pulmonary edema can develop with interstitial and perivascular edema noted first at the lung bases and then subsequently throughout the chest x ray. Slight congestion (pulmonary capillary wedge pressure >15 but <20 mm Hg) usually results in redistribution of blood flow from the base of the lungs to the apices. Frank pulmonary edema occurring when the pulmonary capillary wedge pressure is >20 mm Hg can produce linear densities reflecting interstitial edema in the base of the chest. These are sometimes called Kerley's lines. When congestion worsens and, particularly when the pulmonary capillary wedge pressure rises above 25 mm Hg, alveolar fluid accumulation will occur; this produces a hazy appearance concentrated mostly around the hili of the mediastinum, creating a pattern that sometimes has been referred to as a "butterfly."

As mentioned, pleural effusions can be detected quite readily with a simple chest x ray and, although this is a nonspecific finding, it correlates with the overall congested state. One must always consider the possibility that the effusion is due to something other than heart failure and, if this is an active consideration, thoracentesis should be performed to exclude exudative processes.

Obviously, pleural, parenchymal, and mediastinal masses should be searched for on chest x ray.

Electrocardiogram

Like chest roentenography, the electrocardiogram is an important and cost-effective test to perform in patients presenting with the heart failure. Although there are no specific ECG findings that diagnose presence or absence of heart failure, many different patterns give insight into cardiac dysfunction (Table 32.7). By combining ECG findings with chest x-ray observations, insight into the degree of myocardial impairment can be gained.[24]

Determination of heart rate and rhythm is important. Atrial fibrillation or sinus rhythm with bursts of supraventricular or ventricular arrhythmia portend an adverse prognosis in patients with heart failure, particularly when ischemic heart disease is present. A resting sinus tachycardia also implies substantive cardiac decompensation and can be a helpful observation. Bursts of paroxysmal supraventricular tachycardia may suggest digitalis intoxication. Arrhythmia induction in patients on an antiarrhythmic agent is always possible. Utilization of prolonged ambulatory ECG monitoring may be required to clarify rhythm disturbances. Although this technique can also provide information regarding ST segment changes associated with silent myocardial ischemia, most patients with substantive heart failure and LV dysfunction have ECGs that are uninterpretable from this standpoint.

Evidence of ventricular hypertrophy can be important in patients with hypertensive heart disease and clinical heart failure. Common criteria to diagnose LV hypertrophy rely on an increase in QRS voltage with or without concomitant T-wave changes. Commonly, when the sum of the V-2 S wave and V-5 R wave is greater than 35 mV, LV hypertrophy should be suspected. T-wave inversion in limb lead V-1, AVF, and precordial leads V-4 through V-6, is commonly present but can be caused by a variety of metabolic disturbances as well as ischemic heart disease. The presence of prominent R waves in V-1 suggests right ventricular hypertrophy. Again, these findings, although helpful, are not necessarily sensitive or specific.[25]

Bundle branch block is frequently noted in patients with cardiomyopathy as well as ischemic heart disease and myocardial infarction. The presence of left bundle branch block often is associated with structural LV abnormality, whereas isolated right bundle block can be a normal finding. Patients with left bundle branch block have a higher risk of adverse events when heart failure is present. Incomplete bundle branch block or slightly increased QRS width is much less specific for an adverse outcome, yet can suggest ventricular hypertrophy or fibrotic myocardial infiltration. Left axis deviation alone is not helpful since frequently it may be seen in individuals aged 50 years or greater. In a young patient with left axis deviation and nonspecific QRS widening, myocardial disease usually is present.

Certain ECG findings should imply ischemic heart disease. Most notably, Q waves are characteristic of coronary artery disease causing acute myocardial infarction.[26] It should be noted, however, that patients with idiopathic dilated cardiomyopathy (IDC) also can present with Q waves, particularly in association with QRS prolongation and left bundle branch block. Inferior Q waves are associated much more frequently with substantive coronary artery disease and myocardial infarction, but still, approximately 20% of patients will lose Q waves after having suffered an infarct.

Certain P-wave patterns suggest enlarged atria. P mitrale is a characteristic enlarged "m"-shaped P wave that suggests left atrial enlargement secondary to mitral valve disease. P pulmonale is a peaked or "tented" P wave suggesting right atrial abnormality and enlargement. A biphasic or S-shaped P wave suggests biatrial enlargement.

Many metabolic changes may affect, often in nonspecific fashion, the ECG. Hypokalemia can produce T-wave flattening and U waves in the precordial leads or prolongation of the Q-T interval and QRS. A serum potassium less than 2.6 mEq/l is almost always accompanied by ECG changes. Moderate levels of potassium elevation can cause tall, peaked, narrow T waves in the precordium. This can progress to QRS widening with a reduction in QRS in amplitude, wide P waves, and in severe cases, sine wave formation.

Digitalis, even when not present in intoxicating doses, produces a smooth downward coving of the ST segment that is characteristic but not specific for this medication. Class IC antiarrhythmic drugs (e.g., quinidine and procainamide) can cause widening of the QRS complex with prolongation of the QT interval.

All of these findings are subtle, nonspecific, and sometimes insensitive, but when coupled with chest roentenography, clinical history, and physical examination, provide a great deal of data regarding a patient's clinical situation and prognosis.

Combined Chest X Ray and Electrocardiographic Analysis

Since the chest x ray provides an index of LV volume and the ECG can reflect ventricular mass, LV systolic function can be predicted by combining observations readily available from routine ECG and chest x ray. Indeed, a reasonably accurate, simple, inexpensive, noninvasive method of determining ejection fraction has been developed utilizing precordial R-wave summation and LV volume estimated by chest roentgenography. The formulae enlarged can be utilized to provide an independent index of myocardial performance for clinical use since it reflects the amount of contractile tissue per unit of LV volume.[24] Figure 32.4 graphically describes this technique.

Echocardiography

M-mode, two-dimensional, and Doppler echocardiography, particularly when performed in combined transcutaneous and transesophageal fashion, can provide the greatest amount of noninvasive information concerning etiology and severity of heart failure (Table 32.7). If possible, in any patient with symptoms or physical

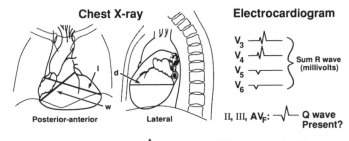

Chest X-ray

Posterior-anterior   Lateral

Electrocardiogram

V_3
V_4
V_5
V_6

Sum R wave (millivolts)

II, III, AV$_F$:   Q wave Present?

1. Heart volume index ($\hat{V}$) = l · w · d · (.38)/patient weight (kg).
2. Heart mass index ($\dot{m}$) = Σ R wave V_{3-6} (millivolts).
3. Q code = pathologic inferior Q present = 1 or absent = 0.

Ejection fraction index = 67.30 − (1.56 · $\hat{V}$) + (0.23 · $\dot{m}$) − (14.18 · Q code)

FIGURE 32.4. A formula was derived after multiple linear regression analysis of certain chest x-ray and ECG findings was performed to estimate LV performance by calculating ejection fraction. The formula is based on the concept that routine chest x ray can provide an estimate of heart volume (V) and the ECG heart mass (M). The formula was found more accurate when an assessment of the presence or absence of inferior Q waves was done (anterior Q waves are factored into the equation by a low R wave sum in V_{3-6}). Inferior Q waves and low sum of R in V_{3-V6} would suggest myocardial scar and therefore diminished myocardial mass. The formula works best when compulsive chest x-ray technique (patient 6 ft from x-ray tube, for example) occurs so that chest x-ray heart voluminometry calculations (V) can be most accurate. Heart length (l), width (w), and diameter (d) measurements are made in centimeters. The heart volume index is normalized per kilogram body weight. An estimated ejection fraction can then be calculated using the linear regression equation EF = 67.30 − (1.56.V) + (0.23.M) − (14.18.Q code). Inferior Q waves are coded 1 when present and 0 when not present.

findings suggesting heart failure, echocardiography should be attempted. Although this is an expensive proposition, we believe the information worthwhile. This is not to say that all patients with heart disease should undergo echocardiography. One drawback relates to technical limitations. High quality echocardiograms may not be obtained in 10% to 20% of patients studied. With improved technology and more readily available trained support personnel, this difficulty seems to be decreasing. Indeed, a completely uninterpretable echocardiogram is rarely seen today.

As echocardiography has become more sophisticated, M-mode studies are less frequently performed. Still, however, much useful information can be gleaned from M-mode images. Although M-mode studies can estimate heart volume and ejection fraction, problems with accurate identification of endocardial surface and tangential views create potential for error.[27] Fractional shortening of the LV (simply, the difference between the end-diastolic and end-systolic dimension divided by the end-diastolic dimension) gives significant information about LV systolic function when it is depressed.

Another gross technique for assessing LV function is determination of the distance between the E point of the mitral valve and the interventricular septum. Upper limits of normal for this E point-septal separation is approximately 8 mm; when this is increased it implies LV dilatation with diminished ejection fraction. Obviously, regional LV wall motion abnormalities will impair one's ability to use this technique and they will adversely affect accurate estimate of shortening fraction. However, when LV filling pressures are elevated, a characteristic protrusion or delay in mitral valve closure occurs on the AC line of the M-mode mitral valve recording. This so-called B hump is a delay in anterior mitral valve coaptation to the posterior mitral valve leaflet and correlates with high LV filling pressure. Obviously, mitral valve disease such as mitral stenosis will alter normal patterns of motion and attenuate the prognostic significance of this observation. Still, however, the finding of valvular or congenital pathology by M-mode echocardiography can be important. M-mode studies do allow precise measurement of septal and posterior LV wall width so that indices of hypertrophy, mass, and wall stress can be calculated. Again, tangential angling creates difficulties but by combining M-mode observations with two-dimensional study some of these problems can be attenuated.

Two-Dimensional Echocardiography

Two-dimensional echocardiography not only increases the number of observation sights but also the degree of spatial orientation that one has when performing the study.[27] Assessment of cardiac chamber dimension can now be performed much more accurately and therefore determination of ventricular systolic performance is more precise with this technique. Although several geometric formulae have been suggested to calculate LV volume accurately, all have a variety of attributes and detriments. Furthermore, these formulae have been correlated with the so-called gold standard of contrast ventriculography performed at the time of cardiac catheterization. Clearly, this method is reliable when done in laboratories with consistent and skilled personnel performing and interpreting the studies.

Transesophageal Echocardiography

Transesophageal echocardiography has been demonstrated to be advantageous in individuals in whom transcutaneous imaging has been less than satisfactory.[28] This technique has provided increased resolution in terms of determining chamber dimension, valve motion, and structural identification. For example, identification of left atrial thrombi or vegetations can be done with much greater accuracy utilizing the transesophageal technique. Obviously, the negative side of this test is the fact that the patient must be sedated and the probe swallowed.

Doppler Studies

Doppler echocardiography has added an interesting dimension by allowing accurate recording of flow across valves; in the ascending aorta this can subsequently be related to ejection volumes and, therefore, to output and systolic performance[29] (Table 32.7). Although M-mode echocardiographic parameters can estimate the rate of LV relaxation, Doppler echocardiography has supplanted this when LV diastolic dysfunction is being quantified.[30] Doppler flow patterns through the mitral valve can be characterized and when diastolic dysfunction is present, early diastolic flow through the mitral valve is reduced with substantive augmentation noted after atrial contraction. This observation can be quantified and provides useful information when evaluating patients with heart failure primarily due to diastolic dysfunction. Examples would include patients with hypertrophic cardiomyopathy and severe LV hypertrophy. Doppler echocardiography is also useful to obtain noninvasive estimates of hemodynamic parameters. The determination of pulmonary artery pressure can be an extraordinarily important guide to therapy. By calculating the velocity of transvalvular blood flow after measuring the integral of the Doppler recording (the area under the recording) and by relating this to the cross-sectional area of the valve orifice, gradients across stenotic valves and pressures can be estimated.[31] Valvular orifice size can be estimated by direct measurement of two-dimensional or M-mode echocardiographic images. The major limitation to Doppler echocardiographic-derived indices relates to the necessity for compulsive technique and attention to the many variables required in making these predictions.

General Echocardiographic Interpretation Concepts

All three types of echocardiographic studies can be done to evaluate most completely the cardiovascular condition of patients presenting with heart failure. Not only can insight be gained into etiology of the problem, but staging of disease therapy can occur after observing parameters such as chamber dilatation, depression of ejection fraction, and degree of wall stress. Furthermore, the demonstration of complications of heart failure, such as clot formation in the left atrium, is possible. Finally, echocardiography can be used during diagnostic procedures, such as endomyocardial biopsy to guide bioptome placement, confirming the fact that tissue will be removed from areas of the right ventricle having generous musculature.[32] Obviously, the compulsive echocardiographic assessment of patients will be helpful in identifying congenital cardiac abnormalities that may be causing the difficulties.

Exercise Echocardiography

Although sometimes difficult to perform, echocardiography done immediately before and then after stress exercise testing can demonstrate exercise-induced regional wall motion abnormalities in patients with coronary artery disease and LV dysfunction.[33] When combined with aortic Doppler assessment of flow, changes in LV systolic function during stress also can be quantitated. This type of stress echocardiography evaluation also can be done during pharmacologic or pacing studies. It may be an alternative to certain radionuclide imaging techniques and offer additional methods to quantify syndrome severity.[34]

Ultrasound Tissue Characterization

Echocardiography can be useful in some clinical situations commonly causing heart failure, such as amyloidosis.[35] The characteristic shimmering and scintillating pattern noted on two-dimensional echocardiography suggests this diagnosis. Fibrosis and scar also may be noted after myocardial infarction. These regions of the myocardium are denser and therefore produce greater echogenicity. Furthermore, they tend to be thinner than normal LV muscle and do not thicken. In addition to amyloid heart disease and scar, a characteristic alteration of myocardial echoes also has been recorded in patients with hypertrophic cardiomyopathy. It should be emphasized, however, that these assessments are highly qualitative visual assessments and, therefore, lack sensitivity and specificity.

Radionuclide Studies

Radionuclide studies performed on patients with heart failure also can give insight into the etiology of a problem as well as help stage its severity.[36] These procedures can be grouped into either perfusion scans designed to delineate the extent of coronary artery obstruction and subsequent tissue ischemia or scar, or performance studies that will characterize cardiac chamber size, shape, and indices of contraction and relaxation. Additionally, exercise, pharmacologic, or pacing stress interventions can be combined to give additional insight into the heart's reaction to increased metabolic demand. Although a major disadvantage to these techniques is their cost, they can be performed on virtually any patient. Unlike echocardiography, there do not seem to be tremendous limitations based on the patient's physical characteristics. Very obese men and large-breasted women may attenuate scintigraphic imaging, but this is uncommon. Furthermore, the accuracy of these studies in determining systolic LV performance probably is greater than with the echocardiogram. For detection and quantification of coronary disease, perfusion studies offer some advantage over echocardiography since these tests provide objective measurements of perfusion defects resulting from myocardial scar or ischemia. Echocardiographic analysis of ischemia is generally based on wall motion abnormality detection at rest or during stress. Ischemia is suspected when new wall motion abnormalities develop after stress and in this sense echocardiographic studies parallel some radionuclide tests. With respect to identification of the etiology of heart failure, radionuclide imaging primarily focuses on ischemic heart disease.[36]

Quantification of Heart Failure Severity

Qualitative and quantitative assessment of cardiac performance with a variety of radiopharmaceuticals can be performed by either analyzing the first transit of a radionuclide through the heart (first-pass radionuclide angiocardiography) or by analyzing a labeled blood pool of radionuclide by equilibrium-gated technique (Table 32.8). Grossly, these techniques allow identification of enlarged ventricles as well as impairment of systolic performance. Although an estimate of aortic regurgitation and mitral regurgitation is also possible, quantification of these abnormalities is not accurate. By creating time activity curves of left or right ventricular radionuclide activity, ejection fraction can be determined after assessment of background radionuclide counts. Quantitative analysis also allows identification and severity assessment of cardiac shunts.

Equilibrium studies are performed after scintigraphic

TABLE 32.8. First-pass versus equilibrium radionuclide studies.

First-pass radionuclide angiocardiography	Gated equilibrium radionuclide angiocardiography
Advantages	*Advantages*
Rapidly performed	Many studies performed over several hours
Upright exercise	Regional wall motion assessed in many views and many interventions
Individual chamber size assessment	
Best RV function assessment	
Best shunt ID/Quant assessment	High count density for analysis (better image creation)
Disadvantages	Can view entire cardiac blood pool simultaneously
Regional wall motion in one view only	Less prone to arrhythmia difficulties
Multiple measurements require multiple injections (short-lived isotopes)	Portable scintillation cameras
	Allows diastolic dysfunction assessment
Only few cardiac cycles sampled (arrhythmias cause problems)	
Low count density data	*Disadvantages*
Needs impeccable injection technique/good veins	Overlapping cardiac radionuclide pool can occur
Big/heavy multicrystal scintillation camera	Long duration of examination
Assessment of diastolic dysfunction difficult	Generally requires supine exercise
	Evaluation of right ventricular performance less accurate

RV = right ventricle; ID/Quant = identification/quantification.

labeling of the blood pool. This increases the number of counts and improves resolution. As opposed to a first-pass angiographic study, the radionuclide must reach equilibrium within the entire blood pool before imaging. All four cardiac chambers can be seen with this technique, but the liver and spleen also will be visualized, sometimes creating difficulties when trying to separate the right and left side of the heart. Gating is required to differentiate systole from diastole during analysis. This technique does offer the advantage of creating a radionuclide cineangiographic display, which is a recurring loop of sequential frames of data that visually allows inspection of systolic and diastolic right and left ventricular performance in multiple views. Several hundred cardiac cycles are usually analyzed as opposed to the two or three cycles analyzed during first-pass studies. During this relatively prolonged data accumulation period, the patient must remain still and the radionuclide must have remained stable in the intravascular and cardiac space. Since the blood pool will be labeled for a longer period of time, many studies can be performed over several hours. This allows regional wall motion assessment in many different views and after many different types of exercise or pharmacologic interventions. Furthermore, the high count density produced during this imaging technique creates a better view of the left and right ventricle provided that there is adequate separation of these cardiac blood pools. Still, the simultaneous viewing of the entire central cardiac blood pool offers some advantages to this technique by allowing simultaneous assessment of right and left ventricular function in a qualitative sense and estimates of atrial as well as ventricular chamber size. Cardiac arrhythmias produce less of a problem with equilibrium studies since many hundred beats are gated and imaged as opposed to the few beats imaged during first-pass radionuclide angiocardiography. Additionally, the scintillation cameras used to collect data during equilibrium studies are generally portable and can allow the performance of these studies at a patient's bedside. Disadvantages of the gated equilibrium technique when compared to first-pass radionuclide angiocardiography (Table 32.8) include the potential for overlapping cardiac blood pool images as well as overlap of hepatic and splenic radionuclide activity. Additionally, the duration of the examination is longer and if exercise studies are to be performed, they generally must be done in the supine position. Finally, evaluation of right ventricular performance seems less accurate when performed by gated equilibrium imaging technique.

Ventricular Performance Assessment

Both techniques can be utilized to evaluate systolic LV performance at rest and during exercise or after pharmacologic or pacing stress tests (Table 32.8). Calculation of ejection fraction and analysis of poorly contracting segments will give insight into patients' complaints when heart failure symptoms are experienced. Furthermore, ventricular shape can give clues to the formation of an aneurysm or pseudoaneurysm after myocardial infarction. Rather precise measurement of ventricular volumes can be done after interventions with inotropic or vasodilating medication. Also, radionuclide angiocardiography can provide insight into etiology of certain forms of heart failure because of characteristic findings associated with, primarily, congestive cardiomyopathy, hypertrophic cardiomyopathy, and ischemic cardiomyopathy. Dilated congestive cardiomyopathy patients demonstrate biventricular enlargement with diffuse hypokinesis. Hypertrophic cardiomyopathy demonstrates small cavity appearance with obliteration of radioisotope image during systole. Ischemic cardiomyopathy will demonstrate pronounced segmental wall motion abnormality. Exercise stress as well as pharmacologic stress can be helpful in identifying patients who develop wall motion abnormality or whose ejection fraction fall with exercise.

Diastolic Function

Because fewer counts are available for analysis and changes in cycle length occur in diastole, creating time-volume curves for the diastolic portion of the cardiac cycle is more difficult than for the systolic portion. Still, diastolic function can be assessed during equilibrium radionuclide ventricular angiocardiography.[36] By utilizing high sensitivity and high temporal resolution techniques, peak filling rate and time-to-peak filling rate can be measured. By normalizing these measurements to end-diastolic volume, an index of diastolic function can be generated, although the precise relationship to more traditional pressure-volume assessments of diastolic performance is not entirely known. As greater insight into the pathophysiology of diastolic left and right ventricular function is gained, quantification of these parameters may prove useful in the management of patients with heart failure. Indeed, it has been suggested that diastolic dysfunction determined by radionuclide imaging may be the best way to predict exercise intolerance in the heart failure milieu.[37]

Myocardial Perfusion Imaging

Determination of relative regional myocardial perfusion may be important in patients with heart failure because of the common problem of ischemic heart disease.[18] Thallium-201 is currently the most common radionuclide tracer used and sequential imaging can help determine if scar or ischemia is present. Biologically, thallium substitutes for ionic potassium and therefore accumulates rapidly within viable myocardial tissues. Scintillation camera detection of isotope can then be performed in a variety of views defining regions of tracer activity in the myocardium. Precise quantification of myocardial thallium uptake can be performed with tomographic imaging techniques that localize defects precisely and measure their extent. At rest, LV dilation can be inferred but the best technique for quantifying this difficulty is first-pass or equilibrium blood pool imaging. Also, LV hypertrophy is suggested by a thickened myocardial wall and decreased cavity size, although echocardiography is better suited for direct visualization of the structures. Absence of thallium uptake in specific regions of the LV at rest implies scar formation. Although the right ventricle usually is not visualized, when there is right ventricular hypertrophy due to volume and pressure overload, this chamber outline can be seen to take up thallium.

When thallium perfusion defects are present at both rest and exercise, scar is apparent. When a defect only manifests with stress testing (exercise, pharmacologic, or pacing stress), ischemia is suspected. Obviously, quantification of the extent and relative contribution of scar and ischemia can be differentiated using these tests. Furthermore, combination of perfusion imaging with functional scintigraphic imaging can provide a great deal of insight into the etiology of the difficulty, anatomic severity, and prognosis.

Positron Emission Tomography

A new, expensive, and not generally available radionuclide imaging technique that can assess myocardial blood flow and metabolism is attracting a great deal of attention. Positron emission tomography (PET) allows three-dimensional display of myocardial radionuclide activity.[38] This display has spatial resolution independent of depth and other attenuation effects. The potential advantage of PET scanning over other radionuclide imaging techniques relates to the fact that radiopharmaceuticals specific for several different metabolic pathways can be utilized as radiolabels to assess myocardial function. Although the clinical application of PET is as yet incompletely defined, the ability to understand myocardial function is great with this technique. This procedure might prove most valuable in defining regions of myocardial viability in ischemic heart disease, or clarifying altered myocardial metabolism in cardiomyopathy patients.[39]

Exercise Testing

In the heart failure milieu, exercise testing is done mostly to evaluate functional capacity by quantification of physical impairment.[40] This is an important procedure to perform on anyone with heart failure, particularly when judgment about therapeutic efficacy is desired. Furthermore, prognostic information that will classify the severity of heart failure mostly relys on ex-

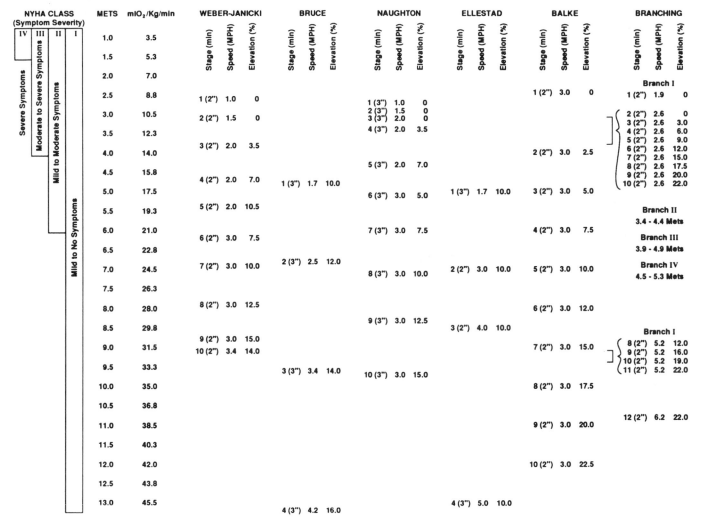

FIGURE 32.5. There are many different exercise protocols that can be used to assess the severity of functional limitations in patients with heart failure. This figure compares six different protocols, demonstrating that best estimates of maximal oxygen utilization can be accomplished with programs that increase physical stress levels gradually (e.g., Weber-Janicki, Naughton, Balke, and Branching protocols). Protocols that rapidly increase stress levels, such as the Bruce and Ellestad, are more suited to screening for ischemic heart disease. Also represented in this figure is the functional classification of heart failure patients that can be utilized to grade the severity of heart failure.

ercise test parameters. Although the test is useful for prognostic stratification of patients after myocardial infarction, and can identify heart failure patients with ischemic heart disease by analyzing stress-induced ST-T changes, this is but a secondary purpose in the heart failure patient. Indeed, frequent baseline ECG abnormalities seen in heart failure patients (digitalis effects, electrolyte effects, presence of bundle branch blocks) attenuate the sensitivity and specificity of this test in patients with ischemic heart disease. Exercise testing also may play a role in uncovering substantive ventricular ectopic activity.

Multiple modes of exercise stress have been proposed. Treadmill protocols are most commonly used (Fig. 32.5). Alternatively, measuring the distance covered during a 6-min hallway walk may provide accurate information about extent of physical limitation and the effect of therapeutic interventions. Most often used treadmill exercise test protocols have as a goal the assessment of peak oxygen utilization[41] (Fig. 32.5). Most protocols are designed to elicit symptoms within 5 to 15 min of exertion. Tests with low initial workload stresses and small workload increments such as the Naughton protocol or branching treadmill exercise test appear to be well suited for quantifying debilitation caused by heart failure (Fig. 32.5). When tests start with relatively high initial workloads and have large subsequent increments (such as with the Bruce protocol), heart failure patients may be unable to exercise long enough to obtain an accurate estimation of peak oxygen uptake. Such tests may be more appropriate for patients with minimal or no symptomatic limitation.

Comparison of treadmill exercise protocols can be done by utilizing metabolic equivalents (METs) and measured peak myocardial oxygen utilization. The MET refers to the energy cost of exertion. One MET is, essentially, the energy expenditure occurring at rest and is approximately 3.5 ml O_2/kg/min (Fig. 32.5). Calculating metabolic equivalents is important when staging a patient's disease severity. Determination of METs and oxygen uptake during exercise can be utilized to mark the boundary between classification grades in the New York Heart Association (NYHA) and Canadian Cardiovascular Society Functional Classification of exercise limitation (Fig. 32.5).

Although values of peak oxygen uptake *estimated* from treadmill exercise workload that are determined by speed of the pathway and grade of walking hill correlate reasonably well with on-line measured values of oxygen consumption, many have encouraged the utilization of respiratory gas analysis techniques to determine functional impairment more accurately in the setting of heart failure.[42] In addition to being able to quantify peak oxygen uptake during exertion, on-line gas analysis can provide the time it takes to reach anaerobic threshold. This measurement possibly gives greater insight into debilitation caused by ventricular dysfunction. Exercise gas analysis, however, requires equipment that can be expensive, needing careful attention for accurate calibration.

Additional observations of importance during exercise testing include the ability to increase heart rate (normal chronotropic response) and the ability to develop an appropriate blood pressure rise. Patients with chronotropic incompetence or a decrease in systolic or mean blood pressure with exercise generally have substantial LV dysfunction. Since dyspnea and fatigue usually are the exercise-limiting factors in patients with heart failure, one needs to monitor carefully at which point these difficulties develop. Although these are subjective complaints, peak heart rate and workloads inducing these symptoms can be reproducible in a given patient. A guide to an appropriate increase in systolic blood pressure is a 10–mm Hg increase over the previous stage. Peak heart rate formulae have been recommended but, again, most heart failure patients when exercising will terminate the protocol because of fatigue or dyspnea before reaching their peak predicted heart rate.

As already mentioned, exercise testing with accompanying echocardiographic wall motion or scintigraphic global LV function assessment also can be useful. Quantification of regions of ischemia and determining at what level of stress wall motion abnormalities develop provides valuable information. Furthermore, a decrease in global ejection fraction with exercise portends a poor prognosis.

Exercise testing also can be useful when determining the ability of certain drugs to control atrial fibrillation rates and identify patients with exercise-induced ventricular tachycardia.

Exercise hemodynamics also have been utilized, although less often, to define high-risk patients with heart failure. By analyzing the ventricular filling pressure response to supine exercise in the cardiac catheterization laboratory, individuals with heart failure and arrhythmias can be identified who are at risk of antiarrhythmic drug-induced difficulties.[43] This approach also may be helpful in patients with borderline symptoms and findings.

As mentioned, classification of the severity of heart failure utilizing respiratory gas exchange techniques during exercise allows patients' symptoms and overall disease state to be stratified precisely based on maximum oxygen consumption. Normal patients (class I) can achieve >20 ml O_2/min/kg at maximum exertion (VO_2 max); 16 to 20 ml O_2/min/kg places a patient in class II with class III patients achieving 10–15 ml O_2/min/kg; class IV patients are able to achieve only <10 ml O_2/min/kg.[44] In this latter group of patients there is an inability to increase stroke volume and cardiac output during exercise. It is important to understand, however, that although response to exercise is determined substantially by cardiac output, other parameters must be considered such as gas exchange and metabolic issues in the skeletal muscles and peripheral vascular beds themselves. Also, motivation is important in patients with heart failure. It is not at all unusual to see individuals with severely depressed ejection fraction exercising substantially and, conversely, to find that some patients with relatively modest impairment in LV function achieve a relatively low maximal workload. This serves to emphasize the need to obtain multidimensional tests to characterize the heart failure milieu most completely.

Cardiac Catheterization

Cardiac catheterization, including the performance of coronary angiography and contrast left ventriculography, has formed the cornerstone on which our understanding of heart failure and LV dysfunction has been based. A great deal of insight regarding mechanics of atrial, ventricular, and valvular performance can be gleaned from routine procedures in the cardiac catheterization laboratory. With respect to ventricular function and the mechanics of contraction, most of these observations focus on determination of chamber volume and pressure changes over time. The major drawback to performing cardiac catheterization is the fact that it is an invasive, operative procedure requiring specialized equipment and expertise and it is expensive. This has limited, somewhat, its applicability but many of the observations made at the time of the invasive

TABLE 32.9. Significance of hemodynamic data in heart failure patients.

Data obtained	Significance
Cardiac output	Oxygen delivery
Systemic vascular resistance	Systemic arteriolar area/volume
Systemic pressure	Systemic perfusion pressure/afterload
Pulmonary capillary wedge pressure	Left ventricular filling and pressure gradient in lung
Pulmonary vascular resistance	Pulmonic arteriolar area/volume
Pulmonary pressure	Pulmonic perfusion pressure/afterload
Right atrial pressure	Right ventricular filling

study can now be obtained with noninvasive techniques. Still, however, it is extraordinarily important to consider cardiac catheterization in any patient suffering heart failure to understand thoroughly cardiac difficulties, stage disease severity, and determine response to medications.[45] It is also important to differentiate information gleaned from hemodynamic monitoring (Table 32.9) versus that available from angiography. Furthermore, one must remember that long-term observation of pump performance indices and intracardiac pressure can be obtained with right heart catheterization utilizing balloon-tipped pulmonary artery catheters having thermal dilution and oxygen saturation sensors. Monitoring patients with heart failure decompensation in intensive care unit settings can allow precise parenteral and oral medication adjustment.

Angiography during cardiac catheterization allows identification and quantification of obstructive coronary pathology. In addition, the degree of aortic or mitral valvular regurgitation can be determined and with single or biplane left ventriculography, volumes calculated such that ejection fraction is defined precisely and regurgitant fraction estimated. Obviously, right and left ventricular chamber shape can be determined as well. More difficult and challenging during LV contrast angiography is the determination of diastolic function. Still, frame-by-frame cineangiographic analysis utilizing simultaneous pressure and volume determination can be done to characterize ventricular filling properties.

Specific hemodynamic observations should include calculation of cardiac output by either indicator dilution methods or angiographic stroke volume determination. By determining flow and pressure, computation of performance indices easily can be done. Table 32.9 summarizes the significance of hemodynamic data in heart failure. Many computer programs and algorithms are available to assist with these calculations. Obviously, the presence of shunts or congenital heart disease should be excluded by oxygen saturation measurement, catheter placement, hemodynamic evaluation, and angiography.

Hemodynamics during exercise sometimes can be helpful when these measurements are normal at rest.[45] Exercise of a patient during cardiac catheterization is most frequently performed in the supine position but with Swan-Ganz catheterization of the pulmonary artery done via internal jugular approach, upright bicycle exercise is possible. Exercise level can be determined by calculating oxygen consumption and METs, as already discussed. In the supine position cardiac output should increase mainly by heart rate rise with only minimal stroke volume augmentation. The arterial venous oxygen content difference will rise in patients with heart failure and intracardiac pressures during exercise can change dramatically. Normally, the LV end-diastolic pressure or pulmonary capillary wedge pressure should not increase to >15 to 18 mm Hg during exercise. Heart failure patients with normal resting hemodynamics may demonstrate a dramatic rise in this pressure. Exercise hemodynamics therefore can quantitate some of the limitations created by a heart failure patient's disease milieu. It should be pointed out, however, that insight into pulmonary artery pressure also may be determined fairly accurately with Doppler echocardiography.[46]

Finally, quantification of hemodynamic response to medication therapy can be determined by cardiac catheterization.[47] It is extraordinarily important, for example, to demonstrate that pulmonary hypertension is not fixed or severe in patients who are being considered for orthotopic cardiac transplantation. By measuring decrement in LV filling and pulmonary artery pressures during vasodilator infusion, appropriate patient selection or exclusion can occur.[48]

Endomyocardial Biopsy

Endomyocardial biopsy can be an important diagnostic procedure in evaluating patients with heart failure (Table 32.10). The procedure is now commonly performed in the cardiac transplantation setting, and the technique has been demonstrated to be safe when performed judiciously. Application of this technique in widespread fashion to patients with heart failure is, however, unwarranted. This procedure should not be performed in everyone with heart failure, rather when information obtained is likely to render a diagnosis or influence therapy. Consensus suggests that endomyocardial biopsy can be useful in the detection of myocarditis, in monitoring anthracycline drug toxicity during chemotherapy, and in confirming etiology of some cardiomyopathies such as hemochromatosis, amyloidosis, and sacoidosis.[69]

In the future, sophisticated biochemical and morphometric analysis of biopsy specimens may allow more accurate prognostication in patients with LV dysfunction, and discriminate between patients likely to im-

TABLE 32.10. When endomyocardial biopsy may be helpful.

Disorders diagnosed
Amyloid heart disease
Anthracycline cardiotoxicity
Carcinoid heart disease
Endocardial fibroelastosis
Fabry's heart disease
Glycogen storage disease
Heart transplantation rejection
Hemochromatosis
Myocarditis
Radiation-induced myocardial fibrosis
Sarcoidosis of the heart
Tumors of the heart

prove with certain therapy and those who probably will not. Furthermore, endomyocardial biopsy may provide an extraordinarily important tool for understanding the molecular genetics of the failing myocardium.

Today, disposable bioptomes with flexible cutting jaws can be inserted percutaneously via central venous (usually the internal jugular) or arterial access sites. Right ventricular endomyocardial biopsy is performed most often but LV biopsy also can be done safely if the operator is skilled and judicious.

Routine histochemical staining methods are utilized with hematoxylin-eosin, Mason's trichome stain for fibrosis, Congo red stain for amyloidosis, and Prussian blue stain for hemochromatosis. Specimens also may be obtained and frozen quickly for immunofluorescent staining protocols. Samples can be placed directly into viral culture medium, although rarely are these cultures productive. Reasonable diagnostic sensitivity can be noted in diseases that affect both right and left ventricular myocardium in symmetrical fashion. Certain conditions that primarily cause changes in the LV dictate biopsy approach to this site. These would include suspected hypertrophic cardiomyopathy, endomyocardial fibrosis, and scleroderma heart disease. When biopsy is performed on patients with asymmetrical hypertrophy or cardiac tumors, echocardiographic guidance can be useful to define the region of biopsy interest. Infiltrative, diffuse cardiomyopathies such as those caused by amyloidosis, sarcoid heart disease, and hematomocrosis can be diagnosed readily by right ventricular endomyocardial biopsy. Again, echocardiographic guidance may be useful to ensure that diffuse, random sampling of the ventricle has occurred. It should be emphasized that in many conditions, sarcoidosis for example, a negative biopsy does not exclude the disorder or cardiac involvement. The presence of sarcoidosis on heart biopsy, however, generally dictates steroid therapy.

Although complications are rare, they can be serious. The usual complications associated with catheterization of any central arterial or venous structure can occur during endomyocardial biopsy. Furthermore, induction of arrhythmias during the biopsy can be seen with rapid atrial fibrillation or even ventricular tachycardia causing hemodynamic deterioration in patients with already compromised ventricular function. Cardiac tamponade occurs when perforation of the right ventricle with biopsy occurs, and it may be fatal. Air embolus can develop with catheterization of the internal jugular vein, and hoarseness secondary to recurrent laryngeal paralysis from lidocaine infusion and Horner's syndrome have been noted. When left heart biopsy is performed systemic embolization is a possibility.

Ambulatory Monitoring

Ambulatory ECG monitoring has been utilized to characterize precisely cardiac arrhythmias and ST-T wave alterations associated with ischemia.[49] Long-term analysis of an ECG has proved much more sensitive and specific for arrhythmias whereas simple resting studies give a great deal of information regarding hypertrophy, ischemia, and metabolic effects.[50] Unfortunately, ST- and T-wave analysis for ischemia is much less sensitive in the heart failure population as the frequency of nonspecific ST- and T-wave changes caused by electrolyte abnormalities, drug effects (digitalis and quinidine for example), and frequent bundle branch blocks preclude accurate estimation of ST segment shifts.

Arrhythmia analysis can be extremely important, however, with ambulatory monitoring identifying highrisk subsets of patients suffering potentially malignant ventricular dysrhythmias, bradycardia, or heart block. Although it is controversial what to do with these patients, it is uniformly believed that improvement in medical therapy for heart failure will lessen the risk of a disastrous difficulty.

Phonocardiology and Pulse-Wave Recording

Although not used with the frequency they once were, pulse-wave recordings can be helpful in heart failure patients. Recording techniques such as apex cardiography, pulse-wave transmission, and phonocardiography can help integrate physical findings with more objective parameters.[51] Timing of heart sounds precisely with apex or venous pulse recording, particularly when combined with M-mode echocardiography, allows measurement of systolic and diastolic function indices. Although not a technique with high sensitivity or specificity, these elegant, but simple, tests should not be forgotten.

Carotid pulse tracings can demonstrate attenuation of the normal rapid upstroke and pathologic exacerbation of the dicrotid notch, giving a bifed-appearing pulse in severe cardiomyopathy and heart failure.[52] Exaggeration of this dicrotid wave, sometimes referred to as a "dicrotid pulse" or "dicrotism," reflects low cardiac output and high peripheral resistance. With a simultaneously recorded phonocardiogram, ECG, and carotid pulse tracing, ejecting time indices can be determined and if they are prolonged, suggest significant obstruction to the aortic valve. On the other hand, shortening of ventricular ejection time suggests diminution of stroke volume due to LV dysfunction or mitral regurgitation.

Jugular venous pressure recordings reflect pressure changes in the right atrium.[53] Right ventricular hypertrophy, tricuspid stenosis, pulmonary valve stenosis, and pulmonary hypertension can cause impaired right atrial emptying and prominent jugular venous A waves. Irregularly appearing, large, exaggerated A waves also can be seen when atrioventricular dissociation is present and right atrial contraction occurs when the tricuspid valve is closed. In patients with heart failure and prominent tricuspid regurgitation, the X descent of the jugular venous pulse is generally exaggerated and the V wave becomes abnormal. If tricuspid regurgitation is particularly pronounced, the V wave merges into an abnormal regurgitant wave that can produce a dramatic neck wave recording and physical finding. Indeed, jugular venous pulsation can be forceful enough in some patients with heart failure and tricuspid regurgitation that a lateral head bob can be noted.

Apex cardiography records the precordial movements reflecting the heart beat.[54] Diastolic events that are usually not perceptible during palpation can be recorded utilizing this technique. As with recordings of the carotid pulse and jugular veins, a normal apex cardiogram can provide an accurate template for cardiac events during systole and diastole. The apex cardiogram frequently demonstrates a high amplitude A wave recorded immediately before S-1 when LV filling pressures are elevated. LV volume overload causes a hyperdynamic apex impulse and LV hypertrophy a very sustained horizontal plateau after the E point.

A variety of combinations of pulse-wave recordings have been utilized to characterize more precisely events related to LV dysfunction. Despite the fact that all of these techniques are relatively subjective, they can be a useful means of augmenting the physical examination.

Magnetic Resonance Imaging

Magnet resonance imaging (MRI) holds great promise for defining and quantifying cardiac pathology in patients with heart failure.[55] Although expensive, the technique can provide detailed information regarding three-dimensional structure in patients with congenital heart disease as well as estimates of biventricular function, valve area, and shunts. The site and extent of myocardial infarction can be surmised as well as the presence of ventricular aneurysm or thrombi. Right and left ventricular ejection fraction can be calculated and cardiac output estimated. Ventricular mass can be determined precisely with this technique and myopathic versus reactive ventricular hypertrophy differentiated. Specifically, with respect to heart failure, the important functional heart information that can be obtained with dynamic MRIs includes chamber volumes, biventricular ejection fraction, cardiac output determination, and regurgitant volume determination.[56,57,58] When MRI is compared to echocardiography (Table 32.11), a major disadvantage seems to be the expense and complexity of the equipment. Furthermore, the inability to estimate stenotic valve pressure gradients and determine pulmonary artery pressure are strikes against this technique. Furthermore, the resolution of contrast ventriculography is better than that obtained with MRI and be-

TABLE 32.11. Noninvasive imaging techniques in heart failure patients.

Observation	M-Mode echo	2D echo	Doppler echo	First-pass RNVG	Equilibrium RNVG	MRI	CT
Anatomic relationships	+	+++	0/+	0/+	+	++++	+++
Tissue characterization	++	++	0	0	0	+++	+++
Wall motion	+	++++	0	++	++++	+++	+++
Hypertrophy	+++	++++	0	0	0/+	++++	+++
Wall thickening	+++	+++	0	0	0	++++	++
Valvular pathology	++	++++	0	0	0	+++	++
Valvular regurgitation and stenosis	++	++	++++	0	0	++	+
Hemodynamics	+	+	++++	0	0	0	0
Diastolic function	++	+++	++++	++	++	+	0
Stress exercise	++++	++++	++++	++++	++++	0	0
Pharmacologic stress	++++	++++	++++	++++	++++	+++++	++++
Lower cost/ Easy availability	++++	++++	+++	+++	+++	+	++

2D = Two-dimensional; RNVG = radionuclide ventriculography; MRI = magnetic resonance imaging; CT = Computerized tomography. 0–++++ represents the relative utility of the different techniques in the authors' opinion.

cause of the equipment size and patient configuration in the scanning machine, MRI cannot evaluate ventricular function under exertional stress as can be done with echocardiography, equilibrium blood pool scanning, or first-pass radionuclide ventriculography. It is possible, however, to consider the use of pharmacologic stress.

Computerized Axial-Tomographic Heart Imaging

Computed tomographic (CT) imaging of the heart has as its major limitation the fact that required exposure times are too long to allow clear and well defined images of the heart. Motion artifact is great. Gating the images based on the ECG has been somewhat helpful with this difficulty, and future developments with ultra-fast CT may obviate this limitation.[59] The major advantage of CT of the heart lies in the fact that cross-sectional images with spatial and density orientation can be produced that seem better than ECG or radionuclide imaging. Furthermore, this technique can provide precise images of the great vessels. Because of the difficulty with gating, CT imaging of the heart has not been performed commonly in patients with heart failure. It seems that the development of MRI procedures may overshadow CT imaging attempts. Still, the speed of CT performance is greater than MRI, and noise is not a detrimental factor. Exercise tests theoretically could also be performed during CT imaging. The overall value of CT imaging of heart failure patients remains to be determined.

Pulmonary Function Testing

Since dyspnea is both a prime component of the heart failure syndrome as well as a variety of other diseases, it is extremely important to differentiate symptoms produced by primary pulmonary, muscular, skeletal, or neurologic abnormalities from those caused by heart failure. Pulmonary function testing, which should include spirometry evaluation, measurement of lung volumes, and determination of carbon dioxide diffusing capacity, can be helpful when questions regarding the etiology of dyspnea persist.[60] An advantage of pulmonary function testing is that it is relatively inexpensive and essentially noninvasive. Furthermore, the combination of information from an exercise protocol with measurement of a variety of pulmonary function parameters can quantify precisely the extent of a patient's physical impairment. It is important to remember, however, that these tests do not assess cardiac function per se and that if testing procedures are not compulsively performed, reproducibility can be a problem.

Changes in pulmonary function noted in patients with chronic CHF generally relate to the production of restrictive defects on spirometry with a diminution in total lung capacity and decreased lung recoil at low volumes.[61] This results in an increased residual volume with subsequent diminution in vital capacity. Although chronic interstitial edema accounts for this problem, when heart failure is aggressively treated some patients with chronic pulmonary congestion do not have complete normalization of their pulmonary function tests.

In abnormalities of small airway function, such as reduced forced expiratory volume and forced expiratory fraction, lung volumes may still be diminished but compliance remains relatively normal. Bronchial spasm can cause frank reactive airway disease that resolves with diminution of pulmonary congestion. Pulmonary function tests, however, are mainly useful in differentiating intrinsic airway disease from gas exchange difficulties produced by congestion and diminution of compliance.[62]

Ancillary Laboratory Analysis

By analyzing a variety of laboratory values, important precipitating or concomitant disease states can be excluded or, if present, addressed. It is extremely important to characterize, for example, the hematologic profile of a heart failure patient. Anemia can present as heart failure when it slowly develops, is substantive, or produces a high output metabolic state. Likewise, leukemias and lymphomas can present with dyspnea and weakness on exertion. In addition to white and red blood cell counts and analyses, measurement of prothrombin and partial thromboplastin times are important. When hepatic congestion is substantive, abnormalities of these clotting indices can be seen and this portends a poor prognosis.

Electrolyte levels, particularly of serum sodium, reflect activation of the neurohormonal axis, particularly via arginine vasopressin, angiotensin, and aldosterone mechanisms. Hyponatremia is associated with severe chronic heart failure and when present portends a poor prognosis.[63] Potassium and magnesium levels also should be assessed. Hypokalemia is frequently noted in patients being diuresed and it is known that hypokalemia can contribute to malignant arrhythmia as well as digitalis intoxication. Hypomagnesemia also is seen in patients receiving diuretics.[64] Furthermore, heart failure can interfere with absorption of magnesium in the gastrointestinal tract, and like potassium, low levels of magnesium have been purported to play a role in arrhythmia induction.

Renal function analysis with determination of blood urea nitrogen, serum creatinine, and creatinine clearance is important in assessing heart failure severity as well as reversibility of prerenal azotemia. Proteinuria is seen in patients with heart failure, but other causes also must be considered. Since the heart failure milieu is frequently seen in patients with diabetes and renal insufficiency due to primary nephrologic causes, proteinuria should always be explored. Furthermore, characterization of renal function is important because of the many nephrotoxic drugs patients with heart failure often receive.

Analysis of hepatic function is helpful when assessing severity and extent of passive congestion of the liver. It is important to differentiate between primary hepatic disease and passive congestion.[65] This has previously been discussed.

A nutritional evaluation also is important in heart failure patients because of the cachexia and negative nitrogen balance that develop.[66] Assessment of lipids may be important. In more advanced stages of the heart failure milieu, hypolipoproteinemia invariably is seen. This abnormality is caused by relative starvation, difficulty in absorbing lipids across a congested, hypoperfused bowel wall, and abnormalities in lipid synthesis pathways.[67]

The appropriate integrity of the pituitary–thyroid axis also should be insured to exclude diseases that can cause LV dysfunction or appear as heart failure.

Determination of catecholamine levels, particularly epinephrine and nonepinephrine, may help determine a patient's prognosis. It has been well demonstrated that elevation of catecholamines correlates with the severity and long-term presence of substantive heart failure.[68]

Integration of Diagnostic Evaluation

In the end, results of the aforementioned procedures of evaluation need to be integrated so that the following questions can be answered:

Does the patient suffer from heart failure?
What is the etiology of the syndrome?
What precipitated the patient's deterioration?
How severe is the heart failure?
What is the patient's long-term prognosis?
How should the patient be treated acutely?
How should the patient be treated chronically?
Can the disease process be cured and can the state of heart failure be ameliorated or attenuated?

We know, for example, that certain parameters predict high mortality in patients with heart failure. For example, individuals having ongoing and active ischemia with low ejection fraction and high left heart filling pressure accompanied by an inability to achieve a VO_2 max greater than 10 ml O_2/kg/min have dismal short-term prognoses. Efforts should be made to correct the ischemic process, increase ejection fraction, and lower filling pressure, thereby improving exercise tolerance, ameliorating symptoms, and prolonging life.

It would not be correct to suggest that all of the tests and procedures mentioned here should be done on every patient with, or suspected of having, heart failure.

Unfortunately, a precise algorithm for ordering procedures is impossible to devise because of the extraordinary patient heterogeneity suggested by Figure 32.2. But by understanding the pathophysiology of heart failure and having insight into the information various clinical procedures might provide (as well as their disadvantages), a patients' diagnostic evaluations can be individually planned. It should be evident from the foregoing discussion that sophisticated cardiac imaging or endomyocardial biopsy is rarely required. However, when LV dysfunction or heart failure is suspected, patients should undergo some form of testing to quantify ejection fraction, assess myocardial perfusion, identify regional wall motion abnormalities, define coronary anatomy, and differentiate ischemia from scar. Arrhythmias should be controlled only when they produce symptoms, are life-threatening, or are known to be associated with high morbidity. Treatable causes of the syndrome of heart failure should be excluded and toxins eliminated. Staging of exercise capacity is mandatory in each patient by some means or another and understanding a patient's hemodynamics will guide drug dispensation. The importance of a thorough and integrated evaluation of the patient with the heart failure syndrome cannot be overemphasized. The etiology and precipitating factors must be known, as well as the patient's prognosis and likelihood of response to therapy.

Acknowledgments. The authors would like to express their appreciation to Kathryn Pruitt-Bruun and Marlane Kayfes for their editorial skills and patience during manuscript preparation.

References

1. Lewis T. *Diseases of the heart.* New York: MacMillan; 1933.
2. Braunwald E. *Heart disease. A textbook of cardiovascular medicine.* 3rd ed. Philadelphia: Saunders; 1988.
3. White PD. *Heart disease.* 3rd ed. New York: MacMillan; 1947.
4. Kannel WB. Epidemiologic aspects of heart failure. In Weber KT, ed. *Heart failure; current concepts and management cardiology. Cardiology Clinic Series.* Philadelphia: Saunders; 1989.
5. Hope JA. *Treatise on the diseases of the heart and great vessels.* London: William Kidd; 1832.
6. Braunwald E. Clinical Manifestation of heart failure. In Braunwald E, ed. *Heart disease: a textbook of cardiovascular medicine.* 3rd ed. Philadelphia: Saunders; 1988.
7. Mackenzie J. *Disease of the heart.* 3rd ed. London: Oxford University Press; 1913.
8. Rushmer RF. Cardiac compensation, hypertrophy, and myopathy, and congestive heart failure. In Rushmer RF, ed. *Cardiovascular dynamics.* Philadelphia: Saunders; 1976.

9. Gibson GR. Enalapril-induced cough. *Arch Intern Med.* 1989;149:2701–2703.

10. The SOLVD Investigators. Effect of enalapril on survival in patients with reduced left ventricular ejection fractions and congestive heart failure. *N Engl J Med.* 1991; 325:293–302.

11. Poole-Wilson PA, Buller NP. Cases of symptoms in chronic congestive heart failure and implications for treatment. *Am J Cardiol.* 1988;62:31A.

12. Braunwald E, Grossman W. Clinical aspects of heart failure. In Braunwald E, ed. *Heart disease: a textbook of cardiovascular medicine.* 4th ed. Philadelphia: Saunders; 1991.

13. Cohn JN, Rector TS. Prognosis of congestive heart failure and predictors of mortality. *Am J Cardiol.* 1988;62:25A.

14. Fuster V, Steele PM, Edwards WD, et al. Primary pulmonary hypertension; natural history and the importance of thrombosis. *Circulation.* 1984;70:580.

15. Rees PJ, Clark TJH. Paroxysmal nocturnal dyspnea and periodic respiration. *Lancet.* 1979;2:1315.

16. McKee PA, Costelli WP, McNamara PM, Kannel WB. The natural history of congestive heart failure. The Framingham Study. *N Engl J Med.* 1971;285:1441.

17. Chakko S, Woska D, Marinez H, DeMarchena E, Futterman L, Kessler K. Clinical radiographic and hemodynamic correlations in chronic congestive heart failure: conflicting results may lead to inappropriate care. *Am J Med.* 1991;90:353.

18. Marantz PR, Alderman MH, Tobin JN. Diagnostic heterogeneity in clinical trials for congestive heart failure. *Ann Intern Med.* 1988;109:55.

19. Packer M, Lee WH, Kessler PD, Gottlieb SS, Barnstein JL, Kukin ML. Role of neurohormonal mechanism in determining survival in patients with severe chronic heart failure. *Circulation.* 1987:75(Suppl 4):80.

20. Packer M. Potential role of potassium as a determinate of morbidity and mortality in patients with systemic hypertension and congestive heart failure. *Am J Cardiol.* 1990;65;45E.

21. Wolke AM, Brooks KM, Schaffauer F. The liver in congestive heart failure. *Primary Cardiol.* 1982;8:130.

22. Haber HL, Leary JA, Kessler PD, Kukin ML, Gottlieb SS, Packer M. The erythrocyte sedimentation rate in congestive heart failure. *N Engl J Med.* 1991;324:353.

23. Glover L, Boxley WA, Dodge HT. A quantitative evaluation of heart size measurements from chest roentgenograms. *Circulation.* 1973;47:1289.

24. Ostojic M, Young JB, Hess KR. Prediction of left ventricular ejection fraction using a unique method of chest x-ray and ECG analysis: a non-invasive index of cardiac performance based on the concept of heart volume and mass interrelationships. *Am Heart J.* 1989;117:590.

25. Reichek N, Devereaux RB. Left ventricular hypertrophy: relationship of anatomic, echocardiographic and electrocardiographic findings. *Circulation.* 1981;63;1391.

26. Sullivan W, Vlodaver Z, Tunor N, Long L, Edwards JE. Correlation of electrocardiographic and pathologic findings in healed myocardial infarction. *Am J Cardiol.* 1978;42;724.

27. Feigenbaum H. Echocardiography. In Braunwald E, ed. *Heart disease. A textbook of cardiovascular medicine.* 4th ed. Philadelphia: Saunders; 1991.

28. Seward JB, Khandheria BK, Oh JK, et al. Transesophageal echocardiography: technique, anatomic correlations, implementation, and clinical applications. *Mayo Clin Proc.* 1988;63:649.

29. Strok TV, Muller RM, Piske GJ, Ewart CO, Hochrein H. Non-invasive measurement of left ventricular filling pressures by means of transmitral pulsed Doppler ultrasound. *Am J Cardiol.* 1989;64:655.

30. Rokey R, Kuo LC, Zoghbi WA, Limacher MC, Quinones MA. Determination of parameters of left ventricular diastolic filling with pulsed Doppler echocardiography: comparisons with cineangiography. *Circulation.* 1985;71:543.

31. Zoghbi WA, Farmer JL, Soto JG, Nelson JG, Quinones MA. Accurate non-invasive quantification of stenotic aortic valve area by Doppler echocardiography. *Circulation.* 1986;73:452.

32. Young JB, Leon CA, Weilbaecher DA. Endomyocardial biopsy in critically ill patients. The procedure and diagnostic and prognostic potential. *Prob Crit Care (Adv Intervent Cardiol).* 1988;2:433–462.

33. Sugishita Y, Kosekt S. Dynamic exercise echocardiography. *Circulation.* 1979;60:743.

34. Presti CF, Armstrong WF, Feigenbaum H. Comparison of echocardiography at peak exercise and after bicycle exercise in evaluation of patients with known or suspected coronary artery disease. *J Am Soc Echo.* 1988;1:119.

35. Borer JS, Henry WL, Epstein SE. Echocardiographic observations in patients with systemic infiltrative disease involving the heart. *Am J Cardiol.* 1977;39:184.

36. Zaret BL, Wackers FJ, Soufer R. Nuclear Cardiology. In Braunwald E, ed. *Heart disease. A textbook of cardiovascular medicine.* 4th ed. Philadelphia: Saunders; 1991.

37. Cohn JN, Johnson G, and The Veterans Administrative Study Group. Heart failure with normal ejection fraction. *Circulation.* 1990;81(Suppl III):4A.

38. Chan SY, Brunken RC, Buxton DB. Cardiac positron emission tomography. The foundations and clinical applications. *J Thorac Imag.* 1990;5:9.

39. Schelbert HR, Buxton D. Insights into coronary artery disease gained from metabolic imaging. *Circulation.* 1988;78:496.

40. Morris CK, Veshna K, Kawaguchi T, Hideg A, Froelich V. The prognostic value of exercise capacity: a review of the literature. *Am Heart J.* 1991;122:1423.

41. Jette M, Sidney K, Blumchen G. Metabolic equivalent (METs) in exercise testing, exercise prescription, and evaluation of functional capacity. *Clin Cardiol.* 1990;13:555.

42. Weber KT, Janicki JS. *Cardiopulmonary exercise testing: physiologic principles and clinical applications.* Philadelphia: Saunders; 1986.

43. Pratt CM, Francis MJ, Seals AA, Zohgbi W, Young JB. Antiarrhythimic and hemodynamic evaluation of indecainide and procainamide in nonsustained ventricular tachycardia. *Am J Cardiol.* 1990;66:68.

44. Rouse RA, Kusimi F, Hosmer D. Maximal oxygen intake and nomographic assessment of functional aerobic im-

pairment in cardiovascular disease. *Am Heart J.* 1973; 85:546.

45. Grossman W, Bain DS. *Cardiac catheterization, angiography, and intervention.* 4th ed. Philadelphia: Lea & Feibiger; 1991.

46. Maeda M, Yokoto M, Iwase M, Miyahara T, Hayashi H, Sotobata I. Accuracy of cardiac output measured by continuous wave Doppler echocardiography during dynamic exercise testing in the supine position in patients with coronary artery disease. *J Am Coll Cardiol.* 1989;13:76.

47. Gollub SV, Elkayam U, Young JB, Miller LW, Haffey KA, for the Dopexamine Investigators and their associates. Efficacy and safety of the short term (six hours) intravenous infusion of dopexamine in patients with severe congestive heart failure: a randomized, double-blind, parallel, placebo-controlled multi-centered study. *J Am Coll Cardiol.* 1991;18:383.

48. Young JB, Leon CA, Lawrence EC, Whisennand HH, Noon GP, DeBakey ME. Heart replacement for terminal cardiac disease: cardiac transplantation and mechanical sustenance of the cardiovascular system (Parts I and II). *Baylor Cardiology Series.* 1989;12:4.

49. Langer A, Freeman MR, Armstrong PW. ST segment shift in unstable angina; pathophysiology in association with coronary anatomy in hospital outcome. *J Am Coll Cardiol.* 1989;13:1495.

50. Kennedy HL. Long term (Holter) electrocardiogram recordings. In Zipes DP, Jalif J, eds. *Cardiac electrophysiology. From cell to bedside.* Philadelphia: Saunders; 1990.

51. Dressler W. Pulsations of the cervical veins and liver. In Dressler W, ed. *Clinical aids in cardiac diagnosis.* New York: Grune and Stratton; 1970.

52. Constant J. *Bedside cardiology.* 3rd ed. Boston: Little, Brown. 1985.

53. Swartz MH. Jugular venous pressure pulse: its value in cardiac diagnosis. *Primary Cardiol.* 1982;8:197.

54. Cohen MV. *Correlative atlas of adult cardiac disorders. Noninvasive diagnostic techniques.* Mt. Kisco, NY: Futura Publishing. 1980.

55. Sechtem U, Sommerhoff BA, Markiewicz W. Assessment of regional left ventricular wall thickening by magnetic resonance imaging. Evaluation in normal persons and patients with global and regional dysfunction. *Am J Cardiol.* 1987;57:154.

56. Busser PT, Aufferman W, Holt WW, et al. Non-invasive evaluation of global left ventricular function with use of sine nuclear magnetic resonance. *J Am Coll Cardiol.* 1989;13:1294.

57. Sechtem U, Pflugfelder P, Gould R. Measurement of right and left ventricular volumes in healthy individuals with sine MR imaging. *Radiology.* 1987;163:697.

58. Higgins CB, Byrd BF, McNamara MT. Magnetic resonance imaging of the heart: a review of the variance in 172 subjects. *Radiology.* 1985;15:671.

59. Rumberger JA, Feiring AJ, Reiter SJ. Ultra-fast computed tomography: evaluation of global left ventricular anatomy and function. In Pohost GM, ed. *New concepts in cardiac imaging.* Chicago: Year Book. 1988.

60. Poole-Wilson PA, Buller NP. Causes of symptoms in chronic congestive heart failure and implications for treatment. *Am J Cardiol.* 1988;62:31A.

61. Petermann W, Barth J, Entzian P. Heart failure in airway obstruction. *Int J Cardiol.* 1987;17:207.

62. Wasserman D. Dyspnea on exertion: is it the heart or the lungs? *JAMA.* 1982;248:2042.

63. Szatalowicz VL, Arnold PE, Chaimovitz C, Bichet D, Beri T, Schrier RW. Radioimmunoassay of plasma arginine vasopressin in hyponatremic patients with congestive heart failure. *N Engl J Med.* 1981;305:263.

64. Birch GE, Giles TD. The importance of magnesium deficiency in cardiovascular disease. *Am Heart J.* 1977; 94:649.

65. Blasco VV. Features of hepatic involvement in congestive heart failure. *Cardiovasc Rev Ret.* 1983;4:963.

66. Berkowitz D, Croll MN, Likoff W. Malabsorption as a complication of congestive heart failure. *Am J Cardiol.* 1963;11:43.

67. Pittman JG, Cohen P. The pathogenesis of cardiac cachexia. *N Engl J Med.* 1964;27:403.

68. Cohn JN, Rector TS. Prognosis of congestive heart failure and predictors of mortality. *Am J Cardiol.* 1988;62:25A.

69. Mason JW, O'Connell JB. Clinical merit of endomyocardial biopsy. *Circulation.* 1989;79:971.

33
Prognosis in Congestive Heart Failure

Michael J. Domanski, Rekha Garg, and Salim Yusuf

Congestive heart failure (CHF) is a common affliction that is increasing in both incidence and prevalence. In this chapter the prognosis of CHF is examined. The epidemiology will be discussed first. Etiology is then considered with special reference to changes that have occurred. Modes of death and predictors of outcome also are considered. This is followed by an examination of the effect of treatment on prognosis.

Epidemiology

CHF affects approximately 3 million people in the United States (approx 1% of the population) and it is estimated that 400,000 new cases appear each year.[1] There has been a continued increase in both incidence and prevalence of this condition. The number of deaths due to CHF has increased four-fold in the last 20 years, during a period of decline in myocardial infarction and stroke.[2] The age-adjusted death rate for CHF also has increased two-fold,[2] suggesting that not all of the increase in CHF mortality is due to aging of the population.

CHF becomes more common with advancing age,[1,3,4] affecting about 10% of individuals over 75 years of age.[1] Men are affected more commonly than women,[2,4] being diagnosed 1.6 times more often at any given age. CHF mortality is 1.5 times higher in blacks than whites overall, although blacks experienced a 17% decline in age-adjusted CHF mortality between 1968 and 1978 at a time when whites experienced a 32% increase.[2] Interestingly, in whites less than 45 years old and in blacks less than 74 years old there was a decline in mortality rates, whereas in older individuals in both groups there was an increase.[2] The reasons for the differences in mortality rates from CHF between whites and blacks are not clear.

In the United States, the rate of hospitalization for CHF also has increased,[2] and CHF is now the most common discharge diagnosis in patients older than 65 years.[1] Ghali et al.[5] studied trends in hospitalization for heart failure in the United States for the years 1973 to 1986. During this period, the number of patients with CHF as a discharge diagnosis more than doubled. Hospitalization rates were 33% higher for nonwhite than white men and 50% higher for nonwhite than white women. Hospitalization rates remained constant for individuals between 35 and 54 years old over the period of the study but increased substantially for older patients. The steepest rise occurred in the oldest patients (>74 years old). The increase in hospitalization rates in the elderly parallels the data on mortality in the elderly.

These data indicate that CHF is an important medical and public health problem and emphasize the need for continuing efforts to improve therapy.

Etiology

Results from the Framingham study published in 1971 suggested that the most common etiologic factor for CHF was hypertension.[4] In this study, 75% of CHF patients had hypertension. Coronary artery disease was present in 38.7% but was associated with hypertension in all but 10%. Although population-based data are not available, it appears that there has been a significant change in the etiology of CHF. As shown in Figure 33.1, most cases are now the result of coronary artery disease,[6] with cardiomyopathy being the second most common etiology.[1] Data from the SOLVD Registry,[7] which collected information on patients seen during a 14-month period in 1988 and 1989, showed that 74% of patients with left ventricular ejection fractions (EF) <45% had ischemic heart disease as the underlying cause of ventricular dysfunction. In 4% of patients, hypertension was considered to be the etiology. The Digitalis Investigation Group (DIG) study[8] showed similar results. In this study, 71% of patients with an EF <45% had ischemic heart disease and 7% had

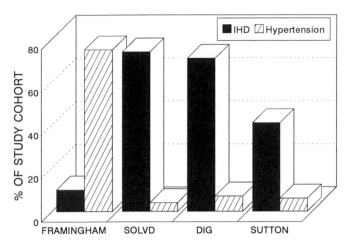

FIGURE 33.1. In contrast to the Framingham study, later studies have demonstrated that the most common cause of heart failure is ischemic heart disease.

hypertension as the primary cause of their left ventricular (LV) dysfunction. A study by Sutton et al.[9] also reported that coronary disease was the most frequent cause of CHF.

Cause of Death

The mortality rate for CHF is about 50% over 5 years.[3] In the Studies of Left Ventricular Dysfunction (SOLVD) Treatment Trial[10] of patients with an EF <35% and CHF that required drug therapy [a randomized trial of 2569 patients comparing angiotensin-converting enzyme (ACE) inhibitor to placebo], 90% of deaths were classified as being cardiovascular, with 49% of all deaths being classified as being due to progressive heart failure and 21% classified being sudden (Table 33.1). Ten percent of deaths were due to myocardial in-

TABLE 33.1. Numbers and percent of deaths in SOLVD patients in the placebo group (mean follow-up 42 months).

	N	%
Randomized patients	1284	(100)
Deaths	510	(39.7)
Cardiovascular deaths	461	(35.9)
Cardiac	441	(34.3)
Arrhythmia	113	(8.8)
Heart failure or arrhythmia with worse CHF	251	(19.5)
Myocardial infarction	53	(4.1)
Other	24	(1.9)
Stroke	11	(0.9)
Other vascular or unknown	9	(0.7)
Noncardiovascular deaths	49	(3.8)

CHF = congestive heart failure.

farction and 2% were due to stroke. In the Veterans Administration study,[11] men with chronic heart failure and EF <45%, cardiothoracic ratio ≥.55, or LV diastolic internal diameter >2.7 cm/m² of body surface area were enrolled. In this patient population the sudden death rate was 45%. Hence, the most common cause of death is progressive heart failure but sudden death also is a common terminal event.

The relative frequency of different causes of sudden death in CHF remains to be completely defined. Ventricular tachycardia and ventricular fibrillation are likely common causes. A study by Luu et al.[12] suggests that electromechanical dissociation or severe brachycardia may not be unusual.

Predictors of Outcome

Clinical (Table 33.2)

Although men have been reported to have a worse prognosis than women (60% 5-yr mortality vs. 45%)[1] in one study, in another study the opposite findings were observed.[7] However, after adjustment for risk factors the mortality differences between sexes disappear.[7]

Data from the SOLVD Registry[7] suggest that a number of other clinical parameters have prognostic significance. Older patients fare worse than younger ones. For instance, patients 21 to 55 years old had a 16.6% 1-yr mortality, whereas patients older than 76 years had a 38.4% 1-yr mortality. Diabetes, presence of atrial fibrillation, history of smoking, alcohol consumption,

TABLE 33.2. Predictors of poor prognosis in CHF patients.

Clinical	Neurohumoral
Old age	↑ Plasma renin activity
Diabetes	↑ Atrial natriuretic factor
Atrial fibrillation	↑ Plasma norepinephrine
Smoking history	levels
Alcohol consumption	
Pulmonary disease	
Higher NYHA class	
Left ventricular function	
Reduced ejection fraction	
CT ratio >.52	
Increased end-systolic or end-diastolic volume	
Functional capacity	
MVO₂ < 10 ml/kg/min	
Reduced distance walked on 6-min walk test	
Ventricular dysrhythmia	
Nonsustained ventricular tachycardia	

CT = cardiothoracic; MVO₂ = myocardial oxygen consumption; NYHA = New York Heart Association.

or pulmonary disease are all associated with a worse prognosis.

Several studies have suggested a strong correlation between New York Heart Association (NYHA) functional class and mortality.[7,11,13] In the SOLVD trial,[10] patients in NYHA functional class IV had a 64% mortality over the follow-up period, which averaged 41.4 months compared to 51% for patients in NYHA functional class III, 35% for patients in NYHA functional class II, and 30% for patients in NYHA functional class I.

Measures of LV Function

Resting EF is among the strongest predictors of mortality.[11,14] EF is readily obtained noninvasively by radionuclide ventriculography. For this reason, EF occupies a central place in the assessment of prognosis. In the SOLVD trial patients with an EF 6% to 22% had a 50% mortality over the 41.4-month average follow-up, patients with EF 23% to 29% had a 39% mortality, and those with EF 30% to 35% had a 28% mortality. Similar results have been reported in several other studies.

A chest x ray with a cardiothoracic ratio >0.52 has been associated with a worse prognosis.[7] White et al.[15] studied 605 men under the age of 60 years after at least one myocardial infarction. This group found that LV dilatation (end-diastolic volume and, in particular, end-systolic volume) after myocardial infarction is an important prognostic indicator and adds useful prognostic information to that obtained from measuring ejection fraction.

Functional Capacity

Szlachcic et al.[16] studied the relationship of exercise capacity measured by maximal oxygen consumption ($M\dot{V}O_2$ max) to prognosis. They found that the 1-yr mortality rate was significantly higher in patients with $M\dot{V}O_2$ max <10 ml/min/kg compared to patients with a higher $M\dot{V}O_2$ max. Other studies suggest that long-term (4–12 months) mortality is not well predicted by exercise capacity.[17,18]

Bittner et al.[19] reported a strong correlation between the distance that patients with CHF or EF <.45 could walk in 6 min and their prognosis. For patients who could walk less than 305 m in 6 min, the 1-yr mortality was 11.3%, whereas it was only 3.8% in patients who could walk more than 443 m. The 6-min walk test also was a strong predictor of hospitalization rates at 1 yr.

Ventricular Dysrhythmias

Couplets and multiform premature ventricular contractions occur in most patients with CHF.[20] About 50% of

CHF patients have nonsustained ventricular tachycardia on 24-hr Holter monitoring[20] and the presence of nonsustained ventricular tachycardia confers about a three-fold increase in risk for death.[21]

Neurohumoral Mechanisms

A number of neurohumoral mechanisms, including the sympathetic nervous system, the renin-angiotensin system, atrial natriuretic peptide, and the arginine vasopressin system, are activated in patients with CHF.[1,22–32] Although their role is to compensate for the disturbances that are brought about by reduced contractile function, the effects of excessive activation contribute to worsening the prognosis in CHF.[1,27] Whether this is a cause or effect remains uncertain.

In the SOLVD registry,[7] which included patients in NYHA functional class I and II, plasma renin activity, plasma norepinephrine, and atrial natriuretic peptide level were strongly associated with a poorer prognosis. However, arginine vasopressin levels were not predictive. An association between elevated plasma norepinephrine with mortality also has been shown in patients with advanced heart failure.[27] (NYHA functional class III and IV).

Hyponatremia identifies a group of patients with very high renin levels (and therefore severe heart failure) and poor prognosis. Lee and Packer reported the prognostic implications of serum sodium.[33] They found that if patients were divided into two groups, one with normal serum sodium (>130 mEq/l) and one with serum sodium (<130 mEq/l), there were significant differences in prognosis, with the lower serum sodium associated with a worse prognosis (Fig. 33.2). These data are consistent data from the SOLVD Study,[7] indicating the association-increased renin level with mortality.

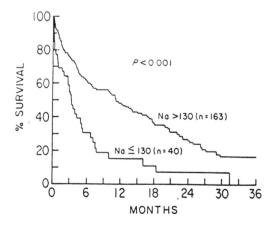

FIGURE 33.2. Hyponatremia is an important risk factor for mortality from CHF with those patients with a serum sodium of less than 130 having a significantly higher mortality. Reproduced, with permission, from *Circulation* 1986;73:257–67. Copyright by the American Heart Association.

Effect of Treatment on Prognosis

Angiotensin-Converting Enzyme Inhibitors

The Cooperative North Scandinavian Study Group (CONSENSUS) study[34] was a randomized placebo-controlled trial that examined the effect of treatment with enalapril on the prognosis of patients with severe heart failure (NYHA functional class IV). The average follow-up in this study was 188 days. Mortality at 6 months was 26% in the enalapril-treated group and 44% in the placebo group ($p = .002$). The reduction in mortality that occurred resulted from a reduction in progressive heart failure. Sudden cardiac death was not altered by enalapril treatment. In addition to a decrease in mortality, there was a significant improvement in functional class in the enalapril-treated group compared to the placebo group. In SOLVD, enalapril treatment was compared to placebo in patients with chronic heart failure and a LVEF ≤35%. Unlike the CONSENSUS study in which only NYHA functional class IV patients were entered, patients with milder heart failure also were studied in SOLVD. During an average follow-up of 41.4 months, the mortality was 39.7% in the placebo group compared to 35.2% in the enalapril-treated patients ($p = .0036$). Most of the decrease in mortality was seen in the first 2 yrs, with the benefit persisting through the end of the study. There also was a favorable effect of enalapril on total hospitalizations for heart failure. Reductions in mortality and hospitalizations were greatest among patients with the lowest EFs. As in the CONSENSUS trial, the mortality reduction was largely confined to the patients with progressive heart failure with little effect on arrhythmic death. From these data it can be concluded that the angiotensin-converting enzyme inhibitors reduce mortality and morbidity.

Other Vasodilators

The Veterans Administration conducted a placebo controlled randomized trial[11] to evaluate the effect on mortality and exercise tolerance of the different vasodilator regimens and placebo in 642 men. Patients with CHF were randomized to receive placebo, prazosin, or a combination of hydralazine and isosorbide dinitrate and were followed for an average of 2.3 yr. Patients treated with hydralazine and isosorbide dinitrate had a trend toward lower mortality ($p = .093$) compared to prazocin over an average of 2.3 yr. The failure of prazosin to improve survival is consistent with hemodynamic tachyphylaxis or failure of alpha receptor blockade to affect the prognosis favorably.

Comparison of Vasodilators

Cohn and his associates[35] compared treatment of chronic CHF with enalapril to treatment with hydralazine and isosorbide dinitrate. In this study 804 men receiving digitalis and diuretics for heart failure were randomly assigned to enalapril or to the combination of hydralazine and isosorbide dinitrate. Two-year mortality was significantly better in the enalapril group than in the hydralazine isosorbide dinitrate group and there was a similar trend that nearly reached significance over the entire follow-up period.

In this study, in contrast to the SOLVD study, the favorable effect on mortality of enalapril relative to hydralazine–isosorbide dinitrate appears to have been related to a reduction in sudden death. The reasons for the apparent discrepancy between this study and SOLVD V-Heft-II results may be related to differences in study design or differences in the classification of deaths. Interestingly, in the Veterans Administration study the hydralazine-nitrate combination had a more beneficial effect on LVEF than did enalapril. This surprising result suggests that EF changes with drug therapy may not necessarily correlate with its effect on prognosis.

From these data it can be concluded that there is a favorable effect of certain vasodilators in the treatment of heart failure and that enalapril is probably superior to the combination of hydralazine and isosorbide dinitrate.

Inotropic Agents

Digitalis

The most commonly used inotropic agent is digitalis, the effect of which was first described by Withering in 1785.[1] Although the mechanism of action remains to be completely defined, a major effect is inhibition of Na-K ATPase, which results in enhanced calcium entry into the cell with an increase in inotropy. Digitalis improves systolic performance in the failing heart[36,37] and the improvement is sustained over time. The improvement appears to be most marked in patients with the worst cardiac function.[38]

The effect of digitalis on mortality remains unclear, despite a number of uncontrolled studies that have addressed the issue.[39] A large randomized, placebo-controlled trial cosponsored by the National Heart, Lung and Blood Institute and the Department of Veterans Affairs is now underway to answer this important question.

Other Inotropic Agents

Since the principal problem in patients with CHF is systolic dysfunction, it would be reasonable to suppose that drugs that enhance contractile function would positively impact survival. As noted above, this remains to be demonstrated in the case of digitalis.

In a recently reported trial[40] the effect of the phosphodiesterase inhibitor, milrinone, on mortality in patients with CHF was examined. In this study, 1088 patients with severe heart failure were randomized to receive either milrinone or placebo. All patients received digitalis, diuretics, and a converting enzyme inhibitor. Compared to placebo, milrinone caused a 28% increase in mortality and significantly increased the number of hospitalizations.

Indeed, all of the other nondigitalis inotropic agents studied have been associated with excessive mortality.[41] A randomized trial of xamoterol[42] was terminated early because of excessive mortality in the xamoterol-treated group (9.1% vs. 3.1% in the placebo group within 100 days of randomization). Dobutamine also has been associated with an increase in mortality.[43]

The role of digitalis in treatment of heart failure should be clarified by the study in progress. The use of the nondigitalis inotropic agents probably should be limited to situations in which acute hemodynamic decompensation has occurred.

Summary

CHF is a common problem and the prevalence is increasing. Mortality and hospitalization rates are high. Ischemic heart disease appears to be the most common cause of heart failure. A number of prognostic factors including, importantly, resting EF, are useful in risk stratification. The cause of death usually is cardiovascular with progressive heart failure being most common. Sudden death is also a relatively common mode of death. Vasodilator therapy with angiotensin-converting enzyme inhibitors is the only form of treatment that has been proved to reduce mortality and hospitalization rates. Further efforts are needed to improve treatment of CHF.

References

1. Parmely W. Pathophysiology and current therapy of congestive heart failure. *J Am Coll Cardiol.* 1989;13:771–785.
2. Yusuf S, Thom T, Abbott R. Changes in hypertension treatment and in congestive heart failure morbidity in the United States. *Hypertension.* 1989;13(Suppl I):I-74.
3. McFate-Smith. Epidemiology of congestive heart failure. *Am J Cardiol.* 1985;55:3A.
4. McKee P, Castelli W, McNamara P, Kannel W. The natural history of congestive heart failure: the Framingham study. *N Engl J Med.* 1971;285:1441–1446.
5. Ghali J, Cooper R, Ford E. Trends in hospitalization rate for heart failure in the United States, 1973–1986. Evidence for increasing population prevalence. *Arch Intern Med.* 1990;150:769–773.
6. Applefeld M. Chronic congestive heart failure: where have we been? *Am J Med.* 1986;80(Suppl 2B):73–77.
7. Nicklas J, Benedict C, Johnstone D, et al. Relationship between neurohumoral profile and one year mortality in patients with CHF and/or LV dysfunction. *Circulation.* 1991;84(Suppl II):II-468.
8. Gorg R, Yusuf S. Epidemiology of congestive heart failure. In Barnett S, Pouleur H, eds. *The changing face of heart failure: pathophysiology, treatment and prevention.* New York: Marcel Dekker. In press.
9. Sutton G. Epidemiologic aspects of heart failure. *Am Heart J.* 1990;120:1538–1540.
10. The SOLVD investigators. Effect of enalapril on survival in patients with reduced left ventricular ejection fractions and congestive heart failure. *N Engl J Med.* 1991; 325:294–302.
11. Cohn J, Archibald D, Ziesche S, et al. Effect of vasodilator therapy on mortality in chronic congestive heart failure. *N Engl J Med.* 1986;314:1547–1552.
12. Luu M, Stevenson W, Stevenson L, et al. Diverse mechanism of unexpected cardiac arrest in advanced heart failure. *Circulation.* 1989;80:1675–1680.
13. Braunwald E, Grossman W. Clinical aspects of heart failure. In Braunwald E, ed. *Heart disease: a textbook of cardiovascular medicine.* 4th ed. Philadelphia: Saunders; 1992.
14. Gradman A, Deedwania P, Cody R, et al. Predictors of total mortality and sudden death in mild to moderate heart failure. *J Am Coll Cardiol.* 1989;14:564–570.
15. White H, Norris R, Brown M. Left ventricular end-systolic volume as the major determinant of survival recovery from myocardial infarction. *Circulation.* 1987;76: 44–51.
16. Szlachic J, Massie B, Kramer B, et al. Correlates and prognostic indicators of exercise capacity in chronic congestive heart failure. *Am J Cardiol.* 1985;55:1037–1042.
17. Franciosa J, Wilen M, Baker B. Functional capacity and long-term survival in chronic left ventricular failure. *Circulation.* 1983;68(Suppl III):III-149. Abstract.
18. Wilson J, Schwartz J, St John Sutton M, et al. Prognosis in severe heart failure: relation to hemodynamic measurements and ventricular ectopy. *J Am Coll Cardiol.* 1983;2:403–410.
19. Bittner V, Rogers W, Weiner D, et al. The six minute walk test predicts morbidity and mortality in patients with left ventricular dysfunction. *Circulation.* 1991;84:II-6. Abstract.
20. Chakko S, de Nadena E, Kessler K, Myerburg R. Ventricular arrhythmias in congestive heart failure. *Clin Cardiol.* 1989;12:525.
21. Bigger T. Why patients with congestive heart failure die: arrhythmais and sudden cardiac death. *Circulation.* 1987;75:IV-28.
22. Levine T, Francis G, Goldsmith S, et al. Activity of the sympathetic nervous system and renin-angiotensin system assessed by plasma hormone levels and their relationship to hemodynamic abnormalities in congestive heart failure. *Am J Cardiol.* 1982;49:1659–1666.
23. Goldsmith S, Francis G, Cowley A, et al. Increased plasma arginine vasopressin levels in patients with congestive heart failure. *J Am Coll Cardiol.* 1983;1:1385–1390.

24. Cohn J, Levine T, Francis G, et al. Neurohumoral control mechanisms in congestive heart failure. *Am Heart J*. 1981;102:509–514.

25. McCall D, O'Rourke R. Congestive heart failure. *Mod Conc Card Dis*. 1985;52:55–60.

26. Packer M, Lee W, Hessler P, et al. Role of neurohumoral mechanisms in determining survival in patients with severe chronic heart failure. *Circulation*. 1987;75(Suppl 14):IV-80.

27. Thomas J, Marks B. Plasma norepinephrine in congestive heart failure. *Am J Cardiol*. 1978;41:233–243.

28. Francis G, Goldsmith S, Cohn J. Relationship of exercise capacity to resting left ventricular performance and basal plasma norepinephrine levels in patients with congestive heart failure. *Am Heart J*. 1982;104:725–731.

29. Withering W. An account of the foxglove and some of its medical uses with practical remarks on dropsy and other diseases. In Willis F, Keys T, eds. *Classics of cardiology*. New York: Henry Schuman; 1941, 1943.

30. Yamane Y. Plasma ADH levels in patients with chronic congestive heart failure. *Jpn Circ J*. 1968;1:745–759.

31. Goldsmith S, Francis G, Cowley A, et al. Increased plasma arginine vasopressin levels in patients with congestive heart failure. *J Am Coll Cardiol*. 1983;1:1385–1390.

32. Reigger G, Leibau G, Koeshiek K. Antidiuretic hormone in congestive heart failure. *Am J Med*. 1982;72:49–52.

33. Lee W, Packer M. Prognostic significance of serum sodium concentration and its modification by converting enzyme inhibition in patients with severe chronic heart failure. *Circulation*. 1986;73:257–267.

34. The CONSENSUS trial study group. Effects of enalapril on mortality in severe congestive heart failure. *N Engl J Med*. 1987;316:1429–1435.

35. Cohn J, Johnson G, Ziesche S, et al. A comparison of enalapril with hydralazine-isosorbide dinitrate in the treatment of chronic congestive heart failure. *N Engl J Med*. 1991;325:303–310.

36. Arnold S, Byrd R, Meister W, et al. Long-term digitalis therapy improves left ventricular function in heart failure. *N Engl J Med*. 1980;303:1443.

37. Smith T. Medical treatment of advanced congestive heart failure: digitalis and diuretics. In Braunwald E, Moch M, Watson J, eds. *Congestive heart failure*. New York: Grune and Stratton; 1982:261–278.

38. Griffiths B, Penny W, Lewis M, et al. Maintenance of the inotropic effect of digoxin on long term treatment. *Br Med J*. 1982;284:1819–1822.

39. Yusuf S, Wittes J, Bailey K, Furberg C. Digitalis—a new controversy regarding an old drug: the pitfalls of inappropriate methods. *Circulation*. 1986;73:14–18.

40. Parker M, Carver J, Rodeherrer R, et al. Effect of oral milrinone on mortality in severe heart failure. *N Engl J Med*. 1991;325:1468–1475.

41. Yusuf S. Obtaining reliable information from randomized controlled trials in congestive heart failure and left ventricular function. In: Dietz R, Kubler W, Brachman W, eds. *Ventricular arrhythmias and heart failure*. Berlin: Springer-Verlag, 1990;147.

42. The Xamoterol in Severe Heart Failure Study Group. Xamoterol in severe heart failure. *Lancet*. 1990;336:1–6.

43. Miller L. Ambulatory isotropic therapy as a bridge to cardiac transplantation. *J Am Coll Cardiol*. 1987;9:89A.

34
The Medical Management of Chronic Congestive Heart Failure

Barry H. Greenberg

The medical management of patients with chronic congestive heart failure (CHF) has evolved considerably over the last two decades. In addition to the availability of new agents with proven clinical efficacy, we now know a great deal more about where and when to use (or sometimes avoid) traditional drugs like digoxin and diuretics. It is not happenstance that changes in therapeutics were preceded by and, in some instances developed in tandem with, advances in our understanding of the pathogenesis of myocardial dysfunction and the integrated series of events that give rise to the clinical syndrome of CHF. In addition, within the past 5 yr the results of a remarkable series of well designed clinical trials have provided guidelines for the medical management of a wide variety of patients with left ventricular (LV) dysfunction. Although CHF remains an extremely serious illness, the advances in our understanding of the pathophysiology and treatment described in this text have resulted in both longer and more enjoyable lives for patients who suffer from this syndrome.

The goal of this chapter is to provide an integrated approach to the medical management of patients with chronic CHF. Since other sections in this text include extensive reviews of the pathophysiology, prognosis, and drugs used to treat CHF, this chapter focuses on selected segments of these topics as they relate to the practical aspects of therapeutics. Since a rational approach to therapy requires an understanding of the pathophysiologic framework, the chapter begins with a brief overview of mechanisms involved in the development and progression of CHF. This is followed by an overview of the three classes of drugs (digoxin, diuretics, and angiotensin-converting enzyme inhibitors) that are the cornerstones of therapy. The results of a series of (mostly) recent clinical trials will be emphasized since the information derived from these studies has provided extremely important guidelines for the management of patients with CHF. Practical aspects of therapy also are covered in this section. At the conclusion of the chap-

ter, an integrated therapeutic approach to patients with varying stages of CHF is presented.

Pathophysiology

To approach the patient with CHF effectively, it is first necessary to define the problem. This is not as easy a task as it initially appears or that it may have been 20 years ago. By necessity, CHF is viewed according to the perspective of the observer. Although there is fortunately a good deal of interdisciplinary cross-talk and a robust cadre of physician-scientists who work and practice in the area, the clinician who must treat patients with rales, edema, and cardiomegaly usually is occupied with something quite different from the molecular biologist who is interested in the genetic control of critical myocardial functions. However, a working definition that should function for the practicing physician and basic scientist alike is that "CHF is a syndrome in which the inability of the heart to provide adequate amounts of oxygenated blood to vital tissue at normal levels of ventricular filling pressure provokes a widespread and progressive response throughout the organism." One key aspect of this definition is that CHF is a syndrome that can result from a variety of different diseases that may or may not primarily affect the heart. Furthermore, it is a dynamic process that depends on the altered function of more than a single organ.

As outlined in Table 34.1, the syndrome of CHF can be due to both cardiac and noncardiac causes. Among the cardiac etiologies, myocardial dysfunction is the most common. Although the two often are related in the same disease process, myocardial abnormalities that primarily affect systolic function and those that predominantly affect diastolic function can both give rise to the syndrome of CHF. Valvular heart disease, congenital or acquired structural abnormalities, and pericardial disease are all nonmyocardial causes of CHF.

TABLE 34.1. Conditions resulting in the syndrome of CHF.

Noncardiac disease
  (e.g., anemia, hemoglobinipathy, A-V fistula, thyroid disease)
Cardiac disease
  Structural (due to intracardiac shunts, valvular lesions, or
    pericardial abnormalities)
    Congenital
    Acquired
  Myocardial
    Congenital (e.g., inborn errors of metabolism)
    Acquired
      Ischemic
      Cardiomyopathic
      Toxic (e.g., alcohol)

CHF = congestive heart failure; A-V = arteriovenous.

The pathogenesis and management of CHF on the basis of myocardial diastolic dysfunction and extracardiac and nonmyocardial causes is covered elsewhere in the text. Thus, the discussion in this chapter is confined to CHF that develops on the basis of abnormalities in systolic myocardial function. However, recognition of the fact that CHF is a syndrome with multiple etiologies brings up one of the most important principles of management. That is, to decide on a rational course of therapy, it is essential to define the cause of the syndrome. Clearly, the approach to the patient with CHF due to a noncardiac disease or on the basis of mitral stenosis will be dramatically different than in a patient who develops this syndrome secondary to myocardial infarction or to an idiopathic cardiomyopathy.

A characteristic of CHF that develops as a result of myocardial dysfunction is that at some point, either at rest or during exercise, there is a reduction in cardiac output. Whether it develops on the basis of an ischemic process, exposure to a myocardial toxin, or to a genetic abnormality, low cardiac output stimulates a pathophysiologic response involving the heart and multiple other organs throughout the body.[1] The primary goal of the compensatory changes, which are summarized in Table 34.2, is to augment the delivery of oxygenated blood to vital organs such as the heart and the brain. It is extremely important to recognize that, in addition to providing (mostly short-term) benefits to the organism, these compensatory changes also are associated with a number of deleterious effects that become progressively more important over time. For instance, retention of salt and water increases sarcomere stretch (or LV preload) and, as a result, stroke volume is increased. The associated increases in LV filling pressure and volume, however, predispose to the development of congestive symptoms. They also increase LV wall stress, thereby promoting hypertrophy, dilation, and ultimately, progressive deterioration in systolic pump function. Thus, one of the key features in considering the therapeutic approach to the patient with CHF is to counteract the effects of these compensatory mechanisms as well as to preserve (and, if possible, improve) myocardial function.

An aspect of CHF that has recently received a great deal of attention is the fact that once myocardial damage occurs, abnormalities in myocardial structure and function are not static. Even when the process is initiated by a discrete event such as a myocardial infarction, there is now good evidence that the deterioration in myocardial systolic function can be progressive.[2,3] This

TABLE 34.2. Compensatory changes in chronic CHF.

Compensation	Mechanism(s)	Beneficial effects	Adverse effects
Increased chronotropy	Sympathetic nervous system	Increased CO (CO = HR × SV)	Enhanced myocardial ischemia Proarrhythmic
Increased inotropy	Sympathetic nervous system	Increased CO (CO = HR × SV)	Long-term deterioration in myocardial function
Increased intravascular volume	Salt-water retention by the kidney Neurohormonal activation	Increased SV by the Frank-Starling mechanism	Pulmonary and systemic congestion LV hypertrophy and dilatation 2° to increased loading conditions
Peripheral vasoconstriction	Neurohormonal (sympathetic nervous system, renin-angiotensin system, arginine vasopressin) Structural changes in blood vessels Local pathways (e.g., ↓ EDRF activity)	Increased SV due to venoconstriction Increased arterial pressure (BP = CO × SVR)	Decreased stroke volume due to high afterload Decreased blood flow to some vascular beds LV dilatation and hypertrophy 2° to increased loading conditions
LV dilatation/ hypertrophy	Increased loading conditions ? Neurohormonal factors (sympathetic nervous system, renin-angiotensin system)	Increased SV Dilatation allows increased LV volume at reduced pressure Hypertrophy helps normalize wall stress	Enhanced myocardial ischemia Long-term deterioration in myocardial function

CHF = congestive heart failure; CO = cardiac output; HR = heart rate; SV = stroke volume; LV = left ventricle; EDRF = endothelium-relaxing factor; BP = blood pressure; SVR = systemic vascular resistance.

is due, in large part, to the remodeling of the heart that occurs in response to alteration in both global myocardial and regional loading conditions and to the influence of various neurohormonal systems that are activated.[2-5] It is important to emphasize the connection between the remodeling process and the compensatory mechanisms that are stimulated by the failing heart. The pathways that are involved in this process are summarized in Table 34.2. As discussed in the section that follows, therapy directed toward interrupting some of the compensatory pathways has now been shown to be effective in preventing the progression of LV dysfunction and the development of CHF.

Drugs Used in the Treatment of CHF

There are three classes of drug that form the "cornerstones" of therapy of CHF.[6] These are the diuretics, the digitalis glycosides, and the angiotensin-converting enzyme inhibitors (ACEIs). In the following section, the efficacy of these agents in the treatment of CHF during its various stages is discussed.

In addition, recent studies have provided new information about the safety and efficacy of β-adrenergic receptor antagonists in the treatment of heart failure. The results of these studies will also be described below.

Diuretics

Since patients with CHF almost always have signs and symptoms of pulmonary and/or systemic congestion, diuretic agents play an integral role in the therapeutic approach to this syndrome. Although there is only limited evidence from clinical trials to document their efficacy in patients with advanced CHF and volume overload,[7,8] the obvious impact of these agents demonstrated by extensive clinical experience has confirmed the value of diuretic therapy in this setting in a manner analogous to the way that penicillin has been accepted as a treatment of pneumococcal pneumonia.

As is discussed in a later section of this chapter and elsewhere in the text, there is well founded enthusiasm for the use of ACEIs to treat a broad range of patients with LV dysfunction. One question that has been raised is whether or not diuretic agents are also needed in patients who are already receiving an ACEI. Although the data base is not extensive, there are two small trials that demonstrate that in patients with heart failure and evidence of fluid retention, ACEI therapy alone did not produce an adequate diuresis.[9,10] In both studies, the addition of a diuretic agent was required to achieve this. Thus, the effects of diuretics and the ACEIs in patients with CHF and evidence of volume overload appear to be additive.

Although diuretics are an essential component of the

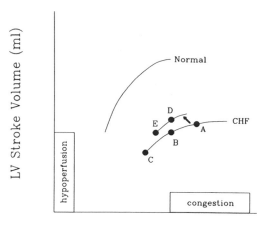

Filling Pressure (mmHg)

FIGURE 34.1. Ventricular function curves in a normal person and in a patient with CHF (see text for explanation).

therapeutic approach to CHF, it is important to keep in mind that they are effective primarily as a means of removing excess salt and water. As indicated in Table 34.2 patients with CHF retain fluid in order to increase LV stroke volume. This response, however, is excessive in most instances. As shown in Figure 34.1, the high levels of LV end-diastolic volume that are usually seen in CHF are no longer effective in enhancing cardiac output since the patient is positioned on the flat portion of the LV function curve. The accompanying increase in LV filling pressure, however, is a major factor in the development of the signs and symptoms of congestion. The predominant impact of diuretic therapy is to reduce filling pressure and relieve congestive symptoms. In this case, the patient moves from point A to point B in the figure. In some instances, diuretic therapy also may increase cardiac output.[11] This is depicted in Figure 34.1 by movement to point D on a new curve that is positioned upward and to the left. There are several mechanisms through which this can occur. Patients with mitral regurgitation on the basis of dysfunction of the subvalvular apparatus may experience considerable improvement in cardiac output with diuretic therapy. In this case, the reduction in LV volume leads to an improvement in valvular competence and there is an increase in forward flow. Cardiac output also can be increased with diuretic therapy when a reduction in ventricular volume helps to reduce LV afterload and when relief of pulmonary congestion leads to a reduction to neurohormonal stimuli, which cause peripheral vasoconstriction.[12]

One important consideration in the use of diuretics is that they can lead to a reduction in cardiac output. This is depicted in Figure 34.1 by movement to point C or point E and is related to the fact that diuresis can move the patient from the flat portion of the LV function curve to the ascending portion. In this position, stroke volume is again responsive to the preload stretch of the sarcomeres and as filling volume is decreased cardiac output goes down. This situation tends to occur when the patient is being diureased aggressively and is more likely to be seen when other agents, such as an ACEI or nitrovasodilator, which also reduce LV filling pressure, are being used. When hypoperfusion occurs, it can be recognized clinically by the complaints of increased weakness and fatigue, a reduction in blood pressure or postural hypotension, and/or an increase in the blood urea nitrogen (BUN) and creatinine (Cr) levels. Although this condition can be treated easily by reducing the dosage of the diuretic (or one of the other agents), it points out a major limitation of the diuretics as monotherapy of CHF.

As a result of their potency and relatively low side-effect profile, the loop diuretics such as furosemide used are most commonly for the treatment of CHF. Diuretics that act on other portions of the nephron may be used in association with one of the loop diuretics to accomplish specific purposes. For instance, a diuretic like metolazone, which acts on the distal collecting tubule, can be used with a loop diuretic to help promote diuresis in otherwise resistant patients.[13] In other instances, a potassium-sparing diuretic can be used with a loop diuretic when potassium supplementation proves inadequate to maintain serum levels within the normal range.

Diuretic agents are associated with a variety of important side effects. The metabolic and electrolyte abnormalities that occur, particularly those involving renal function or serum potassium levels, are a major concern and require careful clinical attention as well as the judicious use of blood chemistry analyses in the follow-up management of patients being maintained on these drugs.

The final remaining issue with the diuretic agents is whether they should be used as monotherapy in patients with CHF. As mentioned previously in this chapter, the predominant effect of these drugs is to relieve congestive symptoms and that if improvements in cardiac function occur, they tend to be modest. There is also information that the use of diuretics activates the renin-angiotensin system.[14] In addition to these theoretical arguments against the use of diuretics as monotherapy, there are now data from clinical trials suggesting that even patients with relatively mild CHF are likely to do better when diuretics are used in combination with another agent like digoxin or an ACEI. This information is presented in greater detail in the next two sections.

Digitalis Glycosides

It remains one of the great oddities of clinical medicine that it has taken more than two centuries to determine whether or not the digitalis glycosides are effective therapy for CHF. The debate has had temporal aspects, with enthusiasm for the drug running high during certain eras but not in others, and there have been geocultural factors leading to widespread acceptance in countries such as Germany and profound skepticism in England. It would seem to be a relatively straightforward process to determine if a particular agent or class of agents does or does not improve the well-being of patients with CHF. After all, these issues were decided in relatively short order for the ACEIs (which are helpful) and for milrinone (which is not). Fortunately, information that has recently become available helps to resolve the question of clinical efficacy. Although the important issue of the effects of the digitalis glycosides on mortality remains unresolved, a trial administered by the National Institutes of Health (NIH) and Veterans Administration (VA), is underway and should provide needed information in this area in the foreseeable future. What follows, then, is a brief description of mostly newer and clinically relevant information regarding this class of drugs. In the remainder of this chapter, I will refer to digoxin alone since this is the most widely used of the digitalis preparations.

Digoxin has well documented inotropic effects[15,16] and it can block impulse transmission across the arteriovenous (AV) node. Atrial fibrillation occurs in 10% to 20% of patients with CHF and digoxin is the drug of choice in this setting. Although verapamil and the beta-blockers also can reduce the ventricular response to atrial fibrillation, these drugs are used less commonly in patients with LV dysfunction since their negative inotropic effects can precipitate worsening CHF. Digoxin, however, has only modest positive inotropic effects. This fact has been used to argue against its use in patients with CHF who have in normal sinus rhythm. The rebuttal to this argument is that whatever inotropic effect is present, it is enough to produce clinical benefits. In fact, more potent inotropic agents actually may have a deleterious effect on patients with CHF.[17] In addition, noncardiac effects of digoxin, such as enhancing baroreceptor sensitivity (which is diminished in CHF), could be related to clinical efficacy. There is recent evidence that digoxin inhibits peripheral sympathetic nervous system activity in patients with CHF.[18] This appears to be due to an intrinsic property of the drug rather than to withdrawal of reflex sympathetic stimulation, since a comparable improvement in cardiac performance with dopamine failed to have the same effect on sympathetic activity. This observation could be clinically relevant since increased activity of the sympathetic nervous system has a number of deleterious effects (such as promoting vasoconstriction and stimulating the renin-angiotensin system) in patients with CHF.

Although several small clinical trials published in the 1980s contained information suggesting that digoxin might be of value in patients with CHF who were in sinus rhythm,[16,19,20] it was not until the latter part of the decade and early 1990s that this point was estab-

TABLE 34.3. Effects of therapy in the digoxin-captopril study.

Study group	n	Change in exercise time (s)	Change (%) in EF	Change in NYHA class	Hospitalizations/ER visits for CHF
Placebo	100	35	0.9	0.02	29
Captopril	104	82[a]	1.8	0.20[a]	17[a]
Digoxin	96	54	4.4[b]	0.09	15[a]

[a] $p < .05$ vs. placebo.
[b] $p < .05$ vs. placebo and captopril.
Values are mean ± SE.
EF = ejection fraction; NYHA = New York Heart Association; ER = emergency room; CHF = congestive heart failure.

lished conclusively by the results from several clinical trials that were specifically designed to evaluate efficacy. One of the first of these trials was a comparison of digoxin, captopril (an ACEI), and placebo.[21] Patients enrolled in this trial were considered to be stable on diuretics alone (which were required in 84%) and 87% were either New York Heart Association (NYHA) functional class I or II. The study design actually biased the trial against finding a positive result in the digoxin group since patients who deteriorated when digoxin was discontinued were excluded from participation. After randomization to either digoxin, captopril, or placebo, patients were followed over a 6-month period.

The major findings that were present at the end of the study period are summarized in Table 34.3. Compared to placebo- and captopril-treated patients, the digoxin-treated group demonstrated a significant increase in LV ejection fraction. The captopril-treated patients experienced a significant increase in treadmill exercise time and NYHA class compared to the placebo group. There were, however, no significant differences in these variables between the captopril- and digoxin-treated patients (who showed an insignificant trends toward improvement in these parameters). The efficacy of the various regimens in preventing hospitalization and emergency room visits also is summarized in Table 34.3. Despite the relatively stable condition of the patients on entry into the study, the brief (6-month) duration of the trial and small numbers involved, there was a significant reduction in clinical events related to CHF in both the captopril and the digoxin groups. This study demonstrates that even in patients with relatively mild CHF, diuretics alone are not adequate therapy. In addition, one can conclude that both digoxin and captopril are effective in this setting.

The effects of digoxin on exercise performance were compared to those of milrinone in another placebo-controlled clinical trial.[22] Patients enrolled in this study had moderately severe CHF and approximately 70% were NYHA class III. All patients were stabilized on furosemide and nearly 25% received captopril. Patients

were randomized to either placebo, digoxin, milrinone (a phosphodiesterase inhibitor with positive inotropic effects), or a combination of digoxin and milrinone. After 12 weeks of therapy there was evidence of a significant increase in exercise capacity in patients receiving either digoxin (+14%) or milrinone (+19%) and little change in the placebo group. The increase in treadmill time in the milrinone group was not significantly greater than in the digoxin-treated group. There was, however, a trend toward decreased survival in the milrinone-treated patients (which was subsequently confirmed in the PROMISE study[17]).

The recently completed RADIANCE (RAndomized, double-blind, placebo-controlled withdrawal study of Digoxin In patients with chronic heart failure treated with Angiotensin-Converting Enzyme inhibitors) trial evaluated the effects of digoxin withdrawal in 178 patients with NYHA class I–III CHF.[23] For entry into the study patients were required to have an ejection fraction below 35% and they had to be in normal sinus rhythm. Patients were stabilized on a regimen of digoxin, diuretics, and ACEIs for 8 weeks before randomization to groups that were either maintained on digoxin (n = 85) or had the drug discontinued (n = 93). During a 12-week period of observation, clinical deterioration occurred more frequently in patients who had digoxin withdrawn (28%) than in patients who had digoxin continued (6%). This was associated with a significantly higher percentage of patients requiring an increase in diuretic dose, emergency room care, or hospitalization for CHF in the withdrawal group compared to the continuation group (25% vs. 5%, $p \le .001$). Patients who had digoxin withdrawn also experienced a 43-s reduction in treadmill exercise time ($p = .003$), a 133-ft reduction in the distance walked over a 6-min period ($p \le .01$), and a 3.3% decrease in LV ejection fraction ($p \le .01$). The results of this study should be widely generalizable since these patients were receiving what would be considered to be "contemporary therapy" for CHF. A similar study done in patients who were not receiving ACEIs reported comparable findings to the RADIANCE trial.[24]

These trials provide us with a clear picture of the clinical effects of digoxin in a fairly wide range of patients with CHF who are in normal sinus rhythm. The results of the trials are generally consistent and they show that in patients with mild to moderate CHF, digoxin increases ejection fraction, enhances exercise capacity, and reduces the incidence of clinical events due to worsening CHF. As demonstrated in the RADIANCE trial, these beneficial effects can be demonstrated even when patients are already receiving diuretics and ACEIs, suggesting that the effects of digoxin are additive to those of the other agents.

One of the advantages of digoxin is that it is relatively easy to use and needs to be given in most patients only once a day. Although the drug is far from innocuous, the incidence of toxicity is probably far below the estimated 15% level that was reported in hospitalized patients in the early 1970s.[25] This is likely due to multiple factors, including the avoidance of longer acting digitalis glycosides, a higher degree of alertness to the signs and symptoms of digoxin toxicity on the part of practicing clinicians, increased recognition of the conditions in which digoxin toxicity is likely to occur, the availability of other agents to treat CHF both acutely and chronically (thus minimizing the need to "push dig" in patients who are doing poorly), greater attention to electrolyte abnormalities that could potentiate digoxin toxicity, and the widespread availability of an assay to determine levels of digoxin in the blood.

The use of digoxin in the acute management of patients with unstable CHF is much less common than in the past, since other more potent inotropic agents that are rapidly acting and that can be carefully titrated are now available. These agents are better suited for use in the acutely ill patient, particularly when treatment is being initiated in an intensive care unit setting. In other, less acutely ill patients, a maintenance dose of digoxin, ranging from 0.125 to 0.375 qd, usually is begun. A stable blood level usually is obtained within 5 to 7 days. Since there is no convincing evidence of a linear relationship between blood levels of drug and clinical efficacy, digoxin levels usually are not obtained as part of routine clinical care. This test appears to be most valuable in situations where it is uncertain whether the patient is actually receiving a full dose of the drug there is suspicion that one of the many factors that can alter digoxin kinetics may be resulting in clinically important increases or decreases in digoxin blood levels, or there is a clinical condition (such as chronic renal failure) that may make decisions about the appropriate dosing regimen difficult to arrive at empirically. Patients with advanced CHF who are doing poorly also might benefit from this test if it is used to adjust their blood levels of digoxin to within the range shown to be efficacious in the clinical trials cited above (i.e., between 0.7 and 2.0 ng/ml). It is important to note, however, that there is little evidence to support this last approach.

Angiotensin-Converting Enzyme Inhibitors

As mentioned in the section on pathophysiology and in other chapters of this text, activation of the renin-angiotensin system plays an important role in the pathogenesis of CHF. In general, elevations in plasma-renin activity correlate with the severity of the condition.[26] A reduction in cardiac output and renal perfusion appears to be a major factor in this process.[14] Patients with asymptomatic LV dysfunction, however,

may have increased levels of plasma-renin activity, particularly if they are being treated with diuretic agents.[26]

As summarized in Table 34.2, the adverse consequences of activation of the renin-angiotensin system provide a rationale for the use of ACEIs in the treatment of CHF. The ACEIs, however, also may have other actions that could account for their clinical efficacy in patients with CHF. Converting enzyme, in addition to blocking the breakdown of angiotensin (A)I to AII, also is involved in the inactivation of bradykinin, substance P, and other vasoactive compounds. The effects on bradykinin may be of particular importance since this substance can stimulate endothelial cells to release prostacyclin and endothelium-derived relaxing factor (EDRF) activity, both of which have vasodilatory properties. Thus, potentiation of the effects of bradykinin by ACEIs could promote vasodilation through a pathway unrelated to the renin-angiotensin system.

As a result of their ability to dilate peripheral vessels and to unload the heart, the ACEIs have been shown to improve cardiac function.[27-29] Initially, there is little impact on exercise capacity despite an increase in cardiac output and a reduction in ventricular filling pressures. However, over a period of weeks to months, exercise duration has been shown to improve in patients with mild to moderate CHF.[30,31] Symptomatic improvement also becomes manifest over time. The reasons for the temporal disparity between the acute cardiac and long-term clinical effects of the ACEIs is uncertain. Enhanced peripheral vasodilation and tissue oxygen extraction during chronic (but not acute) therapy has been demonstrated.[32,33] This could be related to alterations in tissue mechanisms for oxygen extraction, structural changes in blood vessels, or better conditioning (as cardiac function improves). ACEIs also have been shown to enhance EDRF activity in an experimental model of chronic heart failure,[34a] and this factor could help account for the improved peripheral vasodilation and clinical benefits seen during long-term therapy.

One of the most important goals in the management of patients with CHF is to prevent further progression of myocardial dysfunction. There is evidence that after a myocardial infarction, the LV undergoes progressive change in size, structure, and function over time.[2-4] The process is discussed in detail in Chapter 6 of this text. Although increases in wall stress and changes in neurohormonal factors appear to be involved, the precise mechanisms that signal the initiation and then control the rate and extent of this remodeling process are only gradually being unraveled. Patients who survive a myocardial infarction with more than mild myocardial damage experience a progressive increase in chamber size over time. LV dilatation, unfortunately, is strongly related to both late deterioration in LV systolic function and to decreased survival.[35-37]

The fact that ACEIs alter both the mechanical and

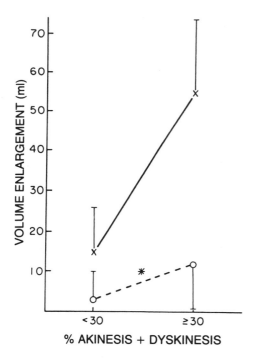

FIGURE 34.2. Increase in LV end-diastolic volume from base line (volume enlargement) in patients with occlusion of the left anterior descending coronary artery at base-line catheterization (n = 36). Reproduced with permission from Pfeffer M, et al. Effect of captopril on progressive ventricular dilatation after anterior myocardial infarction. *N Engl J Med.* 1988;319:80–86.

neurohormonal factors that appear to be major determinants of the remodeling process provided the theoretical basis for evaluating their effects after myocardial infarction. Pfeffer and his colleagues assessed changes in hemodynamic parameters, LV chamber size, and exercise performance over a 1-yr period in a group of 59 patients who had survived an anterior myocardial infarction.[38] Patients were required to have an LV ejection fraction 0.45 or less for entry into the trial. The study population was randomly allocated into groups receiving captopril or placebo. After 1 yr of therapy,

placebo-treated patients demonstrated a significant increase in LV volumes (21 ± 8 ml; $p \leq .02$). Chamber dilation, however, was limited in the captopril-treated group (10 ± 6 ml; p = ns). As shown in Figure 34.2, this effect was most pronounced in patients who had demonstrated the largest amount of myocardial damage. Captopril-treated patients also demonstrated significantly longer exercise times compared to placebo-treated patients. The beneficial effects of ACEIs on LV volumes after myocardial infarction also have been reported by Sharpe et al.[39]

Both of the studies mentioned above were confined to patients who had recently survived a myocardial infarction and involved the early initiation of therapy after the acute event. The effects of ACEI therapy on cardiac structure and function also have been evaluated in a more diverse population, which included both late survivors of a myocardial infarction and patients with cardiomyopathy as the cause of LV dysfunction.[40] Preliminary results of the echocardiography substudy of the SOLVD trial indicate that progressive LV dilation was inhibited by long-term treatment with enalapril. The beneficial effects of therapy in this case appeared to be related to a reduction in LV wall stress.

The effects of ACEIs on survival in patients with CHF has been the focus of several recently reported clinical trials. All of these trials were conducted in double-blind fashion and each contained an adequate control population with which to compare the results from the ACEI-treated group. Although ejection fraction cutoffs and other entry criteria varied somewhat between the trials, all patients had moderate to severe LV systolic dysfunction. The studies included populations in which the severity of CHF ranged from the asymptomatic state to NYHA class IV heart failure. Some of the key features of these trials are summarized in Table 34.4.

The Cooperative North Scandinavian Enalapril Survival Study (CONSENSUS) was the first to provide evidence that ACEI therapy improved survival in patients with CHF.[41] CONSENSUS enrolled patients with

TABLE 34.4. Studies evaluating the effects of ACEI therapy on survival.

Trial	Population	n	Study drugs	EF entry criteria	NYHA class	Mean duration
CONSENSUS	General	253	Enalapril vs. placebo	None	IV	188 days
V-HEFT II	Male U.S. Service Veterans	804	Enalapril vs. hydralazine-isosorbide dinitrate	≤0.45	II–III	30.0 months
SOLVD—treatment	General	2569	Enalapril vs. placebo	≤0.35	II–III	41.4 months
SOLVD—prevention	LV dysfunction not requiring CHF therapy	4228	Enalapril vs. placebo	≤0.35	I–II	37.4 months
SAVE	Survivors of recent myocardial infarction	2231	Captopril vs. placebo	≤0.40	I–III	42 ± 10 months

ACEI = angiotensin-converting enzyme inhibitor; LV = left ventricular.

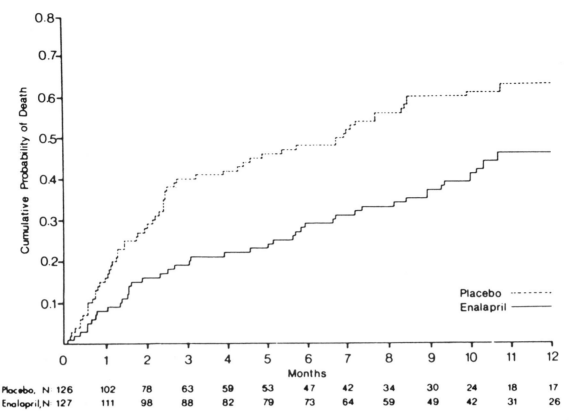

FIGURE 34.3. Cumulative probability of death in the placebo and enalapril groups. Reproduced with permission from The CONSENSUS Trial Study Group. Effects of enalapril on mortality in severe congestive heart failure. *N Engl J Med.* 1987;316:1429–1435.

severe CHF who remained in NYHA functional class IV despite standard medical therapy (including digoxin, diuretics, and in many cases, non-ACEI vasodilators). In this trial, patients were randomized to receive either placebo or enalapril and their clinical course was followed for a period extending up to 20 months. Crude mortality, which was the primary endpoint of the trial, was 44% in the placebo group and 26% in the enalapril-treated group at the end of 6 months. This 40% reduction was highly significant ($p = 0.002$). As depicted in Figure 34.3, the curves showing the life-table analysis for the study groups began to diverge quite early and a highly significant difference between the study groups was seen over the course of the trial. The enalapril group also demonstrated significant improvements in NYHA class, reduction in heart size, and reduced requirement for other therapy for CHF.

Studies Of Left Ventricular Dysfunction (SOLVD) was designed to assess the effects of ACEI therapy on morbidity, mortality, and progression of disease in a broad spectrum of patients with LV dysfunction. Patients enrolled in SOLVD were required to have an LV ejection fraction ≤0.35. Patients who were receiving therapy for heart failure were included in the treatment arm of SOLVD. Those patients with LV dysfunction who met entry criteria but did not require therapy for

CHF were followed in the prevention arm. In contrast to the population followed in the CONSENSUS trial, virtually all of the patients in the treatment arm of SOLVD were NYHA functional class II–III. Approximately two thirds of the prevention arm patients were NYHA class I (with the remainder being class II). In both arms of SOLVD, patients were randomized to either enalapril or placebo and their clinical course was followed over a period of several years. The primary endpoint in both arms of the study was the effects of therapy on all-cause mortality. Important secondary end-points were the effects of treatment on cause-specific mortality, hospitalizations for CHF, functional status, and (in the prevention arm) the development of CHF requiring therapy.

In the treatment arm there was a 16% reduction in risk of dying in the group treated with enalapril ($p = .0036$).[42] As shown in Figure 34.4, the greatest impact was on death due to progressive heart failure and there was relatively little effect on deaths classified as being due to arrhythmia in the absence of worsening pump failure. Furthermore, there was a reduction of 26% in the risk of death or hospitalization for worsening heart failure in the group assigned to enalapril (P ≤.001). Analysis of the effects of therapy on mortality in predefined subgroups based on serum

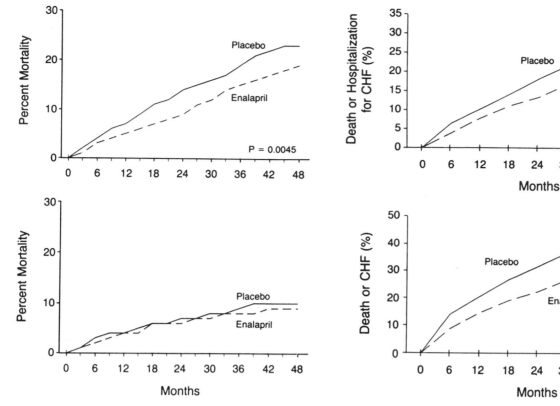

FIGURE 34.4. Mortality due to progressive heart failure (*upper panel*) (p = .0045) and presumed to be due to an arrhythmia but not preceded by worsening CHF (*lower panel*) (p, NS). Reproduced with permission from The SOLVD Investigators. *N Engl J Med.* 1991;325:293–302.

FIGURE 34.5. Death or hospitalization for CHF and death or development of heart failure in the prevention trial. Reproduced with permission from The SOLVD Investigators. *N Engl Med.* 1992;327:685–691.

sodium level, use of non-ACEI vasodilators, presence of ischemic heart disease as the etiology of CHF, and NYHA class at the time of entry failed to demonstrate a significant interaction between any of these variables and the response to therapy. There was, however, a modest effect of prerandomization ejection fraction on the effects of therapy on mortality and on the combined end-points of death and hospitalization, which suggested that patients with lower ejection fractions more the most likely to benefit.

In the prevention arm of SOLVD, enalapril treatment was not associated with a significant reduction in overall mortality (p = .30) and reduction in cardiovascular mortality was marginally reduced (12%, p = .12).[43] There were, however, significant reductions of 29% in death or development of heart failure (p ≤ .001) and 20% in death or hospitalization for heart failure (p ≤ .001). These results are depicted in Figure 34.5. As in the treatment arm of SOLVD, patients with the lowest ejection fractions on entry into the study tended to demonstrate the greatest likelihood of a beneficial effect of therapy.

The results of the Veterans Administration Heart Failure Trial II (VHeFT-II), which were published in

the same issue of the *New England Journal of Medicine* as the results of the SOLVD treatment arm,[44] demonstrated that when compared to the combination of hydralazine-isosorbide, enalapril tended to improve survival in male U.S. service veterans with symptomatic CHF. After 2 yr, the mortality was 25% in the hydralazine-isosorbide group and only 18% in the enalapril group (p = .016). Hydralazine-isosorbide served as a positive control in the study since VHeFT-I, which had enrolled a similar study population, had previously demonstrated that this combination of vasodilators had significantly improved survival compared to a placebo-controlled group.

The <u>S</u>urvival <u>A</u>nd <u>V</u>entricular <u>E</u>nlargement (SAVE) trial (SAVE) evaluated the effects of ACEIs on survival in patients with LV dysfunction as a result of a recent myocardial infarction. In this trial, patients with an ejection fraction of 0.40 or below after myocardial infarction were randomized to either captopril or to placebo between 3 and 16 days of the acute event. Overall mortality was reduced by 19% (p = 0.019) in the captopril group. Cardiovascular events (both fatal and nonfatal), cardiovascular death, development of severe heart failure, and hospitalization for heart failure were also significantly reduced.

These clinical trials provide conclusive evidence that ACEI therapy can improve survival in a broad spectrum of patients with LV dysfunction. Furthermore, there also is good evidence that ACEIs can reduce hospitalizations and prevent the progression of disease. Despite the differences in study design and entry criteria (which are summarized in Table 34.4), the consistency between the results of these trials reinforces the conclusion that this class of drugs is highly effective in treating patients with LV dysfunction whether or not overt manifestations of CHF are present.

The side effects associated with the ACEIs are well known and include hypotension, dizziness and syncope, taste disturbances, worsening renal function, cough, and angioneurotic edema. An initial reduction in blood pressure is expected with the initiation of therapy and in most instances it is of little clinical consequence. Patients at increased risk of developing clinically important hypotensive symptoms can be identified by the following criteria: advanced functional class (i.e., class IV), recent aggressive therapy with diuretics, particularly when there is evidence of volume depletion, use of non-ACEI vasodilators, the presence of low serum sodium levels,[45] and borderline blood pressure when therapy is initiated. Since many of these patients fall into categories that are most likely to benefit from ACEI therapy, the greater incidence of hypotension should not be considered a contradiction to the use of these drugs. In such patients, however, it is prudent to take precautions when initiating therapy. A low dose of an agent with a relatively short half-life (such as captopril) can be started and if well tolerated, the patient can be switched to a higher dose and, perhaps, a longer acting agent over a period of 7 to 10 days. In some instances, it may be necessary to discontinue or lower the dose of diuretics or other vasodilators. When there is a high degree of suspicion that the initiation of an ACEI may provoke symptomatic hypotension, therapy can be initiated in a controlled setting such as an outpatient clinic or during hospitalization. In this way, blood pressure can be monitored frequently and supportive care administered if problems develop. Despite these problems, experience in the SOLVD trials demonstrated that only a small number of patients with LV dysfunction could not be continued on ACEIs because of hypotension.[42,43]

After the initiation of therapy, arterial pressure tends to increase toward pretreatment levels over the first weeks. During this period, patients should be evaluated to assess their clinical status and measure their blood pressure. A blood chemistry screen should be obtained to determine if there is evidence of worsening renal function. Many patients with CHF who are candidates for ACEIs have evidence of mild renal dysfunction before the initiation of therapy. A small "bump" in BUN or Cr levels is common and should not cause undue concern. Increases in BUN greater than 10 to 15 mg% or in Cr greater than 0.3 to 0.5 mg% that persist can be treated by adjusting therapy. In patients receiving diuretics or other non-ACEI vasodilators, a reduction in the dose of these drugs often is sufficient to correct the abnormality. If this tactic fails to bring the measurements back to an acceptable range, one can consider reducing the dose of the ACEI. The abnormalities in renal function are almost always completely reversible. Careful attention, however, is needed to be certain that they are not allowed to persist for prolonged periods of time.

Cough is a frequent complaint in patients with CHF. Although the ACEIs have the capacity to provoke cough (probably on the basis of central mechanisms), this must be differentiated from cough due to the myriad of other causes (including worsening pulmonary congestion!) in patients with CHF. This problem is highlighted by recent information from the treatment arm of the SOLVD study where it was found that 37% of patients treated with enalapril complained of this symptom during the course of the trial.[42] However, it was also noted that 31% of placebo-treated patients had a similar complaint. Thus, cough due to ACEIs is a real problem but the incidence is relatively low. A careful search for other causes of cough should always be undertaken before considering discontinuing ACEI therapy. When the latter step is undertaken, resolution of the problem suggests that it was indeed due to the drug. There is no convincing evidence that one ACEI is more likely to provoke this side effect than an other and, in the author's experience, changing the ACEI is rarely successful in solving the problem. However, when cough does not resolve after the drug is stopped, it is reasonable to conclude that the problem is not a side effect of ACEI. If the original indications for initiating therapy with ACEIs are still present, the drug should then be restarted.

There is a tendency for potassium levels to increase when ACEIs are initiated. As evidenced in both arms of SOLVD,[42,43] the change is small and of little or no clinical consequence in most instances. However, in patients with underlying renal dysfunction and in patients receiving potassium-sparing diuretics or large amounts of potassium supplementation, the increase in serum potassium level can be life-threatening. The condition is quite easy to treat since it responds to a reduction in either the non-ACEI factor or the ACEI itself. Vigilance on the part of the physician is necessary, however, to detect this condition.

An interesting but regrettable phenomenon that has developed with the use of the ACEIs in patients with CHF is that they tend to be used, in many instances, at doses that are lower than those that were used in the studies that provided evidence of efficacy. The obvious reason for this strategy is the desire to avoid side effects. However, SOLVD and other large-scale clinical trials provide strong evidence that the ACEIs tend to be well tolerated. The concern here is that it is uncertain whether the same clinical benefits that were noted in the studies cited earlier in this chapter will be present when the drugs are used at these lower doses. In fact, there is some preliminary information now available that the ACEIs are not as effective at these lower doses. In the absence of any compelling information that the low-dose strategy will be effective, the use of ACEIs in doses similar to those used in the successful clinical trials is strongly recommended.

β-Adrenergic Receptor Antagonists

Activation of the sympathetic nervous system is one of the most important pathophysiologic mechanisms that is responsible for progression of heart failure. This neurohormonal system is activated early in the disease to provide circulatory support, and levels of circulating catecholamines increase in patients with heart failure in proportion to severity of the disease; further, there is a strong association between high plasma levels of norepinephrine and an unfavorable prognosis. These observations suggest that drugs that interfere with the actions of the sympathetic nervous system (e.g., β-blockers) may be useful in the management of heart failure and reduce the risk of disease progression. Previously, such drugs were thought to be contraindicated in this condition because of their negative inotropic properties and short term adverse effects, but controlled clinical trials of a number of different β-blockers have shown they can reduce symptoms and improve left ventricular function. Although numerous small to medication size clinical trials as well as respective analysis of the use of the beta blockers post-myocardial infarction strongly suggest important benefits in heart failure, until recently this promise was not borne out in the few large scale clinical trials that have appeared in the medical literature.

Results of the U.S. Carvedilol Heart Failure Program has changed this situation and provided important information about the beneficial effects of carvedilol on the progression of heart failure. Carvedilol is a non-selective β-blocker. It provides peripheral vasodilation via blockade of α_1-adrenergic receptors and it is also a potent antioxidant. All patients enrolled in the Carvedilol program had chronic symptomatic heart failure (dyspnea or fatigue at rest or on exertion for at least three months) and a left ventricular ejection fraction ≤0.35 despite at least two months of treatment with diuretics and an angiotensin-converting-enzyme inhibitor (if tolerated). Treatment with digoxin, hydralazine and nitrates was allowed but not required. Enrollment was stratified by exercise capacity into one of four treatment protocols by use of a six-minute corridor walk test. Initially, patients

who walked between 425 (later increased to 450) and 550 meters were assigned to the mild heart failure protocol. Those who walked between 150 and 425 meters were assigned either to the moderate heart failure protocol or a dose ranging protocol, and those who walked only less than 150 meters were assigned to the severe heart failure protocol. After establishing ability to tolerate an open-label challenge dose of carvedilol (6.25 mg twice daily), patients were randomly assigned to receive double-blind treatment with placebo or carvedilol in addition to their usual medication. The initial dose, 12.5 mg daily, was increased to the maximum tolerated dose or the maximum dose allowed by the protocol (25 mg twice daily for patients under 85 kg or 50 mg twice daily for heavier patients); in the dose ranging study, patients were randomly assigned to one of four parallel treatment groups: placebo or 6.25 mg, 12.5 mg, or 25 mg of carvedilol twice daily. In all the studies, the initial dose was gradually up-titrated over a period of two to ten weeks, and double-blind therapy was maintained an additional six months (12 months in the mild heart failure protocol). Whenever possible, background therapy with other heart failure medications was held constant.

The overall trial program was terminated early upon the recommendation of the Data Safety Monitoring Board based on the finding that a survival advantage was demonstrated for patients receiving carvedilol. At the time of early termination, the study results showed that in addition to favorable effects on morbidity and mortality, carvedilol can be used safely and produces important hemodynamic and clinical benefits in patients with heart failure when added to standard therapy including digoxin, diuretics and an angiotensin-converting-enzyme inhibitor.

Results of Mild Heart Failure Study[68]

The primary study endpoint, heart failure progression, was defined as death due to heart failure, hospitalization for heart failure, or the need for a sustained increase in heart failure mediation(s). Based on an intent-to-treat analysis, carvedilol treatment reduced the occurrence of clinical progression from 21% to 11%, a decrease of 48% (p = 0.008); the relative risk of heart failure progression was 0.52 (confidence intervals: 0.32, 0.85). The reduction in the overall progression of heart failure endpoint was paralleled by similar reductions in each of the component endpoints. The effect of carvedilol remained significant even if the medication change component was eliminated from the analysis. Furthermore, the effects of carvedilol were independent of patient age, sex, race, etiology of heart failure and baseline left ventricular ejection fraction.

Many secondary study endpoints including left ventricular ejection fraction, NYHA classification heart failure symptom score and both physician and patient global assessments were improved by carvedilol. The congruence of these distinct measures of clinical status strongly supports the conclusion that carvedilol exerted a beneficial effect on clinical symptoms. However, carvedilol had no significant effect on the Minnesota Living with Heart Failure scale, the distance walked in nine minutes on a self-powered treadmill (representing a maximal effort in heart failure patients), or cardiothoracic index. The exercise finding cannot be considered surprising, since heart rate response to exercise, which is an important determinant of maximal exercise capacity, is reduced by β-blockers.

While the number of patients who died was too small to allow conclusions about the effect of carvedilol on mortality in this study, the reductions in mortality due to heart failure and all-cause mortality are qualitatively and quantitatively consistent with the effect of carvedilol observed in the 1,094 patients enrolled in the overall stratified trial program. This observation provides evidence that the improvement in other components of the composite primary endpoint and secondary endpoints did not occur at the expense of an adverse effect on survival.

Finally, carvedilol therapy was well tolerated in the study population. Approximately 4% of patients did not tolerate carvedilol during the open-label challenge. Of the patients randomized to carvedilol, the major adverse effects were related to β-adrenergic blockade and/or α_1-adrenergic blockade including hypotension, bradycardia and dizziness.

Results of Moderate-to-Severe Heart Failure (Prospective Randomized Evaluation of Carvedilol on Symptoms and Exercise: PRECISE) Study[69]

Carvedilol produced a significant improvement in NYHA functional classification and was also associated with an improvement in both the physician and patient global assessment of disease severity. The proportional decrease in the risk of symptomatic deterioration with carvedilol was greater than the proportional increase in the number of patients who showed clinical improvement with the drug. In addition to changes in symptoms, other measures of clinical efficacy were improved by carvedilol. Therapy with the drug was accompanied by an increase in left ventricular ejection fraction (+0.08 on carvedilol versus +0.03 on placebo, $p < 0.001$) which was paralleled by a reduction in cardiovascular morbidity (i.e., hospitalizations). When deaths and cardiovascular hospitalizations were combined in a time-to-first-event analysis to account for competing risks, the probability of a major fatal or non-fatal event was reduced by carvedilol from 31.0% to 19.6% ($p = 0.029$). The favorable effects of carvedilol were similar in patients with ischemic heart disease or idiopathic dilated cardiomyopathy as the cause of heart failure. In contrast, carvedilol therapy had little effect on indirect measures of patient benefit including changes in exercise tolerance or quality of life scores. An important finding in this study was that carvedilol produced clinical improvement in patients both with and without ischemic heart disease as the cause of heart failure.

The most common side effect of initiating therapy with carvedilol was dizziness. During the up-titration and maintenance phases, dizziness and hypotension were the most common side effects of carvedilol, but these generally subsided spontaneously or following adjustment in concomitant therapy and did not require withdrawal of the drug. Heart rate decreased significantly in the carvedilol group as compared with the placebo group (16.3 versus 1.9 beats/minute, $p = 0.0001$), and this was accompanied by small but significant decreases in systolic blood pressure (5.8 versus 0.7 mmHg, $p = 0.002$) and diastolic blood pressure (4.7 versus 0.3mmHg, $p = 0.0001$). Bradycardia was reported as an adverse reaction in 8.3% of the carvedilol group versus 0.7% of the placebo group ($p = 0.002$), whereas hypotension was reported as an adverse reaction in 12.8% of the carvedilol group versus 4.1% of the placebo group ($p = 0.009$).

Concern about the potential adverse effects of β-adrenergic blockade in heart failure has focused especially on patients with severe symptoms whose cardiac function might be critically dependent upon adrenergic stimulation. Although this study of carvedilol was terminated early and patient entry and follow-up were considerably less than had been originally proposed, the results provide useful information with the drug in severe patients (average ejection fraction = 0.22) with marked limitation of exercise capacity. Only 8% of the initially screened group did not tolerate the open-label, low-dose carvedilol challenge; after randomization to double-blind therapy, discontinuation of the drug was infrequent and similar in both the carvedilol and placebo arms. Overall, the incidence of adverse reactions did not differ between the treatment groups. Furthermore, left ventricular ejection fraction and both physician and patient assessment was significantly improved by carvedilol. Though not definitive, these results suggest that carvedilol can be safely administered to patients with severe heart failure.

Results of Dose Ranging Heart Failure (Multicenter Oral Carvedilol Heart Failure Assessment: MOCHA) Study[71]

The primary efficacy parameter was submaximal exercise as measured by the six-minute corridor walk test and the nine-minute self-powered treadmill test. Carvedilol had no detectable effect on submaximal exercise as measured by either technique. Nevertheless, carvedilol was associated with dose-related improvements in left ventricular function (by 5, 6 and 8 ejection fraction units in the low, medium and high dose carvedilol groups, respectively, as compared to 2 units with placebo, p < 0.001) and survival (crude mortality rates of 6.0%, 6.7% and 1.1% with increasing doses of carvedilol as compared to 15.5% with placebo, p < 0.001). All-cause mortality risk was lowered by 73% (all dose groups combined) by carvedilol treatment (relative risk = 0.272; 95% confidence intervals: 0.124, 0.597; p < 0.001). Carvedilol also lowered hospitalization rate (by from 58% to 64%, p = 0.003) with increasing dose and was generally well tolerated.

The increase in left ventricular ejection fraction shown in this study occurred in both ischemic and nonischemic cardiomyopathies. In addition, the reduction in mortality appeared to be present in both ischemic and non-ischemic cardiomyopathies and was observed for both sudden and progressive pump dysfunction classifications of death.

Results of Overall Morbidity and Mortality Analysis[72]

In an intent-to-treat analysis of the results from all 1,094 patients entered into the four treatment protocols of the stratified clinical trial program, the mortality rate was 7.8% in the placebo group and 3.2% in the carvedilol group; the reduction in risk attributable to carvedilol was 65% (95% confidence interval: 39% to 80%; p < 0.001). This finding, as evaluated by a Kaplan-Meier analysis of survival among drug- and placebo-treated patients, was manifest almost immediately after beginning treatment and became highly significant throughout the course of therapy. This effect was consistent in all evaluated subgroups (age, sex, cause of heart failure, ejection fraction, exercise tolerance, systolic blood pressure, heart rate or protocol assignment) and was reflected in a decrease in the risk of death from progressive heart failure as well as in the risk of sudden death. In addition, as compared to placebo, carvedilol therapy was accompanied by a 27% reduction in the risk of hospitalization for cardiovascular causes as well as a 38% reduction in the combined risk of hospitalization or death in a time-to-first-event analysis (24.6% versus 15.8%, p < 0.001).

All of the U.S. Carvedilol Heart Failure Program trials included an open-label challenge phase. Accordingly, those events in the treated group during the two-week period when a patient's ability to tolerate the drug was tested were censored out of the analysis. The seven deaths that occurred during the challenge phase do not appear among the mortality statistics for the carvedilol group, although they would have accounted for 24% of all the deaths in patients receiving therapy; an additional 17 patients (1.4%) were not randomized because of worsening heart failure during the challenge phase. Since patients were selected on the basis of clinical stability, this early morbidity and mortality should not be discounted and cannot be dissociated from a potential

adverse effect of the drug. In contrast, the ongoing Beta-blocker Evaluation Survival Trial (BEST), a study of the effects of bucindolol on survival in 2,800 patients with heart failure who will be followed for at least 18 months, has been designed without a run-in challenge period.

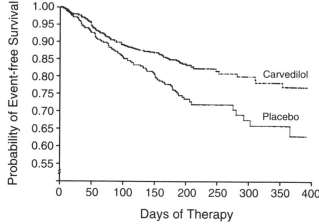

No. at Risk

Placebo	398	336	292	260	134	63	45	35	2
Carvedilol	696	607	529	491	270	117	92	70	9

FIGURE 34.6. Kaplan–Meien Analysis of Survival without Hospitalization for Cardiovascular Reasons (Event-free Survival) in the placebo and Carvedilol Groups. Patients in the carvedilol group had a 38 percent lower risk of death or hospitalization for cardiovascular disease than patients in the placebo group (P<0.001). Reproduced with permission. *N Engl J Med.* 1996; 334: 1353.

Management of Patients with Congestive Heart Failure

The goals for medical management of patients with chronic CHF are relatively straightforward. They include providing symptomatic relief, increasing exercise capacity and sense of well-being, avoiding hospitalization, preventing progression of LV dysfunction, and prolonging life. There is now evidence that, to a certain

TABLE 34.5. Medical management of chronic CHF.

All Patients—identify and treat reversible causes and exacerbating factors
Asymptomatic LV dysfunction
   ACEI (when EF is ≤0.35 or ≤0.45 post-MI)
   Beta-blocker in post-MI patient with EF > 0.45
Mild to moderate CHF
   Diuretic
   ACEI
   Digoxin
   Carvedilol (when EF ≤ 0.35)
Severe CHF
   Diuretic, ACEI, digoxin
   Consider 2nd diuretic increasing dose of ACEI
   Investigational approaches (i.e., experimental drugs, intermittent IV inotropic therapy)

CHF = congestive heart failure; LV = left ventricular; ACEI = angiotensin-converting enzyme inhibitor; EF = ejection fraction; MI = myocardial infraction.

extent, medical therapy is able to accomplish all of these goals. Information summarized in this chapter as well as in many other chapters in this text provide evidence for (and, in some cases, against) the use of the various agents that are available to treat CHF. What follows, then, is a therapeutic approach to the patient with CHF directed toward achieving the goals that are listed above. This approach is outlined in Table 34.5. Certain basic principles that pertain to all patients with CHF will first be discussed.

Since CHF is a syndrome that can develop on the basis of a variety of diseases, it is essential to obtain information about the cause. If, as in most instances, the etiology is cardiac, differentiation between structural or mechanical problems and muscle disease is necessary.

TABLE 34.6. Conditions commonly associated with worsening CHF.

Failure to take adequate dose of prescribed drugs
Dietary indescretion
Uncontrolled hypertension
Concurrent administration of drugs with:
Cardiac effects (i.e., beta-blockers, calcium channel blockers, antiarrhythmics)
Systemic effects (i.e., nonsteroidal antiinflammatory drugs)
Alcohol abuse
Atrial arrhythmias
Infection
Anemia
COPD
Pulmonary emboli
Thyroid disease
Stress
Environmental conditions
Pregnancy

CHF = congestive heart failure; COPD = chronic obstructive pulmonary disease.

Whether muscle disease is due to ischemic or nonischemic causes also should be determined. Although an exact diagnosis of nonischemic cardiomyopathies often is not possible, a search for some of the reversible processes is worthwhile if there are clues that one of these conditions may be present. A carefully performed medical history and examination combined with a chest x ray and electrocardiogram are integral parts of the diagnostic process. Some measurement of LV function also is of considerable value both in confirming the presence or absence of myocardial disease and providing information regarding prognosis. An echocardiogram often is used for this purpose since it provides information about chamber size, the condition of the heart valves and other structures, and an assessment of systolic function. Other tests, which are outlined elsewhere in this text, can be used to define cardiac function and anatomy in the appropriate circumstances.

A carefully performed medical history and physical examination will also help determine if other conditions that exacerbate the cardiac problem or complicate the

therapeutic approach are present. These conditions likewise are discussed in great detail elsewhere. The clinical course of CHF can be variable and, in any given patient, it is rarely predictable. A recent survey, however, points out that worsening CHF often can be ascribed to preventable causes.[46] A list of some of these causes is given in Table 34.6. In a surprisingly large number of cases, patients are found to be doing poorly because they are not taking adequate doses of the drugs that have been prescribed. This situation can have multiple causes including either simple error, forgetfulness, or contrary behavior. Careful explanation to the patient regarding the rationale for the various drugs and description of how frequently they should be taken both initially and during follow-up visits cannot be overemphasized.

Patients with Asymptomatic LV Dysfunction

The goal in this group of patients is to prevent future events and further deterioration in LV performance. The results of the prevention arm of SOLVD showed that in patients with an LV ejection fraction 0.35 or below who did not require therapy for CHF enalapril significantly reduced the progression of disease.[43] Although not all of these patients were entirely asymptomatic, nearly two thirds were considered to be NYHA functional class I at the time of randomization. In addition, post-hoc stratification revealed that symptomatic status had no significant interaction with the response to therapy . Based on SOLVD data, it is estimated that treating 1000 patients who had entry criteria for the prevention arm over 3 years would prevent the onset of CHF in 90 of these patients and hospitalization in 65 of them. ACEI therapy also appears to be effective in modifying the remodeling process that occurs in the LV after myocardial infarction.[38,39] Thus, the point that emerges from these studies is that treatment of LV dysfunction with ACEIs at a relatively early stage has beneficial effects on the subsequent clinical course.

Guidelines for identifying patients who should be started on therapy are based on entry criteria for the SOLVD and SAVE studies and the smaller trial of Pfeffer and colleagues in postinfarction patients.[38,43,43a] Post-hoc stratification based on LV ejection fraction in SOLVD suggests that as the ejection fraction rises, the likelihood of a beneficial effect is somewhat reduced. However, this information is somewhat difficult to apply to an individual patient since EF measurements are subject to considerable biological and technical variability. In addition, some benefits were seen in SOLVD at even the highest EF levels. For instance, patients in the highest tertile of EF (i.e., 33–35%) who were treated with enalapril in the prevention arm of SOLVD demonstrated a 26% reduction in risk for death or development of CHF over the course of the study. Consequently, it is the author's practice to initiate ACEI therapy in patients with asymptomatic LV dysfunction once the LV EF is determined to be in the range of 0.35. In patients who have had a recent myocardial infarction, an EF that is ≤0.40 usually is an indication for starting ACEI therapy.

A question that is often raised in the postinfarction patient is the optimal timing for initiating therapy. It would seem reasonable to start an ACEI within 2 weeks or so of a myocardial infarction (MI) as was done in the SAVE trial. Most patients undergo risk stratification after a MI and information regarding LV EF usually is available fairly early in the postinfarction period. In many cases, the drug can be started while the patient is in the hospital. The results of the CONSENSUS II trial, however, indicate that the initiation of therapy immediately after an infarct adds little benefit and may actually be detrimental in some groups of patients.[46a]

Another issue of some concern is whether to use an ACEI, a beta-blocker, or both in the management of the postinfarction patient. The rationale for the use of beta-blockers is based on a series of clinical trials that demonstrated that these agents could improve survival in postinfarction patients. Post-hoc analysis of the Beta-Blocker Heart Attack Trial (BHAT) suggested that, contrary to what most observers had expected, patients with more severe degrees of LV dysfunction seemed to do well with beta-blocker therapy and, in fact, demonstrated the greatest likelihood of a positive effect of drug on survival.[47] Further support comes from several small trials that showed that the administration of beta-blockers to patients with CHF was associated with improved cardiac function and evidence of increased exercise capacity.[48–50]

This issue is not possible to resolve definitively at the present time since there are no trials available in which the two modes of therapy are directly compared. The following information, however, is helpful in allowing the clinician to make a choice in individual patients. Results of the SOLVD and SAVE trials show that ACEIs improve the clinical course of patients with LV dysfunction and they provide guidelines regarding the extent of LV dysfunction at which the drugs are likely to be effective. The beta-blocker post-MI trials were not specifically designed to look at patient groups with LV dysfunction that was as severe as the groups included in SOLVD and SAVE. Thus, the data base for evaluating the efficacy of beta-blockers in these populations is limited and guidelines for the extent of LV dysfunction at which they are likely to be most useful are lacking. Since beta-blockers have the problem of precipitating worsening heart failure in some patients, and particularly in those with more severe LV dysfunction, they are more difficult to use than the ACEIs. In contrast to the ACEIs, the beta-blockers have a relatively high side effect profile that limits enthusiasm for their use in an asymptomatic population. Based on these considerations, it seems preferable to use an ACEI rather than a beta-blocker in most postinfarction patients with moderate to severe degrees of LV dysfunction. The presence of residual myocardial ischemia would have an important impact on this decision in favor of the use of a beta-blocker. Finally, it is of interest that in both the SOLVD and SAVE trials the beneficial effects of ACEI therapy could be detected in patients who were also receiving a beta-blocker. These latter results suggest that when these two classes of drug are used in combination in the post-MI patient, their effects may be additive.

Although calcium channel blocking agents may be useful in some groups of post-MI patients, their routine use in patients with LV dysfunction must be discouraged at this time. This caution is based on the results of a trial where the effects of diltiazem were compared to those of placebo in a group of patients during the postinfarction period.[51] Overall, the study showed no significant difference between the patients treated with active drug and those treated with placebo. However, in the subgroup of patients with evidence of more severe LV dysfunction, mortality was significantly increased in the patients receiving diltiazem. It is possible that these findings are due to the fact that diltiazem has negative inotropic effects and that the use of calcium channel blockers, which are more specific for the peripheral vasculature or those which are less potent stimulators of the renin-angiotensin system, may have beneficial effects in this population.[51a]

Finally, since digoxin and the diuretic agents have been found to be useful only in relieving symptoms, there is no indication for their use in the truly asymptomatic patient with LV dysfunction.

Symptomatic LV Dysfunction

Patients with CHF should be treated with a combination of three drugs: digoxin, a diuretic, and an ACEI. This approach certainly applies to patients with severe CHF since the available evidence indicates that the effects of these different therapies are additive and complementary. The results of the clinical trials described in the preceding sections indicate that the use of triple therapy also is applicable to patients with less severe amounts of failure. In this subgroup of patients, the ACEIs have been shown to increase exercise capacity, improve NYHA classification, prevent hospitalizations, and prolong survival. However, despite the unquestionable efficacy of the ACEIs in treating patients with CHF, the use of these agents alone usually is not adequate and a diuretic is required to prevent congestive symptoms. The recent information from the RADIANCE study indicates that digoxin will provide additional benefits. Thus, the best approach in symptomatic heart failure appears to be to support the damaged myocardium with a relatively mild inotropic agent and to counteract the compensatory increases in intravascular volume and stimulation of the renin-angiotensin system.

Patients who continue to do poorly even after triple therapy has been initiated present a difficult therapeutic problem to the clinician. After it has been determined that all prescribed medications are being taken correctly and that none of the myriad of factors that are known to exacerbate CHF are present, several steps can be considered. Patients with predominantly congestive symptoms that are refractory to therapy often can be managed successfully by using a combination of diuretics, which affect the nephron at different places. A loop diuretic, such as furosemide, and an agent that acts at the level of the distal tubule, such as metolazone, often are used in conjunction for this purpose. This is an extremely potent combination and great care should be taken to avoid problems related to "over diuresis" and, in particular, the induction of hypokalemia when these two drugs are used together.

As noted previously, ACEIs usually do not produce evidence of clinical improvement until after they have been given for several weeks. If, at that time, the patient remains symptomatic and the blood pressure permits, an increase in the dose of the ACEI can be considered. For instance, increases in the dose of enalapril from the standard dose of 10 mg bid to a regimen of 15 or 20 mg bid is effective in some patients. ACEIs tend to be rather weak vasodilators, and another approach to the patient who remains symptomatic on triple therapy is to add a direct acting vasodilator to the regimen.

Although ACEIs are generally well tolerated, there are some patients who develop side effects that necessitate their discontinuation. When this occurs, thought should be given to treatment with a non-ACEI vasodilator. An alternative is the combination of hydralazine-isosorbide dinitrate. This combination of an arterial dilator with a predominant venodilator has been shown in the VHeFT-I trial to improve survival in patients with NYHA class II–III CHF.[55c] The disadvantage of this combination is that the dosing regimen is somewhat more awkward than that of the ACEIs. It is likely that these two factors resulted in the high percentage of patients who had discontinued one or both of the study drugs by the conclusion of VHeFT-I.

Finally, the results of the U.S. Carvedilol Heart Failure trials show that carvedilol has beneficial effects on the progression of heart failure. Reductions in morbidity and mortality are particularly impressive in patients with mild to moderate heart failure. These results also indicate that carvedilol can be used safely and that it produces important hemodynamic and clinical benefits in patients with chronic heart failure when added to standard therapy including digoxin, diuretics and angiotensin-converting-enzyme inhibitors.

Antiarrhythmics and Anticoagulants

Approximately 40% of patients with CHF die suddenly and the presumed cause of death is a ventricular dysrhythmia.[56] Although the ACEIs have been shown to reduce mortality in patients with CHF, their major impact appears to be on death due to progressive pump failure. Both CONSENSUS and SOLVD showed no apparent significant effects of enalapril on sudden cardiac death. Patients with CHF have frequent ventricular ectopic beats and runs of ventricular tachycardia also are common.[57,58] As noted elsewhere in this text, although these events do appear to be associated with subsequent mortality and are significant predictors of survival in populations with LV dysfunction, they offer little in the way of information in individual patients.[57–60] Although antiarrhythmic agents may successfully treat the ventricular ectopy, there is no convincing evidence that any of the available agents improve survival in patients with CHF . In addition, antiarrhythmic agents tend to have a higher side effect profile, are more likely to be proarrhythmic,[61,62] and may precipitate worsening CHF in patients with LV dysfunction.[63] Thus, their routine use in this population is not indicated. Patients with symptomatic ventricular rhythm disturbances should have these suppressed, preferably with one of the agents that is less likely to adversely affect ventricular function. Electrophysiologic testing can be of value in selecting an appropriate therapeutic regimen in this setting.[64,65]

Patients with LV dysfunction are prone to develop embolic complications.[66,67] The risk appears to increase with increasing severity of LV dysfunction and in patients with large myocardial infarctions, particularly when an LV aneurysm is present. Patients with previous embolic events and those with atrial fibrillation appear to be at the highest risk. There is virtually no information from well designed clinical trials evaluating the effects of anticoagulant therapy in patients with CHF. However, uncontrolled data suggest that this approach is effective.[66] Given the relatively high risk of significant complications with anticoagulation therapy, the approach suggested by Goodnight elsewhere in this text seems reasonable. In this approach, high-risk patients (as defined above) would receive high-intensity warfarin therapy, whereas those who are at low risk would receive low-intensity therapy.

Conclusion

There have been enormous strides in the field of clinical and basic research that have affected the way that patients with CHF are managed. A large body of data from well designed clinical trials that can be used as a guide to decision making in patients seen in clinical practice is now available. This information has enabled us to forge a rational basis of therapy for patients during various stages of the disease. What is most helpful is that there is firm evidence for the efficacy of digoxin, diuretics, and the ACEIs. Carvedilol appears to be a useful new addition to the therapeutic armamentarium. The appropriate timing for interventions with these agents is now much more apparent than in the past. In addition, the clinical efficacy of second-line drugs that can be used as replacements for, or in addition to, standard therapeutic agents also is known.

It must be remembered, however, that CHF remains a common and extremely lethal disease. Despite treatment with enalapril, mortality was still approximately 30% in symptomatic and approximately 13% in asymptomatic patients over a 36-month period in the SOLVD trials. Although there is much work yet to be done, we are on firmer ground in our approach to the medical management of CHF than we were just a decade ago, and it is certain that the recent changes in therapy have resulted in the improved quality and quantity of life of our patients.

References

1. Greenberg B. Mechanical characteristics of the failing left ventricle. *J Cardiovasc Pharm.* 1989;14(Suppl 5):562–568.
2. Pfeffer MA, Pfeffer JM. Ventricular enlargement and survival after myocardial infarction. *Circulation.* 1987;75(Suppl IV):IV-93–IV-97.
3. Jeremy RW, Allman KC, Bautovich G, Harris PJ. Patterns of left ventricular dilatation during the six months after myocardial infarction. *J Am Coll Cardiol.* 1989;13:304–310.
4. Eaton LW, Weiss JL, Bulkley BH, Garrison JB, Weissfeldt ML. Regional cardiac dilatation after acute myocardial infarction: recognition by two-dimensional echocardiography. *N Engl J Med.* 1979;300:57–62.
5. Dzau VJ. Cardiac renin-angiotensin system; molecular and functional aspects. *Am J Med.* 1988;84(Suppl 3A):22–27.
6. Braunwald E. ACE inhibitors—a cornerstone of the treatment of heart failure. *N Engl J Med.* 1991;325:351–353.
7. Biddle TL, Yu PN. Effect of furosemide on hemodynamics and lung water in acute pulmonary edema secondary to myocardial infarction. *Am J Cardiol.* 1979;43:86–90.
8. Hutcheon D, Nemeth E, Quinlan D. The role of furosemide alone or in combination with digoxin in the relief of symptoms of congestive heart failure. *J Clin Pharmacol.* 1980;20:59–68.
9. Dzau VJ, Hollinberg NK. Renal response to captopril in severe heart failure: role of furosemide in natriuresis and reversal of hyponatremia. *Ann Intern Med.* 1984;100:777–782.
10. Anand IS, Kalka KS, Ferrari R, et al. Enalapril as sole treatment in severe chronic heart failure with sodium retention. *Int J Cardiol.* 1990;28:341–346.
11. Stampfer M, Epstein SE, Beiser GD, Braunwald E. Hemodynamic effects of diuresis at rest and during intense upright exercise in patients with impaired cardiac function. *Circulation.* 1968;37:900–911.
12. Wilson JR, Reichek N, Dunkman WB et al. Effect of diuresis on the performance of the failing left ventricle in man. *Am J Med.* 1981;70:234–239.
13. Ghose RR, Gupta SK. Synergistic actions of metolazone with "loop" diuretics. *Br Med J.* 1981;812:1432–1433.
14. Francis GS, Benedict C, Johnstone DE et al. Comparison of neuroendocrine activation in patients with left ventricular dysfunction with and without congestive heart failure: a substudy of the Studies of Left Ventricular Dysfunction (SOLVD). *Circulation.* 1990;82:1729–1739.
15. Sonnenblick EH, Williams JF Jr, Glick G et al. Studies on digitalis XV. Effects of cardiac glycosides on myocardial force-velocity relations in the non-failing human heart. *Circulation.* 1966;34:532–539.
16. Arnold SB, Byrd RC, Meister W et al. Long-term digitalis therapy improves left ventricular function in heart failure. *N Engl J Med.* 1980;303:1443–1448.
17. Parker M, Carver J, Rodeherrer R et al. Effect of oral milrinone on mortality in severe heart failure. *N Engl J Med.* 1991;325:1468.
18. Ferguson DW, Berg WJ, Sanders JS et al. Sympathoinhibilory?? responses to digitalis glycosides in heart failure patients: direct evidence from sympathetic neural recordings. *Circulation.* 1989;80:65–77.
19. Lee DC-S, Johnson RA, Bengham JB et al. Heart failure in outpatients. A randomized trial of digoxin versus placebo. *N Engl J Med.* 1982;306:699–705.
20. Guyatt GH, Sullivan MJJ, Fallen EL, et al. A controlled trial of digoxin in congestive heart failure. *Am J Cardiol.* 1988;61:371–375.
21. The Captopril-Digoxin Multicenter Research Group. Comparative effects of therapy with captopril and digoxin in patients with mild to moderate heart failure. *JAMA.* 1988;259:539–544.
22. DiBianco R, Shabetai R, Kostak et al. A comparison of oral milrinone, digoxin, and their combination in the treatment of patients with chronic heart failure. *N Engl J Med.* 1989;320:677–683.
23. Packer M, Gheorghiade M, Young JB, et al. Randomized double-blind, placebo-controlled, withdrawal study of digoxin in patients with chronic heart failure treated with converting-enzyme inhibitors. *J Am Coll Cardiol.* 1992;19:260A.
24. Young JB, Uretsky BF, Shahidi FE, et al. Multicenter, double-blind, placebo-controlled randomized withdrawal trial of the efficacy and safety of digoxin in patients with mild to moderate chronic heart failure not treated with converting enzyme inhibitors. *J Am Coll Cardiol.* 1992;19:259A.
25. Smith TW. Digitalis—mechanisms of action and clinical use. *N Engl J Med.* 1988;318:358–365.
26. Dzau VJ, Colucci WS, Hollinberg NK, Williams GK. Relation of the renin-angiotensin-aldosterone system to clinical state in congestive heart failure. *Circulation.* 1981;63:645–651.

27. David R, Ribner HS, Keung E, et al. Treatment of chronic congestive heart failure with captopril, an oral inhibitor of angiotensin converting enzyme. *N Engl J Med*. 1979;301:117–121.

28. Ader R, Chatterjee K, Ports T et al. Immediate and sustained hemodynamic and clinical improvement in chronic heart failure by angiotensin-converting enzyme inhibitors. *Circulation*. 1980;61:931–937.

29. Levine TB, Franciosa JA, Cohn JN. Acute and long-term response to an oral converting enzyme inhibitor, captopril, in congestive heart failure. *Circulation*. 1980;63:35–41.

30. Kramer BL, Massie BM, Topic N. Controlled trial of captopril in chronic heart failure: a rest and exercise hemodynamic study. *Circulation*. 1983;67:807–816.

31. Captopril Multicenter Research Group. A placebo-controlled trial of captopril in refractory chronic congestive heart failure. *J Am Coll Cardiol*. 1983;2:755–763.

32. Mancini DM, Davis L, Wexler JP, et al. Dependence of enhanced maximal exercise performance on increased peak skeletal muscle perfusion during long-term captopril therapy in heart failure. *J Am Coll Cardiol*. 1987;845–850.

33. Drexler H, Banhardt U, Meinhertz T, et al. Contrasting peripheral short-term and long-term effects of converting enzyme inhibition in patients with congestive heart failure. A double-blind, placebo controlled trial. *Circulation*. 1989;79:491–502.

34. Ontkean M, Gay R, Greenberg B. ACE inhibition with captopril improves EDRF activity in an experimental model of chronic heart failure. *J Am Coll Cardiol*. 1992;19:207A(abstract).

34a. Greenberg B, Perkinsk, Ontkean M, Gay R. Captopril reverses progressive abnormalities MEDRF activity in chronic heart failure. *J Am Coll Cardiol*. 1993;21:268A(abstract).

35. Hammermeister KE, DeRouen TA, Dodge HT. Variables predictive of survival in patients with coronary disease: selection by univariate and multivariate analyses from the clinical, electrocardiographic, exercise, arteriographic and quantitative angiographic evaluations. *Circulation*. 1979;59:421–430.

36. Norris RM, Barnaby PF, Brandt PWT, et al. Prognosis after recovery from first acute myocardial infarction: determinants of reinfarction and sudden death. *Am J Cardiol*. 1984;53:408–413.

37. White HD, Norris RM, Brown MA, et al. Left ventricular end-systolic volume as the major determinant of survival after recovery from myocardial infarction. *Circulation*. 1987;76:44–51.

38. Pfeffer MA, Lamas GA, Vaughan DE, et al. Effects of captopril on progressive ventricular dilatation after anterior myocardial infarction. *N Engl J Med*. 1988; 319:80–86.

39. Sharpe N, Murphy J, Smith H, Hannan. Treatment of patients with symptomless left ventricular dysfunction after myocardial infarction. *Lancet*. 1988;1:255–259.

40. Greenberg B, Quinones M, Koipillai K, et al. Effects of long-term enalapril therapy on echocardiographic variables in SOLVD patients. *Circulation*. 1992;86:

41. The CONSENSUS Trial Study Group. Effects of enalapril on mortality in severe congestive heart failure. Results of the Cooperative North Scandinavian Enalapril Survival Study (CONSENSUS). *N. Engl J Med*. 1987;316:1429–1435.

42. The SOLVD Investigators. Effects of enalapril on survival in patients with reduced left ventricular ejection fractions and congestive heart failure. *N Engl J Med*. 1991; 325:293–302.

43. The SOLVD Investigators. Effect of enalapril on mortality and the development of heart failure in asymptomatic patients with reduced left ventricular ejection fractions. *N Engl J Med*. 1992;327:685–691.

43a. Pfeffer MA, Braumuald E, Moyé LA, et al. Effects of captopril on mortality and morbidity in patients with left ventricular dysfunction after myocardial infarction. Results of the Survival and Ventricular Enlargement Trial. *N Engl J Med*. 1992;327:669–677.

44. Cohn JN, Johnson G, Zilsche S, et al. A comparison of enalapril with hydralazine-isosorbide dinitrate in the treatment of chronic congestive heart failure. *N Engl J Med*. 1991;325:303–310.

45. Packer M, Medena N, Yushak M. Relationship between serum sodium concentrations and the hemodynamic and clinical response to converting enzyme inhibition with captopril in severe heart failure. *J Am Coll Cardiol*. 1984;3:1035–1043.

46. Ghali JK, Kadakia S, Cooper R, et al. Precipitating factors leading to decompensation of heart failure. *Arch Intern Med*. 1988;148:2013–2016.

46a. Swedberg K, Held P, Kjek Shus J, et al. Effects of the early administration of enalapril on mortality in patients with acute myocardial infarction. Results of the Cooperative Newscandinavian Enalapril Survival Study II (CONSENSUS II), *N Engl J Med*. 1992;327:678–684.

47. B-Blocker Heart Attack Trial Research Group. A randomized trial of propranolol in patients with acute myocardial infarction. I. Mortality results. *JAMA*. 1982;247:1707–1714.

48. Swedberg K, Hjalmaroson A, Waagstein F, et al. Adverse effects of B-blockade withdrawal in patients with congestive cardiomyopathy. *Br Heart J*. 1980;44: 134–142.

49. Engelmeier RS, O'Connell JB, Walsh R, et al. Improvement in symptoms and exercise tolerance by metoprolol in patients with dilated cardiomyopathy. A double-blind, randomized, placebo-controlled study. *Circulation*. 1985;72:536–546.

50. Waagstein F, Caidahl K, Wallentin I, et al. Long-term B-blockade in dilated cardiomyopathy: effects of short- and long-term metoprolol treatment followed by withdrawal and re-administration of metoprolol. *Circulation*. 1989;80:551–563.

51. Moss AJ, Oakes D, Benhorin J, et al. The interaction between diltiazem and left ventricular function after myocardial infarction. *Circulation*. 1989;80(Suppl IV):IV-102–IV-106.

51a. Packer M, Nicod P, Khandheria BR, et al. Randomized multicenter, double-blind, placebo-controlled evaluation of amlodipine in patients with mild-to-moderate heart failure. *J Am Coll Cardiol.* 1991; 17:274A(abstract).

52. Cowley AJ, Wynne RD, Hampton JR. The effects of BTS 4946S on blood pressure and peripheral arteriolar and venous tone in normal volunteers. *J Hypertens.* 1984; 2(Suppl 3):547–549.

53. Elborn J, Stanford C, Nicholls D. Effect of flosequinan on exercise capacity and symptoms in severe heart failure. *Br Heart J.* 1989;61:331–335.

54. Packer M, Narahara KA, Elkayam U, et al. Double-blind, placebo-controlled study of the efficacy of flosequinan in patients with chronic heart failure. *J Am Coll Cardiol.* 1993 (In Press).

55. Pitt B on behalf of the Reflect II Study Group. A randomized, multicenter, double-blind placebo controlled study of the efficacy of flosequinan in patients with chronic heart failure. *Circulation.* 1991;84(Suppl II):II-311 (abstract).

55a. Silke B, Tennet H, Fischer-Hansen J et al. A double-blind, parallel-group comparison of flosequinan and enalapril in the treatment of chronic heart failure. *Eur H J.* 1992;13:1092–1100.

55b. Massie BM, Berk MR, Brozena SC, et al. Can further benefit be achieved by adding a vasodilater to a diuretic, digoxn and angiotensin converting enzyme inhibitor therapy in patients with congestive heart failure? Results of the flosequinan plus ACE inhibitor Trial (FACET). *Circulation.* 1993. (In Press).

55c. Cohn JN, Archibald DG, Ziesche S, et al. Effect of vasodilator therapy on mortality inchronic congestive heart failure: results of a Veterans Administration Cooperative Study. *N Engl J Med.* 1986;314:1547–1552.

56. Franciosa JA, Wilen M, Ziesche S, Cohn JN. Survival in men with severe chronic left ventricular failure due to either coronary heart disease or idiopathic dilated cardiomyopathy. *Am J Cardiol.* 1983;51:831–836.

57. Wilson JR, Schwartz S, St. John Sutton M, et al. Prognosis in severe heart failure: Relation to hemodynamic measurements and ventricular ectopic activity. *J Am Coll Cardiol.* 1983;2:403–410.

58. Maskin CS, Siskind SJ, Lejemtel TH. High incidence of non-sustained ventricular tachycardia in severe congestive heart failure. *Am Heart J.* 1984;107:896–907.

59. Gradman A, Deedwaniap, Cody R, et al. Predictors of total mortality and sudden death in mild to moderate heart failure. *J Am Coll Cardiol.* 1989;14:564–590.

60. Schultz RA, Strauss HW, Pitt B. Sudden death in the year following myocardial infarction. Relation to ventricular premature contractions in the late hospital phase and left ventricular ejection fraction. *Am J Med.* 1977;62:192–199.

61. Slater W, Lambert SL, Podrid PJ, Lown B. Clinical predictors of arrhythmia worsening by antiarrhythmic drugs. *Am J Cardiol.* 1988;61:349–353.

62. Morganroth J, Anderson JL, Gentzkow GD. Clarification of type of ventricular arrhythmia predicts frequency of adverse cardiac events from flecainide. *J Am Coll Cardiol.* 1986;8:607–615.

63. Podrid PJ, Schoeneberger A, Lown B. Precipitation of congestive heart failure by oral disopyramide. *N Engl J Med.* 1980;302:614–617.

64. Poll DS, Marchlinski FE, Buxton AE, et al. Sustained ventricular tachycardia in patients with idiopathic dilated cardiomyopathy: electrophysiologic testing and lack of response to antiarrhythmic drug therapy. *Circulation.* 1984;70:451–456.

65. Liem LB, Swerdlow CD. Value of electrophysiologic testing in idiopathic dilated cardiomyopathy and sustained ventricular tachyarrhythmias. *Am J Cardiol.* 1988;62:611–616.

66. Fuster V, Gersh BJ, Guiliani ER, et al. The natural history of idiopathic dilated cardiomyopathy. *Am J Cardiol.* 1981;47:525–531.

67. Meltzer RS, Visser CA, Fuster V. Intracardiac thrombi and systemic embolization. *Ann Intern Med.* 1986; 104:689–690.

68. Colucci WS, Packer M, Bristow MR, Gilbert EM, Cohn JN, Fowler MB et al. Carvedilol inhibits clinical progression in patients with mild symptoms of heart failure. *Circulation.* 1996; 94: 2800–2806.

69. Packer M, Colucci WS, Sackner-Bernstein JD, Liang C, Goldscher DA, Freeman I. Double-blind, placebo-controlled study of the effects of carvedilol in patients with moderate-to-severe heart failure: The PRECISE Trial. *Circulation.* 1996; 94: 2793–2799.

70. Cohn JN, Fowler MB, Bristow MR, Colucci WS, Gilbert EM. Kinal V. Safety and efficacy of carvedilol in severe heart failure. *Journal of Cardiac Failure.* In Press.

71. Bristow MR, Gilbert EM, Abraham WT, Adams KF, Fowler MB, Hershberger RE. Carvedilol produces dose-related improvements in left ventricular function and survival in subjects with chronic heart failure. *Circulation.* 1996; 94: 2807–2816.

72. Packer M, Bristow MR, Cohn JN, Colucci WS, Fowler MB, Gilbert EM. The effect of carvedilol on morbidity and mortality in patients with chronic heart failure. *N Engl J Med.* 1996;334:1349–55.

35
Arrhythmia in Patients with a Cardiomyopathy and Congestive Heart Failure

Philip J. Podrid, Richard I. Fogel, and Therese Tordjman-Fuchs

Many advances in the treatment of congestive heart failure (CHF) have resulted in improved survival, and a growing number of such patients are being seen by physicians. Although several interventions have reduced the number of patients dying from progressive CHF, sudden cardiac death remains a frequent and important problem in this patient population. It is now well established that ventricular premature beats (VPBs) and complex ventricular arrhythmia, particularly nonsustained ventricular tachycardia (VT), are commonly observed in these patients. It has been proposed that spontaneous ventricular arrhythmia, which results from underlying electrical instability of the myocardium, is a marker of an abnormal substrate capable of generating and sustaining arrhythmia. Additionally, spontaneous arrhythmia may serve as a trigger activating the mechanisms responsible for a sustained ventricular tachyarrhythmia.

This chapter reviews the mechanisms responsible for arrhythmogenesis and the factors that may affect arrhythmia occurrence, especially in patients with CHF. The prevalence of arrhythmia and its role in identifying the patient at risk are discussed fully and the role of other techniques for risk assessment, especially electrophysiologic testing and the signal-averaged electrocardiogram (ECG), are addressed. The benefits and hazards of antiarrhythmic drugs, the role of surgery including transplantation, and the use of the automatic implantable defibrillator conclude this chapter.

Mechanisms for Arrhythmia

Three mechanisms have been proposed to explain the genesis of cardiac arrhythmia: reentry, enhanced automaticity, and triggered automaticity (Fig. 35.1). It is believed that reentry is the predominant mechanism for most clinical ventricular arrhythmias.[1] Evidence to support this claim is derived from (a) the ease of termi-

nation of the arrhythmia by cardioversion in most patients, (b) the ability to entrain the arrhythmia by underdrive and overdrive pacing, (c) the induction of the arrhythmia by electrophysiologic techniques using programmed premature stimulation,[2] (d) direct mapping in isolated and in vitro preparations.[3,4] For reentry to occur, certain preconditions must be met (Fig. 35.2). An appropriate substrate must be present consisting of two limbs or pathways that are anatomically linked, being joined proximally and distally forming a circuit. Each limb must have disparate electrophysiologic characteristics; that is, different conduction velocities and refractory periods. These electrophysiologic properties must be such that a premature impulse, arriving at the proximal portion of the reentrant circuit, finds one limb (B) refractory whereas the other limb (A) is capable of being excited or depolarized. In this way, the premature impulse travels antegradely down the excitable pathway (limb A) while being blocked in the refractory limb B. If the timing is appropriate, upon arriving at the distal junction of the two limbs, the wave of depolarization finds limb B repolarized, excitable, and able to conduct in a retrograde direction. If the time for retrograde conduction in limb B is greater than the time necessary for repolarization of limb A, the impulse reaches the proximal part of the circuit at a time that limb A is capable of being depolarized again. The impulse reenters this pathway, and if this process continues, a reentrant arrhythmia is generated.

Several structural factors present in the ventricular myocardium of the patient with myocardial disease, including those with a cardiomyopathy and CHF, may predispose toward the development of reentrant circuits. Myopathic processes, inflammation, and ischemia as well as the subsequent healing, fibrosis, and remodeling are not uniform. Friedman and colleagues[5] demonstrated the survival of subendocardial Purkinje fibers in areas of extensive infarction in dogs. Since the Purkinje fibers in these areas of nonhomogeneous damage are

MECHANISMS OF ARRHYTHMOGENESIS

FIGURE 35.1. Mechanisms of arrhythmogenesis.

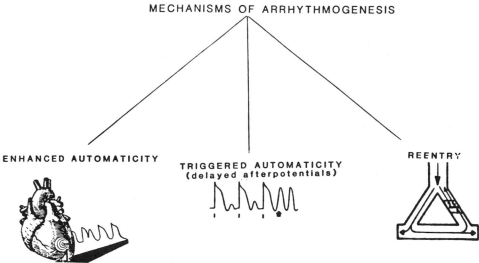

ENHANCED AUTOMATICITY

TRIGGERED AUTOMATICITY
(delayed afterpotentials)

REENTRY

A

NORMAL

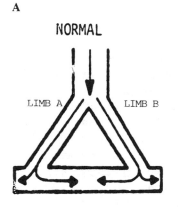

LIMB A   LIMB B

B

UNIDIRECTIONAL BLOCK
REENTRY

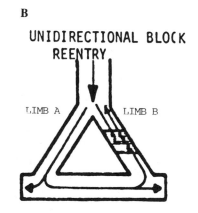

LIMB A   LIMB B

FIGURE 35.2. Mechanism for reentry. In the normal myocardium (Panel **A**) conduction via limbs A and B is uniform. However, in the presence of myocardial disease (Panel **B**) affecting one limb (B) there is block of antegrade impulse conduction (unidirectional block) within this limb. Conduction via limb A is normal. If the impulse is appropriately timed, it will be conducted retrogradely via limb B, and there is the potential for reentry with conduction again down limb A.

viable, their electrophysiologic properties, affected by the underlying disease process, also are not uniform. El-Sherif et al.[6] reported that there is nonuniformity between normal and infarcted tissue, and even within infarcted ventricular myocardium there is electrical inhomogeneity. These authors demonstrated multiple reentrant pathways, functionally dissociated regions, and areas of localized ventricular fibrillation (VF) within the same infarction zone. In a subsequent work[3] these authors demonstrated that the transition from a stable reentrant activation sequence to a more chaotic pattern (VF) was related to the nonhomogeneous shortening of refractoriness in different parts of the infarcted myocardium. Therefore, disease of the myocardium and the resulting inhomogeneity establishes the juxtaposition of tissues with different electrophysiologic properties, creating an arrhythmogenic substrate.

Abnormal automaticity is the second most common etiology for ventricular arrhythmia. In normal atrial and ventricular myocardium, the action potential is generated by the rapid influx of sodium ions.[7] In the sinoatrial and atrioventricular nodes the action potential results from slow inward calcium currents.[8] Under nor-

mal circumstances only pacemaker tissue is capable of generating a spontaneous action potential. After the membrane of the pacemaker tissue has completely repolarized, there is a slow drift of the membrane potential to the threshold level (phase 4) as a result of a leak of sodium and calcium ions into the pacemaker cells. Once the threshold potential is reached in pacemaker tissue, the calcium channels open widely, initiating a slow action potential. Normally, phase 4 spontaneous depolarization occurs more rapidly in pacemaker tissue compared to atrial or ventricular myocardium, in which phase 4 is almost flat. This is because in normal myocardial tissue an active ATPase Na-K pump maintains the balance between intracellular and extracellular ions during phase 4. Normally, the automaticity of myocardial tissue is not apparent, being suppressed by the normal pacemaker tissue. However, under certain pathological situations, non–pacemaker tissue can exhibit enhanced automaticity, and if this automaticity is greater than that of pacemaker tissue, it becomes the dominant focus of impulse generation. Digitalis toxicity is the prototype of this pathology as it poisons and inactivates the ATPase Na-K pump. Ischemia also inactivates the

ATPase pump which is energy dependent and requires oxygen. The increase in circulating catecholamines and activation of the sympathetic nervous system, which occurs in patients with CHF, is another cause of enhanced automaticity.

Triggered automaticity is a third mechanism of arrhythmogenesis. Two forms have been identified. Recordings from intracellular electrodes have demonstrated delayed (late) afterdepolarizations, which are low-amplitude oscillations occurring after the action potential has returned to the resting state.[9] These oscillations are reported to be due to calcium fluxes, and because of a low amplitude, they usually are not manifest and are clinically insignificant. However, under pathological conditions the amplitude of these oscillations increases and may reach threshold, triggering a spontaneous action potential. If this process continues, a sustained tachyarrhythmia will develop. The amplitude of these calcium-mediated oscillations is increased by certain factors such as digoxin and catecholamines. A second form of triggered automaticity, known as early afterdepolarizations, also has been described.[10] Similar to late afterdepolarizations, oscillations during the action potential, occurring during a prolonged phase 2 plateau (i.e., prolongation of repolarization), have been observed. Presumably, these oscillations lead to a nonuniform prolongation of the refractory period and dispersion of impulse conduction through the myocardium. Clinically, early afterdepolarizations are felt to be the etiology of the arrhythmia known as torsade de pointes.

Other factors, often present or activated in the patient with cardiomyopathy and CHF, may interact with these three mechanisms to enhance arrhythmogenesis (Table 35.1). These factors include ischemia, hemodynamic alterations such as left ventricular dilatation and increased intracardiac pressures, electrolyte disturbances, untoward effects of drugs used for the treatment of CHF, and activation of neurohormonal mechanisms, especially the sympathetic nervous system and an increase of circulating catecholamines.

Ischemia, mediated through tissue hypoxia, results in anaerobic metabolites, pH changes, and electrolyte shifts, all of which can significantly alter the electrophysiologic properties of the myocardium.[11] An early notable effect of ischemia on the electrophysiologic properties of the ventricular myocardium is an abbreviation of the phase 2 plateau of the action potential or early repolarization. As a result, there is a shortening of the refractory period.[12] Since ischemia is not uniform, areas of the myocardium will have different refractory periods, resulting in an increase in the temporal dispersion of repolarization. Additionally, there is evidence that ischemic and partially infarcted tissue can exhibit spontaneous automaticity.[13–15]

In a recent report, Dean and Lab[16] summarized

TABLE 35.1. Factors predisposing to arrhythmia in patients with CHF.

Underlying structural disease—abnormal substrate
Electrolyte abnormalities
Potassium
Magnesium
Hemodynamic abnormalities
LV dysfunction and contraction abnormalities
Stretch on myocardium—increased ventricular volume
Increased ventricular pressure
Ischemia
Neurohormonal changes
Digoxin
Sympathetic nervous system
Therapeutic interventions
Digoxin
Diuretics
Beta agonists
Phosphodiesterase inhibitors
Vasodilators
ACE inhibitors

LV = left ventricular; ACE = angiotensin-converting enzyme; CHF = congestive heart failure.

animal and human evidence for what they term "mechanoelectrical feedback". These authors describe mechanical changes of the ventricular myocardium, namely increased wall stress, dilatation, and increased afterload, present in congestive failure, which can alter the electrophysiologic properties of myocardial tissue. Evidence suggests that increased myocardial stretch can lead to shortening of the action potential duration (phases 2 and 3) and the refractory period as well as an increase in membrane spontaneous automaticity. Since the loading conditions in the normal and failing ventricle are not uniform, this mechanism also can create a disparity in the electrical properties of adjacent tissue, predisposing to reentry.

Electrolyte abnormalities, specifically hypokalemia and hypomagnesemia, usually induced by diuretics, have a major role in the etiology of VPBs, VT, and VF in patients with heart disease and CHF.[17] Hypokalemia has several effects on the normal electrophysiologic properties of the myocardium (Table 35.2). Most notably, hypokalemia hyperpolarizes the resting membrane potential, making it more negative. Since the resting potential is further away from the threshold, there is an increase in conduction velocity.[18] Additionally, hypokalemia enhances the rate of spontaneous phase 4 depolarization and causes an increase in membrane automaticity. These effects augment both the excitability and automaticity of myocardial cells and likely have a role in the occurrence of ventricular arrhythmia. Since the therapeutic effects of antiarrhythmic drugs include a reduction in membrane excitability and automaticity, the changes due to hypokalemia may negate the actions of these agents.[19] Animal work has clearly shown a re-

TABLE 35.2. Effects of potassium changes on ventricular myocardial electrophysiologic properties.

Parameter	Effect[a]	
	Low K$^+$	High K$^+$
Resting membrane potential	More negative	Less negative
Velocity of phase 0	Increased	Decreased
Impulse conduction velocity	Increased	Decreased
Action potential amplitude	No change	No change
Action potential duration	Increased	Decreased
Phase 2 duration	Increased	Decreased
Phase 3 duration	Increased	Decreased
Effective refractory period	Increased	Decreased
Phase 4 automaticity	Increased	Decreased

[a]Effects more pronounced in Purkinje fibers compared to ventricular muscle.

TABLE 35.3. Effects of catecholamines on cardiac electrophysiologic properties.

	Conductivity	Refractory period	Automaticity
Sinus node	—	—	Increased
Atrial myocardium	Increased	Shortened	Increased
Atrioventricular node	Increased	Shortened	Increased
His Purkinje system	Increased	Shortened	Increased
Ventricular myocardium	Increased	Shortened	Increased
Accessory pathway	Increased	Shortened	—

duction in the VF threshold with the development of hypokalemia, and its restoration with the repletion of potassium.[20] This experimental work has been supported by a number of human studies involving patients with an acute infarction in which there has been an association between the occurrence of a ventricular tachyarrhythmia and hypokalemia.[21] Although its relationship to arrhythmia is less clear, magnesium repletion in the setting of an acute myocardial infarction has recently been shown to significantly reduce the incidence of tachyarrhythmia and death when compared to placebo.[22]

It is well established that the sympathetic nervous system is activated in patients with CHF. Circulating levels of norephinepherine as well as increased sympathetic neural activity as measured in the peroneal nerve have been demonstrated.[23,24] The sympathetic nervous system and catecholamines can interact with an abnormal myocardium and may enhance arrhythmogenesis by all three proposed mechanisms of arrhythmia formation; that is reentry, afterpotentials, and enhanced automaticity[25,26] (Table 35.3). In an experimental animal model of myocardial infarction, epinephrine increased the automaticity of surviving Purkinje fibers located within the infarction zone or in the periinfarctiion region to a greater extent than in those fibers within the noninfarcted zone.[27] Moreover, Abildskov[28] demonstrated that the distribution of sympathetic nerves within the ventricle is nonhomogeneous and sympathetic stimulation results in nonuniform effects on conduction and refractory period, fostering reentry. Bhagat and co-workers[29] further supported this observation by reporting that in the presence of ischemia, sympathetic stimulation produced a dispersion of refractory periods in adjacent normal and ischemic tissue, creating the potential substrate for reentry.

An additional factor that can enhance inhomogeneity and the amount of dispersion is hypersensitivity to the effect of catecholamine stimulation due to myocardial denervation. It has been reported that in patients with a dilated cardiomyopathy, the underlying disease process results in the disruption of sympathetic neural innervation and the involved parts of the myocardium become denervated. This has been documented by scanning techniques utilizing the labeled tracer I-123 meta-iodobenzylguanidine, which is specifically taken up by the sympathetic nervous system. In patients with a cardiomyopathy, myocardial uptake of the tracer is heterogeneous and reduced when compared to normals. Inoue and Zipes[30] have reported that infarcted myocardial tissue, denervated as a result of disruption of the sympathetic nervous system, demonstrates denervation hypersensitivity to circulating catecholamines and the refractory period of the denervated tissue shortens to a greater degree than that of normal myocardium. During conditions in which circulating catecholamines are elevated, such as CHF and in patients with a cardiomyopathy, there is a substantial amount of heterogeneity of electrophysiologic properties within the myocardium, an important precondition for reentrant arrhythmias.

Delayed afterdepolarizations have been elicited in an in vitro model when isolated Purkinje fibers are perfused with catecholamines. Priori and co-workers,[31] using an in vivo model, reported that stimulation of the left stellate ganglion resulted in the development of delayed afterdepolarizations, which always preceded arrhythmias provoked by this technique.

Finally, the sympathetic nervous system can influence other arrhythmogenic factors such as electrolyte shifts, myocardial mechanoelectrical effects, and ischemia. As a result of β_2 receptor stimulation, catecholamines may enhance potassium entry into cells, resulting in serum hypokalemia.[32] Sympathetic stimulation can increase myocardial contractility and afterload, enhancing the mechanoelectrical feedback mechanism of the myocardium. Last, activation of the sympathetic nervous system may trigger ischemia, which causes important electrophysiologic changes and can augment all three mechanisms of arrhythmogenesis.

In conclusion, there are a number of factors that are responsible for the occurrence of ventricular arrhythmia in patients with CHF, irrespective of its etiology. There is an underlying structural abnormality resulting from an ischemic or nonischemic process. This is acted on by changes in catecholamines and sympathetic neural inputs, shifts in electrolytes, ischemia, activation of neurohormonal systems, and hemodynamic factors.

Hemodynamic Effects of Cardiac Arrhythmias in CHF

It is well established that both atrial and ventricular arrhythmias are more common in patients with CHF. In addition to the underlying CHF, these arrhythmias may produce significant hemodynamic alterations (Table 35.4) These effects may be broadly divided into several categories: those due to changes in heart rate, those due to an abnormal relationship or asynchrony between atrial and ventricular contraction, those due to irregularities in the cardiac cycle, and those due to an abnormal sequence of ventricular activation.[33]

An increased heart rate due to sympathetic stimulation can cause up to a 300% increase in cardiac output. This is due to the elevated rate as well as to an increase in stroke volume resulting from a sympathetically mediated augmentation of ventricular inotropy and ejection fraction. With a non–catecholamine-mediated tachyarrhythmia, including sustained VT or a supraventricular tachyarrhythmia such as atrial fibrillation, changes in heart rate produce variable effects on cardiac output since the inotropy is not affected and stroke volume actually may not be maintained during the increased heart rate due to a decrease in diastolic filling time. In

TABLE 35.4. Factors resulting in hemodynamic changes due to tachyarrhythmia.

Increased heart rate
  Decreased time for diastolic filling
  Reduced stroke volume
  Reduced systolic ejection period
  Increased LV volume
  Development of mitral regurgitation
  Increase expenditure of high energy stores LV dysfunction
Atrioventricular asynchrony due to loss of atrial contraction or atrial-
    ventricular dissociation
  Loss of atrial contribution to LV filling
  Reduced stroke volume and cardiac output
Irregularity of R-R intervals or cycle length
  Reduced end-diastolic volume
  Elevated LV end-diastolic pressure
Loss of normal sequence of ventricular activation
  Contraction pattern disrupted
  Reduced systolic pressure
  Reduced LV ejection fraction
  Reduced stroke volume and cardiac output
  Increased LV volume
  Development of mitral regurgitation

LV = left ventricular.

studies using atrial pacing, stroke volume and systolic ejection period decreased above a certain heart rate.[34,35] There is therefore a relatively constant cardiac index over a physiologic range of paced heart rates.[36,37] With atrial pacing to rates greater than 140 beats per min (bpm), there may actually be a fall in cardiac output due to an abbreviation of the diastolic filling time, a decrease in left ventricular end-diastolic volume, and a further decrease in stroke volume.

From these studies, it is clear that many factors influence the relationship between heart rate and cardiac output, particularly important in patients with CHF. To increase cardiac output at faster rates, there must also be an increase in inotropic stroke volume or left ventricular ejection fraction (LVEF) to offset the decrease in diastolic filling of the left ventricle. The sympathetically mediated sinus tachycardia, often seen in patients with a low LVEF may, in part, be a compensatory mechanism to preserve cardiac output. However, other tachyarrhythmias not mediated by catecholamines may cause hemodynamic compromise by producing a reduction in stroke volume that accompanies the increase in heart rate.

It has been reported by Morady and co-workers[38] that the rate of VT is a major factor in determining the clinical symptoms resulting from the arrhythmia. Among a group of 113 patients with VT, the average VT rate was 163 bpm in asymptomatic patients, 170 bpm in patients who had lightheadedness, 191 bpm when the patient had experienced presyncope, and in patients presenting with syncope the VT rate was 224 bpm ($p < .05$ and $p < .001$). Additionally, compared to those without CHF, patients with CHF were more likely to present with syncope regardless of the VT rate (7% vs. 24%, $p < .05$) and were less likely to be asymptomatic (55% vs. 11%, $p = < .001$).

Not only does a tachyarrhythmia of any etiology further impair LV function and cardiac output when already depressed, but the tachyarrhythmia itself may result in CHF. An incessant or even intermittent tachyarrhythmia present for months to years has been reported to produce a cardiomyopathy in both the pediatric and adult populations.[39,40] Once the tachycardia is controlled, the symptoms of CHF are reversed and LVEF returns to normal. It has been observed clinically that long-standing atrial fibrillation (AF) and a poorly controlled ventricular rate will produce a cardiomyopathy and CHF. A slowing of the ventricular rate results in improvement. It has been postulated that the cause of a tachycardia-mediated cardiomyopathy is reversible depletion of high energy phosphates as a result of the persistently rapid heart rate.[41] There is a reduction in LV contractility, LVEF, and an increase in LV volume.

The function of the atrium is to facilitate transport of blood from the atrium to the ventricle. The loss of atrioventricular synchrony, often seen with ventricular tachycardia, or the loss of atrial contraction, as occurs in AF, also can affect hemodynamics and cardiac output, especially in those patients with CHF. When the timing between atrial systole and ventricular contraction is altered, there are changes in atrial and ventricular volumes that affect the myocardial contractile state. Thus, loss of ventricular filling by atrial contraction may have important implications on ventricular function and cardiac output; the impact depends on the severity of the underlying heart disease. The "atrial kick" has been felt to be responsible for as much as 40% of the cardiac output.[42,43] Unfortunately, much of the data are derived from early studies of patients with rheumatic heart disease and mitral valve involvement in which quinidine was used to convert AF to normal sinus rhythm and their validity are questionable due to the known myocardial effects of quinidine as well as the postulated effects of quinidine on the peripheral circulation. However, Morris et al.[44] studied 11 patients after cardioversion from AF. Cardiac output rose 20% with cardioversion to normal sinus rhythm, although ventricular rate and metabolic demands pre- and postcardioversion, as assessed by oxygen consumption, remained constant. Rodman and co-workers[45] invasively obtained hemodynamic measurements and evaluated 19 patients for 3 hr after cardioversion from AF to normal sinus rhythm. Heart rate was essentially unchanged over the 3 hr. Cardiac index increased progressively over the 3-hr period postcardioversion to an ultimate value which was 12% higher than precardioversion values. Thus, in normal individuals, restoration of atrial contraction and its contribution to ventricular filling was felt to significantly improve LV hemodynamics and cardiac output.

Several authors have suggested that the atrial contribution may play an even more important role in the presence of ventricular dysfunction and CHF, especially when the ventricle is distended and noncompliant and the end-diastolic pressure is elevated.[33,46,47] However, this view has been questioned on theoretical grounds. Because the failing heart generally operates on the flatter portion of the Frank-Starling curve, it has been postulated that the increase in LV filling due to atrial contraction would only minimally increase stroke volume. Greenberg and colleagues[48] assessed the atrial contribution to cardiac output in patients with and without CHF by comparing stroke volume during atrial and ventricular pacing at a constant heart rate. After assessing the atrial contribution at baseline, LV end-diastolic pressure was varied either by volume loading or by sublingual isordil. An inverse relationship between LV filling pressure, as assessed by pulmonary capillary wedge pressure (PCWP), and atrial contribution was seen in the baseline state ($r = 0.53$), as well as when the PCWP was modified ($r = 0.53$). Atrial contribution was substantially greater when the PCWP was less than 20 mm Hg, compared to when the PCWP was greater than 20 mm Hg. Atrial contribution also was greater in patients without a history of CHF compared to those with a history of CHF. The authors concluded that atrial contribution is less important for augmenting cardiac output when the filling pressure is already elevated due to impaired LV function. Another factor is that in those with CHF, the atria often are distended, scarred, and akinetic so that atrial contraction is ineffective and contributes little, if anything, to ventricular filling and cardiac output. However, the rapid rate during AF or loss of atrial ventricular synchrony seen with VT or SVT may be important since this will impact not only on filling due to atrial contraction, but will result in a variable reduction of rapid diastolic filling of the LV.

Another area in which an arrhythmia may affect hemodynamics is irregularity in the cycle length of the arrhythmia. The phenomenon may be observed in AF or when frequent premature beats are present. A premature beat, if conducted, has a shorter diastolic filling period, and as the Frank-Starling relationship predicts, the stroke volume and consequently the peak systolic pressure of the early beat will be diminished. This theoretical effect was confirmed by Braunwald and co-workers,[49] who studied 26 patients with AF undergoing surgery for mitral stenosis. At the time of surgery, LV end-diastolic pressure and systemic arterial pressure were recorded. These authors reported a strong correlation between end-diastolic fiber length, LV end-diastolic pressure, and peak arterial systolic pressure, confirming the Frank-Starling mechanism in humans. When there are frequent VPBs or runs of nonsustained VT, LV function and cardiac output may be substantially reduced.

Last, VT, which originates in the ventricle, activates the myocardium directly, bypassing the His-Purkinje system. This may alter the usual sequence of LV activation and its contraction pattern. The reentrant circuit, which represents the origin of the VT, activates the surrounding myocardium first. Depending on the site of origin of the VT, myocardial activation is abnormal, the usual contraction pattern is disrupted, the LVEF is decreased, and stroke volume and cardiac output may fall. Rosenquist and colleagues,[50] using echocardiography and radionuclide ventriculography, assessed cardiac output and LVEF during atrial demand pacing (AAI) and AV sequential pacing (DDD) at the same rate. These authors found that cardiac output was 11% higher during AAI than during DDD pacing. Similarly, LVEF was 12% greater with AAI pacing compared to DDD pacing. Thus, when the sequence of normal ventricular activation is preserved, hemodynamic function is greater and a normal ventricular activation pattern is a prerequisite for optimal LV function.

In summary, arrhythmias may have significant hemodynamic effects, especially important in patients with CHF. The increase in heart rate may paradoxically decrease cardiac output over a physiologic range of heart rate responses. The loss of the atrial contraction or "kick" with the development of AF, or the absence of atrial ventricular synchrony as in VT, may produce a fall in cardiac index. Frequent premature beats, depending on their timing, may cause significant hemodynamic compromise, particularly if they occur early in diastole or if many runs of nonsustained VT are present. Finally, the loss of the normal ventricular activation sequence and contraction pattern also can contribute to a decrease in cardiac output.

From the preceding analysis, it is clear that many factors contribute to the hemodynamic effects of an arrhythmia and that the clinical manifestations are not related to the etiology of the tachyarrhythmia. Hemodynamic stability during a wide complex tachycardia is commonly, although mistakenly, taken as evidence for a supraventricular mechanism.[51] Because VT produces a wide variety of hemodynamic outcomes, several groups have postulated that variations in adrenergic tone may play a significant role in determining the hemodynamic consequences of VT. Feldman and co-workers,[52] using a dog model, studied the hemodynamic effects of rapid ventricular pacing at baseline, with alpha-blockade, and after beta-blockade. During control conditions, there was an initial marked decline in LV systolic pressure with the onset of simulated VT, but recovery within 20 s. After alpha-blockade, there was persistent hypotension due to failure of vasoconstriction, but LV inotropy was preserved. After beta-blockade, there also was persistent hypotension due to reduction in LV inotropy. The authors concluded that hemodynamic recovery from VT resulted from alpha receptor-mediated vasoconstriction as well as beta receptor-mediated augmentation of contraction.

In a similar human study, 15 patients undergoing programmed electrophysiologic stimulation had forearm blood flow and vascular resistance studied before and after regional intraarterial alpha-blockade with phentolamine.[53] After induction of VT at baseline, mean forearm vascular resistance rose from 32 to 40 units. However, after pretreatment with phentolamine and reinduction of VT, the increase in forearm vascular resistance was 66% less than observed during the baseline induction. The authors concluded that the onset of VT is accompanied by alpha-adrenergic–mediated vasoconstriction and speculated that this effect was modulated by arterial baroreceptors.

These observations have particular relevance to patients with CHF who often have impaired baroreflexes. This impairment may be due to a process intrinsic to CHF[54] or may be secondary to medications including beta-blocking agents or antiarrhythmic agents with alpha-antagonist activity (i.e., quinidine). When VT occurs in these patients, hemodynamic recovery may be blunted, and, therefore, these patients may be more prone to hemodynamic instability and, perhaps, sudden death.

Atrial Arrhythmias and Congestive Heart Failure

Atrial arrhythmias are common in patients with CHF and the most frequent sustained arrhythmia in these patients is AF. In the Framingham Heart Study,[55] CHF was one of the most powerful predictors of AF increasing the risk by 8.5-fold in men and by 14-fold in women. There are many factors responsible for AF in patients with CHF, including an increase in LV end-diastolic pressure and, subsequently, an increase in left atrial pressure. With long-standing CHF, the left atrium becomes dilated, hypertrophied, and damaged by the elevated pressure. As it heals and scars it becomes hypokinetic or even akinetic. LV dilatation may result in mitral regurgitation, an additional factor resulting in left atrial dysfunction and abnormalities of the atrial myocardium. Last, activation of the sympathetic nervous system is important in the genesis of arrhythmia, especially when the substrate is abnormal.[56]

Based on the previously discussed hemodynamic effects of arrhythmia, the onset of AF in patients with CHF may result in a worsening of CHF, pulmonary edema, hypotension, or even cardiogenic shock and death from hypotension. It may cause a serious ventricular tachyarrhythmia or a bradyarrhythmia. It is not certain if AF is an independent predictor of mortality in patients with CHF, but it probably reflects poorer LV function and more significant CHF, which are important predictors of a poorer outcome.

Since AF in these patients usually is symptomatic, it often requires antiarrhythmic therapy for prevention[57,58] (Table 35.5). Drugs that are effective include the 1A agents, quinidine and procainamide. Disopyramide, a potent negatively inotropic drug, is contraindicated in patients with CHF. The 1C agents, propafenone and flecainide, are effective for maintaining sinus rhythm in some patients,[59] but their use may be limited in those with a cardiomyopathy and CHF because of a great risk of serious cardiac side effects, including conduction abnormalities, worsening of CHF, or arrhythmia aggravation. This is discussed in another section. Amiodarone may be of benefit in these patients and often a low dose, associated with less frequent side effects, is effective for maintaining sinus rhythm.[60] Not infrequently, sustained AF will not revert with these agents and electric cardioversion is required. However, the continued use of the antiarrhythmic drug usually is necessary to prevent a recurrence.

TABLE 35.5. Management of atrial fibrillation.

Paroxysmal	Chronic
Acute rate control	Rate control
Digoxin	Digoxin
Beta-blocker	Beta-blocker
Calcium channel blocker	Calcium channel blocker
Reversion	Anticoagulation
Pharmacologic	
Electric cardioversion	
Prevention—antiarrhythmic drugs	
Class 1A: quinidine, disopyramide, procainamide	
Class 1C: flecainide, propafenone	
Class 3: amiodarone, sotaloe	
Anticoagulation	

TABLE 35.6. Total cardiac mortality and sudden death mortality in CHF.

Study	N	Follow-up (mos)	% mortality	% death that was sudden
Francis	159	20	46	63
Huang	35	34	11	50
Sukuri	190	NA	46	22
Wilson	77	12	100	25
Meinertz	74	11	26	63
Maskin	35	NA	71	4
Von Olshausen	60	12	12	43
Holmes	43	14	33	86
Chakko	43	16	37	62
Franciosa	182	12	48	45
Massie	56	13	52	34
Lee	178	36	76	37
Burggraf	28	60	61	53
Cohn	106	1–62	57	47
Gradman	295	16	16	51
Keogh	232	10	33	47
Overall	1793		52	42

CHF = congestive heart failure.

If AF recurs despite antiarrhythmic therapy or if the antiarrhythmic drugs are poorly tolerated, maintaining AF as the rhythm of choice is an alternative. In such patients, controlling the ventricular rate not only at rest, but also during exercise, is of extreme importance[61] (Fig. 35.3). In most patients, ventricular filling and cardiac output are increased and symptoms of CHF better controlled or eliminated when the ventricular rate is slowed. Useful drugs are those that affect atrioventricular nodal properties, including digoxin, verapamil, diltiazem and beta blockers. Although the calcium channel blockers and beta-blockers are negatively inotropic, they may be tolerated in these patients when low doses are used. Importantly, by slowing the ventricular rate, they improve hemodynamics and increase cardiac output.

Another concern is the risk of systemic emboli.[62] During AF, there is an increased risk of thrombus formation in the atria and the atrial appendages; the risk may be even greater in patients with CHF because of the inability of the left atrium to empty during diastole. This is further exacerbated by mitral regurgitation, which results in a great deal of stasis of blood in the atrium and an enhanced risk of clot formation. Anticoagulation is recommended in these patients unless there is a contraindication. The use of warfarin has been reported to reduce significantly the risk of systemic emboli.[63,64]

Total Cardiac and Sudden Death Mortality in Congestive Heart Failure

Patients with cardiomyopathy and CHF have a high total mortality, averaging approximately 50% at 2 yr[65–80] (Table 35.6). Although it has been assumed that the mechanism of death in these patients is progressive CHF, it has now been well established that in a

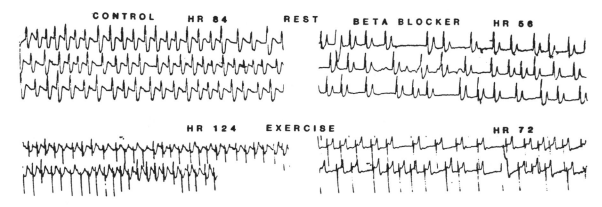

FIGURE 35.3. Rate control of atrial fibrillation (AF). Before therapy, the heart rate during AF is 84, but rapidly accelerates to 124 within 2 min of exercise on a bicycle. After therapy with beta-blocker, heart rate at rest and with exercise is better controlled.

TABLE 35.7. Relationship between ventricular arrhythmia, LV function, and sudden death in patients after a myocardial infarction.

Study	N	Percent sudden death			
		No complex VPBs		Complex VPBs	
		LV intact	LV dysfunction	LV intact	LV dysfunction
Bigger	691	6	22	12	35
Mukharji	533	2	7	7	25
Ruberman	1739	3	7	12	22
Schultz	50	0	0	0	28
Andresen	378	2	4	4	17

LV = left ventricular; VPB = ventricular premature beat.

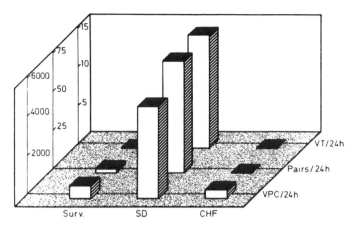

FIGURE 35.4. Relationship between ventricular arrhythmia and outcome among 74 patients with idiopathic cardiomyopathy. Arrhythmia frequency is greater in patients who have sudden death (*SD*) compared to those who survive (*Surv*) or who die from congestive heart failure (*CHF*). Importantly, runs of nonsustained ventricular tachycardia (*VT*) are observed only in those patients who have SD. Reprinted, with permission, from reference 67.

substantial number of these patients, the mechanism is primary sudden cardiac death due to a sustained ventricular tachyarrhythmia. This is defined by WHO as death within 1 hr of symptoms in contrast to sudden death that may result from progressive CHF. This poor prognosis is independent of the nature of the underlying heart disease, i.e., ischemic or nonischemic.[66,67] The etiology of the CHF does not appear to be a factor associated with prognosis in these trials; however, Likoff and co-workers[81] did report an association between the etiology of the cardiomyopathy and survival. At 30 weeks, survival was approximately 36% in patients with an ischemic cardiomyopathy compared with an approximately 60% survival in those with a nonischemic etiology.

A high first-year mortality also has been reported in patients with a recent myocardial infarction who have a reduced LVEF or CHF, and this is independent of ventricular arrhythmia[82-85] (Table 35.7). There are differences, however, in the definition of LV dysfunction. In the study of Ruberman and co-workers,[82] it is clinical CHF; Murkharji and co-workers[83] and Schultz and co-workers[84] define this as a LVEF <40%; Bigger and co-workers[85] defined LV dysfunction as <30%. These last authors also reported that when LVEF is >40%, the 2-yr mortality is approximately 5%, whereas it was 11% when the LVEF was 30% to 39%, 27% when the LVEF was 20% to 29%, and 50% in the group of patients with a LVEF <20%. As with the previous studies, the presence of LV dysfunction was an independent risk factor for sudden cardiac death, especially when runs of nonsustained VT were also documented on ambulatory monitoring (Table 35.7, Fig. 35.4). Thus, in each of the postinfarction studies, the highest mortality from sudden cardiac death is in that group of patients who have both complex ventricular arrhythmia, primarily runs of nonsustained VT, and LV dysfunction or clinical CHF.

Most data about mortality and sudden cardiac death rate are from studies in patients with an ischemic or nonischemic dilated cardiomyopathy and CHF; how-

ever, there are some data in those with other forms of cardiomyopathy, specifically hypertrophic cardiomyopathy, who also have a substantial risk of sudden cardiac death. In a report by Maron and co-workers,[86] 84 patients with a hypertrophic cardiomyopathy treated medically were followed for two yr. During this follow-up period there were seven deaths (8.3%), six of which were sudden. McKenna and co-workers[87] reported a similar incidence of sudden death (8%) among 86 patients with a hypertrophic cardiomyopathy followed for 2.6 yr.

It can be concluded that there is a high yearly mortality in patients with a cardiomyopathy and CHF, regardless of the etiology, and more than 40% of these deaths are sudden. While a bradyarrhythmia has occasionally been documented as the mechanism for sudden death, in the vast majority of patients with class II or III CHF the etiology is a sustained ventricular tachyarrhythmia (i.e., VT or VF). The risk of sudden cardiac death is particularly high in patients with an acute myocardial infarction, especially when LV dysfunction and CHF are present.

Prevalence of Ventricular Arrhythmia in Patients with Cardiomyopathy

Although VPBs are commonly observed in normal individuals as well as those with structural heart disease, they are particularly frequent in patients with a cardiomyopathy and CHF. Many of the earlier studies utilized ambulatory monitoring to document the presence,

TABLE 35.8. Prevalence of ventricular arrhythmia in patients with CHF.

Study	N	% with VPBs or couplets	% with NSVT
Huang	35	93	60
Wilson	77	71	50
Meinertz	74	87	49
Maskin	35	92	71
Von Olshausen	60	95	80
Holmes	31	87	39
Chakko	43	88	51
Frances	346	81	28
Unverferth	69	NA	41
Costanzo-Nordin	55	76	40
Neri	65	95	80
Gradman	295	36	59
Keogh	137	39	41
Overall	1322	78	45

CHF = congestive heart failure; VPB = ventricular premature beat; NSVT = nonsustained ventricular tachycardia.

frequency, and type of ventricular arrhythmia, but in most of these trials only small numbers of patients were evaluated[67–75] (Table 35.8). As reported by Holmes and co-workers,[73] the type and frequency of VPBs were not related to the nature of the underlying heart disease as there was no difference in the frequency or complexity of ventricular arrhythmia between those with an ischemic or nonischemic etiology for the cardiomyopathy. Meinertz and co-workers,[67] Huang and co-workers,[68] and Costanzo-Nordin and co-workers[88] additionally reported that the presence, frequency, and complexity of ventricular arrhythmia were not related to the degree of LV impairment as determined by invasive hemodynamic measurement. Recently, similar data have been reported by larger multicenter trials including V-HeFT,[75] VA Cooperative Study of Captopril, Digoxin and Placebo,[76] and the Australian Transplant Program.[80]

Ventricular arrhythmia is also documented frequently in patients with a hypertrophic cardiomyopathy. McKenna and co-workers[87] reported that frequent VPBs were present in 90% of patients as documented with ambulatory monitoring whereas in 26% runs of nonsustained VT were noted. Exercise testing provoked VPBs in 60% of patients whereas 10% had nonsustained VT. In a report of 100 patients with hypertrophic cardiomyopathy, Savage and co-workers[89] observed that 83% had VPBs on ambulatory monitoring, although they were infrequent (i.e., <30/hr) in 17 patients. Nonsustained VT was observed in 19%. A similar prevalence of ventricular arrhythmia was reported

by Maron and co-workers[86] in 99 patients with hypertrophic cardiomyopathy.

In conclusion, almost 80% of patients with cardiomyopathy have frequent VPBs or couplets whereas 43% will have runs of nonsustained VT. The frequency and complexity of arrhythmia are not related to the etiology of the cardiomyopathy (ischemic or nonischemic) or the type (dilated or hypertrophic).

Relationship Between Arrhythmia and Sudden Cardiac Death in Cardiomyopathy

There have been several studies that have evaluated the relationship between ventricular arrhythmia, primarily runs of nonsustained VT, and the incidence of sudden cardiac death. Unfortunately, this issue is still controversial, as studies have reported conflicting data (Table 35.9). This may be because most of the studies involve small numbers of patients with various types of heart disease and different degrees of LV dysfunction. The small numbers involved in these trials precludes meaningful subset analysis, which would be important as it is likely that the prognostic significance of ventricular arrhythmia is related to these factors.

Holmes and co-workers[73] reported a 25-month follow-up in 31 patients with a congestive cardiomyopathy. At 1 yr, the overall mortality was 59% in those patients with runs of nonsustained VT, whereas the mortality was 11% among patients who had only simple, but frequent, VPBs. These authors observed no relationship between the presence of complex VPBs and nonsustained VT and any invasively obtained hemodynamic variable except for the presence of an

TABLE 35.9. Prognostic significance of NSVT in patients with CHF.

Study	N	Follow-up (mos)	NSVT prognosis of sudden death
Huang	35	34	No
Wilson	77	12	No
Meinertz	74	11	Yes
Von Olshausen	60	12	No
Holmes	43	14	Yes
Chakko	43	16	Yes
Unverferth	61	12	Yes
Costanzo-Nordin	55	16	No
Follansbee	19	19	Yes
Gradman	295	16	Yes
Keogh	137	10	Yes

NSVT = nonsustained ventricular tachycardia; CHF = congestive heart failure.

elevated pulmonary capillary wedge pressure that was observed more commonly in patients who had runs of nonsustained VT. In this trial, there was no excess mortality associated with an elevated LV end-diastolic pressure alone, but the presence of complex VPBs significantly increased mortality independently of filling pressure. In the prospective study of Meinertz and co-workers[67] involving 74 patients with an idiopathic or nonischemic congestive cardiomyopathy, 7 patients died as a result of progressive CHF, whereas 12 patients experienced sudden cardiac death during the mean follow-up of 11 months. Those who died from either cause had abnormal hemodynamics that were significantly different in comparison to those in the survivors. However, there was no difference in LV function or any invasive hemodynamic measurements between the patients who died from CHF and those who died suddenly from arrhythmia. Patients who died suddenly, however, did have a significantly greater incidence of couplets and runs of nonsustained VT when compared to survivors or those dying of CHF (Fig. 35.4). Thus, 75% of patients who died suddenly had repetitive ventricular arrhythmia documented on ambulatory monitoring, although this arrhythmia was not observed in any patient who died of CHF. Similar results were reported by Unverferth and co-workers,[90] Keogh and co-workers,[80] and Gradman and co-workers.[79] This latter report involved 265 placebo patients from the VA Cooperative Trial; using a multiple logistic regression analysis, the presence and frequency of nonsustained VT (>10 runs/day) was significantly associated with a risk of sudden cardiac death as well as total cardiac mortality. The LVEF also was independently associated with sudden cardiac death and total cardiac mortality. However, the presence of frequent runs (>10/day) of nonsustained VT had the strongest association with sudden cardiac death.

In contrast, there have been other studies that have reported no relationship between ventricular arrhythmia and an increased risk of sudden death.[68,70,72] It should be pointed out that most of these studies involved a smaller number of patients with various etiologies for CHF. Indeed, Wilson and co-workers[70] concluded that ventricular arrhythmia was a reflection of the extent of the heart disease and the degree of underlying LV dysfunction, but was not an independent risk factor for sudden cardiac death. However, most of the studies involving larger numbers of patients with a dilated cardiomyopathy and CHF report that the presence of nonsustained VT is associated with an increased risk of sudden death. These trials involve patients with both ischemic and nonischemic etiologies, but it appears that the increased risk is unrelated to the etiology of the heart disease.

In patients with a hypertropic cardiomyopathy, non-

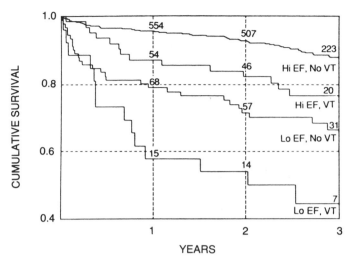

FIGURE 35.5. Survival of patients after a myocardial infarction in relation to nonsustained ventricular tachycardia (*VT*) and left ventricular ejection fraction (*EF*). When nonsustained VT is absent and EF is high (>30%), survival is good. When nonsustained VT and low EF (<30%) are present, survival is poor while it is intermediate when either of these risk factors are present (from the Multicenter Post Infarction Trial). Reprinted, with permission, from Bigger et al. 1986;58:1115. *Am J Cardiol.*

sustained VT has been reported to be a marker of risk. In a study by Maron and co-workers,[86] the annual sudden death mortality in patients with a hypertrophic cardiomyopathy who had nonsustained VT documented on ambulatory monitoring was 8.6% compared to a 1% rate among those without such arrhythmias. Other forms of ventricular arrhythmia, regardless of frequency, complexity, or multiformity, were not predictive of risk.

The largest body of data exist in patients with a recent myocardial infarction (MI). As previously indicated, there have been a number of large-scale epidemiologic studies that have reported an association between complex arrhythmia, primarily nonsustained VT, and an increased risk of sudden cardiac death (by two to five fold).[82–85] However, the highest mortality rate and the strongest association are in those patients who have both complex arrhythmia and LV dysfunction (Fig. 35.5, Table 35.7).

In conclusion, complex arrhythmia, primarily runs of nonsustained VT, is associated with an increased risk of sudden death in patients with a cardiomyopathy and CHF, in patients with hypertrophic cardiomyopathy, and in patients with a recent myocardial infarction, especially those who have LV dysfunction or CHF. Although these studies have identified a high-risk group, they do not offer information about identifying the individual patient at risk.

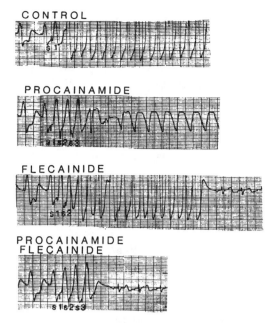

CONTROL

PROCAINAMIDE

FLECAINIDE

PROCAINAMIDE
FLECAINIDE

FIGURE 35.6. Example of electrophysiologic studies in a patient with a cardiomyopathy and sustained ventricular tachycardia (*VT*). In control, one extrastimulus (S_1) induces sustained VT. With procainamide, three extrastimuli (S_1, S_2, S_3) still induce sustained VT, but with a slower rate while during flecainide therapy the VT is nonsustained. When the two drugs are used in combination, arrhythmia is noninducible.

TABLE 35.10. Role of electrophysiologic studies in patients with cardiomyopathy and nonsustained ventricular tachycardia.

Study	No. with cardiomyopathy	No. inducible (%)	Follow-up (mos)	Prediction
Veltri	6	3 (50)	23	No
Sulpizi	9	5 (56)	29	No
Das	24	8 (33)	12	No
Poll	20	1 (5)	18	No
Gomes	10	?	30	Yes
Zheutlin	13	7 (54)	22	Yes[a]
Buxton	18	9 (50)	33	No
Hammill	53 [28 CAD / 25 idiopathic	14 CAD / 1 idiopathic	50	No

[a] Only noninducibility predictive.

Role of Electrophysiologic Testing in Predicting the Patient at Risk for Sudden Cardiac Death

Electrophysiologic testing is an important and useful technique for evaluating and managing patients with serious sustained ventricular tachyarrhythmias, establishing the mechanism, locating the focus or origin of the tachycardia, and for identifying an effective antiarrhythmic drug to prevent recurrence (Fig. 35.6). However, the role of electrophysiologic testing for indentifying the patient with a cardiomyopathy, CHF, and nonsustained VT who is at risk for experiencing a sustained ventricular tachyarrhythmia and sudden cardiac death remains uncertain and controversial (Table 35.10). Unfortunately, there are only a few studies, each involving small numbers, that have addressed this issue in patients with a cardiomyopathy and CHF. It has been reported that the rate of inducibility of arrhythmia among patients with a cardiomyopathy and nonsustained VT is low. Stevenson and co-workers[91] performed electrophysiologic testing in 72 patients with a cardiomyopathy and severe CHF. The etiology was coronary artery disease in 33% and idiopathic in 61%. The remaining patients had valvular disease. Sustained VT was induced in only nine patients (13%).

Prystowsky and co-workers[92] reported that 8 of 15 patients (55%) with a cardiomyopathy and nonsustained VT had sustained VT induced.

Not only is the incidence of inducible arrhythmia in patients with a cardiomyopathy low, but its prognostic significance also is uncertain (Table 35.10). In a study by Gomes and co-workers,[93] 73 patients (10 having a cardiomyopathy) with nonsustained VT documented on ambulatory monitoring underwent electrophysiologic testing. Arrhythmia was induced in 20 patients (group 1) whereas 53 patients (group 2) had no arrhythmia induced. LV dysfunction was more prevalent in group 1 patients and there was a greater proportion who had a LVEF <40% when compared to those in group 2. After a 30-month follow-up, the mortality in group 1 was significantly higher than that of group 2 (32% vs. 2%, $p < .001$). This study concluded that inducibility was predictive of a poorer outcome in patients with nonsustained VT. Unfortunately, it is unknown how many patients with a cardiomyopathy were in each group or how many patients had clinical CHF or reduced LVEF, as these patients were not separately analyzed. Similar results were reported by Zheutlin and co-workers.[94] Although a dilated cardiomyopathy was present in 23 patients, there was no separate analysis of this group. In this trial, the mean LVEF was equivalent in those with and without inducible arrhythmia (37% vs. 36%), as was the number of patients with a clinical history of CHF (39% vs. 45%) and the number of patients who had an LVEF <40% (55% vs. 65%).

A study of Das and co-workers[95] involved 22 patients with a dilated cardiomyopathy. With electrophysiologic testing, 10 patients had either sustained VT or VF induced. During a 12-month follow-up period, three patients experienced sudden cardiac death, but only one of these patients had arrhythmia inducible with electrophysiologic testing. The authors concluded that electrophysiologic testing is not predictive of outcome, although the death rate in this study was low. A lack of association between inducibility and outcome also was reported by Poll and co-workers,[96] Veltri and co-workers,[97] Stevenson and co-workers,[91] and Sulpizi and co-workers.[98] Although inducibility of arrhythmia in patients with cardiomyopathy and nonsustained VT on monitoring was not predictive of an arrhythmic event, Veltri and co-workers did observe an association between LVEF and fatal and nonfatal sustained ventricular arrhythmia. In the study of Stevenson and co-workers,[91] there were 13 sudden deaths among 63 patients (21%) who did not have arrhythmia induced during electrophysiologic testing. The actuarial risk of sudden death in this group was 13% at 6 weeks and 30% at 6 months. Independent predictors of sudden death were pulmonary artery pressure >55 mm Hg, a pulmonary capillary wedge pressure >16 mm Hg, hemodynamic parameters of LV function.

In the study of Sulpizi and co-workers,[98] patients with a cardiomyopathy were not analyzed separately, but there was a separate analysis performed of those patients with reduced LVEF <50% and 13 of 61 had an LVEF of <35%. The induction of nonsustained VT was not related to the LVEF, but the induction of a sustained VT was significantly related to the presence of LV dysfunction. With a multivariate analysis, only LV dysfunction was independently related to inducibility of a sustained VT. The only clinical variable associated with sudden death or cardiac mortality was severe LV dysfunction. In the presence of severe LV dysfunction (LVEF <35%), the incidence of sudden cardiac death was 33% when sustained VT was induced whereas it was only 20% when the patient was noninducible ($p = NS$). Unfortunately, these studies did not analyze separately patients with an ischemic or nonischemic etiology of cardiomyopathy.

Although it has been suggested that electrophysiologic testing may be predictive of risk in those with LV dysfunction due to coronary artery disease, the role of electrophysiologic testing to predict the patient with a nonischemic dilated cardiomyopathy who is at risk for sudden cardiac death is uncertain, but it does not seem to be predictive in this group. Stamato and co-workers[99] prospectively evaluated 15 patients with an idiopathic nonischemic dilated cardiomyopathy who had LV dysfunction (LVEF = 17%), CHF, and nonsustained VT on ambulatory monitoring. Sustained VT was not induced in any patient. These authors concluded that patients with a nonischemic cardiomyopathy respond differently than those with an ischemic etiology and electrophysiologic studies have a limited role in this group of patients. Hammill and co-workers[100] reported on 53 patients with a cardiomyopathy due to coronary artery disease in 28 patients or an idiopathic etiology in 25 patients. In this trial, 15 patients were inducible during

electrophysiologic studies. Coronary artery disease was present in 14 of these patients whereas idiopathic cardiomyopathy was present in 1. After a 50-month follow-up inducibility was not predictive of outcome in either group.

In conclusion, the role of electrophysiologic testing for predicting the risk of sudden cardiac death in patients with a cardiomyopathy and documented runs of nonsustained VT on ambulatory monitoring remains uncertain as data are conflicting. Studies that report an association between inducibility and an increased risk of sudden cardiac death involve patients with a variety of etiologies and severity of heart disease and they do not separately analyze those with cardiomyopathy and CHF. Those studies involving only patients with an idiopathic cardiomyopathy have failed to establish any prognostic role for electrophysiologic testing. Although the results are as yet controversial, only small numbers of patients have been studied and those with an ischemic or nonischemic etiology are not usually analyzed separately. Further investigation with a larger number of patients is required to answer this question. However, at the present time, it does not appear that electrophysiologic studies are predictive of sudden death in patients with a cardiomyopathy and CHF and they remain an investigational technique.

Inducibility in Patients with Cardiomyopathy Who Have Had Sustained VT or VF

Although data are limited, there are a few studies that have reported the role of electrophysiologic testing in patients with an idiopathic dilated cardiomyopathy and CHF who have experienced sustained VT or VF. Naccarelli and co-workers[101] examined the role of electrophysiologic testing in 83 patients with VT who did not have coronary artery disease. A cardiomyopathy was present in 37 patients, 12 of whom had nonsustained VT and 25 of whom presented with sustained VT. Thirteen of these latter patients (52%) had either sustained VT (n = 6) or nonsustained VT (n = 7) induced. Of 12 patients with a cardiomyopathy who had nonsustained VT documented on ambulatory monitoring, sustained VT was not induced in any, although 4 (33%) did have nonsustained VT provoked. Patients with inducible arrhythmia underwent serial drug testing guided either invasively or noninvasively; the authors concluded that for the entire group, suppression of inducible VT predicted effective drug therapy, but those with a cardiomyopathy were not analyzed separately and so no data about long-term outcome in these patients are available from this study. An additional important conclusion was that in patients with a cardiomyopathy and

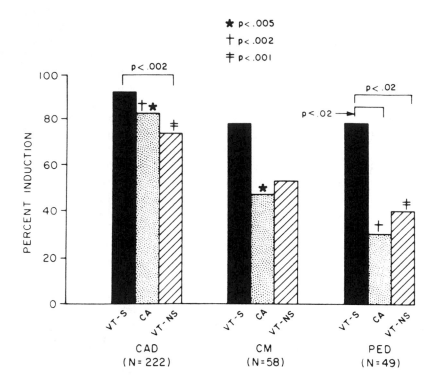

FIGURE 35.7. Relationship between presenting arrhythmia, nature of the underlying heart disease and inducibility with electrophysiologic studies. Regardless of the type of presenting arrhythmia, patients with a cardiomyopathy have a lower rate of induction compared to patients with coronary artery disease (*CAD*). PED = primary electrical disease; VT-S = sustained ventricular tachycardia; CA = cardiac arrest; VT-NS = nonsustained ventricular tachycardia. Reprinted, with permission, from ref. 92. Copyright by the American Heart Association.

a history of CHF who experienced a sustained ventricular tachyarrhythmia, electrophysiologic testing was less likely to induce sustained VT when compared to the results in patients with coronary artery disease who have had a sustained arrhythmia.

In a follow-up study, Prystowsky and co-workers[92] analyzed the results of electrophysiologic testing in 329 consecutive patients with arrhythmia (Fig. 35.7). There were 58 patients who had a cardiomyopathy, 24 of whom presented with sustained VT and 19 of them (79%) were inducible. In contrast, only 9 of 19 (49%) who presented with a cardiac arrest (due to either sustained VT or VF) were inducible, whereas 8 of 15 (53%) with nonsustained VT had VT induced. As with previous reports, patients with a clinical history of sustained VT were significantly more likely to have arrhythmia induced compared to those presenting with a cardiac arrest or nonsustained VT and patients with an idiopathic etiology were less likely to have arrhythmia induced with electrophysiologic testing when compared to those with coronary artery disease.

Signal-Averaged Electrocardiography: Role in the Evaluation of Patients with Cardiomyopathy

Over the past several years, the signal-averaged electrocardiogram (ECG) has emerged as a useful tool in patients with a recent myocardial infarction for a noninvasive assessment of risk for a serious ventricular

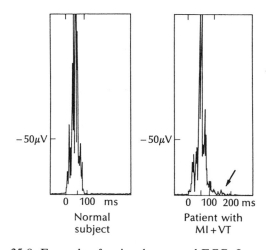

FIGURE 35.8. Example of a signal-averaged ECG. Late potentials are absent in the normal individual whereas they are present (*arrow*) in a patient with a myocardial infarction (*MI*) and ventricular tachycardia (*VT*).

tachyarrhythmia, specifically sustained VT (Fig. 35.8). Work by several groups has demonstrated that conduction through a zone of infarcted tissue is slow, fragmented, and disorganized.[102–106] Josephson and co-workers[107] reported that continuous electric activity occurring at the end of depolarization and indicating delayed activation, is seen in periinfarction tissue. This represents the electrophysiologic substrate for reentrant ventricular tachycardia. This delayed and fragmented conduction theoretically sets up areas of unidirectional block and multiple pathways with varying refractory periods and conduction properties, the precondition for reentry. Unfortunately, these areas of continuous activity are small and the electrical activity they generate is lost in the ambient noise of the routine surface ECG. However, through the computerized averaging of many QRS complexes, their digitalization, and filtering, these high frequency, low amplitude signals can be detected at the end of the QRS complex.

In brief, three standard orthogonal leads from the surface ECG are used and 200 to 300 QRS complexes are recorded. The signals are digitalized, averaged, filtered, and then combined into a root mean square sum. The result is a filtered QRS complex that combines the high frequency content of all three leads. In patients with coronary disease who have had ventricular tachycardia, low amplitude high frequency signals often are present, continuous with the end of the surface QRS complex, and are termed "late potentials." Several criteria have been applied to quantitate these signals. Late potentials are considered to be present when the filtered QRS complex is longer than 120 ms in the absence of a bundle branch block on the surface ECG, the amplitude of the signal in the last 40 ms of the QRS complex is less than 20 to 25 μV, or the terminal filtered QRS complex remains below 40 μV for longer than 38 ms. Most authors use combinations of these criteria to define an abnormal signal-averaged electrocardiogram.

The presence of late potentials has been used to stratify patients after an MI for risk of an arrhythmic event. Much of this work has been based on an early study by Simpson,[108] who reported his findings in 66 post-MI patients, 39 of whom had had VT and 27 who were free of arrhythmia. He reported that patients with VT had a QRS duration or average $2\frac{1}{2}$ times longer than those without VT, and also had a significantly lower voltage in the terminal 40 ms of the filtered QRS complex. Based on this work, he proposed that a duration for the filtered QRS of >120 ms and an amplitude <25 μV in the terminal 40 ms of the QRS complex were criteria to define a late potential. He also suggested that these definitions could be used prospectively to identify patients post-MI at risk for ventricular arrhythmia.

Several other authors have reported that the presence of late potentials will identify a group of patients after MI who are at risk for an arrhythmic event.[109,110] Kuchar and co-workers[111] analyzed the signal-averaged ECG and LV function in 210 post-MI patients. Over a median follow-up of 14 months, there were 15 major arrhythmic events. Using multivariate analysis, the ejection fraction and late potentials on a signal-averaged ECG were both independent variables for predicting outcome and together had a predictive value of 34%. When the ejection fraction was <40%, but late potentials were absent, the risk of an arrhythmic event was only 4%. The authors concluded that in patients with an ischemic cardiomyopathy, an abnormal signal-averaged ECG is strongly predictive of an adverse outcome.

Similar to the infarcted myocardium, the various disease processes that cause cardiomyopathy are non-homogeneous, resulting in a nonuniformity of electrical activity. It has been suggested therefore that the signal-averaged ECG can identify patients with a cardiomyopathy who have an electrically unstable arrhythmogenic substrate and are at risk for sudden death. Several recent articles have addressed this issue. Poll and co-workers[112] obtained a signal-averaged ECG in 41 patients with a nonischemic cardiomyopathy. Twelve had a history of a sustained tachyarrhythmia whereas 29 had no history of arrhythmia. A control group of 55 normal individuals also was studied for comparison. The filtered QRS was significantly longer in those with a history of arrhythmia when compared to patients with cardiomyopathy but no arrhythmia or to normal controls. The voltage in the terminal 40 ms of the QRS complex was not different between the normal group and the group with cardiomyopathy who did not have arrhythmia. In contrast, this voltage in the group with arrhythmia was significantly lower when compared to the other two groups. Eighty-three percent of patients with cardiomyopathy who had VT or VF had an abnormal late potential compared to only 17% of the nonarrhythmic cardiomyopathy group and 7% in the control population. The authors concluded that the presence of late potentials on the signal-averaged ECG could identify patients with nonischemic dilated cardiomyopathy at risk for a sustained ventricular arrhythmia.

Itoh and co-workers[113] assessed the presence of late potentials in a cohort of 80 patients, 40 of whom had a previous MI, 32 of whom had a nonischemic cardiomyopathy, and 8 who had no structural heart disease, but had a history of sustained VT. Patients were divided into three groups: group 1 had a history of sustained VT, group 2 had a history of only nonsustained VT (>5 beats), and group 3 had no VT. In the subset of patients with a cardiomyopathy, the duration of late potentials was significantly longer in group 1 (33.7 ms) when compared to group 2 (20.1 ms) or group 3 (7.1 ms). All group 1 patients and most (83%) of the group 2 patients with cardiomyopathy had abnormal late potentials, whereas only 36% of group 3 patients had abnormal late potentials.

It should be pointed out that both of these studies were retrospective, and provided no information about the predictive value of late potentials in patients with a cardiomyopathy. Ohnishi et al.[114] studied 100 patients with a recent MI and 54 patients with a dilated cardiomyopathy. In the post-MI patients, 31 had positive late potentials and 69 did not. Over a mean follow-up of 18 months, six patients with late potentials died suddenly, and only two patients without late potentials experienced sudden death. Of the patients with dilated cardiomyopathy, there were 5 deaths among the 21 patients with positive late potentials and 2 sudden deaths in the group of 22 patients without late potentials. As a predictor of sudden death in the post-MI population, an abnormal signal-averaged ECG had a sensitivity of 100%, a specificity of 60%, and a predictive accuracy of 63%. However, in the patients with a dilated cardiomyopathy, an abnormal signal-averaged ECG had a sensitivity of 100%, a specificity of 45%, and a predictive accuracy of only 52%. although no patient with a normal signal-averaged ECG had sudden death, many patients with late potentials did not have a serious ventricular arrhythmia. These authors concluded that the signal-averaged ECG may be an effective tool for risk-stratifying patients with a dilated cardiomyopathy.

In contrast, Middlekauff and co-workers[115] did not find that late potentials in patients with a cardiomyopathy were predictive. They obtained a signal-averaged ECG in 62 patients with advanced CHF who were being evaluated for transplantation. No patient had a history of a sustained ventricular tachyarrhythmia. The etiology of CHF was ischemic in 40 patients, whereas 22 had a nonischemic idiopathic cardiomyopathy. Late potentials were present in 16 patients (40%) with an old MI and an ischemic cardiomyopathy, but in only 3 (14%) with an idiopathic cardiomyopathy. The presence and frequency of VPBs and repetitive forms were similar in patients with and without late potentials. After a mean follow-up of 218 days, 18 patients died of a cardiac cause and in 9, death was sudden. The 1-yr cardiac mortality was 37% and for sudden death it was 20%. The risk of sudden death was 12% in patients with late potentials and 21% in those without this abnormality, and this difference was not statistically significant. The authors concluded that the incidence of late potentials in patients with a cardiomyopathy and CHF is related to the etiology of the CHF, but in general, the signal averaged ECG was a poor predictor of sudden death in patients with CHF.

In conclusion, data suggest that the presence of late potentials on a signal-averaged ECG has predictive value for a risk of sudden cardiac death in some groups of patients. In the post-MI patient, late potentials provide prognostic information that is independent of LV function and the presence of nonsustained VT on ambulatory monitoring. Late potentials, also are present in some patients with a dilated cardiomyopathy, but their significance is uncertain and may be related to the nature of underlying disease process. More data are needed, however, before the signal-averaged ECG becomes a useful tool for risk stratification of patients with an ischemic or nonischemic cardiomyopathy. It is possible that late potentials will identify patients who have an appropriate substrate for sustained VT, but not VF. Perhaps of greater importance is that the absence of late potentials may identify a low risk group.

TABLE 35.11. Effect of therapies for CHF on ventricular arrhythmias.

Study	Drug	N	Effect on arrhythmia
Franciosa	Isosorbide dinitrate	32	None
Franciosa	Hydralazine	32	None
Franciosa	Minoxidil	17	Increase
Packer	Amrinone	103	Increase
Anderson	Milrinone	12	Increase
Goldstein	Milrinone	10	Increase
Holmes	Milrinone	15	Increase
DiBianco	Milrinone	230	Increase
Ludmer	Milrinone	74	None
Sharma	Pibuterol	14	Increase
Mettauer	Salbutomol	20	Increase
Digoxin-Captopril	Digoxin	300	None
Multicenter Group	Captopril		None
Cleland	Captopril	14	Decrease
Cleland	Enalapril	20	Decrease
Webster	Enalapril	19	Decrease

CHF = congestive heart failure.

Effect of Therapies for CHF on the Incidence of Ventricular Arrhythmia

Since a large portion of deaths in patients with CHF is sudden, an important question is whether any therapeutic regimen can reduce this sudden death mortality. The two most common approaches have been to improve the hemodynamic abnormalities associated with CHF or to treat the prognostically important ventricular ectopy with antiarrhythmic agents. This section will focus on the first approach.

Investigations of CHF therapy have involved four classes of agents: direct-acting vasodilators, positive inotropic agents, cardiac glycosides, and angiotensin-converting enzyme inhibitors (Table 35.11). Some of these studies have used overall mortality as a primary end-point, whereas others have focused only on the density of ventricular ectopy. Unfortunately, only a few reports have specifically addressed sudden death mortality.

Directing-Acting Vasodilators

Vasodilatory agents used in the treatment of CHF have included nitrates, hydralazine, minoxidil, and nifedipine, among others. In a double-blind crossover study of Franciosa and colleagues,[116] 16 patients received either isosorbide dinitrate or placebo for 8 weeks, and then the other agent for an additional 8 weeks. These authors reported a significant reduction in the number of cardiac events in the nitrate group, but arrhythmia was infrequent in both groups and no conclusions about the effect of these agents on arrhythmia is possible. More recently, Bechler-Lisinska et al.[117] reported that the additional use of isosorbide dinitrate or nifedipine in a group of patients with CHF did not significantly decrease the number of simple or complex VPBs.

Using a double-blind crossover design, Franciosa and co-workers[118] administered minoxidil or placebo to 17 patients. Despite a significant improvement in the invasive hemodynamic measurements in the group receiving minoxidil, a significantly greater number of adverse clinical effects were seen in the treatment group when compared to placebo. In the minoxidil group, two patients developed a new ventricular arrhythmia and two patients died, whereas there were no ventricular arrhythmias or deaths observed in the placebo limb.

In an early trial,[119] hydralazine therapy was compared to placebo but did not significantly increase the exercise capacity or decrease the number of cardiac events among 32 patients with class 3 or 4 symptoms of CHF. However, a more recent study reported that the combined use of hydralazine and isordil in patients with CHF did have a beneficial effect on total cardiac mortality, which included sudden death and death from progressive pump failure.[120] In this study, 642 patients with CHF being treated with digoxin and diuretic were randomly assigned also to receive placebo, prazosin, or isordil and hydralazine in combination. After an average follow-up of 2.3 yr, the mortality rate in the hydralazine and isordil group was reduced by 34% compared to placebo. This difference in mortality persisted for as long as 3 yr. Mortality in the prazosin group was similar to placebo. Unfortunately, this study did not report the percent of death that was either sudden or due to progressive CHF.

In conclusion, the data regarding vasodilator therapy in patients with CHF is inconclusive with respect to its effect on ventricular arrhythmia and sudden death mortality. Although most studies do report that these agents improve LV hemodynamics, none show a significant decrease in VPB density. Only one study reported a reduction in total cardiac mortality, but the mechanism for this effect is uncertain.

Positive Inotropic Agents: Phosphodiesterase Inhibitors and Sympathomimetics

In contrast to studies using vasodilatory agents, the data regarding the new inotropic agents milrinone and amrinone are more substantial. There have been several trials, but the effect of these agents on ventricular arrhythmia is contradictory.

Packer and associates[121] administered oral amrinone (600 mg daily) to 31 patients with CHF. Despite improved hemodynamic indices, 10 patients died within the first 2 weeks of treatment and 16 were dead within 3 months. The mortality rate was felt to be twice as great as that seen in comparable trials with other agents.

Additionally, 4 of the 31 patients (13%) developed symptomatic sustained VT. It was concluded that amrinone may provoke life-threatening ventricular arrhythmia and shorten survival in patients with severe CHF.

Holmes and colleagues[122] reported the results of a 2- to 4-week trial of milrinone therapy in 15 patients. There was a 10-fold increase in the frequency of complex VPBs or the first occurrence of complex VPBs in 47% of patients including sustained VT in 7%. These authors concluded that milrinone therapy was associated with an increase in the complexity of ventricular ectopy and an increase in the density of complex VPBs. Similar results were reported by Goldstein et al.[123] and Anderson and colleagues,[124] who used a 48-hr intravenous infusion of milrinone.

In a long-term outpatient study, Ludmer and co-workers[125] evaluated ventricular arrhythmia frequency, total cardiac mortality, and sudden death mortality in a cohort of 74 patients entered into a trial of oral milrinone. Twenty-four–hour ambulatory monitoring was performed at baseline and after 1 week of milrinone therapy. The end-points of total mortality and mode of death were assessed during a mean follow-up of 6 months. After 1 week of milrinone, 85% of the cohort showed no significant change in arrhythmia, whereas 6% showed a significant decrease in the density of ventricular couplets and the frequency of runs of nonsustained VT and in 9%, the number of runs of nonsustained VT per 24 hr increased from 4 to 15. There was, however, no increased incidence of sudden death or total cardiac mortality in this subset when compared to the other 91% of patients.

In the largest reported study of milrinone to date, DiBianco and colleagues[126] randomly assigned 230 patients with severe heart failure to therapy with placebo, digoxin, milrinone, or both drugs. Although the functional status, as assessed by exercise treadmill time, increased in patients taking digoxin or milrinone, survival analysis according to intention to treat showed an adverse effect from milrinone. After adjustment for an excess of patients with lower LVEF in the milrinone group, this trend toward increased mortality persisted, but was not statistically significant. Eighteen percent of patients receiving milrinone therapy had increased ventricular arrhythmia as compared with 2% receiving either placebo or digoxin. The increase in arrhythmia was primarily VPBs, and no patient showed a change in complex arrhythmia. The authors concluded that although milrinone may increase exercise tolerance, it also increases ventricular arrhythmia and may reduce survival.

Finally, preliminary results from the PROMISE Trial (unpublished data) showed an excess total mortality of 30% ($p = .028$) in the group receiving milrinone compared to those treated with placebo. The mechanism for this excess mortality has not been reported and the effect of milrinone on ventricular arrhythmia frequency or on sudden arrhythmic death in this trial is not known. Taken together, the above data suggest an overall increase in the frequency of ventricular ectopy, and in at least two studies an increase in total mortality among patients treated with amrionone or milrinone.

The effect on arrhythmia of two sympathomimetic agents used in the treatment of CHF has been reported. Sharma and colleagues[127] treated 14 patients with refractory heart failure with one dose of pirbuterol, a beta-2 agonist. Invasive hemodynamic measurements showed a significant improvement in the cardiac index and a reduction of pulmonary artery wedge pressure, but no significant effect on ventricular arrhythmia was observed in this small study.

Mettauer and co-workers[128] reported the hemodynamic and arrhythmogenic effects of salbutamol, another beta-2 agonist, in 20 patients. Acutely, cardiac index increased and pulmonary capillary wedge pressure decreased, but six patients developed recurrent episodes of nonsustained VT (>5 beats) within 48 hr of initiation of drug therapy, which resolved upon discontinuation of the drug. Twelve patients continued to receive salbutamol for 1 month and at the end of this period the effect of the drug on arrhythmia was reevaluated with 36-hr ambulatory monitoring. Six of the 12 had multiple episodes of VT and two required cardioversion. Based on these data, the authors concluded that although salbutamol has beneficial hemodynamic effects, it also may provoke serious ventricular arrhythmias in a substantial number of patients.

Cardiac Glycosides

Two recent studies have evaluated the arrhythmic effects of digoxin in patients with heart failure. In the Captopril-Digoxin Multicentered Research Trial,[129] captopril, digoxin, or placebo was administered in a double-blind fashion to 300 patients. The LVEF increased 4.4% and the mean exercise time on a treadmill adhering to the Bruce protocol increased by 54 s in the digoxin group. However, there was no significant change in mean VPB frequency, which was 63.7/hr before digoxin and 66.0/hr at the completion of the study. During the 6 months of follow-up, there was no difference in the number of deaths among the three groups, although the mechanism of death was not reported. In a recent study from the Russian literature, ambulatory monitoring for 3 days was performed before and after digitalization in 55 patients with CHF.[130] Eight patients had a significant increase in VPB frequency. Taken together, these two studies suggest that whereas digoxin may improve the hemodynamics in patients with CHF, there is no consistent effect on arrhythmia. Its effect on sudden death is also unknown, as there have been no studies that have addressed this issue.

Angiotensin-Converting Enzyme Inhibitors

Perhaps the largest body of data concerning the relationship between the treatment of CHF and ventricular arrhythmia involves therapy with angiotensin-converting enzyme inhibitors. Evidence about this relationship exists in three areas—isolated cell preparations, animal models, and human clinical trials.

Hemsworth and colleagues[131] studied the effects of captopril on the action potential as recorded from guinea pig ventricular and sinoatrial nodal cells. These authors reported that at doses of 1 μM to 100 μM, captopril had no effect on the rate of phase 0 depolarization, the duration of recorded action potentials, or the spontaneous sinus cycle length. They concluded that any antiarrhythmic effects of captopril were unlikely to be due to direct electrical effects on cell membrane properties.

In an in vivo closed chest pig model, myocardial ischemia was induced in 20 animals by inflation of a balloon catheter in the left anterior descending artery.[132] After the production of ischemia, the pigs were divided into two groups: 10 received intravenous (IV) then oral captopril and 10 received placebo. After 2 weeks, programmed electrical stimulation was performed in the 14 surviving animals. Of the eight surviving control animals, six had VT induced. In contrast, none of the six surviving captopril-treated animals had VT induced. The authors concluded that early intervention with captopril in an in vivo ischemia/reperfusion model may reduce the risk for the subsequent development of VT. It was speculated that this protective effect may be due to salvage of ischemic myocardium, improvement in overall LV function, or decreased activity of the sympathetic nervous system resulting from improved LV function and cardiac output.

In another study by deLangen and co-workers,[133] ischemia was induced in 27 pigs by a 60-min occlusion of the left anterior descending artery. Of these 27 animals, 17 survived for 2 weeks and were studied by programmed electrical stimulation. In 8 of these 17, sustained monomorphic VT was reproducibly induced with one or two extra stimuli. Ten minutes after an intravenous bolus of captopril, the identical or more aggressive stimulation protocol was repeated and arrhythmias in five of these eight animals became noninducible. The nine animals originally noninducible received an infusion of angiotensin II, after which programmed electrical stimulation was repeated. In three animals, sustained monomorphic VT was now induced, whereas in three other animals nonsustained VT, which lasted for more than 10 beats, was induced. Additionally, the ventricular refractory period of the pigs with the newly induced arrhythmia was decreased compared to baseline. The authors concluded that modulation of the renin-angiotensin system after myocardial infarction alters the electrophysiologic properties of the heart as well as the inducibility of a malignant ventricular arrhythmia. Data regarding the hemodynamic effects of captopril or angiotensin II were not provided in this study, so the mechanism of these observed effects is not clear.

In the clinical literature, several studies have examined the relationship of therapy with angiotensin converting enzyme inhibitors, CHF, and ventricular arrhythmia. In the Captopril Digoxin Multicenter Research Trial,[129] captopril significantly decreased the number of VPBs/hr from 64.7 in control to 35.3 during therapy. Although captopril resulted in an increase in exercise time on a treadmill and a decrease in New York Heart Association (NYHA) functional class when compared to baseline, over the 6-month follow-up period there was no significant difference in death rate between the captopril, digoxin, and placebo groups.

In another study, Cleland and colleagues[134] evaluated the arrhythmia in 14 patients treated with captopril or placebo using a double-blind design. Exercise tolerance, functional class, and total body potassium content rose significantly, and there was a significant decrease in the frequency of VPBs, couplets per hour, runs of nonsustained VT per hour, and episodes of sustained VT in the captopril group. Over the 12-week study period, there was one death in the group taking placebo. Cleland and co-workers[135] subsequently studied enalapril in 20 patients using a similar double-blind protocol. They again demonstrated an improvement in hemodynamics and a marked decrease in simple VPBs as well as repetitive ventricular extrasystoles compared to placebo. One patient taking placebo died during the 4-month trial.

Webster et al.[136] studied 20 patients with CHF treated with either placebo or enalapril for a 12-week period. The group receiving placebo showed no change in the frequency of any arrhythmia compared to baseline. However, VPBs and couplets decreased fivefold during a 24-hr monitoring period and episodes of nonsustained VT decreased 10-fold in the group receiving enalapril. There were two episodes of sudden death, one in each of the two groups. Compared to placebo, patients receiving enalapril had an increase in potassium levels of 0.33 mol/l, although there was no direct correlation between potassium level and density of ventricular ectopy. The authors concluded that enalapril decreased the frequency of ventricular arrhythmia in patients with CHF, but the mechanism by which this occurs is unknown.

Finally, in the CONSENSUS trial,[137] 253 patients were randomized to receive either placebo or enalapril (2.5–40 mg daily). Over a 6-month follow-up, mortality was 26% in the enalapril group and 44% in the placebo group. Importantly, however, the entire reduction in mortality was due to a decrease in the number of pa-

tients dying from progressive CHF. There was no difference between the two groups in the number of patients who died suddenly.

In conclusion, among the agents used to treat CHF, angiotensin-converting enzyme inhibitors represent the only class that consistently decrease in the density of all forms of VPBs. These agents also have been shown to reduce mortality due to progressive CHF. However, there is no evidence that they reduce sudden cardiac death mortality despite their effect on spontaneous arrhythmia.

Role of Antiarrhythmic Drug Therapy for Preventing Sudden Death in Patients with a Cardiomyopathy and CHF Who Have Nonsustained VT

Although many studies have confirmed that there is an association between the presence of nonsustained VT and an increased risk for a sustained ventricular tachyarrhythmia, there are no well controlled studies that have evaluated the role of antiarrhythmic drugs for preventing sudden death in this group of patients. There are, however, some preliminary data. Hamer and co-workers[138] randomized 34 patients with severe CHF who did not have a history of a sustained ventricular tachyarrhythmia to therapy with low-dose amiodarone (200 mg/day) or placebo. There was a significant reduction in ventricular arrhythmia in the amiodarone-treated group. Runs of nonsustained VT, present in 88% of patients before amiodarone, were observed in only 19% during amiodarone therapy. There was an 11% cardiac mortality in the group receiving amiodarone and only one patient had sudden death. In contrast, the cardiac mortality in the placebo group was 40% and five patients experienced sudden death. Cleland and co-workers[139] prospectively followed 152 patients for a mean of 21 months. In this study, 41 patients were receiving amiodarone and 111 were not, but therapy was based on clinical parameters and patients were not randomized. During the follow-up, 63 patients (41%) died and the mechanism was sudden death in 47 patients. Variables predictive of poor outcome were VPBs, lack of amiodarone therapy, low mean blood pressure, and a diagnosis of coronary artery disease.

Kerin and co-workers[140] prospectively followed 110 patients with structural heart disease, LV dysfunction, and runs of nonsustained VT who were treated with low-dose amiodarone (275 mg/day). The authors observed that survival at 1, 2, 3, and 4 yr was 90%, 85%, 85%, and 85%, respectively, and this was independent of LVEF or suppression of arrhythmia. Although they concluded that amiodarone improves survival of patients with complex ventricular ectopy, there was no placebo group in this trial. Chakko and Gheorghiade (74) randomized 23 patients with a cardiomyopathy who had ventricular arrhythmia documented on ambulatory monitoring to therapy with either procainamide or quinidine while 20 patients did not receive antiarrhythmic therapy. During the follow-up period, there were 16 cardiac deaths, 10 of which were sudden, presumably the result of a sustained ventricular tachyarrhythmia. In this study, mortality was independent of antiarrhythmic therapy. However, the role of drug therapy is uncertain since its use was not based on arrhythmia suppression and there was no attempt to guide therapy by objective criteria. In the report by Unverferth and co-workers[90] involving 69 patients, antiarrhythmic drug therapy was administered to 24 patients. However, the 1-yr mortality was not affected by drug therapy, but as with the study of Chakko and Gheorghiade,[74] no conclusions are possible since the authors did not supply any data about the effect of these agents on the suppression of arrhythmia.

Parmley and Chatterjee[141] reviewed the outcome of 26 patients with CHF and complex arrhythmia who were treated with procainamide, quinidine, or amiodarone. This was not a randomized study and there was no placebo group. The effect of the drugs on ventricular arrhythmia frequency was not commented on by the authors, but sudden death mortality was reduced in the group of patients receiving antiarrhythmic drug therapy. Neri and co-workers[142] reported on 41 patients with a dilated cardiomyopathy who received therapy with amiodarone. In this study, the drug significantly reduced the frequency and complexity of spontaneous ventricular arrhythmias. During the follow-up, there were no sudden deaths in the group receiving amiodarone, in contrast to four sudden deaths among the patients receiving placebo. Keogh and co-workers[80] reported no benefit from amiodarone in their patients who had significant CHF and were awaiting transplantation. However, this was not a randomized trial.

There are only limited data about the role of antiarrhythmic drug therapy in patients with CHF and nonsustained VT who are managed with electrophysiologic testing. Although the role of electrophysiologic testing for identifying the patient at risk for sudden death is still controversial, this technique has been used successfully to guide the selection of antiarrhythmic drugs for long-term therapy. Wilber and co-workers[143] performed electrophysiologic tests on 100 consecutive patients with an ischemic cardiomyopathy (LVEF <40%, mean = 25%) and spontaneous nonsustained VT documented on ambulatory monitoring. Clinical CHF was present in 62% of patients. Serial drug studies (average 2.3 per patient) were carried out in 40 of 43 patients with inducible VT. In 20 patients, an effective agent that prevented the induction of arrhythmia was identified whereas in 20 patients arrhythmia remained inducible, but the agent that resulted in the greatest amount of slowing of the VT rate was selected for long-term use. After a follow-up of 16.7 months, the overall incidence of nonfatal cardiac arrest or sudden death was 9% at 1 yr and 17% at 2 yr (Fig. 35.9). Among the 57 patients who did not have arrhythmia inducible, the 1- and 2-yr incidence of a sustained ventricular tachyarrhythmia was 2% and 6%, respectively. The incidence was 0% and 11%, respectively, among the 20 patients who responded to antiarrhythmic therapy. This was not significantly different from the group without inducible arrhythmia. In contrast, the incidence was 34% and 50% at 1 and 2 yr among the patients with arrhythmia persistently induced on antiarrhythmic therapy. There

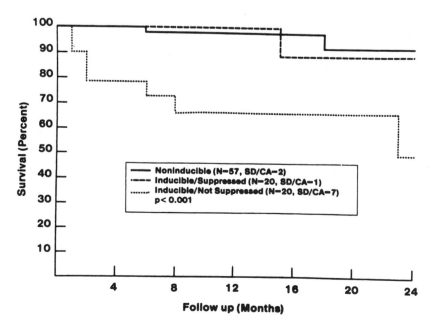

FIGURE 35.9. Results of electrophysiologic testing in patients with coronary artery disease and an ejection fraction <40%. Patients who had no ventricular tachycardia (*VT*) induced or who had inducible sustained (*VT*) that was prevented by an antiarrhythmic drug had an equivalent outcome that was better than patients with VT, which remained inducible despite drug therapy. Reprinted, with permission, from ref. 143. Copyright by the American Heart Association.

was no significant difference in the extent of underlying disease, LVEF, incidence of CHF, or other clinical features between those with or without inducible arrhythmia or between those with or without arrhythmia during the follow-up. There is, unfortunately, no control group as all patients with inducible arrhythmia received therapy.

Although antiarrhythmic drugs have not yet been shown to be of benefit in these patients, there are data suggesting that beta-blockers may have a role. Swedberg and co-workers[144] treated 24 patients who had CHF with metoprolol in addition to conventional CHF therapy. These authors reported a significant improvement in survival when compared to historical controls. Unfortunately, the absence of a placebo control group precludes any meaningful interpretation of these results. Anderson and co-workers[145] randomly assigned 50 patients with CHF to receive standard therapy alone or with metoprolol. Although they reported no difference in outcome between the two groups when analyzed by intention to treat, there was a favorable trend in survival in the group receiving metoprolol when analyzed by actual treatment received.

Data from the Beta Blocker Heart Attack Trial (BHAT) support these observations.[146] In this study, post-MI patients were randomized to receive propranolol or placebo within 3 weeks of the infarction. Propranolol significantly reduced overall mortality. However, Furberg and co-workers[147] reported that the difference in mortality between the placebo- and propranolol-treated groups was more pronounced in patients with decreased LV function. In another analysis of the BHAT data, Chadda and co-workers[148] reported that there was a 47% decrease in sudden death mortality among the propranolol-treated patients who had CHF complicating the MI compared to only a 13% reduction in sudden death mortality among the propranolol-treated patients who did not have CHF. Unfortunately, none of these studies systematically evaluated the effect of the beta-blocker on ventricular arrhythmia so that it is unclear if the beneficial effect of these agents is due to their antiarrhythmic activity or related to their antisympathetic effects in general.

There are limited data about antiarrhythmic therapy in patients with a hypertrophic cardiomyopathy and nonsustained VT. McKenna and co-workers[149] administered amiodarone to 21 such patients and observed elimination of arrhythmia in all patients; after a 5-yr follow-up period, there were no episodes of sudden death. In contrast, Fananapazir and co-workers[150] from the NIH reported that amiodarone therapy was associated with an increased incidence of early sudden death despite the reduction in nonsustained VT and the improvement in functional capacity. In this trial, there were 50 patients with symptoms and 42% had nonsustained VT on monitoring. During a 2.2-yr follow-up,

there were seven sudden deaths and the 1- and 2-yr survival rate was 85% and 80%, respectively. The survival rate of those with nonsustained VT was significantly poorer than those without this arrhythmia (61% vs. 97% at 2 yr) and sudden death occurred despite suppression of nonsustained VT by amiodarone.

In conclusion, there are as yet no well controlled data that antiarrhythmic drugs are of benefit for preventing sudden cardiac death and prolonging life in patients with a cardiomyopathy and CHF who have nonsustained VT, although there are suggestive data about amiodarone. Beta-blockers may have an important role, but the mechanism for this beneficial effect is unknown.

Electrophysiologic Testing for Drug Selection in Patients with Cardiomyopathy Who Have Had Sustained VT or VF

Several studies have evaluated the role of serial electrophysiologic testing for drug selection in patients with cardiomyopathy who have had a sustained ventricular tachyarrhythmia. Poll and co-workers[96] reported on 11 patients with an idiopathic dilated cardiomyopathy who presented with sustained monomorphic VT. Nine of these patients had arrhythmia that was persistently inducible on all drugs tested. After a mean follow-up of 21 months, six of these nine patients experienced arrhythmia recurrence even though in three of these patients the VT rate was significantly slowed by the drug. The other two patients who responded to drug remained free of recurrence. Similar to studies involving patients with coronary artery disease and VT, the authors concluded that in patients with a cardiomyopathy and a clinical history of VT, the arrhythmia often is inducible, but antiarrhythmic drugs are only infrequently effective. However, if an effective drug is identified, recurrence of arrhythmia is prevented. A follow-up study of Poll and co-workers[151] involved 47 patients with a nonischemic cardiomyopathy. Each of the 13 patients who had a clinical history of sustained monomorphic VT had this arrhythmia induced during electrophysiologic testing. There were 14 patients who presented with a cardiac arrest, but in only 5 was arrhythmia inducible. During serial drug testing, arrhythmia became noninducible in only 4 of these 27 patients (15%) and all remained free of recurrence after an 18-month follow-up. In contrast, there were 8 recurrences of arrhythmia among the remaining 23 patients (35%) who did not respond to drug therapy. As with other studies, these authors concluded that sustained monomorphic VT is usually induced in patients with a cardiomyopathy presenting with this arrhythmia, but is provoked less often in patients with a cardiac arrest in whom the mechanism may be VT or VF. Only a few patients respond to anti-arrhythmic drugs when evaluation of efficacy is based on electrophysiologic testing. However, if the patient has no arrhythmia inducible during drug therapy, the outcome is good and recurrence prevented, similar to what has been observed in patients with VT who have underlying coronary artery disease.

Similar results were reported by Rae and co-workers[152] in 38 patients with a dilated cardiomyopathy who presented with a sustained ventricular tachyarrhythmia. Sustained monomorphic VT was induced in 18 patients (47%), VF in 7 (18%), and nonsustained VT in 13 (34%). Drug efficacy, based on repeated electrophysiologic studies, was defined as the induction of <6 repetitive VPBs. At least one effective drug was identified in 20 patients (53%). After a follow-up of 21 months, there were no sudden deaths or nonfatal arrhythmia recurrences in the group who responded to a drug whereas there were five recurrences among the 18 patients (28%) with arrhythmia that was still inducible despite antiarrhythmic therapy.

Constantin and co-workers[153] evaluated 31 patients with a nonischemic cardiomyopathy that was idiopathic or due to valvular disease. The clinical arrhythmia was sustained VT in 16 patients, VF in 11, and 4 patients with syncope of unknown etiology. With electrophysiologic testing, sustained monomorphic VT was induced in 17 patients (55%), 12 of whom had a history of VT (representing 75% of those presenting with VT), 2 had presented with VF (18% of patients with VF), and 3 had syncope. Of these 17 patients, 15 underwent serial drug testing and 13 patients were considered responders to drug. In this group, there were three arrhythmic events during follow-up. As with previous studies, the authors concluded that the induction of a sustained monomorphic VT was related to the arrhythmia the patient presented with clinically and suppression of inducibility predicted freedom from recurrence. Liem and Swerdlow[154] evaluated 64 patients with an idiopathic dilated cardiomyopathy who presented with sustained VT or VF. With electrophysiologic testing, a sustained monomorphic VT was induced in 41 patients (67%). As with other studies, these authors reported that induction of arrhythmia was significantly more common in patients presenting with sustained VT (33 of 44 patients, 75%) compared with the results in patients presenting with VF (8 of 20 patients, 40%). During serial drug testing an effective drug was identified in 15 patients (37% of those inducible, 23% of total population). The remaining patients had an effective drug identified by ambulatory monitoring or in some cases, were not treated. After a mean follow-up of 1.6 yr, there were 32 arrhythmia recurrences, 24 of which were cardiac arrests, whereas in 8, arrhythmia was nonfatal. There were no recurrences among the 15 patients who were treated with a drug predicted to be effective by

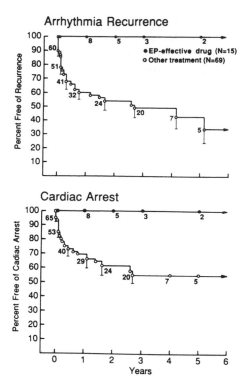

FIGURE 35.10. Electrophysiologic-guided therapy in patients with an idiopathic cardiomyopathy and a sustained ventricular tachycardia. Arrhythmia recurrence and cardiac arrest are significantly reduced ($p = .009$ and $p = .02$, respectively) in patients who had an effective antiarrhythmic drug selected by electrophysiologic (EP) testing. Other treatment includes empiric therapy or ambulatory monitor guided therapy. Reprinted, with permission, from ref. 154.

electrophysiologic testing (Fig. 35.10). In contrast, arrhythmia recurrence (46%) and sudden cardiac death (38%) were significantly greater among the 49 patients treated with a drug selected by ambulatory monitoring, guided by plasma concentration, or those not treated. For patients with class III or IV CHF, the incidence of sudden death was 71% when no effective drug was identified by electrophysiologic testing.

In contrast to these studies, Milner and co-workers[155] reported that in patients with a cardiomyopathy, suppression of arrhythmia during serial drug testing using electrophysiologic techniques did not predict freedom from recurrence. These authors evaluated 19 patients with an idiopathic dilated cardiomyopathy who had a clinical history of sustained VT or VF. The average LVEF was 26%. The clinical arrhythmia was induced in 13 patients (68%), and in 9, arrhythmia became noninducible during therapy with an antiarrhythmic drug selected by electrophysiologic testing. During a 17-month follow-up, five of the nine drug responders (56%) had an arrhythmic recurrence whereas arrhythmia recurred in 5 of the 10 patients who remained inducible despite antiarrhythmic therapy.

In conclusion, electrophysiologic studies have an important role for drug selection in patients with a dilated cardiomyopathy who have a clinical history of sustained VT. The rate of arrhythmia induction in such patients is high, although response to drugs is low. However, similar to other groups of patients, noninducibility of arrhythmia predicts freedom from recurrence. The role of electrophysiologic testing in patients with a cardiomyopathy presenting with sudden death or VF is less well established as the rate of inducibility is lower.

Relationship Between LV Function, CHF, and Response to Drugs

A number of studies have reported that the efficacy of antiarrhythmic drugs in patients with a sustained ventricular tachyarrhythmia is related to LV function and the presence of CHF. In general, it has been observed that antiarrhythmic drugs are less effective in such patients (Table 35.12), likely due to the nonhemogeneity of the substrate, the presence of fibrosis and poor tissue perfusion, and alteration in the ability to bind drug or inability of these drugs to alter sufficiently the electrophysiologic properties of this severely damaged tissue. Hession and co-workers[156] reported that response to the antiarrhythmic drug moricizine was related to the

baseline LVEF. Similar results with moricizine were reported by Pratt and co-workers[157] in a group of 50 patients presenting with frequent VPBs and nonsustained VT. The LVEF was significantly lower (29%) in those patients discontinuing moricizine for inefficacy compared to the LVEF (40%) in those responding to the drug and continuing therapy ($p < .01$). A relationship between LVEF and response to tocainide[158] and encainide[159] also has been reported. Takarada and co-workers[160] correlated the response to drug with several factors. These authors reported a correlation between the presence of repetitive arrhythmia, the degree of LV dilation, and the severity of interstitial myocardial fibrosis. In this study of 42 patients, drug efficacy was unrelated to LV dimension or contractility, but was related to the presence of interstitial myocardial fibrosis, which represented 13% of the myocardium in responders and 26% in the nonresponders ($p < .02$).

The lower response rate in those with poorer LV function has not been a consistent finding with all drugs, however. For example, in a study of patients with a history of serious ventricular arrhythmia evaluated with propafenone, Cueni and Podrid[161] reported that the response rate to the drug was independent of LVEF.

There have been several long-term trials reporting a higher recurrence rate in those with reduced LV function regardless of initial suppression of arrhythmia by antiarrhythmic drugs (Table 35.13). Hohnloser and co-workers[162] evaluated 94 patients presenting with sustained VT (n = 74) or VF (n = 20). Univariate and multivariate analyses demonstrated that only the density of runs of nonsustained VT on baseline ambulatory monitoring and the initial LVEF were independent predictors of short- and long-term drug efficacy (Fig. 35.11). Antiarrhythmic drugs were effective less often in those with LVEF <35%. The LVEF was significantly lower in

TABLE 35.12. Relationship between LV function and response to individual drugs.

	Percent	
	Responders	Nonresponders
Hession et al. (moricizine)		
Overall (n = 102)	33	67
LVEF >40%	35 ⎤ a	65
LVEF <40%	18 ⎦	72
Average LVEF	46 ——— a ——— 31	
Pratt et al. (moricizine)		
Overall (n = 50)	46	54
LVEF >30%	61 ⎤ b	39
LVEF <30%	22 ⎦	78
Average LVEF	42 ——— b ——— 32	
Tordjman et al. (encainide)		
Overall (n = 92)	48	52
LVEF >35%	50 ⎤ c	50
LVEF <35%	29 ⎦	71
Average LVEF	44 ——— c ——— 33	
Hohnloser et al. (tocainide)		
Overall (n = 120)		
Average LVEF	43 ——— a ——— 37	
Cueni et al. (propafenone)		
Overall (n = 92)		
LVEF >50%	55	45
LVEF 30–50%	45	55
LVEF <30%	46	54

[a] $p < .05$; [b] $p < .04$; [c] $p < .03$.
LVEF = left ventricular ejection fraction.

TABLE 35.13. Relationship between LV function and response to drug therapy.

	LVEF (%)		
	>30	<30	p
Hohnloser[20]			
n = 94			
Average LVEF	55	24	.03
% drugs effective	46	34	.03
Total recurrences (%)	16	44	.003
Sudden death (%)	4	16	.003
Lampert[21]			
n = 161			
% controlled	67	33	.05
SCD (%)	7	35	.05
Pratt[19]			
n = 246			
% controlled	36	23	.005
% serious toxicity	2	15	.005

LVEF = left ventricular ejection fraction.

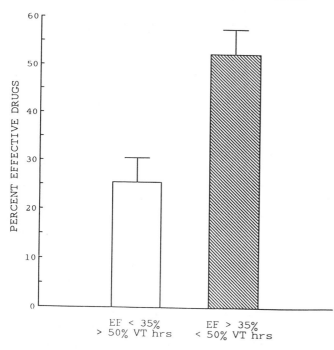

FIGURE 35.11. Relationship between drug efficacy, left ventricular ejection fraction (*EF*), and density of nonsustained ventricular tachycardia (*VT*) on ambulatory monitoring. Drugs are significantly more effective in patients with EF >35% and less frequent runs of VT compared to patients with EF <35% and frequent episodes of VT. Reprinted, with permission, from ref. 162.

patients without successful pharmacologic control of arrhythmia (29% vs. 42%). These data confirmed other studies reporting that drugs are less effective in those with a reduced LVEF and CHF. After a follow-up period of 12.9 months, there were 9 sudden deaths and 19 episodes of nonfatal VT. Patients who had recurrent arrhythmia had a poorer response to drugs and fewer drugs were effective, and they had a lower LVEF (31% vs. 44%). In the group with an LVEF <35%, recurrences of arrhythmia and sudden cardiac death were more frequent compared to those with LVEF >35%. Stepwise logistic regression analysis confirmed that an LVEF <35% was a powerful discriminator of initial drug efficacy and long-term outcome. Pratt and co-workers[163] reported similar results among 246 patients being treated for complex ventricular arrhythmia. In a long-term study of 161 patients with sustained VT or VF followed for up to 9 yr (average 32 months), Lampert and co-workers,[164] using a univariate analysis, reported that predictors of arrhythmia recurrence were a history of CHF, the presence of a third heart sound, a reduced LVEF, and the presence of rales, factors indicating poor LV function. Additionally, the density

and type of VPBs manifest during control monitoring and exercise testing before discharge were of significance. With a multivariate regression analysis, four variables emerged as independent predictors of sudden death including rales, number of VT runs during predischarge exercise testing, number of VPBs on monitoring, and a history of CHF. As with previous studies, a history of CHF and LVEF were significant predictors of arrhythmia suppression by antiarrhythmic drugs. Among patients controlled by a drug, 36% had CHF, 38% had cardiomegaly on chest x ray, and the average LVEF was 40%. In the group of patients with arrhythmia not controlled by antiarrhythmic drugs, 55% had CHF, 63% had cardiomegaly, and the LVEF was 32%. Other than these parameters, there were no other differences between the two groups.

Similar data have been reported when pharmacologic therapy is guided by electrophysiologic testing. Spielman and co-workers[165] retrospectively analyzed data in 84 patients with sustained VT. In only 29 patients (35%) was a successful medical regimen identified. Using a univariate analysis, four factors were associated with pharmacologic success, including age <45, hypokinesis as the only contraction abnormality, the absence of organic heart disease, and LVEF >50%. The strongest variable was LVEF. Swerdlow and co-workers[166] retrospectively analyzed data for 239 patients with sustained VT or VF. Multivariate regression analysis demonstrated that the two strongest predictors for both sudden cardiac death and total cardiac death were failure to identify an effective drug with electrophysiologic testing and NYHA functional class. LVEF also was an important predictor. Although most deaths were sudden, the severity of heart failure was the strongest independent predictor of cardiac mortality and sudden death. Last, Wilber and co-workers[167] retrospectively analyzed the long-term outcome of 166 patients surviving out-of-hospital sudden cardiac death who underwent electrophysiologic testing for drug selection. Using a Cox survival analysis, three variables were significant independent predictors of recurrent sudden death including persistence of inducible ventricular arrhythmia (relative risk 3.97), absence of cardiac surgery (relative risk 4.20) and LVEF <30% (relative risk 2.60). Regardless of the results of drug therapy evaluated electrophysiologically, the presence of a reduced LVEF increased mortality (Fig. 35.12). As reported by other studies, patients who had arrhythmia noninducible during drug therapy had better LV function (LVEF 42% vs. 30% in nonresponders). The LVEF was >50% among 32 patients with inducible arrhythmia and 30 patients (94%) responded to an antiarrhythmic drug. In contrast, only 26 of 45 patients (58%) with LVEF <30% responded. In the group of 50 patients with LVEF between 31% and 50%, 35 patients (70%) responded to drug.

Unfortunately, these many studies do not specifically

FIGURE 35.12. Survival, i.e., without recurrent cardiac arrest (*RCA*), in patients presenting with a RCA is related to the results of electrophysiologic testing and left ventricular ejection fraction (*EF*). Regardless of the results of EP testing and the response to antiarrhythmic drugs, survival rate is lower in patients with a reduced EF compared to those with a higher EF. Reprinted, with permission, from ref. 167. Copyright by the *New England Journal of Medicine*.

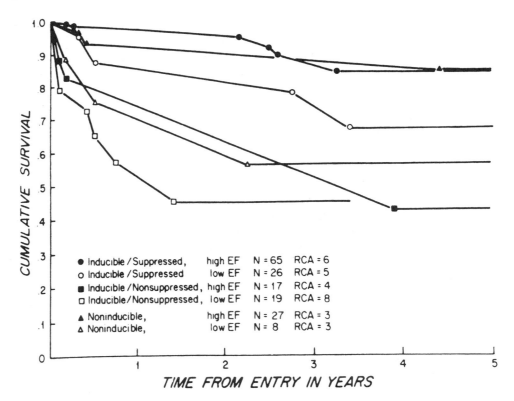

● Inducible / Suppressed,	high EF	N = 65	RCA = 6
○ Inducible / Suppressed	low EF	N = 26	RCA = 5
■ Inducible / Nonsuppressed,	high EF	N = 17	RCA = 4
□ Inducible / Nonsuppressed,	low EF	N = 19	RCA = 8
▲ Noninducible,	high EF	N = 27	RCA = 3
△ Noninducible,	low EF	N = 8	RCA = 3

evaluate the use of electrophysiologic studies or response to drugs in patients with LV dysfunction, reduced LVEF, and CHF as this subgroup is not separately analyzed.

Side Effects of Antiarrhythmic Drugs in Patients with CHF

Further impacting on the usefulness of antiarrhythmic drugs is the increased risk of drug-induced toxicity in patients with poor LV function and clinical CHF (Fig. 35.13). In the presence of CHF, drug pharmacokinetics are altered significantly and this can affect blood levels, metabolism of the agent, and, hence, dose requirements.[168] The plasma concentration of the drug is related to its volume of distribution, which is decreased in patients with CHF as a result of a reduction in tissue perfusion. Therefore, the plasma concentration of the drug at any dose is higher than what is achieved in patients without CHF. The reduction in tissue perfusion in patients with CHF results in changes of drug distribution, metabolism, and clearance largely due to a decrease in renal and hepatic blood flow. Additionally, there is a reduction in hepatic metabolic enzyme activity. As a result, the metabolism and clearance of these agents are impaired, causing an increase in their elimination half-time. Moreover, the time required to reach a steady-state blood level at any given dose of drug administered also is increased. Therefore, the ini-

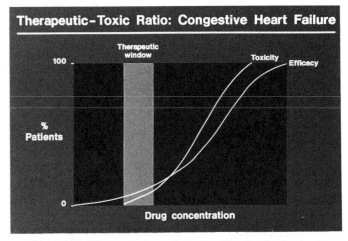

FIGURE 35.13. Therapeutic toxic ratio of antiarrhythmic drugs in patients with CHF. In the presence of CHF, drugs are less effective and tolerated poorly. The therapeutic window is narrow and often toxicity occurs before efficacy is evident.

tial dose of the antiarrhythmic drug administered to those with CHF should be low and upward dose titration carried out slowly and cautiously to avoid excessive blood levels and toxicity.

Another important concern is the potential for drug-drug interactions in patients with CHF who invariably receive polypharmacy. Diuretic drugs usually are prescribed to patients with CHF and the incidence of diuretic-induced hypokalemia and low magnesium is substantial, factors that may be important for the precipitation of ventricular arrhythmia, especially a sustained ventricular tachyarrhythmia, in a vulnerable patient who has underlying myocardial disease and poor LV function.[17] It also has been reported that hypokalemia may interfere with and negate antiarrhythmic drug activity. Low potassium alters the electrophysiologic properties of the myocardium and produces an enhancement of membrane automaticity, excitability, and a reduction in refractory periods. These changes are opposite to those resulting from antiarrhythmic drugs.[19] In some situations, hypokalemia and the associated low magnesium may be a factor increasing the risk of antiarrhythmic drug-induced aggravation of arrhythmia, especially the precipitation of torsade de pointes.[169]

Digoxin also is a commonly administered drug in patients with CHF and a number of drugs have been reported to interact with this agent. Most frequently reported is quinidine, although drug interactions with other antiarrhythmic drugs also have been observed.[170] The combined use of antiarrhythmic drugs with other agents that produce hemodynamic effects and that are used occasionally in patients with CHF such as calcium channel blockers, nitrates, and beta-blockers may result in further exacerbation of CHF or hypotension. Although other drug-drug interactions have not been systematically studied, it is likely that in patients with a cardiomyopathy and CHF, many antiarrhythmic drugs will result in potentially serious drug-drug interactions.

One of the most frequent side effects is aggravation of arrhythmia, which is a serious complication caused by each of the antiarrhythmic drugs[171] (Fig. 35.14). There have been a number of definitions for arrhythmia aggravation[172] (Table 35.14). However, criteria commonly accepted are an exacerbation of a preexisting arrhythmia, the occurrence of a new arrhythmia for the

TABLE 35.14. Definition of arrhythmia aggravation.

Aggravation of existing ventricular arrhythmia
  Increased duration or frequency of arrhythmia
  Increase in numbers of VPBs, couplets, or runs of VT
  Altered rate of arrhythmia
Development of a new arrhythmia
  Supraventricular tachycardia (e.g., atrial tachycardia with block, nonparoxysmal junctional tachycardia)
  Ventricular tachyarrhythmia
    Nonsustained VT converted to sustained VT
    Polymorphic VT
    Torsade des pointes
    Ventricular fibrillation
Bradycardia
  Sinus arrest, sinus exit block, or sinus bradycardia
  AV block

VPB = ventricular premature beat; VT = ventricular tachycardia; AV = arteriovenous.

patient, or a a bradyarrhythmia resulting from depression of sinus or atrioventricular nodal function. The overall incidence of arrhythmia aggravation has been reported to be 9% when noninvasive methods are used to evaluate drug effect, whereas the incidence is 18% when electrophysiologic testing is used for drug selection (Table 35.15).

To establish if there are any predictors of this complication, Slater and co-workers[173] retrospectively analyzed 51 patients who experienced arrhythmia aggravation during in-hospital evaluation of antiarrhythmic drugs and compared these patients to a group of 102 patients who also underwent in-hospital evaluation of drugs, but who never experienced arrhythmia aggravation with any drug evaluated. The only variables that were associated with arrhythmia aggravation were

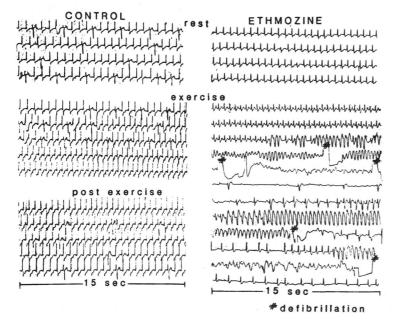

FIGURE 35.14. Example of aggravation of arrhythmia with an antiarrhythmic drug. Before therapy (control) only frequent ventricular premature beats are present at rest and with exercise. During therapy with ethmozine, exercise provokes ventricular fibrillation requiring five shocks before sinus rhythm is restored.

TABLE 35.15. Incidence of arrhythmia aggravation.

	Noninvasive	Invasive
Disopyramide	6	5
Encainide	15	37
Ethmozine	11	14
Flecainide	12	—
Indecainide	19	—
Lorcainide	8	24
Mexiletine	7	20
Procainamide	9	21
Propafenone	8	15
Quinidine	15	20
Tocainide	8	5
Overall	9	18

the nature of the presenting arrhythmia and the presence of LV dysfunction. When patients presented with sustained VT or VF, there was a significantly greater risk of experiencing aggravation when compared to the risk in those presenting with VPBs or runs of nonsustained VT. The average LVEF was 37% in patients who experienced an exacerbation of arrhythmia compared to 43% among those who did not have this side effect. Although this did not quite reach statistical significance, patients with CHF due to systolic dysfunction (LVEF <35%) had a significantly greater likelihood of experiencing aggravation of arrhythmia compared to patients without CHF and a LVEF >35%. No other clinical parameter predicted this complication. Other authors have observed a similar relationship between LV function, the nature of the arrhythmia, and the risk of arrhythmia worsening.[174]

In a study Au and co-workers,[175] no clinical features were associated with an increased risk of arrhythmia aggravation except for a higher frequency of digoxin use, suggesting that patients who develop arrhythmia aggravation were more likely to have LV dysfunction.

In a study of Minardo and co-workers,[176] factors associated with the provocation of VF by antiarrhythmic drugs were digoxin use, diuretic administration, and the presence of hypokalemia. As with the above studies, this study also suggests that the presence of underlying CHF and the need for therapy to control its symptoms are factors associated with an increased risk of arrhythmia aggravation.

Another important and potentially serious cardiac complication due to antiarrhythmic drugs is the precipitation or exacerbation of CHF. Each of the antiarrhythmic drugs is negatively inotropic, especially of concern in patients with underlying LV dysfunction and CHF (Table 35.16). In a retrospective review of 100 patients receiving therapy with disopyramide, Podrid and co-workers[177] reported that exacerbation of CHF occurred in 55% of patients who had a clinical history of heart failure, whereas this complication developed in 5% of those without a previous history of LV decompensation. In another retrospective review of an experience with the newer antiarrhythmic drugs, Ravid and co-workers[178] reported that CHF occurred in 1.8% of patients, but the incidence of worsening CHF was 3.9% among the group of patients who had a clinical history of CHF (Table 35.17). Only 1 of 238 patients (0.4%) without a history of CHF had this complication compared with 19 of 167 patients (11.4%) who had a clinical history of LV decompensation. The only factors predictive of CHF exacerbation were a previous history of CHF, LVEF <35% (indicating systolic dysfunction as the cause of the CHF), and presence of an idiopathic cardiomyopathy.

Although CHF has been reported only infrequently as a complication from the antiarrhythmic drugs, there are a few studies in which the effect of these drugs on LV function have been evaluated. In most of these trials, LV function has been determined by radionuclide scanning, which is used to establish the LVEF. With most drugs, no significant change in LVEF has been

TABLE 35.16. Hemodynamic effects of antiarrhythmic drugs.

Drug	PAP/PCWP	SVR	Contractility	SVI/CI	LVEF	Clinical CHF
Quinidine	0	↓	0 or ↓	0	0	±
Procainamide	0	↓	0 or ↓	0	0	±
Disopyramide	↑	↑	↓ ↓ ↓	↓ ↓	↓	++
Mexiletine	0	sl ↓	0 or ↓	0	0	±
Tocainide	0	sl ↓	0 or ↓	0	0	±
Ethmozine	sl ↑	0	0 or ↓	0	0	+
Encainide	0	↑	↓	↓	0	+
Flecainide	↑	↑	↓ ↓	↓ ↓	↓	++
Propafenone	↑	↑	↓ ↓	↓	0 or ↓	+
Amiodarone	0	↓	0 or ↓	0	0	

PAP = pulmonary artery pressure; PCWP = pulmonary capillary wedge pressure; SVR = systemic vascular resistance; SVI = stroke volume index; CI = cardiac index; LVEF = left ventricular ejection fraction; CHF = congestive heart failure.

TABLE 35.17. Incidence of CHF induction by antiarrhythmic drugs.

Drug	Drug tests (total)	Daily maintenance dose (mg)	Precipitation of CHF n (%)	History of CHF n (%)	CHF aggravation in CHF group n (%)
Encainide	153	75–200	4 (2.6)	70 (46)	4 (5.7)
Ethmozine	125	600–1200	3 (2.4)	62 (50)	3 (4.8)
Lorcainide	144	200–400	1 (0.7)	63 (44)	1 (1.6)
Mexiletine	352	300–1200	3 (0.9)	146 (41)	3 (2.1)
Propafenone	108	450–900	5 (4.7)	43 (40)	4 (9.3)
Tocainide	251	600–2400	4 (6.1)	107 (43)	4 (3.7)
Total	1133	—	20 (1.8)	491 (43)	19 (3.9)

CHF = congestive heart failure.

observed, although worsening of CHF during long-term therapy does occur. Gottlieb and co-workers[179] invasively evaluated 30 class III or IV patients with CHF who had a mean LVEF of 19%. Each patient received a single oral dose of 50 mg of encainide and invasive hemodynamic measurements were obtained before and for 3 hr after receiving the drug. These authors observed that by 90 to 120 min after drug administration, encainide caused a significant deterioration in cardiac performance as determined by a fall in cardiac index by 22%, a decrease in stroke work index by 31%, and an increase in LV filling pressure by 16%. Clinically, 8 of the 30 patients had a clinical worsening of CHF symptoms requiring therapy. In this study, serum levels of encainide and its active metabolites were in the therapeutic range.

In another study, Gottlieb and co-workers[180] again evaluated encainide as well as single oral doses of procainamide (750 mg) and tocainide (600 mg) in 21 patients with severe chronic heart failure; their average LVEF was 21%. As with the previous study, all patients were in functional class III or IV. Invasive hemodynamic variables were obtained before administration of the drug and at each 30-min interval for the subsequent 3 hr (Fig. 35.15). All three drugs caused a decrease in cardiac performance, including a decrease in cardiac index, stroke volume index, and mean arterial pressure and an increase in systemic vascular resistance.

Pratt and co-workers[163] evaluated 246 patients with complex ventricular arrhythmia requiring antiarrhythmic drug therapy. In their population, 42% had LV dysfunction and CHF. These authors utilized eight different antiarrhythmic drugs. In this study, there was a significant relationship between the measured LVEF and clinical CHF and the occurrence of life-threatening complications from the antiarrhythmic drugs, including exacerbation of CHF and arrhythmia aggravation. Life-threatening complications resulting from antiarrhythmic

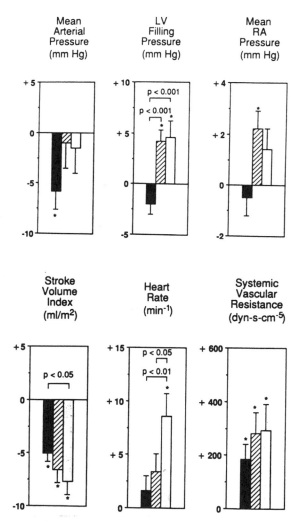

FIGURE 35.15. Effects of procainamide (solid bar), tocainide (striped bar), and encainide (open bar) on invasive hemodynamic parameters in patients with severe left ventricular dysfunction. *indicates significance ($p < .05$) from control value for each drug. p value shown indicates significance between the treatment groups. RA = right atrial; LV = left ventricular. Reprinted, with permission, from ref. 180. Copyright by the American Heart Association.

therapy occurred 7 times more frequently in patients with LVEF <30% compared to those patients with LVEF >30%. Life-threatening complications also occurred 7 times more frequently in patients who had nonsustained VT and an LVEF <30% compared to those patients with LVEF >30%.

In conclusion, antiarrhythmic drugs are more likely to cause side effects in patients with reduced LVEF and CHF. Of most concern is a higher incidence of worsening of heart failure and arrhythmia aggravation in this group. It is recommended that if antiarrhythmic therapy is required, the initial dose be reduced and upward titration be performed more slowly and carefully so as to avoid serious toxicity.

Bradyarrhythmic Death in Patients with CHF

Many studies have reported that the most common mechanism for sudden death is a ventricular tachyarrhythmia. Iseri et al.[181] reviewed the records of 133 patients with prehospital cardiac arrest. Seventy-five percent had sustained VT or VF, whereas only 25% had bradycardia, heart block, or electromechanical dissociation. Nickolic et al.[182] reviewed 21 recordings of patients who experienced sudden death during ambulatory monitoring and reported that the mechanism was sustained VT or VF in 81%. Other authors have reported that in 76% to 92% of patients, sudden death is due to VT or VF as documented by ambulatory monitoring.[183–186] These studies have not established a relationship between the nature and extent of the heart disease and the mechanism of sudden death. CHF is associated with biochemical alterations, activation of the sympathetic nervous system, and neuroregulatory abnormalities and it has been suggested that mechanisms other than a primary ventricular tachyarrhythmia may account for sudden death in this population. Of importance are bradyarrhythmias, conduction abnormalities, and electromechanical dissociation.

Luu and co-workers[187] evaluated the etiology of sudden death in a cohort of 216 hospitalized patients with class III or IV CHF awaiting cardiac transplantation. There were 21 episodes of cardiac arrest occurring in these patients. Sinus bradycardia, high degree heart block, or electromechanical dissociation was the cause of the arrest in 13 patients (62%), and VT or VF was the mechanism in 8 (38%). The patients who had a bradyarrhythmic arrest were similar to those who had a ventricular tachyarrhythmia with respect to age, history of sustained or nonsustained VT, treatment with antiarrhythmic agents, presence of bundle branch block, or first degree AV block and LV function. Only a history of prior MI separated the two groups, being more common in the group with VT or VF (8 of 8), in contrast to those with a bradyarrhythmic cause for the cardiac arrest (6 of 13). No precipitating cause for the arrest could be established in 7 of 13 patients (54%) with a bradycardiac death and 5 of 8 (63%) with VT or VF.

This study is in contrast with the previous reports in which VT or VF was the etiology of sudden death in most patients. Although bradycardiac arrests in heart failure have been anecdotally reported,[188,189] this is the first large series to suggest that bradycardic mechanisms may play a major role in sudden death in the population of patients with serious CHF. However, most of the previous reports involved outpatients who were otherwise stable, whereas the study of Luu and co-workers[187] involved a patient population hospitalized because of severe CHF and end-stage heart disease who were awaiting cardiac transplantation. In the study by Iseril et al.,[181] 75% of all bradyarrhythmic deaths were felt to be the result of an acute process, particularly an acute MI that was documented in two thirds of the patients with a bradyarrhythmia. This in in contrast to the study of Luu in which only 3 of 13 patients with a bradyarrhythmic event had an acute infarction.

The implications of the Luu study are important and suggest that in more than half of patients with severe class III or IV CHF, sudden death is not due to a primary ventricular arrhythmia, and will therefore not respond to any directed antiarrhythmic therapy. A major limitation of the study, however, is the patient selection bias. The patients who required hospitalization and were awaiting transplantation because of the severity of the CHF represent a small subset of patients with cardiomyopathy and CHF. It is not clear that these findings can be generalized to the CHF population as a whole. This criticism aside, it is clear that the issue of bradyarrhythmic arrest in the CHF population deserves further study.

Although the mechanisms responsible for VT and VF are fairly well defined, with reentry in an area of scarred myocardium being most frequent, the mechanism responsible for a serious bradyarrhythmia is less certain. Greenberg[189] has described seven clinical settings in which sudden death can be the result of a bradycardia or asystole: (a) bradycardia after inferior MI, (b) heart block after anterior MI, (c) asystole after infarction, (d) myocardial rupture, (e) drug-induced bradycardia; (f) bradycardia producing VT/VF, and (g) idiopathic sudden bradycardiac-asystolic cardiac arrest. This author suggested that epidemiologically, an idiopathic bradycardic arrest is most important. Three mechanisms have been proposed to explain this syndrome. The first represents an abnormal activation of the Bezold-Jarisch reflex. The Bezold-Jarisch reflex has several characteristics, namely a vagally mediated induction of bradycardia and hypotension, as well as inhibition and withdrawal of sympathetic tone.[190] In a normal individual without heart disease and LV failure, mechanisms are recruited to compensate for and reverse the bradycardia and hypotension. In patients with CHF, LV decompensation can quickly result in a volume-overloaded state, stimulating myocardial stretch receptors and activating the Bezold-Jarisch reflex. Since patients with CHF are often dependent on a high resting sympathetic tone as a compensatory mechanism, inhibition of sympathetic outflow, even if briefly, can have a significantly deleterious effect. An additional factor is that patients with LV dysfunction have been shown to have a selective impairment of baroreflex-mediated vasoconstrictor responses. Ferguson and colleagues[191] studied 11 patients with severe LV dysfunction, subjecting them to a simulated orthostatic stress. They compared the results to similar experiments performed in 17 normal controls. During unloading of baroreceptors, forearm vascular resistance increased appropriately in normal individuals; however, patients with LV dysfunction failed to develop vasoconstriction and paradoxically developed vasodilation. This effect was more pronounced at higher levels of orthostatic stress. The implication is that hypotension in patients with CHF is more dangerous since these patients lack compensatory mechanisms to restore adequate blood pressure.

Kontos and co-workers[192] reported that global hypoxia generated by a decrease in inspired O_2 concentration during constant ventilation resulted in significant bradycardia. Interestingly, severe global hypoxemia did not induce ventricular arrhythmia. The authors postulated that a uniformly hypoxic heart was not an appropriate substrate for reentry, but that regional hypoxia was necessary.

Taken together, these mechanisms suggest a sequence of events that may result in a bradyarrhythmic event and sudden cardiac death in patients with CHF.[189] Exacerbation of CHF causes LV dilatation triggering stretch receptors and the Bezold-Jarisch reflex. This acts to decrease heart rate and inhibits sympathetic tone, resulting in peripheral vasodilation and a fall in mean arterial pressure. As a result of impairment of the baroreceptors, compensatory vasoconstriction does not occur. Additionally, because of progressive pulmonary congestion, hypoxemia develops. Coronary perfusion pressure falls and coronary oxygen delivery is reduced. The heart becomes globally ischemic and myocardial energy stores are utilized and exhausted. Eventually, asystolic cardiac arrest ensues.

Although this sequence of events is based on speculation, it is likely that some combination of these described mechanisms does account for the occurrence of bradycardic cardiac arrest. Further research is needed to define more accurately the epidemiology of this problem, the precise mechanisms, and its prevention.

Surgical Treatment of Ventricular Tachyarrhythmias

Pharmacologic therapy is the cornerstone of therapy for serious ventricular tachyarrhythmia; however, other approaches are required for patients who do not respond to antiarrhythmic drugs or who do not tolerate these agents. This is especially the situation with patients who have a cardiomyopathy, reduced LV function, and CHF. Surgical techniques for the treatment of VT have been available for a decade and are particularly effective in patients with sustained monomorphic VT resulting from ischemic heart disease, especially when an LV aneurysm is present. The literature available unfortunately does not analyze separately patients who have CHF, although most patients who undergo surgery do have significant LV dysfunction. Additionally, there are no reports specifically dealing with patients who have a nonischemic or idiopathic cardiomyopathy and CHF.

The first report of a surgical approach for the treatment of ventricular tachyarrhythmias was in 1959 by Couch,[193] who resected an LV aneurysm in one patient as treatment for a life-threatening ventricular arrhythmia. During the 1970s, several investigators reported that coronary revascularization with resection of the injured myocardium was associated with a high mortality and a low cure rate.[194–196] In 1975, Witting and Boineau[197] and Gallager and co-workers[198] separately reported the use of intraoperative epicardial mapping as a guide to the surgical resection of the tissue responsible for the VT genesis. Although an important step, it was shown that the site of origin of the VT was the endocardium and the epicardial map does not always reflect the VT focus. In 1978, Guiraudon and co-workers[199] introduced another surgical technique known as the encircling endocardial ventriculotomy, which does not require electrophysiologic mapping. With this technique, a surgical incision is made around the entire border of infarcted or aneurysmal tissue guided by visual inspection. As a result, the damaged tissue, the site of origin of the VT, is isolated electrically from the rest of the myocardium and any arrhythmia originating in this area is unable to exit into the normal tissue. Unfortunately, clinical experience has shown that this technique is associated with a high incidence of LV dysfunction and CHF and, therefore has been largely abandoned.[200,201] In 1979, Josephson and co-workers[202] described a surgical technique involving endocardial mapping to localize the site of origin of VT and a subendocardial resection of the arrhythmogenic tissue. This has become the standard technique for the arrhythmia surgery, although this approach has been modified by other investigators. Moran and co-workers[203] described the extended endocardial resection procedure, which involves resection of all the endocardial fibrosis associated with an aneurysm or infarct. Further modifications include the addition of cryoablation or the use of laser as an adjunctive procedure.[204,205]

The surgical technique of endocardial resection has been in wide use and it is often combined with pharmacologic therapy or an (ICD) implantable cardioverter/defibrillator. Simple LV aneurysm resection is not effective for preventing ventricular tachyarrhythmia,[206] whereas many studies have reported that arrhythmic surgery guided by intraoperative mapping is a more effective technique. A report by Zee-Cheng and co-workers[207] described the use of endocardial resection not guided by electrophysiologic mapping, but rather combined with electrophysiologic-guided antiarrhythmic drug therapy. However, when using this technique, there was a 37% recurrence rate. In comparison, Borggrefe and co-workers[208] evaluated the outcome of 665 patients included in a registry and reported only a 17% failure rate when a map-guided approach is used. Efforts to improve the success rate and reduce the time required for intraoperative electrophysiologic mapping include the use of an endocardial sock or plunge electrodes placed through the mitral valve. A computer is used to compile the data and generate an activation sequence map so that the earliest area of LV activation, representing the site of origin of the VT, can be rapidly identified and surgically excised[209-211] (Fig. 35.16). This new technology makes mapping possible even if only a nonsustained VT is induced since only several beats during VT are required.

These surgical approaches have provided new options for the treatment of VT, especially when it is refractory to drug therapy. However, the cumulative experience during the past decade indicates that in patients with significant heart disease and poor LV function, there is a high operative mortality and early post-operative reinducibility is not infrequent. The results are better in patients with intact LV function.[212,213]

Miller and co-workers[213] retrospectively evaluated 100 patients with drug refractory VT who underwent map-guided subendocardial resection. Multivariate analysis identified multiple disparate sites of origin of the VT (>5 cm between the sites) and the absence of a discrete LV aneurysm as the only independent variables associated with failure of subendocardial resection. Two other variables also significantly associated with surgical failure are a site of origin located in the inferior wall and VT with a right bundle branch block morphology. Although not included in the study, patients with a cardiomyopathy, regardless of the etiology, are likely to have these features and are therefore poor candidates for such surgery. In such patients who have significant LV dysfunction, there is not only a substantial failure

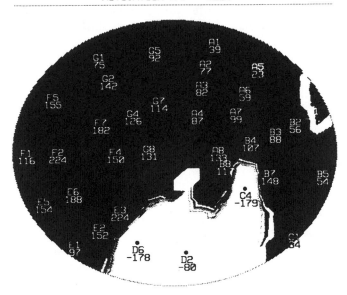

FIGURE 35.16. Example of electrophysiologic mapping during ventricular tachycardia before arrhythmic surgery. Shaded area represents normal activation sequence while white area is region of earliest activation, representing site of origin of VT. Letters and numbers (e.g., A1, F5) represent different electrodes while number below represents time of activation in msec in relation to the reference surface QRS complex. Thus, areas D6, C4, and D2 represent activation before the enscription of the QRS complex and, hence, the site of VT origin.

rate, but the surgery itself is associated with a high mortality. Garan and co-workers[214] analyzed the data on 36 patients with VT who had map-guided endocardial resection. The operative mortality was 17% and the strongest independent predictive factor for operative death was poor systolic function of the nonaneurysmal ventricular segments.

The use of this surgery is problematic in cardiomyopathic patients in whom the myocardium is diffusely damaged, resulting in many potential sites of VT origin. To treat effectively patients with multiple VT site and VT morphologies, Krafcheck and co-workers[215] reviewed a 5-yr experience using a map-guided regional approach in 39 patients with ischemic heart disease. During a 22-month follow-up, recurrence rate was 38% in patients who had a localized resection and only 4% in patients who underwent a regional approach with ablation of multiple sites. Unfortunately, this study included only patients with an ischemic cardiomyopathy and therefore data about the use of this approach in patients who have a nonischemic cardiomyopathy and no localized aneurysm or infarcted tissue are unavailable.

Another modification to this surgical approach was described by Kron and co-workers[216] and Haines and co-workers,[217] who use sequential endocardial resections. After a map-guided endocardial resection is performed, subsequent attempts to induce VT are made with further mapping and resection until VT is no longer inducible. The reported success rate is higher in those undergoing multiple resections (87%) compared to a 73% success rate in a group of patients who have only one area resected.

Other modifications of an endocardial resection to deal with multiple sites of origin of VT include mapping with a balloon catheter that has 112 electrodes permitting more accurate mapping, map-guided cryosurgery for ablation of multiple sites, encircling endocardial cryoablation, and laser photocoagulation.[218–220]

The experience with surgical endocardial resection in patients with nonischemic heart disease is limited, but the results are poor when compared to patients with an ischemic etiology. A report by Frank and co-workers[221] involved 97 patients, 83% of whom had ischemic heart disease and 17% of whom had a nonischemic etiology. The recurrence rate after surgery in the ischemic group was 5% compared with a 45% failure rate in those with a nonischemic etiology. With the availability and growing use of the (ICD),[222] endocardial resection and cryoablation usually are reserved for relatively young patients with underlying coronary artery disease who have a discrete LV aneurysm, myocardial scar, or other anatomic abnormality; who have inducible monomorphic VT; and who are otherwise good operative risks. Surgery for patients who have poor LV function, who are older, who have diffuse and extensive LV scarring and multiple sites of origin of VT is associated with a high mortality and poor outcome. For these patients, surgery may not be the best option.

In conclusion, arrhythmia surgery for therapy of VT has become an accepted and effective approach for management. However, the largest experience and best results are in patients who have sustained monomorphic VT, ischemic heart disease, a discrete LV aneurysm or area of myocardial scar, intact LV function and no CHF, and who are younger. In other groups of patients, the operative mortality is high and recurrences frequent despite surgery. This is no doubt related to the extensive LV damage and the inability to resect successfully all arrhythmogenic tissue. With the emergence of computerized mapping systems, electrophysiologic mapping is more accurate since multiple electrodes are used and there is no longer a need for induction of a sustained arrhythmia as such computerized systems require only several beats of VT for analysis. The ICD has also had an enormous impact on the need for arrhythmia surgery, especially in patients who are high surgical risks and are less likely to have a successful outcome. This includes a substantial number of patients with cardiomyopathy of any etiology, significant LV dysfunction, and CHF. Although the ICD may not replace map-guided techniques in low risk patients, these two methodologies are complementary and often are used together.

Implantable Cardioverter Defibrillator

The ICD is well established as a highly effective treatment for preventing sudden death in patients who have experienced life-threatening ventricular arrhythmia. The device was conceived and developed by Mirowski[222–224] and since the first implants in 1980, the indications for the use of an ICD have evolved. At the present time, the device is recommended in the following groups of patients: (a) those who have experienced sudden cardiac death due to VF or sustained VT, who have not responded to or tolerated antiarrhythmic drugs, and who are not candidates for map guided surgery, (b) those who have had recurrent arrhythmia after arrhythmic surgery, (c) those who have survived a cardiac arrest and do not have inducible arrhythmia during programmed ventricular stimulation and (d) those with a dilated cardiomyopathy who have suffered a cardiac arrest and are awaiting cardiac transplantation.

In some patients, especially those with severe LV dysfunction and CHF, the ICD may be the preferred and initial form of therapy since antiarrhythmic drugs frequently are ineffective and are associated with serious toxicity in such patients. Although there is interest in and potential benefit from the prophylactic use of the ICD in high-risk patients, especially those with a cardiomyopathy, CHF, and nonsustained VT, this is currently an investigational use of the device as it has not been clearly demonstrated as yet that the individual patient at risk can be reliably identified.

In studies involving patients who have experienced sudden cardiac death, the ICD has been associated with an impressive reduction in mortality from a serious ventricular tachyarrhythmia, although there is still a substantial cardiac mortality from progressive CHF. Each of these reports involves patients with diverse heart disease and most have poor LV function and CHF. However, patients with a cardiomyopathy and poor LV function are not separately analyzed. In an earlier report by Mirowski and co-workers[224] involving 52 patients with an ICD, the sudden death rate was 7.2% after a mean follow-up period of 14 months. Echt and co-workers[225] reported on 70 patients treated with the AICD in whom the sudden death rate was 1.9% during a mean follow-up period of 9 months. A similar low sudden death rate has been reported by others.[226–229] In a large series, Kelly and co-workers[228,229] reported on 94 patients who had an ICD implant. The 6- and 12-month survival rates by life-table analysis were 98.7% and 95.4%, respectively, and 46 patients received at least one appropriate shock during the follow-up.

Recently, two large studies have reported a long-term follow-up. Winkle and co-workers[230] reviewed their experience in 270 patients receiving an ICD over a 7-yr period. Coronary artery disease was present in 78% of patients and the average LVEF was 34%. During the follow-up, there were 7 sudden cardiac deaths and 30 nonsudden cardiac deaths, 18 of which were secondary to CHF. The actuarial incidence of sudden death, total cardiac death, and total mortality was 1%, 7%, and 8%, respectively, at 1 yr and 4%, 24%, and 26%, respectively, at 5 yr. Similar results were reported by Tordjman-Fuchs and co-workers[231] in 285 patients with out-of-hospital cardiac arrests.

The role of the ICD in patients with significant LV dysfunction has been reported by several investigators. In a study of 70 patients with LV dysfunction and sustained ventricular tachyarrhythmias, Tchou and co-workers[232] reported a 2-yr survival with the ICD of 93.4% in contrast to a projected survival of 60.3%, based on recurrence of the clinical arrhythmia and the delivery of an appropriate discharge by the ICD. Twenty-five patients with an LVEF of 30% or less were analyzed separately and their survival was 86.7%, in contrast to a projected survival of 56.9%. In contrast, Luceri and co-workers[226] reported that patients with LV dysfunction had a higher sudden death mortality compared to those with better LV function despite the ICD. These authors suggested that most of the cases of sudden death in patients with the AICD resulted from electromechanical dissociation and bradyarrhythmia, for which the ICD is ineffective.

Although the report from Luceri et al. raises important concerns, others have reported improved survival with the ICD in patients with poor LV function. Fogoros and co-workers[233] reported on 119 patients with significant LV dysfunction who received the ICD. Patients were divided into two groups. Group A included 40 patients with an LVEF <30% and Group B included 79 patients with an EF ≥30%. For each group, the cumulative survival was compared with the projected survival if the ICD had not been present, based on the assumption that an appropriate ICD shock represented the occurrence of an arrhythmia that would have resulted in death if the patient did not have the device. For group A, the 3-yr cumulative survival rate was 67% compared to a projected survival of 6% ($p < .001$). For group B, the 3-yr cumulative survival rate was 96% compared to a projected survival rate of 46% ($p < .001$). The authors concluded that the ICD significantly prolonged overall survival even in patients with poor LV function and CHF. Similar results were reported by deMarchena and co-workers[234] in 39 patients with coronary artery disease, LVEF <30% (average = 21%), and sustained VT or VF requiring the ICD (Fig. 35.17). There were no significant clinical differences between survivors and nonsurvivors, although

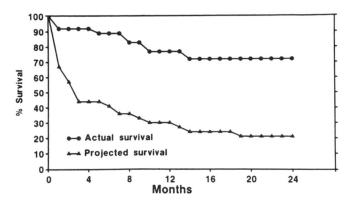

FIGURE 35.17. Actual and projected survival in patients with CHF receiving the automatic implantable cardioverter-defibrillator. The actuarial survival at 1 and 2 yr was 77% and 72% for those with an AICD compared to a projected survival of 30% and 21%, respectively (based on number of patients not receiving any shocks). The difference in survival is significant at 1 yr ($p < .01$) and 2 yr ($p < .05$). Reprinted, with permission, from ref. 234.

there was a trend toward a lower LVEF in those who died.

Although the ICD will prevent sudden death from a tachyarrhythmia, it has no role for preventing sudden death due to a bradyarrhythmia or asystole. This may be an important cause of death in those patients with severe, class IV CHF. Additionally, many of these patients die of progressive CHF. A decision about the ICD in such terminally ill patients, especially those who are older or who are not candidates for transplantation, must consider the potential etiology of death, the risks associated with ICD implantation, the benefit of the ICD, as well as ethical and economic issues involved with its use.

On the basis of these studies, it has been suggested that in patients with a cardiomyopathy and significant CHF, the ICD may be an effective "bridge," preventing sudden cardiac death in patients awaiting cardiac transplantation. It is well recognized that there is a substantial sudden death rate among patients on waiting lists for transplantation. Not infrequently, patients with cardiomyopathy who have experienced sudden cardiac death are appropriate candidates for cardiac transplantation. In some centers, cardiac transplantation is the preferred therapy for such patients who are young. In these patients, the ICD as a bridge to transplantation may be an important intervention for preventing sudden death during the waiting period, especially if there is a delay in obtaining a donor heart. Unfortunately, there have been no studies in which the ICD has been used for this indication. Since a bradyarrhythmia may be the cause of death,[187] the ICD will be ineffective in such cases. Additionally, there may be some cases in which death is due to electromechanical dissociation, for which the ICD is likewise ineffective. An important consideration is the cost of the ICD, which is in addition to the cost for transplantation.

In conclusion, the ICD is a highly effective therapy for preventing recurrent sudden cardiac death in patients who have survived this event or for those with hemodynamically compromising sustained VT. Its use in patients felt to be at high risk for sudden cardiac death has been suggested and there are now ongoing studies evaluating its role in such patients. However, benefit from the ICD in such patients may depend on the ability to identify reliably the individual patient at risk for sudden death. Although the use of the ICD as a bridge to cardiac transplantation in patients with a severe cardiomyopathy is of use, it is a costly procedure that must be considered in addition to the cost of cardiac transplantation itself. Additionally, there are, as yet, no well controlled studies documenting its value for this indication. Appropriate patient selection for this approach is essential.

Recommendations for Antiarrhythmic Therapy of Patients with CHF

Before evaluating the arrhythmia and deciding about antiarrhythmic drug therapy, patients should be stable for several days. LV function should be optimized and CHF compensated. Electrolyte abnormalities must be corrected and active ischemia treated. Once the patient is stable, most arrhythmias resolve. However, if the arrhythmia persists, a decision about therapy must be individualized based on the indication for therapy and the benefits from the antiarrhythmic drug versus the risk of that therapy. In general, arrhythmias are treated because they are associated with symptoms and the suppressing of arrhythmia eliminates them or because the arrhythmia is judged to be potentially serious, associated with an increased risk for sudden death. The rationale for therapy is that arrhythmia suppression will prevent sudden death and prolong life. Although it is well established that antiarrhythmic drug therapy will suppress spontaneously occurring arrhythmias and therefore eliminates symptoms related to them, there are no data that these agents will prevent a sustained ventricular tachyarrhythmia and sudden death. One exception are patients who have already experienced sustained VT or sudden cardiac death due to VF.

Unfortunately, there are many risks associated with these agents, including cardiac toxicity, other organ toxicity, and nuisance and disturbing side effects. It is important, therefore, that a decision regarding antiarrhythmic therapy be individualized, based on a benefit/risk analysis.

For the patient with asymptomatic ventricular arrhythmia, the only benefit of therapy is prevention of sudden death, yet there are no data that drugs are effective. Since there are substantial risks associated with antiarrhythmic drugs, for most of these patients therapy is not recommended, although when there are frequent, rapid, and long runs of asymptomatic nonsustained VT, therapy may prove beneficial. If the patient has symptomatic ventricular or supraventricular arrhythmia, the nature, frequency, and severity of the symptoms and the benefit of their relief must be weighed against the risks of antiarrhythmic drug therapy. For the patient who has had a sustained VT or VF, therapy will prevent a recurrence and it prolongs life. Pharmacologic therapy usually is the first approach despite the risk associated with these drugs, which unfortunately is highest in the patient with CHF. If drugs are ineffective, poorly tolerated, or judged too risky, alternative therapies include the ICD, surgery, or cardiac transplantation. There is a growing belief that in view of the low success rate and high incidence of toxicity, antiarrhythmic drug therapy should not be the first or preferred approach in patients with LV dysfunction, CHF, and serious ventricular tachyarrhythmia. Unfortunately, most of these patients are poor surgical candidates and the success rate is low because of the diffuse nature of the disease. The ICD often is considered to be the best option for such patients. However, many patients with an ICD will still require antiarrhythmic therapy because of long runs of nonsustained VT or supraventricular arrhythmia, which may repeatedly activate the device. When the patient has class IV CHF, sudden death often is due to a bradyarrhythmia and therapy directed against a tachyarrhythmia is not of benefit. Additionally, most deaths in this group are due to progressive CHF even in the patient with a history of sustained VT or VF. For such patients who are not transplant candidates, a decision about the ICD must include ethical and economic considerations. An alternative is empiric amiodarone therapy. Preliminary data suggest that it may prolong life and since the survival in these patients is poor, the risk of amiodarone toxicity during long-term therapy is of less importance.

When using antiarrhythmic drugs in these patients to treat either ventricular or supraventricular arrhythmia,

TABLE 35.18. Antiarrhythmic drugs in patients with CHF—considerations.

Altered pharmacokinetics—lower dose, slower upward titration
Reduced volume of distribution—higher blood levels at any dose
Decreased hepatic and renal clearance—increased half-life
Drugs less effective
Side effects more common
Greater potential for arrhythmia aggravation
Increased risk for CHF
No proven efficacy for preventing sudden death

CHF = congestive heart failure.

the initial dose should be low, often lower than what is recommended, and dose adjustments made at longer intervals (Table 35.18). Patients should be carefully monitored in the hospital for potential side effects. Objective end-points for efficacy must be based on established invasive (electrophysiologic) or noninvasive (ambulatory monitoring and exercise testing) methods.

Future Directions

The management of patients with CHF and arrhythmia is complicated and there is a delicate balance between LV function and arrhythmia. The therapies for either one may offset this balance. Additionally, there is a narrow therapeutic window between drug therapy and toxicity. Although pharmacologic therapy is the first and most frequently used approach in these patients, it is associated with many side effects, especially serious cardiac toxicity.

Before beginning prophylactic drug therapy, it is important to establish if the individual patient is at risk for sudden death. Ambulatory monitoring identifies a higher subgroup; however, it does not identify the individual patient who may be at risk. The signal-averaged ECG and electrophysiologic testing may have a role for risk stratification, but this remains uncertain and they are still investigational techniques. Newer methods are necessary for helping establish risk for the individual patient.

Even if the patient at risk can be identified, there are no data that prophylactic antiarrhythmic therapy will prevent sudden death when efficacy is based on objective criteria (i.e., suppression of spontaneous or inducible arrhythmia). There currently are several randomized trials addressing this question. One of the concerns about therapy is the toxicity of the antiarrhythmic drug and newer drugs that are more effective and safer are necessary. The method for the best measure of efficacy in patients with CHF requires further study. The role of the ICD and surgical and ablative therapy in different subsets requires further exploration. New therapies to treat CHF or prevent its development in high-risk patients would no doubt impact on the incidence of arrhythmia and sudden cardiac death. Last, the prevention of heart disease is the best way to prevent CHF and sudden cardiac death.

References

1. Cranfield PF, Wit AL, Hoffman BF. Genesis of cardiac arrhythmias. *Circulation*. 1973;47:190–195.
2. Brugada P, Wellens HJJ. Programmed electrical stimulation of the heart in ventricular arrhythmia. *Am J Cardiol*. 1985;56:187–190.
3. El Sherif N, Mehra R, Gough WB, Zuber RH. Ventricular activation patterns of spontaneous and induced ventricular rhythms in canine one day old myocardial infarction. Evidence for focal and reentrant mechanisms. *Circ Res*. 1982;51:152–166.
4. Allesse MA, Bonke FM, Schopman FJG. Circus movements in rabbit atrial muscle as a mechanism of tachycardia III. The "leading circle" concept: a new model of arcus movement in cardiac tissue without the involvement of an anatomical obstacle. *Circ Res*. 1977;41:9–18.
5. Friedman PL, Stewart JR, Fenoglio JJ, Wit AL. Survival of subendocardial Purkinje fibers after extensive myocardial infarction in dogs: in vitro and in vivo correlations. *Circ Res*. 1973;33:579–611.
6. El-Sherif N, Scherlag B, Lazzara R, Hope R. Reentrant ventricular arrhythmia in the late myocardial infarction period. 1. Conduction characteristics in the infarction zone. *Circulation*. 1977;55:686–701.
7. Draper MH, Weidman S. Cardiac resting and action potentials recorded with an intracellular electrode. *J Physiol*. 1951;115:74–94.
8. Zipes DP, Fischer JC. Effects of agents which inhibit the slow channel on sinus automaticity and atrioventricular conduction in the dog. *Circ Res*. 1974;34:184–192.
9. Wit AL, Cranefield PF. Triggered activity in cardiac muscle fibers of the simian mitral valve. *Circ Res*. 1976;38:85–98.
10. Wit AL, Cranfield PF, Gadsby DC. Triggered activity. In: Zipes DP, Bailey JC, Elharrar V, eds. *The slow inward current and cardiac arrhythmias*. Boston: Martinus Nijhoff; 1988:437–454.
11. Wit AL, Bigger JT. Possible electrophysiologic mechanisms for lethal arrhythmias accompanying myocardial ischemia and infarction. *Circulation*. 1975;51(Suppl III):96–115.
12. McDonald TF, MacLeod DP. Anoxia-recover cycle in ventricular muscle: action potential duration, contractility and ATP content. *Pfluegers Arch*. 1971;325:305–322.
13. Lazzara R, El-Sherif N, Scherlag BJ. Electrophysiological properties of canine Pukinje cells in one day old myocardial infarction. *Circ Res*. 1973;33:722–734.
14. Kimura S, Bassett AL, Kohya T, Kozlovskis PL, Myerberg RJ. Automaticity, triggered activity and responses to adrenergic stimulation in cat subendocardial Purkinje fibers after healing of myocardial infarction. *Circulation*. 1987,75:651–660.
15. Martins JB. Autonomic control of ventricular tachycardia—sympathetic neural influences in spontaneous tachycardia 24 hours after coronary occlusion. *Circulation*. 1985;72:933–942.
16. Dean JW, Lab MJ. Arrhythmia in heart failure: role of mechanically induced changes in electrophysiology. *Lancet*. 1989;10:1309–1312.
17. Podrid PJ. Potassium and ventricular arrhythmia. *Am J Cardiol*. 1990;65:33E–44E.
18. Gettes L, Surawicz B. Effects of low and high concentrations of potassium on the simultaneously recorded Purkinje and ventricular action potential of the perfused pig moduator band. *Circ Res*. 1968;23:717–726.
19. Singh BN, Vaughan William EM. Effect of altering potassium concentration on the action of lidocaine and

dephenyhydantion in atrial and ventricular muscle. *Circ Res.* 1971;29 286–295.

20. Obeid AI, Verier RL, Lown B. Influence of glucose, insulin, and potassium on the vulnerability to ventricular fibrillation in the canine heart. *Circ Res.* 1978;43:605–608.

21. Hulting J. In hospital ventricular fibrillation and its relations to serum potassium. *Acta Med Scand* (Suppl.). 1981;647:109–166.

22. Schechter M, Hod H, Marks N, Behar S, Kaplinsky E, Rabinowitz B. beneficial effect of magnesium sulfate in acute myocardial infarction. *Am J Cardiol.* 1990;66(3):271–274.

23. Levine TB, Francis GS, Goldsmith SR, Simm AB, Cohn JW. Activity of the sympathetic nervous system and nerve angiotension system assessed by plasma hormone levels and their relationship to hemodynamic abnormalities in congesive heart failure. *Am J Cardiol.* 1982;49:1659–1666.

24. Leimbach WN, Wallen G, Victor RG, Aylward PE, Sundlof G, Mark AL. Direct evidence from intraneural recordings for increased central sympathetic outflow in patients with heart failure. *Circulation.* 1986;73:913–919.

25. Wit AL, Rosen MR. Pathophysiologic mechanisms of cardiac arrhythmias. *Am Heart J.* 1983;106:798–811.

26. Wit AL, Hoffman BF, Rosen MR. Electrophysiology and pharmacology of cardiac arrhythmias 1X. Cardiac electrophysiologic effects of beta-adrenergic receptor stimulation and blockade—part A. *Am Heart J.* 1975;90:521–533.

27. Cameron JS, Han J. Effects of epinephrine on automaticity and the incidence of arrhythmia in Purkinje fibers surviving myocardial infarction. *J Pharmacol Exp Ther.* 1982;223:573–579.

28. Abildskov JA. Neural mechanisms involved in the regulation of ventricular repolarization. *Eur Heart J.* 1985;6(Suppl D):31–39.

29. Bhagat BD, Rao DS, Dhalla NS. Role of catecholamines in the genesis of arrhythmias. *Adv Myocardial.* 1980;2:117–132.

30. Inoue H, Zipes DP. Results of sympathetic denervation in the canine heart. Hypersensitivity that may be arrhythmogenic. *Circulation.* 1987;75:877–887.

31. Priori SG, Mantica M, Schwartz PJ. Delayed afterdepolarizations elected in vivo by left stellate ganglion stimulation. *Circulation.* 1988;78:178–185.

32. Brown MJ, Brown DL, Murphy MB. Hypokalemia from beta-2 receptor stimulation by circulating catecholamines. *N Engl J Med.* 1983;307:1414–1419.

33. Samet P. Hemodynamic sequelae of cardiac arrhythmias. *Circulation.* 1973;47:399–407.

34. Ross J, Linhart JW, Braunwald E. Effect of changing heart rate in man by electrical stimulation of the right atrium. *Circulation.* 1965;32:549–558.

35. Samet P, Castillo C, Berstein WH, Fernandez P. Hemodynamic results of right atrial pacing in cardiac subjects. *Dis Chest.* 1968;53:133–137.

36. Yoshinda S, Ganz W, Donoso R, Marcus HS, Swan HJC. Coronary hemodynamics during successive elevation of heart rate by pacing in subjects with angina pectoris. *Circulation.* 1971;44:1062–1071.

37. Benchimol A, Liggett MS. Cardiac hemodynamics during stimulation of the right atrium, right ventricle and left ventricle in normal and abnormal hearts. *Circulation.* 1966;33:933–944.

38. Morady F, Shen EN, Bhandari A, Schwartz AB, Scheinman MM. Clinical symptoms in patients with sustained ventricular tachycardia. *West J Med.* 1985;142:341–344.

39. Packer DL, Bardy GH, Worley SJ, et al. Tachycardia induced cardiomyopathy: a reversible form of left ventricular dysfunction. *Am J Cardiol.* 1986;57:563–570.

40. McLaran CJ, Gersh BJ, Sugrue DD, Hammill SC, Seward JB, Holmes DR. Tachycardia inducible myocardial dysfunction. A reversible phenomenon. *Br Heart J.* 1985;53:323–327.

41. Coleman HN, Taylor RR, Pool PE, et al. Congestive heart failure following clinical tachycardia. *Am Heart J.* 1971;81:790–798.

42. Killip T, Baer RA. Hemodynamic effect after reversion from atrial fibrillation to sinus rhythm by precordial shock. *J Clin Invest.* 1966;45:658–671.

43. Khaja K, Packer JO. Hemodynamic effects of cardioversion in chronic atrial fibrillation. *Arch Intern Med.* 1972;729:433–440.

44. Morris JJ, Entman M, North WC, Kong Y, McIntosh H. The changes in cardiac output with reversion of atrial fibrillation to sinus rhythm. *Circulation.* 1965;31:670–678.

45. Rodman T, Pastor BH, Figueroa W. Effect on cardiac output of cardioversion from atrial fibrillation to normal sinus mechanism. *Am J Med.* 1966;41:249–258.

46. Benchimol A, Ellis JG, Dimond EG. Hemodynamic consequences of atrial and ventricular pacing in patients with normal and abnormal hearts. *Am J Med.* 1965;39:911–922.

47. Rahimtoola SH, Ehsani A, Sinno MZ, Loeb HS, Rosen KM, Gunnar RM. Left atrial transport function in myocardial infarction. *Am J Med.* 1975;59:686–694.

48. Greenberg B, Chatterjee K, Parmley WW, Werner JA, Holly AN. The influence of left ventricular filling pressure on atrial contribution to cardiac output. *Am Heart J.* 1979;98:742–751.

49. Braunwald E, Frye RL, Aygen MM, Gilbert JW. Studies on Starling's law of the heart. III. Observation in patients with mitral stenosis and atrial fibrillation on the relationship between left ventricular end-diastolic segment length, filling pressure and the characteristics of ventricular contraction. *J Clin Invest.* 1960;39:1874–1884.

50. Rosenquist M, Issaz K, Botvinick EH, et al. Relative importance of activation sequence compared to atrioventricular synchrony in left ventricular function. *Am J Cardiol.* 1991;67:148–156.

51. Steinman RT, Herrera C, Schuger CD, Lehamann MH. Wide QRS tachycardia in the conscious adult. *JAMA.* 1989;261:1013–1016.

52. Feldman T, Carroll JD, Munkenbeck F, et al. Hemodynamic recovery during simulated ventricular tachycardia: role of adrenergic receptor activation. *Am Heart J* 1988;115:576–587.

53. Ellenbogen KA, Smith ML, Tahmes MD, Hoahnty PK.

Changes in regional adrenergic tone during sustained ventricular tachycardia associated with coronary artery disease or idiopathic dilated cardiomyopathy. *Am J Cardiol*. 1990;65:1334–1338.

54. Ferfusuon DW, Abboud FM, Mark A. Selective impairment of baroreflex mediated vasoconstrictor responses in patients with ventricular dysfunction. *Circulation*. 1984;69:451–460.

55. Kannel WB, Abbott RD, Savage DD, McNamara PM. Epidermiologic features of chronic atrial fibrillation. Framingham Study. *N Engl J Med*. 1982;306:1018–1022.

56. Podrid PJ, Fuchs T, Candinas R. Role of the sympathetic nervous system in the genesis of ventricular arrhythmia. *Circulation*. 1990;82(Suppl):103–113.

57. Sodermark T, Yansson B, Olson A, et al. Effect of quinidine on maintaining sinus rhythm after conversion of atrial fibrillation or flutter. A multicenter study from Stockholm. *Br Heart J*. 1975;37:486–492.

58. Boissel JP, Wolf E, Gillett J, et al. Controlled trial of a long acting quinidine for maintenance of sinus rhythm after conversion of sustained atrial fibrillation. *Eur Heart J*. 1981;2:49–55.

59. Berns E, Rinkenberger RL, Yeang MK, Dougherty AH, Yenkins M, Naccarelli GV. Efficacy and safety of flecainide acetate for atrial tachycardia or fibrillation. *Am J Cardiol*. 1987;59:1337–1341.

60. Graboys TB, Podrid PJ, Lown B. Efficacy of amiodarone for refractory supraventricular tachyarrhythmias. *Am Heart J*. 1983;106:870–876.

61. David D, Signi ED, Klein HO, Kaplinsky E. Inefficacy of digitalis in the control of heart rate in patients with chronic atrial fibrillation. Beneficial effect of an added beta adrenergic blocking agent. *Am J Cardiol*. 1979;44:1378–1382.

62. Wolf PA, Dawber TR, Thomas HE, Kannel WB. Epidemiologic assessment of chronic atrial fibrillation and risk of stroke: the Framingham Study. *Neurology*. 1978;28:975–972.

63. Peterson P, Godtfredson J, Boysen G, Anderson ED, Anderson B. Placebo controlled randomized trail of warfarin and aspirin for prevention of thromboembolic complications in chronic atrial fibrillation. *Lancet*. 1989;1:175–179.

64. The Boston Area Anticoagulation Trial for Atrial Fibrillation Investigators. The effect of low dose warfarin in the risk of stroke in patients with nonrheumatic atrial fibrillation. *N Engl J Med*. 1990;323:1505–1511.

65. Burggraf GW, Parker JO. Prognosis in coronary artery disease: angiographic, hemodynamic and clinical factors. *Circulation*. 1975;51:146–156.

66. Franciosa JA, Wilen M, Ziesche JM, Cohn JN. Survival in men with severe chronic left ventricular failure due to either coronary heart disease or idiopathic dilated cardiomyopathy. *Am J Cardiol*. 1983;51:831–836.

67. Meinertz T, Hoffman J, Kasper W, et al. Significance of ventricular arrhythmias in idiopathic dilated cardiomyopathy. *Am J Cardiol*. 1984;53:902–907.

68. Huang SK, Messer JV, Denes P. Significance of ventricular tachycardia in idiopathic dilated cardiomyopathy: observation in 35 patients. *Am J Cardiol*. 1983;51:507–512.

69. Sakurai T, Kawai C. Sudden death in idiopathic cardiomyopathy. *Jpn Cardiol J*. 1983;47:581–586.

70. Wilson JR, Schwartz S, St John Sutton M, et al. Prognosis in severe heart failure: relation to hemodynamic measurements and ventricular ectopic activity. *J Am Coll Cardiol*. 1983;2:403–410.

71. Maskin CS, Siskind SJ, Lejemtel TH. High incidence of nonsustained ventricular tachycardia in severe congestive heart failure. *Am Heart J*. 1984;107:896–907.

72. Von Olshausen K, Schaefer A, Mehmel HC, Schwartz F, Singer J, Jubler WS. Ventricular arrhythmias in idiopathic dilated cardiomyopathy. *Br Heart J*. 1984;51:195–201.

73. Holmes J, Kubo SJ, Cody RJ, Kligfield P. Arrhythmias in ischemic and nonischemic dilated cardiomyopathy: prediction of mortality by ambulatory electrocardiography. *Am J Cardiol*. 1985;55:146–151.

74. Chakko CS, Gheorghiade M. Ventricular arrhythmia in severe heart failure: incidence, significance and effectiveness of antiarrhythmic therapy. *Am Heart J*. 1985;109:497–504.

75. Francis GS. Development of arrhythmia in the patient with congestive heart failure: pathophysiology, prevalence and prognosis. *Am J Cardiol*. 1986;57:3B–7B.

76. Massie B, Ports T, Chatterjee K, et al. Long-term vasodilator therapy for heart failure. Clinical response and its relationship to hemodynamic measurements. *Circulation*. 1981;63:269–278.

77. Lee WH, Packer M. Prognosis value of serum sodium concentration in severe heart failure and its modification by converting enzyme inhibition. *Circulation*. 1984;70(Suppl II):113–118.

78. Cohn JN, Levine TD, Olivari MT, et al. Plasma norepinephrine as a guide to prognosis in patients with chronic congestive heart failure. *N Engl J Med*. 1984;311:819–823.

79. Gradman A, Deedwania P, Cody R, et al. Predictors of total mortality and sudden death in mild to moderate heart failure. *J Am Coll Cardiol*. 1989;14:564–590.

80. Keogh AM, Baron DW, Hickie JB. Prognostic guides in patients with idiopathic or ischemic dilated cardiomyopathy assessed for cardiac transplantation. *Am J Cardiol*. 1990;65:903–908.

81. Likoff MJ, Chandia SL, Kay HK. Clinical determinants of mortality in chronic congestive heart failure secondary to idiopathic dilated or to ischemic cardiomyopathy. *Am J Cardiol*. 1987;59:634–638.

82. Ruberman W, Weinblatt E, Goldberg JD. Ventricular premature complexes and sudden death after myocardial infarction. *Circulation*. 1981;64:297–303.

83. Mukharji J, Rude PE, Poole K, et al. The MILIS Study Group Risk Factors and sudden death following acute myocardial infarction: two year follow-up. *Am J Cardiol*. 1984;54:31–36.

84. Schultz RA, Strauss HW, Pitt B. Sudden death in the year following myocardial infarction. Relation to ventricular premature contractions in the late hospital phase of left ventricular efection fraction. *Am J Med*. 1977;62:192–199.

85. Bigger JT, Fleiss JL, Kleiger R, Miller JP, Rolnitsky LM, The Multicenter Post Infarction Study Group. The

relationship between ventricular arrhythmias, left ventricular dysfunction and mortality in the two years after myocardial infarction. *Circulation*. 1984;69:250–258.

86. Maron BJ, Savage DD, Wolfson JK, Epstein SE. Prognosis significance of 24-hour ambulatory electrocardiographic monitoring in patients with hypertrophic cardiomyopathy: a prospective study. *Am J Cardiol*. 1981;48:252–257.

87. McKenna WJ, Chetty S, Oakley CM, Goodwin JF. Arrhythmia in hypertrophic cardiomyopathy: exercise and 48-hour ambulatory electrocardiographic assessment with and without beta adrenergic blocking therapy. *Am J Cardiol*. 1980;45:1–5.

88. Costanzo-Nordin MR, O'Connell JB, Engelmeier RS, Moran JF, Scanlon PJ. Dilated cardiomyopathy: functional status, hemodynamics, arrhythmias and prognosis. *Cath Cardiovasc Diag*. 1985;11:445–453.

89. Savage DD, Seides S, Maron BJ, Meyer DJ, Epstein SE. Prevalence of arrhythmia during 24-hour electrocardiographic monitoring and exercise testing in patients with obstructive and nonobstructive hypertrophic cardiomyopathy. *Circulation*. 1979;59:866–875.

90. Unverferth DV, Magorien RD, Moeschberger ML, Baker PB, Fetters JK, Heier CJ. Factors influencing the one-year mortality of dilated cardiomyopathy. *Am J Cardiol*. 1984;54:147–152.

91. Stevenson WG, Stevenson LW, Weiss J, Tellisch JH. Inducible ventricular arrhythmias and sudden death during vasodilator therapy of severe heart failure. *Am Heart J*. 1988;116:1447–1454.

92. Prystowsky EN, Miles WM, Evans JJ, et al. Induction of ventricular tachycardia during programmed electrical stimulation: analysis of pacing methods. *Circulation*. 1986;73(Suppl II):32–38.

93. Gomes JA, Hariman RI, Kang PS, El Sherif N, Chowdhry I, Lyons J. Programmed electrical stimulation in patients with high-grade ventricular ectopy: electrophysiologic findings and prognosis for survival. *Circulation*. 1984;70:43–51.

94. Zheutlin TA, Roth H, Chua W, et al. Programmed electrical stimulation to determine the need for antiarrhythmic therapy in patients with complex ventricular ectopic activity. *Am Heart J*. 1986;111:860–867.

95. Das SK, Morady F, DiCarlo L, et al. Prognostic usefulness of programmed ventricular stimulation in idiopathic dilated cardiomyopathy without symptomatic ventricular arrhythmias. *Am J Cardiol*. 1986;58:998–1000.

96. Poll DS, Marchlinski FE, Buxton AE, Josephson ME. Usefulness of programmed stimulation in idiopathic dilated cardiomyopathy. *Am J Cardiol*. 1986;58:992–997.

97. Veltri EP, Platia EV, Griffith LSC, Reid PR. Programmed electrical stimulation and long-term follow-up in asymptomatic, nonsustained ventricular tachycardia. *Am J Cardiol*. 1985;56:309–314.

98. Sulpizi AM, Friehling TD, Kowey PR. Value of electrophysiologic testing in patients with nonsustained ventricular tachycardia. *Am J Cardiol*. 1987;59:841–845.

99. Stamato NJ, O'Connell JB, Murdock DK, Miran JF, Loeb HS, Scanlon PJ. The response of patients with compex ventricular arrhythmia secondary to dilated cardiomyopathy to programmed electrical stimulation. *Am Heart J*. 1986;112:505–508.

100. Hammill SC, Tresty JM, Wood DL, et al. Influence of ventricular function and presence or absence of coronary artery disease on results of electrophysiologic testing for asymptomatic nonsustained ventricular tachycardia. *Am J Cardiol*. 1990;65:722–728.

101. Naccarelli GV, Prystowsky EN, Jackman WM, Higer JJ, Rahilly GT, Zipes DP. Role of electrophysiologic testing in managing patients who have ventricular tachycardia unrelated to coronary artery disease. *Am J Cardiol*. 1982;50:165–171.

102. Berbari EJ, Scherlag BJ, Hope RR, Lazzara R. Recording from the body surface of arrhythmogenic ventricular activity during the ST segment. *Am J Cardiol*. 1978;41:697–702.

103. Boineau JP, Cox JL. Slow ventricular activation in acute myocardial infarction. A source of reentrant premature ventricular contraction. *Circulation*. 1973;48: 702–713.

104. Waldo AL, Kaiser GA. A study of ventricular arrhythmias associated with acute myocardial infarction in the canine heart. *Circulation*. 1973;47:1222–1228.

105. El-Sherif N, Scherlag BJ, Lazzara R. Electrode catheter recordings during malignant ventricular arrhythmias following an experimental myocardial infarction. *Circulation*. 1975;51:1003–1014.

106. El-Sherif N, Scherlag BJ, Lazzara R, Hope RR. Reentrant ventricular arrhythmias in the late myocardial infarction period: 1. Conduction characteristics in the infarction zone. *Circulation*. 1977;55:686–702.

107. Josephson ME, Horowitz LN, Farshidi A. Continuous local electrical activity: a mechanism of reentrant ventricular tachycardia. *Circulation*. 1978;57:659–665.

108. Simson MB. Use of signals in the terminal QRS complex to identify patients with ventricular tachycardia after myocardial infarction. *Circulation*. 1981;64:235–242.

109. Gomes JA, Mehra R, Barreca P, El-Sherif N, Hariman R, Holtzman R. Quantitative analysis of the high frequency components of the signal averaged QRS complex in patients with acute myocardial infarction: a prospective study. *Circulation*. 1985;72:105–111.

110. Kuchar DL, Thorburn CW, Sammel NL. Late potentials detected after myocardial infarction: natural history and prognostic significance. *Circulation*. 1986;74:1280–1289.

111. Kuchar DL, Thorburn CW, Sammel NL. Prediction of serious events after myocardial infarction: signal averaged electrocardiogram, Holter monitoring and radionuclide ventriculography. *J Am Coll Cardiol*. 1987; 9:531–538.

112. Poll DS, Marchlinski FE, Falcone RA, Josephson ME, Simson MB. Abnormal signal averaged electrocardiograms in patients with nonischemic congestive cardiomyopathy: relationship to sustained ventricular tachyarrhythmias. *Circulation*. 1985;72:1308–1313.

113. Itoh S, Kobayashi K, Yoneda N, et al. Clinical study of late potentials—comparison of late potential is myocardial infarction, cardiomyopathy and idiopathic ventricular tachycardia. *Jpn Circ J*. 1988;52:21–29.

114. Ohnishi Y, Inoue T, Fukuzaki H. Value of the signal averaged electrocardiogram as a predictor of sudden

death on myocardial infarction and dilated cardiomyopathy. *Jpn Circ J*. 1990;54:127–136.

115. Middlekauff H, Stevenson WG, Woo MA, Moser DK, Stevens LW. Comparison of frequency of late potentials in idiopathic dilated cardiomyopathy and ishemic myopathy with advanced congestive heart failure and their usefulness in predicting sudden death. *Am J Cardiol*. 1990;66:1113–1117.

116. Franciosa JA, Nordstrom LA, Cohn JN. Nitrate therapy for congestive heart failure. *JAMA*. 1978;240:443–446.

117. Bechler-Lisinska J, Cholewa M, Gorski L, Markiewicz K. Effect of vasodilator agents on the character and incidence of cardiac arrhythmia in chronic heart failure. *Zeitschrift Gesamte Innere Med Grenzgebiete*. 1990; 45(3):71–76.

118. Franciosa JA, Jordan RA, Wilen MM, Leddy CL. Minoxidil in patients with chronic left heart failure: contrasting hemodynamic and clinical effects in a controlled trial. *Circulation*. 1984;70:63–68.

119. Franciosa JA, Weber KT, Levine TB, et al. Hydralazine in the long term treatment of chronic heart failure: lack of difference from placebo. *Am Heart J* 1982; 104:587–594.

120. Cohn JV, Archibald DG, ziesche S, et al. Effect of vasodilator therapy on mortality in chronic congestive heart failure: results of a Veterans Administration cooperative study. *N Engl J Med*. 1986;314:1547–1552.

121. Packer M, Medina V, Yushak M. Hemodynamic and clinical limitations of long term inotropic therapy with amrinone in patients with severe chronic heart failure. *Circulation*. 1984;70:1038–1047.

122. Holmes JR, Kubo SH, Cody RJ, Kligfield P. Milrinone in congestive heart failure: observations in ambulatory arrhythmias. *Circulation*. 1984;70:II-11. Abstract.

123. Goldstein RA, Geraci SA, Gray EL, Rinkenberger RL, Dougherty AH, Naccarelli GV. Electrophysiologic effects of milrinone in patients with congestive heart failure. *Am J Cardiol*. 1986;57:624–628.

124. Anderson JL, Askins JC, Gilbet EM, Menlove RL, Lutz JR. Occurrence of ventricular arrhythmia in patients receiving acute and chronic infusions of milrinone. *Am Heart J*. 1986;111:461–474.

125. Ludmer PL, Baim DS, Antman EM, et al. Effects of milrinone on complex ventricular arrhythmias in congestive heart failure secondary to ischemic or dilated cardiomyopathy. *Am J Cardiol*. 1987;59:1351–1355.

126. DiBianco R, Shabetai R, Kostuk W, Moran J, Schlant RC, Wright RA. A comparison of oral milrinone, digoxin and their combination in the treatment of patients with chronic heart failure. *N Engl J Med*. 1989; 320:677–683.

127. Sharma B, Hoback J, Francis GS, et al. Pirbuterol: a new oral sympathomimitic amine for the treatment of congestive heart failure. *Am Heart J*. 1981;102:533–541.

128. Mettauer B, Rouleau JL, Burgess JH. Detrimental arrhythmogenic and sustained beneficial hemodynamic effects of oral salbuamol in patients with chronic congestive heart failure. *Am Heart J*. 1985;109:840–847.

129. Captopril-Digoxin Multicenter Research Group. Comparative effects of therapy with captopril and digoxin on patients with mild to moderate heart failure. *JAMA*. 1988;259:539–544.

130. Vangeli RS, Naumov VG, Blank ML, Sergakova LM, Grigoriants RA. Antiarrhythmic and arrhythmogenic actions of digoxin in ventricular rhythm disorders in patients with circulatory insufficiency. *Terapevticheskii Arkhiv*. 1987;59(9):81–86.

131. Hemsworth PD, Pallandi RT, Campbell TJ. Cardiac electrophysiologic actions of captopril: lack of direct antiarrhythmic effects. *Br J Pharmacol*. 1989;98:192–196.

132. deGraeff PA, deLangen CDJ, van Gilst WH, et al. Protective effects of captopril against ischemia/reperfusion induced ventricular arrhythmia *in vitro* and *in vivo*. *Am J Med*. 1988;84(Suppl 3A):67–74.

133. deLangen CDJ, deGraeff PA, van Gilst WH, Bel K, Kingma JH, Wesseling H. Effects of angiotension II and captopril on inducible sustained ventricular tachycardia two weeks after myocardial infarction in the pig. *J Cardiovasc Pharmacol*. 1989;13:186–191.

134. Cleland JGF, Dargie HJ, Hodsman GP, et al. Captopril in heart failure: a double blind controlled trial. *Br Heart J*. 1984;52:530–535.

135. Cleland JGF, Dargie HJ, Ball JG, et al. Effects of enalapril on heart failure: a double blind study of effects on exercise performance, renal function, hormones and metabolic state. *Br Heart J*. 1985;54:305–312.

136. Webster MWI, Fitzpatrick MA, Nicholes MG, Ikram H, Wells JE. Effects of enalapril on ventricular arrhythmias in congestive heart failure. *Am J Cardiol*. 1985; 56:566–569.

137. CONSENSUS Trial Study Group. Effects of enalapril on mortality in severe congestive heart failure. *N Engl J Med*. 1987;316:1429–1435.

138. Hamer AWF, Arkles LB, Johns JA. Beneficial effects of low dose amiodarone in patients with congestive cardiac failure. A placebo controlled trial. *J Am Coll Cardiol*. 1989;121:1768–1774.

139. Cleland JGF, Dargre HJ, Ford I. Mortality in heart failure: clinical variables of prognostic value. *Br Heart J*. 1987;58:572–582.

140. Kerin NZ, Rubenire M, Blevens LD, et al. Long-term efficacy, safety and survival of patients with potentially lethal ventricular arrhythmias treated with low dose amiodarone. *Clin Cardiol*. 1988;11:1131–1140.

141. Parmley WW, Chatterjee K. Congestive heart failure and arrhythmia. An overview. *Am J Cardiol*. 1986; 57:34B–37B.

142. Neri R, Mestroni L, Salvi A, Pandullo C, Camerini F. Ventricular arrhythmia in dilated cardiomyopathy: efficacy of amiodarone. *Am Heart J*. 1987;113:707–715.

143. Wilber DJ, Olshansky B, Moran JF, Scanlon PJ. Electrophysiologic testing in nonsustained ventricular tachycardia. Use and limitations in patients with coronary artery disease and impaired ventricular function. *Circulation*. 1990;82:350–358.

144. Swedberg K, Hjalmarson A, Waagstein F, Wallentin I. Prolongation of survival in congestive cardiomyopathy by beta receptor blockade. *Lancet* 1979;1:1374–1376.

145. Anderson J, Lutz JR, Gilbert EM, et al. A randomized

trial of low dose beta blockade therapy for idiopathic dilated cardiomyopathy. *Am J Cardiol.* 1985;55:471–475.

146. Beta Blocker Heart Arrack Trial Research Group. A randomized trial of propranolol in patients with acute myocardial infarction. I. Mortality results. *JAMA.* 1982;247:1707–1714.

147. Furberg CD, Hawkins CM, Lichstein E, for the Beta Blocker Heart Attack Trial Study Group. Effect of propranolol in post-infarction patients with mechanical or electrical complications. *Circulation.* 1984;69:761–765.

148. Chadda K, Goldstein S, Byington R, Curb JD. Effect of propranolol after acute myocardial infarction in patients with congestive heart failure. *Circulation.* 1986;73:503–510.

149. McKenna WJ, Oakley CM, Krikler DM, Goodwin JF. Improved survival with amiodarone in patients with hypertrophic cardiomyopathy and ventricular tachycardia. *Br Heart J.* 1985;53:412–416.

150. Fananapazir L, Leon MB, Bonow RO, Tracy CM, Cannon RO, Epstein SE. Sudden death during empiric amiodarone therapy in symptomatic hypertrophic cardiomyopathy. *Am J Cardiol.* 1991;67:169–174.

151. Poll DS, Marchlinski FE, Buxton AE, Doherty JU, Waxman HL, Josephson ME. Sustained ventricular tachycardia in patients with idiopathic dilated cardiomyopathy: electrophysiologic testing and lack of response to antiarrhythmic drug therapy. *Circulation.* 1984;70:451–456.

152. Rae AP, Spielman SR, Kutalek BP, Kay HR, Horowitz LN. Electrophysiologic assessment of antiarrhythmic drug efficacy for ventricular tachyarrhythmias associated with dilated cardiomyopathy. *Am J Cardiol.* 1987;59:291–295.

153. Constantin L, Martins JB, Kiengle MG, Brownstein SL, McLue ML, Hopson RC. Induced sustained ventricular tachycardia in nonischemic dilated cardiomyopathy: dependence on clinical presentation and response to antiarrhythmic drugs. *PACE.* 1989;12:776–783.

154. Liem LB, Swerdlow CD. Value of electrophysiologic testing in idiopathic dilated cardiomyopathy and sustained ventricular tachyarrhythmias. *Am J Cardiol.* 1988;62:611–616.

155. Milner PG, DiMarco JP, Lerman BB. Electrophysiologic evaluation of sustained ventricular tachyarrhythmias in idiopathic dilated cardiomyopathy. *PACE.* 1988;11:562–568.

156. Hession MJ, Lampert S, Podrid PJ, Lown B. Ethmozine (moricizine HCL) therapy for complex ventricular arrhythmias. *Am J Cardiol.* 1987;60:59F–66F.

157. Pratt CM, Wierman A, Seals A, et al. Efficacy and safety of moricizine in patients with malignant ventricular tachycardia: results of a placebo-controlled prospective long term clinical trial. *Circulation.* 1986;73:718–726.

158. Hohnloser SH, Lange HW, Raeder EA, Podrid PJ, Lown B. Short and long term tocainide therapy for malignant ventricular tachyarrhythmias. *Circulation.* 1986;75:143–149.

159. Tordjman T, Podrid PJ, Raeder E, Lown B. Safety and efficacy of encainide for malignant ventricular arrhythmias. *Am J Cardiol.* 1986;58:87C–95C.

160. Takarada A, Yokota Y, Fukuzaki H. Analysis of ventricular arrhythmias in patients with dilated cardiomyopathy—relationship between the effects of antiarrhythmic agents and severity of myocardial lesions. *Jpn Circ J.* 1990;54:260–271.

161. Cueni L, Podrid PJ. Propafenone therapy in patients with serious ventricular arrhythmia. Noninvasive evaluation of efficacy. *J Electrophysiol.* 1987;1:548–560.

162. Hohnloser SH, Raeder EA, Podrid PJ, Graboys TB, Lown B. Predictors of antiarrhythmic drug efficacy on patients with malignant ventricular tachyarrhythmias. *Am Heart J.* 1987;114:1–7.

163. Pratt CM, Eaton T, Frances M, et al. The inverse relationship between baseline left ventricular ejection fraction and outcome of antiarrhythmic therapy: a dangerous imbalance in the risk-benefit ratio. *Am Heart J.* 1989;118:433–441.

164. Lampert S, Lown B, Graboys TB, Podrid PJ, Blatt CM. Determinants of survival in patients with malignant ventricular arrhythmia. *Am J Cardiol.* 1988;61:791–797.

165. Spielman SR, Schwartz JS, McCarthy DM, et al. Predictors of the success or failure of medical therapy in patients with chronic recurrent sustained ventricular tachycardia: A discriminant analysis. *J Am Coll Cardiol.* 1983;1:401–408.

166. Swerdlow CD, Winkle A, Mason JW. Determinants of survival in patients with ventricular tachyarrhythmias. *N Engl J Med.* 1983;308:1436–1440.

167. Wilber DJ, Garan H, Finkelstein D, et al. Out of hospital cardiac arrest: Use of electrophysiologic testing in the prediction of long-term outcome. *N Engl J Med.* 1988;318:19–24.

168. Woosley RL. Pharmacokinetics and pharmacodynamics of antiarrhythmic agents in patients with congestive heart failure. *Am Heart J.* 1987;114:1280–1291.

169. Kerin A, Tzivoni D, Garvish D, et al. Etiology, warning signs and therapy of torsade des pointes—a study of ten patients. *Circulation.* 1981;64:1167–1174.

170. Bigger JT, Giardina EGU. Drug interaction in antiarrhythmic therapy. In: Greenberg HM, Dwyer EM, eds. *Clinical aspects of life threatening arrhythmias.* NY Acad Sci 1984:140–161.

171. Velebit V, Podrid PJ, Lown B, Cohen BH, Graboys TB. Aggravation and provocation of ventricular arrhythmias by antiarrhythmic drugs. *Circulation.* 1982;65:886–894.

172. Zipes DP. Proarrhythmic effects of antiarrhythmic drugs. *Am J Cardiol.* 1987;59:26E–31E.

173. Slater W, Lambert SL, Podrid PJ, Lown B,. Clinical predictors of arrhythmia worsening by antiarrhythmic drugs. *Am J Cardiol.* 1988;61:349–353.

174. Morganroth J, Anderson JL, Gentzkow GD. Clarification of type of ventricular arrhythmia predicts frequency of adverse cardiac events from flecainide. *J Am Coll Cardiol.* 1986;8:607–615.

175. Au PK, Bhandari AK, Bream R, Schreck D, Siddiqi R, Rahemtoola SH. Proarrhythmic effects of antiarrhythmic drugs during programmed ventricular stimulation in patients without ventricular tachycardia. *J Am Coll Cardiol.* 1987;9:389–397.

176. Minardo JD, Hager JJ, Miles WM, Zipes DP, Prystows-

ky EN. Clinical characteristics of patients with ventricular fibrillation during antiarrhythmic drug therapy. *N Engl J Med*. 1988;319:257–262.

177. Podrid PJ, Schoeneberger A, Lown B. Precipitation of congestive heart failure by oral disopyramide. *N Engl J Med*. 1980;302:614–617.

178. Ravid S, Podrid PJ, Lambert S, Lown B. Congestive heart failure induced by six of the newer antiarrhythmic drugs. *J Am Coll Cardiol*. 1989;14:1326–1330.

179. Gottlieb SS, Kukin ML, Yushak M, Medina N, Packer M. Adverse hemodynamic and clinical effects of encainide in severe chronic heart failure. *Ann Intern Med*. 1989;110:505–509.

180. Gottlieb SS, Kukin ML, Medina N, Yushak M, Packer M. Comparative hemodynamic effects of procainamide, tocainide and encainide in severe chronic heart failure. *Circulation*. 1990;81:860–864.

181. Iseri LT, Humphrey SB, Siner EJ. Prehospital bradyasystolic arrest. *Ann Intern Med*. 1978;88:741–745.

182. Nickolic G, Bishop RL, Singh JB. Sudden death recorded during Holter monitoring. *Circulation*. 1982;66:218–225.

183. Milner PG, Platia EV, Reid PR, Griffith LSC. Ambulatory electrocardiographic recordings at the time of fatal cardiac arrest. *Am J Cardiol*. 1985;56:588–592.

184. Kempi FC, Josephson ME. Cardiac arrest recorded on ambulatory electrocardiograms. *Am J Cardiol*. 1984;53:1577–1582.

185. deLuna AB, Coumel P, Leclercq JF. Ambulatory sudden cardiac death: mechanisms of production of fatal arrhythmia on the basis of data from 157 cases. *Am Heart J*. 1989;117:151–159.

186. Clark MB, Dwyer EM, Greenberg H. Sudden death during ambulatory monitoring. *Am J Med*. 1983; 75:801–806.

187. Luu M, Stevenson WG, Stevenson LW, Baron K, Walden J. Diverse mechanisms of unexpected cardiac death in advanced heart failure. *Circulation*. 1989;80:1673–1680.

188. Radhakrishnan S, Kaul U, Bahi VK, Talwar KK, Bhatia ML. Sudden bradyarrhythmic death in dilated cardiomyopathy: a case report. *PACE*. 1988;11:1369–1372.

189. Greenberg HM. Bradycardia at onset of sudden death: potential mechanisms. *Ann NY Acad Sci*. 1984;427:241–251.

190. Jarisch A, Zotterman Y. Depressor reflexes from the heart. *Acta Physiol Scand*. 1948;16:31–51.

191. Ferguson DW, Abboud FM, Mark A. Selective impairment of baroreflex mediated vasoconstrictor responses in patients with ventricular dysfunction. *Circulation*. 1984;69:451–460.

192. Kontos HA, Mauck HP, Richardson DW, Patterson JL. Mechanism of circulatory responses to systemic hypoxia in the anesthetized dog. *Am J Physiol*. 1965;209:397–403.

193. Couch DA. Cardiac aneurysm with ventricular tachycardia and subsequent excision of aneurysm. *Circulation*. 1959;20:251–253.

194. Buda AJ, Stenson EB, Harrison DC. Surgery for life

threatening ventricular arrhythmias. *Am J. Cardiol*. 1979;44:1171–1177.

195. Harken AH, Horowitz LN, Josephson ME. Comparison of standard aneurysmectomy and aneurysmectomy with directed endocardial resection for the treatment of recurrent sustained ventricular tachycardia. *J Thorac Cardiovasc Surg*. 1980;80:527–534.

196. Boineau JP, Cox JL. Rationale for a direct surgical approach to control ventricular arrhythmias. *Am J Cardiol*. 1982;49:381–396.

197. Witting JH, Boineau JP. Surgical treatment of ventricular arrhythmias using epicardial transmural and endocardial mapping. *Ann Thorac Surg*. 1975;20:117–126.

198. Gallager JJ, Oldham HN Jr, Wallace AG, Peter RH, Kasell J. Ventricular aneurysm with ventricular tachycardia. Report of a case with epicardial mapping and successful resection. *Am J Cardiol*. 1975;35:696–700.

199. Guiraudon G, Foutaine G, Frank R, Escande G, Etievent P, Cabrol C. Encircling endocardial veutriculotomy: a new surgical treatment of life-threatening ventricular tachycardia resistant to medical treatment following myocardial infarction. *Ann Thorac Surg*. 1978;26:438–444.

200. Cox JL, Callagher JJ, Ungerleider RM. Encircling endocardial veutriculotomy (EEV) for refractory ischemic ventricular tachycardia IV. Clinical implications, surgical technique, mechanism of action, and results. *J Thorac Cardiovasc Surg*. 1982;83:865–872.

201. Ostermeyer J, Breithard G, Borggrefe M, Godehardt E, Seipel L, Bircks W. Surgical treatment of ventricular tachycardias. Complete versus partial encircling endocardial veutriculotomy. *J Thorac Cardiovasc Surg*. 1984;87:517–525.

202. Josephson ME, Harken AH, Horowitz LN. Endocardial excision—a new surgical technique for the treatment of recurrent ventricular tachycardia. *Circulation*. 1979;60:1430–1439.

203. Moran JM, Kehoe RF, Loeb JM, Lichteuthal PR, Sanders JH Jr, Michaelis LL. Extended endocardial resection for the treatment of ventricular tachycardia and ventricular fibrillation. *Ann Thorac Surg*. 1982;34:538–552.

204. Selle JG, Svenson RH, Sealy WC, et al. Successful clinical laser ablation of ventricular tachycardia: a promising new therapeutic method. *Ann Thorac Surg*. 1986;42:380–384.

205. Svenson RH, Gallagher JJ, Selle JG, Zimmern SH, Fedor JM, Robicsek R. Neodymium:YAG laser photocoagulation: a successful new map guided technique for the intraoperative ablation of ventricular tachycardia. *Circulation*. 1987;76:1319–1328.

206. Mason JW, Stinson EB, Winkle RA, Oyer PE, Griffin JC, Ross DL. Relative efficacy of blind left ventricular aneurysm dissection for the treatment of recurrent ventricular tachycardia. *Am J Cardiol*. 1982;49:241–248.

207. Zee-Cheng CS, Kouchoukos NT, Connors JP, Ruffy R. Treatment of life-threatening ventricular arrhythmia with non-guided surgery supported by electrophysiologic testing and drug therapy. *J Am Coll Cardiol*. 1989;13:153–162.

208. Borggrefe M, Podczeck A, Ostermeyer J, Breithardt G,

The Surgical Ablation Registry. Long-term results of electrophysiologically guided antitachycardias: a collaborative report on 665 patients. In: Breithardt G, Borggrefe M, Zipes DP, eds. *Nonpharmacological therapy of tachyarrhythmias.* Mount Kisco, NY: Future Publishing, 1987:109–132.

209. Ideker RE, Smith WM, Wallace AG, et al. A computerized method for the rapid display of ventricular activation during the intraoperative study of arrhythmias. *Circulation.* 1979;59:449–458.

210. Dowmar E, Parson ID, Middleborough LL, Cameron DA, Yao LC, Waxman MB. On-line epicardial mapping of intraoperative experience. *J Am Coll Cardiol.* 1984;4:703–714.

211. Cox JL. Intraoperative computerized mapping techniques: do they help us to treat our patients better surgically? In: Brugada P, Wellens HJJ, eds. *Cardiac arrhythmias: where to go from here.* Mount Kisco, NY: Future Publishing; 1987:613–637.

212. Horowitz LN, Harken AH, Kaston JA, Josephson ME. Ventricular resection guided by epicardial and endocardial mapping for treatment of recurrent ventricular tachycardia. *N Engl J Med.* 1980;302:589–593.

213. Miller JM, Kienzle MG, Harken AH, Josephson ME. Subendocardial resection for ventricular tachycardia: predictors of surgical success. *Circulation.* 1984;70:624–631.

214. Garan H, Nguyen K, McGovern B, Buckley M, Ruskin JN. Perioperative and long-term results after electrophysiologically directed ventricular surgery for recurrent ventricular tachycardia. *J Am Coll Cardiol.* 1986;8:201–209.

215. Krafcheck J, Lawrer GM, Roberts R, Magro SA, Wyndham CR. Surgical ablation of ventricular tachycardia: improved results with map directed regional approach. *Circulation.* 1986,73:1239–1247.

216. Kron IL, Lerman BB, Nolan SP, Flanagan TL, Haines DE, DiMarco JP. Sequential endocardial resection for the surgical treatment of refractory ventricular tachycardia. *J Thorac Cardiovasc Surg.* 1987;94:843–847.

217. Haines DE, Lerman BB, Kron IL, DiMarco JP. Surgical ablation of ventricular tachycardia with sequential map guided subendocardial resection: electrophysiological assessment and long-term followup. *Circulation.* 1988;77:131–141.

218. Middleborough LL, Harris L, Downar E, Parson I, Gray G. A new intraoperative approach for endocardial mapping of ventricular tachycardia. *J Thorac Cardiovasc Surg.* 1988;95:271–280.

219. Caceres J, Akhtar M, Werner P, et al. Cryoblation of refractory sustained ventricular tachycardia due to coronary artery disease. *Am J Cardiol.* 1989;63(5):296–300.

220. Page PL, Cardinal R, Shenasa M, Kaltenbrunner W, Cossette R, Nadeau R. Surgical treatment of ventricular tachycardia. Regional crysablation guided by computerized epicardial and endocardial mapping. *Circulation.* 1989;80(Suppl I):124–134.

221. Frank G, Lowes D, Baumgart D, et al. Surgical alternatives in the treatment of life threatening ventricular arrhythmia. *Eur J Cardiothorac Surg.* 1988;2:207–216.

222. Mirowski M. The automatic implantable cardioverter defibrillator: an overview. *J Am Coll Cardiol.* 1985; 6:461–466.

223. Mirowski M, Reid PR, Mower MM, et al. Termination of malignant ventricular arrhythmias with an implanted defibrillator in human beings. *N Engl J Med.* 1980; 303:322–324.

224. Mirowski M, Reid PR, Winkle RA, et al. Mortality in patients with implanted automatic defibrillators. *Ann Intern Med.* 1983;98:585–588.

225. Echt DS, Armstrong K, Schmidt P, Oyer PE, Stimson EB, Winkle RA. Clinical experience, complications, and survival in 70 patients with the automatic implantable cardioverter—defibrillator. *Circulation.* 1985;71:289–296.

226. Luceri RM, Thurer RJ, Palatianos GM, Fernandez PR, El-Shalakany A, Castellanos A. The automatic implantable cardioverter-defibrillator: results, observations and comments. *PACE.* 1986;9:1343–1348.

227. Marchlinski FE, Flores BT, Buxton AE, Josephson M. The automatic implantable cardioverter-defibrillator: efficacy, complications and device failures. *Ann Intern Med.* 1986;104:481–488.

228. Kelly PA, Cannon DS, Garan H, et al. The automatic implantable cardioverter-defibrillator: efficacy, complications and survival in patients with malignant ventricular arrhythmias. *J Am Coll Cardiol.* 1988;11:1278–1286.

229. Kelly PA, Cannon DS, Garan H, et al. Predictors of automatic implantable cardioverter-defibrillator discharge for life-threatening ventricular arrhythmias. *Am J Cardiol.* 1988;62(1):83–87.

230. Winkle RA, Mead RH, Ruder MA, et al. Long-term outcome with the automatic implantable cardioverter-defibrillator. *J Am Coll Cardiol.* 1989;13(6):1353–1361.

231. Tordjman-Fuchs T, Garan H, McGovern B, et al. Out of hospital cardiac arrest: Improved long-term outcome in patients with automatic implantable cardioverter-defibrillator (AICD). *Circulation.* 1989;80(Suppl II): 121.

232. Tchou PJ, Kadri N, Anderson J, Caceres J, Jazayeri M, Akhtar M. Automatic implantable cardioverter-defibrillators and survival of patients with left ventricular arrhythmias. *Ann Intern Med.* 1988;109(7):529–534.

233. Fogoros RN, Elson JJ, Bonnet CA, Burkholder JA. Efficacy of the automatic implantable cardioverter-defibrillator in prolonging survival in patients with severe underlying cardiac disease. *J Am Coll Cardiol.* 1990; 16(2):381–386.

234. deMarchena E, Chakko S, Fernandez P, et al. Usefulness of the automatic implantable cardioverter-defibrillator in improving survival in patients with severely depressed left ventricular function associated with coronary artery disease. *Am J Cardiol.* 1991;67:812–816.

36
Pathogenesis and Therapy of Thrombosis in Patients with Congestive Heart Failure

Scott H. Goodnight

In the past decade, substantial progress has been made in the rational use of anticoagulant therapy for thrombosis complicating cardiac disease. However, relatively few clinical investigators have specifically examined the problem of thromboembolism in patients with congestive heart failure. Instead, other diagnostic categories of heart disease such as acute myocardial infarction, mechanical or tissue heart valves, or cardiomyopathies have been studied, and these trials often have included patients with left ventricular failure. For the purposes of this review, congestive heart failure will be viewed as an important additional risk factor for thromboembolism in patients with cardiac disease, rather than as a specific, isolated indication for antithrombotic treatment.

In this chapter, the pathogenesis of thrombosis complicating cardiac disease and congestive heart failure (CHF) is discussed. Predisposing factors such as sluggish blood flow, the presence of activated clotting factors or platelets, fibrinolytic defects, and antiphospholipid antibodies are reviewed. A second section examines recently published information concerning the optimal use of heparin and warfarin. An assessment of bleeding risks associated with anticoagulation therapy is included, as well as the potential usefulness of "combination" antithrombotic therapy using both antiplatelet agents and anticoagulants.

Thereafter, the indications and optimal use of antithrombotic therapy in patients with various forms of heart disease complicated by ventricular failure are discussed, including cardiomyopathy, acute myocardial infarction (MI), rheumatic heart disease, mechanical or tissue valves, and nonrheumatic atrial fibrillation. A final section considers the management of anticoagulants in patients with CHF who require surgical procedures. Several excellent publications recently have reviewed the use of anticoagulants in various clinical settings and have made recommendations for the use of antithrombotic therapy in patients with cardiac disease.[1–6]

Pathogenesis of Thrombosis (Table 36.1)

Vascular Injury

An effective defense against intravascular thrombosis involves a dynamic interplay between the vasculature, platelets, the formation of fibrin, and fibrinolysis.[7] Vascular endothelial cells are a particularly important barrier to thrombosis. For example, the endothelial surface contains a key glycoprotein, thrombomodulin, which supports the activation of protein C, a potent natural anticoagulant. Activated protein C is able to rapidly destroy activated factors V and VIII, major participants in the formation of fibrin. Moreover, a glycosaminoglycan, heparan, is widely distributed on the endothelial surface and avidly binds antithrombin III, another natural anticoagulant. When bound to the endothelial surface, antithrombin III rapidly neutralizes the clotting enzyme thrombin, as well as activated factor X and other prothrombotic serine proteases.

Vascular endothelial cells also may inhibit platelet adhesion and platelet aggregation. When the endothelium is activated by local injury, inflammation, or other thrombogenic stimuli, prostacyclin (PGI$_2$), a potent in-

TABLE 36.1. Comparison of antithrombotic and prothrombotic properties of the blood vessels, platelets, and plasma.

	Inhibition of thrombosis	Promotion of thrombosis
Coagulation	Antithrombin III activated protein C	Thrombin, factor Xa, factors Va, VIIIa
Platelet reactivity	Prostacyclin (PGI$_2$)	Thromboxane A$_2$
Fibrinolysis	Tissue plasminogen activator (t-PA)	Plasminogen activator inhibitor (PAI-1)
Vascular tone	Endothelium-derived relaxing factor (EDRF)	Endothelin

hibitor of platelet plug formation, may be released. Finally, under appropriate circumstances, blood vessels may markedly enhance local fibrinolysis via the synthesis and release of tissue plasminogen activator.

Injury to normal vascular endothelium may serve as a potent stimulus to thrombosis. For example, a patient with a transmural MI may develop endothelial cell damage overlying the ischemic area of endocardium. The loss of the protective endothelium with the exposure of a thrombogenic surface may subsequently culminate in a ventricular thrombus. The ultimate size of the intracavitary clot will be limited by the antithrombotic potential of the surrounding intact endothelium. A similar sequence of events may occur after the rupture of an atherosclerotic plaque within a coronary artery. Platelets and fibrin rapidly accumulate at the area of injury, which may lead to acute coronary artery occlusion and, ultimately, infarction of the myocardium.

Reduced Blood Flow

Sluggish or disturbed blood flow as seen in ventricular failure or atrial fibrillation may greatly enhance the likelihood of thrombosis. The supply of inhibitors such as antithrombin III or protein C from blood flowing to an area of local tissue injury will be reduced, and activated clotting factors may tend to accumulate, rather than being flushed away into the circulation where they can be cleared by the liver.

Activated Clotting Factors

Clotting proteins such as prothrombin or factor X normally circulate in their nonactivated (zymogen) configuration. However, a variety of stimuli may convert them to an activated form, greatly increasing the possibility of thrombosis. Examples include surgical procedures, tissue necrosis due to infarction, infections, or inflammatory reactions with the release of thrombogenic cytokines such as interleukin-1 or tumor necrosis factor.

Fibrinolytic Defects

The fibrinolytic balance may be altered in some patients with heart disease, leading to an increased likelihood of thrombosis. For example, young men with MI have been shown to have increased plasma levels of plasminogen activator inhibitor (i.e., PAI-1), an important fibrinolytic inhibitor released by endothelial cells and also found in the circulation.[8] Recently, a newly appreciated atherogenic lipoprotein, Lp(a), has been shown to inhibit fibrinolysis in vitro. Lp(a) has striking structural homology with plasminogen, the precursor to the fibrinolytic enzyme plasmin. Lp(a) has been shown to stimulate the release of PAI-1 from endothelial cells,

and to compete effectively with plasminogen for binding on fibrin or the surface of vascular endothelial cells, inhibiting fibrinolysis.[9,10] Individuals with elevated levels of Lp(a) may develop accelerated atherogenesis, but it is not yet known if they may also be prone to thrombosis. Another risk factor for atherothrombotic disease, homocysteinemia, also may produce inhibition of fibrinolysis.[11,12] Recent reports have suggested that heterozygotes for cystathionine beta-synthase deficiency who have mild to moderate elevations of plasma homocysteine, may have accelerated vascular disease.[13–15]

Vascular Reactivity

Recently, the importance of the level of vascular tone and its relationship to thrombogenesis has become increasingly appreciated. Intense vasoconstriction appears to promote thrombogenesis, whereas vasodilatation may allow increased blood flow and inhibit thrombosis. Although the regulation of vascular tone is a complex process, several new mediators recently have been studied in some detail. These include endothelium-derived relaxing factor (EDRF), which may be released by vascular endothelial cells in response to thrombin or the aggregation of platelets. EDRF promotes local vasodilatation and also may help to reduce platelet reactivity.[16–18] In contrast, the endothelins are a family of small peptides that are potent vasoconstrictors released from vascular cells that also may function as mitogenic peptides.[19]

Heightened Platelet Reactivity

The concept that increased platelet reactivity may contribute to arterial thrombosis has not been thoroughly tested, in part because of the lack of sensitive and specific laboratory assays for platelet activation. However, patients with extensive peripheral atherosclerosis have been shown to have increased platelet-vascular interactions, as evidenced by the excretion of platelet and vascular prostaglandin metabolites in the urine.[20] Transient, but greatly enhanced, platelet reactivity also has been found after fibrinolytic therapy for acute coronary thrombosis.[21] Patients with marked hypercholesterolemia were reported several years ago to have increased platelet reactivity, as measured by an increased sensitivity to platelet-aggregating agents such as epinephrine.[22] Last, several investigators have suggested that a diurnal variation in platelet reactivity may occur, a phenomenon that may contribute to acute coronary occlusion.[23–26]

Antiphospholipid Antibodies

Antiphospholipid antibodies such as the lupus anticoagulant or anticardiolipin antibodies have been associated with both arterial and venous thromboembolism for at least a decade.[27] A Swedish study indicated that a substantial proportion of young males with an acute MI had elevated levels of antiphospholipid antibodies in their blood that persisted for 2 yr.[28] Approximately one third of these men developed additional thromboembolic complications. Other patients with rheumatologic syndromes, such as systemic lupus erythematosus, who have high levels of antiphospholipid antibodies have been reported to develop mitral valve lesions with recurrent cerebral emboli.[29–32] The mechanisms underlying thrombosis in patients with high titers of antiphospholipid antibodies remains unknown, but may involve the inhibition of the protein C anticoagulant system, reduction of prostacyclin release from endothelial cells, or inhibition of fibrinolysis.

Advances in Anticoagulation Therapy

Heparin

Heparin functions as an anticoagulant by accelerating the neutralization of several activated clotting factors by antithrombin III (for review see refs. 4 and 33). When unfractionated heparin is employed, antithrombin III inhibits the prothrombotic enzyme thrombin most strongly, closely followed by activated factor X (Xa). In contrast, low molecular weight heparins that contain fewer than 18 sugar residues stimulate antithrombin III to potently inhibit factor Xa to a much greater degree than that of thrombin. Consequently, the therapeutic effects of the newer low molecular weight heparins (or heparinoids) must be monitored by an anti-Xa assay rather than the activated partial thromboplastin time (aPTT).

In solution, thrombin is rapidly neutralized by the combination of heparin and antithrombin III. However, thrombin that is bound to preexisting fibrin clots has been shown to be substantially more resistant to the effects of heparin.[34] As a consequence, much higher doses of heparin may be required to prevent the extension of a thrombus rather than its initiation. As an example, relatively low doses of heparin have been shown to be effective for the prophylaxis of thrombosis in surgical patients, but much higher heparin concentrations are required for treatment of patients who have an acute deep venous thrombosis or left ventricular (LV) mural thrombus.

It is rapidly becoming clear that effective antithrombotic therapy with heparin depends on attaining an optimal therapeutic concentration of heparin activity. The adequacy of anticoagulation therapy with heparin is currently monitored by the activated partial thromboplastin time test. However, the aPTT reagents and automated equipment currently used in hospital laboratories may vary substantially in their sensitivity to the anticoagulant effects of heparin. Heparin concentrations in the blood ranging from 0.35 to 0.7 U/ml of heparin activity (as measured by an anti-Xa inhibition assay) have been recommended for effective anticoagulation therapy. This concentration of heparin generally corresponds to an aPTT ratio (patient/control) of 1.5 to 2.0. However, it is important that each laboratory specify an optimal therapeutic range of the aPTT for heparin, using their own equipment and reagents.

Clinical trials of heparin in patients with deep venous thrombosis have clearly shown that the aPTT must be rapidly prolonged into the therapeutic range to prevent recurrent thromboembolism. In many cases, larger doses of heparin than ordinarily prescribed will be necessary. For example, investigators studying venous thrombosis have recently used 30,000 to 40,000 units of heparin daily in patients at low risk for bleeding rather than the more commonly prescribed 1000 units/hr.[35] A useful clinical protocol recently has been devised to administer heparin more effectively.[36]

A potentially disastrous complication of heparin therapy is heparin-induced thrombocytopenia, which has been estimated to occur in about 2.5% of patients who have received heparin for more than 7 days.[37] Approximately 10% to 15% of these patients develop severe arterial or venous thrombosis. Hopefully, the use of shorter courses of heparin therapy or more purified heparins or heparinoids may reduce the incidence of this serious clinical problem.[38] Patients who have previously received heparin or those receiving heparin for the first time for more than 3 to 4 days should be monitored with daily platelet counts.

Warfarin

The most commonly used oral anticoagulant in the United States, warfarin, exerts its antithrombotic effect by inhibiting the vitamin K–dependent biochemical addition of a series of gamma carboxyglutamic acid residues to the clotting factors II, VII, IX, and X (reviewed in ref. 5). These amino acid–like residues are essential for the normal functioning of these coagulation proteins as well as for the coagulation inhibitors, protein C and protein S. The presence of the modified glutamic acid moieties allows calcium-mediated binding of the clotting factors to phospholipid surfaces, a process necessary for the formation of fibrin. As a result of pharmacologically induced vitamin K deficiency, warfarin therapy effectively inhibits thrombosis, and has proved extremely useful as an oral anticoagulant.

A major advance in the safety and efficacy of oral anticoagulation therapy has been the institution of the International Normalized Ratio (INR) to standardize therapeutic intensities of coumarin antithrombotic therapy throughout the world.[39] The INR is a *calculated* prothrombin time ratio that takes into account local differences in prothrombin time reagents and equipment. It is determined by the following simple formula:

$$INR = PT \ ratio^{ISI}$$

where the ISI is the International Sensitivity Index of the thromboplastin reagent used for performing the prothrombin time. Note that the PT ratio is raised to the *power* of the ISI, making the relationship an exponential one.

Based on the results of several clinical trials, two general therapeutic ranges for oral anticoagulant therapy have been suggested. "Low intensity" anticoagulation therapy has been defined as an INR ranging from 2 to 3, whereas "high intensity" therapy requires an INR of 3 to 4.5. Recent clinical trials of anticoagulation therapy now carefully define the intensity of anticoagulation that was used in the study by specifying the range of INR employed. Deep venous thrombosis usually is treated with warfarin at low intensity, whereas patients with mechanical heart valves or recurrent thromboembolism are given higher intensity anticoagulation therapy (e.g., INR of 2.5–3.5).

The benefits of antithrombotic therapy with oral anticoagulants must be balanced carefully with the potential risks of bleeding. One advantage of low intensity anticoagulation therapy has been the reduction in both major and minor bleeding events. In general, the overall risk of serious bleeding (as defined by hospitalization, blood transfusions, and the interruption of anticoagulation therapy) is approximately 1% to 2% per year for a general clinic population. Several studies have suggested that these risks are not cumulative, but tend to level off after approximately 2 yr of therapy.[40] The incidence of central nervous system hemorrhage has been estimated to occur at a rate of approximately 0.1% per year. About half of these individuals either will die or develop serious disability. It seems likely that patient reliability, the number and severity of concurrent medical and surgical illnesses, and the use of anticoagulation clinics with highly trained professional staff may substantially modify the risks of bleeding.

When high intensity oral anticoagulation therapy is given along with 600 to 1200 mg of aspirin per day, the risk of gastrointestinal hemorrhage and possibly central nervous system hemorrhage has been shown to be greatly increased.[41] More recently, the possible use of lower doses of aspirin (60 to 160 mg/day) plus low intensity warfarin is being considered. Whether combination therapy with an antiplatelet agent and an anticoagulant will increase the therapeutic benefit with acceptable or even reduced risks of bleeding is not yet known.

Warfarin may interact with several cardiac medications commonly in use in patients with heart failure. For example, a recent study has suggested that amiodarone may substantially increase the anticoagulant effect of warfarin.[42] Patients receiving both warfarin and amiodarone or other cardiac medications should have their prothrombin times monitored frequently to detect possible pharmacologic interactions.

Anticoagulants in Heart Disease Associated with Congestive Heart Failure

Cardiomyopathy

Intracardiac thrombi have been found frequently in patients with cardiomyopathy. One pathologic study indicated that 75% of hearts from patients dying of the disorder contain thrombi.[43] At least initially, the lesions tend to be small and remain localized to the apical portion of the heart. The marked stasis of blood that occurs as a result of the hypokinetic ventricle seems likely to play a major role in the genesis of thrombosis in advanced cardiomyopathy. It also has been suggested that disruption or dysfunction of the endothelium may be found in dilated myocardiopathy, although not to the degree that occurs after a large anterior transmural myocardial infarction.[43] The fibrin clot may remain highly thrombogenic because of the persistence of thrombin absorbed on its surface.[34,44] A recent echocardiographic study suggested that intraventricular thrombi in cardiomyopathy seldom change in size or motion profile if patients are not anticoagulated.[45] However, if anticoagulants are given, the thrombi tend gradually to diminish in size or even disappear over weeks to months.

From a clinical perspective, the rate of systemic cardiogenic emboli in patients with cardiomyopathy approaches 4% to 5% per year.[46,47] However, if one or more embolic events have occurred in the prior 2 yr, then there is a much higher risk of subsequent emboli, up to 10% to 20% in the next 1 to 2 yr.[6]

Two studies have suggested that major pulmonary emboli may occur frequently in patients with dilated cardiomyopathy and CHF. In a report by Hsu et al., pulmonary emboli were quite common in a group of pediatric patients with cardiomyopathy who were awaiting transplantation.[48] A recent review of several previous studies analyzing mortality in patients with cardiomyopathy indicated that 38% of the deaths were due to pulmonary emboli, whereas only 30% occurred as a result of systemic arterial embolization.[49] These data suggest that pulmonary embolism may be much more common in patients with cardiomyopathy than is generally appreciated.

To date, there are no prospective clinical trials to test the efficacy of anticoagulation therapy for the prevention of systemic or pulmonary emboli in patients with cardiomyopathy. However, several uncontrolled trials have shown that the rate of systemic emboli has been dramatically reduced, in some cases to zero, after the institution of anticoagulants.[46]

Most would agree that anticoagulation with warfarin is indicated in patients with dilated cardiomyopathy.[6,50] Patients with a history of thromboembolism in the preceding 2 yr are at highest risk since they are likely to have rates of embolization of more than 6% per year. These patients should be treated with moderate intensity warfarin, with INRs maintained between 2.5 and 3.5. Patients with advanced cardiomyopathy but no prior history of embolization may be at lesser risk. Emboli in these patients approximate 2% to 6% per year, and they should be treated with low intensity (INR 2–3) warfarin therapy. Those individuals who have a chronic LV aneurysm after acute MI, but who do not have a global reduction in ventricular function, probably do not require anticoagulation therapy, since the risk of emboli appears to be quite low.

In a study using medical decision analysis, the survival of cardiomyopathy patients treated with oral anticoagulants was prolonged by 2 to 6 months.[49] However, the authors suggested that the increase in survival was associated with a reduced quality of life, as defined by increased hemorrhagic episodes, and frequent visits to health care facilities for prothrombin time determinations because of the difficulty in maintaining stable anticoagulation in patients with severe heart failure.

Recommendations

1. Patients with dilated cardiomyopathy without a history of systemic embolization have a risk of thromboembolism approaching 2% to 6% per year. They should be treated with low intensity warfarin (INR 2–3).
2. Patients with a history of systemic embolization in the preceding 2 yr should be treated with moderate intensity warfarin (INR 2.5–3.5).
3. Patients with very early cardiomyopathy or those with chronic LV aneurysm remote from acute MIs probably do not require anticoagulation therapy.

Transmural Anterior Myocardial Infarction

A substantial portion of patients who have an anterior MI develop LV thrombi (for review see refs. 6, 50–53). The development of these thrombi is due in part to stasis of the blood, which may be particularly severe in the apical segment of the LV. In addition, infarction of the ventricle may produce substantial endothelial damage and inflammation, which exposes thrombogenic endocardial surfaces to the blood. Some investigators also have suggested that a generalized "hypercoagulable state" may accompany acute MI.[53]

Several studies have indicated that more than 50% of patients suffering a large anterior MI (e.g., CPK >2000 units) will develop a LV thrombus, and of these, 10% will have cerebral emboli. If consecutive patients with an acute MI are considered, 2.5% will develop a cerebral vascular accident within the first month. As many as 6% of patients with an anterior MI, but only 1% of those with inferior MI, will have a stroke. Half of these will occur in the first week after the infarct, one quarter in the second week, and one quarter in the next 2 to 12 weeks.

Pooled echocardiographic data suggest that approximately 4% of patients with inferior MIs and 20% to 40% of patients with anterior MIs will be complicated by a mural thrombus within the ventricle. If extensive anterior infarction occurs, then the risk of developing a mural thrombus may be as high as 60%. A recent study of patients with anterior MIs indicated that 27% of those having a mural thrombus developed systemic emboli. However, if mural thrombi were not present as identified by echocardiography, then only 2% had systemic embolization.[54] Most thrombi form between the second and seventh day after MI. Very few thrombi seem to form within the first 24 hr.[50]

In contrast to patients with acute MI, those developing a chronic LV aneurysm commonly will have thrombi (up to 50%) located within the aneurysm, but systemic embolization occurs quite infrequently, perhaps only once per 100 patient years of observation. However, if global LV dysfunction follows acute MI and the ejection fraction is less than 35%, the risks approximate those of patients with dilated cardiomyopathy due to other causes; for example, 3% to 4% per year. If a thrombus protrudes into the LV cavity or is mobile, then the risk of emboli is greatly increased.

Several studies have shown that anticoagulation therapy effectively reduces both ventricular thrombi and embolization in patients with MI (for reviews see refs. 6, 50–53, 55, 56). Three large clinical trials performed in the last 20 yr have shown that heparin followed by oral anticoagulation with warfarin or other coumarin derivatives decreased the rate of cerebral embolism from approximately 3% to 1%. Four echocardiographic trials performed in the last 5 yr showed that anticoagulants (heparin) decreased LV thrombi by more than 50%.

A recent study compared moderately high (12,000-unit) doses with lower (5000-unit) doses of heparin administered subcutaneously twice daily for 10 days.[57] In this trial, two-dimensional echocardiography was obtained on the tenth day in 221 patients with anterior MI. The results showed that only 11% of patients receiving the larger doses of heparin developed LV thrombi, as compared to 32% of patients who received the smaller doses. Of interest, patients who developed thrombi had lower circulating heparin levels and shorter

PTTs, suggesting that even higher doses of heparin may be required for optimal anticoagulation in these patients.

These data strongly support administering heparin in adjusted doses to patients with large anterior MIs in doses sufficient to prolong the PTT to 1.5 to 2.0 times control. The therapy should be begun as soon as possible after admission to the hospital. Warfarin also should be started early, with a goal of low intensity anticoagulation (i.e., an INR of 2–3). Most authorities suggest that warfarin be continued for 3 months. If CHF, atrial fibrillation, or marked LV dysfunction is present, then anticoagulation probably should be continued indefinitely. However, if patients develop a chronic LV aneurysm but have good global LV function, then anticoagulation therapy could be discontinued after 3 months. This recommendation probably remains valid even if thrombi are documented within an aneurysm.

However, several important questions remain unanswered. For example, it remains uncertain whether low or higher intensity warfarin should be administered after anterior MI. Two long-term (i.e., 2–3 yr) trials of oral anticoagulant therapy in patients with MI favor higher intensity therapy.[58,59] Both of these trials, which used high intensity warfarin, showed that total mortality, stroke, and subsequent MI were significantly reduced. However, higher intensity therapy will almost surely produce increased bleeding, so that prospective controlled trials will be necessary to resolve the important issue of risk versus benefit.

A second question might be raised as to whether it is advantageous to identify, prospectively, LV thrombi using serial echocardiography before instituting heparin therapy.[60] Potential problems with this approach include the need for repeated echocardiograms (which would be quite expensive) and the possibility that some early thromboses may be missed. Finally, questions as to the possible beneficial effects of thrombolytic therapy for coronary artery thrombi and subsequent heparin anticoagulation on the formation of intraventricular thrombi in patients with MI also must be addressed. For example, in one study heparin in a dose of 12,500 units every 12 hr subcutaneously substantially reduced short-term mortality in patients with MI.[61] Sixty percent of these patients received thrombolytic therapy with streptokinase.

Recommendations

1. All patients with a transmural anterior MI should receive prompt heparin therapy with adjustment of the aPTT ratio to 1.5 to 2 times control. Warfarin should be started immediately with a goal of increasing the INR to 2 to 3.
2. Low intensity warfarin therapy should be continued for 3 months. However, if marked LV dysfunction

or atrial fibrillation is present, then anticoagulation should be continued indefinitely.
3. If a chronic LV aneurysm is present but is associated with good LV function, then the anticoagulants could be stopped after 3 months.

Rheumatic Heart Disease

The clinical course of patients with rheumatic heart disease, especially mitral valve disease, frequently is complicated by thromboemboli (for reviews see refs. 6, 51, 53, 62). Thrombi form frequently in the enlarged left atrium or left atrial appendage, most likely as a result of stasis. Stasis, and the risk of systemic embolization, is greatly increased if the patient has chronic atrial fibrillation.

Several studies have indicated that systemic emboli may occur at a rate of 1.5% to 4.7% per year in patients with mitral valve disease. Patients with mitral stenosis have been found to have a slightly higher rate of embolization (1.5 times) than patients with mitral regurgitation. Viewed from another perspective, approximately one out of five patients will develop an embolus during the course of their disease, and 75% of these will involve the cerebral circulation.

The presence of atrial fibrillation dramatically increases the potential for systemic emboli in patients with rheumatic heart disease. The risk may be increased from 6 to 18 times baseline, and emboli may occur as a result of either chronic or episodic atrial fibrillation. The emboli classically begin within the first 1 to 2 months after the onset of atrial arrhythmias. Patients with low ejection fractions (e.g., <35%) have more emboli than those with higher ejection fractions. Also, patients with enlarged left atria that are more than 50 mm in diameter have a greater rate of emboli. It is not clear whether the greater risk relates to an increased propensity to atrial fibrillation due to the enlarged atria or whether it is directly linked in some way to the atrial enlargement. Older individuals are said to be more likely to have emboli than younger patients. Last, after the first embolus, recurrent emboli are very frequent, occurring in 30% to 65% of patients. Most of these events occur in the ensuing year.

In contrast, patients with aortic valvular disease have a much lower incidence of symptomatic emboli. The emboli that have been found in pathologic studies usually were small and calcific, and occurred in up to 19% of patients. However, because of their small size, clinical symptoms of organ infarction often are not reported by the patient. The tiny emboli may be discovered in the retinal vasculature, the brain, the heart, or the kidney. However, if patients with aortic valvular disease have coexisting mitral valve disease or atrial fibrillation, then the risk of embolization rises substantially. In an as yet unpublished trial encompassing 68 patients over 10 years, patients with moderate to severe aortic insufficiency were found to have an embolic rate of 0.83% per 100 patient years.[53] To date, there have been no prospective randomized controlled clinical trials to determine whether anticoagulation therapy is effective in preventing systemic embolization in patients with rheumatic valvular disease. However, several large case series without concurrent controls have clearly shown low rates of systemic embolization in patients treated with anticoagulants. The risk appears to have been diminished by two thirds or more in these series.

Most authorities agree that virtually all patients with chronic mitral valve disease associated with atrial fibrillation should receive warfarin. However, there is disagreement as to the level of intensity of the anticoagulation therapy. Some authors suggest that low intensity therapy is sufficient (INR 2–3), whereas others recommend higher intensity treatment.

Patients who have previously had systemic embolization should certainly receive long-term therapy, with the warfarin administered initially in a moderate intensity (INR 2.5–3.5) range. Some have suggested that anticoagulation could be reduced to a lower intensity after 1 yr of treatment. Most agree that if the left atrial diameter is greater than 50 to 55 mm, the patient should chronically receive warfarin. Last, if globally impaired LV systolic function (e.g., ejection fraction of <35%) occurs in patients with mitral valve disease, then warfarin also should be given.

The remaining group of patients who have mitral valve disease but who do not have a markedly enlarged left atrium, atrial fibrillation, ventricular failure, or a past history of systemic emboli pose a difficult therapeutic problem. Clearly, the risk of systemic embolization will be lower in these patients, and they probably do not require immediate therapy. However, close monitoring is essential to detect changes in the course of their disease (e.g., the onset of atrial fibrillation, the appearance of heart failure) that would mandate antithrombotic treatment.

Another difficult problem is encountered in patients who develop recurring systemic emboli despite optimal oral anticoagulant therapy. Supplemental therapy with dipyridamole in a dose of 225 to 400 mg in divided doses daily should be considered in this circumstance. Alternatively low doses of aspirin (60–160 mg daily) may be added to low intensity warfarin if the patient is at low risk of bleeding. Studies performed several years ago using radioactively labeled platelets suggested that platelet survival was frequently shortened in patients with rheumatic mitral stenosis.[63] Sulfinpyrazone corrected the shortened platelet survival in some patients, but it remained unclear whether antiplatelet therapy without anticoagulants would constitute effective antithrombotic therapy.[64,65]

Recommendations

1. Patients with rheumatic mitral valve disease that is complicated by atrial fibrillation, large left atrial diameter (>50 mm), or globally impaired LV function, should be treated with long-term warfarin (e.g., INR 2–3).
2. Patients with a prior history of systemic embolization should be treated with warfarin in a moderate intensity range (INR 2.5–3.5) for at least 1 yr. Thereafter, the therapeutic intensity could be decreased.
3. Patients with atrial fibrillation, large left atria, or ventricular failure probably should receive low intensity warfarin in the earlier stages of their disease, with an increase to a higher intensity of therapy as heart failure or left atrial enlargement becomes more severe.
4. Patients with recurrent emboli despite optimal oral anticoagulation should receive dipyridamole in a dose of 225 to 400 mg daily or aspirin 60–160 mg daily, as a supplement to warfarin anticoagulation.
5. Patients with rheumatic aortic valvular disease usually will not require anticoagulants. However, if patients have a history of embolization or if the disorder is complicated by CHF or atrial fibrillation, then anticoagulation with warfarin may be indicated.

Mechanical or Tissue Cardiac Valves

Despite major efforts to design mechanical heart valves that have low thrombogenicity, thromboemboli continue to occur (for reviews see refs. 6, 53, 62, 66). The nonbiologic surfaces of the prosthesis may promote platelet adhesion and clot formation, and the presence of atrial fibrillation and LV dysfunction in many of these patients also may contribute to stasis and increase the likelihood of clot formation on the implanted valves or elsewhere in the heart.

Unfortunately, thrombosis and systemic embolization still may occur in patients with mechanical prosthetic heart valves despite optimal anticoagulation. Rates of emboli from large groups of patients with various types of mechanical valve prostheses have been reported over several decades. In one large series of 300 elderly patients with Starr-Edwards ball valves who were followed for 10 to 19 yr, embolization occurred in 34% by 10 yr, and in 42% by 15 yr.[67] The cerebral circulation was the destination for 85% of these emboli. Half of the patients developed permanent neurologic deficits and 10% died. The author calculated the event rates for a Starr-Edwards prosthesis in the mitral position of 3.9 occurrences per 100 patient years, and a rate of 3.7 events per 100 patient years when the valve was inserted in the aortic position. Currently, rates of embolization are somewhat lower. As reported in a recent review of anticoagulated patients, 2.5% per year suffered emboli with

Starr-Edwards valves, 2% per year with Bjork-Shilley valves, and 1.5% with St. Jude valves.[68]

Anticoagulation with warfarin is indicated as soon as possible postoperatively with the goal of attaining an INR of 2.5–3.5. A recent study suggested that this less intense anticoagulation regimen is effective.[69] In this trial, one group of patients who were treated with warfarin to an INR of 2.65 was compared with another group of patients receiving warfarin at a mean INR of 9.0. The rate of thromboembolism was found to be the same in both groups; that is, 4 and 3.7 episodes per 100 patient years, respectively. However, as might be expected, the rate of major bleeding was greater in the high intensity anticoagulation group. Bleeding occurred at a rate of 0.95 episodes per 100 patient years in the low intensity group, but was 2.1 episodes per 100 patients years in the high intensity patients. This trial suggests that "intermediate" intensity warfarin therapy (in this case an INR goal of 3.0) will be adequate antithrombotic protection for patients with mechanical heart valves and would result in lower rates of serious bleeding.[1]

In patients with an increased risk of thromboembolism such as those with older valves or a prior history of embolization, then dipyridamole in a dose of 400 mg/day should be added to the warfarin therapy. Alternatively, low doses of aspirin (60–160 mg daily) can be added to the oral anticoagulant. This strategy may offer increased protection without major increase in the risk of bleeding.[69a]

The rationale for the addition of the antiplatelet agent dipyridamole to warfarin is based on several clinical trials, three of which showed that dipyridamole plus warfarin significantly reduced thromboembolism compared to warfarin alone. The addition of high doses of aspirin to high intensity warfarin is risky because of a marked increase in the incidence of severe gastrointestinal bleeding in these patients.[41] However, the use of lower doses of aspirin in the range of 60 to 160 mg per day may be safer.[1,69a]

If hemorrhage occurs on high intensity warfarin therapy, then patients might be treated by reducing the INR to 2 to 3 and adding dipyridamole at a dose of 400 mg/day. If even low intensity warfarin is not tolerated, then consideration must be given to antiplatelet therapy alone, or removing the mechanical prothesis and replacing it with a tissue valve.

In general, tissue valves have a substantially lower thrombogenicity than mechanical valves. The surfaces of these valves may be less likely to promote platelet and fibrin deposition, and the blood flow through these valves may be more "physiologic" with less turbulence and stasis. The risk of thromboembolism is higher when a tissue valve is located in the mitral rather than the aortic position, and in the presence of atrial fibrillation. LV dysfunction also increases the risk of thromboem-

bolism. Several studies have suggested that the early months after valvular implantation confer additional embolic risk as compared to subsequent intervals.

Patients receiving mitral and probably aortic tissue valves should be anticoagulated immediately with warfarin for 3 months. A recent study of tissue valves compared a group of patients anticoagulated with warfarin at low intensity (INR 2–2.5) for 3 months with a second group receiving more intense anticoagulation (INR 2.5–4).[70] There was no difference in the rate of thromboembolism, although bleeding was substantially higher in the high intensity therapy group. Based on this study, low intensity warfarin will likely suffice for most patients receiving tissue valves for the first 3 months after surgery.

Thereafter, if left atrial enlargement persists or if there is atrial fibrillation, a history of systemic embolization, or LV failure, then the anticoagulants probably should be continued. If none of these indications are present, then the anticoagulants may be discontinued, with consideration being given to the administration of one aspirin tablet per day, although there is no documentation as of yet for the efficacy of this approach.

Recommendations

1. All patients receiving mechanical heart valve prostheses should be treated with warfarin with a goal of attaining an INR of 2.5 to 3.5. Therapy should be continued indefinitely.
2. In patients with an increased risk of thromboembolism such as those with older valves or a history of prior embolization, then dipyridamole at a dose of 400 mg/day or aspirin 60–160 mg/day should be added. If systemic emboli persist despite this therapy, then consideration should be given to reoperation and implantation of a tissue valve.
3. If hemorrhage occurs during the administration of moderate intensity warfarin therapy, then the dose of warfarin could be reduced to an INR of 2–3 with the addition of dipyridamole at a dose of 400 mg/day.
4. For patients receiving tissue valves in the mitral, and most probably the aortic position, anticoagulation with warfarin at a low intensity level (INR 2–3) is probably sufficient. In patients with additional risk factors for thrombosis such as marked left atrial enlargement, atrial fibrillation, ventricular failure, or a history of systemic embolization, then higher intensity warfarin (e.g., 2.5–3.5 INR) should be considered.
5. In patients with tissue valves, anticoagulants may be stopped after 3 months in the absence of thromboembolic complications and ongoing risk factors for thrombosis. Consideration should be given to the administration of one aspirin tablet per day,

FIGURE 36.1. Cumulative rate of primary events for warfarin vs. placebo in patients with non-rheumatic atrial fibrillation. Reprinted, with permission from Stroke Prevention in Atrial Fibrillation Investigators. *Circulation*. 1991;84: 527–539. Copyright by the American Heart Association.

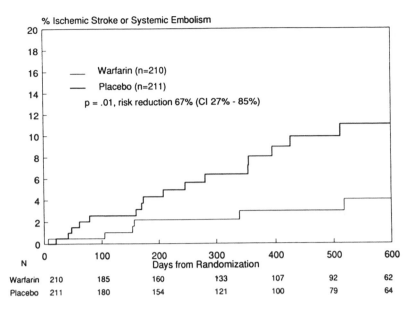

although documentation of efficacy is not yet available.

Nonrheumatic Atrial Fibrillation

Atrial fibrillation complicating cardiac disease greatly increases the risks of thromboembolism (for reviews see refs. 6, 62, 71, 72). As previously discussed, when atrial fibrillation develops in patients with rheumatic mitral valve disease, the risk of thromboembolism increases by 6 to 18 times. The rate of systemic embolization in unselected groups of patients with atrial fibrillation ranges from 3% to 8.5% per year.

Three recent randomized and controlled clinical trials have clearly shown that anticoagulation therapy with warfarin will significantly reduce systemic emboli in patients with atrial fibrillation. In the AFASAK study from Denmark, the rate of thromboembolism was reduced from 5.5% to 2% per year, which translated to a risk reduction of 85%.[73] In the United States SPAF study, the rate of emboli was reduced from 7.4% to 2.3% per year, a risk reduction of 67%[74] (see Fig. 36.1). The Boston-based BAATAF study showed that the rate of embolization decreased from 2.98% to 0.41% per year, a risk reduction of 86%.[75] The reduction in risk in each of these studies was statistically significant and was remarkable in their similarity. Recently, a study was published from Canada showing that low intensity warfarin therapy was associated with a trend toward benefit, with a risk reduction of 37%.[76]

Two of the studies also examined the role of aspirin as compared to warfarin in the prevention of thromboembolism, with conflicting results. The second phase of the SPAF trial (SPAF II) has been designed to answer the question as to whether warfarin or aspirin is superior in preventing systemic emboli in patients with atrial fibrillation.

Each of these studies enrolled patients who had CHF in addition to atrial fibrillation. Subgroup analyses have not yet been reported, which might indicate whether heart failure patients have a higher risk of thromboembolism, and whether warfarin or aspirin was as effective in these patients as in the total group.

In the AFASAK study, 50% to 54% of the patients in the warfarin, aspirin, and placebo groups were reported to have heart failure in addition to atrial fibrillation. In the overall study, warfarin was successful in reducing systemic emboli whereas aspirin, given in a dose of 75 mg once daily, was not. From the data presented, it seems unlikely that low-dose aspirin would provide effective antithrombotic therapy in the subgroup of patients with CHF.

In contrast, the SPAF trial enrolled only 13% of patients with definite CHF in the warfarin or aspirin groups and 17% of patients in the placebo group. In this study, higher dose aspirin (325 mg/day) or warfarin were both effective in the total group of patients as compared to placebo. However, it is unknown whether the subgroup of patients with CHF may have been refractory to either warfarin or aspirin therapy. In the BAATAF study, 24% of the warfarin group and 28% of the control group had CHF. In this study, low intensity warfarin was effective in the prevention of emboli. However, the administration of aspirin in the placebo group was not controlled, and it remains uncertain whether aspirin or low intensity warfarin was effective in patients with CHF.

In these three trials, high intensity warfarin (INR 3–4.5) was used in the AFASAK study, intermediate intensity warfarin (INR 2–3.5) in the SPAF study, and low intensity warfarin (INR 1.5–2.7) in the BAATAF study. Because of the small percentage of patients enrolled in the lower intensity regimens, it seems unlikely that there are enough patients for subgroup analysis to indicate whether warfarin at these doses will benefit patients with heart failure.

Recommendations

1. Low intensity anticoagulation therapy with warfarin is indicated in patients with nonrheumatic atrial fibrillation complicating cardiac disease. If the cardiac disease is mild and uncomplicated, then aspirin (325 mg daily) also may be effective.
2. Patients with significant degrees of uncompensated CHF as well as atrial fibrillation probably should receive low intensity anticoagulation therapy with warfarin.
3. If patients develop excessive bleeding while on low intensity therapy, then oral anticoagulants should be discontinued and aspirin (360 mg daily) used.

Compensated Versus Noncompensated Congestive Heart Failure

Unfortunately, there are no prospective randomized clinical trials to determine whether CHF in the absence of other cardiac risk factors for thrombosis leads to an increased incidence of systemic or pulmonary emboli, or whether the administration of anticoagulation therapy will reduce these events. If heart failure is treated effectively and there are no other risk factors for thrombosis, then it seems likely that there will be little benefit from antithrombotic therapy. However, if heart failure is uncompensated with a substantially reduced cardiac index, then stasis and pooling of blood within the heart may make intracardiac thrombosis more likely. Moreover, low cardiac output and peripheral edema may increase the risk for venous thrombosis and also pulmonary embolism, which could be devastating in the setting of advanced cardiac disease.

In patients with ejection fractions of <35%, chronic anticoagulation therapy must be considered. Low intensity warfarin therapy not only should protect against systemic emboli originating in the heart, but also should reduce the risks of venous thrombosis. However, clinical trials will be required to determine whether the benefits of anticoagulation therapy outweigh the risks of hemorrhage, especially given the difficulty of adjusting doses of anticoagulants in patients with CHF.

Recommendation

1. Patients with moderate or severe uncompensated CHF in the absence of other indications for anticoagulant therapy probably should receive low intensity warfarin therapy (INR 2–3). This therapy should help protect against venous thrombosis as well as systemic thromboemboli.

Management of Surgical Procedures in Patients with Heart Disease Who Are Receiving Anticoagulants

The optimal management of anticoagulation therapy in patients with cardiac disease requiring surgery is a common problem. On one hand, there is an increased risk of systemic or pulmonary emboli during or after a surgical procedure if the anticoagulants are stopped. On the other, there is an excessive risk of bleeding if anticoagulant therapy is continued during the operation.

A number of strategies have been suggested for management of anticoagulants in this clinical situation.[77–80] Several studies have indicated that the risk of systemic embolization in patients with long-term mechanical heart valves is low if oral anticoagulants are withheld for only a few days perioperatively. Therefore, some have recommended simply stopping the anticoagulants several days before surgery, allowing the prothrombin time to return to normal, and then after surgery restarting the anticoagulants.

A second, more aggressive approach has been to admit the patient to the hospital, discontinue the warfarin, and then administer full-dose intravenous heparin anticoagulation after the prothrombin time has fallen to 1.5 times control (an INR of about 3). The heparin is then stopped several hours before surgery and restarted 1 to 2 days postoperatively when the surgical team agrees that it is safe to do so. Warfarin is then restarted. A major problem with this approach is the substantially increased hospital costs as well as a greater chance of postoperative bleeding. A recent study using medical decision analysis suggested that hospitalization for 2 days of postoperative heparin therapy did not excessively increase costs.[80] A third day of heparin therapy in very high risk patients probably is worthwhile. However, if additional days of intravenous inpatient heparin therapy are required, then the costs substantially outweigh the potential benefits.

An important and often overlooked factor in designing antithrombotic strategy for a surgical patient who requires anticoagulants is the propensity of a given surgical procedure to incite thrombosis. For example, a patient undergoing hip replacement surgery will have a very high risk of venous and perhaps systemic thromboembolism. In contrast, dental extractions or other minor surgical procedures probably do not markedly increase the likelihood of thrombosis. In the latter situation, simply stopping anticoagulation therapy temporarily is probably the wisest course of action.

For the exceptionally high risk (e.g., orthopedic) patient, other prophylactic antithrombotic measures can be employed during and after surgery. These include the use of an adjusted dose subcutaneous or intravenous heparin regimen in which the aPTT is maintained at the upper range of normal throughout the operative and postoperative period.[81] An alternative adjusted dose strategy is the use of low doses of warfarin, keeping the prothrombin time prolonged by just 1 to 3 s at the time of surgery. Although there may be a slightly increased rate of wound hematoma or other hemorrhage associated with these prophylactic measures, the bleeding risks seem warranted in patients who are greatly predisposed to thromboembolism. Additional simple prophylactic measures include the routine use of sequential pressure inflatable booties.[82]

Recommendations

1. In patients with strong indications for anticoagulant therapy who are undergoing major surgical procedures, warfarin should be discontinued 5 to 6 days before surgery, and heparin instituted at full dose, either administered twice daily into the subcutaneous fat as an outpatient or by continuous intravenous infusion in the hospital. Before the surgery, the heparin may be discontinued (the $T_{1/2}$ of heparin after intravenous administration is about 1 hr) and adjusted dose heparin administered to keep the aPTT in the upper normal range (e.g., 31–35 s) throughout surgery. The heparin can be administered either every 8 hr by intrafat injection (beginning at 3500 U) or by continuous intravenous infusion beginning at a rate of 400 to 500 units/hr. Beginning 1 to 2 days after surgery, the heparin infusion rate can be increased gradually until the patient is fully anticoagulated. Warfarin therapy may be reinstituted when the patient is able to take oral fluids.
2. Patients with a more moderate risk of thrombosis should have their anticoagulants discontinued before surgery, and prophylactic therapy administered using adjusted dose heparin and pneumatic booties. After surgery, warfarin should be reinstituted.
3. Patients who are not at high risk for thromboembolism and are undergoing minor surgical procedures can simply have their oral anticoagulants discontinued before surgery and restarted shortly thereafter if there is no bleeding.

Conclusions

LV failure is likely to increase the chances of systemic embolization or intracardiac thrombosis in patients with a broad range of cardiac diseases including cardiomyopathy, anterior MI, rheumatic heart disease, mechanical or tissue valves, and nonrheumatic atrial fibrillation (see Table 36.2). Patients with uncompensated CHF should be considered at additional risk of

TABLE 36.2. Risk of embolism in various cardiac diseases.

Disease	Approximate incidence/yr (%)
Cardiomyopathy	4–5
With prior emboli	10–20
Acute MI	
With mural thrombus	27
Without mural thrombus	2
Chronic MI with aneurysm	3–4
Rheumatic mitral disease	
With sinus rhythm	2–5
With atrial fibrillation	12–20
Mechanical valves on warfarin	2–3
Atrial fibrillation	3–9

MI = myocardial infarction.

thromboembolism, and this diagnosis may constitute an indication for antithrombotic therapy.

Few clinical trials have directly addressed the issue of the effects of isolated LV failure as a predisposing factor to systemic or pulmonary thromboembolism. In some instances, subgroup analyses (e.g., in the atrial fibrillation trials) may help determine the magnitude of increased risk and the appropriate therapeutic response for the heart failure patient. However, controlled clinical trials specifically addressing the issue of LV failure and the rates of thromboembolism may be required ultimately to solidify these recommendations.

In the future, the availability of sensitive diagnostic tests to detect circulating activated clotting factors or inhibition of fibrinolysis in vivo may help to determine the need for anticoagulant therapy in either individual patients or groups of patients with various forms of heart disease. Some of these tests are now available, such as an ELISA assay of the prothrombin activation fragment $F_{1.2}$, which is a sensitive measure of thrombin generation within the circulation.[83] Other assays for the activation fragments of factor X and factor IX also are being studied, as are tests for the adequacy of the fibrinolytic response such as plasminogen activator inhibitor and tissue plasminogen activator. Hopefully, these tests can be used to identify patients requiring antithrombotic therapy as well as to suggest appropriate intensities of anticoagulation.

A second area of future promise includes the clinical application of new highly effective antithrombotic agents. Included among these are the highly purified low molecular weight heparins and heparinoids, which inhibit factor Xa to a greater extent than thrombin, and which may lead to an increased ratio of antithrombotic to anticoagulant activity, with reduced rates of bleeding.[33] Several highly specific low molecular weight thrombin inhibitors currently are being studied, including recombinant hirudin (originally from leeches) and chloromethyl ketone (PPACK).[84–86] These inhibitors not only inhibit thrombin, but they also penetrate fibrin clots effectively and have antiplatelet effects. Potent new antiplatelet agents also are now being studied, including monoclonal antibodies or small peptides that neutralize platelet glycoprotein receptors, platelet adhesion, and platelet aggregation.[87–89] Hopefully, the availability of new screening tests to stratify patients as to thrombotic risks coupled with innovative antithrombotic agents will improve the treatment and prognosis of patients with cardiac thromboembolism.

References

1. Dalen JE, Hirsh J. Third ACCP consensus conference on antithrombotic therapy. *Chest.* 1992;102:303S–549S.
2. Stein B, Fuster V, Halperin JL, Chesebro JH. Antithrombotic therapy in cardiac disease. An emerging approach based on pathogenesis and risk. *Circulation.* 1989;80:1501–1513.
3. Hirsh J. Antithrombotic therapy. *Clin Haematol.* 1990;3:1–836.
4. Hirsh J. Drug therapy: heparin. *N Engl J Med.* 1991;324:1565–1574.
5. Hirsh J. Oral anticoagulant drugs. *N Engl J Med.* 1991;324:1865–1875.
6. Ip JH, Stein B, Fuster V, Badimon L. Antithrombotic therapy in cardiovascular diseases. *Ann NY Acad Sci.* 1991;614:289–311.
7. Harker LA. Disorders of hemostasis: thrombosis. In: Williams WJ, Beutler E, Erslev AJ, Lichtman MA, eds. *Hematology.* New York: McGraw-Hill; 1990:1559–1569.
8. Hamsten A, Winman B, de Faire U, Blomback M. Increased plasma levels of a rapid inhibitor of tissue plasminogen activator in young survivors of myocardial infarction. *N Engl J Med.* 1985;313:1557–1563.
9. Hajjar KA, Gavish D, Breslow JL, Nachman RL. Lipoprotein(a) modulation of endothelial cell surface fibrinolysis and its potential role in atherosclerosis. *Nature.* 1989;339:303–305.
10. Etingin OR, Hajjar DP, Hajjar KA, Harpel PC, Nachman RL. Lipoprotein(a) regulates plasminogen activator inhibitor-1 expression in endothelial cells. A potential mechanism in thrombogenesis. *J Biol Chem.* 1991; 266:2459–2465.
11. Coull BM, Malinow MR, Beamer N, Sexton G, Nordt F, De Garmo P. Elevated plasma homocyst(e)ine concentration as a possible independent risk factor for stroke. *Stroke.* 1990;21:572–576.
12. Harpel PC, Chang VT, Borth W. Homocysteine enhances the binding of lipoprotein(a) to plasmin-modified fibrin providing a potential link between thrombosis and atherogenesis. *Blood.* 1990;76:510a.
13. Malinow MR, Kang SS, Taylor LM, et al. Prevalence of hyperhomocyst(e)inemia in patients with peripheral arterial occlusive disease. *Circulation.* 1989;79:1180–1188.
14. Malinow MR. Hyperhomocyst(e)inemia: a common and easily reversible risk factor for occlusive atherosclerosis. *Circulation.* 1990;81:2004–2006.
15. Clarke R, Daly L, Robinson K, et al. Hyperhomocysteinemia: an independent risk factor for vascular disease. *N Engl J Med.* 1991;324:1149–1155.
16. Vanhoutte PM, Shimokawa H. Endothelium-derived relaxing factor and coronary vasospasm. *Circulation.* 1989;80:1–9.
17. Hogan JC, Lewis MJ, Henderson AH. *In vivo* EDRF activity influences platelet function. *Br J Pharmacol.* 1988;94:1020–1022.
18. Sneddon JM, Vane JR. Endothelium-derived relaxing factor reduces platelet adhesion to bovine endothelial cells. *Proc Natl Acad Sci USA.* 1988;85:2800–2804.
19. Randall MD. Vascular activities of the endothelins. *Pharmacol Ther.* 1991;50:73–93.
20. FitzGerald GA, Smith B, Pedersen AK, Brash AR. Increased prostacyclin biosynthesis in patients with severe atherosclerosis and platelet activation. *N Engl J Med.* 1984;310:1065–1068.
21. Fitzgerald DJ, Wright F, FitzGerald GA. Increased thromboxane biosynthesis during coronary thrombolysis: evidence that platelet activation and thromboxane A_2 modulate the response to tissue-type plasminogen activator in vivo. *Circ Res.* 1989;65:83–94.
22. Carvalho ACA, Colman RW, Lees RS. Platelet function in hyperlipoproteinemia. *N Engl J Med.* 1974;290:434–438.
23. Hirsh J. Hyperreactive platelets and complications of coronary artery disease. *N Engl J Med.* 1987;316:1543–1544.
24. Tofler GH, Brezinski D, Schafer AI, et al. Concurrent morning increase in platelet aggregability and the risk of myocardial infarction and sudden cardiac death. *N Engl J Med.* 1987;316:1514–1518.
25. Trip MD, Cats VM, van Capelle FJL, Vreeken J. Platelet hyperreactivity and prognosis in survivors of myocardial infarction. *N Engl J Med.* 1990;322:1549–1554.
26. McCall NT, Tofler GH, Schafer AI, Williams GH, Muller JE. The effect of enteric-coated aspirin on the morning increase in platelet activity. *Am Heart J.* 1991;121:1382–1388.
27. Asherson RA, Khamashta MA, Ordi-Ros J, et al. The "primary" antiphospholipid syndrome: major clinical and serological features. *Medicine (Baltimore).* 1989;68:366–374.
28. Hamsten A, Norberg R, Bjorkholm M, de Faire U, Holm G. Antibodies to cardiolipin in young survivors of myocardial infarction: an association with recurrent cardiovascular events. *Lancet.* 1986;1:113–115.
29. Ford SE, Lillicrap D, Brunet D, Ford P. Thrombotic endocarditis and lupus anticoagulant: a pathogenetic possibility for idiopathic 'rheumatic type' valvular heart disease. *Arch Pathol Lab Med.* 1989;113:350–353.
30. O'Rourke RA. Antiphospholipid antibodies: a marker of lupus carditis. *Circulation.* 1990;82:636–638.
31. Khamashta MA, Cervera R, Asherson RA, et al. Association of antibodies against phospholipids with heart valve disease in systemic lupus erythematosus. *Lancet.* 1990;335:1541–1544.
32. Leung W-H, Wong K-L, Lau C-P, Wong C-K, Liu H-W. Association between antiphospholipid antibodies and cardiac abnormalities in patients with systemic lupus erythematosus. *Am J Med.* 1990;89:411–419.

33. Levine MN, Hirsh J. Clinical potential of low molecular weight heparins. In: Hirsh J, ed. *Bailliere's clinical haematology—antithrombotic therapy*. London: Bailliere Tindall; 1990:545–554.

34. Weitz JI, Hudoba M, Massel D, Maraganore J, Hirsh J. Clot-bound thrombin is protected from inhibition by heparin-antithrombin III but is susceptible to inactivation by antithrombin III-independent inhibitors. *J Clin Invest*. 1990;86:385–391.

35. Hull RD, Raskob GE, Rosenbloom D, et al. Heparin for 5 days as compared with 10 days in the initial treatment of proximal venous thrombosis. *N Engl J Med*. 1990; 322:1260–1264.

36. Cruickshank MK, Levine MN, Hirsh J, Roberts R, Siguenza M. A standard heparin nomogram for the management of heparin therapy. *Arch Intern Med*. 1991;151:333–337.

37. Warkentin TE, Kelton JG. Heparin-induced thrombocytopenia. *Annu Rev Med*. 1989;40:31–44.

38. Chong B, Ismail F, Cade J, Gallus A, Gordon S, Chesterman C. Heparin-induced thrombocytopenia: studies with a new low molecular weight heparinoid, org 10172. *Blood*. 1989;73:1592–1596.

39. Hirsh J, Poller L, Deykin D, Levine M, Dalen JE. Optimal therapeutic range for oral anticoagulants. *Chest*. 1989;95:5–11.

40. Gurwitz JH, Goldberg RJ, Holden A, Knapie N, Ansell J. Age-related risks of long-term oral anticoagulant therapy. *Arch Intern Med*. 1988;148:1733–1736.

41. Chesebro JH, Fuster V, Elveback LR, et al. Trial of combined warfarin plus dipyridamole or aspirin therapy in prosthetic heart valve replacement: danger of aspirin compared with dipyridamole. *Am J Cardiol*. 1983;51: 1537–1541.

42. O'Reilly RA, Trager WF, Rettie AE, Goulart DA. Interaction of amiodarone with racemic warfarin and its separated enantiomorphs in humans. *Clin Pharmacol Ther*. 1987;42:290–294.

43. Roberts WC, Seigel RJ, McNanus BM. Idiopathic dilated cardiomyopathy: analysis of 152 necropsy patients. *Am J Cardiol*. 1987;60:1340–1365.

44. Fuster V, Badimon L, Cohen M. Insights into the pathogenesis of acute ischemic syndromes. *Circulation*. 1988;77:1213–1220.

45. Stratton JR, Nemanich JW, Johannessen KA, Resnick AD. Fate of left ventricular thrombi in patients with remote myocardial infarction or idiopathic cardiomyopathy. *Circulation*. 1988;78:1388–1393.

46. Fuster V, Gersh BJ, Giuliani ER, Tajik AJ, Brandenburg RO, Frye RL. The natural history of idiopathic dilated cardiomyopathy. *Am J Cardiol*. 1981;47:525–531.

47. Meltzer RS, Visser CA, Fuster V. Intracardiac thrombi and systemic embolization. *Ann Intern Med*. 1986;104:689–690.

48. Hsu DT, Addonizio LJ, Hordof AJ, Gersony WM. Acute pulmonary embolism in pediatric patients awaiting heart transplantation. *J Am Coll Cardiol*. 1991;17:1621–1625.

49. Tsevat J, Eckman MH, McNutt RA, Pauker SG. Warfarin for dilated cardiomyopathy: a bloody tough pill to swallow? *Med Dec Making*. 1991;9:162–169.

50. Sherman DG, Dyken ML, Fisher M, Harrison MJG, Hart RG. Antithrombotic therapy for cerebrovascular disorders. *Chest*. 1989;95:140–155.

51. Levine HJ, Pauker SG, Salzman EW. Antithrombotic therapy in valvular heart disease. *Chest*. 1989;95:98–106.

52. Fuster V, Halperin JL. Left ventricular thrombi and cerebral embolism. *N Engl J Med*. 1989;320:392–395.

53. Israel DH, Fuster V, Chesebro JH, Badimon L. Antithrombotic therapy for coronary artery disease and valvular heart disease. In: Hirsh J, ed. *Bailliere's clinical haematology—antithrombotic therapy*. London: Bailliere Tindall; 1990:705–744.

54. Johannessen KA, Nordrehaug JE, von der Lippe G, Vollset SE. Risk factors for embolisation in patients with left ventricular thrombi and acute myocardial infarction. *Br Heart J*. 1988;60:104–110.

55. Editorial. Left ventricular thrombosis and stroke following myocardial infarction. *Lancet*. 1990;335:759–760.

56. Levine MN, Anderson DR. Side-effects of antithrombotic therapy. In: Hirsh J, ed. *Bailliere's clinical haematology—antithrombotic therapy*. London: Bailliere Tindall; 1990:815–829.

57. Turpie AGG, Robinson JG, Doyle DJ, et al. Comparison of high-dose with low-dose subcutaneous heparin to prevent left ventricular mural thrombosis in patients with acute transmural anterior myocardial infarction. *N Engl J Med*. 1989;320:352–357.

58. Report of the Sixty Plus Reinfarction Study Group. A double-blind trial to assess long-term oral anticoagulant therapy in elderly patients after myocardial infarction. *Lancet*. 1980;2:989–993.

59. Smith P, Arnesen H, Holme I. The effect of warfarin on mortality and reinfarction after myocardial infarction. *N Engl J Med*. 1990;323:147–152.

60. Ezekowitz MD, Azrin MA. Should patients with large anterior wall myocardial infarction have echocardiography to identify left ventricular thrombus and should they be anticoagulated? *Cardiovas Clinics*. 1990;21:105–120.

61. SCATTI Group. Randomized controlled trial of subcutaneous calcium-heparin in acute myocardial infarction. *Lancet*. 1989;2:182–186.

62. Oczkowski WJ, Turpie AGG. Antithrombotic treatment of cerebrovascular disease. In: Hirsh J, ed. *Bailliere's clinical haematology—antithrombotic therapy*. London: Bailliere Tindall; 1990:781–814.

63. Steele PP, Weily HS, Davies H, Genton E. Platelet survival in patients with rheumatic heart disease. *N Engl J Med*. 1974;290:537–539.

64. Steele P, Rainwater J. Favorable effect of sulfinpyrazone on thromboembolism in patients with rheumatic heart disease. *Circulation*. 1980;62:462–465.

65. Goodnight SH. Antiplatelet therapy for mitral stenosis? *Circulation*. 1980;62:466–468.

66. Stein PD, Kantrowitz A. Antithrombotic therapy in mechanical and biological prosthetic heart valves and saphenous vein bypass grafts. *Chest*. 1989;95:107–117.

67. Fuster V, Pumphrey CW, McGoon MD. Systemic thromboembolism in mitral and aortic Starr-Edwards prostheses: a long-term follow-up (10–19 years). *Circulation*. 1982;66:157.

68. Fuster V, Badimon L, Badimon JJ, Chesebro JH. Pre-

vention of thromboembolism induced by prosthetic heart valves. *Semin Thromb Hemost.* 1988;14:50–58.

69. Saour JN, Sieck JO, Mamo LAR, Gallus AS. Trial of different intensities of anticoagulation in patients with prosthetic heart valves. *N Engl J Med.* 1990;322: 428–432.

69a. Turpie AGG, Gent M, Laupacis A, et al. Reduction in mortality by adding aspirin (100 mg) to oral anticoagulants in patients with heart valve replacement. *J Am Coll Cardiol.* 1992;19(Suppl A):103A.

70. Turpie A, Gunstensen J, Hirsh J, Nelson H, Gent M. Randomised comparison of two intensities of oral anticoagulant therapy after tissue heart valve replacement. *Lancet.* 1988;1:1242–1245.

71. Dunn MI, Alexander JK, Silva RD, Hildner F. Antithrombotic therapy in atrial fibrillation. *Chest.* 1989; 95:118–127.

72. Rogers KA, Adelstein R. MaxEPA fish oil enhances cholesterol-induced intimal foam cell formation in rabbits. *Am J Pathol.* 1990;137:945–951.

73. Petersen P, Godtfredsen J, Boysen G, Andersen ED, Andersen B. Placebo-controlled, randomised trial of warfarin and aspirin for prevention of thromboembolic complications in chronic atrial fibrillation. *Lancet.* 1989;1:175–179.

74. Stroke Prevent Atrial Fib Inv. Stroke prevention in Atrial Fibrillation Study: final results. *Circulation.* 1991;84:527–539.

75. Boston Area Anticoagulation Trial for Atrial Fibrillation Investigators. The effect of low-dose warfarin on the risk of stroke in patients with nonrheumatic atrial fibrillation. *N Engl J Med.* 1990;323:1505–1511.

76. Connolly SJ, Laupacis A, Gent M, Roberts RS, Cairns JA, Joyner C. Canadian Atrial Fibrillation Anticoagulation (CAFA) study. *J Am Coll Cardiol.* 1991;18:349–355.

77. Evans RW, O'Rourke RA, McGranahan MC. Thromboembolic complications of anticoagulant withdrawal. *Circulation.* 1968;37:74–77.

78. Michaels L. Incidence of thromboembolism after stopping anticoagulant therapy. *JAMA.* 1971;215:595–599.

79. Tinker JH, Tarhan S. Discontinuing anticoagulant therapy in surgical patients with cardiac valve prostheses. *JAMA.* 1978;239:738–739.

80. Eckman MH, Beshansky JR, Durand-Zaleski I, Levine HJ, Pauker SG. Anticoagulation for noncardiac procedures in patients with prosthetic heart valves. Does low risk mean high cost? *JAMA.* 1990;263:1513–1521.

81. Leyvraz PF, Richard J, Bachmann F, et al. Adjusted versus fixed-dose subcutaneous heparin in the prevention of deep-vein thrombosis after total hip replacement. *N Engl J Med.* 1983;309:954–958.

82. Hull RD, Raskob GE, Gent M, et al. Effectiveness of intermittent pneumatic leg compression for preventing deep vein thrombosis after total hip replacement. *JAMA.* 1990;263:2313–2317.

83. Bauer KA, Rosenberg RD. The pathophysiology of the prethrombotic state in humans: insights gained from studies using markers of hemostatic system activation. *Blood.* 1987;70:343–349.

84. Hanson SR, Harker LA. Interruption of acute platelet-dependent thrombosis by the synthetic antithrombin D-phenylalanyl-L-prolyl-L-arginuyl chloromethylketone. *Proc Natl Acad Sci USA.* 1988;85:3184–3188.

85. Cadroy Y, Maraganore JM, Hanson SR, Harker LA. Selective inhibition by a synthetic hirudin peptide of fibrin-dependent thrombosis in baboons. *Proc Natl Acad Sci USA.* 1991;88:1177–1181.

86. Clarke RJ, Mayo G, FitzGerald GA, Fitzgerald DJ. Combined administration of aspirin and a specific thrombin inhibitor in man. *Circulation.* 1991;83:1510–1518.

87. Hanson SR, Pareti FI, Ruggeri ZM, et al. Effects of monoclonal antibodies against the platelet glycoprotein IIb/IIIa complex on thrombosis and hemostasis in the baboon. *J Clin Invest.* 1988;81:149–158.

88. Phillips MD, Moake JL, Nolasco LH, Turner N. Aurin tricarboxylic acid: a novel inhibitor of the association of von Willebrand factor and platelets. *Blood.* 1988;72: 1898–1903.

89. Coller BS. Platelets and thrombolytic therapy. *N Engl J Med.* 1990;322:33–42.

37
Surgical Approaches to Chronic Congestive Heart Failure

Redmond P. Burke and Lawrence H. Cohn

Surgical options in patients with chronic congestive heart failure reflect the diverse etiologies of this disorder. This chapter discusses the preoperative assessment and preparation of the patient, the surgical techniques applicable to the failing heart, postoperative management, complications, and anticipated outcomes. Specific approaches to ischemic cardiomyopathy, ischemic mitral regurgitation, left ventricular aneurysm, and postinfarction ventricular septal defects are defined, followed by a discussion of combined valvular and coronary disease. A discussion of ventricular assist devices and cardiomyoplasty concludes the section on ischemic congestive failure. Surgical approaches to chronic congestive failure due to valvular disease is divided into sections on aortic regurgitation, aortic stenosis, mitral regurgitation and mitral stenosis and, finally, tricuspid insufficiency. In our approach to each patient, we emphasize the need to define the etiology, anatomy, and pathophysiology of the patient's heart failure, establish their functional capacity, and clearly define the therapeutic goals.

Coronary Artery Disease

Ischemic Cardiomyopathy

Ischemic cardiomyopathy, secondary to coronary artery disease (CAD), is caused by multiple infarctions and subsequent diffuse fibrosis. The resulting myocardial dysfunction reduces the left ventricular ejection fraction (LVEF) to ≤30%. This definition excludes patients with ventricular septal defects, aneurysms, and ischemic mitral regurgitation. These patients generally have a poor medical prognosis, which is strongly correlated with their LVEF. They succumb to recurrent infarction, worsening congestive heart failure (CHF), and arrhythmia. LV function is the most important prognostic factor in patients with coronary disease. In the CASS study, patients with single-vessel disease with an LVEF of <35% had a survival rate of 72% at 4 yr, whereas those with three vessel disease and an EF of >0.50 had a 4-yr survival rate of 82%.[1] Better intraoperative myocardial preservation may explain recent improvements in surgical results for these patients. An early mortality of 1.3% to 6.9% can now be achieved after coronary artery bypass in patients with depressed ventricular function, and significantly better survival in patients with EFs <25% with surgical therapy as compared to medical therapy.[2]

The potential for some improvement in contractile function after bypass does exist. Patients with multivessel CAD may have reduced contractility in non-infarcted areas because of chronically reduced coronary perfusion. This "hibernating" myocardium may show improved performance immediately after revascularization.[3] Provocative left ventriculography is an excellent way to perceive the ischemic but not infarcted myocardium.[4] The challenge is to identify patients with ischemic cardiomyopathy who will improve with CABG, and those whose ventricular dysfunction mandates transplantation.

Surgical Technique of Revascularization for Ischemic Cardiomyopathy

We routinely use the left internal mammary artery (LIMA), which is taken down and gently distended with papaverine before grafting to maximize caliber and flow. Bilateral mammary artery grafting is considered in young patients who are not diabetic or obese, but rarely in those with severely depressed ventricular function (LVEF <0.25). IMA grafts may not be used if there is poor runoff in the left anterior descending (LAD) system requiring endarterectomy, or if the operation is urgent. We also consider using the gastroepiploic artery for coronary bypass in patients lacking sufficient internal mammary or saphenous conduit, especially in reoperations.

The aorta and inferior vena cava is cannulated and bypass is instituted. The heart is cooled to 30°C, and fibrillated. The aorta is cross-clamped and hyperkalemic crystalloid cardioplegia at 4°C is infused. Distal anastomoses are constructed using running prolene sutures. The IMA graft, usually to the LAD, is anastomosed last and the aortic clamp is removed. The heart is defibrillated and the proximal anastomoses are placed under a side-biting aortic clamp. Epicardial pacing wires and mediastinal drains are placed routinely.

Patients with preoperative CHF are expected to be volume overloaded and are diuresed appropriately with furosemide and renal-dose dopamine. Patients with severe preoperative CHF from ischemic cardiomyopathy often require pharmacologic inotropic support and intraaortic balloon counterpulsation often is used prophylactically. The use of ventricular assist devices is discussed below.

Supraventricular tachyarrhythmias (SVT) occur in 11% to 40% of postoperative coronary artery bypass grafting (CABG) patients, usually on the second postoperative day, and are particularly truculent in patients with low EF. Elderly patients with a history of atrial arrhythmia, premature atrial contractions on the preoperative electrocardiogram (ECG), and those with a left ventricular end diastolic pressure (LVEDP) of 20 mm Hg or more are at increased risk, but the morbidity of postoperative SVT is minimal and the response to treatment is generally satisfactory.[5] Low dose beta-blockers have become our standard postoperative prophylaxis against SVT, unless the patient has severely depressed ventricular function (EF <15%). Electrocardioversion is used if SVT produces low cardiac output or hypotension.

Outcome of Surgical Reperfusion of Ischemic Cardiomyopathy

Patients with ischemic cardiomyopathy may show functional improvement after CABG despite severe preoperative LV dysfunction. Patients with depressed resting ventricular function (EF <25%) show increased exercise EF after CABG.[6] The mechanisms responsible for this improvement are intricate, but it is clear that complete revascularization and graft patency are essential to revive the hibernating myocardium.

Patients with ischemic cardiomyopathy are at increased risk after CABG. Of the 2144 CASS study patients over 65 years of age, 42% had a cardiothoracic ratio of ≥0.5, and 23% had an LVEDP <20 mm Hg. These findings were associated with increased perioperative mortality. Symptoms and signs of CHF also predicted a higher perioperative mortality.[7] However,

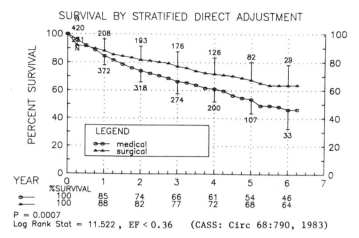

FIGURE 37.1. Percent survival in patients with low EF undergoing CABG. Reproduced, with permission, from Alderman EL, Fisher LD, Litwin P, et al. Results of coronary artery surgery in patients with poor left ventricular function (CASS). *Circulation.* 1983;68(4):785–795. Copyright by the American Heart Association.

good results are achieved after CABG in patients with impaired ventricular function. Patients with EFs <50% had a better 5-yr survival (96%) after CABG than with medical treatment (85%) in the CASS study[8] (Fig. 37.1).

There clearly has been a change in the population of patients we are now operating on for CAD since the CASS study of 1975 to 1978. Jones et al.[9] demonstrate this change by comparing their patients undergoing CABG in 1981 versus 1987. A summary of their findings is presented in Table 37.1.

In 1981, 58% of their patients were in an "optimal group" with no prior cardiac surgery, EF >50% and age <65 yr, whereas only 35% of the patients fit this profile in 1987. There was no difference in the outcomes of patients in the "optimal group" operated on in 1981 versus 1987, and hospital mortality in this group is low (1.1%). We have seen similar changes in our patient population—leading us to speculate that increasing use of percutaneous techniques is altering the outcome after CABG by bringing patients to surgery at a more advanced state of illness with more LV dysfunction from

TABLE 37.1. Change in perioperative complications after CABG from 1981 to 1987.

	% IABP	% MI	% Stroke	% Infection	% Hospital mortality
1981 (n = 1586)	1.4	3.5	1.4	1	1.2
1987 (n = 1513)	4.7 (p < .001)	5.5 (p < .08)	2.8 (p < .08)	3 (p < .01)	3.1 (p < .002)

IABP = intraaortic balloon pump; MI = myocardial infarction.

emboli to distal coronary arteries. Prognosis in ischemic cardiomyopathy is improved if the distal coronary vessels at the time of operation are large and have good runoff, complete revascularization is achieved, and effective intraoperative myocardial preservation is maintained.

Ischemic Mitral Regurgitation

The presence of mitral regurgitation (MR) is a crucial determinant of long-term survival in patients with CAD.[10] review of 11,848 patients having significant CAD defined by catheterization from 1981 to 1987 at Duke showed a 19% incidence of MR, with a 3% incidence of moderate to severe incompetence. Only 0.5% of these patients required a valve procedure. The increased morbidity and mortality of ischemic MR relates to multiple factors: the rapid onset, preoperative multiple system organ failure, prolonged cardiopulmonary bypass for combined valve replacement and coronary bypass, the small left atrium (which may limit operative exposure), the thin annulus (which hold sutures less well), loss of the ventriculoannular apparatus, and the complications of prosthetic valves. Acute valve replacement for ischemic incompetence has been associated with high hospital mortality, leading some surgeons to prefer repair to replacement in this setting.[11] At Duke, mitral valve repair reduced the hospital mortality by 50% over valve replacement in acute ischemic MR.

There is a subgroup of patients with ischemic injury to the mitral valve who develop chronic mitral insufficiency requiring surgery. Posterior infarction can result in posterior papillary muscle dysfunction and patients with multiple infarctions can develop MR due to progressive ventricular and annular dilatation. These patients, combining CAD, LV dysfunction, and mitral incompetence are well known for their dismal prognoses. Hospital mortality after mitral valve replacement and CABG for ischemic incompetence has been 40% when the EF is <35%.[12] Recent data from our institution[13] and others[14] demonstrate that the risk of surgery for MR, with or without CABG, has decreased markedly over the past decade—mortality rates as low as 2.3% can be achieved.

Left Ventricular Aneurysm

LV aneurysm (LVA) is defined as a thinned out segment of LV wall protruding from the normal border of the LV with associated akinesis or dyskinesis. LVA usually is associated with transmural myocardial infarction (MI) in the anterior or apical area where poor collateral flow exists. LVA can present with angina, CHF, ventricular arrhythmia, and/or arterial embolism. Rupture is extremely rare. Thrombus is found in 60% of these aneurysms. Patients with aneurysms involving

20% of the LV usually develop symptoms of CHF. In our series of 303 patients with LVA, 65% presented with CHF.[15]

Patient selection for aneurysm surgery remains controversial. High-risk patients are those with shock, recent infarction (especially within 2 months), EF <20%, and the need for balloon counterpulsation. The contractility of the residual ventricle is a reliable predictor of outcome, making coronary arteriography and ventriculography essential preoperative studies.[16] An ideal candidate has an EF in the residual ventricle above 41% with a graftable proximal LAD lesion. Better than 90% 5-yr survival can be achieved in this group.[17] The distinction between akinetic and dyskinetic aneurysms made by preoperative studies also has prognostic significance.[18] Patients with dyskinetic aneurysms have better postoperative functional improvement and lower operative mortality, probably because the elimination of paradoxical wall motion restores ventricular function toward normal.

LVA and intractable ventricular arrhythmia often coexist. Unfortunately, aneurysm resection is not always sufficient therapy in these patients. Lawrie et al.[19] describe the results of direct ablative operations for drug-refractory ventricular tachycardia (VT) in 80 patients, of whom 55 (68.8%) had LVA. Ablative procedures including endocardial resection, cryothermia, and myocardial excision were associated with high mortality in patients with EFs <20%. They suggest that these patients and those with diffuse hypokinesis and no discrete aneurysm should undergo cardiac transplantation or implantation of automatic implantable cardioverter/ defibrillator (AICD).

Operative Technique

Patients with a history of embolization and who are anticoagulated are converted to heparin preoperatively. Preparation is otherwise the same as for other open heart procedures.

For conventional technique of resection, we perform median sternotomy and commence CPB (at 28–30°C) using cold (4°C) hyperkalemic blood antegrade and retrograde cardioplegia and epicardial irrigation with iced saline. Limited dissection of the ventricles minimizes the risk of embolization. The aneurysm is excised, thrombus removed, and the ventricle closed with horizontal mattress sutures over Teflon pledgets reinforced by a continuous suture. Coronary bypass averaged 2.3 grafts per patient in our series.[15] Associated lesions are addressed: valve repair or replacement, ventricular septal defect (VSD) and atrial septal defect (ASD) repair and intraaortic balloon pump (IABP) insertion may be necessary. If the indication for surgery was refractory VF, mapping and ablation or placement of AICD leads is performed.

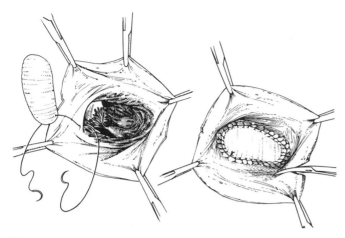

FIGURE 37.2. Technique of ventricular endoaneurysmorrhaphy. Reproduced, with permission, from Cooley DA. Ventricular endoaneurysmorrhaphy: a simplified repair for extensive postinfarction aneurysm. *J Cardiac Surg.* 1989;4(3):200–205.

Endoaneurysmorrhaphy is a new technique designed to avoid the reduction in ventricular volume produced by conventional aneurysm repair, and may improve postoperative ventricular performance (Fig. 37.2), especially in patients with akinetic scars, as we have seen that these patients show the least improvement in ventricular function after conventional aneurysm repair.[20] Our initial results with this technique suggest that early improvement in LVEF can be achieved.[15]

Results of Surgery

In our series of 303 patients with LVA, we had 12 reoperations for bleeding and 4 cases of systemic embolization. The incidence of stroke with LVA in the CASS study was less than 1% per year.[21] Simpson et al. also reported infrequent embolization after aneurysm resection, and they do not routinely anticoagulate.[22]

Early results in patients with LVA in congestive failure were poor, but recent reports suggest that mortalities as low as 8% can be achieved in this group of patients.[23] Cosgrove et al. report a 70% survival at 7 yr in patients operated on for angina, 55% for CHF, 57% for patients with both CHF and angina, and 64% for those with ventricular tachyarrhythmia.[24] Our results showed actuarial 5-yr survival in patients with dyskinetic aneurysms was 63%, and 51% with akinetic aneurysms. Our overall 5- and 10-yr survival was 58% and 34%, respectively.[15]

Functional improvement also can be dramatic in patients with LVAs who present in CHF. Aneurysmectomy and CABG improve CHF and angina in most patients.[25] Louagie et al. describe 49 patients with LVA and CHF who showed improvement from New York Heart Association (NYHA) class 2.9 to 1.6 ($p < .001$),

improvement in Canadian Cardiovascular Society Classification (CCS) anginal class from 1.9 to .9 ($p < .001$), and an increase in EF from 13.7% preoperatively to 30.9% postoperatively ($p < .0001$). Their 5-yr actuarial survival was 70%.[23] Comparative studies suggest that although mortality may not be significantly better, surgically treated patients show more functional improvement and fewer subsequent cardiac complications than those treated medically.[21]

Postinfarction Ventricular Septal Defect

Postinfarction VSD occurs in 1% to 3% of acute MIs, usually in the first week postinfarction. The most common location is the junction of the septum and the anterior or posterior LV wall. Cooley et al. reported the first successful repair in 1957 on a patient 11 weeks postinfarction.[26] Only 20% of these patients will survive past 30 days without surgery.[27]

Postinfarction VSD typically presents as postinfarction cardiogenic shock with a pansystolic left lower sternal border (LLSB) murmur on physical exam. Right heart catheterization shows a left to right shunt that distinguishes VSD from acute MR. Functional status predicts outcome: patients in cardiogenic shock have a 73% mortality.[28] The duration of shock and concomitant multiple system organ failure must be considered before attempting surgical repair. Delaying surgery, anticipating that the infarcted myocardium will scar and anchor sutures more securely, can result in multiple system organ failure and death. Postinfarction VSD should be considered a surgical emergency.

Surgical Repair

Preoperative cardiac catheterization with coronary angiography and ventriculography define the anatomy. Early insertion of IABP is essential to avert the sequelae of a prolonged low output state.

Postinfarction VSD is best approached through a median sternotomy with simultaneous saphenous vein harvest. Cardiopulmonary bypass (CPB) commences with bicaval cannulation. Cold blood antegrade/retrograde cardioplegia is used to cool the heart to 28°C. The approach to the VSD depends on the location of the infarct, but all incisions are through the infarcted LV. If anterior, the infarct is incised and the VSD is repaired with a Dacron patch using pledgetted mattress sutures. If the infarct is apical, we resect the apex. If the infarct is posterior, two patches may be needed. Close attention is paid to maintaining an adequate ventricular volume during the closure. The mitral valve must be evaluated and repaired or replaced as needed. Severely obstructed coronary arteries away from the infarcted VSD are bypassed. After bypass, patients are weaned from the IABP, and monitored for residual left to right shunt. Residual shunt may be present in 10% to 25% of cases and should be re-repaired if the Qp/Qs exceeds 2.[29]

Outcome

The hospital mortality after repair of postinfarction VSD has decreased since 1973 to 18%; before then, hospital mortality had been as high as 47%[30] Long-term follow-up after surgery shows an 8-yr actuarial survival of 63%.[31] Jones et al.[32] report a series of 60 patients treated from 1970 to 1985. There were 23 early deaths and 14 late deaths. Of the 38% long-term survivors, 87% are NYHA class I or II, demonstrating good functional improvement in the survivors. Factors associated with early death include early operation, poor right ventricular (RV) function, and inferior infarction. Good LVEF predicts long-term survival. This study confirms that recent results have improved: from a 58% mortality in the 1970s to a 29% mortality in the 1980s.[32]

Concurrent CAD and Valvular Disease

CAD in patients with valvular disease exacerbates ventricular dysfunction and must be considered in each patient. In the VA Cooperative study, 48% of the patients with valve disease had >50% stenosis of one or more coronary arteries.[33] The indications for coronary angiography in patients with valvular heart disease include age >35 yr, symptoms or signs of CAD, or one or more major risk factors for CAD.[34]

The recognition of concurrent coronary and valvular disease is particularly important in aortic stenosis (AS). The operative mortality of patients with aortic valve disease and associated CAD, who did not undergo CABG with aortic valve replacement (AVR), was increased and the 10-yr survival was reduced[35] (Table 37.2). These results are supported by Lund et al., who found that in 512 patients undergoing AVR for AS, coronary grafting reduced early mortality to a level comparable to that of patients without coronary disease.[36] Angiography should be performed in all adults with symptomatic AS and those with significant CAD should undergo bypass grafting concomitant with valve replacement.

TABLE 37.2. Influence of CAD and CABG on mortality after AVR.

	Operative mortality
AVR	1.4
AVR + CAD + CABG	4.0
AVR + CAD + no CABG	9.4

AVR = aortic valve replacement; CAD = coronary artery disease; CABG = coronary artery bypass grafting.

Ventricular Assist Devices

Congress established the Artificial Heart Program in 1964 with the goal of developing a family of devices to rehabilitate patients effectively with end-stage heart disease. Modern devices can be divided into three categories: tethered total artificial hearts (TTAH), fully implantable total artificial hearts (TAH), and fully implantable LV assist systems (LVAS). Development of such devices adds a powerful option to the physician treating profound ventricular failure, waiting for transplant donor availability, and to the surgeon attempting to wean a failing heart off cardiopulmonary bypass. Current FDA guidelines for patient selection for the use of ventricular assist devices (VADs) are rigid. The patient must be in hemodynamic shock with hypotension (systolic pressure <100 mm Hg), CI <2 L/m^2/min, left atrial pressure (LAP) >20 mm Hg, on full inotropic support and intraaortic balloon counterpulsation. This leaves a narrow time interval for implantation of a device before multiple system organ failure ensues.

VADs as bridges to transplantation have shown promise. In a multicenter trial on 29 patients, reported by Farrar et al., 21 of the patients underwent successful transplantation after 8 hr to 31 days of support using LVADs.[37] These devices were placed in a paracorporeal position on the anterior abdominal wall and connected to the heart and great vessels by cannulas crossing the chest wall. The prosthetic ventricles were driven by a pneumatic drive console providing alternating pulses of pressure and vacuum to empty and fill a blood pump. Complications included infection 6/29, bleeding 11/29, renal failure 2/29, and cerebrovascular accident (CVA) 2/29. Survival after transplantation was good: 92% of the first 12 patients were alive at 1 yr.

The National Heart Lung and Blood Institute is currently funding research on six devices for ventricular support including two LVADs (the Novacor and TCI systems) and four TAHs (Abiomed, Nimbus, Penn State University, and Utah University).[38] Progress continues to be made in addressing the problems of vascular access, patient immobility, infection, thromboembolism, RV failure, and coagulopathy, as well as the broader questions of patient selection and cost.

Dynamic Cardiomyoplasty

The nascent field of cardiomyoplasty holds promise for the treatment of the chronically impaired ventricle.[39] Several configurations of cardiomyoplasty are being explored, each relying on the paced latissimus dorsi muscle to augment cardiac output, either by directly wrapping the LV[40] (Fig. 37.3) or by pumping a bladder as part of an internal counterpulsation system attached to the aorta.[41]

The essential physiologic basis for this technique is

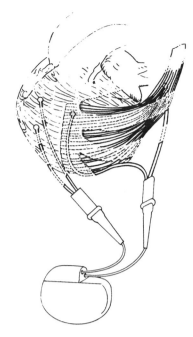

FIGURE 37.3. Cardiomyoplasty technique. Reproduced, with permission, from Magovern GJ, Heckler FR, Park SB, et al. Paced latissimus dorsi used for dynamic cardiomyoplasty of left ventricular aneurysms. *Ann Thorac Surg.* 1987;44:379–388.

the ability of skeletal muscle to be conditioned to become fatigue-resistant by chronic low frequency electrical stimulation. This conditioning results in increased capillary density, oxidative enzymes, and adenosine triphosphate (ATP) production.[42] One drawback to clinical application is that the fiber transformation takes from 4 to 6 weeks. The most efficient skeletal muscle conditioning program has not been defined: the importance of prestimulation with stretch, autotransplantation of the muscle, and postoperative stimulation are being explored.[43]

Skeletal muscle ventricles have been created in animals that have functioned for several weeks, producing effective synchronous diastolic counterpulsation.[44] Carpentier and Chachques reported the first human application of dynamic cardiomyoplasty in 1985, and since then about 100 such procedures have been performed with varying levels of success.[45] Magovern et al. has used paced latissimus dorsi muscle for cardiomyoplasty in humans with ventricular aneurysms with some improvement in cardiac output.[46] Jatene et al.'s results in 13 patients suggest that significant improvements in LV stroke volume and stroke work index can be achieved.[47]

Individual case reports demonstrate that widespread application in the failing heart awaits further understanding of the ideal method for fiber conversion, the timing and duration of skeletal muscle pacing, development of the multiburst pacemaker, and definition of the optimal geometry and technique of skeletal muscle car-

diomyoplasty. The ideal system will maximize cardiac output and minimize the risk of thromboembolism. These biologic and mechanical assist devices are discussed elsewhere extensively in this volume.

Valvular Heart Disease

Aortic Regurgitation

Effective surgical treatment of aortic valvular regurgitation (AR) entails an understanding of the precise etiology, anatomy, and pathophysiology in each patient. AR may be the result of congenital malformations, infectious etiologies, and several inflammatory conditions. Multiple mechanisms produce chronic AR: cuspal perforation, annular dilation, cusp detachment, and scarring preventing diastolic leaflet coaptation. Abnormal flow across valves with underlying deformity results in further scarring, calcification, and degeneration.

The hemodynamic effects of chronic AR have been well described and are critical in defining the optimal timing of surgery. Regurgitation from the aorta into the LV during diastole—which may exceed forward cardiac output by a factor of three times—results in eccentric hypertrophy, where LV wall thickness increases in proportion to the increase in ventricular diameter such that the ratio between wall thickness and chamber radius remains normal. This adaptation allows the patient to maintain a good EF despite an increase in end-diastolic volume.[48] Thus, patients with AR remain well compensated until late in their clinical course. Efforts continue to develop accurate predictors of imminent ventricular dysfunction. Exercise testing is useful but interpretation is complicated by the patient's effective physiologic response to AR.[49]

Chronic volume overload in AR eventually leads to a deterioration in LV systolic function.[50] EF and cardiac output (CO) decline while end-systolic volume rises. Unfortunately, a patient undergoing technically successful AVR after the onset of severe LV decompensation is less likely to improve symptomatically, and the risk of advanced CHF with 5 yr after AVR is markedly increased.[51,52] Asymptomatic patients with AR may progress to irreversible LV dysfunction without symptomatic deterioration. A difficult task is to identify prospectively and follow asymptomatic or minimally symptomatic patients with AR and offer operation before the point at which they develop irreversible LV dysfunction.[53]

Diverse information reflecting the state of the LV is available to the clinician, but the manifestations of deteriorating systolic dysfunction in the patient with chronic AR are subtle. They include increasing LV size, a third heart sound, and the first evidence of reduced exercise capacity.[54] Other variables that correlate with

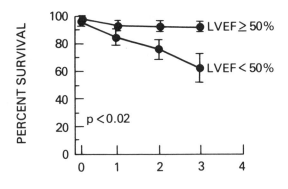

FIGURE 37.4. Long-term survival vs. EF after AVR for AR. Reproduced, with permission, from Forman R, Firth BG, Barnard MS. Prognostic significance of preoperative left ventricular ejection fraction and valve lesion in patients with aortic valve replacement. *Am J Cardiol.* 1980;45:1120–1125.

outcome include LV failure on exam, widened pulse pressure, NYHA functional class, left ventricular hypertrophy (LVH) on electrocardiogram (ECG), and an increased cardiothoracic ratio.[55]

Invasive techniques traditionally have been used as prognostic guides in the patient with AR. EF is highly predictive of postoperative outcome[51] (Fig. 37.4). Survival at 3 yr after AVR for AR in symptomatic patients with normal EF is 30% greater than in those with subnormal EF.[52] An end-systolic volume index <90 ml/m^2 strongly predicts perioperative death in these patients.[56]

In patients with hemodynamically significant AR and symptoms—CHF (NYHA class III or IV), angina, or syncope—we recommend urgent AVR, anticipating symptomatic relief and extended longevity. Minimally symptomatic patients require serial assessments of LV size and function to determine the optimal timing of surgery. An exercise tolerance test will ensure that the patient is not masking symptoms by limiting activity. Asymptomatic patients with LV enlargement (by CXR or Echo) are observed serially as long as LV function remains normal. Surgery is recommended if LV function deteriorates by radionuclide or echocardiographic measure. Noninvasive studies such as serial M-mode echocardiograms are used to follow LV size and function and help predict the onset of LV dysfunction. LV end-systolic diameter >55 mm and fractional shortening $<30\%$ have been shown to predict persistent postoperative LV dysfunction and a poor long-term prognosis.[57] Asymptomatic patients, whose ventricular size is normal, are tested every year for deterioration in resting LV function (EF $<40\%$), increase in the end-systolic diameter to >55 mm, or decrease in LV fractional shortening $<29\%$, understanding that waiting for symptomatic decompensation will compromise the patient's

surgical outcome. We also consider the rate of progression of LV dysfunction, with rapid progression suggesting the need for earlier surgery. Shorter preoperative duration of LV dysfunction predicts the return of normal function postoperatively.[58] Coronary angiography is performed in patients over the age of 45 yr to assess the need for coronary bypass.

Surgical Technique for Aortic Regurgitation

The patient is cannulated via the aorta or femoral artery and venous return is taken from a single cannula in the inferior rena cava (IVC) via the right atrial appendage. CPB is instituted and the patient cooled to 28°C with flows of 1.25 to 1.5 L/min/m^2. The LV is vented through the right superior pulmonary vein to ensure a bloodless operative field. The heart is fibrillated and an oblique aortotomy is made. Inspection of the aortic valve determines the feasibility of valvuloplasty. Heavily calcified and severely deformed leaflets preclude repair and the valve is excised, taking care to preserve the underlying anterior mitral valve leaflet and the atrioventricular (AV) node. Precise and complete calcific debridement prevents perivalvular leaks. The annulus is sized and the appropriate valve chosen. Everting, horizontal mattress sutures are placed through the annulus, using Teflon pledgets if the annular tissue is friable. Free-hand aortic valve homografts require a more elaborate suture technique to restore the natural geometry of the transplanted valve. The aortotomy is closed with two layers of continuous prolene suture. Patients with a dilated aortic root may require reduction aortoplasty or insertion of a one-piece composite valve-graft conduit with reimplantation of the coronary arteries. The latter is mandatory for patients with Marfan's syndrome. Careful attention is paid to deairing the left atrium and ventricle during rewarming, before defibrillation. Appropriate monitoring lines are placed in the atria, epicardial pacing wires are attached, and mediastinal drains inserted. All patients with mechanical valves and those with bioprostheses who have specific indications for anticoagulation, such as chronic atrial fibrillation, are started on coumadin as soon as oral feeding begins, adjusting the prothrombin time (PT), to 1.5 times normal.

Late Postoperative Results for AR

We recently summarized our results after AVR for AR and experienced the following complications in 100 patients (87 porcine valves and 13 mechanical valves) from 1973 to 1982[59] (Table 37.3).

Valve selection requires consideration of several potential complications. The essential problem with bioprosthetic valves remains their lack of durability—95% will function well at 5 yr but as few as 40% will function at 15 yr, because of degenerative failure—

TABLE 37.3. Complications after AVR for AR from 1973 to 1982.

Endocarditis	3/100 (.7%/pt-yr)
Thromboembolism	5/100 (1.2%/pt-yr)
Valve failure	5/100 (1.2%/pt-yr)
Perivalvular leak	3/100 (.7%/pt-yr)
Reoperation	9/100

leaflet tears, and/or calcification of the leaflets. The order of durability of bioprostheses is aortic allograft = 90% (fresh) and 100% (cryopreserved) at 10 yr > porcine xenograft (93% at 7 yr) > pericardial valve (80% at 7 yr). It is hoped that the new "zero-pressure" fixation techniques will preserve some of the stress-reducing properties of aortic valve tissue and improve durability.[60] Results with cryopreserved homografts are encouraging as they minimize the risks of thromboembolism and endocarditis, fit into small aortic roots, and require no anticoagulation. Improved durability and availability would result in an ideal prosthesis. Patients with annular dilatation (i.e., cystic medial necrosis) are poor candidates for homografts as progressive annular dilatation may result in homograft incompetence.

A recent prospective randomized evaluation of prosthetic valves by Bloomfield et al. challenges some of our assumptions about the risks associated with mechanical and bioprosthetic valves. After comparing the Bjork-Shiley, Hancock, and Carpentier-Edwards valves in the aortic and mitral positions, no significant differences in hospital mortality, actuarial survival, incidence of thromboembolism, or need for valve re-replacement were seen.[61]

Outcome After Valve Surgery

Operative mortality ranges from 0 to 17% after AVR for AI.[62] In our series of 100 patients operated on from 1973 to 1982, the operative mortality was 4%, with 1-yr survival of 93% and 5-yr survival of 84%. This group included patients with severe preoperative hemodynamic abnormalities—patients with CI less than 2 (16 patients) and LVEDP above 25 mm Hg (28 patients) are among the operative survivors.

In patients operated on before 1970, the actuarial survival for AVR for severe AR was 84% at 1 yr, 52% at 10 yr, and 40% at 15 yr.[63] This compares favorably to the natural history of medically treated patients where almost 50% of those with LV failure die within 2 yr, and 96% of patients in NYHA functional class III or IV die within 10 yr.[64,65]

Symptomatic improvement after AVR for AI is impressive: 70% to 80% of patients experience improvement and almost 40% have complete symptomatic relief.[63] Ventricular function also improves. Patients with normal preoperative EF usually retain normal function postoperatively, whereas those with moderately reduced ventricular function (EF 0.25–0.49) show improvement about half the time, and one third return to normal. Unfortunately, some patients with poor preoperative EF may have persistently depressed function after AVR and their prognosis is poor,[57] predicting this outcome in specific patients remains uncertain.

Aortic Stenosis

Reduction in aortic valve orifice area is caused most commonly by progressive sclerosis, thickening, and calcification of congenitally bicuspid valves, producing severe stenosis by the fifth decade of life. Senile calcific AS and rheumatic disease also can produce significant obstruction to LV outflow with progressive LV hypertrophy, and eventual dilation and dysfunction. Preoperative noninvasive evaluation with echocardiography delineates the etiology of AS and distinguishes valvular AS from supravalvular obstruction and membranous subvalvular aortic stenosis. Hypertrophic cardiomyopathy also can be discerned with echocardiography.

The average life expectancy after the onset of symptoms in AS is 3 to 5 yr after the occurrence of angina, 3 yr after syncope, and less than 2 yr after the onset of heart failure. An alarming 15% to 20% of the deaths are sudden.[66] In a prospective study of patients with an aortic valve area 0.8 cm² at catheterization, the average survival after onset of symptoms was 23 months, survival after the onset of angina was 45 months, after syncope 27 months, and after the onset of LV failure only 11 months.[67]

We recommend AVR in patients with an aortic valve area index <1.0 cm²/m², and a peak systolic gradient >50 mm Hg, recognizing that this index is dependent on ventricular load (a failing ventricle may produce a deceptively low gradient) and that the variability between the Doppler estimation of the gradient and catheter-derived data can be significant.[68] Natural history studies suggest that mild AS (aortic valve area >1.5 cm²) has a favorable natural history and can be followed, with the recognition that patients with asymptomatic AS are still at risk for sudden death.[69] The natural history of symptomatic AS treated medically has been well described and it is clear that symptomatic AS mandates a surgical solution.[70–72]

Surgical Technique for Aortic Stenosis

The operative exposure, cannulation, and myocardial protection for surgery on stenotic aortic valves are as described for aortic regurgitation. Technical options in AS include valvuloplasty and replacement, although repair is possible less often than in mitral disease. With favorable anatomy, minimal calcific deposits, which do not extend to the ventricular wall, can be gently debrided. Valve competency after debridement is ascertained by fluid competency but most importantly with intraoperative transesophageal echo. Significant rates of restenosis and thromboembolism limit the utility of aortic valve repair in AS. Although Shapira et al. were able to achieve successful repair in 95.8% of their 48 patients with AS, their restenosis rate at a mean of 64 months was 24%.[73] Senile calcific AS appears to be more amenable to repair than rheumatic or bicuspid valve disease, but in our experience valvuloplasty is rarely useful in patients with AS as the restenosis rate remains unacceptably high.

Outcome

In Lund's series of 630 patients undergoing AVR for AS from 1965 to 1986, prosthetic valve complications such as thromboembolism, endocarditis, hemolytic anemia, paravalvular leak, anticoagulant-related hemorrhage, and structural valve failure occurred at a rate of about 5% per year. These complications were fatal in about 15% of instances.[74] Craver et al. report a neurological event rate of 4.2% and a MI rate of 3.5% in 1148 patients undergoing AVR for AS.[75]

Two percent operative mortality after AVR for AS is commonly reported, and late mortality occurs at rates of 3% to 4%/yr with deaths due to CHF (30%), prosthetic valve complications (18%), MI (16%), and arrhythmia (8%). Cumulative 5-, 10-, and 20-yr patient survival rates were 85%, 68%, and 22% in a series of 630 patients reported by Lund.[74] Surgical results after AVR for AS in patients over 70 years of age are good, with hospital mortality between 7% and 12%, and long term survival at 7 yr of 77.2%.[75,76]

Residual hypertrophy late after AVR in AS has been shown to be a prime determinant for impaired LV function, and complete reversibility of hypertrophy after AVR is not the rule.[77,78] In their study of the time course of regression of myocardial hypertrophy after AVR, Monrad et al. show that the process occurs over many years, with continued improvement in ventricular function that may be attributable to remodeling, geometric reconfiguration, and myocardial collagen resorbtion. Early operation for significant AS, even with minimal symptoms, confers normal age- and sex-specific survival up to 20 yr after operation.[74]

Mitral Regurgitation

The technical approaches to chronic MR mandate a clear understanding of the underlying etiology and anatomy. Chronic MR can result from myxomatous degeneration, rheumatic disease, and three types of ischemic injury—posterior papillary muscle dysfunction, papillary muscle rupture, and annular dilatation. Less commonly, infection, hypereosinophilia, and calcification of the mitral annulus can result in chronic MR.

Chronic mitral insufficiency can produce irreversible ventricular injury in relatively asymptomatic patients, making earlier operation desirable. Although prosthetic and bioprosthetic valve devices are hemodynamically sound, each class of device has certain disadvantages. Recent improvements in mitral valvuloplasty for MR may allow earlier surgical intervention so that the 20% to 40% mortality within 5 yr after mitral valve replacement (MVR) in NYHA class IV patients can be avoided. Our indications for mitral valve surgery include symptomatic MR with NYHA class II CHF or worse, evidence of LV dysfunction or increasing LV size, and new-onset atrial fibrillation. The VA Cooperative study on valvular heart disease has defined three variables predicting normal LV size and function after MVR for chronic MR, including an EF >50%, end-systolic volume <50 ml/m^2, and mean pulmonary artery pressure (PAP) <20 mm Hg at rest. We also consider mitral valve repair in minimally symptomatic patients who demonstrate ventricular dilatation (LV end-diastolic diameter >7 cm and end-systolic diameter >5 cm) as these findings portend the risk of irreversible ventricular dysfunction.

Operative Therapy

Dissatisfaction with long-term results after MVR, combined with improved methods for intraoperative myocardial preservation and visualization of the mitral valve via transesophageal echocardiography, has resulted in increase in mitral valvuloplasty (MVP). Repair is strongly considered in patients with ruptured chordae, mild annular dilatation, mitral valve prolapse, endocarditis, and rheumatic valves with slight calcification. Perforations and tears produced by percutaneous balloon procedures also lend themselves to repair. The relative increase in myxomatous MR versus rheumatic mitral disease over the past few decades also has contributed to the resurgence of reparative techniques as repair is possible in most of these patients. Specific techniques have been developed to approach the commonly encountered structural deformities. A dilated annulus can be supported with ring annuloplasty, elongated chordae can be shortened, and ruptured posterior chordae can be replaced with gortex or by transferring normal chordae (Fig. 37.5). Rheumatic involvement of the mitral valve usually produces leaflet retraction, fibrotic thickening, and calcification, making restoration of valve competence more difficult. The long-term results of reconstructive procedures for rheumatic MR have been acceptable, but are probably inferior to those achieved with myxomatous valves.[79,80]

Elegant techniques of mitral valve reconstruction have been developed and described by Carpentier.[81] The essentials of Carpentier's repair include ring annuloplasty, resection of the central portion of the pos-

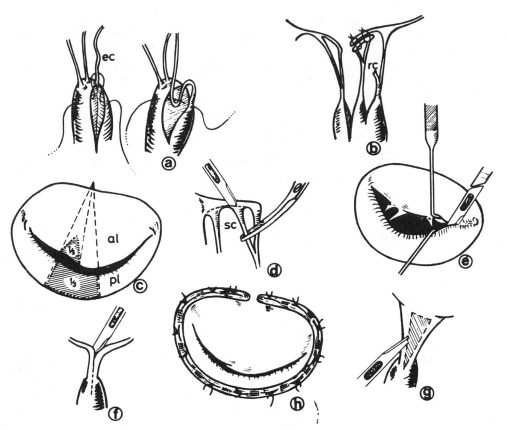

FIGURE 37.5. Mitral valvuloplasty. Reproduced, with permission, from Antunes MJ, Magalhaes MP, Colsen PR, et al. Valvuloplasty for rheumatic mitral valve disease. A surgical challenge. *J Thorac Cardiovasc Surg*. 1987; 94:44–56.

terior leaflet, shortening of elongated chordae, and repair of incidental clefts.[82,83]

Systolic anterior motion (SAM) of the mitral valve with postoperative LV outflow obstruction has been reported after mitral repair using Carpentier's methods.[84,85] Doppler echocardiographic follow-up of patients with postrepair SAM has shown that it tends to resolve with ventricular adaptation during the first year postoperatively Careful attention to the height of the posterior leaflet and avoidance of a large annular plication have been effective in eliminating this complication. Reoperation after valve repair usually is due to unrecognized residual prolapse. Deloche et al. reported a linearized rate of reoperation of 1%/pt-yr in 206 patients undergoing mitral repair.[86] Transesophageal echocardiography (TEE) allows intraoperative recognition of inadequate repair and should decrease the incidence of reoperation.

Operative experiences with mitral valve repair suggest the following contraindications: heavy calcification, severe rheumatic leaflet deformity, submitral calcification, severe damage to the anterior leaflet, and excessively thin leaflets. TEE can be useful in defining the valvular anatomy before attempting repair.

If mitral valve repair is not feasible, the valve is excised, with preservation of the posterior leaflet to avoid the risk of posterior ventricular rupture. Preservation of the anterior leaflet and the chordae to maintain the

functional geometry of the LV is controversial; however, in certain ventricles the totally intact subvalvular structures will enhance LV function.[87] The prosthetic valve ring is sutured and the valve seated in the annulus. The valve is inspected to assure unobstructed leaflet mobility, and the atrium closed. The heart is carefully deaired and monitoring left atrial (LA) and right atrial (RA) lines are placed. TEE is used to assess the effectiveness of repair or the function of a prosthetic valve.

Patients with prosthetic mitral valves are coumadinized when oral intake resumes, maintaining a PT 1.5 times control. Patients in sinus rhythm with bioprosthetic valves are anticoagulated with coumadin for a total of 6 weeks after surgery.

Complications

Complications after mitral valvuloplasty have been reviewed recently by Deloche et al. in 206 consecutive patients[86] (Table 37.4). The incidence of reoperation is significantly ($p < .01$) higher in the rheumatic group than in the patients with degenerative valve disease. This finding is confirmed by Antunes et al., who reported a reoperation rate of 4.3%pt-yr after valve repair in 241 patients with rheumatic mitral disease.[88] Mitral valvuloplasty is proving to be more durable than initially anticipated in degenerative disease. Galloway reports a 5-yr actuarial freedom from late valve replace-

TABLE 37.4. Complications after mitral valvuloplasty.

Complication	Linearized rate
Valve-related mortality	0.9%/pt-yr
Reoperation	1.0%/pt-yr
Thromboembolism	0.4%/pt-yr
Anticoagulation hemorrhage	0.5%/pt-yr
Endocarditis	0.2%/pt-yr

ment of 90%.[89] Our own recent experience with MVP for MR has also been encouraging.[90] Clearly, the risk of thromboembolic and anticoagulant-related complications is lower after repair than replacement, where 10% to 35% of patients have thromboembolic events within 5 to 10 yr after surgery.[91] Endocarditis also is much rarer after mitral repair than replacement, where a 3% to 6% incidence is reported.[92]

Selection of a valve prosthesis for MVR must be individualized. In 253 nonrandomized patients, Perier and colleagues performed 147 CE and 106 Hancock mitral valve replacements, with comparable long-term results. There was no significant difference in the incidence of valve-related deaths: 93% versus 85% free at 10 yr, thromboembolism 0.9% versus 1.1%/pt-yr, and freedom from structural valve deterioration 65% versus 66% at 10 yr. Reoperation was necessary in 64% versus 59% at 10 yr (the mortality for reoperation was 10% in the CE group and 17% in the Hancock group). Freedom from valve failure was 60% versus 59% at 10 yr, from anticoagulant-related hemorrhage 92% versus 85% at 10 yr, and from valve-related mortality and morbidity 50% versus 49% at 10 yr. Several studies confirm the relative immunity from thromboembolic events conferred by bioprosthetic valves; however, durability remains a drawback: at the end of 10 yr 35% of the patients in both groups have undergone reoperation for structural valve deterioration.[93–95]

Outcome

Deloche et al. report 15-yr actuarial survival after mitral repair in 206 patients of 72.4%. Among the 157 survivors, 74% were in NYHA class I or II, whereas 97% of the patients were in classes III and IV preoperatively. Ventricular contractility was normal in 84.5% of patients postoperatively and 91% had minimal or no residual MR by Doppler echocardiographic study.[86] The experience at New York University supports these results: 95% of their patients improved to NYHA class I or II after mitral repair.[89] In our last 200 patients undergoing mitral valve repair, our operative mortality was 2.5%; four of five deaths occurring in patients >70 yr old with combined coronary bypass. Our freedom from reoperation was 85% at 5 yr and the incidences of

thromboembolism (2.5%) and endocarditis (none) were low.

Isolated MVR can be performed with a hospital mortality of 2.0%.[96] Survival at 5 yr is about 80% and at 10 yr 60%, with 45% of patients living 15 yr post-MVR. Half of the late deaths are due to ventricular failure and a fifth are caused by valve-related complications.[97]

Mitral Stenosis

Obstruction to flow across the mitral valve is produced by commissural fusion, decreased leaflet mobility, and shortened rigid chordae. These changes are caused by rheumatic valvulitis. The hemodynamic effects are well known, with gradually increasing left atrial and pulmonary vascular pressures transmitted to the right heart, ultimately producing right heart failure. Physical exam, chest radiography, and echocardiography will establish the presence and significance of MS and distinguish left atrial myxoma, AR, and atrial septal defect, which have similar presentations. Atrial fibrillation, hemoptysis, and systemic emboli are known complications. Since the LV is protected from the valvular deformity, insidious ventricular dysfunction is not a significant factor as in MR. Lacking an ideal prosthetic valve, we recommend valve surgery when patients develop limiting symptoms—NYHA class III or IV—with earlier surgery if repair is considered feasible based on the noninvasive appearance of the valve anatomy.

Preoperative evaluation by Doppler echocardiography helps discern patients whose MS may be amenable to repair. Exposure, cannulation, and myocardial protection are as described above for surgery on MR. Stenotic valves with minimal calcification are repaired by commissurotomy. An open approach allows mitral valve replacement if repair is not possible.

Outcome

MS does not generate the level of ventricular dysfunction seen with regurgitant valves and patients usually have normal ventricular function postoperatively. The nature of the mitral valve dysfunction (stenosis or regurgitation) is not a predictor of mortality after mitral valve replacement except in patients with ischemic mitral regurgitation who have a poorer prognosis.[98,99] Operative morbidity for mitral valve repair for MS runs from 0% to 5%.

Tricuspid Valve Insufficiency

Preoperative Assessment

Acquired isolated tricuspid valve disease is rare, and its causes esoteric—endocarditis from intravenous drug abuse, traumatic rupture after nonpenetrating chest injuries, and carcinoid valve disease. We more frequently see tricuspid regurgitation caused by functionally dilated annulus in association with rheumatic disease involving the mitral and aortic valves. In patients with chronic pure mitral regurgitation, as described by Cohen et al.,[100] 53% had tricuspid regurgitation, which was more likely to be present if the patient had long-standing symptoms of CHF. Tricuspid regurgitation is difficult to quantify but is considered to be present if clinical signs exist and the right atrial pressure is 10 mm Hg or more. Preoperative color Doppler echocardiography has improved our diagnostic accuracy. Digital examination of the tricuspid valve at surgery, with assessment of the annulus size and valve structure, and the appearance of the right atrium can reliably confirm the diagnosis. Intraoperative TEE is developing into a sensitive tool for determining the need for tricuspid valve repair.[101] Preparation for tricuspid surgery is focused on maximal medical treatment of RV failure.

Technique

The optimal approach to tricuspid insufficiency remains controversial. Patients with endocarditis can undergo complete excision of the valve with staged valve replacement when sepsis resolves and the drug abuse stops.[120] Tricuspid valvuloplasty also is an option in right-sided endocarditis.[103]

There are several approaches to patients with hemodynamically significant tricuspid disease. The tricuspid valve can be replaced with stent-mounted heterograft valves, stent-mounted aortic and pulmonary homograft valves, and mechanical prostheses. Repair should most commonly be accomplished using the Carpentier ring annuloplasty, or by the DeVega semicircular suture annuloplasty (Fig. 37.6).[104]

We advocate a systematic approach to combined tricuspid and mitral valve disease. Mild tricuspid regurgitation (TR) with only slightly elevated right heart pressures can be treated simply by correcting the mitral valve lesion. Moderate TR with elevated right heart and pulmonary pressures who have nearly normal valve anatomy can be treated with mitral valve replacement or repair and tricuspid valvuloplasty. Patients with severe TR and abnormal valve anatomy may require combined mitral and tricuspid replacement. Residual or recurrent TR is more likely if the patient has persistent postoperative pulmonary hypertension, making effective treatment of the left sided lesions imperative to ensure successful tricuspid results. Doppler echocardiography is a sensitive method for evaluating preoperative TR and for assessing the success of tricuspid valve repair.[105]

Patients receiving prosthetic valves in the tricuspid position require chronic anticoagulation with coumadin beginning immediately postoperation, as the incidence of thrombosis in this valve position is relatively high. These patients are at risk for late complete heart block and must have continuous ECG monitoring until a stable rhythm is achieved.

Complications

Within the first 5 postoperative weeks, 5% of patients will develop complete heart block after tricuspid valve surgery. Late complete heart block also can occur and is more often seen in patients with combined mitral and tricuspid valve replacement as the atrioventricular node is interposed between the prostheses.

Patients with persistent RV failure postoperation should be evaluated by Doppler echocardiography. In patients with tricuspid valve repair (TVR) using a Carpentier ring, the possibility of inflow obstruction of the RV should be considered.[106]

Outcome

The hospital mortality of tricuspid valve surgery varies from 0 to 33%, depending on the presence of disease in the other valves. Cohen et al. reported 16% operative mortality after tricuspid valve annuloplasty (TVA) and 18% mortality after TVR in patients with pure MR.[100] Survival at 8 yr after MVR alone was 62%; after MVR and nonoperative management of TR, 71%; after MVR and TVA, 40%; and after MVR and TVR, 48%. They compared patients undergoing MVR alone and those undergoing MVR and TVR and found no statistically significant differences in survival at 1, 5, or 8 yr.[98] Func-

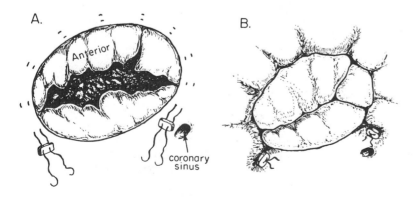

A.   B.

Anterior

coronary sinus

FIGURE 37.6. DeVega suture annuloplasty. Reproduced, with permission, from Rabago G, Fraile J, Martinelli J, et al. Technique and results of tricuspid annuloplasty. *J Cardiac Surg.* 1986;1(3):247–253.

tional improvement is good after tricuspid valve surgery. All but two of the patients surviving in Cohen's series improved by at least one NYHA functional class. McGrath et al. recently reported a 20% actuarial survival rate at 180 months in 530 patients undergoing tricuspid valve surgery, with a 15% incidence of hospital death, demonstrating that the performance of concomitant tricuspid valve procedures in patients with multivalvular disease incurs significant risk.[107]

Conclusion

Advances in myocardial protection, operative technique, and postoperative critical care have expanded the indications for coronary revascularization, especially in patients with poor ventricular function. A renaissance in the use of internal mammary artery grafts may extend the duration of effective revascularization, while we await the development of an effective artificial arterial conduit.

Complex valve repair and replacement have been facilitated by improved intraoperative visualization. Expanded options for valve repair and replacement make earlier surgery feasible, before the onset of ventricular dysfunction. Mechanical and autologous tissue assist devices, capable of supporting the reversibly injured ventricle, or bridging the irretrievably damaged heart to transplant, are approaching clinical availability.

References

1. Mock MB, Ringqvist I, Fisher LD, et al. Survival of medically treated patients in the coronary artery surgery study (CASS) registry. *Circulation.* 1982; 66(3):562–568.
2. Pigott JD, Konchoukkos NT, Oberman A, Culter GR. Late results of surgical and medical therapy for patients with coronary artery disease and depressed left ventricular function. *J Am Coll Cardiol.* 1985;5(5):1036–1045.
3. Topol EJ, Weiss JL Guzman PA, et al. Immediate improvement of dysfunctional myocardial segments after coronary revascularization: detection by intraoperative transesophageal echocardiography. *J Am Coll Cardiol.* 1984;4(6):1123–1134.
4. Cohn LH, Collins JJ Jr, Cohn PF. Use of the augmented ejection fraction to select patients with left ventricular dysfunction for coronary revascularization. *J Thorac Cardiovasc Surg.* 1976;72:835–840.
5. Hashimoto K, Ilstrup DM, Schaff HV. Influence of clinical and hemodynamic variables on risk of supraventricular tachycardia after coronary artery bypass. *J Thorac Cardiovasc Surg.* 1991;101(1):56–65.
6. Hellman C, Schmidt DH, Kamath ML. Bypass graft surgery in severe left ventricular dysfunction. *Circulation.* 1980;62(2 Pt 2)(suppl 1):I:1–103–110.
7. Geresh BJ, Kronmal RA, Frye RL, et al. Coronary arteriography and coronary artery bypass surgery: mor-

bidity and mortality in patients ages 65 years or older. *Circulation.* 1983;67(3):483–491,1.
8. CASS Principal Investigators and Their Associates. Coronary artery surgery study (CASS): a randomized trial of coronary artery bypass surgery: survival data. *Circulation.* 1983;68(5):939–950.
9. Jones EL, Weintraub WS, Craver JM, et al. Coronary bypass surgery: is the operation different today? *J Thorac Cardiovasc Surg.* 1991;101:108–115.
10. Hickey MS, Smith LR, Muhlbaier LH, et al. Current prognosis of ischemic mitral regurgitation: implications for future management. *Circulation.* 1988;78(Suppl 1): 1–51.
11. Rankin JS, Feneley MP, Hickey MS, et al. A clinical comparison of mitral valve repair versus valve replacement in ischemic mitral regurgitation. *J Thorac Cardiovasc Surg.* 1988;95(2):165–177.
12. Radford MJ, Johnson RA, Buckley MJ, et al. Survival following mitral valve replacement for mitral regurgitation due to coronary artery disease. *Circulation.* 1979; 60:(Suppl 1):1–39.
13. Cohn LH, Couper GS, Kinchla NM, Collins JJ. Decreased operative risk of surgical treatment of mitral regurgitation with or without coronary artery disease. *J Am Coll Cardiol.* 1990;16(7):1575–1578.
14. Hendren WG, Nemec JJ, Lytle BW, et al. Mitral valve repair for ischemic mitral insufficiency. Abstract presented at the STS 27th Annual Meeting, San Francisco, CA, Feb. 18–20, 1991.
15. Couper GS, Bunton RW, Birjiniuk V, et al. Relative risks of left ventricular 21. aneurysmectomy in patients with akinetic scars versus true dyskinetic aneurysms. *Circulation.* 1990;82(Suppl 5):IV:248–256.
16. Barratt-Boyes AG, While HD, Agnew TM, Pemberton JR, Wild CJ. The results of surgical treatment of left ventricular aneurysms. *J Thorac Cardiovasc Surg.* 1984;87:87–98.
17. Louagie Y, Alouini T, Lesperance J, Pelletier LC. Left ventricular aneurysm with predominating congestive heart failure: a comparison study of medical and surgical treatment. *J Thorac Cardiovasc Surg.* 1987;94:571–581.
18. Mangschau A. Akinetic versus dyskinetic left ventricular aneurysms diagnosed by gaited scintigraphy: difference in surgical outcome. *Ann Thorac Surg.* 1989;47: 746–751.
19. Lawrie GM, Pacifico A, Kaushik R, et al. Factors predictive of results of direct ablative operations for drug-refractory ventricular tachycardia. *J Thorac Cardiovasc Surg.* 1991;101:44–55.
20. Cooley DA. Ventricular endoaneurysmorrhaphy: a simplified repair for extensive postinfarction aneurysm. *J Cardiac Surg.* 1989;4:200–205.
21. Faxon DP, Myers WO, McCabe CH. The influence of surgery on the natural history of angiographically documented left ventricular aneurysm: the coronary artery surgery study. *Circulation.* 1986;74;1:110–118.
22. Simpson MT, Oberman A, Kouchoukos NT. Prevelance of mural thrombi and systemic embolization with left ventricular aneurysm: effect of anticoagulation therapy. *Chest.* 1980;77(4):463–469.
23. Louagie Y, Alouini T, Lesperance J. Left ventricular

aneurysm with predominating congestive heart failure. A comparative study of medical and surgical treatment. *J Thorac Cardiovasc Surg.* 1987;94(4):571–581.

24. Cosgrove DM, Loop FD, Irarrazaval MJ, et al. Determinants of long term survival after ventricular aneurysmectomy. *Ann Thorac Surg.* 1978;26(4):357–363.

25. Burton NA, Stinson EB, Oyer PE, et al. Left ventricular aneurysm: preoperative risk factors and long-term postoperative results. *J Thorac Cardiovasc Surg.* 1979; 77(1):65–75.

26. Cooley DA, Belmonte BA, Zeis LB, Schnur S. Surgical repair of ruptured interventricular septum following acute myocardial infarction. *Surgery.* 1957;41;930–937.

27. Sanders RJ, Kern WH, Blount SG Jr. Perforation of the interventricular septum complicating myocardial infarction: a report of 8 cases, one with cardiac catheterization. *Am Heart J.* 1956;51:736.

28. Radford MJ, Johnson RA, Daggett WM, et al. Ventricular septal rupture: a review of clinical and physiologic features and an analysis of survival. *Circulation.* 1981;64(3):545–553.

29. Brandt B III, Wright CB, Ehrehaft JL. Ventricular septal defect following myocardial infarction. *Ann Thorac Surg.* 1979;27(6):580–589.

30. Daggett WM, Guyton RA, Mudth ED, et al. Surgery for postinfarction myocardial infarct ventricular septal defect. *Ann Surg.* 1977;186(3):260–271.

31. Keenan DJM, Monro JL Ross JK, Manners JM, Conway N, Johnson AM. Acquired ventricular septal defect. *J Thorac Cardiovasc Surg.* 1983;85(1):116–119.

32. Jones MT, Schofield MB, Dark B, et al. Surgical repair of acquired ventricular septal defect. *J Thorac Cardiovasc Surg.* 1987;93:680–686.

33. Sethi GK, Miller DC, Saxhele J, et al. Clinical, hemodynamic, and angiographic predictors of operative mortality in patients undergoing single valve replacement. *J Thorac Cardiovasc Surg.* 1987;93(6):884–897.

34. ACC/AHA Task Force on assessment of diagnostic and therapeutic cardiovascular procedures. Subcommittee on coronary angiography. Guidelines for coronary angiography. *J Am Coll Cardiol.* 1987;10:935–950.

35. Mullany CJ, Elveback LR, Frye RL, et al. Coronary artery disease and its management: influence on survival in patients undergoing aortic valve replacement. *J Am Coll Cardiol.* 1987;10:66–72.

36. Lund O, Nielsen T, Pilegaard HK, et al. The influence of coronary artery disease and bypass grafting on early and late survival after valve replacement for aortic stenosis. *J Thorac Cardiovasc Surg.* 1990;100:327–337.

37. Farrar DJ, Hill JD, Gray LA, et al. Heterotopic prosthetic ventricles as a bridge to cardiac transplantation. *N Engl J Med.* 1988;318:333–340.

38. Macoviak JA, Dasse KA, Poirier VL. Mechanical cardiac assistance and replacement. *Cardiol Clin.* 1990; 8:(1);39–53.

39. Chiu RCJ, ed. *Biochemical cardiac assist: cardiomyoplasty and muscle-powered devices.* Mt. Kisco, NY: Futura Publishing Co; 1986.

40. Magovern GJ, Heckler FR, Park SB, et al. Paced latissimus dorsi used for dynamic cardiomyoplasty of left ventricular aneurysms. *Ann Thorac Surg.* 1987;44:379–388.

41. Acker MA, Hammond RL, Mannion JD, et al. An autologous biologic pump motor. *J Thorac Cardiovasc Surg.* 1986;92(4):733–746.

42. Walsh GL, Dewar ML, Khalafalla AS, et al. Characteristics of transformed fatigue-resistant skeletal muscle for long term cardiac assistance by extra-aortic balloon counterpulsation. *Surg Forum.* 1986;37:205–207.

43. Sola OM, Dillard DH, Ivey TD, et al. Autotransplantation of skeletal muscle into myocardium. *Circulation.* 1985;71(2):341–348.

44. Acker MA, Anderson WA, Hammond RL, et al. Skeletal muscle ventricles in circulation. *J Thorac Cardiovasc Surg.* 1987;94:163–174.

45. Carpentier A, Chachques JC. Myocardial substitution with a stimulated skeletal muscle. First successful clinical case. *Lancet.* 1985;8440:1267.

46. Magovern GJ, Heckler FR, Park SB, et al. Paced latissimus dorsi used for dynamic cardiomyoplasty of left ventricular aneurysms. *Ann Thorac Surg.* 1987;44:379–388.

47. Jatene AD, Stolf NAG, Moreira LFP, et al. Left ventricular function changes after cardiomyoplasty in patients with dilated cardiomyopathy. *Amer Assoc for Thorac Surg.* 102–103, 70th Ann Mtg, Toronto, Ontario, 1990:7–9.

48. Ross J Jr. Left ventricular function and the timing of surgical treatment in valvular heart disease. *Ann Intern Med.* 1981;94:498–504.

49. Tenenson ME, Frank MF, Schwartz CJ. The effect of rest and physical effort on left ventricular function in mitral and aortic regurgitation. *Am Heart J.* 1970; 80:791–801.

50. Henry WL Bonow RO, Borer JS, Ware JH, et al. Observations on the optimum timing for operative intervention for aortic regurgitation. I. Evaluation of the results of aortic valve replacement in symptomatic patients. *Circulation.* 1980;61:471–483.

51. Cohn PF, Gorlin R, Cohn LH, Collins JJ. Left ventricular ejection fraction as a prognostic guide in surgical treatment of coronary and valvular heart disease. *Am J Cardiol.* 1974;34(2):136–141.

52. Greves J, Rahimtoola SH, McAnulty JH, et al. Preoperative criteria predictive of late survival following valve replacement for severe aortic regurgitation. *Am Heart J.* 1981;101(3):300–308.

53. Bonow RO, Rosing DR, Kent KM, Epstein SE. Timing of operation for chronic aortic regurgitation. *Am J Cardiol.* 1982;50:325–336.

54. Clark DG, McAnulty JH, Rahimtoola SH. Results of valve replacement in aortic incompetence with left ventricular dysfunction. *Circulation.* 1978;58(Suppl II):II-22.

55. Copeland JG, Griepp RB, Stinson EB, Shumway NE. Long term followup after isolated aortic valve replacement. *J Thorac Cardiovasc Surg.* 1977;74:875–885.

56. Borow KM, Green LH, Mann T, et al. End-systolic volume as a predictor of postoperative left ventricular performance in volume overload from valvular regurgitation. *Am J Med.* 1980;68:655–663.

57. Nishimura RA, McGoon MD, Schaff HV, et al. Chronic aortic regurgitation: indications for operation–1988. *Mayo Clin Proc.* 1988;63:270–280.

58. Bonow RO, Rosing DR, Maron BJ. Reversal of left

ventricular dysfunction after aortic valve replacement for chronic aortic regurgitation: influence of duration of preoperative left ventricular dysfunction. *Circulation.* 1984;70:570–579.

59. Cohn LH, DiSesa VJ, eds. *Aortic regurgitation: medical and surgical management.* NY: Marcel Dekker; 1986: 142–152.

60. Vesely I. Analysis of the medtronic intact bioprosthetic valve. *J Thorac Cardiovasc Surg.* 1991;101:90–99.

61. Bloomfield P, Kitchin AH, Wheatly DJ. A prospective evaluation of the Bjork-Shiley, Hancock, and Carpentier-Edwards heart valve prostheses. *Circulation.* 1986;73;6:1213–1222.

62. Bonow RO, Picone AL McIntosh CL, et al. Survival and functional results after valve replacement for aortic regurgitation from 1976 to 1983: impact of preoperative left ventricular function. *Circulation.* 1985;72:1244–1256.

63. McGoon MD, Fuster V, McGoon DC, Pumphrey CW, Pluth JR, Elveback LR. Aortic and mitral valve incompetence: long term followup (10–19 years) of patients treated with the Starr-Edwards prosthesis. *J Am Coll Cardiol.* 1984;3:930–938.

64. Hegglin R, Scheu H, Rothlin M. Aortic insufficiency. *Circulation.* 1968;38(Suppl 5):V77–V92.

65. McGoon MD, Fuster V, Pluth JR, et al. Medical and surgical long term followup (10–21 years) of chronic aortic incompetence. *Circulation.* 1981;64(Suppl 4): IV76. Abstract.

66. Ross J Jr, Braunwald E. Aortic stenosis. *Circulation.* 1968;36(Suppl IV):61–67.

67. Horstkotte D, Loogen F. The natural history of aortic valve stenosis. *Eur Heart J.* 1988;9(Suppl E):57–64.

68. Braunwald E, Morrow AG. Obstruction to left ventricular outflow. Current criteria for the selection of patients for operation. *Am J Cardiol.* 1963;12:53–59.

69. Horskotte D, Loogen F. The natural history of aortic valve stenosis. *Eur Heart J.* 1988;9(Suppl E):57–64.

70. Schwara F, Baumann P, Manthey J, et al. The effect of aortic valve replacement on survival. *Circulation.* 1982;66:1105–1110.

71. O'Keefe JH Jr, Vlietstra RE, Bailey KR, Holmes DR Jr. Natural history of candidates for balloon aortic valvuloplasty. *Mayo Clin Proc.* 1987;62:986–991.

72. Kelly TA, Rothbart RM, Cooper M, Kaiser DL, Smucker ML, Gibson RS. Comparison of outcome of asymptomatic to symptomatic patients older than 20 years of age with valvular aortic stenosis. *Am J Cardiol.* 1988;61:123–130.

73. Shapira N, Lemole GM, Fernandez J. Aortic valve repair for aortic stenosis in adults. *Ann Thorac Surg.* 1990;50:110–120.

74. Lund O. Preoperative risk evaluation and stratification of long term survival after valve replacement for aortic stenosis. *Circulation.* 1990;82:124–139.

75. Craver JM, Weintraub WS, Jones EL et al. Predictors of mortality, complications, and length of stay in aortic valve replacement for aortic stenosis. *Circulation.* 1988;78(Suppl I):I-85–I-90.

76. Bessone LN, Pupello DF, Hiro SP. Surgical management of aortic valve disease in the elderly: a longitudinal analysis. *Ann Thorac Surg.* 1988;46:264–269.

77. Lund O, Jensen FT. Functional status and left ventricular performance late valve replacement for aortic stenosis. Relation to preoperative data. *Eur Heart J.* 1988; 9:1234–1243.

78. Lund O, Jensen FT. Late cardiac deaths after isolated valve replacement for aortic stenosis: relation to impaired left ventricular diastolic performance. *Angiology.* 1989;40:199–208.

79. Antunes MJ, Magalhaes MP, Colsen PR, et al. Valvuloplasty for rheumatic mitral valve disease: a surgical challenge. *J Thorac Cardiovasc Surg.* 1987;94(1):44–56.

80. Duran CG, Revuelta JM, Gaite L, et al. Stability at 10–11 years of the mitral reconstruction surgery. *Circulation.* 1987;76:1775.

81. Carpentier A. Cardiac value surgery—the "French correction." *J Thorac Cardiovasc Surg.* 1983;86:323–337.

82. Carpentier A. A new reconstructive operation for correction of mitral and tricuspid insufficiency. *J Thorac Cardiovasc Surg.* 1971;61(1):1–13.

83. Carpentier A. A reconstructive surgery of mitral valve incompetence—ten year appraisal. *J Thorac Cardiovasc Surg.* 1980;79(3):338–348.

84. Kreindel MS, Schiavone Wa, Lever HM. Systolic anterior motion of the mitral valve after Carpentier ring valvuloplasty for mitral valve prolapse. *Am J Cardiol.* 1986;57(6):408–412.

85. Galler M, Kronzon I, Slater J. Long term followup after mitral valve reconstruction: incidence of postoperative left ventricular outflow obstruction. *Circulation.* 1986;74(3 Pt 2):I99–103.

86. Deloche A, Jebara VA, Relland JRM. Valve repair with Carpentier techniques: the second decade. *J Thorac Cardiovasc Surg.* 1990;99:990–1002.

87. Harpole DH, Rankin JS, Wolfe WG. Effects of standard mitral valve replacement on left ventricular function. *Ann Thorac Surg.* 1990;49:866–874.

88. Antunes MJ, Magalhaes MP, Colsen PR, et al. Valvuloplasty for rheumatic mitral valve disease. *J Thorac Cardiovasc Surg.* 1987;86:553–561.

89. Galloway AC, Colvin SB, Baumann FG, et al. Long term results of mitral valve reconstruction using Carpentier techniques in 148 patients with mitral insufficiency. *Circulation.* 1988;78(Suppl I):I-97–I-105).

90. Cohn LH, Collins JJ Jr, Couper GS. Two hundred consecutive mitral valve repairs for mitral regurgitation: early and late results. *J Am Coll Cardiol.* 1991; 17;2: 40A. Abstract.

91. Edmunds LH Jr. Thrombotic and bleeding complications of prosthetic heart valves. *Ann Thorac Surg.* 1987;44: 430–445.

92. Spencer FC, Baumann FG, Grossi EA, et al. Experiences with 1,643 porcine prosthetic valves in 1,492 patients. *Ann Surg.* 1986;203:691–700.

93. Perier P, Deloche A, Chauvaud S. A 10-year comparison of miral valve replacement with Carpentier-Edwards and Hancock porcine bioprostheses. *Ann Thorac Surg.* 1989;48:54–59.

94. Cohn LH, DiSesa VJ, Collins JJ Jr. The Hancock modified orifice porcine bioprosthetic valve: 1976–1988. *Ann Thorac Surg.* 1989;48(Suppl 3):581–582.

95. Cohn LH, Couper GS, Kinchla NM, Collins JJ Jr. De-

creased operative risk of surgical treatment of mitral regurgitation with or without coronary artery disease. *J Am Coll Cardiol.* 1990;16(7):1575–1578.

96. Ferrazzi P, McGiffin DC, Kirklin JW. Have the results of mitral valve replacement improved? *J Thorac Cardiovasc Surg.* 1986;92:186–197.

97. Teply JF, Grunkemeier GL, Sutherland HD, et al. The ultimate prognosis after valve replacement: an assessment at twenty years. *Ann Thorac Surg.* 1981;32(2): 111–119.

98. Salomon NW, Stinson EB, Greipp RB, et al. Patient related risk factors as predictors of results following isolated mitral valve replacement. *Ann Thorac Surg.* 1977;24(6):519–530.

99. Cohn LH, Allred EN, Cohn LA, et al. Early and late risk of mitral valve replacement. A 12 year concomitant comparison of porcine bioprosthetic and prosthetic disc mitral valves. *J Thorac Cardiovasc Surg.* 1985;90: 6;872–881.

100. Cohen SR, Sell JE, McIntosh CL. Tricuspid regurgitation in patients with acquired, chronic, pure mitral regurgitation. *J Thorac Cardiovasc Surg.* 1987;94:481–487.

101. Goldman ME, Guarino T, Fuster V, Mindich B. The necessity for tricuspid valve repair can be determined intraoperatively by two-dimensional echocardiography. *J Thorac Cardiovasc Surg.* 1987;94:542–550.

102. Robin E, Belamarie J, Thoms NW, Arbulu A, Ganguly SN. Consequences of total tricuspid valvulectomy without prosthetic replacement in treatment of *Pseudomonas* endocarditis. *J Thorac Cardiovasc Surg.* 1974; 68;3:461–465.

103. Yee ES, Ullyot DJ. Reparative approach for right-sided endocarditis: operative considerations and results of valvuloplasty. *J Thorac Cardiovasc Surg.* 1988;96: 133–140.

104. Chidamibaram M, Abdulalis A, Baliga BG, Ionesu MI. Long term results of DeVega's tricuspid annuloplasty. *Ann Thorac Surg.* 1987;43(2):185–188.

105. Wong M, Matsumura M, Kutsuzawa S, et al. The value of Doppler echocardiography in the treatment of tricuspid regurgitation in patients with mitral valve replacement. *J Thorac Cardiovasc Surg.* 1990;99:1003–1010.

106. Lambertz H, Minale C, Flachskampf FA. Long term followup after Carpentier tricuspid valvuloplasty. *Am Heart J.* 1989;117:615–622.

107. McGrath LB, Gonzalez-Lavin L, Bailey BM, Grunkemeier GL, Fernandez J, Laub GW. Tricuspid valve operations in 530 patients: twenty five year assessment of early and late phase events. *J Thorac Cardiovasc Surg.* 1990;99:124–133.

38
Cardiac Transplantation

Jeffrey D. Hosenpud

Over the past 20 years, cardiac transplantation has evolved from a highly experimental procedure performed in a handful of centers to an accepted modality of therapy for the treatment of end-stage heart disease. Cardiac transplantation is now performed on every inhabited continent and in more than 175 centers worldwide. In the last 7 yr, the indications for cardiac transplantation have expanded to include older and higher risk patients. Despite this, the 1-yr survival has increased from 65% to more than 80% at most centers.[1] Unfortunately, despite the expansion of the criteria for acceptable donor organs, the availability of donor hearts remains the limiting factor for this form of therapy. It is estimated that in the United States alone, more than 20,000 patients could benefit from cardiac transplantation, yet the number of donor hearts procured is less than 2000 per year.[2] This chapter reviews the current state of cardiac transplantation, its successes, and the challenges yet to be overcome.

Recipient Selection

The basic tenets expressed in the criteria developed by the Stanford group in the early 1970s[3,4] continue to apply today. Cardiac tranplantation must be reserved for those patients with disabling symptoms of congestive heart failure [CHF; New York Heart Association (NYHA) late functional class III and IV] whose likelihood of survival is poor over the next 6 to 12 months. There have been, however, several modifications of ancillary inclusion and exclusion criteria over the past 20 years. As a result, cardiac transplantation is now being offered to sicker and higher risk patients. Table 38.1 outlines the inclusion and exclusion criteria currently in use at the Oregon Cardiac Transplant Program.

Age

Based on early data from Stanford showing a 20% decrement in 1-yr survival in patients over the age of 50 years, the upper age limit for cardiac transplantation was considered 50 yr.[3] Several studies have now demonstrated that patients between the ages of 50 and 65 yr appear to have comparable outcomes to those in the younger age group.[5–7] An analysis of the data from the Oregon Cardiac Transplant Program investigating not only survival, infection, and rejection but also overall hospitalization and noncardiac morbidity, demonstrated no major differences in these parameters between those patients above and below the age of 55 yr.[8] A more recent study performing similar analyses in patients above and below the age of 65 yr did, however, demonstrate that those over 65 yr of age had prolonged

TABLE 38.1. Recipient selection criteria.

Inclusion criteria
Severe, symptom limiting heart failure (NYHA III and IV) on full
  medical management
At substantial risk for cardiac death within 1 yr
No alternative treatment options
Age usually less than 65 yr
History of medical compliance/good psychosocial environment

Exclusion criteria
Irreversible renal or hepatic disease (relative)
Severe pulmonary parenchymal disease (absolute)
Irreversible elevated pulmonary vascular resistance >6 Wood units
  (absolute)
Diabetes with important end organ damage (relative)
Peripheral or cerebral vascular disease (relative)
Active systemic or organ parenchymal infection (absolute)
Cardiac involvement as part of systemic disease, e.g., amyloidosis,
  sarcoidosis (relative)
Chronic viral infection, e.g., hepatitis B, HIV (absolute)
High titers of cytotoxic antibodies to multiple HLA antigens (relative)
Active medical noncompliance or substance abuse (absolute)

hospitalizations, longer rehabilitations, and a trend toward reduced survival that did not reach statistical significance.[9] Based on these data, it appears that it is reasonable from a medical standpoint to offer cardiac transplantation to patients up to the age of 65 yr if they meet other medical criteria.

Pulmonary Vascular Resistance

Severe and irreversible (nonreflex) pulmonary hypertension has been demonstrated consistently to be a risk factor for poor outcome after cardiac transplantation.[3,10] The reason for this is the inability of the transplanted right ventricle to adapt acutely to elevated pulmonary artery pressures. The transplanted right ventricle usually is procured from a donor with normal pulmonary vascular resistance and hence is of normal thickness. In addition, it is extremely susceptible to preservation injury and perioperative dysfunction because of rapid rewarming during the implantation procedure. Potential recipients who have pulmonary artery hypertension on routine cardiac catheterization receive intravenous vasodilators (sodium nitroprusside, prostaglandin E) to determine if the elevation in pulmonary pressures are secondary to pulmonary vasoconstriction or irreversible disease. Frequently, pulmonary artery pressures and resistance will fall into the acceptable range with pharmacologic intervention acutely. A small number of patients, however, with reversible pulmonary hypertension will require several days of intensive medical management before pulmonary pressures fall to within a range that is acceptable for transplantation. Those patients who persist in having elevated pulmonary vascular resistance despite intensive medical management may be candidates for heart-lung transplantation.

Infection

Patients in severe CHF are at increased susceptibility to infection, especially those waiting in intensive care units for cardiac transplantation. Given the immediate requirements for immunosuppression after cardiac transplantation, patients must be adequately treated for any recent infection and free of infection at the time of transplantation. In general, upper respiratory viral infections and uncomplicated bactiuria have not been considered a contraindication for proceeding to transplantation.

Noncardiac Organ System Dysfunction

Severe CHF is frequently associated with prerenal azotemia and passive hepatic congestion.[11,12] It is therefore important to separate these abnormalities from intrinsic organ dysfunction as several of the commonly used immunosuppressive agents have either renal or hepatic toxicity.[13,14] Patients with a serum creatinine of >2 mg/dl or hepatic enzyme abnormalities greater than twice normal should therefore have careful evaluations to exclude intrinsic organ dysfunction. In addition, severe heart failure frequently impacts pulmonary function. In a series of 17 patients studied with spirometry before and several months after cardiac transplantation, the principal spirometric abnormality was a reduction in lung volumes (restrictive pattern) before transplantation, which was completely reversible after transplantation.[15] The reduction in lung volumes was strongly correlated to the increase in cardiac volume, and obstructive physiology if present before transplantation was unchanged after cardiac replacement and normalization of hemodynamics. These data would suggest that severe obstructive pulmonary physiology before transplantation would be unlikely to improve substantially after cardiac transplantation. Therefore, those patients with a forced vital capacity of <50% of predicted with obstructive physiology would be extremely high risk for postoperative pulmonary complications.

Systemic Diseases and Prior Malignancies

Diabetes initially had been considered a contraindication to cardiac transplantation because of the corticosteroids required as part of the immunosuppressive regimen. With the advent of lower dose steroid protocols utilizing cyclosporine-based immunosuppression, the inclusion of diabetics as candidates for cardiac transplantation has gradually increased. Diabetics with endorgan damage are still for the most part excluded as candidates. Otherwise, it appears that patients with controlled diabetes have acceptable outcomes after cardiac transplantation.[16]

Although definitive studies have not been performed, patients with prior malignancies who are considered "cured" are now being considered for and have undergone cardiac transplantation.[17] Several of these patients were treated with doxorubicin and have cardiomyopathy and heart failure on this basis.[18] Whether these patients are at a higher risk for the development of recurrent or new malignancies is yet to be determined.

Finally, other systemic diseases such as amyloidosis and sarcoidosis have been traditionally considered contraindications for cardiac transplantation because of the concern that these would recur in the allografted organ. The initial small experience with amyloidosis suggested that the prognosis post-transplantation was good with seven patients having equivalent intermediate-term survial compared with an age- and sex-matched control group.[19] However, a longer follow-up of these patients has demonstrated that despite the favorable intermediate prognosis, most patients developed progressive amyloid involvement in major organ systems and ultimately a reduced survival.[20] Anecdotal reports of patients with cardiac sarcoidosis undergoing cardiac transplantation are available.[21,22] Sarcoid granulomas can, however, recur in the allograft.[22]

Medical Compliance, Substance Abuse, and Psychosocial Support

The complexity of the pre-, peri-, and postoperative care in cardiac transplantation necessitates that the patient understand his or her disease and is willing to comply with the recommendations made by the transplant team. Active substance abuse clearly threatens this compliance. The potential emotional stress in all aspects before and after transplantation may be coped with better if social support is available for the patient. It is interesting, however, that it is extremely difficult to predict medical outcome and compliance using standard psychosocial evaluation parameters.[23]

Recipient Evaluation

Table 38.2 outlines the typical evaluation performed for a patient referred for cardiac transplantation. The principal goals of this evaluation are (a) to determine the underlying cardiac disease and if possible delineate alternative treatment strategies, (b) to quantify cardiovascular function, degree of symptoms *attributable to the cardiac function*, and pulmonary vascular resistance, (c) to determine whether immunologic barriers, such as preformed antibodies to HLA antigens, are present either precluding transplantation or modifying post-transplant treatment approaches, and (d) to evaluate other organ function and disease that might impact post-transplant outcome.

The Cardiac Donor

The passage of the Uniform Anatomical Gift Act in 1968,[22] the general acceptance of criteria for brain death,[25] and an increasing public awareness have brought about an increase in the number of available organs. Despite this, as alluded to earlier, the current need, especially with expanded recipient criteria, has not been met by the pool of organ donors. For principally this reason, hearts are now accepted from donors that in prior years had been turned down for transplantation.

Brain Death

Neither the organ procurement agency nor the transplant teams have any involvement in the patient until brain death is declared and consent for organ donation

TABLE 38.2. Recipient evaluation.

Complete history and physical examination

Cardiovascular evaluation
    Coronary angiography (if indicated)
    Endomyocardial biopsy (to r/o myocarditis, amyloidosis, etc. if indicated)
    Quantitative left ventricular ejection fraction
    Quantitation of pulmonary vascular resistance by catheterization
    Ambulatory electrocardiography (if indicated)
    Lipid studies

Noncardiac organ function evaluation
    Pulmonary function studies
    Chemistries for renal and hepatic function
    Urinalysis
    Hematology
    Coagulation studies
    Peripheral or cerebral vascular studies (if indicated)
    Pregnancy testing

Infection surveillance evaluation
    Skin testing for myobacteria and systemic fungi
    Cytomegalovirus serology
    Toxoplasma gondii serology
    Bacterial cultures (if indicated)
    Hepatis B, C serology
    HIV serology
    Dental examination

Systemic disease surveillance evaluation
    Thyroid function
    Rheumatologic screening
    Mammography and PAP screening (if indicated)
    Serum protein electrophoresis
    Stool for hemoglobin

Immunologic evaluation
    Blood type and screen
    Panel reactive antibody screen (detection of HLA antibody)

Psychosocial evaluation

TABLE 38.3. Brain death.

Absence of cortical function
    No spontaneous movement
    No response to external stimuli
    No response to pain

Absence of brain stem function
    No spontaneous respirations
    Absent pupillary and corneal reflexes
    Absent oculocephalic reflexes
    Absent vestibuloocular reflexes

Absence of activity on electroencephalogram

Absence of cerebral blood flow

is obtained. Table 38.3 presents the clinical and laboratory findings in brain death. In general, there is absence of cortical function as assessed by spontaneous movement, response to stimuli, or response to pain. There is absence of brain stem function including a host of brain stem reflexes and spontaneous respiration. Finally, the electroencephalogram has no activity and if measured, there is no cerebral blood flow.[26,27]

Screening for Organ Donation

Aspects of screening of potential donors can be divided into those required for screening the donor for any and all organ donation and those specific for cardiac donation. Generalized donor screening centers around excluding transmissible diseases such as infections and malignancy. Screening now routinely carried out includes a careful medical and social history to eliminate patients whose exposure or lifestyles might increase the likelihood of viral diseases such as hepatitis B and C or human immunodeficiency virus (HIV), specific serology for hepatitis B and C, HIV and HTLV-1, and surveillance bacterial cultures. Patients with active sepsis usually are not considered for organ donation. Localized infection in the lung or urinary tract may allow for the donation of organs not directly involved. Likewise, despite malignancy being a contraindication for organ donation, patients with localized central nervous system malignancy generally are considered acceptable organ donors.

Heart Donation

Once the potential organ donor has been screened for the general contraindications to organ donation, specific issues dealing with cardiac donation can then be addressed. The issues relate primarily to two questions: the function of the heart and the possibility of occult or overt coronary disease. Initially, cardiac donors were strictly age-limited to males 30 yr or less and females 35 yr or less, specifically to reduce the likelihood of occult coronary disease.[28] With the progressive shortage of donors, this age limit was increased to 40 and 45 yr, respectively,[29] and currently, many centers will consider organ donors to the age of 50 yr and beyond depending on the age and stability of their recipients. In general, most centers will attempt to obtain coronary angiography on the older aged donors, but in some smaller hospitals, this is not always achievable. With the same concerns, insulin-requiring diabetics generally are excluded from cardiac donation, and those with other coronary risk factors are carefully evaluated. The electrocardiogram can be extremely helpful in this regard if pathologic Q waves are present. ST segment shifts, T-wave changes, and arrhythmias are generally not helpful as all of these are not infrequently associated with brain stem herniation and brain death.[30,31]

Assessment of Cardiac Function

The first indication of the integrity of cardiac function is the degree of inotropic support required to maintain

TABLE 38.4. Screening criteria for cardiac donation.

General organ donation screening
Absence of infection
Hepatitis B and C, HIV, and HTLV-1 serology
Negative blood cultures
Psychosocial/lifestyle screening
Absence of malignancy (excluding primary CNS tumors)
Screening for coronary disease
Age usually less than 50 yr
Coronary angiography if possible:
Males >40 yr
Females >45 yr
No pathologic Q waves on ECG
No history of insulin-requiring diabetes
No other prior cardiac history
Screening for normal cardiac function
No requirement for high dose inotropic support (after volume replacement)
No prolonged resuscitation
Normal echocardiogram (mild segmental wall motion or mitral prolapse not a contraindication)

stable vital signs in the donor. This, however, can be extremely misleading because before brain death, the goal of the physicians (neurosurgeons or neurologists) caring for the patient is to minimize cerebral edema. This usually is accomplished by aggressive diuresis and fluid restriction. It is not unusual to find a potential organ donor receiving high-dose inotropic and vasopressor support that can be weaned rapidly with aggressive fluid replacement. Most cardiac transplant programs will evaluate a potential donor further if inotropic support (usually either dobutamine or dopamine) can be reduced to <10 μg/kg/min. The echocardiogram is now utilized frequently to evaluate cardiac function in the donor. Gilbert and colleagues demonstrated that echocardiography identified a full 29% of their successful cardiac donors who would have otherwise been excluded using electrocardiogram (ECG) and clinical findings alone.[32] Table 38.4 reviews the current screening criteria for cardiac organ donation.

Myocardial Preservation

The techniques of cold cardioplegia have been developed in cardiovascular surgery over the past 20 yr. There appears to be adequate preservation of the myocardium at temperatures below 20°C in standard cardioplegic (high potassium) solutions.[33] Most centers use standard Euro-Collins solutions for myocardial preservation, although several centers are now switching to solutions containing antioxidants such as the preservation solution developed at the University of Wisconsin (UW solution). UW solution has been demonstrated to have a profound effect on both renal and liver preservation for transplantation. Although there are animal studies demonstrating improved cardiac preservation with

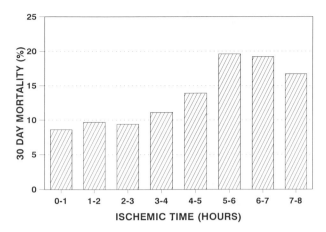

FIGURE 38.1. Ischemic time relates directly to early survival after cardiac transplantation. Reproduced, with permission, from Dr. Michael P. Kaye and the Registry of the International Society for Heart and Lung Transplantation.

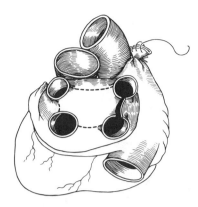

FIGURE 38.2. Donor heart preparation. From Cobanoglu A, in Hosenpud JD, Cobanoglu A, Norman DJ, Starr A, eds. *Cardiac transplantation*. New York: Springer-Verlag; 1991.

these solutions,[34,35] the benefits to human cardiac transplantation are as yet unclear. As shown in Figure 38.1, it is absolutely clear that ischemic time (the time from aortic cross-clamp in the donor to cross-clamp release and restoration of coronary flow in the recipient) is a strong and independent determinant of early survival.[36,37] Most centers, therefore, will, not exceed 4 hr of ischemic time unless their recipient is extremely unstable. Unfortunately, it is the sicker recipients who in general need a well functioning allograft in the early post-transplant period. Methods for improving myocardial preservation, thus allowing for greater ischemic times, are currently under active investigation. One would hope that with improved preservation, better immunologic matching of donors and recipients and a greater use of donated cardiac organs could be achieved.

The Transplant Operation

The cardiac transplant operation is in fact two operations: the donor cardiectomy and the recipient operation. The technical aspects of the cardiac transplant operation are essentially those initially described by Lower and Shumway in 1960.[38] As discussed above, to minimize the total ischemic time, especially when the donor operation is occurring in a city remote from the transplant center, timing and coordination of the two operations is critical. This is especially the case as at least 50% of transplants are now performed on recipients with prior cardiac surgery.

The Donor Cardiectomy

The donor heart is reached through a standard midline sternotomy. The heart is inspected visually to evaluate

chamber size and wall motion, and palpably to detect the degree of chamber filling and the presence of coronary calcification. Once the heart is considered appropriate for transplantation, the transplant center is notified and the recipient operation begins. While other organs are being harvested, the aorta and pulmonary artery are dissected free and controlled with tapes, as is the superior vena cava. Just before harvest, heparin is administered, the superior vena cava is ligated, inferior vena cava cross-clamped, and cold cardioplegic solution is administered into the aorta. The aorta is then cross-clamped and the various cardiac structures transected in the following order: (a) the superior vena cava (between double ligations), (b) inferior vena cava and right lower pulmonary vein, (c) aorta and pulmonary artery, and (d) the remaining pulmonary veins. The pulmonary veins are connected to form the left atrial cuff and the heart is packaged for transport. Figure 38.2 demonstrates the preparation of the donor heart.

The Recipient Operation

The recipient is brought to the operating room and central venous (or pulmonary artery) and intraarterial catheters are placed. The operation is via a midline sternotomy, usually started when communication from the donor team indicates the donor heart is suitable for transplantation. After dissection and control of the great veins and arteries, heparin is administered and the patient is cooled and placed on cardiopulmonary bypass (usually not before the donor heart has arrived at the transplant center). The native heart is excised with incisions transecting the various cardiac structures in the following order: (a) the lateral wall of the right atrium continuing inferiorly and medially to and across the intraatrial septum, (b) the aorta and pulmonary artery, and (c) the left lateral wall of the left atrium. The nearly completed cardiectomy is shown in Figure 38.3. The allograft implantation is then carried out using running

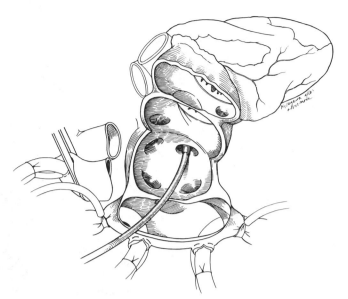

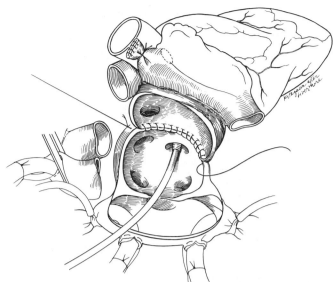

FIGURE 38.3. Recipient cardiectomy. From Cobanoglu A, in Hosenpud JD, Cobanoglu A, Norman DJ, Starr A, eds. *Cardiac transplantation*. New York: Springer-Verlag; 1991.

FIGURE 38.4. Allograft implantation, initial left atrial anastomosis. From Cobanoglu A, in Hosenpud JD, Cobanoglu A, Norman DJ, Starr A, eds. *Cardiac transplantation*. New York: Springer-Verlag; 1991.

suture with anastomoses in the following order: (a) left atrial free wall, (b) intraatrial septum, (c) right atrium, (d) pulmonary artery, and (e) aorta. The early and late stages of the allograft implantation are demonstrated in Figures 38.4 and 38.5, respectively.

Perioperative Care

Immunosuppression Induction

Although immunosuppression is discussed in depth later in this chapter, a few comments are appropriate at this time. The induction of immunosuppression varies widely from center to center but in general these differences do not appear to impact outcome substantially.[1] The protocol used by the Oregon Cardiac Transplant Program is to administer cyclosporine (8 mg/kg) and azathioprine (5 mg/kg) preoperatively and use high-dose corticosteroids (1 g of methylprednisolone) intraoperatively. In the postoperative period intravenous corticosteroids, azathioprine, and cyclosporine are administered until the patient is able to take oral feedings. In patients who have important renal impairment preoperatively, cyclosporine is not administered and the monoclonal antibody to the T-cell receptor (anti-CD3) OKT3 is administered for the first 14 days after transplantation. This allows for the gradual institution of cyclosporine as renal function improves.

Allograft Hemodynamic Support

It is critically important to understand several aspects of allograft physiology early posttransplantation to pro-

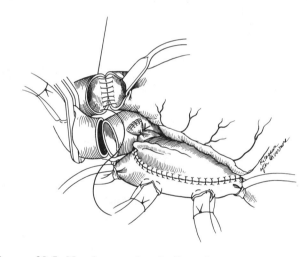

FIGURE 38.5. Nearly completed allograft implantation. From Cobanoglu A, in Hosenpud JD, Cobanoglu A, Norman DJ, Starr A, eds. *Cardiac transplantation*. New York: Springer-Verlag; 1991.

vide appropriate postoperative support. Despite careful attempts at myocardial preservation and limiting total ischemic times, the allograft is ischemically damaged immediately after transplantation. This, coupled with mild to moderate elevations in pulmonary vascular resistance in the recipient,[39] the denervated state of the allograft,[40,41] and the ischemic damage to the sinus node,[42] result in need of support for the heart and predominantly the right ventricle. As one might anticipate, acute right ventricular failure is the most common nonimmunologic cause of perioperative death after cardiac transplantation.[43] The ischemic damage to the

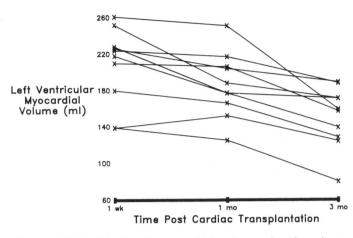

FIGURE 38.6. Calculated myocardial volumes in 10 patients after cardiac transplantation demonstrating a serial decline in myocardial volume (mass), from 1 week to 3 months. Reprinted, with permission, from Hosenpud et al.[45]

allograft, in addition to being manifest as reduced systolic function and sinus node activity, is also manifest by a reduction in ventricular compliance associated with myocardial edema, which can be present for up to 3 months after transplantation.[44,45] Figure 38.6 demonstrates that left ventricular myocardial volumes measured by echocardiogram in 10 allograft recipients are still not normal by 1 month after transplantation. Stinson and colleagues investigated hemodynamics in 10 allograft recipients immediately postoperatively and for the first 7 days.[46] Cardiac function was severely depressed initially (cardiac index 1.8 L/min/m^2, stroke volume index 21 ml/m^2) and then gradually improved. Isoproterenol was extremely effective in providing both inotropic as well as chronotropic support and is now, in most centers, the initial catecholamine of choice after transplantation. If additional inotropic support is required, it is important to choose agents that directly stimulate β-1 receptors such as dobutamine or epinephrine or inhibit cyclic adenosine monophosphate (cAMP) breakdown by phosphodiesterase (amrinone). Agents that indirectly provide inotropic support by releasing stored norepinephrine (dopamine) will be effective for the first several hours after transplantation but will lose their effectiveness because of the denervated state. Elevations in pulmonary vascular resistance exacerbated by the use of blood products can be treated using vasodilators such as sodium nitroprusside or prostaglandin E$_2$.[47] Most often, inotropic, chronotropic, and vasodilator support can be discontinued successfully between 3 and 5 days after transplantation.

Infection Control

Although early experience had most transplant centers using some form of protective isolation, the efficacy of these measures has never been demonstrated. As a result, the general trend has been to relax these measures to a considerable degree. Most patients receive prophylactic antibacterial agents effective against skin organisms for several days after transplantation. At centers where pneumocystis and cytomegalovirus infections have produced substantial morbidity, patients receive prophylactic hyperimmune globulin and/or ganciclovir or acyclovir (cytomegalovirus) and trimethoprim-sulfamethoxazole (pneumocystis). The efficacy of these measures, although suggestive, are not clearly proven.[48-50]

Immunosuppression/The Diagnosis and Treatment of Rejection

It is clear to all involved in the field of heart transplantation that with the advances in surgical care, the procedure itself is now only a minor part of the therapy of transplantation. The immunologic barrier between donor and recipient continues to be a substantial challenge. Figure 38.7 demonstrates a schematic representation of the immune response to alloantigens and the effects on this response by the current commonly used immunosuppressive agents. As stated previously, the specific immunosuppression protocols used vary substantially from center to center, but most use a combination of agents. Table 38.5 lists these agents, their usual dosages, and their principal side effects.

Cyclosporine

Cyclosporine has clearly revolutionized the field of transplantation in its 15 yr of clinical use. First discovered in 1972 and recognized as a potent inhibitor of T-

TABLE 38.5. Commonly used immunosuppressive drugs.

Drug	Average dose	Side effects
Cyclosporine	4–8 mg/kg	Hypertension Nephrotoxicity Hepatotoxicity Neurotoxicity Gingival hyperplasia Hyperglycemia Hirsuitism
Azathioprine	1–3 mg/kg	Bone marrow suppression Hepatotoxicity Pancreatitis
Prednisone	0.1–0.5 mg/kg	Cushingoid habitus Hypertension Bone demineralization Hirsuitism Gastric irritation Mood changes Hyperlipidemia Hyperglycemia

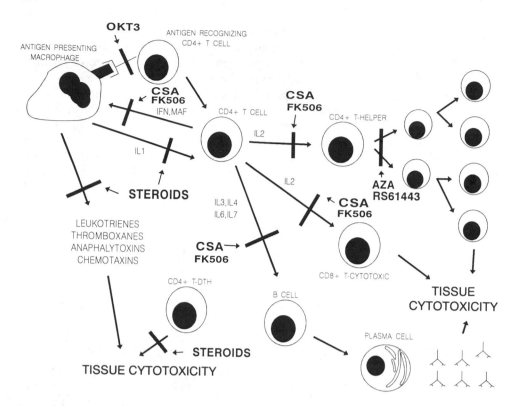

FIGURE 38.7. A schematic representation of the immune response and the effects of the commonly used and newer immunosuppressive agents. CSA = cyclosporine; AZA = azathioprine; IL-1–7 = interleukins 1–7; IFN = interferon-γ; MAF = macrophage activating factor. From Salomon D and Limacher M, in Hosenpud JD, Cobanoglu A, Norman DJ, Starr A, eds. *Cardiac transplantation.* New York: Springer-Verlag; 1991.

cell function by Jean Borel,[51,52] it is now the mainstay of cardiac transplant immunosuppression. Cyclosporine is a T cell–specific drug that inhibits the gene transcription of multiple lymphokines including interferon-γ, interleukin-2, and probably interleukins-3–7.[53,54] These cytokines are extremely important for activation and recruitment of the various components of the immune system. For example, interleukin-2 is the primary signal for T-cell proliferation and clonal expansion.[55] Interferon-γ may be primarily responsible for increasing target cell surface expression of major histocompatibility antigens necessary for recognition by the immune system.[54] In clinical use, in most instances, a loading dose of between 5 and 10 mg/kg is administered preoperatively and the maintenance dose ranges from 3 to 8 mg/kg in divided doses. The specific dose for a given patient is determined by blood or serum levels and can vary considerably from patient to patient and even within a given patient because of the complex metabolism of the drug. In addition, there are several drugs that interact with cyclosporine metabolism, both increasing and decreasing its metabolism.[56] The major toxicities of cyclosporine are the induction or exacerbation of hypertension and renal impairment, both of which occur in most patients taking the drug.[57] Other less common side effects include hepatotoxicity, neurotoxicity and seizures, gingival hyperplasia, hirsuitism, and hyperglycemia. Most side effects are dose-related and will not preclude its use.

Azathioprine

The initial discovery that the purine analogue 6-mercaptopurine was an effective immunosuppressive agent was made by Calne in 1960 in an animal model of renal transplantation.[58] The nitroimidazole derivative of 6-MP, azathioprine, was synthesized in 1975 and subsequently shown to be effective in clinical renal transplantation.[59,60] The mechanism of action of azathioprine is to inhibit de novo purine biosynthesis, which ultimately blocks cell proliferation.[61] Although cardiac transplantation went through a period where azathioprine-prednisone protocols were replaced with cyclosporine-prednisone protocols, the combination of all three agents has been shown to improve outcomes.[62] The usual dose of azathioprine is 1.5 to 2.5 mg/kg. It is not clear whether the immunosuppressive effects of azathioprine relate to the suppression of total white blood count or are independent of the marrow suppression. This has led primarily to two philosophies regarding its dosing: the philosophy of using a standard dose (usually 2 mg/kg) unless toxicity intervenes, or the philosophy that the dose should be increased progressively to reduce total white count to a target level (usually around 5000). As one might expect, the principal toxicity of azathioprine is bone marrow suppression. This is readily reversible with reducing the dose. Other less common side effects are hepatic toxicity, an unusual form of hepatic venoocclusive disease, and pancreatitis.[13,63] Finally, prolonged use has been associated with the development of malignancy and, specifically, skin cancers.[64] This risk brings into question the philosophy of using higher doses of azathioprine to control total white blood cell counts.

Corticosteroids

The first reported use of adrenocorticotropin hormone (ACTH) in renal allograft recipients in 1960[63] soon led to corticosteroids becoming standard therapy for maintenance immunosuppression. The mechanisms of action of corticosteroids are both immunosuppressive and antiinflammatory. The specific immunosuppressive activity is due to (a) the inhibition of the release of the recruiting and inflammatory monokines, interleukin-1 (responsible for initial helper T-cell activation), interleukin-6, and tumor necrosis factor,[64,65]) and (b) their direct lymphocytotoxic effects. Their antiinflammatory effects are mediated by inhibiting the release of inflammatory mediators such as the leukotrienes and anaphalotoxins and chemotoxins from macrophages.[66] Thus, in contrast to cyclosporine, corticosteroids are quite nonspecific in their effects on the alloimmunologic response. Their use clinically in heart transplantation varies from center to center but almost all transplant programs use intravenous methylprednisolone in the intra- and perioperative periods. Once the patient can take oral medications, prednisone is used initially in doses of approximately 0.5 mg/kg and tapered over time. Several centers are now maintaining patients on cyclosporine and azathioprine alone to avoid the many side effects of chronic corticosteroid administration including obesity, cushingoid features, hyperlipidemia, hyperglycemia, hirsuitism, bone demineralization, gastric irritation, and mood changes, all well known to clinicians. It is not yet clear, however, that the elimination of corticosteroids from maintenance immunosuppression will not have adverse long-term effects for the allograft.

Antilymphocyte Antibodies

The use of antilymphocyte preparations, either polyclonal or monoclonal, are restricted to either early posttransplant prophylaxis against rejection or in the treatment of acute rejection. Polyclonal antilymphocyte or antithymocyte preparations are produced by inoculating human lymphocytes (or thymocytes) into animals, usually rabbit or horse, allowing a humoral response to occur and collecting and purifying the antibody fraction from animal serum. These antibodies are by design directed against a whole host of antigens on the human lymphocytes and, hence, the term "polyclonal." The hybridoma technique developed by Kohler and

Milstein,[67] of fusing a single plasma cell clone to a malignant cell line led to the development of specific "monoclonal" antibodies directed at unique antigens. The advantages of polyclonal preparations are their diversity in potentially blocking the immune response at multiple sites, but the disadvantage given their method of synthesis is the extreme variability from lot to lot. This is not the case with monoclonal preparations, where specific antibody titers can be controlled for. Neither antibody preparation has a role in ongoing maintenance immunosuppression because of the requirement that they be given parenterally and because of the development of host antibodies against the animal protein. A solution to the second of these problems may be forthcoming with the development of chimeric or fusion antibodies, which are primarily human in structure. One of the first controlled trials using polyclonal antilymphocyte serum was reported by Sheil and colleagues in cadavaric renal allograft recipients in 1971.[68] The first available monoclonal antibody directed against the T-cell receptor (CD3 antigen) was OKT3 and was initially studied in renal transplantation for the treatment of acute rejection by Cosimi and colleagues in 1981.[69] The mechanism of action of both the polyclonal preparations as well as OKT3 is to deplete T lymphocytes during the course of their administration; hence, they are extremely effective in halting acute rejection. Despite lymphocyte levels tending to revert to normal soon after the discontinuation of these agents, it was hoped that if administered in the early posttransplant period that the immune response would be permanently altered, leading to a greater partial tolerance.[70] Subsequent studies comparing protocols adding antilymphocyte preparations to initial immunosuppression induction have not demonstrated a substantial change in rejection patterns.[71,72] In addition, there are now studies suggesting that the prophylactic use of these agents may increase both early infection rates and severity, as well as the risk of developing malignancy.[73,74]

Methotrexate

Methotrexate, a folic acid analogue that inhibits DNA synthesis and cell division by binding competitively to dihydrofolic reductase, is a potent cytostatic drug that has been used at high dose in malignancies characterized by rapid cellular proliferation, and at lower doses in nonmalignant states characterized by rapid cell turnover like psoriasis. The effectiveness of methotrexate in this and other diseases such as rheumatoid arthritis, polymyositis, and graft versus host disease is attributable both to inhibition of rapid turnover of inflammatory cells and to suppression of cellular and humoral immunity. There are now three reports demonstrating the efficacy of low-dose methotrexate in the treatment of ongoing acute cardiac allograft rejection.[75–77]

Newer Agents and Immunosuppressive Strategies

A whole host of immunosuppressive agents directed toward unique aspects of the immune response are currently under investigation. These include agents similar to cyclosporine such as FK506 and Rapamycin, purine analogues, which are more specific to lymphocyte cell lines such as mycophenolate mofetil (RS61443), agents that block pyrimidine synthesis such as brequinar sodium, and unrelated agents such as deoxyspergualine and prostaglandin analogues. In addition, new monoclonal antibodies directed to specific T-cell subtypes, chimeric molecules, and hybrid molecules coupled to cell toxins are under investigation. Finally, nonpharmacologic mechanisms to alter the immune response such as lymphoid irradiation and photochemical therapy may be potential tools in the therapy of allograft recipients. The days of being limited to azathioprine and prednisone, and even cyclosporine, are rapidly vanishing.

Acute Rejection, Diagnosis, and Treatment

One of the most important advances in cardiac transplantation, equivalent in import to the development of cyclosporine, was the use of transvenous endomyocardial biopsy for monitoring allograft rejection. The application of this technique to cardiac transplantation was reported by Caves and colleagues at Stanford in 1973.[78] Up until this time, rejection was monitored by changes in ECG volume, reflecting myocardial edema, and changes in allograft function. Not only were these early methods at times inaccurate (lacking both sensitivity and specificity) but in addition, by the time many of these features were manifest, rejection was already advanced. Endomyocardial biopsy monitoring allowed for the early detection of rejection, thus improving the chances for effective therapy. The typical monitoring protocol calls for weekly endomyocardial biopsies for the first month to 2 months after transplantation, with the frequency of biopsies declining with increasing time from transplantation. If rejection is present and requires treatment, endomyocardial biopsy is performed to assess efficacy of treatment again at short intervals until the rejection episode is completed.

The currently accepted histologic grading scale developed and supported by the International Society for Heart and Lung Transplantation is presented in Table 38.6.[79] Figure 38.8 demonstrates an endomyocardial biopsy with moderate acute rejection (ISHLT grade 3A). There is a multifocal intense inflammatory infiltrate with evidence of myocyte damage present.

The intensity of the rejection response and the pro-

TABLE 38.6. International Society for Heart and Lung Transplant Biopsy Grading Scale.

Grade	Definition
No rejection	
0	No rejection
Mild rejection	
1A	Focal, perivascular, or interstitial infiltrate without myocyte necrosis
1B	Diffuse, sparse interstitial infiltrate without myocyte necrosis
Moderate rejection	
2	Focal (single), active (lymphoblasts, plasma cells) infiltrate with myocyte necrosis
3A	Multifocal interstitial active infiltrate with myocyte necrosis
3B	Diffuse (involving all areas) active infiltrate with myocyte necrosis
Severe rejection	
4	Diffuse aggressive infiltrate (lymphoblasts, polymorphonuclear cells, and eosinophils) with myocyte necrosis, edema, and hemorrhage

ximity of the rejection episode to transplantation usually guides the intensity of antirejection therapy. In general, rejection grades of only moderate or greater are treated with intensification of immunosuppression (outlined below) as lesser grades may resolve spontaneously[56] or with minor increases in maintenance immunosuppression. The alterations of immunosuppression can include stepwise increases in corticosteroids, courses of antilymphocyte antibodies (monoclonal or polyclonal), or drugs like methotrexate. The algorithm used in the Oregon Cardiac Transplant Program (OCTP) is demonstrated in Figure 38.9.

Chronic Rejection/Cardiac Allograft Vasculopathy

The principal factor limiting long-term survival after cardiac transplantation is a unique form of obliterative coronary artery disease termed "cardiac allograft vasculopathy" (CAV[80]). The incidence of the disease is as high as 15% per year with a 5-yr prevalence of as high as 45%.[80] Figure 38.10 demonstrates the OCTP incidence of CAV. It is most certainly a form of chronic rejection as the disease is limited solely to the allograft. Whether humoral or cellular mechanisms are more important are still under investigation. Additional evidence for an alloimmunologic role in this disease process is the association with cytomegalovirus,[81] the association with cytotoxic B-cell antibodies,[82] the correlation with immunoglobulin in the allograft,[83] and the association with the recipient's developing anti-HLA antibodies post-transplantation.[84]

The histopathology is unique as well. In contrast to

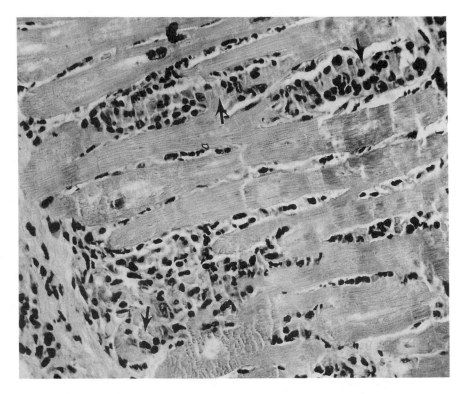

FIGURE 38.8. Endomyocardial biopsy showing moderate acute rejection with interstitial inflammation and myocyte necrosis (*arrows*). Hemotoxylin-eosin, ×675. From Ray J and Hosenpud JD, in Hosenpud JD, Cobanoglu A, Norman DJ, Starr A, eds. *Cardiac transplantation*. New York: Springer-Verlag; 1991.

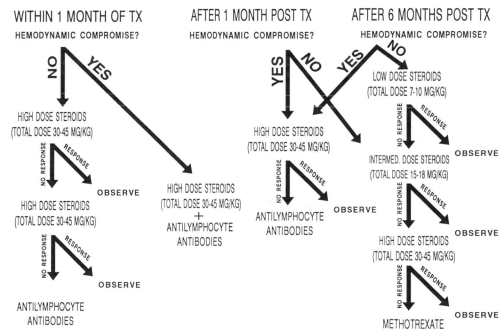

FIGURE 38.9. Algorithm used at the Oregon Cardiac Transplant Program for the treatment of acute rejection. Parameters used in the decision process are time post-transplantation, presence or absence of hemodynamic compromise, and the prior treatment history.

traditional atherosclerosis, which is focal and proximal in nature, CAV is a diffuse process involving the entire length of the coronary tree.[80] Only later do the lesions become more complex with differential areas of narrowing.[85] There is concentric myointimal proliferation (see Fig. 38.11) in CAV, in contrast to the frequently eccentric involvement characteristic of traditional CAD. The internal elastic lamina usually is intact and there is rarely calcium deposition until late in the disease.[80] Although many lesions are bland, without evidence of an inflammatory infiltrate, scattered mononuclear cells can at times be identified throughout the

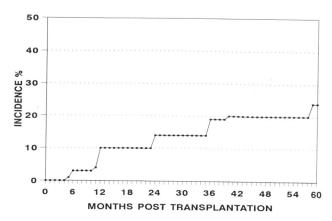

FIGURE 38.10. The risk of developing cardiac allograft vasculopathy (chronic rejection) increases over time with a 5-yr risk of 22% based on data from the Oregon Cardiac Transplant Program. In other series this risk has been reported as high as 45%.[83]

myointima. Libby and colleagues pointed out the presence and close association of mononuclear cells just below the endothelial layer suggesting a role for cell-mediated immunity.[86]

It is ironic that although the major late complication after cardiac transplantation is the development of CAV, the vast majority of patients (with exceptions) have no chest pain, because of afferent denervation of the heart. For this reason, most centers perform routine annual coronary angiography to screen for the development of CAV. Unfortunately, because of its diffuse nature, if CAV is discovered, treatment cannot be approached by traditional methods such as coronary bypass grafting. Although angioplasty has been attempted for high-grade lesions superimposed on the diffuse disease,[87] the long-term outcome of this intervention is unknown. At this juncture, repeat transplantation is currently the only available treatment option.

Medical Complications after Cardiac Transplantation

Most medical complications after cardiac transplantation are a direct result of the immunosuppression required to preserve allograft function. These can be divided into acute and chronic complications, with the common acute complications being infection, acute renal dysfunction, hypertension, diabetes, and neurologic complications. The more chronic complications include malignancy, chronic renal dysfunction, and bone disease.

Infection

The increased incidence of important infection is directly related to immunosuppression. This is illustrated in Figure 38.12, which demonstrates the incidence of acute rejection requiring augmentation of immunosuppression over time, and the parallel incidence of infection. In

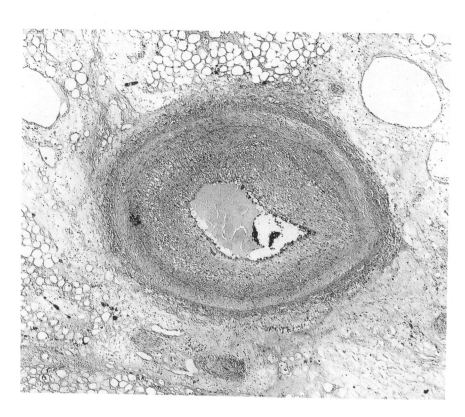

FIGURE 38.11. Concentric myointimal hyperplasia of cardiac allograft vasculopathy. Hemotoxylin-eosin, ×58. From Ray J and Hosenpud JD, in Hosenpud JD, Cobanoglu A, Norman DJ, Starr A, eds. *Cardiac transplantation*. New York: Springer-Verlag; 1991.

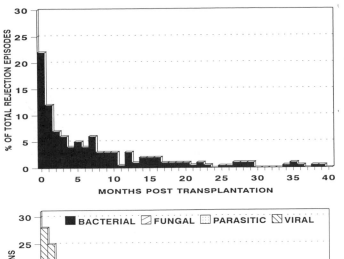

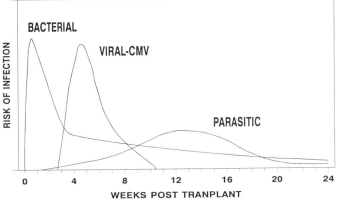

FIGURE 38.13. The specific types of organisms responsible for infection vary over time with bacterial infections largely a complication of surgery and the most common important viral infection, cytomegalovirus (*CMV*), occurring between 4 and 8 weeks after transplantation.

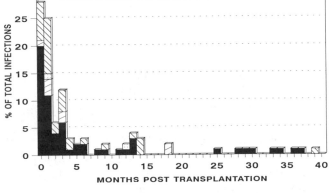

FIGURE 38.12. The incidence of rejection (*top*) and infection (*bottom*) over time after transplantation is presented (based on OCTP data). The parallels result from the requirement to augment immunosuppression to treat rejection, thus increasing infection risk.

addition, certain infections are more or less likely at certain times post-transplantation (Fig. 38.13). The incidence of serious infection dropped substantially after the introduction of cyclosporine and the reduction of corticosteroids in the maintenance immunosuppression protocols. Hofflin and colleagues reported a 72% reduction in infectious death in cyclosporine-based immunosuppression compared to azathioprine/prednisone maintenance.[88] In a recent meta-analysis, cyclosporine contributed to a 50% reduction in serious infection and a shift from predominantly bacterial infections to a higher percentage of viral infections in the cyclosporine-treated patients.[89]

Bacterial infections continue, however, to be an important problem after cardiac transplantation, with those due to surgical complications being most common in the early post-transplant period. Intravascular catheter bacteremias, mediastinitis, and pneumonias account for most of these. Frequent changes in vascular access and aggressive pulmonary toilet after early extubation may be helpful. Mediastinitis, fortunately least common of these infectious complications, requires urgent and aggressive therapy with surgical drainage, debridement, and irrigation. Because of the delayed healing with cor-

ticosteroid use and the relatively avascular sternum, plastic procedures such as the use of a skeletal muscle flap are frequently required.[90,91]

Although allograft recipients are suseptible to all of the usual pathogens, serious infection after the transplant hospitalization is not infrequently due to opportunistic agents. Examples of opportunistic agents transmitted via the donor organ or blood products include cytomegalovirus and *Toxoplasma gondii*. Opportunistic infections transmitted by environmental exposure include organisms such as *Legionella*, *Pneumocystis*, *Listeria*, *Norcardia*, *Candida*, and *Aspergillus*.

Cytomegalovirus (CMV) is clearly the most common opportunistic infection seen after transplantation. Depending on demographics, up to 80% of the general population has been exposed to CMV. After transplantation, it is transmitted almost exclusively by the donor organ or is reactivated in a recipient with prior exposure. Those patients with no prior exposure as evidenced by negative serology for CMV who receive an organ from a donor who is also CMV seronegative will not develop CMV infection or disease.[92] Those patients who are CMV seronegative who receive a heart from a seropositive donor will almost always develop a primary CMV infection, which usually produces the most severe disease. Those with prior CMV exposure whether or not they receive a heart from a seropositive donor will likely develop recurrent CMV infection (secondary infection), albeit with usually milder symptoms than those accompanying primary disease.[93] The manifestations of CMV disease are variable, ranging from a mononucleosis-like syndrome with viremia to important tissue invasion with pneumonitis, hepatitis, or gastrointestinal invasion. Mortality from tissue-invasive CMV disease and especially pneumonia (the most common cause of post-transplant interstitial pneumonia) after

TABLE 38.7. Post-transplant lymphomas/sarcomas.

Age (yr)	Sex	Mos post-treatment	Site	Therapy	Outcome
37	M	7	CNS	Immunosuppression Local irradiation	Remission
62	M	3	Lung	Immunosuppression Local irradiation	Remission
41	F	11	Abdomen	Chemotherapy	Died
59	M	14	Perinephric	Immunosuppression Local irradiation	Remission
55	M	18	Subcutaneous	Immunosuppression Local irradiation	Remission
52	M	13	Cutaneous[a]	Immunosuppression Local irradiation	Remission

[a] Kaposi's sarcoma.

transplantation has been reported as high as 80%.[93,94] With the introduction of the guanine analogue, ganciclovir, this mortality has dropped substantially.[95,96] Possibly as disturbing as the acute infectious morbidity caused by CMV is the previously mentioned association with the development of cardiac allograft vasculopathy. There appears to be an even stronger association with CAV in patients who are persistently culture positive for CMV.[97] Whether these patients should receive ganciclovir therapy is unclear.

It is extremely important that the approach to the febrile allograft recipient be an aggressive one. Full evaluation including bacterial, viral, and fungal blood cultures should be obtained. If there are respiratory symptoms with or without associated x-ray findings, early adequate pulmonary culturing (usually bronchoscopy with brushings but with a low tolerance to proceed to lung biopsy) are critical to direct appropriate therapy to the wide range of potential pathogens in this population. In the early postoperative period, computerized tomographic studies of the chest are extremely helpful to evaluate collections of fluid and rule out mediastinitis, which can present much less acutely than in the nonimmunocompromised host. Finally, knowing the possible etiologic agents based on preoperative infection screening (CMV and toxoplasma serology, myobacterial and systemic fungal skin testing, etc.) and the temporal occurrence post-transplantation also will assist in making the appropriate diagnostic and therapeutic decisions in these complex patients.

Malignancy

The most common immunosuppression-related malignancies are skin cancers and lymphoproliferative disorders. The overall risk of developing a post-transplant malignancy is between 6% and 10%, which is 100-fold greater than the population at large.[98] The lymphomas that develop post-transplantation are unique in several aspects. First, they are generally of B-cell origin, associated with Epstein-Barr virus, and can present both a polyclonal lymphoproliferative disorder or a more traditional monoclonal lymphoma.[99,100] Second, they frequently present extranodally with the central nervous system, the gastrointestinal tract, and the lung being common sites. Finally, chemotherapy does not appear to be beneficial, and aggressive reduction of immunosuppression coupled with local therapy with or without the use of acyclovir has resulted in remissions.[100] Table 38.7 summarizes five cases of post-transplant lymphoma seen in the OCTP population and their clinical outcomes. One additional case of Kaposi's sarcoma is also included. All of the survivors were treated with local irradition and reduction of immunosuppression. The one fatality was treated with chemotherapy.

Miscellaneous

Most other medical complications relate to side effects directly attributable to the specific immunosuppressive agents used post-transplantation. Diastolic hypertension is an almost uniform side effect of cyclosporine and is contributed to by corticosteroids. It is poorly controlled with conventional antihypertensive agents, although the calcium antagonists, and in particular, nifedipine, are reasonably effective. Diabetes and hyperlipidemia are primarily secondary to corticosteroids but are also complications of cyclosporine. Bone disease and particularly compression fractures are corticosteroid related and can be especially severe if osteoporosis predates the transplant. A more unusual form of bone disease, also secondary to steroids, is osteonecrosis, most commonly of the hip followed in frequency with the knees and shoulders. This has a reported incidence as high as 20% in renal allograft recipients.[101] Finally, renal dysfunction is a major complication of cyclosporine therapy.[57]

Physiology of the Transplanted Heart

Despite the similarities, there are substantial differences in the function of the transplanted cardiac allograft compared to the normal heart. The factors that can substantially influence allograft function can be divided into three major categories: (a) mechanical, including loss of normal atrial transport, donor-recipient size matching, and preservation injury, (b) denervation and denervation hypersensitivity, and (c) effects of acute and chronic rejection.

Mechanical Factors

Normally, the atrial contribution to total stroke volume is between 15% and 20%.[102] As previously described, the reconstruction of the left and right atria, as a consequence of the transplant operation, results in a larger atrial chamber with both recipient and donor atrial components and usually two sinus nodes. Only the donor sinus node is electrically coupled to the donor ventricle, as electrical impulses will not traverse the suture line. Stinson and colleagues demonstrated that with synchrony of the donor and recipient atria, atrial contraction contributed between 2 and 4 mm Hg to left ventricular filling.[42] Unfortunately, this coatrial synchrony is the exception rather than the rule, as demonstrated by Figure 38.14, which shows both recipient and donor P waves. In this case, it is unlikely that random recipient atrial contractions have a meaningful contribution to ventricular filling and when completely out of phase with donor atrial contractions may actually hinder ventricular filling.

Cardiac transplantation is unique in that the heart size is not explicitly matched to the circulation. Most centers use body weights to match a given donor organ to a given recipient and allow for as much as a 30% discrepancy between the two. This donor-recipient size mismatch can play an important role in allograft function, especially if there are inadequate compensatory changes. If a patient receives a relatively smaller heart, in order to maintain cardiac output, attempts to maintain stroke volume will result in higher filling pressures. If stroke volume is inadequate an increase in heart rate will be required. Conversely, if the recipient receives a relatively larger heart, filling pressures will be lower,

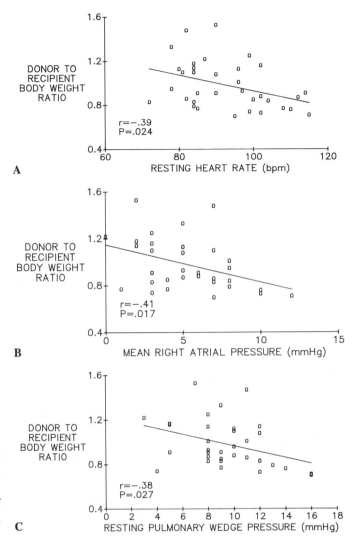

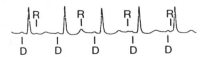

FIGURE 38.14. Electrocardiogram from a cardiac allograft recipient demonstrating both recipient (*R*) and donor (*D*) P waves. Note that the recipient P wave rate is slower and the P waves are not associated with the donor QRS complexes.

FIGURE 38.15. Three months after cardiac transplantation there is a negative correlation between the donor/recipient body weight ratio and heart rate (**A**), right atrial (**B**), and pulmonary wedge (**C**) pressures in 34 patients. This would suggest that relatively smaller hearts require increased heart rates and filling pressures to maintain cardiac output. Reprinted, with permission, from Hosenpud et al.[103]

stroke volume will be greater, and a slower heart rate will meet cardiac output needs. This is exactly what is demonstrated in 34 allograft recipients studied 3 months after transplantation (Fig. 38.15, ref. 103).

Denervation

With the transection of the aorta, pulmonary artery, and atria, the donor heart is completely separated from both sympathetic and parasympathetic innervation. The loss of both afferent and efferent autonomic innervation results in a variety of reflexes summarized in Figure 38.16. There is loss of efferent vagal tone to the sinus node, resulting in an increase in resting heart rate, and

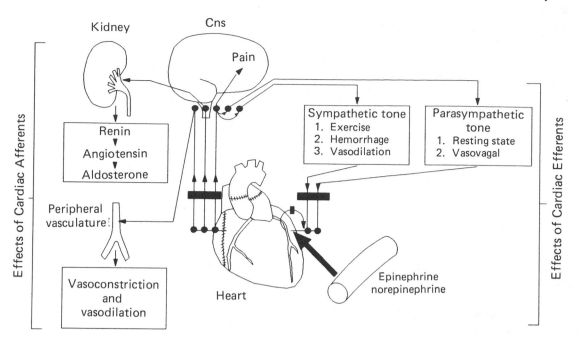

FIGURE 38.16. The effects of cardiac denervation involve the loss of both the cardiac afferents and efferents. The cardiac afferents have potential roles in salt and water regulation via the renin-angiotensin-aldosterone system, in reflex control of the peripheral vasculature, and in the sensation of cardiac pain. The cardiac efferents are responsible for the rapid changes in heart rate and contractility associated with changes in the physiologic state. In addition, central reflexes are transmitted to the heart via the vagal efferent nerves. Finally, cardiac denervation results in hypersensitivity to circulating catecholamines caused by the lack of adrenergic neuronal uptake. From Hosenpud JD and Morton MJ, in Hosenpud JD, Cobanoglu A, Norman DJ, Starr A, eds. *Cardiac transplantation*. New York: Springer-Verlag; 1991.

a loss of sympathetic tone to mediate reflex increases in heart rate and contractility brought about by exercise, hemorrhage, or acute vasodilation. A loss of cardiac afferents affects cardiorenal reflexes important in salt and water handling and reflexes that influence peripheral vascular tone.[104] Although gross clinical and histologic observations had led to the conclusion that reinnervation did not occur in the human allograft, recent data suggests that partial reinnervation can and does occur.[105] Using tyramine-induced release of norepinephrine across the cardiac bed, Wilson and colleagues demonstrated that late following transplantation, functioning sympathetic neurons are present in the allograft. In the patients with this partial reinnervation, a sympathetic reflex loop also can be demonstrated and many of these patients have a slightly greater heart rate response to exercise.[105] We and others have noted that some patients exhibit typical angina in response to ischemia consistent with partial afferent innervation.[106] Despite these interesting recent findings, the changes noted are subtle and for the most part after cardiac transplantation patients are functionally denervated.

In the normally innervated heart, resting heart rate is slow because of resting vagal tone. With the onset of exercise, vagal tone is released and heart rate increases rapidly and proportionally to the level of exercise. The increase in cardiac output associated with exercise is primarily due to the increase in heart rate, with stroke volume playing only a minor role.[107-109] Stinson and colleagues defined the exercise response in allograft recipients 1 and 2 yr after cardiac transplantation.[110] They demonstrated that the allograft heart had a resting heart rate approximately 30% higher than the normally innervated heart. With the onset of exercise, heart rate increased gradually, with a rapid increase in filling pressures. The substantial increase in cardiac output was mediated predominantly via an increase in stroke volume. Susequent studies demonstrated that the increase in heart rate paralleled an increase in circulating catecholamines.[111] Table 38.8 demonstrates resting and exercise hemodynamics in 23 allograft recipients 1 yr after cardiac transplantation and contrasts these to normal values.[112] One can therefore summarize these data as follows. Individuals with cardiac innervation rely on heart rate primarily to increase cardiac output with exercise. Cardiac allograft recipients rely primarily on stroke volume mediated via the Starling mechanism and pay for this increase with substantial increases in filling pressures. Only with increasing circulating catecholamines does heart rate add to the exercise response.

Another important aspect of allograft denervation is the altered response to commonly used cardiovascular

TABLE 38.8. Rest and exercise hemodynamics 1 yr post-transplantation.

Parameter	Normal[a]	Rest	Exercise
Right atrial (mm Hg)	0–8	6 ± 2	14 ± 7
Pulm artery mean (mm Hg)	9–16	18 ± 3	32 ± 9
Pulmonary wedge (mm Hg)	1–10	10 ± 3	20 ± 6
Cardiac output (L/min)	—	5.0 ± 0.9	9.9 ± 1.7
Cardiac index (L/min/m²)	2.4–4.2	2.5 ± 0.5	5.0 ± 0.8
Stroke volume (ml)	—	55 ± 9	77 ± 13
Stroke index (ml/m²)	30–56	28 ± 6	39 ± 7
Heart rate (bpm)	—	90 ± 11	122 ± 18
Mean arterial (mm Hg)	70–105	91 ± 12	102 ± 14
SVR (Wood U)	10–19	17.7 ± 4.0	9.3 ± 2.4

[a] Data from Grossman WH. *Cardiac catheterization and angiography.* Philadelphia; Lea & Febiger; 1986. From Hosenpud JD and Morton MJ, in Hosenpud JD, Cobanoglu A, Norman DJ, Starr A, eds. *Cardiac transplantation.* New York: Springer-Verlag; 1991.
SVR = systemic vascular resistance.

TABLE 38.9. Cardiovascular drugs after cardiac transplantation.

Drug	Effect in recipient	Mechanism
Digitalis	Normal increase in contractility, minimal AV nodal effect	Denervation
Atropine	None	Denervation
Epinephrine	Increased contractility and chronotropy	Denervation hypersensitivity
Norepinephrine	Increased contractility and chronotropy	Denervation hypersensitivity
Isoproterenol	Normal increase in inotropy and chronotropy	No neuronal uptake
Quinidine	No vagalytic effect	Denervation
Verapamil	Normal AV block	Direct effect
Nifedipine	No reflex tachycardia	Denervation
Hydralazine	No reflex tachycardia	Denervation
Beta blockers	Increased antagonist effect during exercise	Denervation

From Hosenpud JD and Morton MJ, in Hpsenpud JD, Cobanoglu A, Norman DJ, Starr A, eds. *Cardiac transplantation.* New York: Springer-Verlag; 1991.
AV = arteriovenous.

controlling atrial fibrillation, and atropine, which has no effect on bradycardias (both responses due to stimulation and inhibition, respectively of vagal efferents).

Cardiac Function in Acute Rejection

Before the introduction of cyclosporine, allograft rejection not infrequently led to acute ventricular dysfunction.[113,114] The combination of earlier detection and the use of cyclosporine have altered the natural history

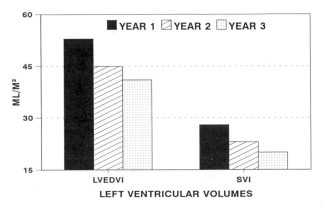
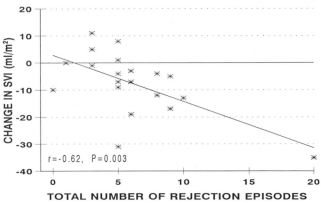

FIGURE 38.17. In 20 stable allograft recipients followed over 3 yr, mean end-diastolic volume and stroke volume fell (*top*). This fall was weakly correlated with the total number of rejection episodes over the 3-yr period (*bottom*).

of rejection in that systolic dysfunction is rare and, if present, often is a premorbid event.[115,116] Several investigators have reported that although systolic function may be normal, abnormalities in diastolic function may be present with rejection. Dawkins et al. demonstrated that mean isovolumic relaxation time fell with progressively severe rejection.[115] Paulsen and colleagues demonstrated rejection was associated with a prolonged rapid filling period.[117] In addition to alterations in allograft function acutely, there may also be alterations that occur over the longer term. In 20 patients followed serially over 3 yr after cardiac transplantation, resting and exercise pressures and flows remained fairly stable, with the exception of a gradually falling resting cardiac output. This fall in cardiac output was associated with a gradual fall in left ventricular end-diastolic volume and stroke volume measured by radionuclide ventriculography and was weakly correlated with the total number of rejection episodes over the 3-yr period (Fig. 38.17). No other clinical factor was associated with this fall in ventricular volumes. These data would suggest that although therapy may reverse the acute alterations in allograft function, repeated rejection episodes can have lasting effects on the allograft.

Outcomes

Survival

Survival after cardiac transplantation has steadily improved over the past 25 yr. Based on data from the Registry of the International Society for Heart and Lung Transplantation, patients transplanted through 1979 had a 1- and 5-yr survival of 50% and 30%, respectively; those transplanted through the subsequent 5 yr, a 70% and 55% survival, respectively; those transplanted from 1985 through 1990, an 81% and 70% survival, respectively.[1] Other factors that appear to be related to outcome include age of less than 1 yr, which has a substantially higher operative mortality, in the range of 20% (compared to 9% overall), and retransplantation, which has a 1-yr survival of approximately 50% and a 5-yr survival of under 40%.[1] Use of different immunosuppressive protocols, specifically those with and without antilymphocyte antibody prophylaxis has no impact on survival.[1] Figure 38.18 presents survival of four groups of heart failure patients, those most recent 181 patients undergoing cardiac transplantation at the OCTP, patients from the SOLVD placebo group who where NYHA functional class II and III,[118] reported patients undergoing skeletal myoplasty,[119] and a series of severely ill NYHA functional class IV patients not candidates for cardiac transplantation. Figure 38.19 outlines the cause of death based on time post-transplantation in a large registry population.[1] Early death within the first month is predominantly surgical; this is later followed by death from infection and rejection, with chronic rejection (CAV) responsible for most rejections after 1 yr. Finally, deaths from malignancies gradually increase over time.

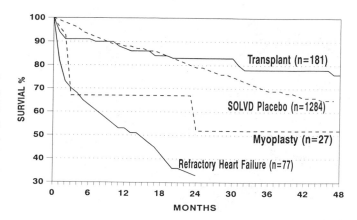

FIGURE 38.18. Survival of four groups of heart failure patients: 1) cardiac transplant recipients (OCTP data), 2) SOLVD placebo group,[122] 3) skeletal myoplasty,[123] and 4) NYHA functional class IV patients.

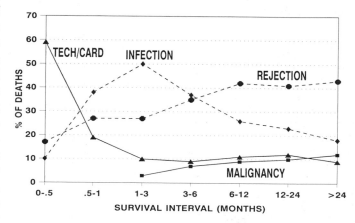

FIGURE 38.19. Cause of death after cardiac transplantation based on time post-transplant. Reprinted, with permission, from ref. 1.

Rehabilitation and Quality of Life

Outcome other than survival has been the topic of several investigations. It is the general perception that most patients are medically rehabilitated after cardiac transplantation and that it is usually social impediments (loss of insurance and disability income, inability to acquire employment due to health risk) that prevent full rehabilitation and return to productive lives. Gaudiani reported the Stanford experience, which demonstrated an 86% rehabilitation rate in 143 transplant recipients.[120] Lough reported that the principal negative factors after transplantation were related to side effects from immunosuppression. Nonetheless, 89% of patients were rehabilitated.[121] More recently, Bunzel and colleagues evaluated 35 patients after cardiac transplantation. A variety of factors were graded including physical, emotional, financial, etc., and an overall satisfaction parameter was calculated. Based on an improvement

scale from 0 to 50, the average overall improvement in the total score was 25.[122] Most recently, a multicenter study investigating parameters that predicted post-transplant return to work was reported. Those patients who were male, with a good educational background, who felt they were physically able to work, who would not lose health insurance or disability income, and who were at least 6 months post-transplant had the greatest likelihood of returning to gainful employment. The overall return to work rate in this series of 250 patients was 45%.[123]

One can conclude from these data that both survival and quality of life are acceptable after cardiac transplantation, with a high percentage of patients being fully rehabilitated and becoming productive members of society.

Conclusions

Cardiac transplantation is now a viable and proven therapy for the treatment of end-stage heart disease. Acute and subacute survival is now at acceptable levels; however, long-term survival continues to remain a major challenge. This has become increasingly evident as infants and children have begun to make up an increasing percent of patients transplanted. In contrast to the adult population, 5- and even 10-yr survivals in this population will not be considered acceptable. Despite its current success, the other principal limitation to cardiac allograft transplantation is the restricted ability to apply this therapy to only 10% of patients who could benefit. Even with the continued expansion of donor criteria, the number of allograft organs will never meet the demand. Other technologies must therefore be actively sought, including the use of artificial devices and hopefully ultimately xenograft transplantation. Only then can the successes in the field of transplantation be fully appreciated.

References

1. Kriet JM, Kaye MP. The registry of the international society for heart and lung transplantation: eighth official report—1991. *J Heart Lung Transplant*. 1991;10:491–498.
2. Evans RW. The economics of heart transplantation. *Circulation*. 1987;75:63–75.
3. Baumgartner WA, Reitz BA, Oyer PE, et al. Cardiac transplantation. *Curr Probl Surg*. 1979;16:2–61.
4. Copeland JG. Stinson EB. Human heart transplantation. *Curr Probl Cardiol*. 1979;4:1–51.
5. Miller LW, Vitale-Noedel N, Pennington DG, et al. Heart transplantation in patients over age 55. *J Heart Transplant*. 1988;7:254–257.
6. Olivari MT, Antolick A, Kaye MP, et al. Heart transplant in elderly patients. *J Heart Transplant*. 1988;7:258–264.
7. Carrier M, Emery RW, Riley JE, et al. Cardiac transplantation in patinets over the age of 50 years. *J Am Coll Cardiol*. 1986;8:285–288.
8. Hosenpud JD, Pantely GA, Norman DJ, Cobanoglu AM, Hovaguimian H, Starr A. A critical analysis of morbidity and mortality as it relates to recipient age following cardiac transplantation. *Clin Transplant*. 1990;4:51–54.
9. Heroux AL, O'Sullivan EJ, Kao WG, et al. Should cardiac transplantation be a treatment option after 65 years of age? *J Heart Lung Transplant*. 1992;11:220.
10. Griepp RB, Stinson EB, Dong E, et al. Determinants of operative risk in human heart transplant. *Am J Surg*. 1971;122:192–197.
11. Pastan SO, Braunwald E. Renal disorders and heart disease. In: Braunwald E, ed. *Heart disease*. Philadelphia: Saunders; 1988:1828–1835.
12. Kubo SH, Walter BA, John DHA, et al. Liver function abnormalities in chronic heart failure. Influence of systemic hemodynamics. *Arch Intern Med*. 1987;147:1227–1230.
13. Kaplan SR, Calabresi P. Immunosuppressive agents. *N Engl J Med*. 1973;289:1234–1236.
14. Moran M, Tomlanovich S, Myers BD. Cyclosporine-induced chronic nephropathy in human recipients of cardiac allografts. *Transplant Proc*. 1985;17(4, Suppl 1):185–190.
15. Hosenpud JD, Stibolt TA, Atwal K, Shelley. Abnormal pulmonary function specifically related to congestive heart failure: comparison of patients before and after cardiac transplantation. *Am J Med*. 1990;88:493–496.
16. Rhenman MJ, Rhenman B, Icenogle T, et al. Diabetes and heart transplantation. *J Heart Transplant*. 1988;7:356–358.
17. Armitage JM, Griffith BP, Kormos RL, et al. Cardiac transplantation in patients with malignancy. *J Heart Transplant*. 1989;8:89. Abstract.
18. Minow RA, Benjamin RS, Lee ET, Gottlieb JA. Adriamycin cardiomyopathy—risk factors. *Cancer*. 1977;39:1397–1402.
19. Hosenpud JD, Uretsky BF, O'Connell JB, et al. Cardiac transplantation for amyloidosis. Results of a multicenter survey. *J Heart Transplant*. 1989;8:99. Abstract.
20. Hosenpud JD, DeMarco T, Frazier OH, et al. Progression of systemic disease and reduced long-term survival in patients with cardiac amyloidosis undergoing heart transplantation. *Circulation*. 1991;84(Suppl III):III338–III343.
21. Valantine HA, Tazelaar HD, Macoviak J, et al. Cardiac sarcoidosis: response to steoids and transplantation. *J Heart Transplant*. 1987;6:244–250.
22. Oni AA, Hershberger RE, Norman DJ, et al. Recurrence of sarcoidoisis in a cardiac allograft: control with augmented corticosteroids. *J Heart Lung Transplant*. 1992;11:367–369.
23. Maricle RA, Hosenpud JD, Norman DJ, Pantely GA, Cobanoglu AM, Starr A. The lack of predictive value of preoperative psychologic distress for postoperative medical outcome in heart transplant recipients. *J Heart Lung Transplant*. 1991;10:942–947.
24. Sadler AM, Sadler BL, Statson EB. The Uniform Anatomical Gift Act. *JAMA*. 1968;206:2501.
25. Black PM. Brain death. *N Engl J Med*. 1978;299:338.
26. Pallis C. Prognostic significance of a dead brain stem. *Br Med J*. 1981;282:533.
27. Powner DJ, Fromm GH. The electroencephalogram in the determination of brain death. *N Engl J Med*. 1979;300:502.
28. Griepp RB, Stinson EB, Clark DA, et al. The cardiac donor. *Surg Gynecol Obstet*. 1971;133:792.
29. Copeland JG. Cardiac transplantation. *Curr Probl Cardiol*. 1988;13:159.
30. Fentz V, Gormsen J. Electrocardiographic patterns in patients with cerebrovascular accidents. *Circulation*. 1962;25:22.
31. Novitzky D, Wicomb WN, Cooper KDC, et al. Electrocardiographic, hemodynamic and endocrine changes

occuring during experimental brain death in the chacma baboon. *J Heart Transplant.* 1984;4:63.

32. Gilbert EM, Krieger SK, Murray JL, et al. Echocardiographic evaluation of potential cardiac transplant donors. *J Thorac Cardiovasc Surg.* 1988;95:1003.

33. Hearse DJ, Stewart DA, Braimbridge MV. Cellular protection during myocardial ischemia: the development and characterization of a procedure for the induction of reversible ischemic arrest. *Circulation.* 1976;54:193.

34. Gott JP, Pan-Chih, Dorsey LMA, et al. Cardioplegia for transplantation: failure of extracellular solution compared with Stanford or UW solution. *Ann Thorac Surg.* 1990;50:348–354.

35. Gott JP, Brown WM III, Pan-Chih, Dorsey LMA, Walker B, Guyton RA. Cardioplegia for heart transplantation: unmodified UW solution compared with Stanford solution. *J Heart Lung Transplant.* 1992;11:353–362.

36. Heck CF, Shumway SJ, Kaye MP. The registry of the international society for heart transplantation: sixth official report—1989. *J Heart Transplant.* 1989;8:271–276.

37. Bourge RC, Naftel DC, Costanzo-Nordin M, Kirklin JK, Young J, and the Transplant Cardiologists' Research Database Group. Risk factors for death after cardiac transplantation: a multi-institutional study. *J Heart Lung Transplant.* 1992;11:191.

38. Lower RR, Shumway NE. Studies on orthotopic homotransplantation of the canine heart. *Surg Forum.* 1960;11:18–19.

39. Lewin W. Factors in the mortality of closed head injuries. *Br Med J.* 1953;1:1239.

40. Cannom DS, Graham AF, Harrison DL. Electrophysiological studies in the denervated transplanted human heart: response to atrial pacing and atropine. *Circ Res.* 1973;32:268–278.

41. Cannom DS, Rider AK, Stinson EB, et al. Electrophysiologic studies in the denervated transplanted human heart. II. Response to norepinephrine, isoproterenol and propranolol. *Am J Cardiol.* 1975;36:859–866.

42. Stinson EB, Schroeder JS, Griepp RB, et al. Observations on the behavior of recipient atria after cardiac transplantation in man. *Am J Cardiol.* 1972;30:615–622.

43. Cobanoglu A. Operative techniques and early postoperative care in cardiac transplantation. In: Hosenpud JD, Cobanoglu A, Norman DJ, Starr A, ed. *Cardiac transplantation.* New York: Springer-Verlag; 1991:95–114.

44. Davies RA, Koshal A, Walley V, et al. Temporary diastolic noncompliance with preserved systolic function after heart transplantation. *Transplant Proc.* 1987;19:3444–3447.

45. Hosenpud JD, Norman DJ, Cobanoglu MA, Floten HS, Conner RM, Starr A. Serial echocardiographic findings early after heart transplantation: evidence for reversible right ventricular dysfunction and myocardial edema. *J Heart Transplant.* 1987;6:343–347.

46. Stinson EB, Caves PK, Griepp RB, Oyer PE, Rider AK, Shumway NE. Hemodynamic observations in the early period after human heart transplantation. *J Thorac Cardiovasc Surg.* 1975;69:264–270.

47. Pascual JMS, Fiorelli AI, Bellotti GM, Stolf NAG, Jatene AD. Prostacyclin in the management of pulmonary hypertension after heart transplantation. *J Heart Transplant.* 1990;9:644–651.

48. Syndman DR, Werner BG, Heinze-Lacey B, et al. Use of cytomegalovirus immune globulin to prevent cytomegalovirus disease in renal-transplant recipients. *N Engl J Med.* 1987;317:1049–1054.

49. Balfour HH, Chace BA, Stapleton JT, et al. A randomized, placebo-controlled trial of oral acyclovir for the prevention of cytomegalovirus disease in recipients of renal allografts. *N Engl J Med.* 1989;320:1381–1387.

50. Higgins RM, Bloom SL, Hopkin JM, et al. The risks and benefits of low-dose cotrimoxazole prophylaxis for Pneumocystis pneumonia in renal transplantation. *Transplantation.* 1989;47:558–560.

51. Borel JF, Feurer C, Bugler HU, et al. Biological effects of cyclosporin A: a new antilymphocytic agent. *Agents Actions.* 1976;6:468–475.

52. Borel JF, Feurer C, Magnee C, et al. Effects of the new anti-lymphocytic peptide cyclosporin A in animals. *Immunology.* 1977;32:1017–1025.

53. Cohen DJ, Loertscher R, Rubin MF, et al. Cyclosporine: a new immunosuppressive agent for organ transplantation. *Ann Intern Med.* 1984;101:667–682.

54. Kalman VK, Klimpel GR. Cyclosporin A inhibits the production of gamma interferon (IFN gamma) but does not inhibit production of virus induced IFN alpha/beta. *Cell Immunol.* 1983;78:122–129.

55. Grey HM, Chestnut R. Antigen processing and presentation to T cells. *Immunol Today.* 1985;6:101–106.

56. Salomon DR, Limacher MC. Chronic immunosuppression and the treatment of acute rejection. In: Hosenpud JD, Cobanoglu A, Norman DJ, Starr A, ed. *Cardiac transplantation.* New York: Springer-Verlag; 1991:139–168.

57. McGiffin DC, Kirklin JK, Naftel DC. Acute renal failure after heart transplantation and cyclosporine therapy. *J Heart Transplant.* 1985;4:396–399.

58. Calne RY. Rejection of renal homografts: inhibition in dogs by 6-mercatopurine. *Lancet.* 1960;1:417–418.

59. Murray JE, Merrill JP, Harrison JH, et al. Prolonged survival of human kidney homografts by immunosuppressive therapy. *N Engl J Med.* 1963;268:1315–1323.

60. Woodruff MFA, Robson JS, Nolan B, et al. Homotransplantation of kidney in patients treated by preoperative local irradiation and postoperative administration of an antimetabolite (Imuran): report of six cases. *Lancet.* 1963;2:675–682.

61. McCormack JJ, Johns DG. Purine antimetabolites. In: Chabner B, ed. *Pharmacologic principles of cancer treatment.* Philadelphia: Saunders; 1982:213–228.

62. Shumway SJ, Kaye MP. The international society for heart transplantation registry. In: Terasaki P, ed. *Clinical transplant 1988.* Los Angles: UCLA Tissue Typing Laboratory; 1988:1–5.

63. Merrill JP, Murray JE, Harrison JH, et al. Successful homotransplantation of the kidney between nonidentical twins. *N Engl J Med.* 1960;262:1251–1260.

64. Durum SK, Schmidt JA, Oppenheim JJ. Interleukin-1: an immunological perspective. *Annu Rev Immunol.* 1985;3:263–288.

65. MacDonald HR, Habholz MT. T-cell activation. *Annu Rev Cell Biol*. 1986;2:231–253.

66. Russell SW, Salomon Dr. Macrophage effector and regulatory functions. In: Reif AE, Mitchell MS, eds. *Immunity to cancer*. New York: Academic Press; 1985: 205–216.

67. Köhler G, Milstein C. Continuous cultures of fused cells secreting artibody of predefined specificity. *Nature*, Lond. 1975;256:495–497.

68. NACB/AACC Task Force on Cyclosporine Monitoring. Critical issues in cyclosporine monitoring. *Clin Chem*. 1987;33:1269–1288.

69. Cosimi AB, Burton RC, Colvin RB. Treatment of acute renal allograft rejection with OKT3 antibody. *Transplantation*. 1981;32:535–539.

70. Bristow MR, Gilbert EM, Renlund DG, et al. Use of OKT3 in heart transplantation; review of the inital experience. *Transplant Proc*. 1988;7:1–11.

71. Kriett JM, Kaye MP. The registry of the international society for heart transplantation: seventh official report—1990. *J Heart Transplant*. 1990;9:323–330.

72. Johnson MR, Martin Mullen G, O'Sullivan EJ, et al. The risk/benefit ratio of perioperative OKT3 in cardiac transplantation. *J Heart Lung Transplant*. 1992;11:207.

73. Hooks MA, Wade CS, Millikan WJ Jr. Muromonab CD-3: a review of its pharmacology, pharmacokinetics, and clinical use in transplantation. *Pharmacotherapy*. 1991; 11:26–37.

74. Swinnen LJ, Costanzo-Nordin MR, Fisher SG, et al. Increased incidence of lymphoproliferative disorder after immunosuppression with the monoclonal antibody OKT3 in cardiac-transplant recipients. *N Engl J Med*. 1990;323:1723–1728.

75. Costanzo-Nordin MR, Grusk BB, Silver MA, et al. Reversal of recalcitrant cardiac allograft rejecton with methotrexate. *Circulation*. 1988;78(Suppl III):III47–57.

76. Olsen SL, O'Connell JB, Bristow MR, Renlund DG. Methotrexate as an adjunct in the treatment of persistent mild cardiac allograft rejection. *Transplantation*. 1990; 50:773–775.

77. Hosenpud JD, Hershberger RE, Ratkovec RM, et al. Methotrexate for the treatment of patients with multiple episodes of acute cardiac allograft rejection. *J Heart Lung Transplant*. 1992;11:739–745.

78. Caves PK, Stinson EB, Billingham M, Shumway NE. Percutaneous transvenous endomyocardial biopsy in human heart recipients. Experience with a new technique. *Ann Thorac Surg*. 1973;16:325–336.

79. Billingham ME, Cary NRB, Hammond ME, et al. A working formulation for the standardization of nomenclature in the diagnosis of heart and lung rejection: heart rejection study group. *J Heart Transplant*. 1990;9:587–601.

80. Hosenpud JD, Shipley DG, Wagner CR. Cardiac allograft vasculopathy: current concepts, recent developments, and future directions. *J Heart Lung Transplant*. 1992;11:9–23.

81. Grattan MT, Moreno-Cabral CE, Starnes VA, Oyer PE, Stinson EB, Shumway NE. Cytomegalovirus is associated with cardiac allograft rejection and atherosclerosis. *JAMA*. 1989;261:3561–3566.

82. Hess JL, Hastillo A, Mohanakumar T, et al. Accelerated atherosclerosis in cardiac transplantation: role of cytotoxic B-cell antibodies and hyperlipidemia. *Circulation*. 1983;68(Suppl 2):94–101.

83. Hammond EH, Yowell RL, Nunoda S, et al. Vascular (humoral) rejection in heart transplantation: pathologic observations and clinical implications. *J Heart Transplant*. 1989;8:430–443.

84. Rose EA, Smith CR, Petrossian GA, Barr ML, Reemtsma K. Humoral immune responses after cardiac transplantation: correlation with fatal rejection and graft atherosclerosis. *Surgery*. 1989;106:203–207.

85. Billingham ME. Cardiac transplant atherosclerosis. *Transplant Proc*. 1987;19(Suppl 5):19–25.

86. Libby P, Salomon RN, Payne DD, Schoen FJ, Pober JS. Functions of the vascular wall cells related to development of transplantation-associated coronary arteriosclerosis. *Transplant Proc*. 1989;21:3677–3684.

87. Vetrovec GW, Cowley MJ, Newton CM, et al. Applications of percutaneous transluminal angioplasty in cardiac transplantation. Preliminary results in five patients. *Circulation*. 1988;78(Suppl III):III83–86.

88. Hofflin JA, Potasman I, Baldwin JC, et al. Infectious complications in heart transplant recipients receiving cyclosporine and corticosteroids. *Ann Intern Med*. 1987; 106:209–216.

89. Hosenpud JD, Norman DJ, Pantely GA, Cobanoglu AM, Starr A. Low morbidity and mortality from infection following cardiac transplantation using maintenance triple therapy and low-dose corticosteroids for acute rejection. *Clin Transplantation*. 1988;2:201–206.

90. Trento A, Dummer GS, Hardesty RL. Mediastinitis following heart transplantation: incidence, treatment, and results. *Heart Transplant*. 1984;3:336–340.

91. Miller R, Ruder J, Karwande SV, et al. Treatment of mediastinitis after heart tranplantation. *J Heart Transplant*. 1986;5:477–479.

92. Chou S, Norman DJ. The influence of donor factors other than serologic status on transmission of cytomegalovirus to transplant recipients. *Transplantation*. 1988; 46:89–93.

93. Dummer JS, White LT, Ho M, et al. Morbidity of cytomegalovirus infection in recipients of heart or heartlung transplants who received cyclosporine. *J Infect Dis*. 1985;152:1182–1191.

94. Smith CB. Cytomegalovirus pneumonia state of the art. *Chest*. 89;95(Suppl):182S–187S.

95. Watson FS, O'Connell JB, Amber IJ, et al. Treatment of cytomegalovirus pneumonia in heart transplant recipients with 9(1,3-dihydroxy-2-proproxy-methyl)-guanine (DHPG). *J Heart Transplant*. 1988;7:102–105.

96. Keay S, Petersen E, Icenogle T, et al. Ganciclovir treatment of serious cytomegalovirus infection in heart and heart-lung transplant recipients. *Rev Infect Dis*. 1988; 10(Suppl 3):S563–S572.

97. Everett JP, Hershberger RE, Norman DJ, et al. Prolonged cytomegalovirus infection with viremia is associated with development of cardiac allograft vasculopathy. *J Heart Lung Transplant*. 1992;11:S133–S137.

98. Penn I. Malignancies associated with immunosuppressive or cytotoxic therapy. *Surgery*. 1978;83:492–502.

99. Cleary ML, Sklar J. Lymphoproliferative disorders in cardiac transplant recipients are multiclonal lymphomas. *Lancet.* 1984;2:491–493.

100. Hanto DW, Gajl-Peczalska KJ, Balfour HH, et al. Acyclovir therapy of Epstein-Barr virus-induced post-transplant lymphoproliferative diseases. *Transplant Proc.* 1985;17:89–92.

101. Ibels LS, Alfrey AC, Huffer WE, Weil R. Aseptic necrosis of bone after renal transplantation: experience in 194 transplant recipients and review of the literature. *Medicine.* 1978;57:25–45.

102. Rahimtoola SH, Ehsani A, Sinno MZ, et al. Left atrial transport function in myocardial infarction: importance of its booster pump function. *Am J Med.* 1975;59:686–694.

103. Hosenpud JD, Pantely GA, Morton MJ, Norman DJ, Cobanoglu AM, Starr A. Relationship between recipient: donor body size matching and hemodynamics 3 months following cardiac transplantation. *J Heart Transplant.* 1989;8:241–243.

104. Hosenpud JD, Morton MJ. Physiology and hemodynamic assessment of the transplanted heart. In: Hosenpud JD, Cobanoglu A, Norman DJ, Starr A, eds. *Cardiac transplantation.* New York: Springer-Verlag; 1991:169–189.

105. Wilson RF, McGinn AL, Laxson DD, Christensen BV, Johnson TH, Kubo SH. Regional differences in sympathetic reinnervation after cardiac transplantation. *Circulation.* 1991;84(Suppl II):489.

106. Vora KN, Hosenpud JD, Ray J, et al. Angina pectoris in a cardiac allograft recipient. *Clin Transplant.* 1991;5:20–22.

107. Thadani U, Parker JO. Hemodynamics at rest and during supine and sitting bicycle exercise in nomal subjects. *Am J Cardiol.* 1978;41:52–59.

108. Pflugfelder PW, Purves PD, McKenzie FN, Kostuk WJ. Cardiac dynamics during supine exercise in cyclosporine-treated orthotopic heart transplant recipients: assessment by radionuclide angiography. *J Am Coll Cardiol.* 1987;10:336–341.

109. Ross J, Linhart JW, Braunwald E. Effects of changing heart rate in man by electrical stimulation of the right atrium. Studies at rest, during exercise and with isoproterenol. *Circulation.* 1965;32:549–558.

110. Stinson EB, Griepp RB, Schroeder JS, Dong E Jr, Shumway NE. Hemodymanic observations one and two years after cardiac transplantation in man. *Circulation.* 1972;45:1183–1193.

111. Pope SE, Stinson EB, Daughters GT, Schroeder JS, Ingels NB, Alderman EL. Exercise response of the denervated heart in long-term cardiac transplant recipients. *Am J Cardiol.* 1980;46:213–218.

112. Grossman WH. *Cardiac catheterization and angiography.* Philadelphia: Lea & Febiger; 1986.

113. Griepp RB, Stinson EB, Dong E Jr, Clark DA, Shumway NE. Acute rejection of the allografted human heart. *Ann Thorac Surg.* 1971;12:113–126.

114. Leachman RD, Cokkinos DVP, Rochelle DG, et al. Serial hemodynamic study of the transplanted heart and correlation with clinical rejection. *J Thorac Cardiovasc Surg.* 1971;61:561–569.

115. Dawkins KD, Oldershaw PJ, Billingham ME, et al. Changes in diastolic function as a noninvasive marker of cardiac allograft rejection. *J Heart Transplant.* 1984;3:286–294.

116. Haverich A, Kemnitz J, Fieguth HG, et al. Non-invasive parameters for detection of cardiac allograft rejection. *Clin Transplant.* 1987;1:151–158.

117. Paulsen W, Magid N, Sagar K, et al. Left ventricular function of heart allografts during acute rejection: an echocardiographic assessment. *J Heart Transplant.* 1985;4:525–529.

118. The SOLVD Investigators. Effect of enalapril on survival in patients with reduced left ventricular ejection fractions and congestive heart failure. *N Engl J Med.* 1991;325:293–302.

119. Carpentier A, Chachques JC, Grandjean P. *Cardiomyoplasty.* M. Kisco, NY: Futura Publishing Co; 1991.

120. Gaudiani VA, Stinson EB, Alderman E, et al. Longterm survival and function after cardiac transplantation. *Ann Surg.* 1981;194:381–385.

121. Lough ME, Lindsey AM, Shinn JA. Life satisfaction following heart transplantation. *J Heart Transplant.* 1985;4:446–449.

122. Bunzel B, Grundbock, A, Laczkovics A, Holzinger C, Teufelsbauer H. Quality of life after orthotopic heart transplantation. *J Heart Lung Transplant.* 1991;10:455–459.

123. Paris W, Woodbury A, Thompson S, et al. Return to work after cardiac transplantation. *J Heart Lung Transplant.* 1992;11:195.

Part VII
Future Directions

39

The Diagnosis and Management of Congestive Heart Failure: What Does the Future Hold?

Jeffrey D. Hosenpud and Barry H. Greenberg

The approach to the patient with severe congestive heart failure (CHF) has changed dramatically over the past decade. Better definition of the etiology of CHF, stratification of risk using variables readily available in clinical practice, the use of vasodilator therapy (particularly, the angiotensin-converting enzyme inhibitors), improvements in surgical techniques for intervention in both acute and chronic disease, and cardiac replacement via cardiac transplantation and mechanical ventricular assistance are all responsible for a substantial improvement in the quality and quantity of life in patients with this syndrome. With the advent of new diagnostic techniques, new classes of pharmaceuticals, implantable defibrillators, molecular technology, and advances in cardiac replacement, the future appears to be quite promising. In this closing chapter of the text, modalities of diagnosis and treatment that are likely to alter the way in which patients with CHF are managed in the future are briefly discussed.

Diagnostic Modalities

Since coronary artery disease is by far the most common etiology of CHF, advances in the early diagnosis and successful treatment of this disease will have an enormous impact on the incidence of heart failure. Improved methods for risk stratification, identification of new risk factors (i.e., lipoprotein a and homocysteine), and early recognition of established disease by noninvasive imaging techniques are all necessary steps in limiting myocardial damage due to ischemic disease.

A major challenge of the next decade will be an attempt to understand the diseases that have been broadly characterized as the cardiomyopathies. We now have several new tools that may be of assistance in understanding better both mechanisms generic to heart failure as well as those that might be specific to individual disease states.

Magnetic Resonance Technology

Magnetic resonance imaging (MRI) already has made its impact in the diagnosis of cardiovascular diseases. It is being used regularly in the assessment of structure and function of the heart and pericardium and has several advantages over other imaging techniques. These include excellent contrast between different soft tissues, very high spatial resolution, the ability to sample over multiple tomographic sections in any number of orientations, and the potential for dynamic (cine) presentation. Although MRI may be quite helpful in individual patients, it is a further refinement of other imaging techniques and, thus, is not likely to provide major advances in understanding cardiovascular pathophysiology. In contrast, magnetic resonance spectroscopy has the potential of providing information not available by other techniques. By analysis of spin characteristics of individual elements, the concentrations of a variety of molecules such as hydrogen, phosphorus, fluorine, and carbon within the heart can be measured in vivo. In this way, energy utilization and a variety of metabolic pathways can be evaluated in the normal and cardiomyopathic heart.

The current emphasis of magnetic resonance spectroscopy has been on determining concentrations of high energy phosphate compounds in the normal heart and various disease states.[1] One could likewise apply this technology to the analysis of carbon-containing compounds. For instance, ^{13}C-glutamate currently is being investigated in experimental heart models to analyze substrate utilization by the tricarboxylic acid cycle.[2] The major limitation of this technology is the requirement for a substantial concentration of the specific compound of interest to be present within the heart and in the proper state. For example, free adenosine triphosphate (ATP) can be measured but the substantial fraction of ATP bound to magnesium will not be detected. As the technology advances, the concentration requirements are being reduced and the ability for specific localization of the area of interest (e.g., endocardium vs. epicardium) is improving.

Positron Emission Tomography

The ability to assay positron emitters such as C^{11} or N^{13} enables one to synthesize organic compounds that can be utilized in almost all human metabolic pathways. This, coupled with the ability to image tracer amounts of these compounds, makes this technology ideal for studying metabolic pathways within the heart. The measurement of ^{18}fluorodeoxyglucose for the analysis of an intact glycolytic pathway, which presumably is a sign of viable myocardium, is just one example of the use of this methodology.[3] One could envision screening for enzymatic defects in energy utilization, amino acid biosynthesis, and degradation or fatty acid metabolism.

Molecular Biologic Techniques

With the advent of endomyocardial biopsy, cardiac histology could be obtained from the living patient safely for the first time. This resulted in the appreciation that inflammatory heart disease could masquerade clinically as a dilated cardiomyopathy.[4] Other less common diseases also were being diagnosed during life rather than at autopsy.[5] Unfortunately, because of the extremely small sample size obtained by this technique, little other than routine histology evaluation has been attempted. A limited amount of receptor pharmacology and other metabolic studies have been performed, but only with the use of large numbers of samples.[6]

The technique of nucleic acid amplification using the polymerase chain reaction (PCR) has opened up new vistas for tissue analysis and, hopefully, diagnosis. This technique, expanded elsewhere in this text, relies on a heat-stable DNA polymerase isolated from a species of algae and automated temperature cycling. By repeatedly heating and cooling the sample in the presence of this enzyme (to denature double-stranded DNA and to anneal and synthesize new DNA, respectively), a single copy of DNA or mRNA (following reverse transcription to complementary DNA) can be exponentially amplified to the level of detection and quantification. Any gene or segment of RNA can be amplified (providing that the nucleotide sequence is known); given the amplification power, extremely small samples of tissue (i.e., endomyocardial biopsies) can be assayed.

To date, PCR has been used in several studies, including the identification of variants of G proteins,[7] the identification of mutations in cardiac sodium channel subunits,[8] the quantification of contractile protein mRNA in normal and pressure-loaded hearts,[9] the quantification of age-dependent deletions in cardiac mitochondrial DNA,[10] the activation of tissue-specific cardiac angiotensin-converting enzyme,[11] the assay of interleukin and interleukin receptor mRNA using endomyocardial biopsies from patients with myocarditis and cardiomyopathy,[12] and the identification of viral mRNA in cardiac tissue.[13] It is obvious, even at this early date, that the potential applications of this technique are numerous and could yield extremely important and novel information in poorly understood diseases such as the cardiomyopathies.

Evaluation of mRNA levels also is likely to provide important clues regarding the expression of genes in the heart and in peripheral tissue that are involved in the pathogenesis of CHF. The mechanisms by which these genes are activated or "deactivated" and that control transcription of DNA to mRNA and translation of mRNA to proteins during various stages of the disease also are an area of research that promises to provide information that, ultimately, could be important in directing therapeutic interventions. A word of caution is in order, however. The extreme power of the PCR to amplify genetic material can provide misleading information. For instance, the technique is capable of detecting minute quantities of DNA or mRNA and could, therefore, yield misleading information about the importance of a particular gene or metabolic pathway. Methods of quantifying PCR recently have become available and their widespread use should increase the validity of the technique.[14]

Therapeutic Advances

Disease Prevention

As mentioned previously, the most common cause of CHF is ischemic heart disease due to coronary atherosclerosis. Thus, meaningful modification of risk factors involved in the growth and development of atherosclerotic plaques is of upmost importance. The last decade has resulted in the development of new classes of lipid-lowering agents, antihypertensives, and antiplatelet agents. A better understanding of specific molecular defects in lipid metabolism, vascular reactivity, and coagulation will likely provide the templates for specific and effective pharmacologic, substrate, or genetic therapy.

In addition to better control of risk factors, advances in prevention of myocardial infarction and preservation and salvage of heart muscle during ischemic episodes should reduce myocardial damage in patients with established atherosclerotic disease. These latter advances, however, may have the paradoxical effect of increasing the incidence of CHF as more patients with serious cardiac damage are able to survive a myocardial infarction.

Treating the Diseased Heart

Modification and extension of existing approaches to CHF are certain to occur. Newer vasodilating agents that are either more potent or have fewer side effects likely will come available. Newer classes of vasodilators such as the angiotensin II receptor antagonists currently are under development and could provide additional benefits used either by themselves or in combination with other vasodilating agents.[15] The use of combinations of vasodilators to inhibit homeostatic compensatory mechanisms that develop when specific classes of agents are used by themselves, such as the angiotensin-converting enzyme inhibitors, appears to be a promising approach to patients with CHF.

Despite the disappointing results reported by the milrinone trial,[16] other oral inotropic agents continue to be developed. Although sharing some similarities to milrinone, many of these agents have substantially different pharmacologic effects and thus may yield different outcomes. One such agent, vesnarinone (OPC 8212), is released for use in Japan and has demonstrated extremely positive early results in studies in this country.[17] A large multicenter trial has just concluded in New York Heart Association (NYHA) functional class III and IV patients and these results should be available soon.

After more than 200 years of debate, the role of the digitalis glycosides is on the verge of being definitively decided on. Data from several well designed clinical trials, which are outlined in various chapters of the text, demonstrate that digoxin can improve exercise tolerance, relieve symptoms, and prevent hospitalizations in heart failure patients who are in sinus rhythm. These effects appear to be manifest even in relatively mild heart failure[18] and are additive to those of the angiotensin-converting enzyme inhibitors.[19] A major outstanding issue, however, is the effect of digoxin on mortality. This question currently is being addressed by a large clinical trial that is cosponsored by the VA and the NIH. The results of this study should provide important information regarding the use of digoxin in CHF.

Although the adverse effects of activation of the sympathetic nervous system in CHF are well documented and there is some information that beta-blockade actually may benefit patients,[20] there currently is no clear-cut direction in this field. Whether or not beta-blockage will improve the clinical course and survival of heart failure patients, at what stage they should best be given, and whether "designer" drugs (i.e., those possessing properties in addition to beta-blockade, such as intrinsic sympathomimetic activity or direct vasodilating

activity) will be effective are all unanswered questions. This is clearly a field that is ripe for well designed clinical trials to address these issues.

It is entirely realistic to expect that with the expanded use of molecular biology in the investigation of heart failure etiologies, that specific substrate abnormalities or deficiencies will be elucidated. A well known example of a specific defect is the congenital cardiomyopathy associated with carnitine deficiency.[21] Direct replacement of deficient substrates to provide normal metabolic function hopefully will be a treatment approach to a greater number of patients. Alternatively, incorporation of specific genes into myocardial cells, already shown possible,[22] may lead to correction of metabolic defects directly and permanently at the molecular level.

Other Approaches to Reducing Morbidity and Mortality Associated with CHF

Sudden cardiac death accounts for between 30% and 50% of the mortality in patients with CHF. As extensively reviewed elsewhere in this text, predicting and treating those at risk for this complication has been a major challenge. The automatic implantable cardiac defibrillator may prove to be a major advance in the approach to these patients.[23] Further refinements in this technology, including less invasive placement (transvenous venous approach) defibrillator units, and combined antitachycardic and antibradycardic capabilities, are already in clinical trials. As the use of this technology becomes more widespread, the costs associated with these devices hopefully should fall. It is not entirely clear, however, that preventing sudden death in this patient population will have a major overall effect on long-term outcome, as those patients may have been at higher risk for other complications that will now have the opportunity to become manifest when the rhythm disturbance is successfully treated.

Another major complication of patients with severe CHF is thromboembolism. Many patients receive long-term anticoagulation with agents such as warfarin. Difficulties with this class of agents in patients with severe CHF include variabilities in absorption due to alterations in mesenteric flow and intestinal venous engorgement, marked variabilities in metabolism due to changes in hepatic function associated with heart failure, and variabilities in action due to alterations in levels of vitamin K–dependent clotting factors, again due to changes in hepatic function. As a result, these patients require extremely close monitoring and have an increased incidence of bleeding complications. It is anticipated that agents that have more specific actions in the coagulation pathway such as the highly purified low molecular weight heparins and heparinoids or the newer thrombin inhibitors will have a greater therapeutic index and require less stringent monitoring.

Replacement

Cardiac transplantation has evolved from an experimental curiosity to an accepted clinical modality in a matter of 15 yr. It is likely that with continued understanding of the allogeneic response that more targeted immunosuppression and ultimately true graft tolerance will be possible. This will minimize the need and risks of global immunosuppression. Despite these advances, the number of available human organ donors will never meet the demand, which currently stands at between 20,000 and 50,000 per year in the United States alone. Alternatives to allogeneic transplantation therefore must be developed.

The evolving field of skeletal muscle pumps may for a segment of the heart failure population provide an alternative to transplantation.[24] As better techniques and patient selection are developed, outcomes are likely to improve. The better understanding of differences between skeletal and cardiac muscle may allow for its modification beyond the currently used and rather primitive training protocols. Conceivably, the direct molecular manipulation of skeletal muscle to make it express genes normally found in cardiac muscle may be achievable.

Artificial ventricular assistance is rapidly becoming a reality. There are already several systems used as bridges to transplantation and some patients have remained on these devices for several months. Totally implantable systems maintaining cutaneous integrity are already under development and in early clinical trials. These devices will continue to evolve with better and longer life power sources, less thrombogeneic potential, and greater ease of implantation. Societal costs, however, will be a major limiting feature as there will be no self-limited cap on the number of patients who could receive these devices, as there is with allogeneic transplantation.

Finally, a major thrust in the field of organ replacement is in xenotransplantation. Although the immunologic barriers to overcome are substantially less with concordant xenografts (primate to primate transplantation), the ethical aspects of using larger primates as human organ donors make this an unlikely solution. Discordant xenotransplantation probably would achieve societal acceptance given that the most likely candidate as a human cardiac donor is the pig (size and structure). In addition to attempts to manipulate the recipient immune system using a variety of techniques, the same molecular techniques are being applied in attempts to develop transgenic animals that would express human rather than animal cell-surface antigens.[25,26] Major centers are now devoting considerable resources to overcoming the immunologic barriers to discordant xenotransplantation and substantial strides are being made.

Conclusions

As much as the past decade has resulted in substantial advances in the diagnosis and treatment of CHF, the next is likely to be equally as profitable. Prevention of CHF by the identification of patients at high risk for developing CAD and positive modification of risk factors known to be important in the development of atherosclerosis is clearly the most cost effective means of approaching the problem. Ongoing improvements in pharmacologic therapy for heart failure with new classes of agents and agents with fewer side effects will likely lead to improved survival and quality of life in patients with CHF. Cardiac replacement and assistance is advancing at a rapid rate, although the costs of this technology will likely be far too high to be applied broadly in the short and intermediate terms. Finally, the advances in molecular biologic techniques alone have dramatically altered the potential avenues that might be approached in diagnosis, therapy, and even replacement of the diseased heart.

References

1. Weiss RG, Bottomley PA, Hardy CJ, Gerstenblith G. Regional myocardial metabolism of high-energy phosphates during isometric exercise in patients with coronary artery disease. *N Engl J Med.* 1990;323:1596–1600.
2. Malloy CR, Thompson JR, Jeffrey MH, Sherry AD. Contribution of exogenous substrates to acetyl coenzyme A: measurement by 13C NMR under non-steady-state conditions. *Biochemistry.* 1990;29:6756–6761.
3. Shtern F. Positron emission tomography as a diagnostic tool. *Invest Radiol.* 1992;27:165–168.
4. Mason JW, Billingham ME, Ricci DR. Treatment of acute inflammatory myocarditis assisted by endomyocardial biopsy. *Am J Cardiol.* 1980;45:1037–1042.
5. Hosenpud JD. Usefulness of endomyocardial biopsy in tertiary care. *West J Med.* 1989;15043–15045.
6. Bristow MR, Ginsburg R, Fowler M, et al. β_1- and β_2-adrenergic receptor subpopulations in normal and failing ventricular myocardium: Coupling of both receptor subtypes to muscle contraction and selective b1 receptor down-regulation in heart failure. *Cir. Res.* 1986;59:297–308.
7. Holmer SR, Homcy CJ. G proteins and the heart. *Circulation.* 1991;84:1891–1902.
8. Satin J, Kyle JW, Chen M, et al. A mutant of TTX-resistant cardiac sodium channels with TTX-sensitive properties. *Science.* 1992;256:1202–1205.
9. McAuliffe JJ, Robbins J. Troponin T expression in normal and pressure-loaded fetal sheep heart. *Pediatr Res.* 1991;29:580–585.
10. Hattori K, Tanaka M, Sugiyama S, et al. Age-dependent

increase in deleted mitochondrial DNA in the human heart: possible contributory factor to presbycardia. *Am Heart J*. 1991;121:1735–1742.

11. Hirsch AT, Talsness CE, Schunkert H, Paul M, Dzau VJ. Tissue-specific activation of cardiac angiotensin converting enzyme in experimental heart failure. *Circ Res*. 1991;69:475–482.

12. Han RO, Ray PE, Baughman KL, Feldman AM. Detection of interleukin and interleukin-receptor mRNA in human heart by polymerase chain reaction. *Biochem Biophys Res Commun*. 1991;181:520–523.

13. Ross RS, Chien KR. Of molecules and myocardium. PCR diagnosis of viral myocarditis in cardiac biopsies (editorial). *Circulation*. 1990;82:294–295.

14. Wang, AM, Doyle MV, Mark OF. Quantitation of mRNA by the polymerase chain reaction. *Proc Natl Acad Sci USA*. 1989;86:9717–9721.

15. Munafo A, Christen Y, Nussberger J, et al. Drug concentration response relationships in normal volunteers after oral administration of losartan, angiotensin II receptor antagonist. *Clin Pharmacol Ther*. 1992;51:513–521.

16. Packer M, Carver JR, Ivanhoe RJ, et al. Effect of oral milrinone on mortality in severe chronic heart failure. *N Engl J Med*. 1991;325:1468–1475.

17. Nanto S, Kodama K, Kimura Y, et al. Effect of OPC-8212 (2(1H)—quinolinone), a new inotropic agent, on myocardial energy metabolism in patients with coronary heart disease. *Jpn Circ J*. 1988;52:155–161.

18. The Captopril-Digoxin Multicenter Research Group. Comparative effects of therapy with captopril and digoxin in patients with mild to moderate heart failure. *JAMA*. 1988;259:539–544.

19. Packer M, Gheorgheade M, Young JB, et al. Randomized double-blind, placebo-controlled, withdrawal study of digoxin in patients with chronic heart failure treated with converting enzyme inhibitors. *J Am Coll Cardiol*. 1992;19:260A.

20. Waagsteen F, Caidahl K, Wallentin I, et al. Long-term B-blockade in dilated cardiomyopathy—effects of short-term and long-term metoprolol treatment followed by withdrawal and re-administration of metoprolol. *Circulation*. 1989;80:551–563.

21. Rebouch CJ, Engel AG. Carnitine metabolism and deficiency syndromes. *Mayo Clin Proc*. 1983;58:533–540.

22. Shubeita HE, Thorburn J, Chien KR. Microinjection of antibodies and expression of vectors into living myocardial cells. Development of a novel approach to identify candidate genes that regulate cardiac growth and hypertrophy. *Circulation*. 1992;85:2236–2246.

23. Hargrove WC, Miller JM. Risk stratification and management of patients with recurrent ventricular tachycardia and other malignant ventricular arrhythmias. *Circulation*. 1989;79:I178–I181.

24. Chachques JC, Grandjean PA, Pfeffer TA, et al. Cardiac assistance by atrial or ventricular cardiomyoplasty. *J Heart Transplant*. 1990;9:239–251.

25. Bieberich C, Yoshioka T, Tanaka K, Jay G, Scangos G. Functional expression of a heterologous major histocompatibility complex class I gene in transgenic mice. *Mol Cell Biol*. 1987;7:4003–4009.

26. Auchincloss H Jr, Moses R, Conti D, et al. Xenograft rejection of class I-expressing transgenic skin is CD4-dependent and CD8-independent. *Transplant Proc*. 1990;22:2335–2336.

Index